Melatonin in the Promotion of Health

Second Edition

Edited by Ronald Ross Watson

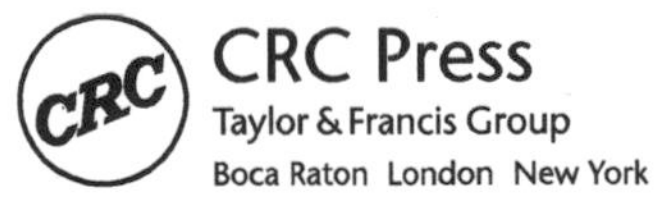

CRC Press is an imprint of the
Taylor & Francis Group, an **informa** business

CRC Press
Taylor & Francis Group
6000 Broken Sound Parkway NW, Suite 300
Boca Raton, FL 33487-2742

First issued in paperback 2017

Version Date: 20110427

ISBN-13: 978-1-4398-3979-9 (hbk)
ISBN-13: 978-1-138-11218-6 (pbk)

Library of Congress Cataloging-in-Publication Data

Melatonin in the promotion of health, second edition / [edited by] Ronald Ross Watson. -- 2nd ed.
p. ; cm.
Includes bibliographical references and index.
ISBN 978-1-4398-3979-9 (hardback : alk. paper)
1. Melatonin--Physiological effect. 2. Melatonin--Health aspects. I. Watson, Ronald R. (Ronald Ross)
[DNLM: 1. Melatonin--physiology. 2. Melatonin--therapeutic use. WK 350]

QP572.M44M46 2012
612.4'92--dc22 2011011807

Visit the Taylor & Francis Web site at
http://www.taylorandfrancis.com

and the CRC Press Web site at
http://www.crcpress.com

Contents

SECTION III Treatment of Disease and Physiological Disorders with Melatonin

Preface

Melatonin is a small molecule, a derivative of the amino acid tryptophan, *N*-acetyl-5 methoxytryptamine. It is a potent hormone with well-recognized activities and the potential to influence many bodily functions. It is produced by the pineal gland in the brain and is secreted when the body recognizes darkness. Melatonin has intense effects on the timing of the sleep/awake cycle, regulating the circadian rhythms of several biological functions. This is its most studied biological activity. Melatonin, as a multifunctional hormone, appears to regulate or modulate other functions in humans through the activation of its receptors and works as a strong antioxidant that protects the DNA. Melatonin's antioxidant activity may reduce Parkinson's disease development, prevent cardiac arrhythmia, and, in animals, promote longevity. Studies on human disease prevention and treatment are more limited and will be a major area of review in this book. Aging involves many changes in our physiology, and only a few are understood. It has been recognized that melatonin levels decline with age and may play a role in many age-related changes. Melatonin is a powerful antioxidant with numerous effects on the metabolism and health of older people. Melatonin has been available as a dietary supplement in the United States since 1993 as well as in Canada and some European countries. In moderate doses, melatonin has routinely been found to be safe, with very low toxicity in animals and humans. There is evidence that melatonin supplementation or level in human affect headaches, fertility, attention deficit–hyperactivity disorder, mood disorders, cancer, gall stones, circadian rhythm disorders (sleep). They help prevent ischemic damage, autism, immune regulation, dreaming, oxidant removal, as well as recent but more limited evidence of roles in other human health conditions. The editor selected researchers with experience in studying the role of melatonin in various disease and physiological states primarily in humans. Thus, this book has a wide variety of expert reviews on the biology of melatonin relevant to health in humans. The editor, Dr. Watson, has done research with melatonin as a modulator of immune function and regulator of AIDS in mice.

Section I reviews key areas of melatonin, including a history of melatonin and its use in various therapies, as well as melatonin and circadian rhythms. The focus of Section II relates to melatonin's action in the prevention of diseases such as cardiovascular diseases, reproductive diseases, solar skin damage, diabetes, immune function, uveitis, and gut function, among others. There are three other sections with clinical potential importance and varying levels of study. The key section, Section III, relates to melatonin's action in the treatment of diseases and physiological disorders such as surgery, bone, breast cancer, gastrointestinal function, reproduction, and pancreas diseases. In some cases, the role of melatonin is still controversial in certain human health conditions, and the researchers define what is known for the various conditions being treated. Section IV describes melatonin in the context of sleep and circadian rhythm regulation. Finally, Section V describes how melatonin's actions on physiological functions in humans focus on the effects of loss of pineal function and the subsequent reduction in melatonin production as well as its replacement as a therapy. These include neuroendocrine effects, inflammation, age-related degeneration, collagen synthesis, vascular structure, DNA protection, oxidation, and traumatic stress, among others. Understanding melatonin is critical, as it is a hormone that is sold over the counter as a dietary supplement and is thus readily available to consumers in many countries.

Acknowledgments

Special thanks are extended to Bethany L. Stevens, the editorial assistant to Dr. Ronald Ross Watson. She spent many hours working with the publisher and with the authors of this book. She made it possible for Dr. Watson to function as the editor by lightening his load and taking responsibility for routine questions, format, and style. Support for editorial assistance was provided by Southwest Scientific Editing and Consulting, LLC. The help of Mari Stoddard, an Arizona Health Sciences Librarian, was crucial to finding all the authors and topics that appear in the book.

Editor

Ronald R. Watson attended the University of Idaho but graduated from Brigham Young University in Provo, UT, with a degree in chemistry in 1966. He earned his PhD in biochemistry from Michigan State University in 1971. His postdoctoral schooling in nutrition and microbiology was completed at the Harvard School of Public Health, where he gained two years of postdoctoral research experience in immunology and nutrition.

From 1973 to 1974, Dr. Watson was assistant professor of immunology and performed research at the University of Mississippi Medical Center in Jackson. He was assistant professor of microbiology and immunology at the Indiana University Medical School from 1974 to 1978 and associate professor at Purdue University in the Department of Food and Nutrition from 1978 to 1982. In 1982, Dr. Watson joined the faculty at the University of Arizona Health Sciences Center in the Department of Family and Community Medicine of the School of Medicine. He is currently professor of health promotion sciences in the Mel and Enid Zuckerman Arizona College of Public Health.

Dr. Watson is a member of several national and international nutrition, immunology, cancer, and alcoholism research societies. Among his patents, with more pending, is a dietary supplement using passion fruit peel extract. He has done melatonin research on its effects on mouse AIDS and immune function for 20 years. He edited a previous book on melatonin, *Melatonin in the Promotion of Health* (CRC Press, 1998, 224 pp.). For 30 years, he was funded by the Wallace Research Foundation to study dietary supplements in health promotion. Dr. Watson has edited more than 35 books on nutrition, dietary supplements and over-the-counter agents, and 53 other scientific books. He has published more than 500 research and review articles.

Contributors

Marco Antonioli
Section of Perinatal Psychiatry and Stress
King's College London
London, United Kingdom

Andreas Gunter Bach
Clinic for Diagnostic Radiology
Martin Luther University of Halle-Wittenberg
Halle, Germany

Soyhan Bağci
Department of Neonatology
University of Bonn
Bonn, Germany

Mariano Bizzarri, MD, PhD
Department of Experimental Medicine
University "La Sapienza"
Rome, Italy

Petr Bob
Department of Psychiatry
Charles University
Prague, Czech Republic

Gregory M. Brown
Department of Psychiatry
University of Toronto
Toronto, Ontario, Canada

Iwona Brzozowska
Department of Physiology
Jagiellonian University Medical College
Cracow, Poland

Tomasz Brzozowski
Department of Clinical Physiology
Jagiellonian University Medical College
Cracow, Poland

George A. Bubenik
Department of Integrative Biology
University of Guelph
Guelph, Ontario, Canada

Daniel P. Cardinali
Department of Teaching and Research
Pontifical Catholic University of Argentina
Buenos Aires, Argentina

Livia A. Carvalho
Department of Life Sciences
Roehampton University
London, United Kingdom

Marek Cegielski
Department of Histology and Embryology
Wrocław Medical University
Wrocław, Poland

Krzysztof Celinski
Department of Gastroenterology
Medical University of Lublin
Lublin, Poland

Mónica Chianelli
Department of Human Biochemistry
University of Buenos Aires
Buenos Aires, Argentina

Indrajit Chowdhury
Department of Obstetrics and Gynecology
Morehouse School of Medicine
Atlanta, Georgia

William P. Clafshenkel
Graduate School of Pharmaceutical Sciences
Duquesne University
Pittsburgh, Pennsylvania

Alessandra Cucina
Department of Surgery "P. Valdoni"
University "La Sapienza"
Rome, Italy

Fabrizio D'Anselmi
Department of Surgery "P. Valdoni"
University "La Sapienza"
Rome, Italy
and
Italian Space Agency
Rome, Italy

Vicki L. Davis
Graduate School of Pharmaceutical Sciences
Duquesne University
Pittsburgh, Pennsylvania

Simona Dinicola
Department of Experimental Medicine
University "La Sapienza"
Rome, Italy

Balasunder R. Dodda
Graduate School of Pharmaceutical Sciences
Duquesne University
Pittsburgh, Pennsylvania

Piotr Dzięgiel
Department of Histology and Embryology
Wrocław Medical University
Wrocław, Poland

Tom S. Edrington
USDA–Agricultural Research Service
College Station, Texas

Pedro A. Fernandes
Laboratory of Chronopharmacology
University of São Paulo
São Paulo, Brazil

Diego C. Fernandez
Department of Human Biochemistry
University of Buenos Aires
Buenos Aires, Argentina

Tobias W. Fischer
Department of Dermatology
University of Lübeck
Lübeck, Germany

Eleonora Foglio
Department of Biomedical Sciences and Biotechnologies
University of Brescia
Brescia, Italy

José Luis Guzmán
Department of Agroforestry Sciences
University of Huelva
Huelva, Spain

Khek-Yu Ho
University Medicine Cluster
National University Health System
and
Department of Medicine
National University Hospital
Singapore
and
Department of Medicine
National University of Singapore
Singapore

Dan-Ning Hu
Tissue Culture Center
The New York Eye and Ear Infirmary
New York, New York
and
New York Medical College
New York, New York

Salah A. Ismail
Department of Anesthesia
Suez Canal University
Ismailia, Egypt

Ilona Iżykowska
Department of Histology and Embryology
Wrocław Medical University
Wrocław, Poland

Jolanta Jaworek
Department of Medical Physiology
Jagiellonian University School of Medicine
Cracow, Poland

Birgit C. P. Koch
Erasmus Medical Center
Rotterdam, The Netherlands

Masayuki Kondo
Human Life R&D Institute
Sekisui House, Ltd.
Kyoto, Japan

Peter C. Konturek
Department of Internal Medicine
University Erlangen–Nuremberg
Erlangen, Germany

Stanislaw J. Konturek
Department of Clinical Physiology
Jagiellonian University School of Medicine
Cracow, Poland

Mary P. Kotlarczyk
Graduate School of Pharmaceutical Sciences
Duquesne University
Pittsburgh, Pennsylvania

Mauro Labanca
Department of Biomedical Sciences and Biotechnologies
University of Brescia
Brescia, Italy

Theodore Lialiaris
Laboratory of Genetics
Demokrition University of Thrace University
Alexandroupolis, Greece

Saumen Kumar Maitra
Department of Zoology
Visva-Bharati University
Santiniketan, West Bengal, India

Maria D. Maldonado
Department of Medical Biochemistry and Molecular Biology
University of Seville Medical School
Seville, Spain

Benoît Malpaux
Joint Research Unit:
National Institute of Agronomic Research
National Center for Scientific Research
Universite de Tours, and Haras Nationaux
Nouzilly, France

Regina P. Markus
Laboratory of Chronopharmacology
University of São Paulo
São Paulo, Brazil

Takeshi Morita
Department of Living Environmental Science
Fukuoka Women's University
Fukuoka, Japan

Hany A. Mowafi
Department of Anesthesia
Dammam University
Dammam, Saudi Arabia

María José Munuce
Laboratory of Reproductive Studies
University of Rosario
Rosario, Argentina

J. Elsbeth Nagtegaal
Meander Medical Center
Amersfoort, The Netherlands

David J. Nisbet
USDA–Agricultural Research Service
College Station, Texas

V. Haktan Ozacmak
Department of Physiology
Zonguldak Karaelmas University
Zonguldak, Turkey

Seithikurippu R. Pandi-Perumal
Somnogen Inc.
New York, New York

Alessia Pasqualato
Department of Basic and Applied Medical Sciences
University G. d'Annunzio
Chieti-Pescara, Italy

Ming Pei
Stem Cell and Tissue Engineering Laboratory
West Virginia University
Morgantown, West Virginia

Maria A. Pérez-San-Gregorio
Department of Personality, Evaluation and Psychological Treatment
University of Seville
Seville, Spain

Elmar Peschke
Institute of Anatomy and Cell Biology
Martin Luther University of Halle-Wittenberg
Halle, Germany

Carlos Ponce
Program of Anatomy and Developmental Biology
University of Chile
Santiago, Chile

Sara Proietti
Department of Experimental Medicine
University "La Sapienza"
Rome, Italy

Rita Rezzani
Human Anatomy Section
University of Brescia
Brescia, Italy

Joan E. Roberts
Division of Natural Sciences
Fordham University
New York, New York

Luigi Fabrizio Rodella
Department of Biomedical Sciences and Biotechnologies
University of Brescia
Brescia, Italy

Héctor Rodríguez
Program of Anatomy and Developmental Biology
University of Chile
Santiago, Chile

Richard B. Rosen
New York Eye and Ear Infirmary
New York, New York
and
New York Medical College
New York, New York

Ruth E. Rosenstein
Department of Human Biochemistry
University of Buenos Aires
Buenos Aires, Argentina

Marije Russcher
Resident in Hospital Pharmacy
Meander Medical Center
Amersfoort, The Netherlands

Joanna Rybka
Department of Biochemistry
Nicolaus Copernicus University
Toruń, Poland
and
Ludwik Rydygier Collegium Medicum
Bydgoszcz, Poland
and
Section of Perinatal Psychiatry and Stress
King's College London
London, United Kingdom

Daniel A. Sáenz
Department of Human Biochemistry
University of Buenos Aires
Buenos Aires, Argentina

Alexander Samel
Division of Flight Physiology
Institute of Aerospace Medicine
Cologne, Germany

Pablo H. Sande
Department of Human Biochemistry
University of Buenos Aires
Buenos Aires, Argentina

Luis Sarabia
Program of Anatomy and Developmental Biology
University of Chile
Santiago, Chile

Shalini Sethi
Graduate School of Pharmaceutical Sciences
Duquesne University
Pittsburgh, Pennsylvania

Andrzej T. Slominski
Skin Cancer Division
University of Tennessee
Memphis, Tennessee
and
Department of Pathology and Laboratory Medicine
University of Tennessee Health Science Center
Memphis, Tennessee

Radomir Slominski
Department of Pathology and Laboratory Medicine
University of Tennessee Health Science Center
Memphis, Tennessee

D. Warren Spence
Sleep and Alertness Clinic
Toronto, Ontario, Canada

Ioannis A. Taitzoglou
Faculty of Veterinary Medicine
Aristotle University of Thessaloniki
Thessaloniki, Greece

John E. Tidwell
Department of Orthopaedics
West Virginia University
Morgantown, West Virginia

Ilya Trakht
Department of Medicine
Columbia University
New York, New York

Maria P. Tsantarliotou
Faculty of Veterinary Medicine
Aristotle University of Thessaloniki
Thessaloniki, Greece

G. C. Verster
Department of Psychiatry
University of Stellenbosch
Cape Town, South Africa

Tomoko Wakamura
Department of Human Health Sciences
Kyoto University
Kyoto, Japan

Allan F. Wiechmann
Department of Cell Biology
University of Oklahoma Health Sciences Center
Oklahoma City, Oklahoma

Paula A. Witt-Enderby
Graduate School of Pharmaceutical Sciences
Duquesne University
Pittsburgh, Pennsylvania

Jennie Wong
Department of Medicine
National University of Singapore
Singapore

Mustafa Yildiz
Kosuyolu Heart Center
Istanbul, Turkey

Luis Ángel Zarazaga
Department of Agroforestry Sciences
University of Huelva
Huelva, Spain

1 Melatonin Time Line: From Discovery to Therapy

Indrajit Chowdhury and Saumen Kumar Maitra

CONTENTS

1.1 INTRODUCTION

Discovery of an active substance in any component of a living system has never been so exciting as what happened with the isolation, purification, and characterization of an indole compound from extracts of the pineal gland, which has long been considered as a functional relic of the brain [1]. The credit of such breakthrough research goes to a group led by an American dermatologist, Dr. Aaron Bunsen Lerner, in the Yale University School of Medicine, who extracted only a few milligrams of *N*-acetyl-5-methoxy-serotonin from more than 100,000 cattle pineal glands nearly 53 years ago [2,3]. They named this purified pineal substance melatonin (MEL) in recognition of an initial observation that treatment with crude acetone extract of bovine pineal glands to *Rana pipens* tadpole caused a pronounced lightening (blanching) of their skins (i.e., melanophore-contracting hormone; Greek: μελαζ = black; τονζ = tension, in the sense of contraction), resulting in clear visibility of the larger viscera through the dorsal body wall [4]. Nevertheless, the functional implication of pineal has a history way back to the 19th century, when Huebner [5] reported for the first time that tumor of the human pineal altered pubertal development, indicating a possible role of some factor(s) of pineal origin in influencing reproductive functions. This observation led many scientists in the first half of the 20th century to experimentally examine the association of the pineal with the reproductive status in a variety of animal species with limited compelling evidences [6] (Table 1.1).

TABLE 1.1
Melatonin Time Line

Year	Critical Findings
1898	• Tumor of human pineal is found to be associated with altered pubertal development.
1917	• Injection of bovine pineal extract to *Rana pipens* causes pronounced lightening of their skin.
1958	• MEL is isolated from bovine pineal gland.
1961	• *O*-Methylated by hydroxyindole-*O*-methyltransferase (*S*-adenosyl L-methionine: hydroxyindole *O*-methyltransferase; EC 2.1.1.4; HIOMT) is isolated and characterized.
1964	• L-Aromatic amino acid decarboxylase (aromatic L-amino acid carboxylase, EC 4.1.1.28, AAAD/AADC) is isolated and characterized.
1964	• Role of MEL as an antigonadotropic factor is demonstrated.
1967	• Trp-5-monooxygenase/hydroxylase (L-tryptophan, tetrahydropterin-dine: oxygen oxidoreductase (EC 1.14.16.4, TPH) is isolated and characterized.
1974	• The location of the biological clock, the mind's clock, in mammals is identified in the SCN.
1984	• Arylalkylamine-*N*-acetyltransferase (acetyl CoA: arylalkylamine-*N*-acetyltransferase/serotonin *N*-acetyltransferase; EC 2.3.1.87; AA-NAT) is isolated and characterized.
1982	• Possible role of MEL in breast cancer is demonstrated.
1991	• The antioxidant properties of MEL are demonstrated.
1991	• MEL is suggested as dietary supplement for beneficiary role.
1993	• The MEL rhythm is described as both clock and calendar.
1993	• The increase in MEL secretion in the evening is found correlated with an increase in sleep propensity.
1994	• MEL receptors (MT_1 and MT_2) are cloned.
1996	• The circadian rhythm of MEL production is found regulated by SCN of the anterior hypothalamus.
1999	• MT_1 dual signaling mechanism is identified.
2000	• MEL receptor MT3 is demonstrated as the enzyme quinine reductase 2.
1995–2002	• MEL is found in a wide spectrum of organisms including bacteria, fungi, plants, protozoa, invertebrates, and vertebrates and also in extrapineal sites like the retina, Harderian gland, gut, bone marrow, platelets, and skin in vertebrates.
2005	• MEL agonist agomelatine and ramelteon are launched as an orally active hypnotic for the treatment of transient and chronic insomnia in human.

Note: See text for details and references.

In the past 50 years since the discovery of MEL, we have witnessed an emergence of a plethora of information from studies on a wide group of animals, including vertebrates and invertebrates, and plants subjected to MEL, the most unique and wonder molecule among all the known substances in areas covering endocrinology, pharmacology, physiology, psychology, chronobiology, and environmental biology. The most remarkable feature of this pineal hormone is its synthesis in the synchronization with the environmental light/dark (LD) conditions. In all the animals investigated so far, irrespective of their habit, MEL synthesis in a 24-hour cycle reaches peak during the dark phase. As a hormone, MEL afforded the first opportunity for its use as a chronobiological marker, particularly for those who are engaged in circadian studies. It plays a central role in primary circadian pacemaker (suprachiasmatic nucleus, SCN) to synchronize the body functions to LD cycle of the environment. Accordingly, this hormone is considered as a "chronobiotic molecule," or the "hormone of darkness." Molecular biology study dealing with its biosynthetic enzymes and their genes, molecular regulators, degradation byproducts, and the mechanisms of signaling in a cell has opened up a new chapter in circadian research. Carefully controlled studies in different animals, including the human, have implicated MEL in the control of a wide variety of body functions ranging from aging to aggression, hibernation to hypertension, jet lag to seasonal affective disorders, sleep to stress, and reproduction to tissue regeneration. More recent studies revealed that MEL, because of its lipophilic nature, can cross the plasma membrane of any cell and thereby has free access to all the tissues, organs, and systems in the living body and by acting as a potent scavenger of free radicals may play an important role in combating oxidative stress in a metabolically active cell [7]. Moreover, MEL is known to be involved in complex processes of cellular protection and apoptosis. A rapidly expanding body of literature suggests that MEL as a biomarker of circadian dysfunctions may play pivotal roles in various neurodegenerative or neurological diseases. As a result, MEL has become a potent candidate for investigation in several disciplines of experimental biology and pathophysiology signifying its importance in clinical and therapeutic research. The aim of this review is to track the progress in research from discovery of MEL to its potential use in therapy by focusing the most fascinating, and arguably important, data gathered in recent past. We emphasize mostly on recent review articles, including ours [8], as they included many original findings that contributed to the current state of knowledge.

1.2 UBIQUITOUS DISTRIBUTION

MEL is ubiquitously distributed in the living system and is suggested to represent one of the most primitive biological signals on earth [9]. It is found not only in vertebrates but in all major phylogenetically distant taxa, including bacteria, unicellular eukaryotes, in different parts of plants (including the roots, stems, flowers, and seeds), and in invertebrate as well [10–13]. In vertebrates, MEL is produced predominantly by the pinealocytes of the pineal gland [14]. Additionally, it is produced in several extrapineal tissues and cells including the Harderian gland, extraorbital lachrymal gland, retina, bone marrow cells, platelets, lymphocytes, skin, enterochromaffin cells of gastrointestinal (GI) tract, and in bile in a variety of animal species [15–21]. In the retina, it is produced by photoreceptor cells [14,18]. MEL is released from extrapineal sites, either only poorly or in high amounts (by order of magnitude), as in the case of the GI tract, but without profound chronological consequences [10,15,22]. In bile, MEL concentration is about 1000 times higher than its daytime concentrations in the blood [23].

1.3 BIOSYNTHESIS

In all vertebrates investigated so far, MEL is primarily synthesized in the pinealocytes of pineal gland [20] at night regardless of the diurnal or nocturnal activity of the concerned animals. Biosynthesis of MEL is a four-step phenomenon (Figure 1.1). First, its precursor L-tryptophan (Trp) is taken up by the pinealocyte from the circulation (blood) and is converted to 5-hydroxy-Trp (5-HTP) in the mitochondria by Trp-5-monooxygenase/hydroxylase (L-tryptophan, tetrahydropterin-dine:

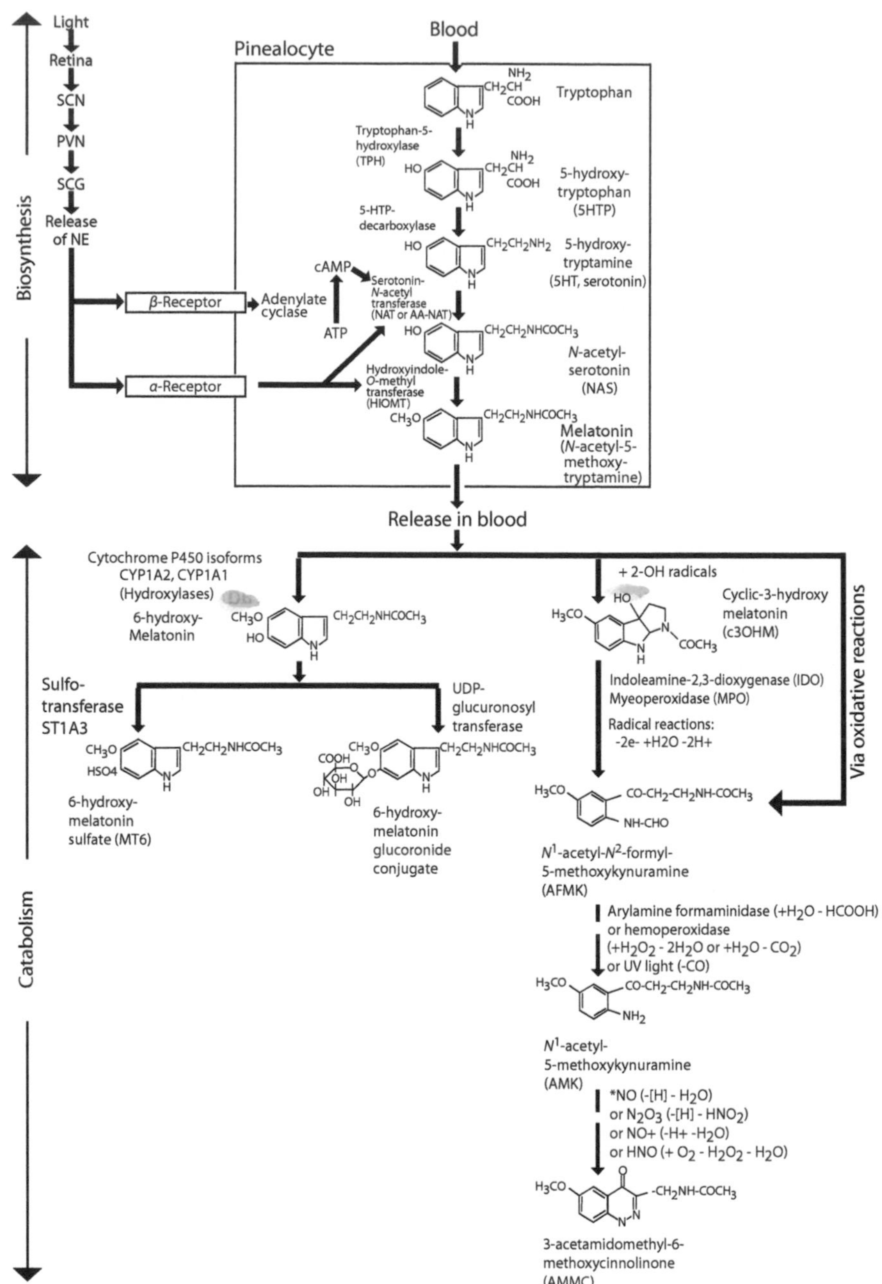

FIGURE 1.1 Schematic representation of the pathway of synthesis, secretion, and catabolism of MEL (from tryptophan to kynurenine). The hormone MEL is synthesized from tryptophan in a four-step pathway, which are under the control of the enzymes tryptophan 5-hydroxylase (TPH), 5-hydroxytryptophan-(5HTP)-decarboxylase, serotonin-*N*-acetyltransferase (NAT), or AA-NAT, and hydroxyindole-*O*-methyl transferase (HIOMT) in the pinealocytes of pineal gland. The rate of MEL formation depends on the multiple molecules that act through multiple mechanisms at different steps of its synthesis. The formation and secretion of AA-NAT and HIOMT are influenced by suprachiasmatic nucleus (SCN) activity via seasonal and circadian timing mechanisms. Under natural environment, MEL is secreted during the night in the healthy human. The catabolism of MEL is through the classical hydroxylation pathway or by kynuric pathway through oxidation of indole core of MEL. During catabolism, various catabolites are formed, which includes N^1-acetyl-5-methoxykynuramine (AMK), N^1-acetyl-N^2-formyl-5-methoxykynuramine (AFMK), glucuronides, etc. (see text for details).

oxygen oxidoreductase, EC 1.14.16.4, TPH) [24] and is then decarboxylated to form serotonin (5-hydroxytryptamine, 5-HT) in the cytosol by L-aromatic amino acid decarboxylase (aromatic L-amino acid carboxylase, EC 4.1.1.28, AAAD/AADC). A fraction of 5-HTP may be methylated into 5-methoxytryptophan [25].

Serotonin is the initial substrate of three different synthetic pathways [26]: (a) 5-HT can be directly *O*-methylated by hydroxyindole-*O*-methyltransferase (*S*-adenosyl L-methionine: hydroxyindole *O*-methyltransferase; EC 2.1.1.4; HIOMT) into 5-methoxytryptamine [27]. (b) 5-HT can be deaminated by monoamine oxidase (amine: oxygen oxidoreductase; EC 1.4.3.4; MAO) into 5-hydroxyindole-acetaldehyde (5-HIAL). This compound is then either successively oxidized into 5-hydroxyindole acetic acid (5-HIAA) by an aldehyde dehydrogenase (aldehyde: NAD^+ oxidoreductase; EC 1.2.1.3) then *O*-methylated by HIOMT to form 5-methoxyindole acetic acid (5-MIAA), or successively reduced into 5-hydroxytryptophol (5-HL) by an alcohol dehydrogenase (alcohol: NAD^+ oxidoreductase; EC 1.1.1.1) then *O*-methylated by HIOMT to form 5-methoxytryptophol (5-ML). (c) The most physiologically important metabolic pathway of 5-HT leads to the synthesis of MEL [28]. 5-HT is first acetylated (*N*-acetylation) by arylalkylamine-*N*-acetyltransferase (acetyl CoA: arylalkylamine-*N*-acetyltransferase/serotonin *N*-acetyltransferase; EC 2.3.1.87; AA-NAT) into *N*-acetyl serotonin (NAS) [29], which plays a key role in MEL biosynthesis. Finally, *N*-acetyl serotonin is *O*-methylated by hydroxyindole-*O*-methyltransferase (*S*-adenosyl-L-methionine: *N*-acetylserotonin-*O*-methyltransferase, EC 2.1.1.4, HIOMT) to form MEL [30].

1.4 REGULATORS OF MEL BIOSYNTHESIS

The rate of MEL formation depends on the multiple molecules that act through multiple mechanisms at different steps of its synthesis. The most important among them are endogenous circadian clock and environmental light, the activity of AA-NAT [18,31], and, to a lesser extent, TPH (which controls the availability of serotonin) [32], HIOMT, noradrenergic regulators, and different peptidergic regulators. AA-NAT switched MEL synthesis on and off with photoperiodic variations in duration, whereas HIOMT tunes the amplitude of the nocturnal MEL synthesis with photoperiodic variation in magnitude. In a few species, nutritional factors such as the availability of tryptophan, folate, and vitamin B6 could also influence MEL synthesis [33–35].

1.4.1 Endogenous Circadian Clock and Environmental Light

The levels of MEL are high during the dark phase of any natural or imposed LD illumination cycle [36]. Studies performed so far in different mammalian models including humans revealed that the magnitude and duration of the nocturnal increase in MEL synthesis is dependent upon the length of the dark phase in a photoperiodic cycle or external geophysical cycle that acts as a "clock" and "calendar" for the entrainment of other biological activities [37], regardless of whether a given species is active during daytime (diurnal), nighttime (nocturnal), or exhibits a crepuscular activity pattern.

The rate and pattern of the nocturnal increase in MEL production depend on species and tissues, among other factors. Light is the dominant environmental factor that controls MEL biosynthesis both in the pineal gland and in the retina. A light signal/pulse of suitable intensity and duration [38] perceived by the retina is transmitted primarily through the retinohypothalamic tract to the SCN, circadian oscillator/master pacemaker of the anterior hypothalamus in brain [39]. Otherwise, constant darkness is sufficient to phase-shift and to synchronize the MEL rhythm in animal species to 24 hours via SCN, which is considered as the major central rhythm-generating system or "clock" in mammals [37,40]. Nerve fibers from the SCN subsequently conveys the signal to the pineal via multisynaptic descending pathways, the subparaventricular zone or paraventricular nucleus, the dorsomedial hypothalamic nucleus, the upper thoracic cell columns of the spinal cord, the superior cervical ganglia, and, finally, the postganglionic adrenergic fibers innervating the pineal gland [41], which itself is a self-sustaining "clock" in some species except in lower vertebrates [42]. The SCN clock is set to a 24-hour day by the natural LD cycle via retinal light input that then sends circadian signals over a neural pathway including sympathetic nerve terminals that project from the superior cervical ganglia to the pineal gland. Changes in the levels of noradrenaline (NA) released from these fibers ensure proper translation of the light information (via the circadian clock) and thereby driving rhythmic MEL synthesis by the pineal gland [43].

The main photoreceptor pigment for circadian timing appears to be melanopsin in the retinal ganglion cells. Specifically, SCN is the major regulatory site of the activity of AA-NAT, which is the ultimate and key enzyme in the synthesis of MEL from tryptophan (Figure 1.1). Furthermore, the prolonged duration of the night leads to a longer duration of secretion of MEL in most animal species [44]. Ocular light serves to entrain/synchronize the rhythm to 24 hours and suppress secretion at the beginning and/or the end of the dark phase. The amount of light required to suppress MEL secretion during the night varies from species to species, with the time of night, and with the previous light exposure [45]. The amplitude of nocturnal MEL secretion exhibits considerable interindividual differences and is believed to be genetically determined.

1.4.2 Tryptophan Hydroxylase

The mitochondrial enzyme TPH transforms tryptophan to 5-HT and requires a pteridine cofactor, tetrahydrobiopterin (BH4) for its catalytic action. The localization of TPH is restricted to serotonin-synthesizing tissues, including the pineal gland and retina [46,47]. TPH exists in two isoforms, TPH1 found in the pineal and gut, whereas TPH2 is exclusively expressed in the brain [47,48]. The rat pineal *Tph* gene codes for two transcripts of 1.8 and 4 kb [49] with same coding sequences but differ by their 3′ noncoding region length. The promoter region does not have a canonical CRE motif [50], but an inverted CCAAT box and a GC-rich region that binds the transcription factors NF-Y and Sp1, both being essential for *Tph* gene transcription at the basal level and following cyclic adenosine monophosphate (cAMP) treatment [51]. In the pineal gland and retina, *Tph* gene expression (TPH mRNA) and/or TPH enzyme activity display daily variations, low (20%) during the day [52] and high (100%) during the night [53], through post-transcriptional/post-translational mechanisms [53,54]. Thus, TPH represents clock-driven circadian rhythms [47,55,56]. The nocturnal increase in the enzyme activity requires de novo protein synthesis [56]. Exposure to light during the night causes a rapid reduction in nocturnal TPH activity [56–57]. The TPH protein has short half-life (~75 minutes) [58] and is activated through the phosphorylation by the cAMP-dependent protein kinase A (PKA) [59], a Ca^{2+} calmodulin (CaM)-dependent protein kinase (PKCa^{2+}/CaM) and PKC [60].

1.4.3 Aromatic Amino Acid Decarboxylase

AAAD is present in large quantities in the cytosolic fraction of the pinealocytes for the synthesis of 5-HT [61]. However, it is not a rate-limiting enzyme, since it is not a specific enzyme to the pineal gland only.

1.4.4 Monoamine Oxidase

MAO activity is detectable in the pinealocytes and in the noradrenergic nerve endings [62]. This differential distribution reflects two types of MAO: type A in the nerve terminals and type B in the pinealocytes. These two types of MAO are characterized by different biochemical properties and sensitivity to inhibitors. It appears that MAO-A is mainly involved in 5-HT oxidation [61]. Consequently, 5-HT exits the pinealocytes for oxidation in the noradrenergic nerve terminals and then returns to the pinealocytes. MAO activity displays day/night variations, with higher values during the day [61].

1.4.5 Alcohol and Aldehyde Dehydrogenases

Neither alcohol nor aldehyde dehydrogenase is saturated by 5-HIAL. Pineal titers of 5-HIAA and 5-HL vary similar to that of 5-HT. The 5-HIAA/5-HL ratio is around 1:6 and is probably related to the lower affinity of alcohol dehydrogenase for its substrate [61].

1.4.6 Arylalkylamine-*N*-Acetyltransferase (Serotonin-*N*-Acetyltransferase)

N-Acetyltransferase, which was first identified as the arylamine-*N*-acetyltransferase (EC 2.3.1.5; NAT), catalyzes *N*-acetylation of 5-HT and is considered as the "rate-limiting enzyme" for the synthesis of MEL, although serotonin availability is one of the major factors that play an important regulatory role in this process [63]. There are two types of *N*-acetyltransferase found in the pineal gland, the arylamine-*N*-acetyltransferase (ANAT) and the arylalkylamine-*N*-acetyltransferase (AA-NAT) named after their best substrates [29]. The affinity of 5-HT is much higher for AA-NAT than A-NAT and only the former enzyme is involved in the rhythmic synthesis of MEL. The cDNA coding for *Aa-nat* has been isolated first in the rat [64,65], then in sheep [66], human [67,68], monkey [69,70], mouse [71], cow [72], Syrian hamster [73], and grass rat [74], with few interspecies differences in the *Aa-nat* gene sequence [69]. A single *Aa-nat* gene has been found in mammalian, avian, and anuran genomes [75]. Teleost fish have two genes: *Aa-nat-1* (homologous to the non-fish *Aa-nats*) and *Aa-nat-2*, primarily expressed in the retina and pineal gland, respectively [76,77]. The *Aa-nat* gene is located on chromosome 11 (position E1.3-2.3) in the mouse, on chromosome 10q32.3 in the rat [78], and on chromosome 17q25 in the human [67].

Aa-nat gene has four exons separated by three introns and encodes for only one transcript (size varies between 1.0 and 1.7 kb according to species). In most species, *Aa-nat* gene expresses in several tissues with a high level in the pineal and the retina and with a much lower level in different nervous tissues (including the pars tuberalis [PT], SCN, hippocampus) and peripheral tissues (including testis and ovaries) [64,67,69,79]. The rat gene has been widely studied. The rat promoter region of the *Aa-nat* gene has one CRE-like sequence (differing by one base from the perfect CRE sequence and named natCRE), an inverted CCAAT box, and an activating protein 1 (AP-1) site [80]. The natCRE site is capable of binding the phosphorylated form of CREB (pCREB), whereas CCAAT box activation by specific binding proteins (CATBP) also appears necessary for large activation of *Aa-nat*. cAMP-induced *Aa-nat* gene transcription requires activation of a CRE–CCAAT complex and appears critical to achieve full stimulation of *Aa-nat* gene expression [81]. Another *cis*-DNA sequence named E-box (able to mediate transcriptional up-regulation via the action of the BMAL1/CLOCK heterodimer) has been identified in the first intron of the rat *Aa-nat* gene [82]. However, transfection of pinealocytes with *Bmal1/Clock* was unable to induce *Aa-nat* transcription, whereas the same kind of transfection in retinal cells led to activation of *Aa-nat* gene expression [82]. The pineal *Aa-nat* gene promoter contains a pineal regulatory element (PIRE) that binds the transcription factor cone–rod homeobox (CRX), which is exclusively expressed in photoreceptors and pinealocytes [83]. Northern blot analysis revealed the presence of high AA-NAT mRNA levels in the pineal glands and retinas in vertebrates [18,84]. In the retina, AA-NAT mRNA has been observed primarily in photoreceptor cells [70,85] and at significantly lower levels in the inner nuclear layer and the ganglion cell layer [85,86]. These findings suggest that, in addition to photoreceptors, other retinal cells may also possess a limited capacity to produce MEL [18].

The vertebrate AA-NATs belong to a superfamily of GCN5-related *N*-acetyltransferases (GNAT), an approximately 23-kDa soluble cytosolic protein with a catalytic core and regulatory regions. The rat AA-NAT protein structure is globular, made of eight β-sheets and five α-helices [87]. Based on the deduced amino acid sequence homology, human AA-NAT is 97% homologous with the monkey, 84% with the sheep, and 90% with the rat. The N-terminal area involved in the binding of the arylalkylamines as an acetyl group donor and facilitates the transfer of the acetyl group, while the C-terminal area with two well-preserved motifs, named A and B, which bind the cofactor acetyl coenzyme A (AcCoA) and contains phosphorylation sites critical for activation and stabilization of the catalytic core [31,75]. Several well-preserved putative phosphorylation sites for the PKA, the PKC, and the casein kinase of type II are present across species [69]. Phosphorylation on the Thr31 residue of AA-NAT promotes binding with the chaperone protein 14-3-3 proteins with a ratio of 1:1 (AA-NAT/14-3-3 protein). This protein–protein interaction yields a relatively stable complex and leads to conformational changes with the unfolding of the binding site of the two substrates onto the AA-NAT protein [88–91], which reduces the K_m for the arylalkylamine substrates and also protects the enzyme from proteosomal proteolysis [75,76]. Additionally, an intramolecular disulfide bond between the Cys61 and Cys177, formed upon oxidation and cleaved upon reduction, is proposed to act as a catalytic switch for AA-NAT activation [92]. The enzyme has a high affinity for arylalkylamines, such as tryptamine and serotonin, and has a very low activity with regard to arylamines, such as phenylamine [93].

1.4.7 Molecular Mechanism of AA-NAT Regulation

The dynamic changes of AA-NAT synthesis and activity are regulated by complex control systems at different stages of enzyme synthesis and processing, and such systems consist of two basic elements: an autonomous circadian clock and turn-off mechanisms [31,94] (Figure 1.2). The circadian clock is composed of transcriptional/translational feedback loops and is entrained to the environmental lighting conditions. Turn-off mechanisms are responsible for the rapid suppressive effects of light on AA-NAT levels and activity [38,76,96]. At the transcriptional level, the control is through posttranscriptional processes (such as phosphorylation and binding to chaperone proteins) and through regulation of protein degradation velocity by proteosomal proteolysis [18,31,43,89].

The sympathetic neurotransmitter, NA, released from postganglionic fibers that innervate the pineal, is central to rhythmic AA-NAT fluctuations. At night, when the activity of these fibers increases, NA is released and stimulates postsynaptic β_1- and α_1-adrenergic receptors located on pinealocytes. In a process termed *biochemical "AND" gate*, an increase in intracellular Ca^{2+} concentration (resulting from α_1-adrenoceptor stimulation) results in the activation of adenylate cyclase (AC), resulting from β_1-adrenoceptor stimulation by a mechanism involving protein kinase C and calcium/calmodulin protein kinase. This activation causes a rapid and large increase (~100-fold in the rat) of intracellular cAMP level [84,96]. Elevated levels of cAMP, the second messenger that controls MEL biosynthesis in mammals, subsequently activate PKA and exert dual actions on AA-NAT. Thus, during the night or darkness (when cAMP levels are high), AA-NAT is phosphorylated by PKA and forms a complex with 14-3-3 proteins. Within this complex, AA-NAT is catalytically activated and protected from dephosphorylation and degradation [31,90,97]. In humans, the AA-NAT is regulated primarily at a post-transcriptional level, whereas in rodents, the key event appears to be cAMP-dependent phosphorylation of a transcription factor that binds to the AA-NAT promoter [98]. In rhesus monkey and human, the quantity of *Aa-nat* mRNA is high and displays no daily variations, while the enzyme activity increases by up to 10-fold at night [70]. Due to change in MEL content and secretion reflect oscillation in AA-NAT activity, it is also known as "the MEL rhythm-generating enzyme" [31,64,99,100].

The magnitude of the light evoked changes in nocturnal AA-NAT activity and dependent on the duration and intensity of the light pulse, its wavelength (blue and red light being the most and least potent, respectively), tissue, and species examined [101–103]. Studies performed on humans and nonhuman mammals indicate that a novel photoreceptor system that is distinct from the classical visual photoreceptors (cones and rods) and sensitive to the blue portion of visible light (λ_{max} between 446 and 484 nm), primarily involved in MEL-related and other non-image–forming light responses [101–102,104–106]. It is suggested that melanopsin, a newly discovered photo pigment [107–108], plays a primary role in light-induced MEL suppression [108].

Light pulses beginning late in the subjective day and early in the subjective night delay the phase of the MEL/AA-NAT activity circadian rhythm, while pulses beginning during the second half

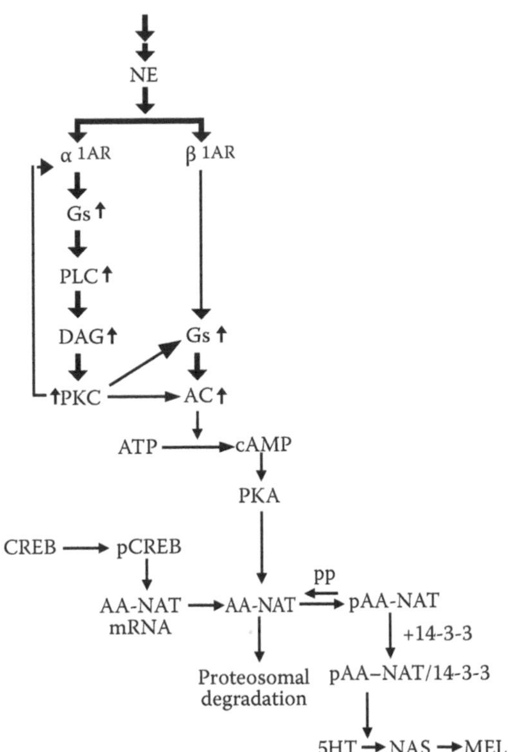

FIGURE 1.2 Schematic representation of the pathway of synthesis and degradation of AA-NAT. The dynamic changes of AA-NAT synthesis and activity are regulated by complex control systems at different stages of enzyme synthesis and processing. At night, NE is released from sympathetic nerves in the perivascular space in the pineal gland. NE interacts with adrenergic receptors on the pinealocyte membrane to increase intracellular levels of cAMP, results in activation of cAMP dependent PKA and phosphorylation of cAMP response element binding protein (CREB), thereby promoting transcription of AA-NAT. Moreover, PKA phosphorylates the AA-NAT protein that increases the affinity of the AA-NAT protein for 14-3-3 proteins. The phosphorylated AA-NAT (pAA-NAT)/14-3-3 regulatory complex protects the pAA-NAT against dephosphorylation by protein phosphatase (PP) and destruction by proteasomal proteolysis. In addition, complex (pAA-NAT)/14-3-3 has higher affinity for serotonin (5-HT) and increases *N*-acetylation of 5-HT resulting in an increase in *N*-acetylserotonin (NAS), which in turn enhances MEL production (see text for details).

of the subjective night produce a phase advance of the rhythm [109–114]. These time-dependent effects can be summarized as a phase response curve (PRC) [115]. The human PRC to light [111] is about 12 hours out of phase with the PRC to MEL [116]. In some reports, pulses of light given during the subjective day did not produce phase shifts [109,117]. However, it remains controversial whether such a "dead zone" exists in humans [116], in which clear evidence is available for the participation of two "oscillators" in the production of phase shifts [118]. The phase-advancing morning light has a greater affect on the MEL/AA-NAT rhythm decline, while evening phase-delaying light has a greater effect on the MEL/AA-NAT rise [119–120].

Exposure to light lowers cAMP, which leads to dephosphorylation of AA-NAT and disruption of the AA-NAT/14-3-3 complex, with a concomitant drop in AA-NAT catalytic activity and rapid proteasomal proteolysis of the enzyme [97,99,121–124]. This is the only cellular mechanism known to control AA-NAT activity in primates [31]. The rapid decline in the activity of AA-NAT with light treatment at night [38] appears to be complex and associated with the control of catabolism through various phosphorylation of AA-NAT by PKA, rho kinase, checkpoint protein 1 (CHK1)

[125], and subsequent association of the phosphorylated AA-NAT with the chaperone-like 14-3-3 protein [89]. This dimerization either drives the complex to a proteasomal mediated proteolysis or protects the complex from breakdown [126]. The retinal AA-NAT enzyme appears to be protected against breakdown during the day [127].

1.4.8 Hydroxyindole-*O*-Methyltransferase

HIOMT catalyzes the final step of MEL synthesis and other 5-methoxyindoles. This enzyme transfers a methyl group from the cofactor *S*-adenosyl-L-methionine to its indolic substrate. HIOMT represents 2%–4% of the pineal protein fraction [128]. The mean daily level of pineal HIOMT activity is about 4.3 ± 0.1 nmol/h/mg protein in humans [129] and ~9 nmol/h/mg protein in rhesus monkey [70], with no significant day/night variation.

The cDNA coding for *Hiomt* was first isolated in the cow [130], then in chicken [131], human [132], rat [133], and monkey [71], indicating large species differences. The rat cDNA displays low homologies with the cDNA of the cow (65%), human (63%), and chicken (59%). The whole cDNA sequence in the rat is 1728 bp long: the coding region contains 1101 bp, the 5′-noncoding region 184 bp and 3′-noncoding region 444 bp [133]. The human *Hiomt* gene is the best studied so far [129,132,134]. It is located in the pseudoautosomal region of the X chromosome and codes for three transcripts containing a transposable long interspersed element 1 (LINE-1) fragment. Two promoters, containing different *cis*-regulatory elements, have been characterized: one promoter A, whose expression appears restricted to the retina (contains the CCAATTAG sequence able to recognize transcription factors specific for the retina), and one promoter B, containing a CRE and an AP-1 site, whose strong expression is induced by a pineal specific regulatory element [134] like CRX. Indeed, PIRE and the CRX binding site have been reported in the promoter of human *Hiomt* [83]. The putative amino acid sequence of the rat HIOMT displays 60% homology with human. In the rat, the translated protein is made of 367 amino acids with putative sites of phosphorylation for PKC, type II casein kinase, and tyrosine kinase [133]. In different species studied so far, the enzyme displays a high molecular mass (76–78 kDa) and is made up of two similar subunits of about 39 kDa each. Immunochemical studies have revealed a large heterogeneity in the protein structure and enzymatic properties [135]. The HIOMT is very stable ($t_{1/2}$ > 24 hours) protein [129,136].

HIOMT activity has also been measured in the retina and the Harderian gland, although at much lower levels [129–134,137,138]. A very weak HIOMT activity has been demonstrated in the duodenum and colon (enterochromaffin cells) [139], in the human retinoblastoma Y79 cell line [129,136], and in ovaries [140]. RT-PCR experiments have also shown the presence of HIOMT mRNA in human platelets and the testis [141]. In contrast to AA-NAT, the nocturnal increase in pineal HIOMT activity is very low. In rats, pineal HIOMT activity displays a weak but significant nocturnal increase (by 40%–50%) [142]. This increase activity persists in constant darkness (D/D) and is inhibited in constant light (L/L) [142].

Hiomt gene expression is already high during the day but still displays a twofold increase at night that persists in D/D [133,142]. Light exposure at night rapidly decrease ($t_{1/2}$ = 20 minutes) the level of *Hiomt* mRNA [142]. A β-adrenergic receptor (β-AR) agonist stimulates daytime levels of *Hiomt* mRNA, whereas a β-AR antagonist inhibits it [133,142]. The short-term regulation of the enzyme appears to involve Ca^{2+} and PKC-dependent mechanisms [143], suggesting the activity and expression of HIOMT is regulated by different neurotransmitters using different mechanisms [144]. The decrease in enzyme activity corresponds to a reduction of the quantity of protein and decrease can be abolished by daily injections of a noradrenergic agonist [143,145]. The long-term regulation of HIOMT activity is due to the high stability of the protein ($t_{1/2}$ > 24 hour) [128,136,146] and depends upon noradrenergic control of *Hiomt* gene expression [142].

Demonstration of specific regulation of HIOMT activity in different mammalian species strongly suggests that HIOMT is involved in the rhythmic synthesis of MEL, especially the long term/seasonal rhythm in the nocturnal MEL peak pattern, which is an important indicator of the transmission of photoperiodic information. During the day, AA-NAT activity is lower than HIOMT activity and would be the limiting factor for the synthesis of MEL. The increase in AA-NAT activity at the beginning of the night thus induces the increase in MEL synthesis. During the night, however, HIOMT activity is lower than AA-NAT activity and would thus become the limiting enzyme for MEL production. Consequently, any variation in nighttime HIOMT activity should modulate the rate of MEL synthesis (the amplitude of the nocturnal MEL peak) [26]. Thus, HIOMT displays an important role in the photoperiodic control of pineal metabolic activity.

1.4.9 Noradrenergic and Other Regulators

Studies have shown that the pattern of MEL synthesis and secretions (the duration and amplitude of the nocturnal peak) coincide with target sensitivity, suggesting a complex control supported by the presence of multiple transmitters/neurotransmitters and their receptors in the pinealocyte/pineal gland. Therefore, the pinealocyte is orchestrating the functions of numerous neurotransmitters in the regulation of MEL synthesis. A dense noradrenergic innervation of postganglionic sympathetic nerve fibers that ends at the pineal gland release norepinephrine (NE) and plays a crucial role in the control of MEL synthesis [147]. Noradrenergic regulation of MEL synthesis in mammalian species (including Syrian hamsters, Siberian hamsters, European hamsters, mice, sheeps, cows, monkeys, and humans) has been well studied [26]. A marked species difference exists in the nocturnal NE stimulation of MEL synthesis. Limited studies in humans and monkeys suggest a "sheep-like" regulation. In humans, there is a large interindividual variability in the daily pattern of MEL synthesis, which also varies depending on age [148]. The nocturnal elevations in noradrenergic (NA) stimulation, via β- and α_1-adrenergic receptor of pinealocytes, increase the intracellular concentration of cAMP, which in turn activates AA-NAT [98], with the resulting MEL rhythm characterized by high levels at night. Stimulation of α-adrenergic receptors potentiates β-stimulation and requires the participation of other molecules such as calcium ions, phosphatidyl-inositol, diacyl-glycerol, and protein kinase C [149]. Thus, the synthesis and release of MEL are stimulated by darkness (~80% synthesis of MEL) and are inhibited by light. There is an immediate increase in circulating MEL at the onset of darkness [109]. Daytime β1-AR stimulation does not stimulate MEL synthesis [150], but its nocturnal synthesis can be inhibited by a β1-AR antagonist [151]. These findings suggest that NE is probably an important neurotransmitter regulating daily MEL synthesis. Since different mammalian species are not fully responsive to NE, it appears possible that other transmitters like 5-hydroxytryptamine, monoamine oxidase, cortisol, corticosterone, aldosterone, testosterone, and estradiol might play role to obtain a full MEL response, but their exact molecular mechanisms are not yet well characterized. Notably, the majority of the studies are restricted in the rat, mice, hamsters, and cell lines.

MEL synthesis, secretions, and catabolism are also regulated by a wide range of peptides including vasoactive intestinal peptide (VIP), pituitary adenylate cylcase (PACAP), histidine isoleucine peptide (HIP), neuropeptide Y (NPY), vasopressin, oxytocin, substance P, calcitonin gene related peptide (CGRP), secretoneurin (SN), hypocretin, natriuretic peptides (atrial, ANP; brain, BNP, and C-type, CNP), angiotensin, opiate peptide, and gonadotropin-releasing hormone (GnRH) [26]. However, most of this information emerged from the studies on nonprimates or cell lines.

1.5 SECRETION

Under natural environment, MEL is secreted during the night in the healthy human, as in all other species. MEL, being a lipophilic molecule, it is not stored but directly released by diffusion out of the pineal gland and released into the cerebrospinal fluid and the circulation. Although the eye contributes significantly to circulating MEL levels in a few species (sea bass, frog, quail, pigeon), retinal MEL acts primarily within the eye [18,152]. In humans, serum concentrations of MEL is low during the day (10–20 pg/ml) and is significantly higher at night (80–120 pg/ml), with peak between 02:00 and 04:00 h, when measured with high-specificity assay. The onset of secretion usually takes place around 21:00–02:00 h and the offset around 07:00–09:00 h in adults in the temperate zone [109]. The concentrations of MEL in saliva are approximately one third of those in plasma. Minimum concentrations in both fluids are usually below 5 pg/ml. The most striking characteristic of the human MEL is its reproducibility from day to day and from week to week in normal individuals, rather like a hormonal fingerprint [109]. A large variability in the amplitude of the rhythm between subjects and the nighttime production of hormone can differ by three orders of magnitude among individuals.

1.5.1 Factors Affecting the MEL Rhythm

The concentration of MEL varies in relation to the stage of development, puberty, menstrual cycle, and age of the individuals. Its peak values in blood may also vary from one individual to the other and depend on their age, sex, and disease [20]. Just after birth, very little MEL or 6-sulfatoxymelatonin (MT6s) is detectable in body fluids. A robust MEL rhythm appears around 6 to 8 weeks of age [153]. The development of MEL production is markedly delayed in premature infants [153,154]. The amplitude of serum level of MEL increases rapidly thereafter and reaches a highest peak in between 1 and 3 years of age [95,155]. The increment is much greater at night (54–75 pg/ml). Subsequently, a steady decrease (80%) occurs, reaching a mean adult concentration in mid to late teens, with a major decline before puberty, becomes relatively stable until 35 to 40 years, and a final decline in amplitude doesn't take place until low levels (16–40 pg/ml) are seen in old (~70 years) age [45,156,157]. During childhood, the decline in MEL production may be due to the increasing size of the human body [158,159].

Although MEL concentration is low during precocious puberty, higher MEL is noted in delayed puberty and hypothalamic amenorrhea compared with age-matched control [155] and abnormal MEL secretion in patients with premenstrual tension [160]. Low MEL is associated with cardiovascular diseases and diabetic autonomic neuropathology [161]. A potent reduction in nocturnal MEL together with an increase in daytime levels has been found in patients with Alzheimer's disease (AD), and these pathomorphological processes include dysfunction of SCN innervation to the pineal gland, degenerative changes in the SCN [162], and insufficient environmental illumination [163], a life condition frequently found in older residents of nursing homes. The plasma MEL profiles in blind people also fluctuate and may be categorized into three groups: (a) entrained with a normal phase, (b) entrained with an abnormal phase, and (c) free-running, with a circadian period (tau) different from 24 hours [164]. The majority of totally blind subjects have free running circadian rhythms and cyclic (non–24-hour) sleep/wake disorders. These are characterized by a period of good sleep followed by a period of poor sleep (short night-sleep duration) when the MEL rhythm is in an abnormal phase position (e.g., peaks during the day) [164,165]. This has been associated with increased napping and reduced alertness and performance during the day [164,166]. Appropriately timed daily doses of MEL have been shown to improve night sleep and reduce daytime napping as well as to entrain the free-running circadian rhythms [167–169].

1.6 CATABOLISM

Pineal MEL is released in the cerebrospinal fluid in the third ventricle via the pineal recess and attains levels up to 20–30 times higher than in blood but rapidly diminishes with increasing distance from the pineal gland [170]. This observation suggests that MEL is taken up by brain tissues. In the blood, 50%–75% of total MEL is bound reversibly to albumin and glycoproteins. The half-life of MEL is biexponential, with a first distribution half-life of 2 minutes and a second of 20 minutes [9,171] in the bloodstream [172]. The half-life of exogenous MEL is about 12–48 minutes [173–175].

The mechanism of catabolism of MEL is less understood, with the exception of the conjugation steps that account for ~70% of the ingested dose. MEL in all cells is metabolized nonenzymatically and also by free radicals as an oxidant. It is converted into cyclic 3-hydroxymelatonin (c3OHM) when it directly scavenges two hydroxyl radicals [176]. More than 90% of circulating MEL is primarily metabolized through the classical hydroxylation pathway in human and rodent liver by microsomal enzymes, cytochrome P_{450} monooxygenases (isoenzymes CYP1A2, CYP1A1, or CYP1B1) to 6-hydroxy-MEL [177,178], which undergoes further conjugation with either sulfate, catalyzed by sulfotransferase ST1A3, to form 6-sulfatoxy-MEL (aMT6s), and eliminated in the urine [109,179], or glucuronic acid, catalyzed by UDP-glucuronosyltransferase, to form 6-hydroxymelatonin glucuronide (in mouse) [9,171,180]. Urinary aMT6s excretion closely reflects the plasma MEL profile and is frequently used for evaluation of MEL rhythm in humans [109,181]. The magnitude of the light evoked changes in nocturnal aMT6s concentration is dependent on the duration and intensity of the light pulse, its wavelength (blue and red light being the most and least potent, respectively), tissue, and the species examined [94]. The appearance and peak plasma levels of aMT6s are delayed by 1 to 2 hours, and the morning decline by 3 to 4 hours [182]. In urine, 50%–80% of aMT6s appears in overnight sample (2400 to 0800 h), and levels are low but rarely undetectable in the afternoon and early evening [109]. In healthy full-term infants, rhythmic aMT6s excretion in urine is detected at 5–12 weeks of life [154,183]. At 24 weeks of age, total aMT6s excretion is 25% of adult levels [183]. Several other metabolites (approximately 30% of overall MEL) are also formed by the oxidative pyrrole ring cleavage [125]. Within the brain, MEL is degraded via oxidative catabolism by indoleamine-2,3-dioxygenase (IDO; EC 1.13.11.1.7) and/or myeloperoxidase (MPO; EC 1.11.1.7) leads to the formation of unstable intermediary kynurenine derivative, N^1-acetyle-N^2-formyl-5-methoxy-kynurenine (AFMK). IDO and MPO have micromolar range affinity with MEL. AFMK is further deformylated to the more stable metabolized either spontaneously or enzymatically by kynunerine formamidase (arylamine formamidase or hemoperoxidase) to N^1-acetyl-5-methoxy-kynunerine (AMK) [181,184,185]. AFMK is the primitive and primary active metabolite of MEL [185] (Figure 1.1).

Metabolic breakdown of retinal MEL is different from that of the MEL synthesized by the pineal gland. Initially, aryl acylamidase (aryl-acylamide amidohydrolase) catalyzes the deacetylation of MEL to 5-methoxytryptamine. Subsequently, 5-methoxytryptamine is metabolized via the same pathway as indoleamines and catecholamines, with deamination by monoamine oxidase to form 5-methoxyindole acetaldehyde, and its further oxidation to 5-methoxyindoleacetic acid or reduction to 5-methoxytryptophol [186]. Thus, 90% clearance rate of MEL is associated with excretion in the urine in metabolized form and in small quantities (~10%) in unmetabolized form.

1.7 MEL RECEPTORS

Being a lipophilic molecule, MEL has free access to all cells, all tissues, and all organs of the body. MEL has in addition acquired autocoid (act like local *hormones* near the site of synthesis, have a short half-life, and one that is not waste), paracoid, and hormonal properties [187]. The response of a cell to MEL may be due to receptor mediated, protein mediated (activate endogenous antioxidant enzymes) or non-protein–mediated (interact with different cations and metals) actions (see later section of this review). The development of high affinity radioligand binding assays of 2-[^{125}I] iodo-MEL, autoradiography, and studies with putative MEL receptor agonist and antagonists have allowed to identify, characterize, and demonstrate distribution patterns of MEL receptors in various central and pheripheral tissues [188–190]. The first MEL receptor was cloned from *Xenopus laevis* immortalized melanophore (dermal melanophore) mRNAs by using a cDNA library construct [191], but expressed only in nonmammalian species (birds and fish). Subsequently, human MEL receptors have been cloned [192].

Two forms of high-affinity MEL receptors have been identified on the basis of pharmacological and kinetic differences in 2-[^{125}I] iodo MEL binding assay [192,193]. According to the classification of nomenclature committee of IUPHAR (http://www.iuphar-db.org/iuphar-rd) [194], the high-affinity MT receptors are designated as MT_1 and MT_2, corresponding to the subtypes previously known as Mel_{1a} and Mel_{1b}, respectively [191,192,195]. In humans, MT_1 receptor is mapped to chromosome 4q35.1 and consists of 350 amino acids [196]. The gene for MT_2 receptor is located into chromosome 11q21-22 and cDNA encodes a protein containing 362 amino acids. Human MT_1 and MT_2 receptors show high homology at the amino acid level (60% overall and 70% within transmembrane [TM] domain) and have similar affinity for MEL [192,195,197]. These membrane-bound receptors (MT_1 and MT_2) belong to the superfamily of guanidine triphosphate binding proteins or G protein-coupled receptors (GPCR) containing the typical seven TM α-helices (TMI– TMVII) domains linked by three alternating intracellular (IC1–IC3) and three extra cellular (EC1–EC3) loops [198,199], and share high (~55%) homology in their amino acid sequences [193,200–202] (Figure 1.3). Glycosylation sites have been detected in the N-terminal region and, more importantly, the fourth IC loops of either receptor contain palmitoylable cystein residues [203], and the C-terminal domains putative phosphorylation sites for PKA and PKC as well as casein kinases I and II (CK I and II) [193]. Site-directed and chimeric receptor mutagenesis studies have identified residues critical for MEL binding to the MT_1 and MT_2 receptors [96,204,205]. Moreover, site-directed mutagenesis study [203] showed that neither the replacement of the palmitoylation site by alanine nor the truncation of the C-terminal domain containing the phosphorylation sites altered receptor affinity. However, the presence of both the lipid anchor and the C-terminal tail are required for G protein interaction, as judged from the lack of the cAMP response. The phosphorylation, but not the palmitoylation, sites are required for internalization indicating the unusual internalization process via phosphorylation and β-arrestin binding. In the brain, SCN is the main target of MEL, but the receptor density is ~4 fmol/mg protein, which is ~100 times lower than 5-HT receptors in other brain areas [206].

The human MT_2 has a lower affinity (K_d = 160 pmol/l) for ^{125}I-MEL as compared with the human MT_1 (K_d = 20–40 pmol/l), but the binding characteristics of the two are generally similar, such as, both are of high affinity and the agonist binding is guanosine triphosphate-sensitive [193]. MT_1 and MT_2 differ in their affinities to the natural ligand. For the human MT_1 and MT_2 receptors, K_i values are 80.7 and 383 pM, respectively [207]. However, higher inhibition or dissociation constants for MT receptors are also known [208]. Based on $MT_{1/2}$ receptors analogy to other GPCRs, it is suggested that MEL receptors form both homo- and heterodimers [209].

An additional cloned MEL-related receptor (GPR50) has around 40% sequence identity with $MT_{1/2}$ receptors, but is incapable of binding MEL [210]. At present, this receptor is classified as an orphan GPCR cytosolic enzyme, quinone reductase 2 (QR2, NRH-quinone-oxidoreductase 2, NQO_2; NRH, dihydronicotinamide riboside) and represented by MT_3 (previously known as Mel1c) [211,212]. Unlike $MT_{1/2}$ receptors, MT_3 is not a GPCR. MT_3 belongs to a group of reductase that participates in the protection against oxidative stress by preventing electron transfer reactions of quinines.

MEL is also ligand for transcription factors belonging to the retinoid-related orphan nuclear hormone receptor superfamily. These receptors are cloned and named retinoid Z receptor (RZR) and retinoid acid receptor (ROR)–related orphan receptor [213,214]. The RZR/ROR family consists of three subtypes: α, β, and γ. The ROR-α1, ROR-α2, and RZR/ROR-β have low affinity with MEL (K_d values in the lower nano molar range), and are widely expressed in the central and peripheral nervous systems and cancer tissues [213,215–217]. In addition, at elevated concentration of MEL interacts weakly with several intracellular proteins such as calmodulin (CaM) [218,219], calreticulin [220,221], or tubulin [222] and antagonizes the binding of Ca^{2+} to calmodulin [223].

1.7.1 Receptor Distribution

MT_1 and MT_2 are expressed both singly and together in various cells and tissues of the body [193,195] (Table 1.2). The density of MEL receptors not only varies with species and location, but also with the lighting regime, time of the day, tissues, developmental, or endocrine status of the species, MEL concentration in the plasma and aging or disease [224]. In birds and lower vertebrates, MEL

(a)

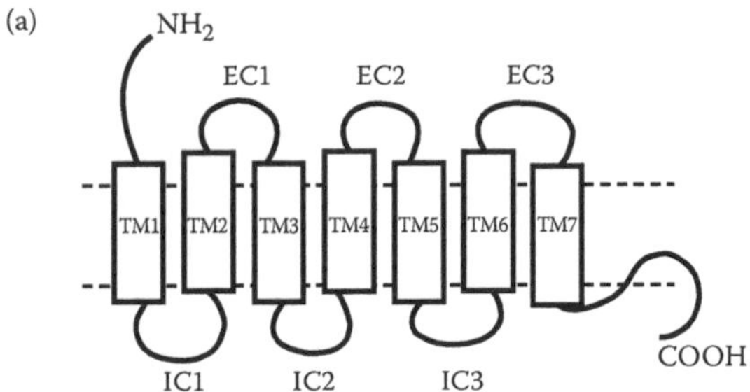

(b)

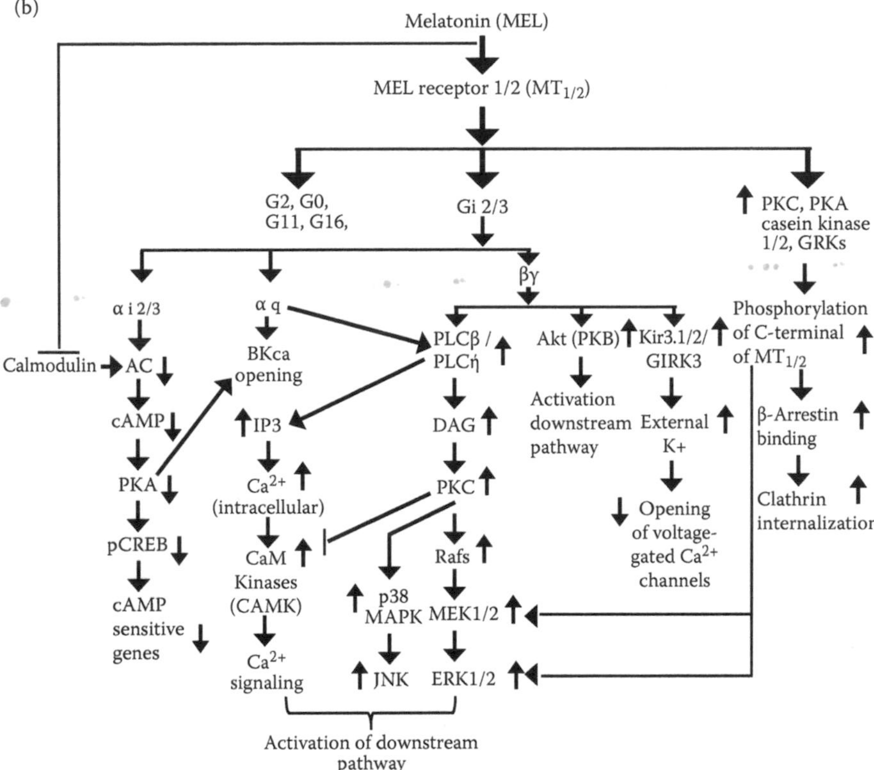

FIGURE 1.3 (a) Schematic representation of the structure of MEL receptors (MT_1 and MT_2). The membrane-bound MT_1 and MT_2 receptors belong to the superfamily of guanidine triphosphate–binding proteins or GPCR containing the typical seven transmembrane (TM) α-helices (TMI–TMVII) domains linked by three alternating intracellular (IC1–IC3), three extra cellular (EC1–EC3) loops, an extracellular N-terminal tail and a cytosolic C-terminal tail. (b) An overview of parallel and cross-signaling pathways of MT_1 and MT_2 receptors. In relationship with the function of MT_1 and MT_2 receptors, MEL influences second messenger cascades that vary in cell, tissue, and species-specific ways. These cascades include AC/cAMP/PKA/cAMP response element-binding protein (CREB) pathway, phospholipase C (PLC) β and PLC-η pathway, Ras/Rafs/MEK1/2/ERK1/2 pathway, PI3K/Akt (PKB) pathway, Kir3 (GIRK) inward rectifier potassium channels, GC/cGMP/PKG pathway, and receptor-independent signaling through Ca^{2+} binding proteins (see text for details). Abbreviations: Gα subunits and Gβγ dimers are depicted for Gi and Gq proteins; AC, adenylyl cyclase; Akt, homolog of kinase from retrovirus AKT8; Ca^{2+}, intracellular calcium; CaM, calmodulin; cAMP, cyclic adenosine 3′,5′-monophosphate; cGMP, cyclic guanosine 3′,5′-monophosphate; DAG, diacyl glycerol; ERK, extracellular signal-regulated kinase; IP3, inositol 1,4,5-tris-phosphate; MAP kinase: mitogen-activated protein kinase; MEK, MAP ERK kinase; pCREB, phosphorylated cAMP/Ca^{2+} response element-binding protein; PI3K, phosphoinositide 3-kinase; PLC, phospholipase C; PK, protein kinase; Raf, homolog of retroviral kinase, the product of oncogene v-raf; ↑, up-regulation or rise; ↓, down-regulation or decrease.

TABLE 1.2
Functional Attribute to Activation of Different Types of MEL Receptors in Humans

Site of Activity	Activation of MT_1 Receptor	Activation of MT_2 Receptor
SCN	• Inhibition of neuronal firing rate that modulates (entrains) the circadian rhythm (phase shift) and induce sleep • Inhibition of the cAMP response element-binding protein phosphorylation	• Induction of phase shifts in circadian rhythms
PT	• Inhibition of prolactin secretion	–
Central dopaminergic system	• Modulation of dopamine synthesis, release, and activation of dopamine receptors	–
Hippocampus	• Memory, excitation, and inhibition of neuronal activity; enhancement of seizure threshold via depression of GABAa receptor	• Same as MT_1 receptors
Cerebellum	• Interactions with glutamatergic synapses	• Same as MT_1 receptors
Retinal cells	• Inhibition of stimulation evoked release of dopamine, modulation of rod phototransduction pathways and photoreceptor functions, adaptation to low light intensities	• Same as MT_1 receptors
Cardiac ventricular wall	• Modulation of β-adrenergic receptor mediated cAMP signaling and stimulate voltage-activated calcium current	• Same as MT_1 receptors
Coronary, cerebral, and systemic artery	• Induction of vasoconstriction	• Induction of vasodilation
Prostate epithelial cells	• Suppression of DNA synthesis	–
Prostate cancer cells (LNCaP)	• Antiproliferative effect	–
Breast cancer cells	• Inhibition of proliferation in ER-α-positive cells (MCF-7)	–
Myometrium	• Modulation of uterine contraction, lower expression of MT_1 receptors in pregnant woman	• Same as MT_1 receptors, lower expression of MT_2 receptors
Granulosa cells	• Increase in LH receptor mRNA levels (luteal phase) and hCG stimulated progesterone levels; decrease in GnRH receptor levels	• Same as MT_1 receptors
Gallbladder epithelia	• Gallbladder contraction	• Same as MT_1 receptors
Pancreatic cancer cell lines (MIA, PANC)	• Regulation of acid/base homeostasis (stimulation of HCO_3 secretion)	
Skin and skin cells	• Antiproliferative effects on melanoma cells and normal cells	• Same as MT_1 receptors
Duodenal enterocytes	–	• Stimulation of HCO_3 secretion via neural stimulation
Adipocytes	• Lowering of GLUT4 mRNA and glucose uptake	• Same as MT_1 receptors
Choriocarcinoma	• Antiproliferative effects	
Immune system	–	• Increase splenocyte proliferation • Inhibition of leukotrine B4-induced leukocyte adhesion

Note: See text for details and references.
Activation of MT_3 (QR2) receptors: immunostimulatory effects.
Protection against a potential toxification mechanism.

receptors are widely distributed in the central nervous system (CNS) [195,225–227]. On the other hand, the distribution of MEL receptors is more restricted in mammals, and the level of expression is markedly weaker than in nonmammalian species. In mammals, most of the [^{125}I] MEL binding observed by in vitro autoradiography and physiological responses to MEL reflect MT_1 receptors, and MT_1 is more prevalent than the MT_2. The highest expression of MEL receptors in mammals (including human) has been found in the PT of the anterior pituitary (adenohypophysis).

Functional MT_1 receptors have been widely localized in the SCN [193,228], cerebellum [229], hippocampus [230], central dopaminergic pathways (including substantia nigra, ventral tegmental area, nucleus accumbens, caudate–putamen) [231], PT, ovary [232,233], testis [234], mammary gland [235], retina [236], coronary blood vessels and aorta [237,238], liver and kidney [239], gallbladder [240], skin [241], adrenal gland, and the immune system (T and B lymphocytes) [242]. The presence of MT_1 mRNA has also been demonstrated in the cerebral cortex, thalamus, hippocampus, cerebellum, cornea, and retina [198,243,244].

MT_2 receptors are more restrictedly expressed, being found mainly in the brain (hippocampus, SCN, and cerebellum of human) and retina, although their presence has also been detected in the lung, cardiac, aortic and coronary tissue, myometrium and granulosa cells, immune cells, duodenum, and adipocytes [21,193,198,239,243,246–248]. Moreover, both MT_1 and MT_2 receptors have been reported in the retina, cornea, ciliary body, lens, choroids, and sclera [243,249]. Both MT_1 and MT_2 receptors are widely distributed in the cancer tissues and cells, including breast, ovarian, endometrial, colon, hepatoma, melanoma, and prostate cancers [224].

The MT_3 receptor is expressed in the liver, kidney, brain, heart, lung, intestine, muscle, brown adipose tissue, and eye [250,251]. *In situ* hybridization studies have demonstrated mRNA expression of the RZR/ROR-β receptors in the rat brain, pineal, and neurons of several sensory regions including the dorsal horn of the spinal cord, but not in regions involved in motor control [252].

1.7.2 Mechanism of Action of MEL at Cellular Level

The SCN is the putative site of circadian action of MEL, and the hypophyseal PT is the putative site for its reproductive effects (Figure 1.3). In the SCN, MEL affects under both *in vivo* and *in vitro* conditions, circadian phase, and amplitude. MT_1 acts by suppressing neuronal firing activity by mediating a pertussis toxin (an inhibitor of Gαi)-sensitive vasoconstriction through BKca, whereas MT_2 inducing phase shifts by mediating vasodilatation [193,253,254]. However, the receptor subtypes are complementary in their actions and can, to a limited extent, mutually substitute for each other. In the extreme, one of these receptors can be exceptionally missing, as shown in two Siberian hamsters, *Phodopus sungorus* and *Ph. campbelli*, which lack active MT_2 receptors [255].

Depending on the tissue and species, MEL can activate different second messenger cascades acting on the same receptor subtype. By using recombinant MEL receptors, it has been shown that the predominant cellular effect of the MEL is the inhibition of forskolin-stimulated cAMP accumulation in the SCN and PT [256]. This effect of MEL is pertussis toxin sensitive, indicating coupling of the receptor to a G_i protein [257]. However, a cholera toxin (inhibitor of Gsα subunit)–sensitive component also mediates the inhibition of forskolin-stimulated cAMP accumulation [258], implying coupling through a G_0 protein. Thus, the classical effect of MT_1 and MT_2 receptors are primarily coupled, in an inhibitory manner, to the AC → cAMP → PKA signaling pathway, via a pertussis toxin sensitive G_i protein [193,195,198,254,255,260]. The decrease in cAMP production reduces the uptake of linoelic acid, an essential and major fatty acid, by specific fatty acid transporters. Co-precipitation experiments showed that the MT_1 receptor is coupled to different G proteins that mediate AC inhibition and phopholipase Cβ activation. Thus, MT_1 receptor activation leads to activation of a large variety of G proteins including $G_{i\alpha2}$, $G_{i\alpha3}$, and $G_{\alpha q/11}$ proteins [261], and $G_{i\alpha s}$, $G_{\alpha z}$, and $G_{\alpha16}$ [262,263]. Moreover, activation of MT_1 receptors leads to activation of phospholipase Cβ (PLC-β), with a concomitant increase of inositol-(1,4,5)-triphosphate (IP3), cytosolic Ca^{2+} and 1,2-diacylglycerol [198,243,253,264]. In addition, activated MT_1 receptors inhibit cAMP responsive element binding protein (CREB) phosphorylation, a nuclear transcriptional activator of cAMP-sensitive gene factor [265–268], and also inhibit the formation of immediate early gene products, c-Fos and Jun B [269]. The functional significance of this differential G protein coupling has further deciphered that G_{i2} and G_{i3} proteins mediate AC inhibition through a pertussis toxin–insensitive $G_{q/11}$ protein and are coupled to phospholipase Cβ activity in cell lines (HEK293, Cos-7, CHO cells) through stably expressing MT_1 receptors [261,264]. Parallel signaling processes are observed through other G proteins, including G_0, G_z, or G_{16}. This stimulatory effect is independent of an interaction with G_i or G_s proteins and associated with a calcium–calmodulin (CaM) signal transduction pathway and c-Jun N-terminal kinase activation [263,272].

Furthermore, stimulation of recombinant human MT_1 receptors causes not only the inhibition of forskolin-induced cAMP accumulation [259,261,264], but also potentiates the prostaglandin $F_{2\alpha}$–induced release of arachidonate and hydrolysis of phosphoinositide [259]. Activation of the MT_1 receptor induces a transient elevation in cytosolic calcium ion concentration and in inositol phosphate accumulation [261,264]. Stimulation of the MT_1 receptor is associated further with increased phosphorylation of mitogen-activated protein kinase (MEK1/2) and extracellular signal–regulated kinase (ERK1/2) [263,271]. In addition, MT_1 receptors regulate other ion fluxes and specific ion channels, such as increase in potassium conductance by activating inward rectifier potassium channels (Kir3/GIRK or Ca^{2+} activated K^+ channel, BKca) [272], and potentiate prostaglandin $F_{2\alpha}$- and ATP-mediated stimulation of PLC activity [259,264]. Both processes may involve activation of membrane-bound βγ-subunits released by G_i proteins. Thus, MEL restores the metabolic functions of cells with improvement in several aspects of Ca^{2+}-signaling such as the amplitude and frequency, the size of intracellular Ca^{2+} pool, capacitative Ca^{2+} entry, and the mitochondrial potential [273,274].

Activation of the recombinant MT_2 receptor couples to a number of signal transduction pathways including phosphoinositide production, inhibition of the formation of cAMP via the AC, and cGMP levels following the soluble guanylate cyclase pathway. Additionally, MEL increases the PKC activity through MT_2 receptor in rat SCN [253,275]. Expression of human MT_1 and MT_2 receptors in COS-7 cells demonstrates that activation of these receptors stimulates c-Jun N-terminal kinase (JNK) activity via pertussis toxin–sensitive and insensitive G proteins [263]. Moreover, despite the low expression of both MT_1 and MT_2 receptors in peripheral tissues/cells, they inhibit AC through αi, and activate other parallel signaling cascades through different G-protein subforms and also βγ heterodimers [193,198,224,259,261,268,276]. A critical step in MEL action through $MT_{1/2}$ is increased intracellular Ca^{2+} that leads to activation of PKCα [259,277,278]. PKC activation by MEL attenuates specific cellular functions such as androgen-dependent gene expression in prostate cell [279]. Furthermore, MEL blocks calmodulin (CaM) interactions with its target enzymes through induction of CaM phosphorylation by PKCα [280]. CaM Kinase II plays a regulatory role in the maintenance of CREB phosphorylation in the spinal cord [281].

A third mechanism of the biological effects of MEL is through MT_3 receptor, which is identified with lower MEL affinity, very rapid ligand association/dissociation kinetics, and widely distributed in various tissues of the body [282]. Mass spectrometry and enzymatic data confirmed that MT_3 is quinine reductase 2 (QR2), a known detoxifying enzyme [283]. The MT_3 receptor modulates calcium and CaM activity. Calcium-activated CaM is involved in the initiation of the S and M phases of the cell cycle, cell cycle–related gene expression, and the reentry of quiescent cells from G_0 back into the cell cycle [282]. Becker-Andre et al. [213] demonstrated that beside MT receptors, MEL has genomic action through a novel class of orphan nuclear receptors of the retinoic acid receptor family. ROR-α1 and ROR-α2 receptors are involved in immune modulation and inflammatory reactions [284]. MEL also acts as an intracrine, paracrine, or an autocrine manner in the pineal gland, eye, lymphocytes, gut, bone marrow, skin, and gonads for the local coordination [15,17,200,249,251,285–287]. The role of RZR/ROR-β as a transcription factor in sensory system is also suggested. The mechanism of actions of MEL at the cellular level has been schematically presented in Figure 1.3.

1.8 PHYSIOLOGICAL DIVERSITY AND THE THERAPEUTIC POTENTIALS

The amphiphilic (lipophilic and hydrophilic) character and pleiotropic nature of MEL with wide range of distributions of its receptors ascribe for multipotent physiological or pathophysiological functions of this hormone in humans. Although most of the studies in order to provide experimental evidence for the roles of MEL in human have used pharmacological doses of MEL (1 μM and above), a few studies confirmed these functions clinically or perfect experimentally as opposed to physiological doses (below the nanomolar range) of MEL [201,288]. Since several recent publications including ours [8] have reviewed the current status on multiple physiological functions including the autocrine–paracrine role of MEL, the current treatise emphasizes only a few of them, which proved important in the context of human health.

1.8.1 Synchronization of Rhythmic Body Functions with the Environment

Biological rhythmicity is fundamental to various physiological processes, and these rhythms are described according to frequency, period length, amplitude, and phase [289]. Circadian frequency implies that one repetition occurs every 24 hours. In humans, a few physiological variables (ACTH, cortisol, FSH, LH, MEL, prolactin, TSH, lymphocytes, and eosinophil counts) attain peak levels during sleep. Catecholamines and blood pressure surges occur during the transition from sleep to wakefulness. Other variables (blood viscosity, platelet adhesiveness, erythrocyte count, body temperature, blood levels of insulin and cholesterol, fifth Ewing variant [FEV], an E-twenty-six [ETS] transcription factor) that are assumed to be involved in the transcription of gene(s) in the serotonergic pathway and to play a role in early brain development attain peak activity during wakefulness, while gastric secretion and WBC count peak during the transition from wakefulness to sleep [289]. Circadian rhythms are generated by the SCN in the hypothalamus and are influenced by a variety of factors including sleep, cyclical hormone secretion, and daily rhythms of core body temperature [290]. Chronobiological disorders are the result of these rhythms failing to remain synchronized with environmental rhythms or discrepancy occurs when external time cues are removed. In human circadian periodicity has a frequency of 23.8 to 27.1 hours (~24.2 hours/cycle) with the body functions and is an inherited characteristic. This circadian frequency is closely related to diurnal preference and the early or late timing of the circadian system (MEL, cBT) in a normal entrained situation [291] (Figure 1.4).

The most important entrainment factor is environmental light and others include food, hormones (MEL, thyroid, and adrenal cortex hormones), social factors, and physical activity, although these are not as potent as photic stimulation [289,292]. MEL acts as an endogenous synchronizer either in stabilizing rhythms (circadian) of body functions or in reinforcing them. Hence, MEL is called a "chronobiotic" molecule [293]. It is also considered as a "neuroendocrine transducer" or "hormone of darkness" or "biological night," which is exclusively involved in signaling the "length of night" or "time of day" and "time of year" to all tissues. In humans, the exogenous administration of MEL changes the timing of rhythms by increasing sleepiness, wake electroencephalogram (EEG) theta activity, rapid eye movement (REM) sleep propensity, sleep propensity, endogenous MEL, and decreasing core body temperature, which ultimately leads to sleep [44,294,295]. This phase-shifting effect of MEL depends upon its time of administration. MEL phase-advances the circadian clock when given during the evening and the first half of the night, whereas the circadian rhythms are phase-delayed during the second half of the night or at early daytime. Thus, the exogenous administration of MEL at night (23:30 h) has a sedative effect, but earlier administration (18:00 h) causes the effect of temazepam [296]. The magnitude of phase advance or phase delay depends on the dose of MEL [297]. As MEL crosses the placenta, it plays an active role in synchronizing the fetal biological clock [9]. Thus, a practical definition of MEL would be "a substance that adjusts the timing of internal biological rhythms" or more specifically "a substance that adjusts the timing of the central biological clock" as chronological pacemaker or *zeitgeber* (time cue) as calendar function

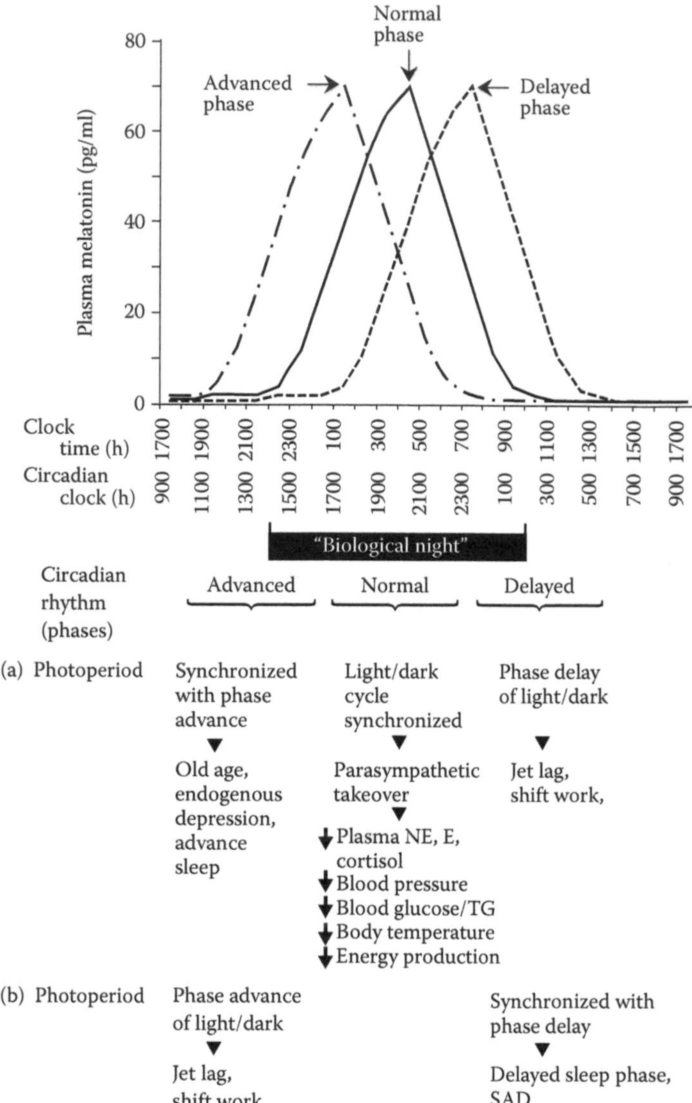

FIGURE 1.4 Schematic representation of the normal endogenous profile of plasma MEL secretions defining biological night, phase advance and delays, based on published data on phase response curves. (a) and (b) represent normal circadian rhythm disorders in relations to photoperiod (see text for details).

[298], although the appropriate zeitgeber circadian oscillators are found in every organ and indeed in every cell in the body [299].

The chronobiotic effect of MEL is caused by its direct influence on the electrical and metabolic activity of the SCN as shown by *in vitro* as well as *in vivo* experiments [293,300]. MEL, through various receptors, induces a differential influence on clock genes. All of the currently known mammalian clock genes have been cloned during the last two decades (1987–2005). These include the three mammalian homologues of *period* (*Perl*, *Per2*, and *Per3*), circadian locomotors output cycles kaput (*clock*), brain and muscle ARNT-like 1 (*Bmal*1/Mop3), the two homologues of *Drosophila cryptochrome* (*Cryl* and *Cry2*) and casein kinase 1ε (CK1ε). Human clock genes show high similarity to those of other mammalian clock genes. *Perl, Per2, Per3, clock, Bmall* (*Mop3*), *Cryl*, and

Cry2 genes are expressed in all peripheral tissues [301,302]. The clock genes are observed from flies to humans, but the functional roles played by some of their corresponding products differ between insects and mammals. In humans, the PT and SCN clock genes expression pattern show 24-hour rhythmicity. *Per1* is activated at the beginning of the light phase and Cry1 at the onset of the dark phase. Long or short photoperiod information is encoded within the SCN. Thus, synthesis of MEL is driven by the SCN and conveys the photoperiodic information to the PT by virtue of its secretion pattern. This phenomenon, in turn, influences the pattern of expression of the clock genes *Per1* and *Cry1* within the PT, providing a means of translating the MEL signal for the control of body rhythm or rhythmic synthesis and secretions of hormones [303]. However, amplitude modulation is unrelated to clock gene expression in the SCN [190,303]. The circadian regulation is determined by and interacts with neurotransmitter functions too. The highest concentrations of serotonin in the CNS is in the SCN [304,305], and its turnover exhibits marked circadian and seasonal rhythmicity, which is rapidly stimulated by light exposure [305].

At the cellular level, circadian rhythms of other clock genes are driven by the interlocking self-regulatory interaction. The positive arm of the circuit is the heterodimer of the proteins CLOCK:BMAL1. This complex binds E-box elements (CACGTG/T) at the promoter region of *Per1–2* and *Cry1–2*, including their transcription. The negative regulators are the translated CRY and PER proteins that complex with CK1ε and translocate into the nucleus, interacting with the CLOCK:BMAL1 complex, thus blocking their own transcription. Phosphorylation of PER and CRY proteins by CK1ε controls their proteosomal degradation, delaying the formation of CRY:PER complex and determining the length of the cycle. Additional regulators are negative loop generated by the transcription of the differentiated embryo chondrocyte (*dec1/sharp2/stra13*) and *dec2* (*sharp1*) genes, which are driven by CLOCK:BAML1 via E-boxes in their promoters. The basic helix–loop–helix proteins differentiated embryo chondrocyte 1 (DEC1) and DEC2 may block circadian gene expression, in part by the formation of a nonfunctional heterodimer with BMAL1, which inhibits the expression of all genes dependent on an E-box as well as plays a role in light induction of genes in the SCN. The circadian oscillation of clock gene expression controls the expression of genes involved in multiple cellular functions in a 24-hour cycle (clock control genes, CCGs) by at least two mechanisms, the direct interaction with E-boxes in the promoters of these genes and the regulation of other CCGs that in turn regulate transcription factors, like albumin D site-binding protein [306]. These studies reveal that MEL is an effective chronobiotic molecule that synchronizes rhythmic body functions with the environmental variables and clock genes.

1.8.2 Regulation of Sleep/Wakefulness Cycle

Two-process model of sleep regulation considers the timing and architecture of sleep to be a consequence of a homeostatic process of rising sleep pressure and the duration of prior wakefulness that is dissipated during the sleep period and is a function of circadian pacemaker [307]. Over the past decade, two important protocols have been developed to understand circadian and sleep homeostatic processes in human [308]. Based on these protocols, a strong relationship has been found between sleep and MEL levels [294]. Several epidemiological studies have confirmed the concept of the need for 7–8 hours of sleep per night, as this amount of sleep is associated with the lowest mortality and morbidity [309]. Both nocturnal MEL levels and the quality of sleep decline at puberty and in older people [310] (Table 1.3). The nocturnal peak is almost lost with age, which contributes to the homeostatic sleep drive decrease and need for daytime naps with poor nighttime sleep (mainly due to circadian loss). The period of sleep tends to become shorter and the quality of sleep poorer with decrease amplitude of the circadian rhythm and waking in a 12-hour light/12-hour dark cycle and, some time with phase advancement of circadian rhythm, caused delayed sleep phase syndrome, advance sleep phase syndrome, irregular sleep wake pattern, and non–24-hour sleep–wake syndrome [308,311,312]. Even a short period of sleep deprivation causes abnormal endocrine responses, leading to further complications such as impaired glucose tolerance, increased blood

TABLE 1.3
Relationship among Human Age, Plasma Concentrations of MEL, and Duration of Sleep per Day

Age	Plasma MEL (pg/ml)	Average sleep / day (hour)
Newborn–1 month	~5–10	Up to 18
1–12 month	~110	14–18
1–3 years	~110	12–15
3–5 years	~130	11–13
5–10 years	~160–170	9–11
10–18 years	~80–105	9–11
18–40 years	~85	7–8
41–50 years	~80	7–8
51–65 years	~60–75	7–8
65–70 years	~60	7–8
>70 years	~28–40	Irregular

Note: See text for details and references.

pressure, sympathetic activation, reduced levels of leptin, and increased inflammatory markers [309]. Similarly, cross-meridian flights involve disorganization of biological rhythm (jet lag) caused by the rapid change of environment and associated LD cues. Eastward travel affects sleep latency, while westward travel affects sleep maintenance. Delays in the LD cycle produce fewer symptoms, and therefore, westward flights tend to be less disruptive [312–314]. Jet lag exacerbates existing mood disorders (depressed mood) with reduced alertness, loss of appetite, poor psychomotor coordination, and reduced cognitive skills.

The clock genes in the SCN gradually adapt to phase-shift of the LD cycle (as found in shift work, trans-meridian flight). Peripheral clocks in the muscle, liver, pancreas, kidney, heart, lung, and mononuclear leukocytes are entrained directly by the SCN through some neurohormonal signals, glucocorticoids, retinoic acid, growth factors, and other zeitgeber, such as body temperature and feeding time, which resynchronize their clock genes at their own rates [315,316]. Circadian clocks in peripheral tissues/cells are resynchronized on their own. This results in a "double desynchronization"—"internal desynchronization" between different clocks in the body and brain and "external desynchronization" between the timing of body rhythms with respect to the LD cycle. This temporal orchestra of "jet lags" (sleep disturbance, mental inefficiency, or daytime fatigue) can be corrected by MEL taken at local bedtime only after arrival (between 10 pm and midnight), and effectiveness could be attenuated by the appropriate use of bright light [317]. Moreover, patient or animal model with primary insomnia (wakefulness and inability to fall asleep before 02:00 to 03:00 am), narcolepsy (a disorder of disturbed circadian sleep/wake rhythm and REM (sleep deficit), and sleep disorders in children (hyperactivity disorder) can be successfully corrected by treating or using wide pharmacological doses (0.5–50 mg) of MEL, but 5 mg seems to be the most effective dose and should be taken close to the target bedtime at the destination (22:00–24:00 h) [318]. Doses higher than 5 mg appear to have no further benefits, although higher secretion of MEL causes maximum sleepiness and fatigue at night [312,314,319]. Thus, MEL can be used at local bedtime to help in resynchronization of the circadian oscillator with the new environment for coordination of circadian rhythms and sleep function [318,319]. These studies indicate that application of MEL in optimum dose and schedule can successfully solve sleep-related problems in different age group of human.

1.8.3 Regulation of Mental State, Behavior, and Brain Functions

The pineal gland promotes homeostatic equilibrium through MEL and acts as a "tranquilizing organ" in stabilizing electrical activity of the CNS and causes rapid synchronization of the EEG. The classic endogenous, or nonseasonal, depression is characterized by insomnia (early morning awakening), appetite suppression, weight loss, and advanced onset of nocturnal MEL release, which begins in the spring and persists through the summer or through the winter during the period of light-phase shortening [320] (Figure 1.4). Similarly seasonal affective disorder (SAD) is characterized by late sleep, morning hypersomnia, increased appetite, and retarded onset of nocturnal MEL release, which peaks in the fall and spring [295]. Such phenomena are associated with individuals with low nocturnal MEL levels and major depressive/panic disorders [321]. Some patients experience major depressive disorder with seasonal pattern (MDD-SP), which is characterized by depressive episodes that occur at the same time every year [322,323]. The mood usually worsens as the duration of light hours is reduced in the winter. The circadian rhythms in these patients are usually in a phase-delay status. A supposition of strong link among MEL levels, pineal function, and mood disorders in these patients is strengthened by epidemiologic and chronobiological evidences. Moreover, in patients with depression, disrupted sleep is of major significance [324,325] with an increase in cortisol and temperature, and decrease in MEL amplitude [326,327]. In practice, between 40%–95% of subjects with depression have poor sleep quality [324,326,327]. These finding have been corroborated by physiological criteria from polysomnographic studies. About 40%–60% of outpatients and 90% of inpatients with depression exhibit polysomnographic abnormalities [326]. There is a casual relationship between insomnia and depression such as insomnia increases the risk of onset of depression and persistent insomnia is associated with a 40-fold increase in risk of depression. Moreover, insomnia increases the risk of recurrence of depression, whereas a stable sleep/wake rhythm and good sleep habits are essential in the prevention of further relapses in depressed patients [324]. Insomnia could also contribute to worse in the symptoms already caused by depression, such as irritability, decreased cognitive functioning, and poor executive functioning [290]. The treatment with different doses (>1 mg/day) of MEL in mentally depressed individuals at night prolongs the nocturnal MEL rise and helps in recovering SAD by changing the expression of clock gene and by changing the expression of *Per2* gene in bipolar or classic depression [321,328] and finally changing the quality and duration of sleep. However, the use of large doses of MEL in morning or early afternoon represents no clear effects [329]. In children, MEL is well tolerated and does appear to reduce the time to sleep onset as well as in minimizing nighttime awakening [290]. MEL is effective in hyperactive and neurologically compromised children and developmental gains have been reported after treatment with MEL (2.5–5 mg approximately 30–60 minutes before bedtime) [330].

Phototherapy as an adjuvant may accelerate responses to antidepressants among patients with depression [331]. MEL secretion has been shown to be wavelength-dependent as exposure to monochromatic light at 460 nm produced a twofold greater circadian phase delay [105]. These results are further confirmed by measuring brain 5-HT and Trp levels which rise after MEL administration and are directly linked with an array of neuropsychiatric phenomenon [332]. The diminished central 5-HT, as indicated by low levels of serotonin marker 5-hydroxy indole acetic acid (5-HIAA) in cerebrospinal fluid, is associated with impulsiveness, aggression and autoaggregation, alcoholism, compulsive gambling, overeating, and other obsessive–compulsive behaviors [333]. Moreover, the requirement of intact β-receptor function for MEL synthesis and stimulatory effect of norepinephrine on MEL synthesis and release demonstrate a direct relation of MEL to depression [334].

Administration of tricyclic antidepressants (TCA) at night also exerts sedative effects with increased MEL synthesis through binding with β-adrenergic receptors of pinealocyte and increased cAMP production, which in turn activates AA-NAT and enhanced MEL rhythm amplitude. TCA also inhibits cytochrome p450 enzyme CYP1A2, which metabolizes MEL in the hepatocytes and increases endogenous MEL levels [335,336]. Finally, it supports the serotonergic system to change or elevate mood, reduce aggression, increase the pain threshold, reduce anxiety, relieve insomnia, improve impulse control, and ameliorate obsessive–compulsive syndromes. However, higher doses or long term use of TCA has side effects by blocking muscarinic, histaminergic, and adrenergic receptors because of its joined benzene ring structure. In consideration to the quality of sleep and inducing onset of sleep with negligible daytime consequences, a schedule of treatment of insomnia patients with 2 mg MEL at night has been found to be equal to the treatment with zopiclone 5 mg at night [337]. Unfortunately, exogenous MEL has a very short half-life and is quickly cleared from the circulation.

Collectively, available information suggests that appropriate exogenous MEL administration can restore human neurological disorders with direct impact on general health of elderly people [338]. However, in some isolated cases, it has been demonstrated that a long-term use of MEL causes psychomotor disturbance, increased seizure risk, blood clotting abnormalities, headache, insomnia, GI tract effects, delayed puberty, and hypogonadism [339]. High doses of MEL in healthy subjects also cause drowsiness, decreased attention, and prolonged reaction time [322].

1.8.4 Scavenger of Free Radicals

The amphiphilic character of MEL helps it to cross both in the lipid and aqueous subcellular compartments in all morphological and physical barriers or hemato-encephalic barrier (blood–brain barrier [BBB], placenta) and reaches all tissues of the body within a very short period [9,340,341]. Therefore, the antioxidant properties of MEL appear to effect and perform a very important receptor-independent metabolic function as a multifaceted scavenger of free radicals. The antioxidant effects of MEL have been well described and included both direct and indirect effects with equal efficiency in multiple sites (nucleus, cytosol, and membranes) of the cell [305]. MEL is a more potent antioxidant than vitamins C (exclusively water soluble) and E (exclusively lipid soluble) [342]. Free radicals are defined as molecules or molecular fragments containing one or more unpaired electrons in their atomic or molecular orbital. Radicals and their nonradical related species are referred to as reactive oxygen and nitrogen species (ROS and RNS, respectively) and are products of normal cellular metabolism. The first indication that MEL may be a direct free radical scavenger was reported by Ianas et al. [343]. Two years later, Tan et al. [344,345] provided strong evidence that MEL is highly effective in detoxifying the highly reactive hydroxyl radical (•OH). MEL detoxifies a variety of free radicals and reactivates oxygen intermediates including the hydroxyl radical (•OH), hydrogen peroxide (H_2O_2), peroxy radicals (LOO•), peroxynitrite anion ($ONOO^-$), singlet oxygen ($^1O_2$), nitric oxide (NO•), superoxide anions (O_2•–), and lipid peroxidation. MEL neutralizes H_2O_2 by three different ways, through directly interacting with H_2O_2, by enhancing H_2O_2-catabolizing enzymes, or through its catabolic products (Figure 1.5).

MEL is itself not a direct free radical scavenger, but catabolites of MEL that formed during these interactions (namely AFMK and with considerably higher efficacy, AMK) [346,347] are excellent scavengers of toxic reactants. AFMK is produced by both enzymatic and non-enzymatic mechanisms [22] and mainly by myeloperoxidase (MPO) [125]. AFMK is capable of donating two electrons and, therefore, acts as a direct free radical scavenger in its own capacity [340]. The potent scavenger, AMK, consumes additional radicals in primary and secondary reactions [348]. Interestingly, AMK interacts not only with ROS but also with RNS [349]. MEL scavenges •OH by contributing an electron and, thereby rendering the radical nonreactive, becomes itself a radical, the indolyl cation radical [350]. This product is not very reactive and is, therefore, nontoxic to the cell [351]. The indolyl cation radical then scavenges the O_2–• forming AFMK, which is excreted in the urine. Each MEL molecule also scavenges two •OHs and generates the product, cyclic-3-hydroxyMEL and is directly excreted in the urine [352] as the classic antioxidant. The ratio of scavenger to radicals neutralized is 1:1.

The evidence that MEL neutralizes $^1O_2$ was first provided by Cagnoli et al. [353]. Subsequent study revealed that this function is performed through the formation of AFMK [354]. MEL scavenges the LOO•, which is produced during lipid peroxidation and able to propagate the chain reaction.

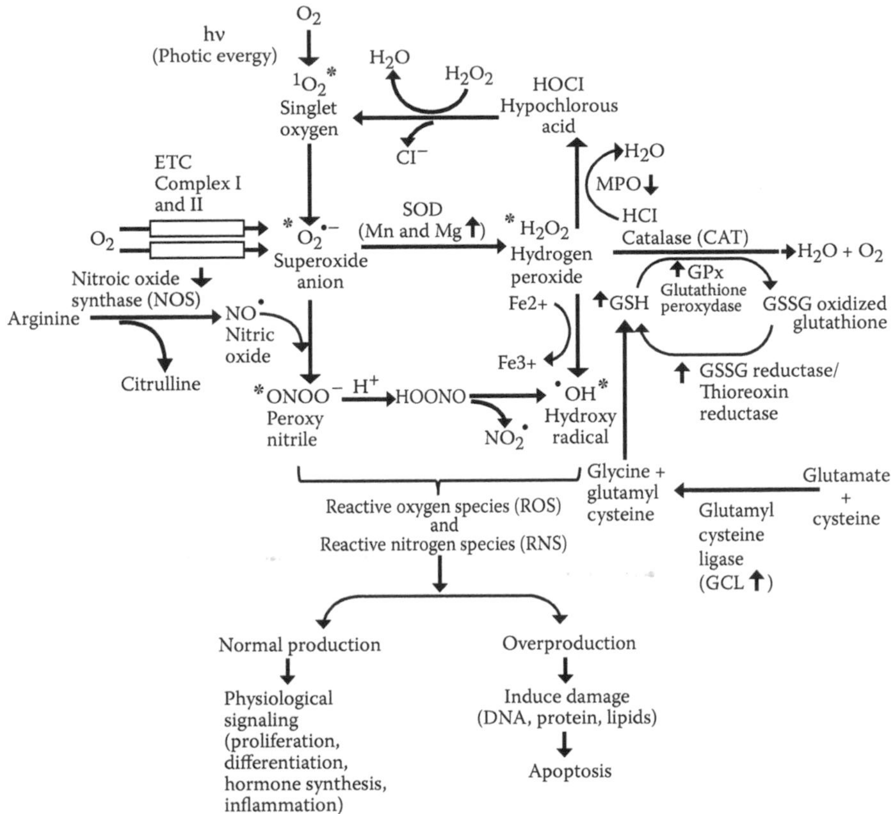

FIGURE 1.5 Schematic representation of the pathways of generation and neutralization of ROS and RNS by MEL. The main cellular source of ROS and RNS and the interrelationship between the antioxidant defenses by MEL. MEL directly scavenges the reactants marked with an asterisk. Abbreviations: •OH, hydroxyl radical; H_2O_2, hydrogen peroxide; LOO•, peroxy radicals; $ONOO^-$, peroxynitrite anion; $^1O_2$, singlet oxygen; NO•, nitric oxide; $O_2^{\bullet-}$, superoxide anions; GPx, glutathione peroxidise; GRd, glutathione reductase; G6PD, glucose-6-phosphate dehydrogenase; SOD, superoxide dismutase, both MnSOD and CuZnSOD, CAT, catalase; NOS, nitric oxide synthase; GSH, glutathione (see text for details).

Moreover, MEL is more effective than vitamin E in neutralizing LOO• and inhibiting lipid peroxydation [355]. Furthermore, MEL protective effects are a consequence of its ability to reduce NO• formation and scavenge $ONOO^-$ and associated oxidants. Although, inherently nonreactive, NO• quickly couples with O_2–• to form $ONOO^-$ [356]. Thus, by scavenging NO•, MEL reduces its generation under some circumstances by inhibiting the activity of its rate-limiting enzyme, nitric oxide synthases (c) [357,358]. The role of MEL in this process supports its anti-inflammatory ability.

The broad spectrum antioxidant activity of MEL also includes an indirect effect by up-regulating several antioxidative enzymes, and down-regulating pro-oxidant enzymes and 5- and 12-lipo-oxygenases [359], glutathione peroxidase (GPx) [360,361], glutathione reductase (GRd) [361], glucose-6-phospahte dehydrogenase (G6PD) [340,362], superoxide dismutase (SOD, both manganese–superoxide dismutase, MnSOD, and CuZnSOD) [363–365], catalase (CAT) [340,362] NOS [176] in particular. SOD plays a role in the dismutation of O_2–• from cells, thereby lowering the formation of highly reactive and damaging $ONOO^-$ [356]. GPx and catalase enzymes are involved in converting H_2O_2 to nontoxic products (water) in the body [366]. However, reduced glutathione (GSH) is oxidized to its disulfide, GSSG. GSSG is rapidly reduced back to GSH by GRd, thereby helping to maintain high levels of reduced glutathione [367].

MEL acts as a metal chelator. Limson et al. [368] demonstrated that MEL forms complexes with aluminum (III), cadmium (II), copper (II), iron (III), lead, and zinc. It forms complexes with lithium, potassium, sodium, and calcium [369]. The metal chelating ability of MEL increases with increasing concentrations of MEL. Thus, as a metal chelator, MEL acts as a neuroprotector agent.

MEL via AFMK pathway is highly efficient; a single MEL molecule scavenges up to 10 ROS or RNS. During oxidative stress, MEL level declines as it is metabolized by interaction with different reactive species [370]. More AFMK is produced during high oxidative stress along with cyclic-3-hydroxyMEL [370]. Likewise, AMK is 25% more potent than MEL in the inhibition of neuronal NOS (nNOS) [370]. Moreover, 6-OH-MEL (6-OHM) is also an effective free radical scavenger [371] as it binds with iron (III) and converts to iron (II), which is a more biologically usable form of iron [372].

Due to its strong antioxidant property, MEL protects membrane lipid, cytosolic proteins, nuclear DNA, and mitochondria from free radical damages. In mitochondria, MEL accumulates in high concentrations and stabilizes inner mitochondrial membrane thereby improving electron transport chain (ETC) activity [373–376]. It increases the activity of the brain and liver mitochondria respiratory complex I and IV, whereas the activities of complex II and III are not affected [377]. The high redox potential of MEL (0.94 V) suggests that it may interact with the respiratory complexes of the ETC and may donate and accept electrons, thereby increasing electron flow, an effect not possessed by other antioxidants [355,378]. MEL interacts, at high affinity (K_i = 150 pM) with a binding site at the amphipathic ramp of Complex I, thereby presumably modulating electron flux [276]. Thus, MEL protects the mitochondria from oxidative damage, reducing oxygen consumption concomitantly with its concentration, inhibits any increase in oxygen flux in the presence of an excess of ADP, reduces the membrane potential and consequently inhibits the production of superoxide anion and H_2O_2 [355]. At the same time, MEL maintains the efficiency of oxidative phosphorylation and ATP synthesis while increasing the activity of the respiratory complexes.

The protective effects of MEL and catabolic products on lipid peroxidation are induced by oxidative stress in mitochondrial membrane. MEL at micromolar concentration prevents the oxidation depletion of cariolipin (CL), which is particularly rich in unsaturated fatty acids (~80% represented by linoleic acid in heart tissue), and in addition CL is located near to the sites of ROS production. CL molecules are particularly susceptible to peroxidation by LOO• [355]. MEL prevents Ca^{2+}/peroxidized CL-dependent mitochondrial permeability transition pore (MPTP) opening and mitochondrial cytochrome c release. It also exerts antiapoptotic actions by up-regulating anti–apoptotic B-cell lymphoma (Bcl-) proteins, preventing Bax translocation, and directly inhibiting the MPTP at low affinity (K_i = 0.8 μM) [276]. This effect of MEL may have important implications in those pathophysiological situations that are characterized by alterations of Ca^{2+} homeostasis and accumulation of peroxidized CL in mitochondria [355]. Further, the functional alterations of the mitochondrial ETC complexes, as noted in heart ischemia/ reperfusion, and in the heart and brain of old animals, may increase the electron leak from the ETC, generating more O_2–• and perpetuating a cycle of oxygen radical–induced damage that ultimately leads to mitochondrial dysfunction because of oxidation/depletion of CL molecules [355]. AMK exerts its effects on electron flux through the respiratory chain and improves ATP synthesis in conjugation with the rise in complex I and IV activities [379]. Thus, MEL can be used in the treatment of several neurodegenerative diseases such as Alzheimer's disease (AD), Parkinson's disease, Huntington's chorea, amyotrophic ateral sclerosis, and aging, which are caused by three major and frequently interrelated processes, namely glutamate excitotoxicity, free radical–mediated nerve injury, and mitochondrial dysfunction [347,380–382]. These studies showed disruption of nocturnal surge of MEL in ischaemic stroke patients and patients with acute cerebral hemorrhage and reduction in the degree of tissue damage against ischemic injury through direct free radical scavenging or by indirect antioxidant activities in these patients following exogenous administration of MEL, which is suggested to have the neuroprotective role in MEL in strokes [383].

The oxidative stress is an important hallmark in disorganizing the cortical actin cytoskeletal assembly and disruption of accompanied subcellular intricate fibrous network composed of microtubules, microfilaments, and intermediate filaments (IF) as well as by associated proteins [384]. MEL prevents cytoskeletal structure disruption followed by cell shape changes and increased lipid peroxidation or apoptosis induced by okadaic acid of physiological plasma and cerebrospinal fluid [385]. In this process, PKC participates as an important signaling molecule as demonstrated by a PKC inhibitor (bisindolylmaleimide) abolished cytoskeltal re-establishment elicited by MEL, while the PKC agonist (PMA) reorganized microtubules and microfilaments [386]. Thus, MEL may be a suitable compound in the treatment of neurodegenerative diseases as a cytoskeletal modulator and also as a free radical scavenger [332,387].

The antioxidant properties of MEL help in reducing blood cholesterol (~38%) mainly by inhibiting copper-induced oxidation of low-density lipoprotein (LDL), with reduction in blood pressure and catecholamine levels via relaxation of smooth muscles in the aortic walls, thereby potentially contributing to an antiatherosclerotic effect on the cardiovascular system [388]. Likewise, exogenous MEL administration causes vasodilatation, decreasing internal artery pulsatile index, increases the cardiac vagal tone, decreases circulating norepinephrine levels, and finally reduces blood pressure in hypertensive patients [389]. MEL's antioxidant properties can also be additive to the treatment of gastric ulcer, bowel syndrome, ulcerative colitis, diarrhea, and glycerol-induced renal failure [390,391]. Taken together, MEL may act as a potent free radical scavenger, by neutralizing hydroxyl and peroxyl radicals among others, preventing lipid membrane peroxidation, apoptosis, and protecting the DNA from the damage induced by free radicals [392].

1.8.5 Antinociceptive, Anti-Inflammatory, and Immunomodulatory Function

The role of MEL as an immunomodulator in the regulation of proliferation, differentiation, and functions of lymphoid tissues has been known for nearly the past three decades [285,393–395]. The nocturnal rise in blood MEL levels in human is associated with increased production of interleukins (IL, including IL-1, IL-2, IL-6, IL-12), thymosin 1a, thymulin, and tumor necrosis factor-alpha (TNF-α). MEL production has been identified in lymphocytes and associated with IL-2 secretions [17,395]. The IL-2 is required for T-cell proliferation and clonal expansion, secretion of interferon γ (IFN γ), B-cell maturation and differentiation, and natural killer (NK) cell activation. All these factors are involved in allorecognition and responses [396]. In humans, MEL represents an inflammatory stimulus to monocytes, and it is suggested that monocyte function is directed toward an inflammatory phenotype during the night, when production of IL-12 is increased and IL-10 is decreased [397]. Furthermore, MEL implants enhance a defined T helper 2 (Th2)-based immune response under *in vivo* conditions and MEL supplementation enhances antigen presentation from antigen-presenting cells (APC) to T-cells via the specific up-regulation of major histocompatibility complex (MHC) class II molecules, and further increases TNF-α and IL-1 secretions [398]. MEL augments peripheral blood mononuclear cell (PBMC) proliferation *in vitro*, via the inhibition of production of T-helper type 2 (Th2) cytokines (IL-10) [399]. MEL may increase chemotaxis via the up-regulation of the chemokine production at the sites of inflammation, a process that may be synergistic with TNF-α [400]. In rodents, postnatal pinealectomy suppresses immunity and thymic atrophy, whereas exogenous MEL treatment increases cell-mediated immune function by increasing NK cell activity [401]. MEL limits the expression and activity of matrix metalloproteinases (MMP-2 and MMP-9) through the regulation of MAPK, JNK, ERK1/2, and the high-mobility group box 1 protein expression (HMGB1), thereby, reducing proinflammatory effects of TNF-α [402,403]. Collectively, these studies suggest potential role of MEL as a novel adjuvant immunomodulatory agent, in the adaptive processes of allo-recognition and allo-response [404]. Thus, MEL can be used as a potent therapeutic molecule to prevent graft rejection after organ transplantation. Since all organ transplant recipients are treated with continuous and permanent immunosuppression, this in turn increases the risk of infection and neoplasia formation [396].

MEL acts on immunocompetent cells (monocytes, B-lymphocytes, NK lymphocytes, T-helper lymphocytes, cytotoxic T lymphocytes) through MT_1 and RZR/ROR-α orphan nuclear receptor family and enhances cytokine production/secretions, cell proliferation, or oncostasis [405,406]. In B-lymphocytes, MEL binds to the RZR/ROR-α receptors to down-regulate the gene expression of 5-lipoxygenase (5-LOX), which is an important enzyme in allergic and inflammatory diseases like asthma and arthritis [284,407]. Immunomodulatory effects of MEL are observed in humans with bronchial asthma. On the other hand, exogenous MEL has an adverse effect in patients with asthma [347]. The nocturnal asthma is associated with elevation and phase delay of peak serum MEL levels [408]. In adjuvant-induced arthritis, both prophylactic and therapeutic MEL administrations inhibit the inflammatory response [409].

MEL also plays a role in pain modulation through $MT_{1/2}$ receptors as activation induces an antinociceptive effect at spinal and supraspinal levels under conditions of acute and inflammatory pain [410]. This effect agrees with localization of $MT_{1/2}$ receptors in thalamus, hypothalamus, dorsal horn of the spinal cord, spinal trigeminal tract, and trigeminal nucleus. The activation of $MT_{1/2}$ receptors leads to reduced cAMP formation and reduced non-reception. In addition, MEL is able to activate opioid receptors indirectly, to open several K^+ channels and to inhibit expression of 5 lipoxygenase, and cyclooxygenase 2 [410]. Thus, MEL and the immune system are linked by complex bidirectional communication. The immune system, in turn, appears to reciprocally regulate the pineal gland functions, mainly via cytokines produced by activated immune cells and depends on age, sex, and species [285,393–395].

1.8.6 Influences on Endocrine Network

MEL affects the synthesis, secretion, and action of steroid as well as nonsteroid hormones. It influences the adenohypophysial activity, which is dependent on the age and sex of the species, as well as the concentration of the hormone. There are substantial in favor of the conjecture that MEL modifies synthesis and secretion of different adenohypophysial hormones such as growth hormone/somatotrophin (GH), thyrotropin (TSH), and adrenocorticotropin (ACTH) either by directly influencing the secretory activity of the cells in the anterior pituitary or indirectly by influencing the hypothalamic neurons producing the respective neurohormones that stimulate or inhibit the release of adequate adenohypophysial hormones [411,412]. MEL has a positive phase relation with the synthesis of prolactin and negative with GH [411–413] and is involved in the regulation of calcium and phosphorus metabolism by stimulating the parathyroid gland or inhibiting calcitonin release and prostaglandin synthesis [414]. A similar change in prolactin levels is observed with the nocturnal increase and morning decrease as MEL levels. Administration of MEL also stimulates prolactin secretion [415]. However, the relationship between MEL and GH are poorly understood.

MEL affects the activity of pituitary–adrenal axis by modulating the peripheral action of corticoids [411,412]. Pinealectomy leads to adrenal hypertrophy, which is reversed by administration of exogenous MEL [339]. Therefore, it is proposed that MEL acts as a corticotrophin-releasing factor inhibitor with disinhibition of the pituitary–adrenal axis in major depression, since pineal MEL levels are low and unable to modulate its influence on adrenal gland [416]. Similar phenomenon (low MEL level) is found in patients with Cushing diseases (hyperadrenocorticism) [417] and hypercortisolemia, which is further linked to several aspects of aging and age-associated phenomena, including glucose intolerance, atherogenesis, impaired immune functions, and cancer [418]. Nocturnal MEL levels decline or are almost completely lost with age in humans [157,419]. This close reciprocal relation of MEL and corticoids or loss of MEL rhythmicity may be responsible for the pituitary/adrenal axis disinhibition that has been described as a characteristic of aging. The adrenals of elderly humans are apparently hypersensitive to adrenocorticotropic hormone, and midnight corticoid levels (low in young) are markedly elevated at old age [420]. Thus, MEL has phasic inhibitory effects on both the release of corticoids and their peripheral actions by immune depression, hypercatabolism, thymic involution, and adrenal suppression [421], which finally delays aging. However, there are no sufficient direct experimental evidences to demonstrate a relationship between MEL and hypothalamic–pituitary–adrenal axis.

There is a strong relationship between the functions of pineal gland and hypothalamic–hypophysial–thyroid axis [422]. But there are no sufficient data on the existence of such relationship in humans. Most of the studies in relation to thyroid and MEL are in other mammalian or nonmammalian vertebrate species.

The sex steroid production at different stages of ovarian follicular maturation is influenced by MEL. Adriaens et al. [423] have demonstrated that MEL (100 μM) increased progesterone (P) and androstenedione (A) production in mouse preantral follicles after incubation for 12 days, and MEL at a dose (100 ng/ml) stimulates P and A production in 30-hour cultures of porcine antral follicles, whereas estradiol (E_2) levels are not changed [424]. MEL also inhibits CYP 11A and CYP 17 expression but not that of CYP 19. Despite an increase in P production, the expression of CYP 11A is significantly inhibited. Further studies suggested that, at the time point studied, CYP 11A is transcriptionally inhibited as a result of feedback inhibition by high levels of P secreted into the culture medium. In contrast, MEL (0.1–10 ng/mL) decreases P, E_2, and cAMP production by hamster preovulatory follicles after 24 hours of incubation with hCG [425]. When theca cells and granulosa cells (GCs) are separated, MEL reduces P production by theca, whereas it does not influence the GCs. MEL may directly suppress follicular (thecal) steroidogenesis at an early stage in the steroid synthesis pathway through cAMP modulation. Moreover, MEL blocks the expression of steroidogenic acute regulatory protein (StAR) [426]. It is believed that StAR protein determines the translocation of cholesterol across the intermembrane space into the inner membrane where P450scc cleaves cholesterol into pregnenolone. MEL (10 nM) treatment for 3 hours reduces the StAR protein expression stimulated by hCG in mouse Leydig tumor cells. An *in vitro* study clearly demonstrated that MEL accelerates the action of maturation inducing hormone (MIH) in denuded fish oocytes [427]. However, the direct action of MEL on follicular steroid production is complicated; it seems to depend on the cell type (theca cell or GC), duration of treatment (acute- or long-term response), experimental model (cell culture or follicle culture), species, and the dose of hormone [428].

Locally produced growth factors, such as the insulin-like growth factors (IGFs, and members of the transforming growth factor β (TGF-β)) superfamily (inhibins, activins, and bone morphogenetic proteins, BMPs), work in concert with gonadotropins (FSH, LH) throughout the follicular growth continuum [428]. Insulin-like growth factors are produced by GCs and theca cells during follicle development [429]. Insulin-like growth factors are mitogenic and anti-apoptotic peptides which promote differentiation and also cause insulin-like metabolic effects mediated by binding to specific high-affinity membrane receptors. The IGF-I and IGF-II stimulate DNA synthesis and E_2 and P secretion by human GCs and granulosa–luteal cells [434]. Insulin-like growth factor I is an anti-apoptotic in ovarian follicles, whereas ovarian apoptosis is enhanced by IGF binding protein [430]. MEL (0.01-10 μg/mL) stimulates IGF-I production by cultured human GCs [431]. Recently, Picinato et al. [432] demonstrated that MEL (0.1 μM) induces IGF-I receptor and activates two intracellular signaling pathways: the PI3 K/AKT, which is mainly involved in cell metabolism, and MEK/ERKs that participate in cell proliferation, growth, and differentiation.

The TGF-β superfamily is expressed by ovarian cells and oocytes in a developmental, stage-related manner and functions as intra-ovarian regulators of follicle development. In humans, TGF-β is produced by both thecal cells and GCs [433]. The TGF-β stimulates FSH receptor expression [434], amplifies FSH-induced aromatase activity, and P production and LH receptor induction in GCs [435-437]. Interestingly, MEL enhances synthesis of TGF-β1 in human benign prostate epithelial cells [438]. Similarly, TGF-β1 immunostaining of multinuclear chondrocytes are dramatically increased in degenerated intervertebral disk tissue after exogenous MEL treatment (30 mg/kg of body weight daily at 5 pm to 6 pm for 4 weeks) in rats [439]. MEL treatment (5 mg/kg intraperitoneal injection) upregulates the level of gene expression of TGF-β in mouse peritoneal cells [406]. There is increasing evidence to support a critical role of TGF-β superfamily members BMP and growth and differentiation factor-9 (GDF-9) in growing antral follicles. BM-15 and GDF-9, exclusively produced by oocytes, may exert their effects by regulating the actions of gonadotropins. The BMP-15 has been shown to attenuate FSH actions on rat GCs by suppressing FSH receptor expression [440]. The GDF-9 reduced FSH-stimulated P and E_2 production and attenuated FSH-induced LH receptor formation [441]. These studies suggest an important interaction between MEL and BMP-15 and GDF-9 in the growing follicle.

1.8.7 Influences on Reproduction

The role of MEL in the regulation of reproduction is one of the major areas that received wide attention for different mammalian–nonmammalian animal species as well as in humans [7,428,442–444]. Obviously, MEL is per se neither antigonadotrophic nor progonadotrophic. Rather, the changing duration of the nocturnal MEL message is a passive signal that provides the hypothalamic–pituitary–gonadal axis information as to the time of year (calendar information) [445]. The reproductive axis uses the seasonally dependent MEL rhythm to adjust testicular and ovarian physiology accordingly. MEL has an inverse relationship with the hypothalamic GnRH, which is a decapeptide, released in pulsatile fashion from neurosecretory cells in the hypothalamus and acts on GnRH-receptors (GnRH Rs) in the pituitary to regulate the production and release of gonadotropins (follicle stimulating hormone, FSH; luteinizing hormone, LH) from the anterior pituitary. Traditionally, LH has been used as a surrogate marker of GnRH pulse generator activity in the human, based on its validation in animal models as a faithful mirror of GnRH secretions [446]. GnRH has been detected in human embryonic brain extracts as early as 4–5 weeks [451]. By 9 weeks gestation, GnRH neurons have been demonstrated in the fetal hypothalamus, although functional connections between these neurons and the portal system are not established until 16 weeks [451]. LH and FSH, being first detectable in the pituitary at 10 weeks, are measurable in peripheral blood by 12 weeks, reach a peak in midgestation, and then decreased toward term with the development of functioning gonadal negative feedback mechanisms [452].

During the neonatal period, there is a clear evidence of GnRH secretion in the study showing the persistence of pulsatile secretions of gonadotropins (FSH and LH) [453] followed by a decrease by approximately 6 months postnatal life in boys and 1–2 year in girls to the low levels that are present until the onset of puberty [454,455] (Table 1.4), whereas in neonatal period (~1–12 months), both boys and girls exhibit very low levels of plasma MEL (~5–10 pg/ml). The ultrasensitive LH assays have revealed that pulsatile GnRH secretion continues throughout the childhood period, albeit at a markedly reduced amplitude [456], when MEL level (~110–130 pg/ml) reaches its peak at night. The precise mechanism responsible for reversibly restraining the hypothalamic GnRH pulse generator at this time has not yet been elucidated. However, it is likely to involve a process that inhibits GnRH release rather than its synthesis as demonstrated in primates that abundant GnRH mRNA and protein are present within the appropriate hypothalamic neurons at an equivalent developmental stage [457]. In contrast, it has demonstrated that MEL down-regulates GnRH gene expression in a cyclical pattern over a 24-hour period through MEL receptors MT_1, MT_2, ROR-α, and RZR-β [458]. In neonatal pituitary cells, MEL inhibits GnRH-induced calcium signaling and gonadotropin (FSH, LH) secretion through MT_1 and MT_2 receptors. Further, MEL (1 nM) treatment in GT1/7 cells results in significant down-regulation of rat GnRH (rGnRH)-I mRNA rhythmic expression in a 24 h-cycle [459]. The potential regulator elements of MEL are localized to five regions, including -1827 to -1819 bp, -1780 to -1772 bp, -1746 to -1738 bp, -1736 to -1728 bp, and -1697 to -1689 bp, within the rGnRH-I enhancer [460]. These regions have been found to bind a number of transcription factors, such as Oct-1, GATA-4, and Otx2. In addition, two direct repeats of consensus binding sites for orphan nuclear receptors, including retinoic acid receptor-related orphan receptor/retinoid Z receptor, and COUP-TFI, and also other consensus binding sites for AP-1 and CCAAT-enhancer-binding protein (C/EBPb), are found within the -1736 to -1728 bp region [461]. Super-shift assays have demonstrated that only COUP-TFI and C/EBPb bind to this enhancer region of the rGnRH-I gene. Thus, the hypothalamic–pituitary–gonadal axis, which is already active during fetal life, remains quiescent until the age of ~10 years due to high levels of MEL (~160–170 pg/ml at night). This inhibitory

TABLE 1.4
Relationship between Human Age and Plasma Concentrations (UI/l) of Gonadotropins (FSH and LH)

	Male		Female	
Age	**LH**	**FSH**	**LH**	**FSH**
Day 1 to 1 month	~0.21–3.0	~0.25–1.50	~0.10–0.50	~0.20–6.70
1–3 months	~0.10–0.60	~0.10–0.90	~0.15–0.65	~1.10–2.50
4–6 months	~0.10–0.60	~0.10–0.90	<0.07–0.31	~0.50–1.60
7–24 months	~0.10–0.60	~0.10–0.90	<0.07–0.11	~0.40–0.75
2–10 year	~0.10–0.60	~0.10–0.90	<0.07	<0.10–0.50
Puberty				
Tanner stage I (preadolescent: elevation of papilla only, B1)	~0.30–1.00	~0.70–1.50	~0.30–1.00	<0.07–0.15
Tanner stage II (breast bud stage: elevation of breast and papilla, enlargement of areola diameter, B2)	~2.00–3.00	~1.10–1.70	~0.80–2.50	~1.30–4.20
Tanner stage III (further enlargement and elevation of breast and areola, without separation of contours, B3)	~4.50–5.50	~2.00–3.5	~3.50–5.80	~4.50–6.80
Tanner stage IV (projection of areola and papilla to form a secondary mound above levels of the breast, B4)	~4.00–8.00	~3.00–7.00	~5.00–11.00	~3.30–6.00
Tanner stage V (mature stage, projection of papilla only, recession of the areola to the general contour of the breast, B5)	~4.00–5.00	~1.50–4.50	~2.00–6.00	~3.00–5.00
18–40 years	~2.00–6.00	~3.5–5.00	a. Follicular phase ~2.40–12.60 b. Midcycle ~14.00–95.60 c. Luteal phase ~1.00–11.5	a. Follicular phase ~3.50–12.50 b. Midcycle ~4.70–21.50 c. Luteal phase ~1.70–7.50
>40 years	~0.80–8.00	~0.70–11.00	Menopause ~7.00–40.00 Postmenopause ~8.00–58.00	Menopause ~11.00–>20.00 Postmenopause ~25.00–134.00

Note: For details, see the works of Seminara et al. [446], Bergada et al. [447], Chada et al. [448], Phillips et al. [449], and Resende et al. [450].

role of MEL on the hypothalamus is responsible for sexual inhibition. However, other peptidergic regulators are also involved in this process.

Commensurate with the onset of puberty, there is a sleep-entrained reactivation of the reproductive axis characterized by a marked increase in amplitude of GnRH-induced LH pulse with much more modest changes in frequency with decrease in MEL levels (~80–105 pg/ml) [446]. This nocturnal augmentation of LH secretion stimulates secretion of sex steroids and inhibin from gonads at night with subsequent decrease to pubertal levels during the day [462]. As puberty progresses, secretion of gonadotropins occurs during both day and night. Moreover, the decline of plasma MEL below a threshold value (~115 pg/ml) may constitute the activation of signals for the hypothalamic pulsatile (increase in the amplitude and frequency of GnRH pulses) secretion of GnRH and reactivation of the pulsatile secretion of LH and FSH that are crucial subsequent pubertal changes (~10 years age onward) [411,412,463]. Furthermore, the inhibitory effects of MEL on GnRH action gradually decline due to decreased expression of functional MEL receptors [464]. The low concentration of MEL would result in premature activation of the hypothalamic GnRH secretion and the occurrence of precocious puberty [465]. These effects are further clinically demonstrated in humans showing that acute oral doses of MEL amplify LH pulses in early follicular phase, stimulate prolactin secretion and vasopressin secretions [283].

In adulthood, both sexes secrete gonadotropins in a pulsatile fashion, but in different patterns. In the adult male, wide variations in LH interpulse interval (2-hour frequency) have been reported with parallel changes in sex steroids [446]. In the female, the reproductive axis is under more dynamic regulation, with a complex series of changes in GnRH pulse frequency occurring throughout the menstrual cycle [446]. In the early follicular phase, the GnRH pulse frequency starts at approximately 90 minutes, shifts to 60 minutes in the mid- and late-follicular phases and, with the appearance of P secretions in the luteal phase, shows to cyclic changes approximately every 4–6 hours. By the late luteal phase, the GnRH pulse generator is active only at interval of 6–8 h, but accelerates once again during the luteal–follicular transition to approximately hourly intervals during the day, acquiring the sleep-induced slowing typical of the early follicular phase [446,466]. Furthermore, administration of exogenous MEL in combination with P to women reportedly induces a reduction in LH secretion, blocks ovulation, and in the luteal phase increases P without affecting FSH or inhibiting E_2 [467]. Acute suppression of LH levels is also observed in men after MEL treatment [468]. These effects may be mediated by MEL's ability to influence hypothalamic gonadotropin release [469]. Thus, decrease in MEL levels at the pubertal phase promotes GnRH dependent pubertal maturation and sexual development.

In contrast to hypothalamic action of MEL, a direct effect as an autocrine/paracrine manner on reproductive axis is also known [470]. Studies in human GCs showed that both types of MEL receptors (MT_1 and MT_2) are present, and MEL up-regulates LH mRNA-receptor too [470,471]. LH is essential for the initiation of leuteinization. Furthermore, MEL treatment enhances the human chorionic gonadotropin (hCG) stimulated P secretion with an inhibition of GnRH and GnRH receptor (GnRH-R) expressions. In the female reproductive tract P plays key roles in ovulation, implantation, and the maintenance of pregnancy by regulating GC function and follicle rupture during ovulation [472]. Ovulation is a complex process by which a preovulatory follicle ruptures and releases a fertilizable oocyte into the oviductal lumen. This process occurs as a result of a dynamic interaction between the LH surge and local factors including steroids, NO, prostaglandins, and peptides in a time-dependent manner. The LH surge triggers structural and biochemical changes that lead to rupture of the Graafian follicles, resulting in expulsion of the oocyte and subsequent development of a CL. After hCG injection, follicular steroidogenesis quickly shifts from E_2 dominance to P dominance by the inhibition of 17α-hydroxylase-C_{17-20} lyase activity [473]. This acute increase of P production is essential for luteinization and ovulation. Progesterone and E_2 concentrations are significantly higher in the large follicles (size > 18 mm, P ~10 μg/ml; E_2 ~512 ng/ml; T ~5ng/ml) than in the small follicles (size < 10 mm, P ~3.3 μg/ml; E_2 ~299 ng/ml; T ~7.5 ng/ml) of humans, and likewise, MEL concentrations are also higher in the large follicles (MEL ~123 pg/ml) compared with smaller follicles (~54 pg/ml) [428]. Interestingly, there is a positive correlation between follicular P and MEL concentrations [474]. Elevated concentrations of MEL in preovulatory follicle may be involved in P production, resulting in luteinization and ovulation.

Activation of the LH receptor in follicular cells by the preovulatory LH surge causes ovulation and rapidly initiates a program of terminal differentiation of the ovulated follicle into a CL through a process termed luteinization. Formation of the CL is initiated by a series of morphological and biochemical changes in cells of the theca interna and granulosa of the preovulatory follicle. Remarkably, transformation of GCs into luteal cells occurs within a few hours [475]. Not only structural changes, but genomic alterations also lead to the terminal differentiation of follicular cells into P-producing luteal cells. Progesterone receptor (PR) and cyclooxygenase 2 (COX-2) gene expression are induced after LH/hCG surge in GCs of ovulating follicles [476,477]. Ovulation is similar to a local inflammatory response [478], with both RNS and ROS being generated in this process. Both endothelial NO synthase (eNOS) and inducible NO synthase (iNOS) are present in the oocytes and thecal cells of the mouse [479]. The major source of ROS appears to be inflammatory cells including macrophages and neutrophils, as they are present in the ovary at ovulation [480,481] and they generate tremendous numbers of free radicals. These radicals act not only in the regulation of ovulation but also induce apoptosis of ovarian cells [482,483]. Thus, MEL, as well as its metabolites, acts as broad-spectrum antioxidants and exhibit free radical scavenger properties. Further, MEL concentrations in human ovarian follicular fluid (FF) obtained from the antra of Graafian follicles are significantly higher (>112 pg/ml) than those in simultaneously collected plasma samples [474]. Therefore, MEL and its metabolites quench ROS as well as RNS (see section MEL role as scavenger). Elevated MEL in preovulatory follicles is likely to protect GCs and the oocyte from free radicals that are induced during ovulation. MEL also prevents ovarian GnRH induced regression of corpus luteum [411,412,484]. Additionally, MEL's epigenetic efficacy through nuclear MEL receptor inhibits DNA methyl transferase by masking target sequences or by blocking the active site of the enzyme protects ovarian follicles [485].

In males, sperm are also protected from oxidative damage by MEL or its metabolites. Diazinon is a widely used organophosphorus pesticide that is toxic to sperm acting via free radical mechanisms. Exposure of any species to this toxin results in abnormal spermatogenesis. MEL has been found to be protective against many other free radical–generating toxic molecules [486]. In mouse, MEL treatment preserved spermatogenesis that was interrupted due to diazinon exposure [487]. Under other conditions in which testicular free radical generation is accelerated, MEL markedly reduces the level of gonadal oxidative stress [487,488]. For mammalian spermatozoa to be capable of fertilizing an oocyte, they must be capacitated and thereafter undergo an acrosome reaction and hyperactivation, which is a specialized movement of the flagellum of the sperm that permits it to penetrate the zona pellucidum. Human seminal fluid contains MEL [489] and spermatozoa reportedly possess membrane MEL receptors [490]. In hamsters, the addition of nighttime serum MEL (1 nM) resulted in significant hyperactivation of sperm within 1–2 hours [491]. This activation response was inhibited by the addition of the MTNR1A/MTNR1B MT receptor antagonist luzindole to the incubation medium, while the addition of specific MTNR1B antagonists was incapable of altering the hyperactivation response to MEL. The ability of MEL to stimulate flagellar motility is important given that this response is a requirement for the successful penetration of the zona pellucidum and fertilization of the egg. The physiological MEL concentrations in the seminal fluid of humans do not correlate with sperm motility. Further studies are needed to clarify the role of MEL in sperm activation and function in humans and other species.

MEL is also involved in myometrial cell functions. Human births occur more frequently at night when MEL levels are at their maximum than during the day. Schlabritz-Loutsevitch et al. [492] demonstrated that the two events are related and that myometrial cell possesses MEL receptors. Use of RT-PCR and *in situ* hybridization methods revealed that human myometrial cell membranes of uterine tissues have both MTNR1A and MTNR1B membrane receptors, and they are G_i protein linked to AC as in other cells. These receptors are also present in rat myometrial cells [493]. In myometrial cells collected from women during labor, the expression levels of the MTNR1B MEL receptor are markedly up-regulated. Moreover, in these cells, the actions of MEL synergize with those of oxytocin to promote muscle contractions and gap junction activity that is important in the coordination of myometrial contractions [494]. These observations are confirmed further by the study on cultured uterine cells in which the interactive effects of oxytocin and MEL are coordinated and lead to forceful myometrial contractions that enhance successful parturition [494]. These studies demonstrate a strong role of MEL in the maintenance of the hypothalamic–pituitary–gonadal axis.

1.8.8 Oncostatic Effects

The study on the influences of MEL on cancer has a long history. Cohen et al. [495] first put forward the theory on the possible role of the pineal gland on the etiology of breast cancer and suggested that a decrease in pineal function (reduction in MEL secretion) could induce a state of relative hyperestrogenism and the early and prolonged exposure of the breast tissue to the estrogens could be involved in the etiology of breast carcinogenesis. A few years later, Tamarkin et al. [496] described a relationship between plasma MEL concentration and breast cancer. There are also low incidences of breast cancer in blind women [497,498]. Subsequent studies have shown reduced levels of MEL in patients with certain types of cancers compared with normal healthy people of the same age [499–501]. The nighttime plasma MEL levels are lower in women with estrogen receptor–positive breast cancer than in estrogen receptor negative breast cancer and even lower than in healthy control women. Notably, women with the lowest peak MEL concentrations have the highest concentrations of estrogen receptors [496]. These oncostatic effects of MEL are evident further from the study showing consequent reduction of hormones such as prolactin and to a large extent estradiol, which are responsible for normal and pathological growth of the mammary epithelium [502]. Later, it has been demonstrated that MEL has antiproliferative effect through receptors MT_1 and MT_2 on various types of cancers including breast, lung, metastatic renal cell carcinoma, hepatocellular carcinoma, brain metastases from solid tumors, ovarian carcinoma, human neuroblastoma cells, bladder carcinoma, and erythroleukemia with tumor growth [500,503,504]. In these studies, the incidence of metastases has shown physiological to pharmacological effects of MEL. The antiproliferative effects of MEL are related to its modulatory effects on the cell cycle. In MCF-7 human breast cancer cells, MEL, in the presence of normal serum or estradiol, has been shown to retard or block the progression of cells from G_0–G_1 into S phase [505,506]. It has been demonstrated that exposure of rats with hematomas or human breast cancer xenografts to light during each 12 hours of dark phase resulted in a dose-dependent suppression of nocturnal MEL levels in blood and a stimulation of tumor growth [503]. Similarly, the treatment of prostate cancer cells with pharmacological doses of MEL significantly reduces the number of prostate cancer cells and stopped cell cycle progression in both androgen-dependent (LNCaP) and androgen-independent (PC3) epithelial prostate cancer cells and induced cellular differentiation [507]. Thus, it is evident that MEL not only reduces cell proliferation but also their metastatic capacity. MEL, at nanomolar concentrations, increases the expression of p53 and p21WAF1 [508,509], cell surface adhesion proteins (E-cadherin and β-integrin [510], and increases gap junctional intercellular communication between adjacent epithelial cells [511].

It has been demonstrated further that MEL through the action on the neuroendocrine reproductive axis may down-regulate the expression of estrogen receptor α (ER-α) and finally inhibits the binding of estradiol–ER complex to the estrogen response element (ERE) on DNA [506,512], and these effects depend on its binding to a high-affinity membrane-bound receptor coupled to G_i proteins [235,513,514]. MEL also shifts forskolin- and estrogen-induced elevation of cAMP levels by 57% and 45%, respectively, thereby affecting signal transduction mechanisms in human breast cancer cells [515]. cAMP and other protein kinase activators have been documented to synergize with steroid hormone–occupied receptors, leading to enhanced ER-mediated transcription through phosphorylation of the ER or associated transcription factors [516]. Estrogen-activated AC markedly increases the concentration of cAMP in ER-responsive breast cancer cells in culture in a manner that does not require new mRNA or protein synthesis, and is mediated by a high-affinity hormone binder (possibly ER). MEL, after its binding to $MT_{1/2}$ receptors, inhibits the AC and decreases cAMP, thus counteracting the effects of estrogens [508].

Another possible link between MEL and the estrogen signaling pathway is calmodulin (CaM). ER-α (not ER-β) has a CaM binding site and interacts with CaM [517]. The binding of CaM to ER-α stimulates the phosphorylation of the receptor, thus facilitating the binding of the estrogen as well as the binding of the estradiol–ER complex to the ERE [517,518]. MEL modulates the Ca^{2+}/CaM signaling pathway either by changing the intracellular Ca^{2+} concentration via activation of its G-protein coupled $MT_{1/2}$ receptors or through a direct interaction with CaM [218,519]. This is an antiestrogenic effect of MEL [506].

MEL treatment also showed MT_1/MT_2-dependent inhibition of uptake of fatty acids in general and of linoleic acid in particular, thereby preventing the formation of its mitogenic metabolite, 13-hydroxyoctadecadienonic acid [250]. At the same time, MEL also inhibits the fatty acid growth-factor uptake by cancer cells, inhibits telomerase activity by reducing telomere length, which causes apoptosis in cancer cells, inhibits endothelin-1 synthesis, an angiogenic factor that promotes blood vessel growth in tumors and finally modulates the expression of tumor suppressor gene, *TP53*, or inhibit transcriptional expression of cyclin D1. The action of MEL at different levels of signaling pathways in a tumor cell collectively promotes the idea that MEL may be considered as a supportive anticancer drug in the prevention and treatment of cancer, but the exact mechanisms of MEL action on cancer remain unknown.

1.9 MEL AS DIETARY SUPPLEMENT

Available literature providing evidence that various age-related or different physiological changes may be modulated by the decrease in MEL led few researchers and physician to suggest a beneficiary role of MEL as a dietary supplement against general age-related deterioration of health [520]. Degenerative conditions such as Alzheimer's disease and deterioration of cognitive function and behavior are strongly associated with low levels of MEL [311]. An obvious outcome of such observations is the suggestion that the required amount of MEL can be obtained from various plant sources (root, leaves, fruits, and seeds) in different species [19] (Table 1.5). It is expected that an efficient uptake of MEL from food should influence plasma MEL concentration, which is basically very high at night and is below the level of 10pg/ml during the day [22].

1.10 PHARMACOLOGICAL STRATEGIES IN USING MEL AS A THERAPEUTIC AGENT

Even though the MEL is a pleiotropic molecule that mediates the induction of a wide variety of physiological processes, a major constrain in the therapeutic use of MEL is its short half-life. Thus, pharmacological strategies need to be developed to overcome this shortcoming. The most effective tool of such development may be the strategy of slow-release of MEL preparations or the use of a MEL analog with a longer half-life ($t_{1/2}$ = 8–10 hours) than endogenous MEL, which might have greater effect on melatoninergic receptors in the SCN and other regions of the brain and can mimic the physiological profile with improvement in sleep quality, daytime alertness, sleep-onset latency, and general quality of life [311,532]. In the current scenario, there are only two applications for an improved therapeutic use of MEL: agomelatine (Valdoxan®, Melitor®), for the treatment of depression [533], and ramelteon (Rozerem®), approved by the Food and Drug Administration (FDA) for the treatment of primary chronic insomnia characterized by difficulty with sleep onset [534]. In addition, at present, phase II and III studies on tasimelteon (VEC-162, a high-affinity agonist of human MT_1 and MT_2 receptors) are in progress to demonstrate that the drug may have therapeutic potential for transient insomnia in circadian rhythm sleep disorders in general and for improved sleep latency, sleep efficiency, and sleep maintenance in particular [535]. These MEL agonists appear to be the most successful in clinical applications in chronobiology to date.

A more targeted therapeutic use of MEL is attempted in the form of ramelteon, which is synthesized by Takeda Chemical Industrial Ltd. (Osaka, Japan). Ramelteon has a very high affinity for

TABLE 1.5
Sources of MEL in Plants, Which May Be Used for Humans as Dietary Supplement

Source	MEL Content (pg/g)	References
White mustard seed	189,000	Manchester et al., 2000 [521]
Black mustard seed	129,000	Manchester et al., 2000 [521]
Turmeric	120,000	Chen et al., 2003 [522]
Wolf berry seed	103,000	Manchester et al., 2000 [521]
Fenugreek seed	43,000	Manchester et al., 2000 [521]
Almond seed	39,000	Manchester et al., 2000 [521]
Sunflower seed	29,000	Manchester et al., 2000 [521]
Fennel seed	28,000	Manchester et al., 2000 [521]
Alfalfa seed	16,000	Manchester et al., 2000 [521]
Green cadamone seed	15,000	Manchester et al., 2000 [521]
Tart cherries	2060–13,460	Burkhardt et al., 2001 [523]
Fax seed	12,000	Manchester et al., 2000 [521]
Anise seed	7,000	Manchester et al., 2000 [521]
Coriander seed	7,000	Manchester et al., 2000 [521]
Celery seed	7,000	Manchester et al., 2000 [521]
Poppy seed	6,000	Manchester et al., 2000 [521]
Tall fescue	5,288	Hattori et al., 1995 [524]
Walnuts	3,500	Reiter et al., 2005a,b [525,526]
Milk thistle seed	2,000	Manchester et al., 2000 [521]
Oat	1,796	Hattori et al., 1995 [524]
Sweet corn	1,366	Hattori et al., 1995 [524]
Tomato	1,067–1399	Pape and Luning, 2006 [527]
Rice	1,006	Hattori et al., 1995 [524]
Grape skin	5–965	Iriti et al., 2006 [528]
Japanese radish	657	Hattori et al., 1995 [524]
Japanese ashitaba	624	Hattori et al., 1995 [524]
Ginger	584	Hattori et al., 1995 [524]
Banana	466	Dubbels et al., 1995 [529]
Chungiku	417	Hattori et al., 1995 [524]
Barley	378	Hattori et al., 1995 [524]
Wheat	125	Hernandez-Ruiz et al., 2005 [530]
Olive oil	71–119 (pg/ml)	De La Puetra et al., 2007 [531]
Chinese cabbage	113	Hattori et al., 1995 [524]
Cabbage	107	Hattori et al., 1995 [524]
Welsh onion	86	Hattori et al., 1995 [524]
Cucumber	86	Dubbels et al., 1995 [529]
Carrot	55	Hattori et al., 1995 [524]
Tarro	55	Hattori et al., 1995 [524]
Japanese butterbur	50	Hattori et al., 1995 [524]
Apple	48	Hattori et al., 1995 [524]
Indian spinach	39	Hattori et al., 1995 [524]
Pineapple	36	Hattori et al., 1995 [524]
Canary grass	27	Hernandez-Ruiz et al., 2005 [530]
Strawberry	12	Hattori et al., 1995 [524]
Asparagus	10	Hattori et al., 1995 [524]

human MT_1 and MT_2 receptors, and a negligible affinity for MT_3 binding sites and for a large number of other receptors, including NA, GABA, glutamate, serotonin, histamine, acetylcholine, dopamine, and opioid receptors [207]. The half-life of circulating ramelteon is in the range of 1–2 hours, which is much longer than that of endogenous human MEL [536]. Ramelteon is metabolized in the liver by hepatic cytochrome p450 monooxygenases (CYP1A2, CYP2C, and CYP3A isoforms). Four distinct metabolites (M-I, M-II, M-III, and M-IV) of ramelteon are formed [536]. Among these, the metabolite M-II exerts a selective action on MT_1 and MT_2 as does the parent compound, but with an affinity of only 10% of ramelteon itself. Since, the metabolite M-II circulates at much higher concentrations than ramelteon resulting in a 20- to 100-fold greater mean systemic exposure, it is likely to most effectively contribute to biological action of the drug [536]. Ramelteon does not appear to significantly alter sleep architecture [537]. It reduces the evening circadian arousal signal and thus enhances the ability to fall asleep and stay asleep during the early part of the night [538,539]. The improvement in sleep-onset latency with ramelteon treatment is similar to that of MEL; however, ramelteon does not improve the patient's perceived sleep quality and next-day performance compared with placebo [534]. Ramelteon shows no evidence of accumulation after multiple dosing [536] and does not produce next-day residual effects [537]. It may be used at a dose of 8 mg at night as an approval of FDA for long-term use in adults. In contrast to commonly uses hypnotic drugs, ramelteon lacks abuse liability and does not impair motor and cognitive function. Ramelteon also has benign side effect profile, but some hormonal changes such as reduced testosterone have been reported [539].

Agomelatine is another pharmaceutical agent that is a potent and novel antidepressant agonist of MEL MT_1 and MT_2 receptors [540] and an antagonist of the serotonin 5-HT2c receptor subtype [541] and is endowed with antidepressant properties [311,327,542–545]. Like MEL, agomelatine causes inhibition of SCN neuronal activity, but its action is more prolonged than that of MEL due to its higher binding affinity to MT_1 receptor in the SCN [546]. Clinical studies of patients with MDD have demonstrated that the symptoms of depression are significantly improved with agomelatine compared with placebo, and agomelatine appears to be quite efficacious in treating MDD as other antidepressants but with fewer adverse effects [533,543,545]. Rapid onset of improved REM sleep quality without daytime sedation is achieved with oral administration (agomelatine ~5 or 100 mg/day) together with effective antidepressant and anxiolytic activity. In addition, polysomnographic studies have shown that agomelatine reduces sleep latency, decreases waking after sleep onset, and improves sleep stability, as measured by changes in the cyclic alternating pattern [543,547,548]. No significant discontinuation symptoms are known [327]. Agomelatonin has proven antidepressant effects with rapid efficacy in improving subjective sleep compared with several commonly used antidepressants [327,543]. Chronic treatment with agomelatonin leads to increased cell proliferation and neurogenesis in the ventral dentate gyrus in animals, suggesting similar effects in humans [327]. Agomelatonin has a strong restoring effect on the disrupted circadian rhythm in SAD [312].

1.11 CONCLUSIONS

MEL, a tiny tryptophan derivative in the bovine pineal extract discovered by a dermatologist just 53 years back, drew first scientific attention for its ability of blanching the skin in tadpole. Since then, the data already gathered from carefully controlled studies in a large number of animals and even plants have clearly implicated this wonder molecule in the control mechanisms of a wide variety of physiological and psychological activities of human beings. As an obvious outcome, MEL is now considered as a potent candidate for therapeutic use in the treatment of a diverse range of diseases mostly because of its recognition as a chronobiotic pleiotrophic molecule with multifaceted effects. Convincing reports do suggest that MEL causes modulation of body functions at various levels of hierarchy. The daily rhythm in MEL may have synchronized all physiological functions. But information on MEL synthesis in extrapineal sites at low or almost no circadian dynamics also indicate its additional noncircadian functions by the formation of bioactive metabolites and/or by specific subcellular actions. Although the roles and signaling mechanisms of tissue MEL are poorly understood to date, it seems that the coexistence of endocrine, paracrine, autocrine, and intracrine actions of MEL goes beyond local feedback effects common to other hormones, which are mostly mediated by the same receptors, or variants of them, as found in the respective target organs [276]. Additional binding sites different from membrane receptors may be of importance particularly for extrapineal MEL. As a whole, MEL displays a remarkable contextual diversity of functions, reaching from the control of circadian pacemakers and hypothalamic/pituitary axes to vasomotor effects and exhibits various facets of immunomodulation, antioxidant actions (expression of genes relevant to redox metabolism), direct and indirect antiapoptotic effects, interference with NO signaling, other antiexcitatory actions via ion channels and neurotransmitter systems, and modulation of mitochondrial electron flux. Its efficacy and safety may eventually drive its use in universally effective clinical applications and an adjuvant therapy for future treatment of different diseases as a supportive molecule to act together with other medicine. Moreover, melatoninergic agonists have a longer half-life than MEL and are widely useful in the modulation of sleep and depression.

In some countries (United States, China, Argentina, Poland), MEL is sold as a dietary supplement in health food and grocery stores/drug stores, but not as a drug, since all potential risks and/or advantages of MEL are yet to be clearly known. The effects of MEL at clinically relevant concentrations or under pathological situations are also required to be demonstrated in appropriate studies. Further detailed clinical investigation of the crosstalk and transactivation of different pathways would certainly help in understanding the mechanisms of action of MEL as a drug, allowing the design of powerful therapeutic agents for pathophysiological healing. Collectively, the current state of knowledge extends strong support to the contention of Ebadi et al. in 1989 [549] that, "the research for and discovery of how MEL, with its apparent omnipotent effects, brings forth a wide range of functions may raise the exciting prospect of providing new avenues of treating numerous diseases, thus replacing old treatments which sustain life but diminish its quality."

REFERENCES

1. Vollrath, L., The pineal organ, in *Handbuch Der Mikroskopischen Anatomie Des Menschen* (Oksche, A., Vollrath, L., eds.), vol. 7. Berlin: Springer, 1981.
2. Lerner, A.B., Takahashi, Y., Lee, T.H., Mori, W., Isolation of melatonin, the pineal gland factor that lightens melanocytes. *J Am Chem Soc*, 80, 2587, 1958.
3. Lerner, A.B., Case, J.D., Heinzelman, R.U., Structure of melatonin. *J Am Chem Soc*, 81, 6084–6085, 1959.
4. McCord, C.P., Allen, F.B., Evidence associating pineal gland function with alterations in pigmentation. *J Exp Zool*, 23, 207–224, 1917.
5. Huebner, O., Tumor des Glandula pinealis. *Dtsch Med Wochenschr*, 24(pt 2), 214–215, 1898.
6. Kitay, J.I., Altschule, M.D., *The Pineal Gland.* Cambridge, MA: Harvard University Press, 1954.
7. Reiter, R.J., Tan, D.X., Manchester, L.C., Paredes, S.D., Mayo, J.C., Sainz, R.M. Melatonin and reproduction revisited. *Biol Reprod*, 81, 445–56, 2009.
8. Chowdhury, I., Sengupta, A., Maitra, S.K., Melatonin: Fifty years of scientific journey from the discovery in bovine pineal gland to delineation of functions in human. *Indian J Biochem Biophys*, 45, 289–304, 2008.
9. Claustrat, B., Brun, J., Chazot, G., The basic physiology and pathophysiology of melatonin. *Sleep Med Rev*, 9, 11–24, 2005.
10. Hardeland, R., Poeggeler, B. Non-vertebrate melatonin. *J Pineal Res*, 34, 233–41, 2003.
11. Hardeland, R., Melatonin, hormone of darkness and more: Occurrence, control mechanisms, actions and bioactive metabolites. *Cell Mol Life Sci*, 65, 2001–18, 2008.
12. Hardeland, R., Backhaus, C., Fadavi, A., Reactions of the NO redox forms NO+, *NO and HNO (protonated NO-) with the melatonin metabolite *N*1-acetyl-5-methoxykynuramine. *J Pineal Res*, 43, 382–388, 2007.
13. Reiter, R.J., Tan, D.X., Melatonin: An antioxidant in edible plants. *Ann N Y Acad Sci*, 957, 341–344, 2002.
14. Korf, H.W., Schomerus, C., Stehle, J.H., The pineal organ, its hormone melatonin and the photoneuroendocrine system. *Adv Anat Embryol Cell Biol*, 146, 1–100, 1998.

15. Bubenik, G.A., Gastrointestinal melatonin: Localization, function, and clinical relevance. *Dig Dis Sci*, 47, 2336–2348, 2002.
16. Bubenik, G.A., Thirty four years since the discovery of gastrointestinal melatonin. *J Physiol Pharmacol*, 59(Suppl 2), 33–51, 2008.
17. Carrillo-Vico, A., Calvo, J.R., Abreu, P., Lardone, P.J., García-Mauriño, S., Reiter, R.J., Guerrero, J.M., Evidence of melatonin synthesis by human lymphocytes and its physiological significance: Possible role as intracrine, autocrine, and/or paracrine substance. *FASEB J*, 18, 537–539, 2004.
18. Iuvone, P.M., Tosini, G., Pozdeyev, N., Haque, R., Klein, D.C., Chaurasia, S.S., Circadian clocks, clock networks, arylalkylamine *N*-acetyltransferase, and melatonin in the retina. *Prog Retin Eye Res*, 24, 433–456, 2005.
19. Kandil, T.S., Mousa, A.A., El-Gendy, A.A., Abbas, A.M., The potential therapeutic effect of melatonin in gastro-esophageal reflux disease. *BMC Gastroenterol*, 10, 7, 2010.
20. Karasek, M., Melatonin in human physiology and pathology, in *Frontiers in Chronobiology Research* (Columbus, F., ed.), pp.1–43. Haupage, NY: Nova Science, 2006.
21. Slominski, A., Tobin, D.J., Zmijewski, M.A., Wortsman, J., Paus, R., Melatonin in the skin: Synthesis, metabolism and functions. *Trends Endocrinol Metab*, 19, 17–24, 2008.
22. Hardeland, R., Pandi-Perumal, S.R., Melatonin, a potent agent in antioxidative defense: Actions as a natural food constituent, gastrointestinal factor, drug and prodrug. *Nutr Metab (Lond)*, 10, 2–22, 2005.
23. Konturek, P.C., Konturek, S.J., Majka, J., Zembala, M., Hahn, E.G., Melatonin affords protection against gastric lesions induced by ischemia-reperfusion possibly due to its antioxidant and mucosal microcirculatory effects. *Eur J Pharmacol*, 322, 73–77, 1997.
24. Lovenberg, W., Jequier, E., Sjoerdsma, A., Tryptophan hydroxylation: Measurement in pineal gland, brain stem and carcinoid tumor. *Science (Washington, DC)*, 155, 217–219, 1967.
25. Balemans, M.G.M., Bary, F.A.M., Legerstee, W.C., van Benthem, J., Estimation of the methylating capacity in the pineal gland of the rat with special reference to the methylation of *N*-acetylserotonin and 5-hydroxytryptophol separately. *Experientia*, 34, 1434–1435, 1978.
26. Simonneaux, V., Ribelayga, C., Generation of the melatonin endocrine message in mammals: A review of the complex regulation of melatonin synthesis by norepinephrine, peptides, and other pineal transmitters. *Pharmacol Rev*, 55, 325–395, 2003.
27. Axelrod, J., Weissbach, H., Purification and properties of hydroxyindole-*O*-methyl transferase. *J Biol Chem*, 236, 211–213, 1961.
28. Axelrod, J., Shein, H.M., Wurtman, R.J., Stimulation of C14-melatonin synthesis from C14-tryptophan by noradrenaline in rat pineal in organ culture. *Proc Natl Acad Sci USA*, 62, 544–549, 1969.
29. Voisin, P., Namboodiri, M.A.A., Klein, D.C., Arylamine *N*-acetyltransferase and aryl-alkylamine *N*-acetyltransferase in the mammalian pineal gland. *J Biol Chem*, 259, 10913–10918, 1984.
30. Axelrod, J., Weissbach, H., Enzymatic O-methylation of *N*-acetylserotonin to melatonin. *Science*, 131, 1312, 1960.
31. Klein, D.C., Arylalkylamine *N*-acetyltransferase: "the timezyme." *J Biol Chem*, 282, 4233–4237, 2007.
32. Thomas, K.B., Brown, A.D., Iuvone, P.M., Elevation of melatonin in chicken retina by 5-hydroxytryptophan: Differential light/dark responses. *Neuroreport*, 9, 4041–4044, 1998.
33. Fournier, I., Ploye, F., Cottet-Emard, J.M., Brun, J., Claustrat, B., Folate deficiency alters melatonin secretion in rats. *J Nutr*, 132, 2781–2784, 2002.
34. Luboshitzky, R., Ophir, U., Nave, R., Epstein, R., Shen-Orr, Z., Herer, P., The effect of pyridoxine administration on melatonin secretion in normal men. *Neuroendocrinol Lett*, 23, 213–217, 2002.
35. Zawilska, J.B., Lorenc, A., Berezińska, M., Vivien-Roels, B., Pévet, P., Skene, D.J., Daily oscillation in melatonin synthesis in the Turkey pineal gland and retina: Diurnal and circadian rhythms. *Chronobiol Int*, 23, 341–350, 2006.
36. Reiter, R.J., Melatonin: The chemical expression of darkness. *Mol Cell Endocrinol*, 79, C153–8, 1991.
37. Illnerová, H., Borbély, A.A., Wirz-Justice, A., Prasko, J., Circadian rhythmicity: From basic science to clinical approach. *Suppl Clin Neurophysiol*, 53, 339–47, 2000.
38. Maitra, S.K., Huesgen, A., Vollrath, L.,The effects of short pulses of light at night on numbers of pineal "synaptic" ribbons and serotonin *N*-acetyltransferase activity in male Sprague–Dawley rats. *Cell Tissue Res*, 246, 133–136, 1986.
39. Moore, R.Y., Neural control of the pineal gland. *Behav Brain Res*, 73, 125–130, 1996.
40. Liu, C., Weaver, D.R., Strogatz, S.H., Reppert, S.M., Cellular construction of a circadian clock: Period determination in the suprachiasmatic nuclei. *Cell*, 91, 855–860, 1997.
41. Buijs, R.M., Hermes, M.H., Kalsbeek, A., The suprachiasmatic nucleus-paraventricular nucleus interactions: A bridge to the neuroendocrine and autonomic nervous system. *Prog Brain Res*, 119, 365–382, 1998.

42. Cassone, V.M., Natesan, A.K., Time and time again: The phylogeny of melatonin as a transducer of biological time. *J Biol Rhythms*, 12, 489–497, 1997.
43. Karolczak, M., Korf, H.W., Stehle, J.H., The rhythm and blues of gene expression in the rodent pineal gland. *Endocrine*, 27, 89–100, 2005.
44. Ekmekcioglu, C., Melatonin receptors in human: Biological role and clinical relevance. *Biomed Pharmacother*, 60, 97–108, 2006.
45. Arendt, J., Melatonin in humans: It's about time. *J Neuroendocrinol*, 17, 537–538, 2005.
46. Malek, Z.S., Dardente, H., Pévet, P., Raison, S., Tissue specific expression of tryptophan hydroxylase mRNAs in the rat midbrain: Anatomical evidence and daily profiles. *Eur J Neurosci*, 22, 895–901, 2005.
47. Sudgen, D., Comparison of circadian expression of tryptophan hydroxylase isoform mRNAs in the rat pineal gland using real-time PCR. *J Neurochem*, 86, 1308–1311, 2003.
48. Sakowski, S.A., Geddes, T.J., Thomas, D.M., Levi, E., Hatfield, J.S., Kuhn, D.M., Differential tissue distribution of tryptophan hydroxylase isoforms 1 and 2 as revealed with monospecific antibodies. *Brain Res*, 1085, 11–18, 2006.
49. Darmon, M.C., Guibert, B., Leviel, V., Ehret, M., Maitre, M., Mallet, J., Sequence of two mRNAs encoding active rat tryptophan hydroxylase. *J Neurochem*, 51, 312–316, 1988.
50. Boularand, S., Darmon, M.C., Mallet, J., The human tryptophan hydroxylase gene. An unusual splicing complexity in the 5′-untranslated region. *J Biol Chem*, 270, 3748–3756, 1995.
51. Cote, F., Schussler, N., Boularand, S., Peirotes, A., Thevenot, E., Mallet, J., Vodjdani, G., Involvement of NF-Y and Sp1 in basal and cAMP-stimulated transcriptional activation of the tryptophan hydroxylase (TPH) gene in the pineal gland. *J Neurochem*, 81, 673–685, 2002.
52. Besancon, R., Simonneaux, V., Jouvet, A., Belin, M.F., Fevre-Montange, M., Nycthemeral expression of tryptophan hydroxylase mRNAs in the rat pineal gland. *Mol Brain Res*, 40, 136–138, 1996.
53. Ehret, M., Pevet, P., Maıtre, M., Tryptophan hydroxylase synthesis is induced by 3′,5′-cyclic adenosine monophosphate during circadian rhythm in the rat pineal gland. *J Neurochem*, 57, 1516–1521, 1991.
54. Sun, X., Deng, J., Liu, T., Borjigin, J., Circadian 5-HT production regulated by adrenergic signaling. *Proc Natl Acad Sci USA*, 99, 4686–4691, 2002.
55. Chong, N.W., Cassone, V.M., Bernard, M., Klein, D.C., Iuvone, P.M., Circadian expression of tryptophan hydroxylase mRNA in the chicken retina. *Mol Brain Res*, 61, 243–250, 1998.
56. Thomas, K.B., Iuvone, P.M., Circadian rhythm of tryptophan hydroxylase activity in the chicken retina. *Cell Mol Neurobiol*, 11, 511–527, 1991.
57. Florez, J.C., Takahashi, J.S., Regulation of tryptophan hydroxylase by cyclic AMP, calcium, norepinephrine, and light in cultured chick pineal cells. *J Neurochem*, 67, 242–250, 1996.
58. Sitaram, B.R., Lees, G.J., Diurnal rhythm and turnover of tryptophan hydroxylase in the pineal gland of the rat. *J Neurochem*, 31, 1021–1026, 1978.
59. Johansen, P.A., Jennings, I., Cotton, R.G.H., Kuhn, D.M., Phosphorylation and activation of tryptophan hydroxylase by exogeneous protein kinase A. *J Neurochem*, 66, 817–823, 1996.
60. Ehret, M., Etudes de la régulation de la synthèse de la sérotonine dans divers modèles chez l'animal: Aspects transcriptionnels, posttranscriptionnels et posttraductionnels de la régulation de l'expression de la tryptophane hydroxylase. Thèse de doctorat de l'Université Louis Pasteur. 1994.
61. King, T.S., Steinlechner, S., Pineal indolalkylamine synthesis and metabolism: Kinetic considerations. *Pineal Res Rev*, 3, 69–113, 1985.
62. Yang, H.Y.T., Goridis, C., Neff, N.H., Properties of monoamine oxydases in sympathetic nerve and pineal gland. *J Neurochem*, 19, 1241–1250, 1972.
63. Klein, D.C., Evolution of the vertebrate pineal gland: The AANAT hypothesis. *Chronobiol Int*, 23, 5–20, 2006.
64. Borjigin, J., Wang, M.M., Snyder, S.H., Diurnal variation in mRNA encoding serotonin *N*-acetyltransferase in pineal gland. *Nature (Lond)*, 378, 783–785, 1995.
65. Roseboom, P.H., Coon, S.L., Baler, R., McCune, S.K., Weller, J.L., Klein, D.C., Melatonin synthesis: Analysis of the more than 150-fold nocturnal increase in serotonin *N*-acetyltransferase mRNA in the rat pineal gland. *Endocrinology*, 137, 3033–3044, 1996.
66. Coon, S.L., Roseboom, P.H., Baler, R., Weller, J.L., Namboodiri, M.A.A., Koonin, E.V., Klein, D.C., Pineal serotonin *N*-acetyltransferase: Expression cloning and molecular analysis. *Science*, 270, 1681–1683, 1995.
67. Coon, S.L., Mazuruk, K., Bernard, M., Roseboom, P.H., Klein, D.C., Rodriguez, I.R., The human serotonin *N*-acetyltransferase (EC 2.3.1.87) gene (AANAT): Structure, chromosomal localization and tissue expression. *Genomics*, 34, 76–84, 1996.

68. Coon, S.L., McCune, S.K., Sugden, D., Klein, D.C., Regulation of pineal alpha1B adrenergic receptor mRNA: Day/night rhythm and β-adrenergic receptor/cyclic AMP control. *Mol Pharmacol*, 51, 551–557, 1997.
69. Klein, D.C., Coon, S.L., Roseboom, P.H., Weller, J.L., Bernard, M., Gastel, J.A., Zatz, M., Iuvone, P.M., Rodriguez, I.R., Begay, V., Falcón, J., Cahill, G.M., Cassone, V.M., Baler, R., The melatonin rhythm-generating enzyme: Molecular regulation of serotonin *N*-acetyltransferase in the pineal gland. *Recent Prog Horm Res*, 52, 307–358, 1997.
70. Coon, S.L., Del Olmo, E., Young, W.S. III, Klein, D.C., Melatonin synthesis enzymes in *Macaca mulatta*: Focus on arylalkylamine *N*-acetyltransferase (EC 2.3.1.87). *J Clin Endocrinol Metab*, 87, 4699–4706, 2002.
71. Roseboom, P.H., Namboodiri, M.A.A., Zimonjic, D.B., Popescu, N.C., Rodriguez, I.R., Gastel, J.A., Klein, D.C., Natural melatonin "knockdown" in C57BL/6J mice: Rare mechanism truncates serotonin *N*-acetyltransferase. *Mol Brain Res*, 63, 189–197, 1998.
72. Craft, C.M., Murage, J., Brown, B., Zhan-Poe, X., Bovine arylalkylamine-Nacetyltransferase activity correlated with mRNA expression in pineal and retina. *Mol Brain Res*, 65, 44–51, 1999.
73. Gauer, F., Poirel, V.J., Garidou, M.L., Simonneaux, V., Pevet, P., Molecular cloning of the arylalkylamine-*N*-acetyltransferase and daily variations of its mRNA expression in the Syrian hamster pineal gland. *Mol Brain Res*, 71, 87–95, 1999.
74. Garidou, M.L., Gauer, F., Vivien-Roels, B., Sicard, B., Pevet, P., Simonneaux, V., Pineal arylalkylamine *N*-acetyltransferase gene expression is highly stimulated at night in the diurnal rodent, Arvicanthis ansorgei. *Eur J Neurosci*, 15, 1632–1640, 2002.
75. Coon, S.L., Klein, D.C., Evolution of arylalkylamine *N*-acetyltransferase: Emergence and divergence. *Mol Cell Endocrinol*, 252, 2–10, 2006.
76. Falcón, J., Gothilf, Y., Coon, S.L., Boeuf, G., Klein, D.C., Genetic, temporal and developmental differences between melatonin rhythm generating systems in the teleost fish pineal organ and retina. *J Neuroendocrinol*, 15, 378–382, 2003.
77. Zilberman-Peled, B., Benhar, I., Coon, S.L., Ron, B., Gothilf, Y., Duality of serotonin-*N*-acetyltransferase in the gilthead seabream (*Sparus aurata*): Molecular cloning and characterization of recombinant enzymes. *Gen Comp Endocrinol*, 138, 138–147, 2004.
78. Yoshimura, T., Nagabukuro, A., Matsuda, Y., Suzuki, T., Kuroiwa, A., Iigo, M., Namikawa T., Ebihara, S., Chromosomal mapping of the gene encoding serotonin *N*-acetyltransferase to rat chromosome 10q32.3 and mouse chromosome 11E2. *Cytogenet Cell Genet*, 79, 172–175, 1997.
79. Uz, T., Manev, H., Chronic fluoxetine administration increases the serotonin *N*-acetyltransferase messenger RNA content in rat hippocampus. *Biol Psychiatry*, 45, 175–179, 1999.
80. Baler, R., Covington, S., Klein, D.C., The rat arylalkylamine *N*-acetyltransferase gene promoter. cAMP activation via a cAMP-responsive element-CCAAT complex. *J Biol Chem*, 272, 6979–6985, 1997.
81. Burke, Z., Wells, T., Carter, D., Klein, D.C., Baler, R., Genetic targeting: The serotonin *N*-acetyltransferase promoter imparts circadian expression selectively in the pineal gland and retina of transgenic rats. *J Neurochem*, 73, 1343–1349, 1999.
82. Chen, W., Baler, R., The rat arylalkylamine *N*-acetyltransferase E-box: Differential use in a master vs. a slave oscillator. *Mol Brain Res*, 81, 43–50, 2000.
83. Li, X., Chen, S., Wang, Q., Zack, D.J., Snyder, S.H., Borjigin, J., A pineal regulatory element (PIRE) mediates transactivation by the pineal/retina-specific transcription factor CRX. *Proc Natl Acad Sci USA*, 95, 1876–1881, 1998.
84. Schomerus, C., Korf, H.W., Mechanisms regulating melatonin synthesis in the mammalian pineal organ. *Ann NY Acad Sci*, 1057, 372–383, 2005.
85. Liu, C., Fukuhara, C., Wessel, J.H. 3rd, Iuvone, P.M., Tosini, G., Localization of Aa-nat mRNA in the rat retina by fluorescence in situ hybridization and laser capture microdissection. *Cell Tissue Res*, 315, 197–201, 2004.
86. Bernard, M., Iuvone, P.M., Cassone, V.M., Roseboom, P.H., Coon, S.L., Klein, D.C., Avian melatonin synthesis: Photic and circadian regulation of serotonin *N*-acetyltransferase mRNA in the chicken pineal gland and retina. *J Neurochem*, 68, 213–224, 1997.
87. Hickman, A.B., Klein, D.C., Dyda, F., Melatonin biosynthesis: The structure of serotonin *N*-acetyltransferase at 2.5 angström resolution suggests a catalytic mechanism. *Mol Cell*, 3, 23–32, 1999.
88. Coon, S.L., Weller, J.L., Korf, H.W., Namboodiri, M.A., Rollag, M., Klein, D.C., cAMP regulation of arylalkylamine *N*-acetyltransferase (AANAT, EC 2.3.1.87): A new cell line (1E7) provides evidence of intracellular AANAT activation. *J Biol Chem*, 276, 24097–24107, 2001.
89. Ganguly, S., Coon, S.L., Klein, D.C., Control of melatonin synthesis in the Mammalian pineal gland: The critical role of serotonin acetylation. *Cell Tissue Res*, 309, 127–137, 2002.

90. Ganguly, S., Gastel, J.A., Weller, J.L., Schwartz, C., Jaffe, H., Namboodiri, M.A., Coon, S.L., Hickman, A.B., Rollag, M., Obsil, T., Beauverger, P., Ferry, G., Boutin, J.A., Klein, D.C., Role of a pineal cAMP-operated arylalkylamine *N*-acetyltransferase/14–3–3-binding switch in melatonin synthesis. *Proc Natl Acad Sci USA*, 98, 8083–8088, 2001.
91. Klein, D.C., Ganguly, S., Coon, S., Weller, J.L., Obsil, T., Hickman, A., Dyda, F., 14–3–3 proteins and photoneuroendocrine transduction: Role in controlling the daily rhythm in melatonin. *Biochem Soc Trans*, 30, 365–373, 2002.
92. Tsuboi, S., Kotani, Y., Ogawa, K., Hatanaka, T., Yatsushiro, S., Otsuka, M., Moriyama, Y., An intramolecular disulfide bridge as a catalytic switch for serotonin *N*-acetyltransferase. *J Biol Chem*, 277, 44229–44235, 2002.
93. Ferry, G., Loynel, A., Kucharczyk, N., Bertin, S., Rodriguez, M., Delagrange, P., Galizzi, J.P., Jacoby, E., Volland, J.P., Lesieur, D., Renard, P., Canet, E., Fauchère, J.L., Boutin, J.A., Substrate specificity and inhibition studies of human serotonin *N*-acetyltransferase. *J Biol Chem*, 275, 8794–8805, 2000.
94. Zawilska, J.B., Debra, J.S., Josephine, A., Physiology and pharmacology of melatonin in relation to biological rhythms. *Pharmacol Rep*, 61, 383–410, 2009.
95. Stokkan, K.A., van Oort, B.E., Tyler, N.J., Loudon, A.S., Adaptations for life in the Arctic: Evidence that melatonin rhythms in reindeer are not driven by a circadian oscillator but remain acutely sensitive to environmental photoperiod. *J Pineal Res*, 43, 289–293, 2007.
96. Kokkola, T., Foord, S.M., Watson, M.A., Vakkuri, O., Laitinen, J.T., Important amino acids for the function of the human MT1 melatonin receptor. *Biochem Pharmacol*, 65, 1463–1471, 2003.
97. Pozdeyev, N., Taylor, C., Haque, R., Chaurasia, S.S., Visser, A., Thazyeen, A., Du, Y., Fu, H., Weller, J., Klein, D.C., Iuvone PM., Photic regulation of arylalkylamine *N*-acetyltransferase binding to 14–3–3 proteins in retinal photoreceptor cells. *J Neurosci*, 26, 9153–9161, 2006.
98. Ackermann, K., Stehl, J.H., Melatonin synthesis in the human pineal gland: Advantages, implications, and difficulties. *Chronobiol Int*, 23, 369–379, 2006.
99. Schomerus, C., Korf, H.W., Laedtke, E., Weller, J.L., Klein, D.C., Selective adrenergic/cyclic AMP-dependent switch-off of proteasomal proteolysis alone switches on neural signal transduction: An example from the pineal gland. *J Neurochem*, 75, 2123–2132, 2000.
100. Stehle, J.H., von Gall, C., Schomerus, C., Korf, H.W., Of rodents and ungulates and melatonin: Creating a uniform code for darkness by different signaling mechanisms. *J Biol Rhythms*, 16, 312–325, 2001.
101. Brainard, G.C., Hanifin, J.P., Greeson, J.M., Byrne, B., Glickman, G., Gerner, E., Rollag, M.D., Action spectrum for melatonin regulation in humans: Evidence for a novel circadian photoreceptor. *J Neurosci*, 21, 6405–6412, 2001.
102. Thapan, K., Arendt, J., Skene, D.J., An action spectrum for melatonin suppression: Evidence for a novel non-rod, non-cone photoreceptor system in humans. *J Physiol*, 535, 261–267, 2001.
103. Zawilska, J.B., Derbiszewska, T., Sek, B., Nowak, J.Z., Dopamine-dependent cyclic AMP generating system in chick retina and its relation to melatonin biosynthesis. *Neurochem Int*, 27, 535–543, 1995.
104. Cajochen, C., Münch, M., Kobialka, S., Kräuchi, K., Steiner, R., Oelhafen, P., Orgül, S., Wirz-Justice, A., High sensitivity of human melatonin, alertness, thermoregulation, and heart rate to short wavelength light. *J Clin Endocrinol Metab*, 90, 1311–1316, 2005.
105. Lockley, S.W., Brainard, G.C., Czeisler, C.A., High sensitivity of the human circadian melatonin rhythm to resetting by short wavelength light. *J Clin Endocrinol Metab*, 88, 4502–4505, 2003.
106. Revell, V.L., Skene, D.J., Light-induced melatonin suppression in humans with polychromatic and monochromatic light. *Chronobiol Int*, 24, 1125–1137, 2007.
107. Berson, D.M., Phototransduction in ganglion-cell photoreceptors. *Pflugers Arch*, 454, 849–855, 2007.
108. Hankins, M.W., Peirson, S.N., Foster, R.G., Melanopsin: An exciting photopigment. *Trends Neurosci*, 31, 27–36, 2008.
109. Arendt, J., *Melatonin and the Mammalian Pineal Gland*. London: Chapman & Hall (eds.), 1995.
110. Cahill, G.M., Besharse, J.C., Circadian rhythmicity in verterate retinas: Regulation by a photoreceptor oscillator. *Prog Retin Eye Res*, 14, 267–291, 1995.
111. Khalsa, S.B., Jewett, M.E., Cajochen, C., Czeisler, C.A., A phase response curve to single bright light pulses in human subjects. *J Physiol*, 549, 945–952, 2003.
112. Lewy, A.J., Bauer, V.K., Ahmed, S., Thomas, K.H., Cutler, N.L., Singer, C.M., Moffit, M.T., Sack, R.L., The human phase response curve (PRC) to melatonin is about 12 hours out of phase with the PRC to light. *Chronobiol Int*, 15, 71–83, 1998.
113. Warman, V.L., Dijk, D.J., Warman, G.R., Arendt, J., Skene, D.J., Phase advancing human circadian rhythms with short wavelength light. *Neurosci Lett*, 342, 37–40, 2003.

114. Zawilska, J.B., Lorenc, A., Berezińska, M., Regulation of serotonin *N*-acetyltransferase activity in the chick pineal gland by UV-A and white light: Role of MK-801- and SCH 23390-sensitive retinal signals. *Pharmacol Rep*, 59, 408–413, 2007.
115. Johnson, C.H., *An Atlas of Phase Responses Curves for Circadian and Circatidal Rhythm*. Nashville, TX: Department of Biology, Vanderbilt University, 1990.
116. Burgess, H.J., Revell, V.L., Eastman, C.I., A three pulse phase response curve to three milligrams of melatonin in humans. *J Physiol*, 586, 639–647, 2008.
117. Illnerová, H., Sumová, A., Photic entrainment of the mammalian rhythm in melatonin production. *J Biol Rhythms*, 12, 547–555, 1997.
118. Daan, S., Albrecht, U., van der Horst, G.T., Illnerová, H., Roenneberg, T., Wehr, T.A., Schwartz, W.J., Assembling a clock for all seasons: Are there M and E oscillators in the genes? *J Biol Rhythms*, 16, 105–116, 2001.
119. Illnerová, H., Sumová, A., Photic entrainment of the mammalian rhythm in melatonin production. *J Biol Rhythms*, 12, 547–555, 1997.
120. Wehr, T.A., Aeschbach, D., Duncan, W.C. Jr., Evidence for a biological dawn and dusk in the human circadian timing system. *J Physiol*, 535, 937–951, 2001.
121. Falcón, J., Galarneau, K.M., Weller, J.L., Ron, B., Chen, G., Coon, S.L., Klein, D.C., Regulation of arylalkylamine *N*-acetyltransferase-2 (AANAT2, EC 2.3.1.87) in the fish pineal organ: Evidence for a role of proteasomal proteolysis. *Endocrinology*, 142, 1804–1813, 2001.
122. Iuvone, P.M., Brown, A.D., Haque, R., Weller, J., Zawilska, J.B., Chaurasia, S.S., Ma, M., Klein, D.C., Retinal melatonin production: Role of proteasomal proteolysis in circadian and photic control of arylalkylamine *N*-acetyltransferase. *Invest Ophthalmol Vis Sci*, 43, 564–572, 2002.
123. Rosiak, J., Iuvone, P.M., Zawilska, J.B., UV-A light regulation of arylalkylamine *N*-acetyltransferase activity in the chick pineal gland: Role of cAMP and proteasomal proteolysis. *J Pineal Res*, 39, 419–425, 2005.
124. Seth, M., Maitra, S.K., Importance of light in temporal organization of photoreceptor proteins and melatonin producing system in the pineal of carp *Catla catla*. *Chronobiol Int*, 27, 463–486, 2010.
125. Ferry, G., Ubeaud, C., Lambert, P.H., Bertin, S., Coge, F., Chomarat, P., Delagrange, P., Serkiz, B., Bouchet, J.P., Truscott, R.J., Boutin, J.A., Molecular evidence that melatonin is enzymatically oxidized in a different manner than tryptophan: Investigation with both indoleamine 2, 3-dioxygenase and myeloperoxidase. *Biochem J*, 388, 205–215, 2005.
126. Gastel, G.A., Roseboom, P.H., Rinaldi, P.A., Weller, J.L., Klein, D.C., Melatonin production: Proteosomal proteolysis in serotonin *N*-acetlytransferase regulation. *Science*, 279, 1358–1360, 1998.
127. Garbarino-Pico, E., Carpentieri, A.R., Contin, M.A., Sarmiento, M.I., Brocco, M.A., Panzetta, P., Rosenstein, R.E., Caputto, B.L., Guido, M.E., Retinal ganglion cells are autonomous circadian oscillators synthesizing *N*-acetylserotonin during the day. *J Biol Chem*, 279, 51172–51181, 2004.
128. Sugden, D., Cena, V., Klein, D.C., Hydroxyindole-*O*-methyltransferase. *Methods Enzymol*, 42, 590–596, 1987.
129. Bernard, M., Donohue, S.J., Klein, D.C., Human hydroxindole-*O*-methyltransferase in pineal gland, retina and Y79 retinoblastoma cells. *Brain Res*, 696, 37–48, 1995.
130. Ishida, I., Obinata, M., Deguchi, T., Molecular cloning and nucleotide sequence of cDNA encoding hydroxyindole-*O*-methyltransferase of bovine pineal glands. *J Biol Chem*, 262, 2895–2899, 1987.
131. Voisin, P., Guerlotte, J., Bernard, M., Collin, J.P., Cogne, M., Molecular cloning and nucleotide sequence of a cDNA encoding hydroxyindole-*O*-methyltransferase from chicken pineal gland. *Biochem J*, 282, 571–576, 1992.
132. Donohue, S.J., Roseboom, P.H., Illnerova, H., Weller, J.L., Klein, D.C., Human hydroxyindole-*O*-methyltransferase: Presence of LINE-1 fragment in a cDNA clone and pineal mRNA. *DNA Cell Biol*, 12, 715–727, 1993.
133. Gauer, F., Craft, C.M., Circadian regulation of hydroxyindole-*O*-methyltransferase mRNA levels in rat pineal and retina. *Brain Res*, 737, 99–109, 1996.
134. Rodriguez, I.R., Mazuruk, K., Schoen, T.J., Chader, G.J., Structural analysis of the human hydroxyindole-*O*-methyltransferase gene. *J Biol Chem*, 269, 31969–31977, 1994.
135. Nakane, M., Yokoyama, E., Deguchi, T., Species heterogeneity of pineal hydroxyindole-*O*-methyltransferase. *J Neurochem*, 40, 790–796, 1983.
136. Bernard, M., Voisin, P., Klein, D.C., Hydroxyindole-*O*-methyltransferase in Y-79 cells: Regulation by serum. *Brain Res*, 727, 118–124, 1996.
137. Djeridane, Y., Vivien-Roels, B., Simonneaux, V., Pevet, P., Evidence for melatonin synthesis and release from rodent Hardarian gland. A dynamic in vitro study. *J Pineal Res*, 25, 54–64, 1998.

138. Ribelayga C., Gauer F., Pevet, P., Simonneaux, V., Distribution of hydroxyindole- O-methyltransferase in the rat brain: An in situ hybridization study. *Cell Tissue Res*, 291, 415–421, 1998.
139. Quay, W.B., Ma, Y.H., Demonstration of gastrointestinal hydroxindole-*O*-methyltransferase. *Med Sci*, 4, 563, 1976.
140. Itoh, M.T., Ishizuka, B., Kudo, Y., Fusama, S., Amemiya, A., Sumi, Y., Detection of melatonin and serotonin *N*-acetyl-transferase and hydroxyindole-*O*-methyltransferase activities in rat ovaries. *Mol Cell Endocrinol*, 136, 7–13, 1997.
141. Champier, J., Claustrat, B., Besancon, R., Eymin, C., Killer, C., Jouvet, A., Chamba, G., Fevre-Montange, M., Evidence for tryptophan hydroxylase and hydroxyindole-*O*-methyltransferase mRNAs in human blood platelets. *Life Sci*, 60, 2191–2197, 1997.
142. Ribelayga, C., Gauer, F., Pevet, P., Simonneaux, V., Photoneural regulation of rat pineal hydroxyindole-*O*-methyltransferase (HIOMT) messenger ribonucleic acid expression: An analysis of its complex relationship with HIOMT activity. *Endocrinology*, 140, 1375–1384, 1999.
143. Ribelayga, C., Pevet, P., Simonneaux, V., Adrenergic and peptidergic regulations of hydroxyindole-*O*-methyltransferase in rat pineal gland. *Brain Res*, 777, 247–250, 1997.
144. Ribelayga, C., Gauer, F., Pevet, P., Simonneaux, V., Ontogenesis of hydroxyindole-*O*-methyltransferase gene expression and activity in the rat pineal gland. *Dev Brain Res*, 110, 235–239, 1998.
145. Sugden, D., Klein, D.C., Beta-adrenergic receptor control of rat pineal hydroxyindole-*O*-methyltransferase. *Endocrinology*, 113, 348–353, 1983.
146. Janavs, J.L., Pierce, M.E., Takahashi, J.S., *N*-acetyltransferase and protein synthesis modulate melatonin production by Y79 human retinoblastoma cells. *Brain Res*, 540, 138–144, 1991.
147. Moore, R.Y., Klein, D.C., Visual pathways and the central neural control of a circadian rhythm in pineal serotonin *N*-acetyltransferase activity. *Brain Res*, 71, 17–33, 1974.
148. Baskett, J.J., Wood, P.C., Broad, J.B., Duncan, J.R., English, J., Arendt, J., Melatonin in older people with age-related sleep maintenance problems: A comparison with age matched normal sleepers. *Sleep*, 24, 418–424, 2001.
149. Sugden, D., Melatonin biosynthesis in the mammalian pineal gland. *Experientia*, 45, 922–932, 1989.
150. Berlin, I., Touitou, Y., Guillemant, S., Danjou, P., Puech, A., Beta-adrenoceptor agonists do not stimulate daytime melatonin secretion in healthy subjects. A double blind placebo controlled study. *Life Sci*, 56, 325–331, 1995.
151. Cowen, P.J., Bevan, J.S., Gosden, B., Elliot, S.A., Treatment with β-adrenoceptor blockers reduces plasma melatonin concentration. *Br J Clin Pharmacol*, 19, 258–260, 1985.
152. Rada, J.A., Wiechmann, A.F., Melatonin receptors in chick ocular tissues: Implication for a role of melatonin in ocular growth regulation. *Invest Ophthalmol Vis Sci*, 47, 25–33, 2006.
153. Kennaway, D.J., Stamp, G.E., Goble, F.C., Development of melatonin production in infants and impact of prematurity. *J Clin Endocrinol Metab*, 75, 367–369, 1992.
154. Ardura, J., Gutierrez, R., Andres, J., Agapito, T., Emergence and evolution of the circadian rhythm of melatonin in children. *Horm Res*, 59, 66–72, 2003.
155. Waldhauser, F., Boepple, P.A, Schemper, M., Mansfield, M.J., Crowley, W.F. Jr., Serum melatonin in central precocious puberty is lower than in age-matched prepubertal children. *J Clin Endocrinol Metab*, 73, 793–796, 1991.
156. Arendt, J., Melatonin: Characteristics, concerns and prospects. *J Biol Rhythms*, 20, 291–303, 2005.
157. Karasek, M., Melatonin, human aging, and age-related diseases. *Exp Gerontol*, 39, 1723–1729, 2004.
158. Bojkowski, C.J., Arendt, J., Factors influencing urinary 6-sulphatoxymelatonin, a major melatonin metabolite, in normal human subjects. *Clin Endocrinol (Oxf)*, 33, 435–444, 1990.
159. Waldhauser, F., Kovács, C.S., Reiter, E., Age-related changes in melatonin levels in humans and its potential consequences for sleep disorders. *Exp Gerontol*, 33, 759–772, 1998.
160. Parry, B.L., Berga, S.L., Mostofi, N., Klauber, M.R., Resnick, A., Plasma melatonin circadian rhythms during the menstrual cycle and after light therapy in premenstrual dysphoric disorder and normal control subjects. *J Biol Rhythms*, 12, 47–64, 1997.
161. Scheer, F.A., Kalsbek, A., Buijs, R.M., Cardiovascular control by the suprachiasmatic nucleus: Neural and neuroendocrine mechanisms in human and rat. *Biol Chem*, 384, 697–709, 2003.
162. Zimmermann, R.C., McDougle, C.J., Schumacher, M., Olcese, J., Mason, J.W., Heninger, G.R., Price, L.H., Effects of acute tryptophan depletion on nocturnal melatonin secretion in humans. *J Clin Endocrinol Metab*, 76, 1160–1164, 1993.
163. Mishima, K., Okawa, M., Shimizu, T., Hishikawa, Y., Diminished melatonin secretion in the elderly caused by insufficient environmental illumination. *J Clin Endocrinol Metab*, 86, 129–134, 2001.

164. Lockley, S.W., Skene, D.J., Tabandeh, H., Bird, A.C., Defrance, R., Arendt, J., Relationship between napping and melatonin in the blind. *J Biol Rhythms*, 12, 16–25, 1997.
165. Arendt, J., Aldhous, M., Wright, J., Synchronisation of a disturbed sleep-wake cycle in a blind man by melatonin treatment. *Lancet*, 331, 772–773, 1988.
166. Lockley, S.W., Dijk, D.J., Kosti, O., Skene, D.J., Arendt, J., Alertness, mood and performance rhythm disturbances associated with circadian sleep disorders in the blind. *J Sleep Res*, 17, 207–216, 2008.
167. Hack, L.M., Lockley, S.W., Arendt, J., Skene, D.J., The effects of low-dose 0.5-mg melatonin on the free-running circadian rhythms of blind subjects. *J Biol Rhythms*, 18, 420–429, 2003.
168. Lockley, S.W., Skene, D.J., James, K., Thapan, K., Wright, J., Arendt, J., Melatonin administration can entrain the free-running circadian system of blind subjects. *J Endocrinol*, 164, R1–6, 2000.
169. Sack, R.L., Brandes, R.W., Kendall, A.R., Lewy, A.J., Entrainment of free-running circadian rhythms by melatonin in blind people. *N Engl J Med*, 343, 1070–1077, 2000.
170. Tricoire, H., Malpaux, B., Moller, M., Cellular lining of the sheep pineal recess studied by light-, transmission-, and scanning electron microscopy: Morphologic indications for a direct secretion of melatonin from pineal gland to the cerebrospinal fluid. *J Comp Neurol*, 456, 39–47, 2003.
171. Ma, X., Chen, C., Krausz, K.W., Idle, J.R., Gonzalez, F.J., A metabolomic perspective of melatonin metabolism in the mouse. *Endocrinology*, 149, 1869–1879, 2008.
172. Gibbs, F.P., Vriend, J., The half-life of melatonin elimination from rat plasma. *Endocrinology*, 109, 1796–1798, 1981.
173. Fourtillan, J.B., Brisson, A.M., Gobin, P., Ingrand, I., Decourt, J.P., Girault, J., Bioavailability of melatonin in humans after day-time administration of D(7) melatonin. *Biopharm Drug Dispos*, 21, 15–22, 2000.
174. Lane, E.A., Moss, H.B., Pharmacokinetics of melatonin in man: First pass hepatic metabolism. *J Clin Endocrinol Metab*, 61, 1214–1216, 1985.
175. Vijayalaxmi, Thomas, C.R. Jr., Reiter, R.J., Herman, T.S., Melatonin: From basic research to cancer treatment clinics. *J Clin Oncol*, 20, 2575–2601, 2002.
176. Hardeland, R., Antioxidative protection by melatonin: Multiplicity of mechanisms from radical detoxification to radical avoidance. *Endocrine*, 27, 119–130, 2005.
177. Ma, X., Idle, J.R., Krausz, K.W., Gonzalez, F.J., Metabolism of melatonin by human cytochromes P450. *Drug Metab Dispos*, 33, 489–494, 2005.
178. Skene, D.J., Papagiannidou E, Hashemi E, Snelling J, Lewis DF, Fernandez M, Ioannides, C., Contribution of CYP1A2 in the hepatic metabolism of melatonin: Studies with isolated microsomal preparations and liver slices. *J Pineal Res*, 31, 333–342, 2001.
179. Skene, D.J., Timbers, S.E., Middleton, B., English, J., Kopp, C., Tobler, I., Ioanides, C., Mice convert melatonin to 6-sulphatoxymelatonin. *Gen Comp Endocrinol*, 147, 371–377, 2006.
180. Kennaway, D.J., Voultsios, A., Varcoe, T.J., Moyer, R.W., Melatonin in mice: Rhythms, response to light, adrenergic stimulation, and metabolism. *Am J Physiol Regul Integr Comp Physiol*, 282, R358–365, 2002.
181. Arendt, J., Melatonin and human rhythms. *Chronobiol Int*, 23, 21–37, 2006.
182. Bojkowski, C.J., Arendt, J., Shih, M.C., Markey, S.P., Melatonin secretion in humans assessed by measuring its metabolite, 6-sulfatoxymelatonin. *Clin Chem*, 33, 1343–1348, 1987.
183. Kennaway, D.J., Rowe, S.A., Impact of light pulses on 6-sulphatoxymelatonin rhythms in rats. *J Pineal Res*, 16, 65–72, 1994.
184. Rozov, S.V., Filatova, E.V., Orlov, A.A., Volkova, A.V., Zhloba, A.R., Blashko, E.L., Pozdeyev, N.V., *N*1-acetyl-*N*2-formyl-5-methoxykynuramine is a product of melatonin oxidation in rats. *J Pineal Res*, 35, 245–250, 2003.
185. Tan, D.X., Manchester, L.C., Terron, M.P., Flores, L.J., Tamura, H., Reiter, R.J., Melatonin as a naturally occurring co-substrate of quinone reductase-2, the putative MT3 melatonin membrane receptor: Hypothesis and significance. *J Pineal Res*, 43, 317–320, 2007.
186. Grace, M.S., Cahill, G.M., Besharse, J.C., Melatonin deacetylation: Retinal vertebrate class distribution and *Xenopus laevis* tissue distribution. *Brain Res*, 559, 56–63, 1991.
187. Tan, D.X., Manchester, L.C., Hardeland, R., Mayo, J.C., Sainz, R.M., Reiter, R.J., Melatonin: A hormone, a tissue factor, an autocoid, a paracoid and an antioxidant vitamin. *J Pineal Res*, 34, 75–78, 2003.
188. Dubocovich, M.L., Takahashi, J.S., Use of 2-[125I]-iodomelatonin to characterize melatonin binding sites in chicken retina. *Proc Natl Acad Sci USA*, 84, 3916–3920, 1987.
189. Poirel, V.J., Cailotto, C., Streicher, D., Pevet, P., Masson Pevet, M., Gauer, F., MT1 melatonin receptor mRNA tissular localization by PCR amplification. *Neuroendocrinol Lett*, 24, 33–38, 2003.

190. Witt-Enderby, P.A., Bennett, J., Jarzynka, M.J., Firestine, S., Melan, M.A., Melatonin receptors and their regulation: Biochemical and structural mechanisms. *Life Sci*, 72, 2183–2198, 2003.
191. Ebisawa, T., Karne, S., Lerner, M.R., Reppert, S.M., Expression cloning of a high-affinity melatonin receptor from *Xenopus* dermal melanophores. *Proc Natl Acad Sci USA*, 91, 6133–6137, 1994.
192. Reppert, S.M., Godson, C., Mahle, C.D., Weaver, D.R., Slaugenhaupt, S.A., Gausella, J.F., Molecular characterization of a second melatonin receptor expressed in human retina and brain: The Mel1b melatonin receptor. *Proc Natl Acad Sci USA*, 92, 8734–8738, 1995.
193. Dubocovich, M.L., Markowska, M., Functional MT1 and MT2 melatonin receptors in mammals. *Endocrine*, 27, 101–110, 2005.
194. Dubocovich, M.L., Cardinali, D.P., Delagrange, P., Krause, D.N., Strosberg, D., Sugden, D., Yocca, F.D., Melatonin receptors, in *The IUPHAR Compendium of Receptor Characterization and Classification*, 2nd edn. (IUPHAR, ed.), pp. 271–277. London: IUPHAR Media, 2000.
195. Reppert, S.M., Weaver, D.R., Cassone, V.M., Godson, C., Kolakowski, L.F. Jr., Melatonin receptors are for the birds: Molecular analysis of two receptor subtypes differentially expressed in chick brain. *Neuron*, 15, 1003–1015, 1995.
196. Slaugenhaupt, S.A., Roca, A.L., Liebert, C.B., Altherr, M.R., Gusella, J.F., Reppert, S.M., Mapping of the gene for the Mel1a-melatonin receptor to human chromosome 4 (MTNR1A) and mouse chromosome 8 (Mtnr1a). *Genomics*, 27, 355–357, 1995.
197. Audinot, V., Mailliet, F., Lahaye-Brasseur, C., Bonnaud, A., Le Gall, A., Amossé, C., Dromaint, S., Rodriguez, M., Nagel, N., Galizzi, J.P., Malpaux, B., Guillaumet, G., Lesieur, D., Lefoulon, F., Renard, P., Delagrange, P., Boutin, J.A., New selective ligands of human cloned melatonin MT1 and MT2 receptors. *Naunyn Schmiedebergs Arch Pharmacol*, 367, 553–561, 2003.
198. Dubocovich, M.L., Rivera-Bermudez, M.A., Gerdin, M.J., Masana, M.I., Molecular pharmacology, regulation and function of mammalian melatonin receptors. *Front Biosci*, 8, d1093-d1108, 2003.
199. Reppert, S.M., Melatonin receptors: Molecular biology of a new family of G protein-coupled receptors. *J Biol Rhythms*, 12, 528–531, 1997.
200. Boutin, J.A., Audinot, V., Ferry, G., Delagrange, P., Molecular tools to study melatonin pathways and actions. *Trends Pharmacol Sci*, 26, 412–419, 2005.
201. Delagrange, P., Boutin, J.A., Therapeutic potential of melatonin ligands. *Chronobiol Int*, 23, 413–418, 2006.
202. Zlotos, D.P., Recent advances in melatonin receptor ligands. *Arch Pharmacol*, 338, 229–247, 2005.
203. Sethi, S., Adams, W., Pollock, J., Witt-Enderby, P.A., C-terminal domains within human MT1 and MT2 melatonin receptors are involved in internalization processes. *J Pineal Res*, 45, 212–218, 2008.
204. Barrett, P., Conway, S., Morgan, P.J., Digging deep–structure-function relationships in the melatonin receptor family. *J Pineal Res*, 35, 221–230, 2003.
205. Gerdin, M.J., Mseeh, F., Dubocovich, M.L., Mutagenesis studies of the human MT2 melatonin receptor. *Biochem Pharmacol*, 66, 315–320, 2003.
206. Gauer, F., Masson-Pevet, M., Stehle, J., Pevet, P., Daily variations in melatonin receptor density of rat pars tuberalis and suprachiasmatic nuclei are distinctly regulated. *Brain Res*, 641, 92–98, 1994.
207. Kato, K., Hirai, K., Nishiyama, K., Uchikawa, O., Fukatsu, K., Ohkawa, S., Kawamata, Y., Hinuma, S., Miyamoto, M., Neurochemical properties of ramelteon (TAK-375), a selective MT1/MT2 receptor agonist. *Neuropharmacology*, 48, 301–310, 2005.
208. Von Gall, C., Stehle, J.H., Weaver, D.R., Mammalian melatonin receptors: Molecular biology and signal transduction. *Cell Tissue Res*, 309, 151–162, 2002.
209. Levoye, A., Jockers, R., Ayoub, M.A., Delagrange, P., Savaskan, E., Guillaume, J.L., Are G protein-coupled receptor heterodimers of physiological relevance? Focus on melatonin receptors. *Chronobiol Int*, 23, 419–426, 2006.
210. Reppert, S.M., Weaver, D.R., Ebisawa, T., Mahle, C.D., Kolakowski, L.F. Jr., Cloning of a melatonin-related receptor from human pituitary. *FEBS Lett*, 386, 219–224, 1996.
211. Mailliet, F., Ferry, G., Vella, F., Berger, S., Cogé, F., Chomarat, P., Mallet, C., Guénin, S.P., Guillaumet, G., Viaud-Massuard, M.C., Yous, S., Delagrange, P., Boutin, J.A., Characterization of the melatoninergic MT3 binding site on the NRH: Quinone oxidoreductase 2 enzyme. *Biochem Pharmacol*, 71, 74–88, 2005.
212. Nosjean, O., Ferro, M., Coge, F., Beauverger, P., Henlin, JM., Lefoulon, F., Fauchere, J.L., Delagrange, P., Canet, E., Boutin, J.A., Identification of the melatonin-binding site MT3 as the quinone reductase 2. *J Biol Chem*, 275, 31311–31317, 2000.
213. Becker-André, M., Wiesenberg, I., Schaeren-Wiemers, N., André, E., Missbach, M., Saurat, J.H., Carlberg, C., Pineal gland hormone melatonin binds and activates an orphan of the nuclear receptor superfamily. *J Biol Chem*, 269, 28531–28534, 1994.

214. Giguere, V., Orphan nuclear receptors: From gene to function. *Endocrine Rev*, 20, 689–752, 1999.
215. Carlberg, C., Gene regulation by melatonin. *Ann N Y Acad Sci*, 917, 387–396, 2000.
216. Karasek, M., Carrillo-Vico, A., Guerrero, J.M., Winczyk, K., Pawlikowski, M., Expression of melatonin MT(1) and MT(2) receptors, and ROR alpha (1) receptor in transplantable murine colon 38 cancer. *Neuroendocrinol Lett*, 23, 55–60, 2002.
217. Weissenberg, I., Missbach, M., Kahlen, J.P., Schrader, M., Carlberg, C., Transcriptional activation of the nuclear receptor RZR alpha by the pineal gland hormone melatonin and identification of CGP 52608 as a synthetic ligand. *Nucleic Acid Res*, 23, 327–333, 1995.
218. Benítez-King, G., Huerto-Delgadillo, L., Antón-Tay, F., Binding of 3H-melatonin to calmodulin. *Life Sci*, 53, 201–207, 1993.
219. Benítez-King, G., Antón-Tay, F., Calmodulin mediates melatonin cytoskeletal effects. *Experientia*, 49, 635–641, 1993.
220. Macías, M., Escames, G., Leon, J., Coto, A., Sbihi, Y., Osuna, A., Acuña-Castroviejo, D., Calreticulin-melatonin. An unexpected relationship. *Eur J Biochem*, 270, 832–40, 2003.
221. Turjanski, A.G., Vaqué, J.P., Gutkind, J.S., MAP kinases and the control of nuclear events. *Oncogene,* 26, 3240–3253, 2007.
222. Meléndez, J., Maldonado, V., Ortega, A., Effect of melatonin on beta-tubulin and MAP2 expression in NIE-115 cells. *Neurochem Res*, 21, 653–658, 1996.
223. Benítez-King, G., Melatonin as a cytoskeletal modulator: Implications for cell physiology and disease. *J Pineal Res*, 40, 1–9, 2006.
224. Pandi-Perumal, S.R., Trakht, I., Srinivasan, V., Spence, D.W., Maestroni, G.J., Zisapel, N., Cardinali, D.P., Physiological effects of melatonin: Role of melatonin receptors and signal transduction pathways. *Prog Neurobiol*, 85, 335–353, 2008.
225. Mazurais, D., Brierley, I., Anglade, I., Drew, J., Randall, C., Bromage, N., Michel, D., Kah, O., Williams, L.M., Central melatonin receptors in the rainbow trout: Comparative distribution of ligand binding and gene expression. *J Comp Neurol*, 409, 313–324, 1999.
226. Natesan, A., Geetha, L., Zatz, M., Rhythm and soul in the avian pineal. *Cell Tissue Res*, 309, 35–45, 2002.
227. Park, Y.J., Park, J.G., Jeong, H-B., Takeuchi, Y., Kim, S.J., Lee, Y.D., Takemura, A., Expression of the melatonin receptor Mel1c in neural tissues of the reef fish *Siganus guttatus. Comp Biochem Physiol A: Mol Integr Physiol*, 147, 103–111, 2007.
228. Liu, C., Weaver, D.R., Jin, X., Shearman, L.P., Pieschl, R.L., Gribkoff, V.K., Reppert, S.M., Molecular dissection of two distinct actions of melatonin on the suprachiasmatic circadian clock. *Neuron*, 19, 91–102, 1997.
229. Al-Ghoul, W.M., Herman, M.D., Dubocovich, M.L., Melatonin receptor subtype expression in human cerebellum. *Neuroreport*, 9, 4063–4068, 1998.
230. Savaskan, E., Olivieri, G., Meier, F., Brydon, L., Jockers, R., Ravid, R., Wirz-Justice, A., Muller-Spahn, F., Increased melatonin 1a-receptor immunoreactivity in the hippocampus of Alzheimer's disease patients. *J Pineal Res*, 32, 59–62, 2002.
231. Uz, T., Arslan, A.D., Kurtuncu, M., Imbesi, M., Akhisaroglu, M., Dwivedi, Y., Pandey, G.N., Manev, H., The regional and cellular expression profile of the melatonin receptor MT1 in the central dopaminergic system. *Brain Res Mol Brain Res*, 136, 45–53, 2005.
232. Clemens, J.W., Jarzynka, M.J., Witt-Enderby, P.A., Down-regulation of MT1 melatonin receptors in rat ovary following estrogen exposure. *Life Sci*, 69, 27–35, 2001.
233. Chattoraj, A., Seth, M. and Maitra, S.K., Localization and dynamics of Mel1a melatonin receptor in the ovary of carp *Catla catla* in relation to serum melatonin levels. Comp. Biochem, Physiol, 152, 327–333, 2009.
234. Frungieri, M.B., Mayerhofer, A., Zitta, K., Pignataro, O.P., Calandra, R.S., Gonzalez- Calvar, S.I., Direct effect of melatonin on Syrian hamster testes: Melatonin subtype 1a receptors, inhibition of androgen production, and interaction with the local corticotropin-releasing hormone system. *Endocrinology*, 146, 1541–1552, 2005.
235. Ram, P.T., Dai, J., Yuan, L., Dong, C., Kiefer, T.L., Lai, L., Hill, S.M., Involvement of the MT1 melatonin receptor in human breast cancer. *Cancer Lett,* 179, 141–150, 2002.
236. Scher, J., Wankiewicz, E., Brown, G.M., Fujieda, H., MT1 melatonin receptor in the human retina: Expression and localization. Investig. *Ophthalmol. Vis Sci*, 43, 889–897, 2002.
237. Ekmekcioglu, C., Haslmayer, P., Philipp, C., Mehrabi, M.R., Glogar, H.D., Grimm, M., Leibetseder, V.J., Thalhammer, T., Marktl, W., Expression of the MT1 melatonin receptor subtype in human coronary arteries. *J Recept Signal Transduct Res*, 21, 85–91, 2001.

238. Ekmekcioglu, C., Haslmayer, P., Philipp, C., Mehrabi, M.R., Glogar, H.D., Grimm, M., Thalhammer, T., Marktl, W., 24 h variation in the expression of the MT1 melatonin receptor subtype in coronary arteries derived from patients with coronary heart disease. *Chronobiol Int*, 18, 973–985, 2001.
239. Naji, L., Carrillo-Vico, A., Guerrero, J.M., Calvo, J.R., Expression of membrane and nuclear melatonin receptors in mouse peripheral organs. *Life Sci*, 74, 2227–2236, 2004.
240. Aust, S., Thalhammer, T., Humpeler, S., Jager, W., Klimpfinger, M., Tucek, G., Obrist, P., Marktl, W., Penner, E., Ekmekcioglu, C., The melatonin receptor subtype MT1 is expressed in human gallbladder epithelia. *J Pineal Res*, 36, 43–48, 2004.
241. Slominski, A., Pisarchik, A., Zbytek, B., Tobin, D.J., Kauser, S., Wortsman, J., Functional activity of serotoninergic and melatoninergic systems expressed in the skin. *J Cell Physiol*, 196, 144–153, 2003.
242. Pozo, D., Garcia-Maurino, S., Guerrero, J.M., Calvo, J.R., mRNA expression of nuclear receptor RZR/RORalpha, melatonin membrane receptor MT, and hydroxindole-*O*-methyltransferase in different populations of human immune cells. *J Pineal Res*, 37, 48–54, 2004.
243. Alarma-Estrany, P., Pintor, J., Melatonin receptor in the eye: Location, second messengers and role in ocular physiology. *Pharmacol Ther*, 113, 507–522, 2007.
244. Wu, Y.H., Zhou, J.N., Balesar, R., Unmehopa, U., Bao, A., Jockers, R., Van Heerikhuize, J., Swaab, D.F., Distribution of MT1 melatonin receptor immunoreactivity in the human hypothalamus and pituitary gland: Colocalization of MT1 with vasopressin, oxytocin, and corticotropin-releasing hormone. *J Comp Neurol*, 499, 897–910, 2006.
245. Masana, M.I., Doolen, S., Ersahin, C., Al-Ghoul, W.M., Duckles, S.P., Dubocovich, M.L., Krause, D.N., MT2 melatonin receptors are present and functional in rat caudal artery. *J Pharmacol Exp Ther*, 302, 1295–1302, 2002.
246. Richter, H.G., Torres-Farfan, C., Garcia-Sesnich, J., Abarzua-Catalan, L., Henriquez, M.G., Alvarez-Felmer, M., Gaete, F., Rehren, G.E., Seron-Ferre, M., Rhythmic expression of functional MT1 melatonin receptors in the rat adrenal gland. *Endocrinology*, 149, 995–1003, 2008.
247. Sallinen, P., Saarela, S., Ilves, M., Vakkuri, O., Leppäluoto, J., The expression of MT1 and MT2 melatonin receptor mRNA in several rat tissues. *Life Sci*, 76, 1123–1134, 2005.
248. Ting, K.N., Blaylock, N.N.A., Sugden, D., Delagrange, P., Scalbert, E., Wilson, V.G., Molecular and pharmacological evidence for MT1 melatonin receptor subtype in the tail artery of juvenile Wistar rats. *Br J Pharmacol*, 127, 987–995, 1999.
249. Thomas, L., Purvis, C.C., Drew, J.E., Abramovich, D.R., Williams, L.M., Melatonin receptors in human fetal brain: 2-[(125)I]iodomelatonin binding and MT1 gene expression. *J Pineal Res*, 33, 218–224, 2002.
250. Nosjean, O., Nicolas, J.P., Clupsch, S., Delagrange, P., Canet, E., Boutin, J.A., Comparative pharmacological studies of melatonin receptors: MT1 MT2 and Mt3/QR2. Tissue distribution of MT3/QR2. *Biochem Pharmacol*, 61, 1369–1379, 2001.
251. Pintor, J., Pelaez, T., Hoyle, C.H., Peral, A., Ocular hypotensive effects of melatonin receptor agonists in the rabbit: Further evidence for an MT3 receptor. *Br J Pharmacol*, 138, 831–836, 2003.
252. Park, H.T., Kim, Y.J., Yoon, S., Kim, J.B., Kim, J.J., Distributional characteristics of the mRNA for retinoid Z receptor beta (RZR beta), a putative nuclear melatonin receptor, in the rat brain and spinal cord. *Brain Res*, 747, 332–337, 1997.
253. Hunt, A.E., Al-Ghoul, W.M., Gillette, M.U., Dubocovich, M.L., Activation of MT (2) melatonin receptors in rat suprachiasmatic nucleus phase advances the circadian clock. *Am J Physiol Cell Physiol*, 280, C110-C118, 2001.
254. Jin, X., Von Gall, C., Pieschl, R.L., Gribkoff, V.K., Stehle, J.H., Reppert, S.M., Weaver, D.R., Targeted disruption of the mouse Mel(1b) melatonin receptor. *Mol Cell Biol*, 23, 1054–1060, 2003.
255. Weaver, D.R., Liu, C., Reppert, S.M., Nature's knockout: The Mel1b receptor is not necessary for reproductive and circadian responses to melatonin in Siberian hamsters. *Mol Endocrinol*, 10, 1478–1487, 1996.
256. Vaněcek, J., Vollrath, L., Melatonin inhibits cyclic AMP and cyclic GMP accumulation in the rat pituitary. *Brain Res*, 505, 157–159, 1989.
257. Morgan, P.J., Williams, L.M., Barrett, P., Lawson, W., Davidson, G., Hannah, L., MacLean, A., Differential regulation of melatonin receptors in sheep, chicken and lizard brains by cholera and pertussis toxins and guanine nucleotides. *Neurochem Int*, 28, 259–269, 1996.
258. Morgan, P.J., Barrett, P., Hazlerigg, D., Milligan, G., Lawson, W., MacLean, A., Davidson, G., Melatonin receptors couple through a cholera toxin-sensitive mechanism to inhibit cyclic AMP in the ovine pituitary. *J Neuroendocrinol*, 7, 361–369, 1995.

259. Godson, C., Reppert, S.M., The Mel1a melatonin receptor is coupled to parallel signal transduction pathways. *Endocrinology*, 138, 397–404, 1997.
260. Morgan, P.J., Barrett, P., Howell, H.E., Helliwell, R., Melatonin receptors: Localization, molecular pharmacology and physiological significance. *Neurochem Int*, 24, 101–146, 1994.
261. Brydon, L., Roka, F., Petit, L., de Coppet, P., Tissot, M., Barrett, P., Morgan, P.J., Nanoff, C., Strosberg, A.D., Jockers, R., Dual signaling of human Mel1a melatonin receptors via Gi2, Gi3, and Gq/11 proteins. *Mol Endocrinol*, 13, 2025–2038, 1999.
262. Ho, M.K., Yung, L.Y., Chan, J.S., Chan, J.H., Wong, C.S., Wong, Y.H., Galpha(14) links a variety of G(i) and G(s)-coupled receptors to the stimulation of phospholipase C. *Br J Pharmacol*, 132, 1431–1440, 2001.
263. Chan, A.S., Lai, F.P., Lo, R.K., Voyno-Yasenetskaya, T.A., Stanbridge, E.J., Wong, Y.H., Melatonin MT1 and MT2 receptors stimulate c-Jun N-terminal kinase via pertussis toxinsensitive and -insensitive G proteins. *Cell Signal*, 14, 249–257, 2002.
264. Roka, F., Brydon, L., Waldhoer, M., Strosberg, A.D., Freissmuth, M., Jockers, R., Nanoff, C., Tight association of the human Mel1a-melatonin receptor and Gi: Precoupling and constitutive activity. *Mol Pharmacol*, 56, 1014–1024, 1999.
265. McNulty, S., Ross, A.W., Shiu, K.Y., Morgan, P.J., Hastings, M.H., Phosphorylation of CREB in ovine pars tuberalis is regulated both by cyclic AMP-dependent and cyclic AMP-independent mechanisms. *J Neuroendocrinol*, 8, 635–645, 1996.
266. Kopp, M., Meissl, H., Korf, H.W., The pituitary adenylate cyclase-activating polypeptide-induced phosphorylation of the transcription factor CREB (cAMP response element binding protein) in the rat suprachiasmatic nucleus is inhibited by melatonin. *Neurosci Lett*, 227, 145–148, 1997.
267. von Gall, C., Duffield, G.E., Hastings, M.H., Kopp, M.D., Dehghani, F., Korf, H.W., Stehle, J.H., CREB in the mouse SCN: A molecular interface coding the phase-adjusting stimuli light, glutamate, PACAP, and melatonin for clockwork access. *J Neurosci*, 18, 10389–10397, 1998.
268. von Gall, C., Garabette, M.L., Kell, C.A., Frenzel, S., Dehghani, F., Schumm-Draeger, P.M., Weaver, D.R., Korf, H.W., Hastings, M.H., Stehle, J.H., Rhythmic gene expression in pituitary depends on heterologous sensitization by the neurohormone melatonin. *Nat Neurosci*, 5, 234–238, 2002.
269. Ross, A.W., Barrett, P., Mercer, J.G., Morgan, P.J., Melatonin suppresses the induction of AP-1 transcription factor components in the pars tuberalis of the pituitary. *Mol Cell Endocrinol*, 123, 71–80, 1996.
270. Schuster, C., Williams, L.M., Morris, A., Morgan, P.J., Barrett, P., The human MT1 melatonin receptor stimulates cAMP production in the human neuroblastoma cell line SH-SY5Y cells via a calcium-calmodulin signal transduction pathway. *J Neuroendocrinol*, 17, 170–178, 2005.
271. Witt-Enderby, P.A., MacKenzie, R.S., McKeon, R.M., Carroll, E.A., Bordt, S.L., Melan, M.A., Melatonin induction of filamentous structures in non-neuronal cells that is dependent on expression of the human mt1 melatonin receptor. *Cell Motil Cytoskeleton*, 46, 28–42, 2000.
272. Nelson, C.S., Marino, J.L., Allen, C.N., Melatonin receptor activate heterotrimeric G-protein coupled Kir3 channels. *Neuroreport*, 7, 717–720, 1996.
273. Camello-Almaraz, C., Gomez-Pinilla, P.J., Pozo, M.J., Camello, P.J., Age-related alterations in Ca2+ signals and mitochondrial membrane potential in exocrine cells are prevented by melatonin. *J Pineal Res*, 45:191–198, 2008.
274. Jou, M.J., Peng, T.I., Yu, P.Z., Jou, S.B., Reiter, R.J., Chen, J.Y., Wu, H.Y., Chen, C.C., Hsu, L.F., Melatonin protects against common deletion of mitochondrial DNA-augmented mitochondrial oxidative stress and apoptosis. *J Pineal Res*, 43, 389–403, 2007.
275. McArthur, A.J., Hunt, A.E., Gillette, M.U., Melatonin action and signal transduction in the rat suprachiasmatic circadian clock: Activation of protein kinase C at dusk and dawn. *Endocrinology*, 138, 627–634, 1997.
276. Hardeland, R., Melatonin: Signaling mechanisms of a pleiotropic agent. *BioFactors*, 183–192, 2009.
277. Gerdin, M.J., Masana, M.I., Rivera-Bermúdez, M.A., Hudson, R.L., Earnest, D.J., Gillette, M.U., Dubocovich, M.L., Melatonin desensitizes endogenous MT2 melatonin receptors in the rat suprachiasmatic nucleus: Relevance for defining the periods of sensitivity of the mammalian circadian clock to melatonin. *FASEB J*, 18, 1646–1656, 2004.
278. Rimler, A., Jockers, R., Lupowitz, Z., Sampson, S.R., Zisapel, N., Differential effects of melatonin and its downstream effector PKCalpha on subcellular localization of RGS proteins. *J Pineal Res*, 40, 144–152, 2006.
279. Rimler, A., Jockers, R., Lupowitz, Z., Zisapel, N., Gi and RGS proteins provide biochemical control of androgen receptor nuclear exclusion. *J Mol Neurosci*, 31, 1–12, 2007.

280. Soto-Vega, E., Meza, I., Ramírez-Rodríguez, G., Benitez-King, G., Melatonin stimulates calmodulin phosphorylation by protein kinase C. *J Pineal Res*, 37, 98–106, 2004.
281. Fang, L., Wu, J., Lin, Q., Willis, W.D., Calcium-calmodulin-dependent protein kinase II contributes to spinal cord central sensitization. *J Neurosci*, 22, 4196–204, 2002.
282. Blask, D.E., Sauer, L.A., Dauchy, R.T., Melatonin as a chronobiotic/anticancer agent: Cellular, biochemical and molecular mechanisms of action and their implication for circadian-based cancer therapy. *Curr Top Med Chem*, 2, 113–132, 2002.
283. Juszczak, M., Stempniak, B., Melatonin inhibits the substance-P induced secretion of vasopressin and oxytocin from the rat hypothalamo-neurohypophyseal system: *In vitro* studies. *Brain Res Bull*, 59, 393–397, 2003.
284. Steinhilber, D., Brungs, M., Werz, O., Weisenberg, I., Danielsson, C., Kahlen, J.P., Naveri, S., Schrader, M., Carlberg, C., The nuclear receptor for melatonin represses 5- lipoxygenase gene expression in human B lymphocytes. *J Biol Chem*, 270, 7037–7040, 1995.
285. Skwarlo-Sonta, K., Majewski, P., Markowska, M., Ocbalp, R., Olszanska, B., Bidirectional communication between the pineal gland and the immune system. *Can J Physiol Pharmacol*, 81, 342–349, 2003.
286. Conti, A., Conconi, S., Hertens, E., Skwarlo-Sonta, K., Markowska, M., Maestroni, J.M., Evidence for melatonin synthesis in mouse and human bone marrow cells. *J Pineal Res*, 28, 193–202, 2000.
287. Slominski, A., Fischer, T.W., Zmijewski, M.A., Wortsman, J., Semak, I., Zbytek, B., Slominski, R.M., Tobin, D.J., On the role of melatonin in skin physiology and pathology. *Endocrine*, 27, 137–148, 2005.
288. El-Sherif, Y., Witt-Enderby, P., Li, P.K., Tesoriero, J., Hogan, M.V., Wieraszko, A., The action of a charged melatonin receptor ligand, TMEPI, and an irreversible MT2 receptor agonist, BMNEP, on mouse hippocampal evoked potentials in vitro. *Life Sci*, 75, 3147–3156, 2004.
289. Burns, R.E., Sateia, M.J., Lee-Chiong, T.L., Basic principles of chronobiology and disorders of circadian sleep–wake rhythm, in *Sleep Medicine*, 1st ed. (Lee-Chiong, T.L., Sateia, M.J., Carskadon, M.A., eds.), pp. 245–252, Philadelphia: Hanley & Belfus, 2002.
290. Vester, G.C., Melatonin and its agonists, circadian rhythms and psychiatry. *Afr J Psychiatry*, 12, 42–46, 2009.
291. Atkinson, G., Edwards, B., Reilly, T., Waterhouse, J., Exercise as a synchroniser of human circadian rhythms: An update and discussion of the methodological problems. *Eur J Appl Physiol*, 99, 331–341, 2007.
292. Boivin, D.B., James, F.O., Insomnia due to circadian rhythm disturbances, in *Insomnia: Principles and Management*, 1st ed. (Szuba, M.P., Kloss, J.D., Dinges, D.F., eds.), pp. 155–191. Cambridge, MA: Cambridge University Press, 2003.
293. Pevet, P., Agez, L., Bothorel, B., Saboureau, M., Gauer, F., Laurent, V., Masson-Pevet, M., Melatonin in the multi-oscillatory mammalian circadian world. *Chronobiol Int*, 23, 39–51, 2006.
294. Rajaratnam, S.M., Middleton, B., Stone, B.M., Arendt, J., Dijk, D.J., Melatonin advances the circadian timing of EEG sleep and directly facilitates sleep without altering its duration in extended sleep opportunities in humans. *J Physiol*, 561, 339–351, 2004.
295. Scheer, F.A., Czeisler, C.A., Melatonin, sleep, and circadian rhythms. *Sleep Med Rev*, 9, 5–9, 2005.
296. Turek, F.W., Circadian rhythms: From the bench to the bedside and falling asleep. *Sleep*, 27, 1600–1602, 2004.
297. Cajochen, C., Krauchi, K., Wirz-Justice, A., Role of melatonin in the regulation of human circadian rhythms and sleep. *J Neuroendocrinol*, 15, 432–437, 2003.
298. Stehle, J.H., Von Gall, C., Korf, H.W., Melatonin: A clock output, a clock input. *J Neuroendocrinol*, 15, 383–389, 2003.
299. Schibler, U., Ripperjer, J., Brown, S.A., Peripheral circadian oscillators in mammals: Time and food. *J Biol Rhythms*, 18, 250–260, 2003.
300. Ko, C.H., Takahashi, J.S., Molecular components of the mammalian circadian clock. *Hum Mol Genet Spec*, (2), R271–277, 2006.
301. Lamont, E.W., James, F.O., Bovin, D.B., Cermakian, N., From circadian clock gene expression to pathologies. *Sleep Med*, 8, 547–556, 2007.
302. Kudo, T., Horikawa, K., Shibata, S., Circadian rhythms in the CNS and peripheral clock disorders: The circadian clock and hyperlipidemia. *J Pharmacol Sci*, 103, 139–143, 2007.
303. Poirel, V.J., Boggio, V., Dardente, H., Pevet, P., Masson-Pevet, M., Gauer, F., Contrary to the other non photic cues, acute melatonin injection does not induce immediate changes of the clock gene mRNA expression in the rat suprachiasmatic nuclei. *Neuroscience*, 120, 745–755, 2003.
304. Lambert, G.W., Reid, C., Kaye, D.M., Jennings, G.L., Esler, M.D., Effects of sunlight and season on serotonin turnover in the brain. *Lancet*, 360, 1840–1842, 2002.

305. Moore, R.Y., Speh, J.C., Serotonin innervation of the primate suprachiasmatic nucleus. *Brain Res*, 1010, 169–173, 2004.
306. Seron-Ferre, M., Valenzuela, G.J., Torres-Farfan, C., Circadian clocks during embryonic and fetal development. *Birth Defect Res*, 81, 204–214, 2007.
307. Daan, S., Beersma, D.G., Borbely, A.A., Timing of human sleep: Recovery process gated by a circadian pacemaker. *Am J Physiol*, 246, 161–183, 1984.
308. Fahey, C.D., Zee, P.C., Circadian rhythm sleep disorders and phototherapy. *Psychiatr Clin North Am*, 29, 989–1007, 2006.
309. Alvarez, G.G., Ayas, N.T., The impact of daily sleep duration on health: A review of the literature. *Prog Cardiovasc Nurs*, 19, 56–59, 2004.
310. Pandi-Perumal, S.R., Zisapel, N., Srinivasan, V., Cardinali, D.P., Melatonin and sleep in aging population. *Exp Gerontol*, 40, 911–925, 2005.
311. Turek, F.W., Gilette, M.U., Melatonin, sleep, and circadian rhythms: Rationale for development of specific melatonin agonists. *Sleep Med*, 5, 523–532, 2004.
312. Srinivasan,V., Pandi-Perumal, S.R., Warren Spence D., Hardeland, R., Melatonin and melatonergic drugs on sleep: Possible mechanisms of action. *Int J Neurosci*, 119, 821–846, 2008.
313. Edwards, B.J., Atkinson, G., Waterhouse, J., Reilly, T., Godfrey, R., Budgett, R., Use of melatonin in recovery from jet-lag following an eastward flight across 10 time-zones. *Ergonomics*, 43, 1501–1513, 2000.
314. Herxheimer, A., Petrie, K.J., Melatonin for the prevention and treatment of jet lag. *Cochrane Database Syst Rev*, (1), CD001520, 2001.
315. Sharkey, K.M., Fogg, L.F., Eastman, C.I., Effects of melatonin administration on daytime sleep after simulated night shift work. *J Sleep Res*, 10, 181–192, 2001.
316. Badiu, C., Genetic clock of biologic rhythms. *J Cell Mol Med*, 7, 408–416, 2003.
317. Bergiannaki, J.D., Soldatos, C.R., Paparrigopoulos, T.J., Syrengelas, M., Stefanis, C.N., Low and high melatonin excretors among healthy individuals. *J Pineal Res*, 18, 159–164, 1995.
318. Cardinali, D.P., Brusco, L.I., Lloret, S.P., Furio, A.M., Melatonin in sleep disorders and jet-lag. *Neuroendocrinol Lett*, 1, 9–13, 2002.
319. Arendt, J., Importance and relevance of melatonin to human biological rhythms. *J Neuroendocrinol*, 15, 427–431, 2003.
320. Wehr, T.A., Rosenthal, N.E., Seasonality and effective illness. *Am J Psychiatry*, 46, 829–839, 1989.
321. Srinivasan, V., Smits, M., Spence, W., Lowe, A.D., Kayumov, L., Pandi-Perumal, S.R., Parry, B., Cardanali, D.P., Melatonin in mood disorders. *World J Biol Psychiatry*, 7, 138–151, 2006.
322. Pacchierottim, C., Iapichino, S., Bossini, L., Pieraccini, F., Castrogiovanni, P., Melatonin in psychiatric disorders: A review on the melatonin involvement in psychiatry. *Front Neuroendocrinol*, 22, 18–32, 2001.
323. Shiloh, R., Nutt, D., Weizman, A., *Atlas of Psychiatric Pharmacotherapy*, revised ed., pp. 98–99. London: Martin Dunitz, 2000.
324. Wade, A.G., Sleep problems in depression: How do they impact treatment and recovery? *Int J Psychiatry Clin Pract*, 10(Suppl 1), 38–44, 2006.
325. Thase, M.E., Depression and sleep: Pathophysiology and treatment. *Dialogues Clin Neurosci*, 8, 217–226, 2006.
326. De Los Reyes, V., Guilleminault, C., Sleep disorders as a major clinical manifestation of disturbed circadian rhythms in depression. *Medicographia*, 29, 28–36, 2007.
327. Zupancic, M., Guilleminault, C., Agomelatine—A preliminary review of a new antidepressant. *CNS Drugs*, 20, 981–992, 2006.
328. Paul, M.A., Gray, G., MacLellan, M., Pigeau, R.A., Sleep-inducing pharmaceuticals: A comparison of melatonin, zaleplon, zopiclone, and temazepam. *Aviat Space Environ Med*, 75, 512–519, 2004.
329. Szymanska, A., Rrabe-Jablonska, J., Karasek, M., Diurnal profile of melatonin concentrations in patients with major depression: Relationship to the clinical manifestation and antidepressant treatment. *Neuroendocrinol Lett*, 22, 192–198, 2001.
330. Buck, M.L., The use of melatonin in children with sleep disorders. *Pediatr Pharm*. 9, 1–4, 2003.
331. Sewerynek, E., Melatonin and the cardiovascular system. *Neurolendocrinol Lett*, 1, 79–83, 2002.
332. Young, S.N., Tye clinical psychopharmacology of tryptophan. *Nutr Brain*, 7, 49–88, 1986.
333. Roy, A., Virkkunen, M., Guthrie, S., Linnoila, M., Indices of serotonin and glucose metabolism in violent offenders, arsonists, and alcoholics *Ann. N Y Acad Sci*, 487, 202–220, 1986.
334. Maestroni, G.J., Conti, A., Beta-endorphin and dynorphin mimic the circadian immunoenhancing and anti-stress effects of melatonin. *Int J Immunopharmacol*, 11, 333–340, 1989.

335. von-Bohr, C., Ursing, C., Yasui, N., Tybring, G., Bertilsson, L., Röjdmark, S., Fluvoxamine but not citalopram increases serum melatonin in healthy subjects—An indication that cytochrome p450 CYP1A2 and CYP2C19 hydroxylate melatonin. *Eur J Clin Pharmacol*, 56, 123–127, 2000.
336. Yeleswaram, K., Vachharajani, N., Santone, K., Involvement of cytochrome P450 isoenzymes in melatonin metabolism and clinical implications. *J Pineal Res*, 26, 190–191, 1999.
337. Pandi-Perumal, S.R., Srinivasan, V., Maestroni, G.J., Cardinali, D.P., Poeggeler, B., Hardeland, R., Melatonin: Nature's most versatile biological signal? *FEBS J*, 273, 2813–2838, 2006.
338. Souêtre, E., Salvati E, Belugou, J.L., Pringuey, D., Candito, M., Krebs, B., Ardisson, J.L., Darcourt, G., Circadian rhythms in depression and recovery: Evidence for blunted amplitude as the main chronobiological abnormality. *Psych Res*, 28, 263–278, 1989.
339. Malhotra, S., Sawhney, G., Pandhi, P., The therapeutic potential of melatonin: A review of the science. *Medscape Gen Med*, 6, 46, 2004.
340. Reiter, R.J., Tan, D.X., Sainz, R.M., Mayo, J.C., Lopez-Burillo, S., Melatonin: Reducing the toxicity and increasing the efficacy of drugs. *J Pharm Pharmacol*, 54, 1299–1321, 2002.
341. Macchi, M.M., Bruce, J.N., Human pineal physiology and functional significance of melatonin. *Front Neuroendocrinol*, 25, 177–195, 2004.
342. Montilla–Lopez, P., Munoz-Aqueda, M.C., Feijoo-Lopez, M., Munoz-Castaneda, J.M., Bujalance-Arenas, I., Tunez-Finana, I., Comparison of melatonin versus vitamin C on antioxidative stress and antioxidant enzyme activity in Alzheimer's disease induced by okadaic acid in neuroblastoma cells. *Eur J Pharmacol*, 451, 237–243, 2002.
343. Ianăş, O., Olinescu, R., Bădescu, I., Melatonin involvement in oxidative processes. *Endocrinologie*, 29, 147–53, 1991.
344. Tan, D.X., Chen, L.D., Poeggeler, B., Manchester, L.C., Reiter, R.J., Melatonin: A potent, endogenous hydroxyl radical scavenger. *Endocrine J*, 1, 57–60, 1993.
345. Tan, D.X., Pöeggeler, B., Reiter, R.J., Chen, L.D., Chen, S., Manchester, L.C., Barlow-Walden, L.R., The pineal hormone melatonin inhibits DNA-adduct formation induced by the chemical carcinogen safrole in vivo. *Cancer Lett*, 70, 65–71, 1993.
346. Tan, D.X., Manchester, L.C., Burkhardt, S., Sainz, R.M., Mayo, J.C., Kohen, R., Shohami, E., Huo, Y.S., Hardeland, R., Reiter, R.J., *N*1-acetyl-*N*2-formyl-5-methoxykynuramine, a biogenic amine and melatonin metabolite, functions as potent antioxidant. *FASEB J*, 15, 2294–2296, 2001.
347. Mayo, J.C., Sainz, R.M., Tan, D.X., Hardeland, R., Leon, J., Rodriguez, C., Reiter, R.J., Anti-inflammatory actions of melatonin and its metabolites, *N*1-acetyl-*N*2-formyl-5-methoxykynuramine (AFMK) and *N*1-acetyl-5-methoxykynuramine (AMK), in macrophages. *J Neuroimmunol*, 165, 139–49, 2005.
348. Than, N.N., Heer, C., Laatsch, H., Hardeland, R., Reactions of melatonin metabolite *N*-acetyl-5-methoxy kynuramine (AMK) with ABTS cation radical: Identification of new oxidation products. *Redox Rep*, 11, 15–24, 2006.
349. Guenther, A.l., Schmidt, S.I., Laatsch, H., Fotso, S., Ness, H., Ressmeyer, A.R., Poeggeler, B., Hardeland, R., Reactions of melatonin metabolite AMK (*N*1-acetyl-5-methoxykynuramine) with reactive nitrogen species: Formation of novel compounds, 3-acetamidomethyl-6-methoxycinnolinone and 3-nitro AMK. *J Pineal Res*, 39, 251–260, 2005.
350. Reiter, R.J., Pablos, M.I., Agapito, T.T., Guerrero, J.M., Melatonin in the context of the free radical theory of aging. *Ann NY Acad Sci*, 786, 362–378, 1996.
351. Lewis, A.J., Kerenyi, N.A., Feuer, G., Neuropharmacology of pineal secretions. *Rev Drug Metab Drug Interact*, 8, 247–312, 1990.
352. Tan, D.X., Manchester, L.C., Reiter, R.J., Plummer, B.E., Hardies, L.J., Weintraub, S.T., Vijayalaxmi, Shepherd, A.M., A novel melatonin metabolite, cyclic 3-hydroxymelatonin: A biomarker of in vivo hydroxyl radical generation. *Biochem Biophys Res Commun*, 253, 614–620, 1998.
353. Cagnoli, C.M., Atabay, C., Kharlamova, E., Manev, H., Melatonin protects neurons from singlet oxygen-induced apoptosis. *J Pineal Res*, 18, 222–226, 1995.
354. de Almeida, E.A., Martinez, G.R., Klitzke, C.F., de Medeiros, M.H., Di Mascio, P., Oxidation of melatonin by singlet molecular oxygen (O2(1deltag)) produces *N*1-acetyl-*N*2-formyl-5-methoxykynurenine. *J Pineal Res*, 35, 131–137, 2003.
355. Paradies, G., Petrosillo, G., Paradies, V., Reiter, R.J., Ruggiero, F.M., Melatonin, cardiolipin and mitochondrial bioenergetics in health and disease. *J Pineal Res*, 48, 297–310, 2010.
356. Beckman, J.S., Beckman, T.W., Chen, J., Marshall, P.A., Freeman, B.A., Apparent hydroxyl radical production by peroxynitrite: Implications for endothelial injury from nitric oxide and superoxide. *Proc Natl Acad Sci USA*, 87, 1620–1624, 1990.

357. Pozo, D., Delgado, M., Fernandez-Santos, J.M., Calvo, J.R., Gomariz, R.P., Martin-Lacave, I., Ortiz, G.G., Guerrero, J.M., Expression of the Mel1a-melatonin receptor mRNA in T and B subsets of lymphocytes from rat thymus and spleen. *FASEB J*, 11, 466–473, 1997.
358. Crespo, E., Macias, M., Pozo, D., Escames, G., Martin, M., Vives, F., Guerrero, J.M., Acuna-Castroviejo, D., Melatonin inhibits expression of the inducible NO synthase II in liver and lung and prevents endotoxemia in lipopolysaccharide-induced multiple organ dysfunction syndrome in rats. *FASEB J*, 13, 1537–1546, 1999.
359. Zhang, H., Akbar, M., Kim, H.Y., Melatonin an endogenous negative modulator of 12 lipoxygenation in the rat pineal gland. *Biochem J*, 344, 487–493, 1999.
360. Barlow-Walden, L.R., Reiter, R.J., Abe, M., Pablos, M., Menéndez-Peláez, A., Chen, L.D., Poeggeler, B., Melatonin stimulates brain glutathione peroxidase activity. *Neurochem Int*, 26, 497–502, 1995.
361. Pablos, M.I., Guerrero, J.M, Ortiz, G.G., Agapito, M.T., Reiter, R.J., Both melatonin and a putative nuclear melatonin receptor agonist CGP 52608 stimulate glutathione peroxidase and glutathione reductase activities in mouse brain in vivo. *Neuroendocrinol Lett*, 18, 49–58, 1997.
362. Rodriguez, C., Mayo, J.C. Sainz, R.M., Antolin, I., Herrara, F., Martin, V., Reiter, R.J., Regulation of antioxidant enzymes: A significant role for melatonin. *J Pineal Res*, 36, 1–9, 2004.
363. Antolin, I., Rodriguez, C., Sainz, R.M., Mayo, J.C., Uria, H., Kotler, M.L., Rodriguez-Colunga, M.J., Tolivia, D., Menéndez-Peláez, A., Neurohormone melatonin prevents cell damage: Effect on gene expression for antioxidant enzymes. *FASEB J*, 10, 882–890, 1996.
364. Kotler, M., Rodriquez, C., Sainz, R.M., Antolin, I., Menedez-Pelaez, A., Melatonin increases gene expression for antioxidant enzymes in rat brain cortex. *J Pineal Res*, 24, 83–89, 1998.
365. Albarran, M.T., Lopez-Burillo, S., Pablos, M.I., Reiter, R.J., Agapito, M.T., Endogenous rhythms of melatonin, total antioxidant status and superoxide dismutase activity in several tissues of chick and their inhibition by light. *J Pineal Res*, 30, 227–233, 2001.
366. Chance, B., Sies, H., Boveris, A., Hydroperoxide metabolism in mammalian organs. *Physiol Rev*, 59, 527–605, 1979.
367. Hara, M., Yoshida, M., Nishijima, H., Yokosuka, M., Iigo, M., Ohtani-Kaneko, R., Shimada, A., Hasegawa, T., Akama, Y., Hirata, K., Melatonin, a pineal secretory product with antioxidant properties, protects against cisplatin-induced nephrotoxicity in rats. *J Pineal Res*, 30, 129–138, 2001.
368. Limson, J., Nyokong, T., Daya, S., The interaction of melatonin and its precursors with aluminium, cadmium, copper, iron, lead, and zinc. An adsorptive voltammetric study. *J Pineal Res*, 24, 12–21, 1998.
369. Lack, B., Nyokong, T., Daya, S., Interaction of serotonin and melatonin with sodium, potassium, calcium, lithium, and aluminium. *J Pineal Res*, 31, 102–108, 2001.
370. Tan, D-X., Manchester, L.C., Terron, M.P., Flores, L.F., Reiter, R.J., One molecule, many derivatives: A never-ending interaction of melatonin with reactive oxygen and nitrogen species? *J Pineal Res*, 42, 28–42, 2007.
371. Maharaj, D.S., Anoopkumar-Dukie, S., Glass, B.D., Antunes, E.M., Lack, B., Walker, R.B., Daya, S., Identification of the UV degradants of melatonin and their ability to scavenge free radicals. *J Pineal Res*, 32, 257–261, 2002.
372. Maharaj, D.S., Limson, J.L., Daya, S., 6-Hydroxymelatonin converts iron (III) to iron (II). *Life Sci*, 72, 1367–75, 2003.
373. Martin, M., Macias, M., Escames, G., Leon, J., Acuna-Castroviejo, D., Melatonin but not vitamins C and E maintains glutathione homeostasis in t-butyl hydroperoxide-induced mitochondrial oxidative stress. *FASEB J*, 14, 2128, 2000.
374. Martin, M., Macias, M., Escames, G., Reiter, R.J., Agapito, M.T., Ortiz, G.G., Acuna-Castroviejo, D., Melatonin-induced increased activity of the respiratory chain complexes I and IV can prevent mitochondrial damage induced by rethenium red invivo. *J Pineal Res*, 28, 242–248, 2000.
375. Garcia-Maurino, S., Pozo, D., Carrillo-Vicco, A., Calvo, J.R., Guerrero, J.M., Melatonin activates Th 1 lymphocytes by increasing IL –12 production. *Life Sci*, 65, 2143–2150, 1999.
376. Acuna-Castroviejo, D., Martin, D., Macias, M., Escames, G., Leon, J., Khaldy, H., Reiter, R.J., Melatonin, mitochondria, and cellular bioenergetics. *J Pineal Res*, 30, 65–74, 2001.
377. Martin, M., Macias, M., Leon, J., Escames, G., Khaldy, H., Acuna-Castroviejo, D., Melatonin increases the activity of the oxidative phosphorylation enzymes and the production of ATP in rat brain and liver mitochondria. *Int J Biochem Cell Biol*, 34, 348–357, 2002.
378. Tan, D.X., Manchester, L.C., Reiter, R.J., Qi, W.B., Karbownik, M., Calvo, V.R., Significance of melatonin in antioxidative defense system: Reactions and products. *Biol Signals Recept*, 9, 137–159, 2000.
379. Leon, J., Acuna-Castroviejo, D., Escames, G., Tan, D.X., Reiter, R.J., Melatonin mitigates mitochondrial malfunction. *J Pineal Res*, 38, 1–9, 2005.

380. Srinivasan, V., Maestroni, G.J.M., Cardinali, D.P., Esquifino, A.I., Pandi-Perumal, S.R., Miller, S.C., Melatonin, immune function and aging. *Immun Ageing*, 2, 17, 2005.
381. Feng, Z., Oin, C., Chang, Y., Zhang, J.T., Early melatonin supplementation alleviates oxidative stress in a transgenic mouse model of Alzheimer's disease. *Free Radic Biol Med*, 40, 101–109, 2006.
382. Lee, C.O., Complementary and alternative medicine patients are talking about: Melatonin. *Clin J Oncol Nurs*, 10, 105–107, 2006.
383. Lee, Y.M., Chen, Y.R., Hsiao, G., Sheu, J.R., Wang, J.J., Yen, M.H., Protective effect of melatonin on myocardial ischemia/reperfusion injury in vivo. *J Pineal Res*, 33, 72–80, 2002.
384. Milzani, A., Dalledonne, I., Colomlso, R., Prolonged oxidative stress on actin 3. *Arch Biochem Biophys*, 339, 267–274, 1997.
385. Benitez-King, G., Tunez, I., Bellon, A., Ortiz, G.G., Anton-Tay, F., Melatonin prevents cytoskeletal alterations and oxidative stress induced by okadaic acid in *N*1E-115 cells. *Exp Neurol*, 182, 151–159, 2003.
386. Benitez-King, G., Ortiz-Lopez, L., Jimenez-Rubio, G., Melatonin precludes cytoskeletal collapse caused by hydrogen peroxide: Participation of protein kinase C. *Therapy*, 2, 767–778, 2005.
387. Anisimov, S.V., Popovic, N., Genetic aspects of melatonin biology. *Rev Neurosci*, 15:209–230, 2004.
388. Altun, A., Ugur-Altun, B., Melatonin: Therapeutic and clinical utilization. *Int J Clin Pract*, 61, 835–845, 2007.
389. Nishiyama, K., Yasue, H., Moriyama, Y., Tsunoda, R., Ogawa, H., Yoshimura, M., Kugiyama, K., Acute effects of melatonin administration on cardiovascular autonomic regulation in healthy men. *Am Heart J*, 141, E9, 2001.
390. Bandyopadhyay, D., Biswas, K., Bhattacharyya, M., Reiter, R.J., Banerjee, R.K., Involvement of reactive oxygen species in gastric ulceration: Protection by melatonin. *Indian J Exp Biol*, 40, 693–705, 2002.
391. Ferraz, F.F., Kos, A.G., Janino, P., Homsi, E., Effects of melatonin administration to rats with glycerol-induced acute renal failure. *Renal Fail*, 24, 735–746, 2002.
392. Majsterek, I., Gloc, E., Blasiak, J., Reiter, R.J., A comparison of the action of amifostine and melatonin on DNA-damaging effects and apoptosis induced by idarubicin in normal and cancer cells. *J Pineal Res*, 38, 254–263, 2005.
393. Skwarlo-Sonta, K., Melatonin in immunity: Comparative aspects. *Neuroendocrinol Lett*, 23, 67–72, 2002.
394. Skwarlo-Sonta, K., Majewski, P., Markowska, M., Jakubowska, A., Waloch, M., Bi-modal effect of melatonin on inflammatory reaction in young chickens, in *Treatise on Pineal Gland and Melatonin* (Haldar, C., Singaravel, M., Maitra, S.K. ed.), pp. 225–238. Enfiled, NH: Science Publishers, 2002.
395. Carrillo-Vico, A., Reiter, R.J., Lardone, P.J., Herrera, J.L., Fernandez-Montesinos, R., Guerrero, J.M., Pozo, D., The modulatory role of melatonin on immune responsiveness. *Curr Opin Invest Drugs*, 7, 423–431, 2006.
396. Fildes, J.E., Yoran, N., Keevil, B.G., Melatonin-apleotropic molecule involved in pathophysiological process following organ transplantation. *Immunology*, 127, 443–449, 2009.
397. Lange, T., Dimitrov, S., Fehm, H.L., Westermann, J., Born, J., Shift of monocyte function toward cellular immunity during sleep. *Arch Intern Med*, 166, 1695–700, 2006.
398. Pioli, C., Caroleo, M.C., Nistico, G., Doria, G., Melatonin increases antigen presentation and amplifies specific and non specific signals for T-cell proliferation. *Int J Immunopharmacol*, 15, 463–468, 1993.
399. Kuhlwein, E., Irwin, M., Melatonin modulation of lymphocyte proliferation and Th1/Th2 cytokine expression. *J Neuroimmunol*, 117, 51–57, 2001.
400. Luo, F., Liu, X., Li, S., Liu, C., Wang, Z., Melatonin promoted chemotaxins expression in lung epithelial cell stimulated with TNFα. *Respir Res*, 5, 20, 2004.
401. Mayo, J.C., Sainz, R.M., Tan, D.X., Antolin, I., Rodriquez, C., Reiter, R.J., Melatonin and Parkinson's disease. *Endocrine*, 27, 169–178, 2005.
402. Esposito, E., Mazzon, E., Riccardi, L., Caminiti, R., Meli, R., Cuzzocrea, S., Matrix metalloproteinase-9 and metalloproteinase-2 activity and expression is reduced by melatonin during experimental colitis. *J Pineal Res*, 45, 166–173, 2008.
403. Esposito, E., Genovese, T., Caminiti, R., Bramanti, P., Meli, R., Cuzzocrea, S., Melatonin reduces stress-activated/mitogen-activated protein kinases in spinal cord injury. *J Pineal Res*, 46, 79–86, 2009.
404. Regodon, S., Martin–Palomino, P., Fernandez Montesinos, R., Herrera, J.L., Carroscosa- Salmoral, M.P., Piriz, S., Vadillo, S., Guerrero, J.M., Pozo, D., The use of melatonin as a vaccine agent. *Vaccine*, 23, 5321–5327, 2005.
405. Winczyk, K., Pawlikowski, M., Karasek, M., Melatonin and RZR/ROR receptor ligand CGP52608 induce apoptosis in the murine colonic cancer. *J Pineal Res*, 31, 179–182, 2001.

406. Liu, F., Ng, T.B., Fung, M.C., Pineal indoles stimulate the gene expression of immunomodulating cytokines. *J Neural Transm*, 108, 397–405, 2001.
407. Garcia-Maurino, S., Pozo, D., Calvo, J.R., Guerrero, J.M., Correlation between nuclear receptors expression and enhanced cytokine production in human lymphocytic and monocytic cell lines. *J Pineal Res*, 29, 129–137, 2000.
408. Sutherland, E.R., Ellison, M.C., Kraft, M., Martin, R.J., Elevated serum melatonin is associated with the nocturnal worsening of asthma. *J Allergy Clin Immunol*, 112, 513–517, 2003.
409. Maestroni, G.J.M., Cardinali, D.P., Esquifino, A.I., Pandi-Perumal, S.R., Does melatonin play a disease promoting role in rheumatoid arthritis? *J Neuroimmunol*, 158, 106–111, 2005.
410. Ambriz-Tututi, M., Rocha-Gonzalez, H.I., Cruz, S.L., Granados-Stoco, V., Melatonin: A hormone that modulates pain. *Life Sci*, 84, 489–498, 2009.
411. Juszczak, M., Michalska, M., The effect of melatonin on prolactin, luteinizing hormone (LH), and follicle stimulating hormone (FSH) synthesis and secretion. *Postepy Hig Med Dosw*, 60, 431–438, 2006.
412. Juszczak, M., Michalska, M., The role of the pineal gland and melatonin in the regulation of adenohypophysial hormone synthesis and secretion. *Postepy Hig Med Dosw*, 60, 653–659, 2006.
413. Karasek, M., Pawlikowski, M., Lewinski, A. Hyperprolactinemia: Causes, diagnosis, and treatment. *Endokrynol Pol*, 57, 656–662, 2006.
414. Kelly, R.W., Amato, F., Seamark, R.F., *N*-Acetyl-5-methoxy kynorenamine, brain metabolite of melatonin, is a potent inhibitor of prostaglandin biosynthesis. *Biochem Biophys Res Commun*, 121, 372–379, 1984.
415. Webley, G.E., Bohle, A., Leidenberger, F.A., Positive relationship between the nocturnal concentrations of melatonin and prolactin, and a stimulation of prolactin after melatonin administration in young men. *J Pineal Res*, 5, 19–33, 1988.
416. Vondrasova-Jelinkova, D., Hajek, I., Illnerova, H., Adjustment of the human melatonin and cortisol rhythms to shortening of the natural summer photoperiod. *Brain Res*, 816, 249–253, 1999.
417. Wetterberg, L., The relationship between the pineal gland and the pituitary-adrenal axis in health, endocrine and psychiatric conditions. *Psychoneuroendocrinology*, 8, 75–80, 1983.
418. Sorenson, D., An adventitious role of cortisol in degenerative process due to decrease opposition by insulin: Implication of aging. *Med Hypotheses*, 7, 315–331, 1981.
419. Wu, Y.H., Swaab, D.F., The human pineal gland and melatonin in aging and Alzheimer's disease. *J Pineal Res*, 38, 145–152, 2005.
420. Selmaoui, B., Touitou, Y., Reproducibility of the circadian rhythms of serum cortisol and melatonin in healthy subjects: A study of three different 24-h cycles over six weeks. *Life Sci*, 73, 3339–3349, 2003.
421. Maestroni, G.J., Adrenergic modulation of dendritic cells function: Relevance for the immune homeostasis. *Curr Neurovasc Res*, 2, 169–73, 2005.
422. Lewiniski, A., Karbownik, M., Melatonin and the thyroid gland. *Neuroendocrinol Lett*, 23, 73–78, 2002.
423. Adriaens, I., Jacquet, P., Cortvrindt, R., Janssen, K., Smitz, J., Melatonin has dose-dependent effects on folliculogenesis, oocyte maturation capacity and steroidogenesis. *Toxicology*, 228, 333–43, 2006.
424. Tanavde, V.S., Maitra, A., In vitro modulation of steroidogenesis and gene expression by melatonin: A study with porcine antral follicles. *Endocrinol Res*, 29, 399–410, 2003.
425. Tamura, H., Nakamura, Y., Takiguchi, S., Kashida, S., Yamagata, Y., Sugino, N., Kato, H., Melatonin directly suppresses steroid production by preovulatory follicles in the cyclic hamster. *J Pineal Res*, 25, 135–141, 1998.
426. Wu, C.S., Leu, S.F., Yang, H.Y., Huang, B.M., Melatonin inhibits the expression of steroidogenic acute regulatory protein and steroidogenesis in MA-10 cells. *J Androl*, 22, 245–254, 2001.
427. Chattoraj, A., Bhattacharya, S., Basu, D., Bhattacharya, S., Bhattacharya, S., Maitra, S.K., Melatonin accelerates maturation inducing hormone (MIH)–induced oocyte maturation in carps. *Gen Comp Endocrinol*, 140, 145–155, 2005.
428. Tamura, H., Nakamura, Y., Korkmaz, A., Manchester, L.C., Tan, D.X., Sugino, N., Reiter, R.J., Melatonin and the ovary: Physiological and pathophysiological implications. *Fertil Steril*, 92, 328–343, 2009.
429. Poretsky, L., Cataldo, N.A., Rosenwaks, Z., Giudice, L.C., The insulin-related ovarian regulatory system in health and disease. *Endocrinol Rev*, 20, 535–582, 1999.
430. Chun, S.Y., Billig, H., Tilly, J.L., Furuta, I., Tsafriri, A., Hsueh, A.J., Gonadotropin suppression of apoptosis in cultured preovulatory follicles: Mediatory role of endogenous insulin-like growth factor I. *Endocrinology*, 135, 1845–1853, 1994.
431. Schaeffer, H.J., Sirotkin, A.V., Melatonin and serotonin regulate the release of insulin-like growth factor-I, oxytocin and progesterone by cultured human granulosa cells. *Exp Clin Endocrinol Diabetes*, 105, 109–112, 1997.

432. Picinato, M.C., Hirata, A.E., Cipolla-Neto, J., Curi, R., Carvalho, C.R., Anhe, G.F., Carpinelli, A.R., Activation of insulin and IGF-1 signaling pathways by melatonin through MT1 receptor in isolated rat pancreatic islets. *J Pineal Res*, 44, 88–94, 2008.
433. Knight, P.G., Glister, C., TGF-beta superfamily members and ovarian follicle development. *Reproduction*, 132, 191–206, 2006.
434. Dunkel, L., Tilly, J.L., Shikone, T., Nishimori, K., Hsueh, A.J., Follicle-stimulating hormone receptor expression in the rat ovary: Increases during prepubertal development and regulation by the opposing actions of transforming growth factors beta and alpha. *Biol Reprod*, 50, 940–948, 1994.
435. Hutchinson, L.A., Findlay, J.K., de Vos, F.L., Robertson, D.M., Effects of bovine inhibin, transforming growth factor-beta and bovine activin-A on granulosa cell differentiation. *Biochem Biophys Res Commun*, 146, 1405–1412, 1987.
436. Chen, Y.J., Hsiao, P.W., Lee, M.T., Mason, J.I., Ke, F.C., Hwang, J.J., Interplay of PI3K and cAMP/PKA signaling, and rapamycin-hypersensitivity in TGF beta1 enhancement of FSH-stimulated steroidogenesis in rat ovarian granulosa cells. *J Endocrinol*, 192, 405–419, 2007.
437. Johnson, A.L., Bridgham, J.T., Woods, D.C., Cellular mechanisms and modulation of activin A- and transforming growth factor beta-mediated differentiation in cultured hen granulosa cells. *Biol Reprod*, 71, 1844–1851, 2004.
438. Rimler, A., Matzkin, H., Zisapel, N., Cross talk between melatonin and TGFbeta 1 in human benign prostate epithelial cells. *Prostate*, 40, 211–217, 1999.
439. Turgut, M., Oktem, G., Uslu, S., Yurtseven, M.E., Aktug, H., Uysal, A., The effect of exogenous melatonin administration on trabecular width, ligament thickness and TGF-beta(1) expression in degenerated intervertebral disk tissue in the rat. *J Clin Neurosci*, 13, 357–363, 2006.
440. Otsuka, F., Yao, Z., Lee, T., Yamamoto, S., Erickson, G.F., Shimasaki, S., Bone morphogenetic protein-15. Identification of target cells and biological functions. *J Biol Chem*, 275, 39523–39528, 2000.
441. Vitt, U.A., Hayashi, M., Klein, C., Hsueh, A.J., Growth differentiation factor-9 stimulates proliferation but suppresses the follicle-stimulating hormone-induced differentiation of cultured granulosa cells from small antral and preovulatory rat follicles. *Biol Reprod*, 62, 370–377, 2000.
442. Kennaway, D.J., Rowe, S.A., Melatonin binding sites and their role in seasonal reproduction. *J Reprod Fertil Suppl*, 49, 423–435, 1995.
443. Maitra, S.K., Chattoraj, A., Role of photoperiod and melatonin in the regulation of ovarian functions in Indian carp *Catla catla*: Basic information for future application. *Fish Physiol Biochem*, 33, 367–382, 2007.
444. Wojtowicz, M., Jakiel, G., Melatonin and its role in human reproduction. *Ginekol Pol*, 73, 1231–1237, 2002.
445. Hazlerigg, D.G., What is the role of melatonin within the anterior pituitary? *J Endocrinol*, 170, 493–501, 2001.
446. Seminara, S.B., Hayes, F.J., Crowley, W.F. Jr., Gonadotropin-releasing hormone deficiency in the human (idiopathic hypogonadotropic hypogonadism and Kallmann's syndrome): Pathophysiological and genetic considerations. *Endocr Rev*, 19, 521–539, 1998.
447. Bergadá, I., Milani, C., Bedecarrás, P., Andreone, L., Ropelato, M.G., Gottlieb, S., Bergadá, C., Campo, S., Rey, R.A., Time course of the serum gonadotropin surge, inhibins, and anti-Müllerian hormone in normal newborn males during the first month of life. *J Clin Endocrinol Metab*, 91, 4092–4098, 2006.
448. Chada, M., Průsa, R., Bronský, J., Kotaska, K., Sídlová, K., Pechová, M., Lisá, L., Inhibin B, follicle stimulating hormone, luteinizing hormone and testosterone during childhood and puberty in males: Changes in serum concentrations in relation to age and stage of puberty. *Physiol Res*, 52, 45–51, 2003.
449. Phillips, D.J., Albertsson-Wikland, K., Eriksson, K., Wide, L., Changes in the isoforms of luteinizing hormone and follicle-stimulating hormone during puberty in normal children. *J Clin Endocrinol Metab*, 82, 3103–3106, 1997.
450. Resende, E.A., Lara, B.H., Reis, J.D., Ferreira, B.P., Pereira, G.A., Borges, M.F., Assessment of basal and gonadotropin-releasing hormone-stimulated gonadotropins by immunochemiluminometric and immunofluorometric assays in normal children. *J Clin Endocrinol Metab*, 92, 1424–1429, 2007.
451. Kaplan, S.L., Grumbach, M.M., Clinical review 14: Pathophysiology and treatment of sexual precocity. *J Clin Endocrinol Metab*, 71, 785–789, 1990.
452. Kaplan, S.L., Grumbach, M.M., The ontogenesis of human foetal hormones. II. Luteinizing hormone (LH) and follicle stimulating hormone (FSH). *Acta Endocrinol (Copenh)*, 81, 808–829, 1976.
453. Waldhauser, F., Weissenbacher, G., Frisch, H., Pollak, A., Pulsatile secretion of gonadotropins in early infancy. *Eur J Pediatr*, 137, 71–74, 1981.

454. Winter, J.S., Faiman, C., Hobson, W.C., Prasad, A.V., Reyes, F.I., Pituitary-gonadal relations in infancy. I. Patterns of serum gonadotropin concentrations from birth to four years of age in man and chimpanzee. *J Clin Endocrinol Metab*, 40, 545–551, 1975.
455. Forest, M.G., Pituitary gonadotropin and sex steroid secretion during the first two years of life, in *Control of the Onset of Puberty* (Grumbach, M.M., Sizonenko, P.C., Aubert, M.L., eds.), pp. 451–478, Baltimore, MD: Williams & Wilkins, 1990.
456. Apter, D., Cacciatore, B., Alfthan, H., Stenman, U.H., Serum luteinizing hormone concentrations increase 100-fold in females from 7 years of age to adulthood, as measured by time-resolved immunofluorometric assay. *J Clin Endocrinol Metab*, 68, 53–57, 1989.
457. Wiemann, J.N., Clifton, D.K., Steiner, R.A., Pubertal changes in gonadotropin-releasing hormone and proopiomelanocortin gene expression in the brain of the male rat. *Endocrinology*, 124, 1760–1767, 1989.
458. Roy, D., Belsham, D.D., Melatonin receptor activation regulates GnRH gene expression and secretion in GT1–7 GnRH neurons: Signal transduction mechanisms. *J Biol Chem*, 277, 251–258, 2001.
459. Roy, D., Angelini, N.L., Fujieda, H., Brown, G.M., Belsham, D.D., Cyclical regulation of GnRH gene expression in GT1–7 GnRH-secreting neurons by melatonin. *Endocrinology*, 142(11), 4711–4720, 2001.
460. Lee, V.H., Lee, L.T., Chow, B.K., Gonadotropin-releasing hormone: Regulation of the GnRH gene. *FEBS J*, 275, 5458–5478, 2008.
461. Gillespie, J.M., Roy, D., Cui, H., Belsham, D.D., Repression of gonadotropin-releasing hormone (GnRH) gene expression by melatonin may involve transcription factors COUP-TFI and C/EBP beta binding at the GnRH enhancer. *Neuroendocrinology*, 79, 63–72, 2004.
462. Boyar, R.M., Rosenfeld, R.S., Kapen, S., Finkelstein, J.W., Roffwarg, H.P., Weitzman, E.D., Hellman, L., Human puberty: Simultaneous augmented secretion of luteinizing hormone and testosterone during sleep. *J Clin Invest*, 54, 609–618, 1974.
463. Vanecek, J., Inhibitory effect of melatonin on GnRH-induced LH release. *Rev Reprod*, 4, 67–72, 1999.
464. Balík, A., Kretschmannová, K., Mazna, P., Svobodová, I., Zemková, H., Melatonin action in neonatal gonadotrophs. *Physiol Res*, 53(Suppl 1), S153–166, 2004.
465. Commentz, J.C., Helmke, K., Percocious puberty and decreased melatonin secretion due to a hypothalamic hamartoma. *Horm Res*, 44, 271–275, 1995.
466. Filicori, M., Butler, J.P., Crowley, W.F. Jr., Neuroendocrine regulation of the corpus luteum in the human. Evidence for pulsatile progesterone secretion. *J Clin Invest*, 73, 1638–1647, 1984.
467. Voordouw, B.C., Euser, R., Verdonk, R.E., Alberda, B.T., De Jong, F.H., Droqendijk, A.C., Fauser, B.C., Cohen, M., Melatonin and melatonin-progestin combinations alter pituitary-ovarian function in women and can inhibit ovulation. *J Clin Endocrinol Metab*, 74, 108–117, 1992.
468. Luboshitzky, R., Shen-Orr, Z., Shochat, T., Herer, P., Lavie, P., Melatonin administered in the afternoon decreases next-day luteinizing hormone levels in men: Lack of antagonism by flumazenil. *J Mol Neurosci*, 12, 75–80, 1999.
469. Luboshitzky, R., Lavie, P., Melatonin and sex hormone interrelationships—A review. *J Pediatr Endocrinol Metab*, 12, 355–362, 1999.
470. Yie, S.M., Niles, L.P., Yopunglai, E.V., Melatonin receptors on human granulosa cell membranes. *J Clin Endocrinol Metab*, 80, 1747–1749, 1995.
471. Woo, M.M., Tai, C.J., Kang, S.K., Nathwani, P.S., Pang, S.F., Lueng, P.C., Direct action of melatonin on human granulose-luteal cells. *Clin Endocrinol Metab*, 86, 4789–4797, 2001.
472. Graham, J.D., Clarke, C.L., Physiological action of progesterone in target tissues. *Endocr Rev*, 18, 502–519, 1997.
473. Roy, S.K., Greenwald, G.S., *In vitro* steroidogenesis by primary to antral follicles in the hamster during the periovulatory period: Effects of follicle-stimulating hormone, luteinizing hormone, and prolactin. *Biol Reprod*, 37, 39–46, 1987.
474. Nakamura, Y., Tamura, H., Takayama, H., Kato, H., Increased endogenous level of melatonin in preovulatory human follicles does not directly influence progesterone production. *Fertil Steril*, 80, 1012–1016, 2003.
475. Richards, J.S., Russell, D.L., Ochsner, S., Espey, L.L., Ovulation: New dimensions and new regulators of the inflammatory-like response. *Annu Rev Physiol*, 64, 69–92, 2002.
476. Natraj, U., Richards, J.S., Hormonal regulation, localization, and functional activity of the progesterone receptor in granulosa cells of rat preovulatory follicles. *Endocrinology*, 133, 761–769, 1993.
477. Lim, H., Paria, B.C., Das, S.K., Dinchuk, J.E., Langenbach, R., Trzaskos, J.M., Dey, S.K., Multiple female reproductive failures in cyclooxygenase-2 deficient mice. *Cell*, 91, 197–208, 1997.

478. Espey, L.L., Current status of the hypothesis that mammalian ovulation is comparable to an inflammatory reaction. *Biol Reprod*, 50, 233–238, 1994.
479. Mitchell, L.M., Kennedy, C.R., Hartshorne, G.M., Expression of nitric oxide synthase and effect of substrate manipulation of the nitric oxide pathway in mouse ovarian follicles. *Hum Reprod*, 19, 30–40, 2004.
480. Nakamura, Y., Smith, M., Krishna, A., Terranova, P.F., Increased number of mast cells in the dominant follicle of the cow: Relationships among luteal, stromal, and hilar regions. *Biol Reprod*, 37, 546–549, 1987.
481. Brannstrom, M., Mayrhofer, G., Robertson, S.A., Localization of leukocyte subsets in the rat ovary during the periovulatory period. *Biol Reprod*, 48, 277–286, 1993.
482. Gupta, R.K., Miller, K.P., Babus, J.K., Flaws, J.A., Methoxychlor inhibits growth and induces atresia of antral follicles through an oxidative stress pathway. *Toxicol Sci*, 93, 382–389, 2006.
483. Korzekwa, A.J., Okuda, K., Woclawek-Potocka, I., Murakami, S., Skarzynski, D.J., Nitric oxide induces apoptosis in bovine luteal cells. *J Reprod Dev*, 523, 353–361, 2006.
484. Stocco, C., Telleria, C., Gibori, G., The molecular control of corpus luteum formation, function, and regression. *Endocr Rev*, 28, 117–149, 2007.
485. Korkmaz, A., Reiter, R.J., Epigenetic regulation: A new research area for melatonin? *J Pineal Res*, 44, 41–44, 2008.
486. Reiter, R.J., Melatonin: Lowering the high price of free radicals. *News Physiol Sci*, 15, 246–250, 2000.
487. Sarabia, L., Maurer, I., Bustos-Obregón, E., Melatonin prevents damage elicited by the organophosphorous pesticide diazinon on the mouse testis. *Ecotoxicol Environ Saf*, 72(3), 938–942, 2009.
488. Semercioz, A., Onur, R., Ogras, S., Orhan, I., Effects of melatonin on testicular tissue nitric oxide level and antioxidant enzyme activities in experimentally induced left varicocele. *Neuroendocrinol Lett*, 24, 86–90, 2003.
489. Bomman, M.S., Oosthuizen, J.M.C., Barnard, H.C., Schulenburg, G.W., Boomker, P., Reif, S., Melatonin and sperm motility. *Andrologia*, 21, 483–485, 1989.
490. Van Vuuren, R.J.J., Pitout, M.J., Van Aswegen, C.H., Theron, J.J., Putative melatonin receptor in human spermatozoa. *Clin Biochem*, 25, 125–127, 1992.
491. Fujinoki, M., Melatonin-enhanced hyperactivation of hamster sperm. *Reproduction*, 136, 533–541, 2008.
492. Schlabritz-Loutsevitch, N., Hellner, N., Middendorf, R., Muller, D., Olcese, J., The human myometrium as a target for melatonin. *J Clin Endocrinol Metab*, 88, 908–913, 2003.
493. Steffens, F., Zhou, X.B., Sausbier, V., Sailer, C., Motejlek, K., Ruth, P., Olcese, J., Korth, M., Weiland, T., Melatonin receptor signaling in pregnant and nonpregnant rat uterine myocytes as probed by large conductance Ca2+-activated K+ channel activity. *Mol Endocrinol*, 17, 2103–2115, 2003.
494. Sharkey, J.T., Puttaramu, R., Ward, R.A., Olcese, J., Melatonin synergizes with oxytocin to enhance contractility of human myometrial smooth muscle cells. *J Clin Endocrinol Metab*, 94, 421–427, 2009.
495. Cohen, M., Lippman, M., Chabner, B., Role of pineal gland in aetiology and treatment of breast cancer. *Lancet*, 2, 814–816, 1978.
496. Tamarkin, L., Danforth, D.N., Lichter, A., DeMoss, E., Cohen, M., Chabner, B., Lippman, M., Decreased nocturnal plasma melatonin peak in patients with estrogen receptor positive breast cancer. *Science*, 216, 1003–1005, 1982.
497. Coleman, M.P., Reiter, R.J., Breast cancer, blindness and melatonin. *Eur J Cancer*, 28, 501–503, 1992.
498. Kliukiene, J., Tynes, T., Andersen, A., Risk of breast cancer among Norwegian women with visual impairment. *Br J Cancer*, 84, 397–399, 2001.
499. Kiefer, T., Ram, P.T., Yuan, L., Hill, S.M., Melatonin inhibits estrogen receptor transactivation and cAMP levels in breast cancer cells. *Breast Cancer Res Treatment*, 71, 37–45, 2002.
500. Mirick, D.K., Davis, S., Melatonin as a biomarker of circadian dysregulation. *Cancer Epidemiol Biomarkers Prev*, 17, 3306–3313, 2008.
501. Sánchez-Barceló, E.J., Cos, S., Mediavilla, D., Martínez-Campa, C., González, A., Alonso-González, C., Melatonin-estrogen interactions in breast cancer. *J Pineal Res*, 38, 217–222, 2005.
502. Sánchez-Barceló, E.J., Cos, S., Fernández, R., Mediavilla, M.D., Melatonin and mammary cancer: A short review. *Endocr Relat Cancer*, 10, 153–159, 2003.
503. Blask, D.E., Brainard, G.C., Dauchy, R.T., Hanifin, J.P., Davidson, L.K., Krause, J.A., Sauer, L.A., Rivera-Bermudez, M.A., Dubocovich, M.L., Jasser, S.A., Lynch, D.T., Rollag, M.D., Zalatan, F., Melatonin depleted blood from premenopausal women exposed to light at night stimulates growth of human breast cancer xenografts in nude rats. *Cancer Res*, 65, 11174–11184, 2005.

504. Mills, W., Wu, P., Seely, D., Guyatt, G., Melatonin in treatment of cancer: A systematic review of randomized controlled trials and meta-analysis. *J Pineal Res*, 39, 360–366, 2005.
505. Cos, S., Blask, D.E., Lemus-Wilson, A., Hill, S.M., Effects of melatonin on the cell cycle kinetics and 'estrogen-rescue' of MCF-7 human breast cancer cells in culture. *J Pineal Res*, 10, 36–43, 1991.
506. García-Rato, A., García-Pedrero, J.M., Martínez, M.A., Del Rio, B., Lazo, P.S., Ramos, S., Melatonin blocks the activation of estrogen receptor for DNA binding. *FASEB J*, 13, 857–868, 1999.
507. Sainz, R.M., Mayo, J.C., Tan, D.X., León, J., Manchester, L., Reiter, R.J., Melatonin reduces prostate cancer cell growth leading to neuroendocrine differentiation via a receptor and PKA independent mechanism. *Prostate*, 63, 29–43, 2005.
508. Mediavilla, M.D., Cos, S., Sanchez-Barcelo, E.J., Melatonin increases p53 and p21WAF1 expression in MCF-7 human breast cancer cells in vitro. *Life Sci*, 65, 415–420, 1999.
509. Brzezinski, A., Melatonin in humans. *N Engl J Med*, 336, 186–195, 1997.
510. Cos, S., Fernández, R., Guezmes, A., Sanchez-Barcelo, E.J., Influence of melatonin on invasive and metastatic properties of MCF-7 human breast cancer cells. *Cancer Res*, 58, 4383–4390, 1998.
511. Cos, S., Fernandez, R., Melatonin effects on intercellular junctional communication in MCF-7 human breast cancer cells. *J Pineal Res*, 29, 166–171, 2000.
512. Reiter, R.J., Mechanisms of cancer inhibition by melatonin. *J Pineal Res*, 3, 213–214, 2004.
513. Jones, M.P., Melan, M.A., Witt-Enderby, P.A., Melatonin decreases cell proliferation and transformation in a melatonin receptor-dependent manner. *Cancer Lett*, 151, 133–143, 2000.
514. Yuan, L., Collins, A.R., Dai, J., Dubocovich, M.L., Hill, S.M., MT1 melatonin receptor overexpression enhances the growth suppressive effects of melatonin in human breast cancer cells. *Mol Cell Endocrinol*, 192, 147–156, 2002.
515. Martín, V., Herrera, F., Carrera-Gonzalez, P., García-Santos, G., Antolín, I., Rodriguez-Blanco, J., Rodriguez, C., Intracellular signaling pathways involved in the cell growth inhibition of glioma cells by melatonin. *Cancer Res*, 66, 1081–1088, 2006.
516. Arónica, S.M., Kraus, W.L., Katzenellenbogen, B.S., Estrogen action via the cAMP signalling pathway: Stimulation of adenylate cyclase and cAMP-regulated gene transcription. *Proc Natl Acad Sci USA*, 91, 8517–8521, 1994.
517. García-Pedrero, J.M., Martínez, M.A., Del Rio, B., Martínez-Campa, C., Muramatsu, M., Lazo, P.S., Ramos, S., Calmodulin is a selective modulator of estrogen receptors. *Mol Endocrinol*, 16, 947–960, 2002.
518. Bouhoute, A., Leclercq, G., Modulation of estradiol and DNA binding to estrogen receptor upon association with calmodulin. *Biochem Biophys Res Commun*, 208, 748–755, 1995.
519. Benítez-King, G., Ríos, A., Martínez, A., Antón-Tay, F., *In vitro* inhibition of Ca2+/calmodulin-dependent kinase II activity by melatonin. *Biochim Biophys Acta*, 1290, 191–196, 1996.
520. Armstrong, S.M., Redman, J.R., Melatonin: A chronobiotic with anti-aging properties? *Med Hypotheses*, 34, 300–309, 1991.
521. Manchester, L.C., Tan, D.X., Reiter, R.J., Park, W., Monis, K., Qi, W., High levels of melatonin in the seeds of edible plants: Possible function in germ tissue protection. *Life Sci*, 67, 3023–3029, 2000.
522. Chen, G., Huo, Y., Tan, D.-X., Liang, Z., Zhang, W., Zhang, Y., Melatonin in Chinese medicinal herbs. *Life Sci*, 73, 19–26, 2003.
523. Burkhardt, S., Tan, D.X., Manchester, L.C., Hardeland, R., Reiter, R.J., Detection and quantification of the antioxidant melatonin in Montmorency and Balaton tart cherries (*Prunus cerasus*). *J Agric Food Chem*, 49, 4898–4902, 2001.
524. Hattori, A., Migitaka, H., Iigo, M., Itoh, M., Yamamoto, K., Ohtani-Kaneko, R., Hara, M., Suzuki, T., Reiter, R.J., Identification of melatonin in plants and its effects on plasma melatonin levels and binding to melatonin receptors in vertebrates. *Biochem Mol Biol Int*, 35, 627–634, 1995.
525. Reiter, R.J., Manchester, L.C., Tan, D.-X., Melatonin in walnuts: Influence on levels of melatonin and total antioxidant capacity of blood. *Nutrition*, 21, 920–924, 2005.
526. Reiter, R.J., Tan, D.X., Maldonado, M.D., Melatonin as an antioxidant: Physiology versus pharmacology. *J Pineal Res*, 39, 215–216, 2005.
527. Pape, C., Lüning, K., Quantification of melatonin in phototrophic organisms. *J Pineal Res*, 41, 157–165, 2006.
528. Iriti, M., Rossoni, M., Faoro, F., Melatonin content in grape: Myth or panacea? *J Sci Food Agric*, 86, 1432–1438, 2006.
529. Dubbels, R., Reiter, R.J., Klenke, E., Goebel, A., Schnakenberg, E., Ehlers, C., Schiwara, H.W., Schloot, W., Melatonin in edible plants identified by radioimmunoassay and by high performance liquid chromatography-mass spectrometry. *J Pineal Res*, 18, 28–31, 1995.

530. Hernandez-Ruiz, J., Cano, A., Arnao, M.B., Melatonin acts as a growth stimulating compound in some monocot species. *J Pineal Res*, 39, 137–142, 2005.
531. De La Puerta, C., Carrascosa-Salmoral, M.P., Garcia-Luna, P.P., Lardone, P.J., Herrera, J.L., Fernandez-Montesinos, R., Guerrero, J.M., Pozo, D., Melatonin is a phytochemical in olive oil. *Food Chem*, 104, 609–612, 2007.
532. Wade, A.G., Ford, I., Crawford, G., McMahon, A.D., Nir, T., Laudon, M., Zisapel, N., Efficacy of prolonged release melatonin in insomnia patients aged 55–80 years: Quality of sleep and next-day alertness outcomes. *Curr Med Res Opin*, 23, 2597–605, 2007.
533. Ghosh, A., Hellewell, J.S., A review of the efficacy and tolerability of agomelatine in the treatment of major depression. *Expert Opin Invest Drugs*, 16, 1999–2004, 2007.
534. Roth, T., Seiden, D., Sainati, S., Wang-Weigand, S., Zhang, J., Zee, P., Effects of ramelteon in patients-reported sleep latency in older adults with chronic insomnia. *Sleep Med*, 7, 312–318, 2006.
535. Rajaratnam, S.M., Polymeropoulos, M.H., Fisher, D.M., Roth, T., Scott, C., Birznieks, G., Klerman, E.B., Melatonin agonist tasimelteon (VEC-162) for transient insomnia after sleep-time shift: Two randomised controlled multicentre trials. *Lancet*, 373, 482–491, 2009.
536. Karim, A., Tolbert, D., Cao, C., Disposition kinetics and tolerance of escalating single doses of ramelteon, a high affinity MT1 and MT2 melatonin receptor agonist indicated for treatment of insomnia. *J Clin Pharmacol*, 46, 140–148, 2006.
537. Zammit, G., Erman, M., Wang-Weigand, S., Sainati, S., Zhang, J., Roth, T., Evaluation of the efficacy and safety of ramelteon in subjects with chronic insomnia. *J Clin Sleep Med*, 3, 495–504, 2007.
538. Richardson, G.S., Zee, P.C., Wang-Weigand, S., Rodriguez, L., Peng, X., Circadian phase-shifting effects of repeated ramelteon administration in healthy adults. *J Clin Sleep Med*, 4, 456–461, 2008.
539. Buysse, D., Bate, G., Kirkpatrick, P., Fresh from the pipeline: Ramelteon. *Nat Rev Drug Discov*, 4, 881–882, 2005.
540. Yous, S., Andrieux, J., Howell, H.E., Morgan, P.J., Renard, P., Pfeiffer, B., Lesieur, D., Guardiola-Lemaitre, B., Novel naphthalenic ligands with high affinity for the melatonin receptor. *J Med Chem*, 35, 1484–1486, 1992.
541. Millan, M.J., Gobert, A., Lejeune, F., Dekeyne, A., Newman-Tancredi, A., Pasteau, V., Rivet, J.M., Cussac, D., The novel melatonin agonist agomelatine (S20098) is an antagonist at 5-hydroxytryptamine 2C receptors, blockade of which enhances the activity of frontocortical dopaminergic and adrenergic pathways. *J Pharmacol Exp Ther*, 306, 954–964, 2003.
542. Bertaina-Anglade, V., la Rochelle, C.D., Boyer, P.A., Mocaër, E.. Antidepressant-like effects of agomelatine (S 20098) in the learned helplessness model. *Behav Pharmacol*, 17, 703–713, 2006.
543. Lemoine, P., Nir, T., Laudon, M., Zisapel, N., Prolonged-release melatonin improves sleep quality and morning alertness in insomnia patients aged 55 years and older and has no withdrawal effects. *J Sleep Res*, 16, 372–380, 2007.
544. Papp, M., Gruca, P., Boyer, P.A., Mocaër, E., Effect of agomelatine in the chronic mild stress model of depression in the rat. *Neuropsychopharmacology*, 28, 694–703, 2003.
545. Olié, J.P., Kasper, S., Efficacy of agomelatine, a MT1/MT2 receptor agonist with 5-HT2C antagonistic properties, in major depressive disorder. *Int J Neuropsychopharmacol*, 10, 661–673, 2007.
546. Ying, S.W., Rusak, B., Delagrange, P., Mocaer, E., Renard, P., Guardiola-Lemaitre, B., Melatonin analogues as agonists and antagonists in the circadian system and other brain areas. *Eur J Pharmacol*, 296, 33–42, 1996.
547. Olié, J.P., Tonnoir, B., Ménard, F., Galinowski, A., A prospective study of escitalopram in the treatment of major depressive episodes in the presence or absence of anxiety. *Depress Anxiety*, 24, 318–324, 2007.
548. Lopes, M.C., Quera-Salva, M.A., Guilleminault, C., Non-REM sleep instability in patients with major depressive disorder: Subjective improvement and improvement of non-REM sleep instability with treatment (agomelatine). *Sleep Med*, 9, 33–41, 2007.
549. Ebadi, M., Hexum, T.D., Pfeiffer, R.F., Govitrapong, P., Pineal and retinal peptides and their receptors. *Pineal Res Rev*, 7, 1–156, 1989.

2 Melatonin and Circadian Rhythms: An Overview

G. C. Verster

CONTENTS

2.1 INTRODUCTION

Day and night, darkness and light: due to the Earth's daily rotation around the sun, these are the most pervasive recurring environmental stimuli to which virtually all living organisms are exposed. Mammals—humans included—have adapted to this phenomenon by organizing their behavior into periods of rest or sleep and activity, depending on the time of day or night. Some animals are more active at night—usually those with enhanced olfactory and auditory senses—whereas most are more active during the day, utilizing vision as their primary sense [1].

Adaptation theories for sleep would explain why humans sleep at night and are active during the day. During most of human evolution, it was much safer to be asleep and at rest in a safe sleep environment when it is dark, rather than wandering outside. Considering that, compared with most animals, humans have a poorly developed sense of smell and hearing and with poor night vision, it would make sense that daytime activity would promote a better chance of survival—relating to both hunting and feeding as well as falling prey to potential predators. Natural selection has therefore promoted the development of internal biological clocks to keep track of time related to day and night and effect appropriate behavioral changes. These clocks ensure that various biological functions are automatically initiated when the timing is most appropriate—e.g., becoming drowsy and falling asleep when it is dark outside [2].

Clock mechanisms also act as seasonal timers, assisting organisms in seasonal rhythmicity regarding fertility and even hibernation. Again, this is an evolutionary function that promotes fertility at a time (e.g., spring) when food is expected to be more readily available in a few weeks from conception, rather than allowing random conception with the possibility of having to provide food for a newborn during winter, when little food is available in a potentially cold and hostile environment.

Individual cells also need to be able to time anabolic and catabolic functions to enhance optimal functioning of the organism. The purpose of this would be to ensure optimal cellular utilization of nutrients after feeding. This results in a complex rhythmical behavioral and hormonal cycle as an integral part of normal human physiology [3].

2.2 BIOLOGICAL RHYTHMS IN VARIOUS SPECIES

The physiology of the *Drosophila* fly has been extensively studied and deserves a special mention in the study of sleep and biological rhythms. These flies emerge from their pupal cases in the early morning when it is cool and moist, so as to ensure maximum chance of survival. This behavior is retained with the timing of expected dawn even when external light/dark stimuli are removed, indicating the presence of an internal clock, developed as a necessity for the survival of the fly. Further circadian patterns in these flies restrict activities such as flying and feeding as well as mating to daytime while they experience relative inactivity at night [2].

In simple organisms such as algae and fungi, clock mechanisms are also present, even though these organisms have no neurons. In more complex organisms like fruit flies and zebrafish, there are clock-containing cells in all parts of the body, but concentration is highest in the retina. In these organisms, light is able to penetrate all tissues. In birds, the pineal gland and retina have light receptive cells, whereas in humans, only the retina is able to transmit the light signal to the central nervous system [4].

Although sleep is the most obvious rhythmic activity in which man partakes, there are various other physiological and behavioral manifestations that also exhibit rhythmic patterns.

2.3 CIRCADIAN RHYTHMS

Circadian (Latin: *circa* = about; *dien* = day) rhythms refer to all biological rhythms that exhibit a daily cyclical pattern. These include sleep cycles and various physiological parameters, including melatonin secretion. Circadian rhythms are generated by the suprachiasmatic nucleus (SCN) in the hypothalamus and are in turn influenced by a variety of factors. Output signals from the SCN modulate not only daily rhythms of sleep and wakefulness but also the rhythms of a number of hormones as well as core body temperature [5–8].

In humans, the following physiological variables attain peak levels during sleep: thyroid-stimulating hormone, prolactin, melatonin, adrenocorticotropic hormone, follicle-stimulating hormone, luteinizing hormone, cortisol, and lymphocyte and eosinophil counts. Other variables, e.g., blood viscosity, platelet adhesiveness, erythrocyte count, forced expiratory volume, core body temperature, blood levels of insulin and cholesterol, attain peak activity or elevation during wakefulness, while gastric acid secretion and white cell count peak during the transition from wakefulness to sleep. Since ablation of the SCN abolishes their circadian rhythmicity, these rhythms depend on the proper functioning of the SCN [8].

Normal functioning circadian rhythms require generation by endogenous pacemakers and regular resetting by environmental stimuli. In a free-running state without external stimuli, the cycles of sleep/wake persist but are not synchronized with exact day/night rhythms. The process of synchronization via external stimuli, e.g., light and darkness, is called *entrainment* [1,5].

In humans, it has been proposed that a number of "oscillators" interact with the SCN to influence sleep, wakefulness, body temperature, and cognitive performance. This concept of peripheral modulation of SCN function becomes even more complex, given the exciting discovery that clock genes are expressed not only in the master circadian clock, but also throughout the body in a circadian fashion [9].

Many organs have cells that retain a rhythmic function and express clock genes with a circadian rhythmicity independent from the SCN, but they lose this function within a few days unless there is daily reinforcement by the SCN [4].

For the SCN-governed clock to function effectively, the following are needed: photoreceptors to record the environmental changes, entrainment pathways to relay the information to the circadian pacemakers, and efferent pathways that link the pacemakers to effector systems [1].

2.4 MELATONIN AND CIRCADIAN RHYTHMS

Melatonin remains an important and accurate marker of the central circadian clock of the SCN, and an understanding of the secretion patterns of melatonin is essential when studying circadian rhythms. Melatonin rhythm is the best peripheral indicator of human circadian rhythms and most humans have a uniquely reproducible melatonin rhythm from day to day [10–12].

The circadian rhythmicity of melatonin is dependent on signals from the SCN, and although these signals persist independently from environmental light, entrainment does happen subsequent to light exposure [13].

Pineal melatonin levels gradually begin to rise with the onset of darkness. The circadian rhythm of plasma melatonin levels closely follows the cycle of core body temperature, with the minimum of the core body temperature rhythm occurring just after the peak of plasma melatonin levels [13,14]. The rate-limiting enzyme in the synthesis of melatonin is arylalkylamine *N*-acetyltransferase (AA-NAT), which increases at night by a factor of 7–150 [15]. Both serotonin and *N*-acetylserotonin, acting as precursors for melatonin synthesis, display dramatic circadian rhythmicity, which persist in the absence of external stimuli, again indicating a circadian clock driving pineal secretion [11].

Photic information from the retina is transmitted via the SCN and the sympathetic nervous system to the pineal gland where synthesis of melatonin is stimulated. The SCN conveys the signal to the pineal gland via the dorsomedial hypothalamic nucleus, the upper thoracic cell columns of the spinal chord, the superior cervical ganglia, and postganglionic adrenergic fibres. Peak secretion is attained in the early morning hours (between 2 and 4 AM).

In lower vertebrates, the pineal gland is photosensitive and is the site of a self-sustaining circadian clock. In humans, the gland has lost direct photosensitivity but responds to light via the previously mentioned multisynaptic pathway [12].

Melatonin exerts chronobiological effects via membrane G-protein–coupled melatonin receptors (MT_1 and MT_2) in the SCN. It inhibits neuronal firing in the SCN via the MT_1 receptor, which is likely to be responsible for the regulation of sleep. The phase-shifting effects of melatonin are mediated via the MT_2 receptor [8].

In the absence of photostimulation, melatonin secretion persists and follows a circadian rhythm in all humans except young infants, as very little melatonin is secreted below 3 months of age. At 24 weeks of age, melatonin concentrations are still only about 25% of adult levels [12].

The adrenal gland has melatonin receptors that inhibit adrenocorticotropic hormone–stimulated cortisol production. This is effected via a direct inhibition of clock genes in the adrenal cortex. The adrenal gland is thus an important site for integrating photic and nonphotic (feeding) signals. Melatonin also has a role as *zeitgeber* in pancreatic β-cells, which demonstrates a circadian insulin secretion pattern [3,16].

2.5 PHOTIC ENTRAINMENT/ZEITGEBERS

In normal individuals exposed to the earth's light/dark cycles, the internal circadian clock is entrained to the 24-hour cycle by light received at the retina. Thus, although the circadian clock has the capability to run autonomously, in its natural state, it regularly receives environmental signals and adjusts its timing in response to these signals in order to maintain a rhythm that is synchronized with the environment [14].

Free-running human circadian rhythms have a frequency of 23,8 to 27,1 hours and not 24 hours exactly. This discrepancy occurs when external time cues are removed, e.g., by putting a test subject in a room that is isolated from external input such as regular light/dark cycles and scheduled activities. This results in rhythms moving out of phase within a few days [1,14].

As mentioned before, repeated entrainment by environmental light is thus needed to synchronize the intrinsic circadian cycle to 24 hours. Bright light in the evening will delay the circadian clock and bright light in the morning is necessary to synchronize the clock to a 24-hour rhythm [1,17].

When resetting the circadian pacemaker on a daily basis, environmental light in the morning acts as a so-called zeitgeber. The circadian pacemaker is reset via glutamatergic inputs to the neurons of the SCN of the hypothalamus via the retinohypothalamic tract [5,18]. This pathway functions independently from the optic nerves, and in experimental models where complete blindness was induced by transaction of the optic nerves, photic entrainment of the circadian rhythms persisted [1].

Nonrod, noncone photoreceptors have been discovered in the ganglion cells of the retina, and these receptors are the essential components needed to initiate the photic registration of daily rhythms. These photoreceptors contain the photopigment melanopsin and are most sensitive to blue wavelength light. This implies that blue light is the most effective wavelength to effect the circadian system and suppress melatonin. Nevertheless, rods and cones can also influence the circadian response, and ordinary white light is therefore also sufficient to produce an effect [6]. The effect of light is also dependent on time of day, that is, light alters pacemaker function in a time-dependent manner. This means that the circadian system is least sensitive to light at midday and most sensitive during nighttime [1,6].

The zeitgebers trigger a cascade of cyclical events into the brain and in the whole organism that will continue during the day, influencing neurotransmitter turnover, hormonal production, rest activity, and sleep/wake cycles [18].

2.6 NONPHOTIC ENTRAINMENT

The behavior of human circadian rhythms functions on two levels: the circadian pacemaker, or so-called SCN oscillator that drives temperature and plasma melatonin rhythms, and the sleep/wake rhythm, or non-SCN oscillator [19].

As mentioned before, circadian rhythmicity needs regular reinforcement. As humans have no light-sensitive organs, except for the retina, synchronization of peripheral clocks is also achieved by entraining factors such as behavior, food intake, hormones, and temperature/energy balance. The hormonal clues include corticoids, insulin, and ghrelin. Conditioned learning responses determined by the timing of photic and feeding/fasting signals can also influence recurring circadian responses [3,4,20].

Physical activity enhances the firing of raphé serotonergic neurons, which, in turn, modifies SCN activity. Brain serotonin (5-HT) turnover, which mediates this nonphotic entrainment of the circadian clock and modulates the response of the SCN to photic inputs, follows a cyclical pattern with the highest activity during behavioral arousal and the lowest during sleep. In a similar way, dopamine turnover follows a circadian pattern influenced by light, while, in turn, signaling mediated by the dopamine D2 receptor potentiates circadian regulation by clock genes. The SCN, in turn, regulates circadian variations in noradrenergic locus ceruleus impulse activity, while norepinephrine provides further circadian regulation of the sleep/wake cycle.

Cholinergic neurons are involved in the generation of REM sleep, and acetylcholine follows a circadian rhythm, playing a role in modulating the photic information reaching the SCN and in entraining the clock.

The circadian behavioral transition from sleep to waking can affect basic cellular functions such as RNA and protein synthesis, neuronal plasticity, neurotransmission, and metabolism [18].

A subdivision of the lateral geniculate complex, the intergeniculate leaflet, has projections to the SCN. This system appears to integrate photic and nonphotic information (e.g., responses to locomotor activity) to further modulate pacemaker functioning [1].

Manipulation of sleep patterns independent of light/darkness can thus lead to entrainment of circadian rhythms. Teenagers and young adults often tend to go to sleep later and wake up later during weekends, and a mere 2 days of this disturbed pattern may lead to subsequent difficulty in initiating sleep [21].

This has further implications when managing conditions like jet lag and sleep disturbances secondary to shift work. Scheduled activity and rest periods independent from day-light cycles may assist in re-entraining these sleep phase disturbances [20].

Other entrainment factors include food and meals, hormones, and social factors, although none of these are as potent as photic stimulation. Various signals indicate to animals when specific food types are available. These include endogenous oscillators as well as environmental cues. This induces animals to have meal-anticipatory behaviors in response to stimuli that reliably indicate food availability. These signals are so strong that they can induce feeding in animals that are already sated [3].

On a behavioral level, rats fed one meal per day increase their daily physical activity regularly prior to the feeding. Further animal studies have shown that daytime restriction of food and water induces phase shifts in the circadian rhythms of corticosteroids and core body temperature. These rhythms have persisted in animals where the SCN was ablated, proving the presence of the non-SCN oscillators [3].

2.7 CIRCADIAN RHYTHMS AND PSYCHIATRY

Circadian rhythms are disturbed in various sleep and sleep phase disorders (jet lag, shift workers) as well as other psychiatric disorders, including mood disorders. Several markers have demonstrated decreased circadian amplitudes as well as phase advances or delays. This may imply changes in the circadian clocks or in sensitivity to environmental factors, such as light or social cues [8,22].

Various nonpharmacological (bright light therapy, sleep deprivation, social rhythm therapy) and pharmacological (lithium, antidepressants, e.g., agomelatine) therapies influence circadian rhythms, further emphasizing the role of biological clocks in the pathogenesis of these conditions [22].

2.8 SLEEP AND CIRCADIAN RHYTHMS

Sleep is regulated by the interplay of different factors, e.g., the interaction between the homeostatic and the endogenous circadian processes. The homeostatic process accumulates with wakefulness, i.e., there is more homeostatic factor the longer you are awake. This factor is believed to be of main importance for sleep quality, that is, the longer you are awake, the deeper the following sleep episode will be (increased slow-wave activity). The circadian factor, on the other hand, plays an important role in sleep quantity, that is, sleep duration is for the most part determined by when you go to bed. In other words, sleep length is not dependent on the sleep homeostatic factor but largely dependent on when you go to sleep according to your own circadian rhythms [23].

Each individual has a favorable sleep window, determined by the circadian rhythm, which affects the quality and quantity of sleep. To determine this circadian time window, the 24-hour profile of melatonin secretion is generally considered to provide the best measure [24].

2.9 GENETIC FACTORS

Individual neurons in the SCN have been shown to exhibit circadian rhythms, implying an intracellular timekeeping mechanism. Subsequently, a number of circadian clock genes have been isolated. These are essential for sustaining rhythms in constant conditions [25].

The study of *Drosophila* has formed the basis for understanding genetic factors involved in circadian rhythmicity. Mutagen-exposed flies exhibited defects in rhythms for locomotor activity, suggesting that specific sets of genes were involved in timing of certain complex behaviors. These findings have also been investigated in rodents and experiments have demonstrated that specific chromosomal mutations in hamsters have induced an advanced sleep phase and changes in timed behavioral patterns. It has subsequently been suggested that in humans with familial advanced sleep phase syndrome, a similar mutation may be involved. Affected humans have phase advances in sleep/wake, temperature, and melatonin rhythms [2,25].

Clock genes and their associated proteins are involved in positive and negative feedback loops to influence circadian periodicity. Expression of the clock genes are activated by the aptly named transcriptional activator *CLOCK* (circadian locomotor output cycles kaput) and *BMAL1* (brain and muscle ARNT-like protein 1), among others [22,25].

As mentioned previously, peripheral clocks can be entrained by feeding rhythms. Changing feeding habits in rodents shifts the phase of clock gene RNA expression in the liver and other peripheral tissues, while gene expression in the SCN remains entrained to the light/dark cycle.

2.10 CHRONOTYPES

There are also some individual variations in responses to zeitgebers. Individuals vary in the time that they would respond to cues, e.g., time between onset of dawn and waking, responses to melatonin onset. This relationship is referred to as *phase of entrainment*, and individual variations in people are referred to as their *chronotypes* [5]. Chronotypes classify individuals according to their preferred timing for activity and sleep [26].

Persons who are phase-advanced are morning types (M types) and would have a preference for going to bed and waking early, whereas evening types (E types) are phase-delayed, going to bed late and waking later in the morning. The majority of people do not fall into either extremes and are classified in the intermediate circadian position (N types).

A person's chronotype would have obvious implications for the duration of their sleep. A person with an E-type chronotype would normally be expected to wake up later. In a normal office-hour work environment, the person would have to wake up earlier than required by the chronotype and this would lead to sleep deficit during the week, as waking time would be determined by work requirements and not by chronotype. Catching up on the sleep deficit over weekends then follows, with the resulting late sleeping perpetuating the chronotype.

Women have a greater tendency toward being M types. This is possibly due to sociocultural influences or biological factors. Adolescents commonly have more delayed sleep times, whereas increased age is associated with a tendency toward being M type [26].

The importance of determination of chronotypes is that it determines daily patterns of behavioral and performance rhythms. E types are less alert in the mornings, have more irregular sleep schedules, and a tendency to compensate for shorter sleep duration over weekends. They also report more attention problems and impairment in academic performance with higher incidences of emotional problems and substance abuse [26].

Industrial societies appear to have wide variations in chronotypes. This may be due to the diluted influence of environmental photic influences on entrainment. An indoors environment during daytime does not expose individuals to the same light intensities they would experience outdoors, and artificial light during nighttime obviously inhibits the effects of environmental darkness. This effect is called *chronodisruption.* Unfortunately, we are people of the 21st century, with markedly different social habits from our early ancestors, although we remain genetically similar. It is currently estimated that two thirds of the world's population live under night sky whose brightness is higher than baseline levels. This is mostly due to urban sky glow [16].

2.11 THERAPEUTIC MANIPULATION OF CIRCADIAN RHYTHMS

Contrary to what might be expected, melatonin is not required for sleep in humans. Patients who have undergone pinealectomies have shown little disturbances in their sleep/wake cycles. Nevertheless, exogenous melatonin has beneficial effects on promotion of sleep. This was first described more than 40 years ago, using very high doses (100 mg). Subsequently, much lower doses have been promoted, and 3–5 mg should be sufficient for adults [12].

When administered late at night (2330 h), it has little sedative properties, but when administered earlier (1800 h), it is comparable to temazepam [8]. It affects the onset of sleep as well as duration and quality of sleep with an increase in REM sleep [13].

Administration of exogenous melatonin to humans in the early evening advances the phase of the circadian rhythm; administration in the early morning delays the phase. This has obvious and proven implications for sufferers from jet lag following travel over time zones. Melatonin given approximately 12 hours before daily core temperature minimum is achieved will lead to phase advance, and when taken 1–4 hours after, phase delay will follow [12,14].

Jet lag develops when the circadian rhythms are not synchronized with local time and subsequent day/night rhythms. Symptoms are tiredness (with cognitive consequences), inability to sleep at the local bed time, generally disturbed sleep, headaches, and gastrointestinal problems. Symptoms are worse in older persons, when more time zones are crossed, and when flying from west to east [15].

The importance of disturbed circadian rhythms in various psychiatric and physical conditions has been well established [8]. Rational use of melatonin or melatonin agonists have been suggested in the management of these conditions. Recent developments have determined the importance of behavioral influences on circadian rhythms, and therefore, it seems plausible that a combination of melatonergic agonism together with behavioral interventions should be an even more powerful option [10].

2.12 CONCLUSION

With recent developments in the understanding of the genetics of clock genes and the influence of gene expression on daily biological rhythms, chronotherapeutics and its role in treatment of various sleep and psychiatric disorders have become an important topic for research and discussion.

Although the role of behavior and other nonphotic factors have been shown to be important in understanding the expanded knowledge in the field of circadian rhythms, melatonin remains a cornerstone in the measuring of sleep phases and the management of circadian rhythm–related disorders.

REFERENCES

1. Moore RY. Circadian rhythms: Basic neurobiology and clinical applications. *Annu Rev Med* 1997; 48:253–266.
2. Panda S, Hogenesch JB, Kay SA. Circadian rhythms from flies to human. *Nature* 2002; 417:329–335.
3. Silver R, Balsam P. Oscillators entrained by food and the emergence of anticipatory timing behaviours. *Sleep Biol Rhythms* 2010; 8:120–136.
4. Buijs RM, Van Eden CG, Goncharuk VD, Kalsbeek A. Circadian and seasonal rhythms. *J Endocrinol* 2003; 177:17–26.
5. Roenneberg T, Kuehnle T, Juda A, Kantermann T, Allebrand K, Gordijn M, Merrow M. Epidemiology of the human circadian clock. *Sleep Med Rev* 2007; 11:429–438.
6. Sack RL, Auckley D, Auger RR, Carskadon MA, Wright KP, Vitiello MV, Zhdanova IV. Circadian rhythm sleep disorders: Part I, basic principles, shift work and jet lag disorders. *Sleep* 2007; 30(11):1460–1483.
7. Saper CB, Scammell TE, Lu J. Hypothalamic regulation of sleep and circadian rhythms. *Nature* 2005; 437:1257–1263.
8. Verster GC. Melatonin and its agonists, circadian rhythms and psychiatry. *Afr J Psychiatry* 2009; 12(1):42–46.
9. Freeman GM, Webb AB, An S, Herzog ED. For whom the bells toll: Networked circadian clocks. *Sleep Biol Rhythms* 2008; 6:67–75.
10. Arendt J. Melatonin and human rhythms. *Chronobiol Int* 2006; 23(1 and 2):21–37.
11. Chattoraj A, Liu T, Zhang LS, Huang Z, Borjigin J. Melatonin formation in mammals: *In vivo* perspectives. *Rev Endocrinol Metab Disord* 2009; 10:237–243.

12. Zawilska JB, Skene DJ, Arendt J. Physiology and pharmacology of melatonin in relation to biological rhythms. *Pharmacol Rep* 2009; 61:383–410.
13. Brzezinski A. Melatonin in humans. *N Engl J Med* 1997; 336(3):186–195.
14. Zee PC, Manthena P. The brain's master circadian clock: Implications and opportunities for therapy of sleep disorders. *Sleep Med Rev* 2007; 11(1):59–70.
15. Berra B, Rizzo AM. Melatonin: Circadian rhythm regulator, chronobiotic, antioxidant and beyond. *Clinics Dermatol* 2009; 27:202–209.
16. Korkmaz A, Topal T, Tan D, Reiter RJ. Role of melatonin in metabolic regulation. *Rev Endocr Metab Disord* 2009; 10:261–270.
17. Nutt D, Wilson S, Paterson L. Sleep disorders as core symptoms of depression. *Dialogues Clin Neurosci* 2008; 10(3):329–336.
18. Benedetti F, Barbini B, Colombo C, Smeraldi E. Chronotherapeutics in a psychiatric ward. *Sleep Med Rev* 2007; 11(6):509–522.
19. Nakao M, Okayama H, Karashima A, Katayama N. Top–down modeling of hierarchical biological clock mechanisms. *Sleep Biol Rhythms* 2010; 8:106–113.
20. Khalsa SB, Jewett ME, Cajochen C, Czeisler CA. A phase response curve to single bright light pulses in human subjects. *J Physiol* 2003; 549.3:945–952.
21. Taylor A, Wright H, Lack L. Sleeping-in on the weekend delays circadian phase and increases sleepiness the following week. *Sleep Biol Rhythms* 2008; 6:172–179.
22. Schulz P, Steimer T. Neurobiology of circadian systems. *CNS Drugs* 2009; 23(Suppl 2):3–13.
23. Bjorvatn B, Pallesen S. A practical approach to circadian rhythm sleep disorders. *Sleep Med Rev* 2009; 13(1):47–60.
24. Van Someren EJ, Nagtegaal E. Improving melatonin circadian phase estimates. *Sleep Med* 2007; 8(6): 590–601.
25. Cermakian N, Boivin DB. The regulation of central and peripheral circadian clocks in humans. *Obes Rev* 2009; 10(suppl 2):25–36.
26. Fernandez-Mendoza J, Ilioudi C, Montes MI, Olavarrieta-Bernardino S, Aguirre-Berrocal A, De la Cruz-Troca JJ, Vela-Bueno A. Circadian preference, nighttime sleep and daytime functioning in young adulthood. *Sleep Biol Rhythms* 2010; 8:52–62.

3 Synthesis and Metabolism of Melatonin in the Skin and Retinal Pigment Epithelium

Radomir Slominski and Andrzej T. Slominski

CONTENTS

3.1 MELATONIN IN THE SKIN: AN OVERVIEW

It has been over 50 years since Lerner has discovered that melatonin (*N*-acetyl-5-methoxytryptamine) is present in the skin (reviewed in [1]). In 1958, Lerner et al. isolated the chemical compound from the beef pineal extract and injected it into the frog melanocytes [2]. He found that this extract causes the lightening of the skin. Although the first experiment to ever show that the pineal gland causes lightening of the frog skin was performed by McCord and Allen in 1917, Lerner was the first to define the structure of melatonin as *N*-acetyl-5-methoxytryptamine and show that it is an antagonist for melanocyte-stimulating hormone [2].

Since then, melatonin has been found to play many roles in the skin (Figure 3.1). These include the removal of free radicals, protection of the skin cells from UV damage, promotion of hair growth, prevention of apoptosis, and even inhibition of skin cancer (reviewed in refs. [1,3,4]). Melatonin mediates its actions through the following: melatonin membrane receptors MT1 and MT2 [5,6], nuclear receptors of the ROR-α family [7], and finally on its own as a metabolic modulator or free radical scavenger [1,8,9].

3.2 SYNTHESIS OF MELATONIN IN THE SKIN

3.2.1 Introduction to the Cutaneous Pathway

Melatonin synthesis is a four-step process that begins with the hydroxylation of the amino acid L-tryptophan to 5-hydroxytryptophan by tryptophan hydroxylase (TPH, EC 1.14.16.4) [10] and is then decarboxylated to serotonin by amino acid decarboxylase (AAD, EC 4.1.1.28) [11]. Serotonin is then acetylated to *N*-acetylserotonin by the enzyme arylalkylamine *N*-acetyltransferase (AANAT, EC 2.3.1.87) [12]. *N*-Acetylserotonin is finally converted to melatonin by hydroxyindole-*O*-methyl transferase (HIOMT, EC 2.1.1.4) [13].

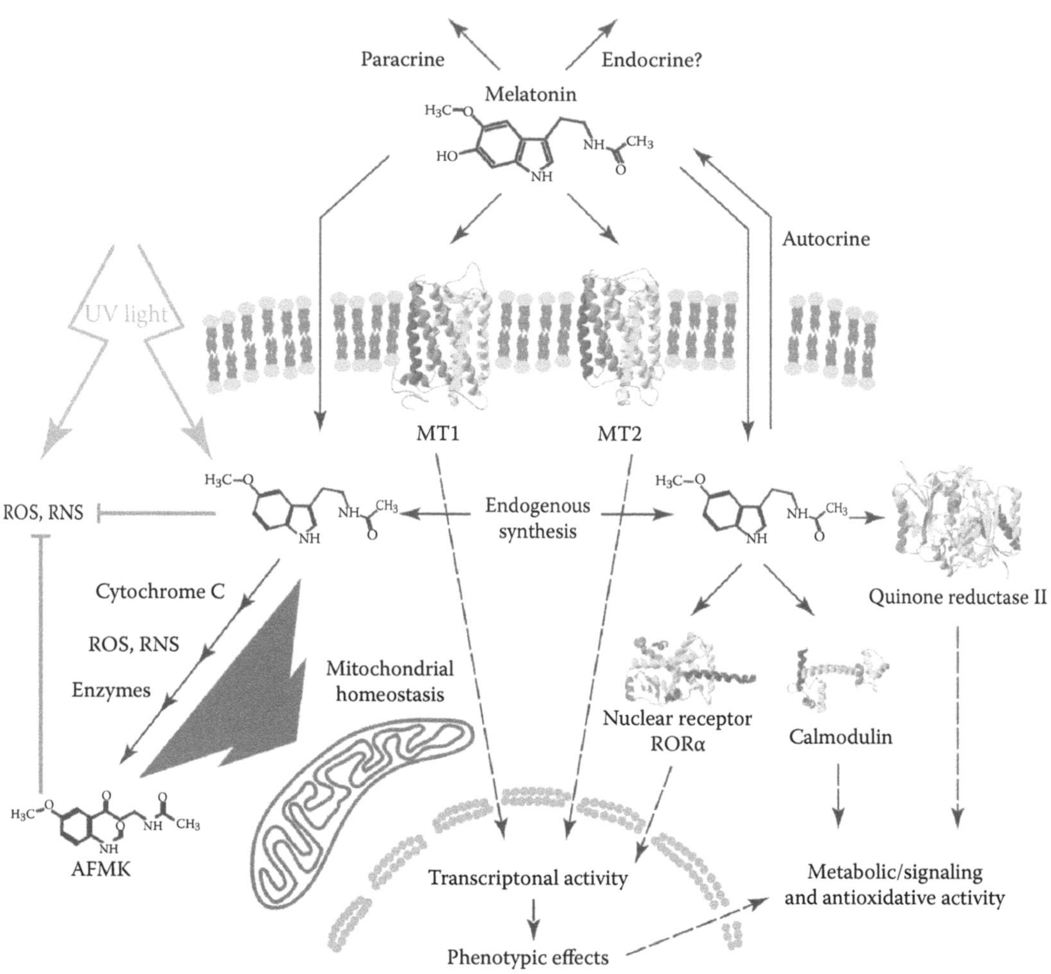

FIGURE 3.1 Diverse effects of melatonin in the mammalian skin cell. Melatonin can regulate skin cell phenotype by interactions with membrane-bound MT1 and MT2 receptors or with nuclear ROR-α/RZR receptor. Nonreceptor actions can be mediated through interactions with quinone reductase 2 or caldmodulin, through regulation of mitochondrial metabolism, through activation of cellular antioxidative stress responses, or through direct free radical scavenging. In skin, melatonin effects can also represent intracrine, paracrine, and autocrine actions to regulate local homeostasis protect against endogenous or exogenous insults, aging, carcinogenesis or other pathology. (Reprinted from *Trends Endocrinol Metab*, 19, Slominski, A. et al., 17–24, Copyright 2009, with permission from Elsevier.)

Melatonin synthesis was originally thought to occur only in the pineal gland; however, evidence proved that it also occurs in the skin (reviewed in [9]). The first piece of evidence that melatonin can be synthesized in the mammalian skin has been the demonstration that serotonin is transformed to melatonin in hamster skin incubated ex vivo [14]. In 1993, researchers found activity of two isoforms of arylamine *N*-acetyltransferase in the hamster skin, e.g., NAT-1 and NAT-2 [15]. Specifically, the skin NAT-2 isoform was involved in the transformation of serotonin to acetylserotonin and interestingly of dopamine to *N*-acetyl-dopamine [15]. Thus, these authors were the first to show that hamster skin contains enzymatic activity characteristic for pineal AANAT, transforming serotonin to *N*-acetylserotonin [15].

A few years later, Slominski et al. have shown actual conversion of serotonin to melatonin in hamster skin organ culture by using radioactively labeled serotonin that was converted to

N-acetylserotonin and, finally, melatonin with its subsequent metabolism [14]. The chemical nature of the outcome in organ culture *N*-acetylserotonin was confirmed by gas chromatography/mass spectrometry [14].

Afterward, it has been found that all steps of melatonin synthesis starting from tryptophan are expressed in human skin and skin cells [16] (Figure 3.2). The melatoninergic pathway has been detected in whole human skin, normal and immortalized epidermal keratinocytes and melanocytes, dermal fibroblasts, squamous cell carcinoma cells, and in a large panel of human melanoma cell lines [16]. This was shown by findings of expression of genes, proteins, and the actual activity of the rate-limiting enzymes TPH, AANAT, and HIOMT in these cells [16]. The human melanoma cells have also been found to express the rate-limiting enzymes in melatonin synthesis but at a higher rate than the normal human skin cells [16]. Actually, all intermediates of the melatoninergic pathway were detected by liquid chromography/mass spectrometry (LC/MS) in human and rodent melanoma lines and keratinocytes [16–19]. These finding were further confirmed by demonstration of melatonin synthesis in rodent and human hair follicles [3].

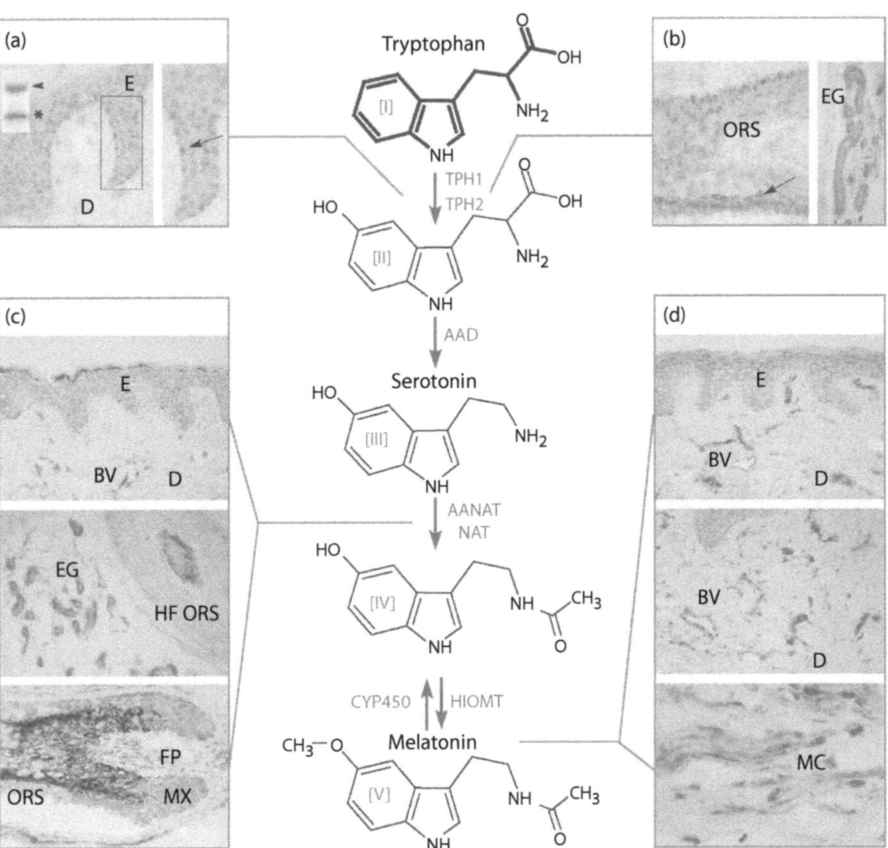

FIGURE 3.2 The biosynthetic pathway for melatonin synthesis. The first step in melatonin synthesis is tryptophan hydroxylation to 5-hydroxytryptophan by TPH. TPH (MW = 50 kD) is shown by the WB insert. TPH can be degraded to a smaller weight, which is shown by the asterisk. (a,b) TPH is found in the epidermis (E), hair follicle (ORS), and eccrine gland (EG). (c) AAD then decarboxylates 5-hydroxytryptophan to produce serotonin, which is then converted to NAS by serotonin-*N*-acetyltransferase. The serotonin-*N*-acetyltransferase group is expressed in the following compartments: epidermal, dermal, and adnexal. (d) NAS is then converted to melatonin by HIOMT. Melatonin is found in the blood vessels, epidermis, hair follicle, and mast cells. (Reprinted from *Trends Endocrinol Metab*, 19, Slominski, A. et al., 17–24, Copyright 2009, with permission from Elsevier.)

In addition, immunofluorescence studies have detected melatonin antigens in the epidermis, keratinocyes of strata spinosum granulosum, hair follicle epithelium, and dermal mast cells (Figure 3.2) [20].

3.2.2 TPH Activity and Serotonin Synthesis

The first step in both serotonin and melatonin synthesis is the conversion of L-tryptophan to 5-hydroxytryptophan by TPH (EC 1.14.16.4) [1]. TPH acts by hydroxylating the fifth position of the indole ring of L-tryptophan [10]. There are two major types of TPH: *TPH1*, which is the predominant type in peripheral tissues [19,21], and *TPH2*, which is found only in the central nervous system [22].

TPH activity requires the presence of cofactor 6-tetrahydropterin (6-BH4) [21], which acts as an electron donor [23]. The creation of 6-BH4 starts from guanosine triphosphate, which undergoes a multistep process [24]. The skin cells that have been found to synthesize 6-BH4 include keratinocytes and melanocytes [23].

The TPH gene and active enzyme have been found to be expressed in normal and pathological rodent and human skin and cultured skin cells [17,25,26]. The *TPH1* gene expression has been found in the following human cells: cultured normal epidermal and follicular melanocytes, normal neonatal and adult epidermal and follicular keratinocytes, and follicular and dermal fibroblasts [16,20,27]. The *TPH1* gene was also found in the following skin cancer cells: basal cell carcinomas, melanoma cell lines (all cell lines tested), and squamous cell carcinoma cells [16].

This was further confirmed by the detection of TPH protein by Western blotting (WB) in extracts from human and rodent skin and skin cells [17,25,26]. Actual enzymatic activity was also detected in skin and skin cell extracts being found predominantly in melanocytes [19,20,26]. Molecular analyses demonstrated that the main form of TPH in the skin cells was *TPH1* [19], while *TPH2* was only expressed in melanocytes and melanoma cells [28]. To define in situ localization of TPH, immunocytochemistry and immunofluorescence techniques were used. The TPH was predominantly localized in the epidermal melanocytes and melanoma cells [19]. Similarly, serotonin was detected in situ in the same cell type by immunocytochemistry [26,29]. Using more sensitive methods (frozen sections of scalp skin) of detection, the above authors have also been able to detect TPH in situ in the keratinocytes of epidermis and hair follicle, as well as in the melanocytes and fibroblasts, eccrine glands, and the blood vessels [20]. These results are consistent with detection of TPH and serotonin production in the breast epithelial cells [30–32].

TPH protein expression was also found in the dermis and epidermis of both the mouse and hamster skin [17,25]. In fact, the hamster *TPH1* was even cloned from the skin cells [17].

5-Hydroxytryptophan is then converted to serotonin (5-hydroxytryptamine) by the enzyme AAD [11], which is ubiquitously expressed through the body. AAD protein expression has been found in human skin cells including melanocytes and keratinocytes [33].

The evidence that serotonin is synthesized by skin cells has been found in human [16], mouse [25], and hamster skin [26]. The evidence that supports this claim includes the conversion of tryptophan to hydroxytryptophan and actual detection of serotonin in skin or skin cells by HPLC and LC/MS [16,17,19,25]. Also by immunocytochemistry, serotonin was detected in skin mast cells, melanocytes, and epithelial cells of the epidermis and hair follicle (Figure 3.2) [20].

Serotonin plays several roles in the skin, including acting as a neurotransmitter, as a vasodilator, as a modulator of the immune system, and it can simulate the actions of the growth factors [27]. Serotonin has also been found to play a role in inflammatory skin disorders and serotonin receptors are widely expressed in skin cells, including melanocytes, keratinocytes, and immune cells [20,26].

3.2.3 Metabolism of Serotonin to Melatonin

There are two pathways of metabolism of serotonin: one pathway is that it becomes melatonin [34] and the other pathway is that serotonin is degraded to 5HIAA (5-hydroxyindoleacetic acid)

[35]. In the second pathway in the skin, serotonin undergoes oxidative deamination by monoamine oxidase to 5-hydroxyindoleacetaldehyde [26,36]. 5-Hydroxyindoleacetaldehyde is then oxidized to either 5HTPOL (5-hydroxytryptophol) or 5HIAA by alcohol dehydrogenase (EC 1.1.1.1) or aldehyde dehydrogenase (EC 1.2.1.3), respectively [36].

The first pathway, synthesis of melatonin, involves the acetylation from serotonin to *N*-acetylserotonin (NAS) by the rate-limiting enzyme AANAT [12]. In 2002, researchers found AANAT gene expression in the following normal human skin cells: cultured normal epidermal and follicular melanocytes, normal neonatal and adult epidermal keratinocytes, and follicular and dermal fibroblasts [16]. AANAT gene expression was also found in normal skin biopsies, skin biopsies containing basal cell carcinomas, in melanoma cell lines (all lines except SKMEL 188), and squamous cell carcinoma [16]. AANAT mRNA can undergo alternative splicing in human samples, with appearance of new spliced forms in pathological skin including basal cell carcinoma (BCC) [16].

AANAT protein and enzyme activity was detected in cultured human normal epidermal melanocytes, normal neonatal and adult epidermal keratinocytes, and dermal fibroblasts as well as in melanoma cell lines (all cell lines tested) and squamous cell carcinoma cells [9,16,27]. The characteristic of AANAT in selected skin samples is shown in Table 3.1.

The AANAT protein was detected by WB in skin cells and in situ by immunofluorescence in the following skin cell compartments: epithelial layers of the epidermis and hair follicle, epithelial cells of sweat glands, wall of blood vessels, and sensory nerve endings [20].

Interestingly, there were differences in AANAT activity between the skin from white and black patients [16]. The AANAT activity in black skin is about twice as much as in white skin [16].

The AANAT enzymatic activity and NAS itself have also been detected in rodent skin including hamster skin, rat skin, and rodent melanoma lines [16,36]. NAS has also been detected in the human melanoma cells by using the tools HPLC and LC/MS [16,18].

Interestingly, while the skin of C57BL/6 mouse was able to acetylate serotonin to *N*-acetyserotonin, the AANAT protein produced in this species was inactive enzymatically because of genetic defect leading to alternative splicing of AANAT message [19,37]. The detailed discussion of this phenomenon is listed below.

C57BL/6 mice express the gene for AANAT but do not produce the active form of AANAT [37]. These authors have suggested that C56BL/6 mice are a natural AANAT knockout strain, and as a result, it is a melatonin-deficient strain of mice. However, in 2003, Slominski et al. [25] found, using HPLC and LC/MS detection techniques, that serotonin has been acetylated to *N*-acetylserotonin in the skin of C57BL/6 mice. They also confirmed the findings of Roseboom et al. [37] by the detection of several alternatively spliced forms of the AANAT that would produce inactive enzyme proteins [25]. However, they have clearly demonstrated transformation of serotonin to NAS in the C57BL/6 mouse skin with a V_{max} of 174 pmol h^{-1} and K_m of 0.56 mM by an enzyme different from the AANAT [20,25]. This was later confirmed by Kobayashi et al., who detected a surprisingly high level of melatonin in the C57BL/6 mice hair follicles [3]. In fact, they found that melatonin levels in

TABLE 3.1
AANAT Activity in Different Human Skin Samples

Tissue	V_{max} (pmol/h)	K_m (mM)
Whole skin	36.64	0.69 ± 0.08
Epidermal melanocytes	40.64	3.96 ± 0.6
Epidermal keratinocytes	44.24	2.71 ± 0.57

Note: For details, see ref. [16].

TABLE 3.2
HIOMT Activity in Different Human Skin Samples

Tissue	HIOMT Activity (pmol/min/mg protein)
White skin	0.179 ± 0.01
Black skin	0.705 ± 0.14
HaCaT keratinocytes	0.825 ± 0.03
SKMEL 188 (melanoma cell line)	3.31 ± 0.15
WM 35 (melanoma cell line)	1.35 ± 0.08

Note: For details, see ref. [16].

the hair follicle are nearly 10 times higher than in the blood serum, giving further evidence of the local production of melatonin in the skin [3].

Thus, in the skin, serotonin can be transformed to NAS by AANAT or an alternative enzyme [16,17,20,25,36]. For example, another enzyme that can acetylate serotonin to *N*-acetylserotonin is the arylamine *N*-acetyltransferase (NAT) [15]. NAT has been discovered in the hamster liver over 25 years ago [38]. Nearly 10 year later, two isozymes of NAT have been found in the hamster skin, of whom only NAT-2 mediates the acetylation of serotonin to NAS [15]. More detailed biochemical analyses on acetylation of serotonin by skin extracts were performed in hamsters and rats using the Cole bisubstrate inhibitor CoA-S-*N*-acetyltryptamine (BSI), an inhibitor of AANAT. These studies demonstrated two enzymatic activates converting serotonin to NAS, one that is sensitive to it (AANAT) and the second one resistant to the inhibitor (apparently NAT) [20,26,36].

The final step of melatonin synthesis is the conversion of NAS to melatonin (*N*-acetyl-5-methoxytryptamine) by the rate-limiting enzyme HIOMT [13]. The HIOMT gene has been expressed in the human skin biopsies and following skin cells in culture: normal epidermal and follicular melanocytes, normal neonatal and adult epidermal and follicular keratinocytes, and follicular and dermal fibroblasts as well as in all melanoma lines and in squamous cell carcinoma [16]. In the human skin, HIOMT enzymatic activity has been found in the skin and in cultured epidermal keratinocytes and malignant melanocytes (melanoma cells) [16]. Interestingly, it has been found that HIOMT activity was the highest in the melanoma cell lines and higher in black than white skin [16] (Table 3.2).

Finally, melatonin was detected by LC/MS in human keratinocytes [16], and it was shown that serotonin can be converted to melatonin in human and hamster melanoma cell lines [17,18]. These have confirmed earlier findings that in normal hamster skin, radioactive serotonin was converted to melatonin by using the HPLC technique [14].

In C57BL/6 mice, the researchers could not detect the HIOMT in corporal skin of these mice; however, it was detected in the ear skin and Cloudman melanoma line, which is of DBA/2J origin [25].

Melatonin synthesis in the pineal gland is regulated in several different ways. The regulatory factors include light, norepinephrine (NE), cAMP, and c-fos [34]. In the skin, melatonin production can be stimulated either by increasing cAMP levels using forskolin [14] or by exogenous NE [3].

3.3 METABOLISM OF MELATONIN

As of 2010, there have been four major melatonin metabolism pathways, of whom three are enzyme-mediated and the other is nonenzymatic. The three enzyme-mediated melatonin metabolic pathways are the classical degeneration pathway, the indolic pathway, and the kynuric pathway. All of these pathways have been detected in human skin (Figure 3.3).

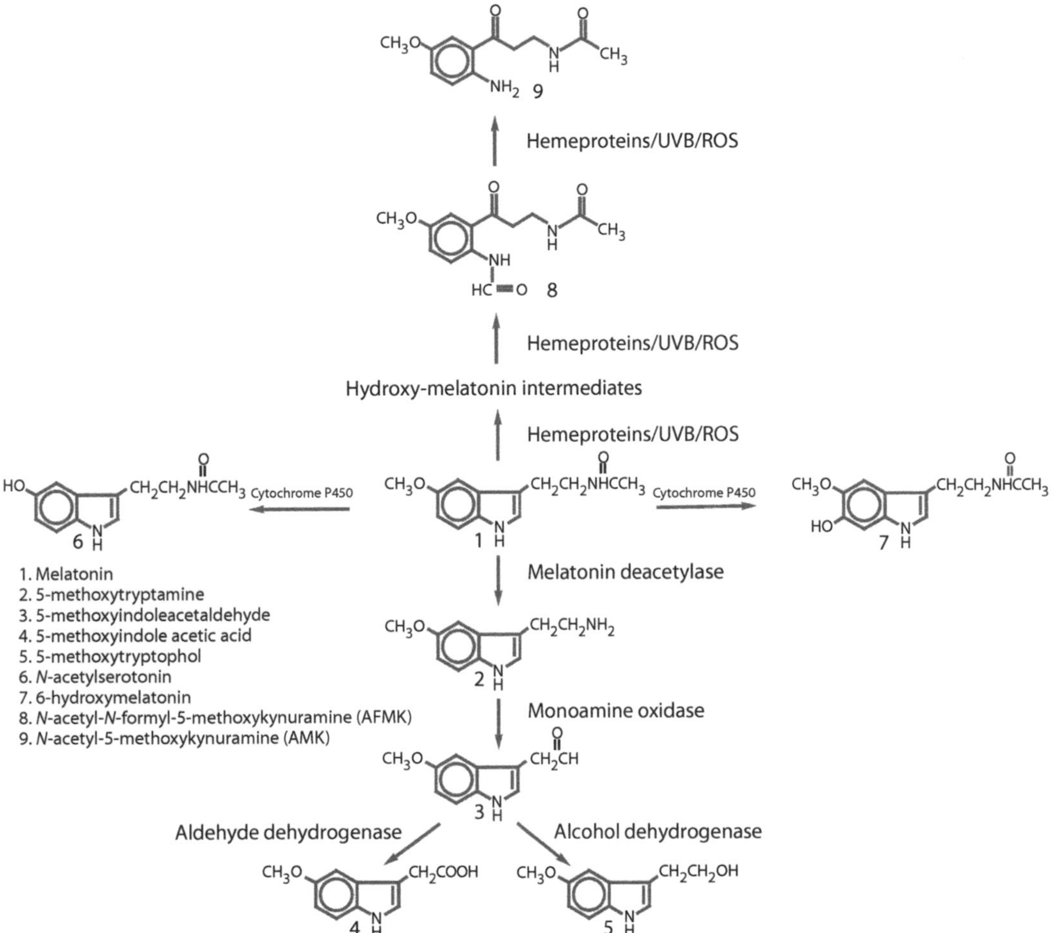

FIGURE 3.3 Metabolism of melatonin. It shows the four possible pathways of melatonin metabolism. These pathways, from top going clockwise, are kynuric, classical, indolic, and classical. The nonenzymatic pathway can also go through the same process as the kynuric pathway.

In the classical pathway, melatonin is metabolized by cytochrome P450 enzymes in the liver to 6-hydroxymelatonin [39]. The specific cytochrome P450 enzymes that metabolize melatonin are CYP1A1, CYP1A2, and CYP1B1 [39]. 6-Hydroxymelatonin is then combined with either a sulfate or glucuronide to make it more polar and is secreted in the urine [40]. Production of 6-hydroxymelatonin has been shown in human keratinocytes [41].

In the indolic pathway, melatonin is metabolized by the enzyme melatonin deacetylase to 5-methoxytryptamine [42]. 5-Methoxytryptamine is then converted to 5-methoxyindoleacetaldehyde by monoamine oxidase. 5-Methoxyindoleacetaldehyde then goes through either one of the two metabolic pathways: it can either by converted to 5-methoxyindole acetic acid (5MIAA) by aldehyde dehydrogenase or it can be metabolized to 5-methoxytryptophol (5MTOL) by alcohol dehydrogenase [43]. The indolic pathway of melatonin degradation has been found in hamster skin by using RP-HPLC and radioactive tracing [14].

The kynuric pathway starts with the metabolism of melatonin by indoleamine 2,3-dioxygenase to produce *N*1-acetyl-*N*2-formyl-5-methoxykynuramine (AFMK) [44]. AFMK is then further degraded by arylamine formamidase to *N*1-acetyl-5-methoxykynuramine (AMK) [44,45]. The

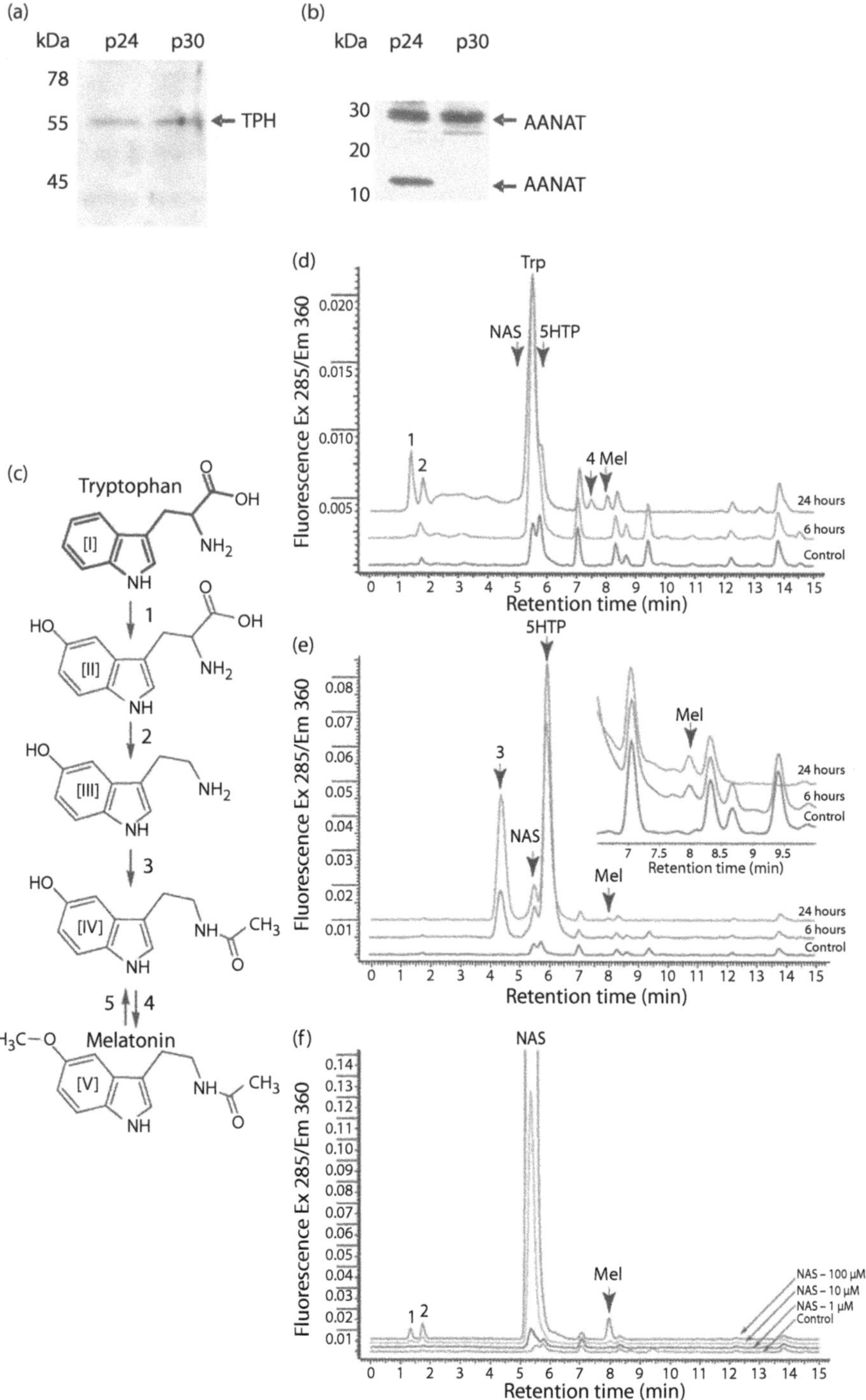

FIGURE 3.4 Evidence of melatonin synthesis in the cultured retinal pigment epithelium cell line. Rate-limiting enzymes (a) TPH and (b) AANAT are present in RPE. (c) Melatonin synthesis pathway. Detection of precursors to melatonin synthesis: (d) tryptophan, (e) serotonin, and (f) NAS. (Reprinted from *Mol Cell Endocrinol*, 307, Smijewski, M.A. et al., 211–216, Copyright 2009, with permission from Elsevier.)

kynuric degradation pathway can also involve the action of different enzymes and pseudoenzymes, including peroxidase, myeloperoxidase, oxoferryl haemoglobin, or free radical species [1]. Fischer et al. [41] have also shown that UV radiation, particularly ultraviolet B, can also promote the kynuric melatonin degradation pathway in the human epidermal keratinocytes.

The first step in the nonenzymatic melatonin degradation pathway in the epidermis starts with melatonin being transformed to AFMK by either ultraviolet B radiation or reactive oxygen species (ROS) [41]. AFMK can also act as a free radical scavenger that plays a key role in protecting the cells from oxidative damage [8]. AFMK mediates its actions on the ROS by donating its electrons, thus acting as a reducing agent [8]. AFMK can even be degraded to AMK by either catalase or ROS [46].

Recently, metabolism of melatonin by cytochrome C in mitochondria was reported by Semak et al. [47]. Melatonin has been found to be converted to *N*1-acetyl-*N*2-formyl-5-methoxykynuramine by cytochrome P450 enzymes in the mitochondria, with the intermediates 2-hydroxymelatonin and 2,3-dihydroxymelatonin being formed before complete reaction [47]. This reaction was shown by using LC/MS [47].

3.4 MELATONIN IN RETINAL PIGMENTAL EPITHELIUM

Melatonin plays numerous roles in the retina. These include regulating dopamine release, acting on the vascular smooth muscle, regulating the GABA transmission release, and modifying the transmission of the light/dark signal from the retina [6,48].

There has been evidence that melatonin can be produced in the retinal pigment epithelium. The first piece of evidence is that the rate-limiting enzymes in melatonin synthesis, TPH, AANAT, and HIOMT, have been found in the retinal pigment epithelium (RPE) cell line. These have been found by using molecular techniques such as RT-PCR and WB analysis [28]. The second piece of evidence that melatonin is locally produced in the RPE is the metabolic transformation of L-tryptophan to serotonin and finally melatonin as shown by HPLC (Figure 3.4) [28]. The functional significance for locally produced melatonin was enhanced by detection of melatonin receptors in the RPE [28]. The membrane receptor MT2, but not MT1, has been detected in the APRE-19 cell type. Both nuclear receptors ROR-α1 and ROR-α4 have also been detected in the same cell line [28].

The clinical implication of melatonin in the RPE are numerous and could include prevention of keratopathies and age-related macular degeneration (AMD), as well as its application in corneal healing and even protecting the retina from UV damage [28].

3.5 CONCLUSION

Both the synthesis and metabolism of melatonin have been shown to occur in the skin. The evidence for this includes finding the rate-limiting enzymes in melatonin synthesis (TPH, AANAT, and HIOMT) and finding melatonin and its precursors localized in the skin. These evidences were found by using molecular biochemical and analytical techniques such as LC/MS, HPLC, radioactive tracing, and immunofluorescence staining.

It is not surprising that melatonin is both synthesized and metabolized in the skin, since melatonin plays numerous roles in this organ, which include acting as a free radical scavenger, protection of fibroblasts and keratinocytes from UV radiation, promotion of hair growth, stimulation or inhibition of keratinocyte proliferation, prevention of premature cell death, and prevention of carcinogenesis [1,3,4,9,49].

Melatonin availability for the above functions can be regulated by precise local synthesis and degradation [1]. Its local synthesis can be stimulated by factors increasing cAMP such as forskolin [14] or by NE [3]. Finally, UV light has been shown to stimulate the melatonin degradation process [41]. The UV effect on serotoninergic and melatoninergic systems still awaits experimental investigation [20].

The clinical implication of discovering melatonin metabolism and synthesis in the skin include its potential as a cancer treatment, treatment for alopecia, skin protection from UV light, and even antiaging and immunomodulatory effects [9,50].

REFERENCES

1. Slominski, A., Tobin, D. J., Zmijewski, M. A., Wortsman, J., and Paus, R. (2008) Melatonin in the skin: Synthesis, metabolism and functions, *Trends Endocrinol Metab* 19, 17–24.
2. Lerner, A. B., Case, J. D., and Takahashi, Y. (1960) Isolation of melatonin and 5-methoxyindole-3-acetic acid from bovine pineal glands, *J Biol Chem* 235, 1992–1997.
3. Kobayashi, H., Kromminga, A., Dunlop, T. W., Tychsen, B., Conrad, F., Suzuki, N., Memezawa, A., Bettermann, A., Aiba, S., Carlberg, C., and Paus, R. (2005) A role of melatonin in neuroectodermal–mesodermal interactions: The hair follicle synthesizes melatonin and expresses functional melatonin receptors, *FASEB J* 19, 1710–1712.
4. Fischer, T. W., Slominski, A., Zmijewski, M. A., Reiter, R. J., and Paus, R. (2008) Melatonin as a major skin protectant: From free radical scavenging to DNA damage repair, *Exp Dermatol* 17, 713–730.
5. Witt-Enderby, P. A., Bennett, J., Jarzynka, M. J., Firestine, S., and Melan, M. A. (2003) Melatonin receptors and their regulation: Biochemical and structural mechanisms, *Life Sci* 72, 2183–2198.
6. Dubocovich, M. L., and Markowska, M. (2005) Functional MT1 and MT2 melatonin receptors in mammals, *Endocrine* 27, 101–110.
7. Becker-Andre, M., Wiesenberg, I., Schaeren-Wiemers, N., Andre, E., Missbach, M., Saurat, J. H., and Carlberg, C. (1994) Pineal gland hormone melatonin binds and activates an orphan of the nuclear receptor superfamily, *J Biol Chem* 269, 28531–28534.
8. Tan, D. X., Manchester, L. C., Burkhardt, S., Sainz, R. M., Mayo, J. C., Kohen, R., Shohami, E., Huo, Y. S., Hardeland, R., and Reiter, R. J. (2001) *N*1-Acetyl-*N*2-formyl-5-methoxykynuramine, a biogenic amine and melatonin metabolite, functions as a potent antioxidant, *FASEB J* 15, 2294–2296.
9. Slominski, A., Fischer, T. W., Zmijewski, M. A., Wortsman, J., Semak, I., Zbytek, B., Slominski, R. M., and Tobin, D. J. (2005) On the role of melatonin in skin physiology and pathology, *Endocrine* 27, 137–148.
10. Mc, I. W., and Page, I. H. (1959) The metabolism of serotonin (5-hydroxytryptamine), *J Biol Chem* 234, 858–864.
11. Lovenberg, W., Weissbach, H., and Udenfriend, S. (1962) Aromatic L-amino acid decarboxylase, *J Biol Chem* 237, 89–93.
12. Lovenberg, W., Jequier, E., and Sjoerdsma, A. (1967) Tryptophan hydroxylation: Measurement in pineal gland, brainstem, and carcinoid tumor, *Science* 155, 217–219.
13. Weissbach, A. (1960) A novel system for the incorporation of amino acids by extracts of *E. coli* B, *Biochim Biophys Acta* 41, 498–509.
14. Slominski, A., Baker, J., Rosano, T. G., Guisti, L. W., Ermak, G., Grande, M., and Gaudet, S. J. (1996) Metabolism of serotonin to *N*-acetylserotonin, melatonin, and 5-methoxytryptamine in hamster skin culture, *J Biol Chem* 271, 12281–12286.
15. Gaudet, S. J., Slominski, A., Etminan, M., Pruski, D., Paus, R., and Namboodiri, M. A. (1993) Identification and characterization of two isozymic forms of arylamine *N*-acetyltransferase in Syrian hamster skin, *J Invest Dermatol* 101, 660–665.
16. Slominski, A., Pisarchik, A., Semak, I., Sweatman, T., Wortsman, J., Szczesniewski, A., Slugocki, G., McNulty, J., Kauser, S., Tobin, D. J., Jing, C., and Johansson, O. (2002) Serotoninergic and melatoninergic systems are fully expressed in human skin, *FASEB J* 16, 896–898.
17. Slominski, A., Pisarchik, A., Semak, I., Sweatman, T., Szczesniewski, A., and Wortsman, J. (2002) Serotoninergic system in hamster skin, *J Invest Dermatol* 119, 934–942.
18. Slominski, A., Semak, I., Pisarchik, A., Sweatman, T., Szczesniewski, A., and Wortsman, J. (2002) Conversion of L-tryptophan to serotonin and melatonin in human melanoma cells, *FEBS Lett* 511, 102–106.
19. Slominski, A., Pisarchik, A., Johansson, O., Jing, C., Semak, I., Slugocki, G., and Wortsman, J. (2003) Tryptophan hydroxylase expression in human skin cells, *Biochim Biophys Acta* 1639, 80–86.
20. Slominski, A., Wortsman, J., and Tobin, D. J. (2005) The cutaneous serotoninergic/melatoninergic system: Securing a place under the sun, *FASEB J* 19, 176–194.
21. Mockus, S. M., and Vrana, K. E. (1998) Advances in the molecular characterization of tryptophan hydroxylase, *J Mol Neurosci* 10, 163–179.

22. Zhang, X., Beaulieu, J. M., Sotnikova, T. D., Gainetdinov, R. R., and Caron, M. G. (2004) Tryptophan hydroxylase-2 controls brain serotonin synthesis, *Science* 305, 217.
23. Schallreuter, K. U., Wood, J. M., Pittelkow, M. R., Gutlich, M., Lemke, K. R., Rodl, W., Swanson, N. N., Hitzemann, K., and Ziegler, I. (1994) Regulation of melanin biosynthesis in the human epidermis by tetrahydrobiopterin, *Science* 263, 1444–1446.
24. Davis, M. D., and Kaufman, S. (1989) Evidence for the formation of the 4a-carbinolamine during the tyrosine-dependent oxidation of tetrahydrobiopterin by rat liver phenylalanine hydroxylase, *J Biol Chem* 264, 8585–8596.
25. Slominski, A., Pisarchik, A., Semak, I., Sweatman, T., and Wortsman, J. (2003) Characterization of the serotoninergic system in the C57BL/6 mouse skin, *Eur J Biochem* 270, 3335–3344.
26. Slominski, A., Pisarchik, A., Zbytek, B., Tobin, D. J., Kauser, S., and Wortsman, J. (2003) Functional activity of serotoninergic and melatoninergic systems expressed in the skin, *J Cell Physiol* 196, 144–153.
27. Nordlind, K., Azmitia, E. C., and Slominski, A. (2008) The skin as a mirror of the soul: Exploring the possible roles of serotonin, *Exp Dermatol* 17, 301–311.
28. Zmijewski, M. A., Sweatman, T. W., and Slominski, A. T. (2009) The melatonin-producing system is fully functional in retinal pigment epithelium (ARPE-19), *Mol Cell Endocrinol* 307, 211–216.
29. Johansson, O., Liu, P. Y., Bondesson, L., Nordlind, K., Olsson, M. J., Lontz, W., Verhofstad, A., Liang, Y., and Gangi, S. (1998) A serotonin-like immunoreactivity is present in human cutaneous melanocytes, *J Invest Dermatol* 111, 1010–1014.
30. Matsuda, M., Imaoka, T., Vomachka, A. J., Gudelsky, G. A., Hou, Z., Mistry, M., Bailey, J. P., Nieport, K. M., Walther, D. J., Bader, M., and Horseman, N. D. (2004) Serotonin regulates mammary gland development via an autocrine–paracrine loop, *Dev Cell* 6, 193–203.
31. Pai, V. P., Marshall, A. M., Hernandez, L. L., Buckley, A. R., and Horseman, N. D. (2009) Altered serotonin physiology in human breast cancers favors paradoxical growth and cell survival, *Breast Cancer Res* 11, R81.
32. Stull, M. A., Pai, V., Vomachka, A. J., Marshall, A. M., Jacob, G. A., and Horseman, N. D. (2007) Mammary gland homeostasis employs serotonergic regulation of epithelial tight junctions, *Proc Natl Acad Sci U S A* 104, 16708–16713.
33. Gillbro, J. M., Marles, L. K., Hibberts, N. A., and Schallreuter, K. U. (2004) Autocrine catecholamine biosynthesis and the beta-adrenoceptor signal promote pigmentation in human epidermal melanocytes, *J Invest Dermatol* 123, 346–353.
34. Reiter, R. J. (1991) Pineal melatonin: Cell biology of its synthesis and of its physiological interactions, *Endocr Rev* 12, 151–180.
35. Knell, A. J., Davidson, A. R., Williams, R., Kantamaneni, B. D., and Curzon, G. (1974) Dopamine and serotonin metabolism in hepatic encephalopathy, *Br Med J* 1, 549–551.
36. Semak, I., Korik, E., Naumova, M., Wortsman, J., and Slominski, A. (2004) Serotonin metabolism in rat skin: Characterization by liquid chromatography–mass spectrometry, *Arch Biochem Biophys* 421, 61–66.
37. Roseboom, P. H., Namboodiri, M. A., Zimonjic, D. B., Popescu, N. C., Rodriguez, I. R., Gastel, J. A., and Klein, D. C. (1998) Natural melatonin 'knockdown' in C57BL/6J mice: Rare mechanism truncates serotonin *N*-acetyltransferase, *Brain Res Mol Brain Res* 63, 189–197.
38. Hein, D. W., Kirlin, W. G., Ferguson, R. J., and Weber, W. W. (1985) Biochemical investigation of the basis for the genetic *N*-acetylation polymorphism in the inbred hamster, *J Pharmacol Exp Ther* 234, 358–364.
39. Ma, X., Idle, J. R., Krausz, K. W., and Gonzalez, F. J. (2005) Metabolism of melatonin by human cytochromes p450, *Drug Metab Dispos* 33, 489–494.
40. Arendt, J. (1988) Melatonin, *Clin Endocrinol (Oxf)* 29, 205–229.
41. Fischer, T. W., Sweatman, T. W., Semak, I., Sayre, R. M., Wortsman, J., and Slominski, A. (2006) Constitutive and UV-induced metabolism of melatonin in keratinocytes and cell-free systems, *FASEB J* 20, 1564–1566.
42. Rogawski, M. A., Roth, R. H., and Aghajanian, G. K. (1979) Melatonin: Deacetylation to 5-methoxytryptamine by liver but not brain aryl acylamidase, *J Neurochem* 32, 1219–1226.
43. Grace, M. S., Cahill, G. M., and Besharse, J. C. (1991) Melatonin deacetylation: Retinal vertebrate class distribution and *Xenopus laevis* tissue distribution, *Brain Res* 559, 56–63.
44. Hirata, F., Hayaishi, O., Tokuyama, T., and Seno, S. (1974) In vitro and in vivo formation of two new metabolites of melatonin, *J Biol Chem* 249, 1311–1313.
45. Hardeland, R., Reiter, R. J., Poeggeler, B., and Tan, D. X. (1993) The significance of the metabolism of the neurohormone melatonin: Antioxidative protection and formation of bioactive substances, *Neurosci Biobehav Rev* 17, 347–357.

46. Tan, D. X., Manchester, L. C., Terron, M. P., Flores, L. J., and Reiter, R. J. (2007) One molecule, many derivatives: A never-ending interaction of melatonin with reactive oxygen and nitrogen species? *J Pineal Res* 42, 28–42.
47. Semak, I., Naumova, M., Korik, E., Terekhovich, V., Wortsman, J., and Slominski, A. (2005) A novel metabolic pathway of melatonin: Oxidation by cytochrome C, *Biochemistry* 44, 9300–9307.
48. Pandi-Perumal, S. R., Trakht, I., Srinivasan, V., Spence, D. W., Maestroni, G. J., Zisapel, N., and Cardinali, D. P. (2008) Physiological effects of melatonin: Role of melatonin receptors and signal transduction pathways, *Prog Neurobiol* 85, 335–353.
49. Fischer, T. W., Slominski, A., Tobin, D. J., and Paus, R. (2008) Melatonin and the hair follicle, *J Pineal Res* 44, 1–15.
50. Fischer, T. W., Burmeister, G., Schmidt, H. W., and Elsner, P. (2004) Melatonin increases anagen hair rate in women with androgenetic alopecia or diffuse alopecia: Results of a pilot randomized controlled trial, *Br J Dermatol* 150, 341–345.

4 Melatonin in Prevention of Mutagenesis, Oxidation, and Other Damage to Cells

Theodore Lialiaris

CONTENTS

4.1 INTRODUCTION

Melatonin is a small amphiphilic indolamine secreted from the pineal gland principally at night. The hormone is involved in sleep regulation as well as in a number of other cyclical bodily activities and circadian rhythm in humans [1]. The concentration of melatonin in the blood of an organism is high at night, as the produced amounts of melatonin are massive during that time and are released into the circulatory system, setting the body ready for slumber. When the night is about to become daytime, blood melatonin levels are reduced.

Melatonin is also produced in other organs and represents, additionally, a normal food constituent found in yeast and plant material, which can influence the level in the circulation. Compared with the pineal tract, the gastrointestinal tract contains several hundred times more melatonin, which can be released into the blood in response to food intake and stimuli by nutrients, especially tryptophan [1].

Synthesis and release of melatonin are stimulated by darkness; thus, melatonin is the "chemical expression of darkness" and inhibited by light. Photic information from the retina is transmitted to the pineal gland through the suprachiasmatic nucleus of the hypothalamus and the sympathetic nervous system [2]. During daylight hours the retinal photoreceptor cells are hyperpolarized and inhibit the release of norepinephrine. With the onset of darkness, the photoreceptors release norepinephrine, thereby activating the system, and a number of a_1- and b_1-adrenergic receptors in the gland increase. The activity of arylalkylamine *N*-acetyltransferase, the enzyme that regulates the rate of melatonin synthesis, is increased, initiating the synthesis and release of melatonin. As the synthesis of melatonin increases, the hormone enters the bloodstream through passive diffusion [1].

Melatonin, or *N*-acetyl-5-methoxytryptamine, is also one of the few maternal hormones that cross the placenta unaltered. Although the fetal pineal gland does not secrete melatonin, the fetus is exposed to melatonin of maternal origin [2].

Melatonin's activity though is not limited to a simple "time index." As seen below, this can expand to various levels such as cell protection, fighting off tumors, and operating as an antioxidant, antimutagenic, anti-inflammatory, and anticancer agent.

4.2 MELATONIN AS A CYTOPROTECTIVE AGENT

4.2.1 Neuroprotective Effect of Melatonin

Spinal cord injury (SCI) can result in severe disability, sensory disorder, paralysis, other neurologic deficits, and even death. Unfortunately, about 250,000 people in the United States suffer from SCI, with almost 11,000 new cases occurring every year. SCI induces numerous cell death cascades, and that is why pharmacotherapy may require either a combination of agents or a single agent with multiple effects. Currently, the only approved treatment for SCI is methylprednisolone, and the efficacy of this therapy has been controversial. A relative scientific search on SCI treatment outlines the use of melatonin as a potential therapy for experimentally induced SCI in rats [3].

The $Ca2^+$-activated neutral protease calpain seems to be involved in the pathogenesis of SCI, and calpain activity has been shown to have great importance in cell injury and tissue destruction after SCI. Although calpain has a role in normal cell functions, overactivation of this protease leads to degradation of cytoskeletal and myelin proteins and also the activation of proapoptotic factors such as Bax, calcineurin, and caspase-3. Overactivation of calpain has been noted in neurons and glial cells exposed to toxins in vitro. Protein degradation after SCI leads to neuronal death and destruction of axons and myelin.

The results indicated that melatonin treatment indeed inhibited inflammation by reducing the activation of astrocytes, microglia, and macrophages. Calpain expression and caspase-3 activation were also significantly reduced, and neuronal death was attenuated after administration of melatonin in acute SCI rats. Furthermore, melatonin treatment was also associated with reduced axonal degeneration in the SCI. These experimental data suggest that melphalan as a single agent or perhaps in combination with other agents may have therapeutic potential for the treatment of SCI [4].

4.3 MELATONIN AS AN ANTIOXIDANT AGENT

4.3.1 Antioxidant Activity

The antioxidant activity of melatonin is ascribed to two different mechanisms:

- Melatonin stimulates radical detoxifying enzymes, such as glutathione peroxidase.
- Melatonin directly scavenges OH^- radicals with an efficacy greater than vitamin E or mannitol [4].

All the mechanisms by which melatonin can be protective of a wide variety of molecules, that is, lipids, proteins, DNA, and so on, and in such widely diverse areas of the cell and different organs are likely not yet identified. Melatonin actions that have been identified include its ability to directly neutralize a number of toxic reactants and stimulate antioxidative enzymes.

Furthermore, several metabolites that are formed when melatonin neutralizes damaging reactants are themselves scavengers, suggesting that there is a cascade of reactions that greatly increase the efficacy of melatonin in stymying oxidative mutilation.

Suggested, but less well defined, processes that may contribute to melatonin's ability to reduce oxidative stress include:

a. Stimulation of glutathione synthesis (an important antioxidant that is at high concentrations within cells),
b. Reduction of electron leakage from the mitochondrial electron transport chain (which would reduce free radical generation),
c. Limiting cytokine production and inflammatory processes (actions that would also lower toxic reactant generation),
d. Synergistic effects with other classic antioxidants (e.g., vitamins C, E, and glutathione) [5].

4.3.2 Melatonin and Oxidative Stress

Oxidative stress plays a key role in the pathogenesis of aging and many metabolic diseases; therefore, an effective antioxidant therapy would be of great importance in these circumstances. Nutritional, environmental, and chemical factors can induce the overproduction of the superoxide anion radical in both the cytosol and mitochondria.

This is the first and key event that leads to the activation of pathways involved in the development of several metabolic diseases that are related to oxidative stress. As oxidation of essential molecules continues, it turns to nitrooxidative stress because of the involvement of nitric oxide in pathogenic processes. Once peroxynitrite forms, it damages via two distinctive mechanisms. First, it has direct toxic effects leading to lipid peroxidation, protein oxidation, and DNA damage. This mechanism involves the induction of several transcription factors leading to cytokine-induced chronic inflammation [6].

Classic antioxidants, including vitamins A, C, and E, have often failed to exhibit beneficial effects in metabolic diseases and aging. Melatonin is a multifunctional indolamine that counteracts virtually all pathophysiological steps and displays significant beneficial actions against peroxynitrite-induced cellular toxicity. This protection is related to melatonin's antioxidative and anti-inflammatory properties. Melatonin has the capability of scavenging both oxygen- and nitrogen-based reactants, including those formed from peroxynitrite, and blocking transcriptional factors, which induce proinflammatory cytokines [6].

Melatonin possesses genomic actions and regulates the expression of several genes, including those for superoxide dismutases and glutathione peroxidase (antioxidant enzymes). Melatonin influences both antioxidant enzyme activity and cellular mRNA levels for these enzymes under physiological conditions and during elevated oxidative stress, possibly through epigenetic mechanisms. The occurrence of these two features in a single molecule is unique for an antioxidant, and both actions protect against pathologically generated free radicals.

4.3.3 An Indolamine-Countering Inflammation

In many inflammatory processes, $ONOO^-$ rather than other reactive molecules is the predominant molecule that determines the fate of cells. Once formed by the coupling of NO and $O_2^{\bullet -}$, $ONOO^-$ cannot be removed or scavenged by vitamins E or C, or by other conventional antioxidants.

As a multifunctional antioxidant, however, melatonin and its metabolites have unique features not shared by the usual antioxidants, including inducible nitric oxide synthase (iNOS) inhibitory and $ONOO^-$ scavenging properties. These features of melatonin, apart from direct antioxidative effects, have been documented in chemical-induced hyperglycemia and other circumstances such as colitis, liver and lung damage, and alkylating-agent toxicity [6].

Melatonin has been shown to ameliorate inflammation by blocking transcriptional factors and tumor necrosis factor α. Evidence confirms that these cytokines induce formation of free radicals and promote iNOS activity and transcriptional factor activation within cells. These events inevitably induce a vicious cycle of cellular damage. It is well documented that NO derived from iNOS during inflammatory processes further potentiates cycloxygenase-2 (COX-2) activity through the NF-κB pathway, thereby exaggerating the inflammatory process. This effect is not unexpected given that $ONOO^-$ directly activates COX-2 as well. Melatonin, on the other hand, inhibits COX-2 and iNOS transcriptional activation.

That being said, melatonin is a nontoxic hormone that might prove an extremely useful treatment because of its ability to block the biohazardous effects of (nitro)oxidative stress and inflammation by itself or in combination with other treatments [6,7].

4.3.4 Effects of Melatonin in Acute Stroke

Stroke (hypoxia/ischemia or ischemia) is the second leading cause of death worldwide. Focal cerebral ischemia is the major form of stroke and is usually caused by thromboembolic occlusion of supplying arteries. In contrast, global ischemia is often caused by cardiac arrest, massive hemorrhage, or carbon monoxide poisoning. In either circumstance, brain damage occurs when cerebral blood flow drops to 25% of its normal value. The longer the duration of occlusion, the greater the damage to the brain; and such impairment is usually irreversible.

The primary therapeutic strategy in treating cerebral ischemia is to restore blood flow so that ischemic tissues can be reperfused (or reoxygenated) in the shortest time possible (ideally within minutes) to preserve neural tissues, which is also in favor of later functional recovery and survival of individuals [8].

The secondary approach is to ameliorate pathophysiological consequences of stroke, including excitotoxicity, apoptosis, inflammation, penumbral depolarization, and diaschisis, caused by free radicals generated during hypoxia/ischemia and reperfusion. For the first strategy, tissue plasminogen activator and other thrombolytic agents are applied. For the second approach, melatonin would be an ideal therapeutic agent since it is a naturally occurring antioxidant, has a known safety profile being virtually nontoxic to humans, and readily crosses the blood-brain barrier when administrated through peripheral routes.

In accordance with the common clinical scenario of stroke, rodent models of focal cerebral ischemia with middle cerebral artery occlusion (MCAO) have been widely studied in the laboratory. Temporary occlusion of MCA is performed for 60–90 minutes, and melatonin is administered either before ischemia or shortly after reperfusion. Several physiological parameters, including pH, pCO_2, pO_2, core temperature, and blood pressure, are monitored during the course of study and are found unchanged upon administration of melatonin. Abundant literature demonstrated that administering melatonin significantly reduces brain infarction, neurological deficits, and a number of outcome measurements, which has been systemically analyzed, and the effect size of melatonin is reported around 0.5 [8].

The protective effects of melatonin in acute stroke (within 2 days from the onset of vessel occlusion) mainly derive from its being a direct and indirect antioxidant and that it promotes mitochondrial functions. Antioxidant actions of melatonin include scavenging of free radicals and increasing activity of antioxidant enzymes as described above. Moreover, melatonin suppresses nitric oxide production by reducing nNOS synthesis in neurons in a calmodulin-dependent pathway and abolishing iNOS expression in macrophages through an NF-κB-mediated mechanism. In addition, melatonin stimulates the activity of NADH-coenzyme Q reductase (Complex I) and cytochrome *c* oxidase (Complex IV) in the electron transport chain of mitochondria and consequently reduces electron leakage and free radical production and maintains normal adenosine triphosphate production. This suggests that administering melatonin in stroke patients could counteract energy shortage to maintain normal cellular function and to decrease brain damage.

The ability of melatonin to reduce oxidative damage caused by ischemia has been reported in other organs, such as heart, liver, and kidney. Moreover, melatonin is capable of reducing cerebral inflammation after stroke. Administering melatonin at the onset of reperfusion decreases microglial/macrophage activation and reduces immune cell infiltration to the ischemic hemisphere without changing the cellular immune response in the blood stream at 2 days post-MCAO. Although such effect could be, at least in part, a result of decreased infarction and other brain damage after melatonin treatment, it has been shown that in an inflammatory rat model of colitis, administering melatonin suppresses the mRNA and protein expression of tumor necrosis factor α and intercellular adhesion molecule-1 in colon tissues. Both membrane and nuclear receptors for melatonin have been identified in peripheral blood mononuclear cells, and melatonin stimulation modulates their differentiation, proliferation, and cytokine production, indicating a direct role of melatonin in controlling immune systems [8].

Melatonin reduces apoptosis after stroke. Administering melatonin before MCAO or at the onset of reperfusion restores the injury-induced reduction in phosphorylated AKT (p-AKT), p-Bad, and Bcl-XL levels and the binding of p-Bad and 14-3-3 as well as decreases caspase-3 activation. Treatment with melatonin also suppresses the immunoreactivity of cytosolic cytochrome *c* oxidase in the ischemic cortex 4 and 24 hours after MCAO.

Cumulatively, in an acute stage of cerebral hypoxia/ischemia, melatonin shows a capacity to reduce brain damage by

1. Reducing oxidative stress,
2. Promoting mitochondrial functions,
3. Decreasing excitotoxicity,
4. Suppressing inflammation, and
5. Diminishing apoptosis [8].

4.4 MELATONIN AS AN ANTITUMOR AGENT

4.4.1 Role of Melatonin in Carcinogenesis

Melatonin has well-established oncostatic properties in experimental in vitro and in vivo models that can be studied in their own right as a potential mediator in disease development or through administration of synthetic melatonin as an adjuvant therapy for light- or melatonin-associated diseases. In addition to melatonin's direct oncostatic properties, the endogenous melatonin signal may thwart cancer development and growth via indirect mechanisms involving its ability to enhance immune activity and mitigate against stress-induced immune suppression [9,10].

Moreover, melatonin has been shown to prevent iron-induced lipid peroxidation. Thus, melatonin may also prevent carcinogenesis. Additionally, once oncogenesis has occurred, melatonin seems to control cancer growth by means other than its antioxidant activity.

Melatonin might inhibit the uptake and metabolism of fatty acid signaling molecules that promote the production of tumoral growth factors, reduce telomerase activity by shortening telomer length, and modulate expression of tumor suppressor genes such as P53. More recent studies report that melatonin significantly suppresses endothelin-1-converting enzyme activity. Endothelin-1 is a potent vasoconstrictor peptide that is involved in angiogenesis and cancer growth. This peptide is usually elevated in the plasma of a patient with various solid tumors and acts to protect cancer cells from apoptosis and promote endothelial and smooth muscle proliferation. Finally, the antiestrogenic activity of melatonin also seems to play a role in its ability to decrease proliferation in some hormone-responsive tumors [9,10].

4.4.2 Importance of Melatonin in Breast Cancer

Manipulation of melatonin levels has been found to affect development of several different cancer types in animals including breast cancer, prostate cancer, and melanoma. In particular, melatonin injection has been reported to inhibit chemically induced mammary tumor development in rats, and pinealectomy enhances it in both the 7,12-dimethylbenz(α)anthracene model [11] and the N-nitroso-*N*-methylurea model [12]. There are several mechanistic interpretations of these observations.

Two of these interpretations—that melatonin may slow development and turnover of the normal mammary cells at risk of malignant transformation and that melatonin may be directly oncostatic—act at opposite ends of the carcinogenic process.

For epidemiological studies, the oncostatic capability of melatonin is far more tractable because recent exposures that lower melatonin level would be relevant; if melatonin slows the development of normal cells that are at risk, exposures in the past would be relevant and correspondingly much more difficult to estimate.

Nighttime plasma melatonin levels have been reported to be lower in women with estrogen receptor–positive breast cancer than in those with estrogen receptor–negative breast cancer and in healthy control women, and lower in cases of primary breast cancer than in women with benign breast disease. In contrast, daytime melatonin was found to be higher in breast cancer patients in one report.

It is difficult to assess the meaning of these findings because of the presence of disease and its possible effect on melatonin levels. It is difficult to determine whether low nocturnal melatonin predisposes to increased risk of breast cancer in women. Clarifying the role of melatonin in normal and malignant growth of breast tissue may provide a better understanding of the roles of estrogen and prolactin in the etiology of breast cancer [13].

4.5 MELATONIN AS AN ANTIMUTAGENIC AGENT

4.5.1 Melatonin versus Mitomycin C

Mitomycin C (MMC) is a quinone-containing antibiotic originally isolated from *Streptomyces caespitosus* in 1958. MMC has been used to treat a wide variety of solid tumors but is also able of generating free radicals when metabolized. According to a scientific research on the effect of melatonin against MMC-induced genotoxicity in polychromatic erythrocytes, melatonin is able of countering the damaging side effects caused by MMC. More specifically, rats (n = 36) were classified into four groups: control, melatonin, MMC, and MMC + melatonin. The number of micronucleated polychromatic erythrocytes (PCE) per 1000 PCE was used as a genotoxic marker. The MMC group showed a significant increase in micronucleated PCE at 24, 48, 72, and 96 hours that was significantly reduced with coadministration of melatonin. The final results of that research indicate that MMC-induced genotoxicity can be reduced by melatonin [10].

4.5.2 Melatonin versus Carbamazepine

The mutagenic potential of carbamazepine (CBZ) therapy has been evaluated both in vivo and in vitro. Based on this, a research program was established to confirm a potential countering effect of melatonin against carbamazepine. Analysis of chromosome aberrations (CA), sister chromatid exchanges (SCEs), mitotic and proliferation indices (MI, PRI) were performed. The in vivo study was carried out on 30 patients with idiopathic epilepsy undergoing treatment with CBZ for different periods starting from 6 months to 15 years. Plasma CBZ levels were also determined for each patient. The results showed that the total CA and SCEs were significantly increased in CBZ-treated patients. There was no significant correlation between CA and either the duration of treatment or the plasma CBZ levels for each patient. The mitotic and proliferation indices were found to be slightly but nonsignificantly decreased compared to control values.

Pretreatment of human lymphocytes with melatonin (0.5 mM) exhibited a significant decrease in the frequencies of CBZ-induced CA and SCEs as compared with nontreated cultures. The depressed mitotic and proliferation indices were also found to be improved in cultures pretreated with melatonin.

In conclusion, these observations suggest that CBZ monotherapy may lead to chromosome damaging effects (genotoxic), and the use of melatonin as an antimutagenic agent for human protection against CBZ-induced chromosome damage should be considered [14].

4.5.3 Melatonin versus Melphalan

Melphalan (MEL), a bis(chloroethyl)amine with potent alkylating properties, is one of the most clinically useful nitrogen mustards used in the treatment of multiple myeloma, breast cancer, non-Hodgkin's lymphoma, testicular seminoma, osteogenic sarcoma, and nonresectable advanced ovarian cancer [15].

Melatonin's antigenotoxic effect was tested against MEL, which encompasses a number of side effects since it is also highly mutagenic and clastogenic and the SCE cytogenetic method was used to determine the antimutagenic properties of this agent. The capability of melatonin to modulate the repair of oxidative and nitrosative lesions, considered as a major side effect of various anticancer drugs and nitrogen mustards specifically, was examined. Melatonin was found to act as an antioxidant-radical scavenger by suppressing MEL-induced genotoxic damage. According to these findings, melatonin alone in concentrations less than 750 μM did not increase the levels of SCEs/cell in human lymphocytes cultures. On the other hand, MEL alone elicited a significant increase in the levels of SCEs/cell, but the combined treatments of melatonin and MEL lead to a remarkably significant reduction of the SCEs levels in cultured human lymphocytes. The protection that melatonin provides to cells is probably due to its capacity to enter the nucleus and interact with chromatin. It interacts with double-stranded DNA and possibly stabilizes it, whereas MEL as an alkylating agent causes distortion of the helix. Since SCEs represent double-strand breaks, melatonin reduces the damaging effect of MEL on lymphocytes [15]. About 1000 research studies (50% of which were performed in vivo) document that melatonin reduces free radical damage. Many researchers believe that melatonin is a potent genoprotector, anticarcinogen, and antitumor compound. It has been suggested that it may play an important role in defending cells from DNA damage induced not only by oxidative mutagens but also by different alkylating agents. It was suggested that it may prove useful in reducing some of the toxic effects associated with certain classes of chemotherapeutic agents. It is a molecule with an intense past, significant present, and hopeful future [15].

4.6 CONCLUSIONS

Melatonin is a hormone responsible for regulating the time of sleep. Its levels in the blood can increase and decrease in virtue of whether it is night or day. This allows us to sleep and wake up, which under regular circumstances occur in the absence and the presence of light correspondingly.

However, melatonin has a number of different activities that makes it a multifunctional agent of great importance. In keeping with several research projects on that matter, it is safe to assert that this indolamine can scavenge free radicals, and fight oxidative stress and inflammation, where other antioxidants seem to fail, counter tumors successfully, and abridge chromosome aberrations while acting as an antimutagenic agent. Finally, melatonin can protect cells and molecules against different kinds of damage.

REFERENCES

1. Grivas Th, Savvidou O. Melatonin the "light of night" in human biology and adolescent idiopathic scoliosis. *Scoliosis*. 2007; 2:6, doi:10.1186/1748-7161-2-6.
2. Torres-Farfan C, Valenzuela FJ, Mondaca M, Valenzuela GJ, Krause B, Herrera EA, Riquelme R, Llanos AJ, Seron-Ferre M. Evidence of a role for melatonin in fetal sheep physiology: direct actions of melatonin on fetal cerebral artery, brown adipose tissue and adrenal gland. *J Physiol*. 2008; 586(16): 4017–4027.
3. Samantaray S, Sribnick EA, Das A, Knaryan VH, Matzelle DD, Yallapragada AV, Reiter RJ, Ray SK, Banik NL. Melatonin attenuates calpain upregulation, axonal damage and neuronal death in spinal cord injury in rats. *J Pineal Res*. 2008 May; 44(4): 348–357. doi:10.1111/j.1600-079X.2007.00534.x.
4. De Salvia R, Fiore M, Aglitti T, Festa F, Ricordy R, Cozzi R. Inhibitory action of melatonin on H2O2- and cyclophosphamide-induced DNA damage. *Mutagenesis*. 1999; 14(1): 107–112.
5. Reiter RJ, Tan D-X, Gitto E, Sainz RM, Mayo JC, Leon J, Manchester LC, Vijayalaxmi, Kilic E, Kilic Ü. Pharmacological utility of melatonin in reducing oxidative cellular and molecular damage. *Pol J Pharmacol*. 2004; 56: 159–170, ISSN 1230-6002.
6. Korkmaz A, Reiter RJ, Topal T, Manchester LC, Oter S, Tan D-X. Melatonin: an established antioxidant worthy of use in clinical trials. *Mol Med*. 2009; 15(1–2): 43–50.
7. Stevens RG, Blask DE, Brainard GC., Hansen J, Lockley SW, Provencio I, Rea MS, Reinlib L. Meeting report: the role of environmental lighting and circadian disruption in cancer and other diseases. *Environ Health Perspect*. 2007; 115(9): 1357–1362.
8. Lin H-Wen, Lee E-J. Effects of melatonin in experimental stroke models in acute, sub-acute, and chronic stages. *Neuropsychiatr Dis Treat*. 2009; 5: 157–162.
9. Hardeland R, Pandi-Perumal SR. Melatonin, a potent agent in antioxidative defense: actions as a natural food constituent, gastrointestinal factor, drug and prodrug. *Nutr Metab* (*Lond*). 2005; 2: 22, doi:10.1186/1743-7075-2-22.
10. Ortega-Gutiérrez S, López-Vicente M, Lostalé F, Fuentes-Broto L, Martínez-Ballarín E, García JJ. Protective effect of melatonin against mitomycin C–induced genotoxic damage in peripheral blood of rats. *J Biomedicine Biotech*. 2009; 2009: 791432, doi:10.1155/2009/791432.
11. Tamarkin L, Cohen M, Roselle D, Reichert C, Lippman M, Chabner B. Melatonin inhibition and pinealectomy enhancement of 7,12-dimethylbenz(a)anthracene-induced mammary tumors in the rat. *Cancer Res*. 1981; 41: 4432–4436.
12. Blask DE, Pelletier DB, Hill SM, Lemus-Wilson A, Grosso DS, Wilson ST, Wise ME. Pineal melatonin inhibition of tumor promotion in the *N*-nitroso-*N*-methylurea model of mammary carcinogenesis: potential involvement of antiestrogenic mechanisms in vivo. J Cancer Res Clin Oncol. 1991; 117: 526–532.
13. Stevens RG, Davis S. The melatonin hypothesis: electric power and breast cancer. *Environ Health Perspect*. 1996; 104(Suppl 1): 135–150.
14. Awara WM, El-Gohary M, El-Nabi SH, Fadel WA. In vivo and in vitro evaluation of the mutagenic potential of carbamazepine: does melatonin have anti-mutagenic activity? *Toxicology*. 1998; 125: 45–52.
15. Lialiaris T, Lyratzopoulos E, Papachristou F, Simopoulou M, Mourelatos C, Nikolettos N. Supplementation of melatonin protects human lymphocytes in vitro from the genotoxic activity of melphalan. *Mutagenesis*. 2008; 23: 347–354.

5 Cardiovascular Protection by Melatonin

Rita Rezzani

CONTENTS

5.1 INTRODUCTION

The pineal gland is the major source of circulating melatonin in all mammalian species, including humans.[1] Secondary sources of melatonin production are the retina, gut, skin, platelets, bone marrow, and different fluids related to reproduction.[2]

Information about the pineal gland or epiphysis cerebri, in reference to its position to the top of the brain in animals mainly, has been known for more than 2000 years. Galen of Pergamon (130–200 AD) appears to have provided the first description of the pineal's location in the human brain, characterizing it as a gland (analogous to lymph glands), and naming it *konareion* (*conarium* in Latin) for its pinecone shape.[3] The organ was subsequently named *glandula pinealis*, hence *pineal*. The central location and singularity of the pineal as an unpaired organ, as well as its extensive vascularization, described by Andreas Vesalius Bruxellensis (1515–1564), are probably the foundation of René Descartes' (1596–1650) conceptualization of the pineal as the "seat of the soul," or as the organ coordinating psychophysiological functions.[4] In this regard, he said: "The reason which persuades me that the soul can have no other place in the whole body but this kernel where she immediately exercises for functions is for that I see: all the other parts of our brain are paired, as also we have two eyes two hands, two ears; lastly, all the organs of our exterior senses are double and forasmuch as we have but one very thing at one and the same time."

Ahlborn (1884) was the first to notice the remarkable resemblance between the pineal/parietal organ (now the "third eye") of some lower vertebrates and the structure of the lateral eyes. This was the crucial observation leading to extensive interest in the evolutionary history of the pineal in this century and to the statement[5] that the photosensory organ of lower vertebrates became the secretory mammalian pineal. Further progress did not occur until the biochemical isolation of melatonin from pineal extracts[6] and the determination of its structure.[7] One of the major advances in pineal researches occurred when it was demonstrated that the pineal gland participates in the regulation of diurnal rhythms.[8] Diurnal activity of the pineal gland itself is mediated by sympathetic nervous system response to light entering through the eyes.[9,10] The synthesis and release of pineal melatonin exhibit a circadian rhythm resulting in low plasma melatonin concentrations at night (dark phase). Seasonal change of melatonin concentration in the pineal gland and plasma is associated with the natural light/dark cycle.[11]

Although it has been recognized that the pineal gland plays an important role in reproductive biology in different species,[12] only recently has it become apparent that melatonin plays a role in regulation of physiological systems,[13,14] including the cardiovascular system.[15–18]

Regarding its different and powerful functions, the main goal of this chapter is to focus on cardiovascular regulatory effects of melatonin in normal and pathological conditions defining the multifactorial nature of the cardiovascular diseases (CVDs). Moreover, the present chapter, before evaluating the potential melatonin–cardiovascular system interactions, will deal with molecular and biochemical mechanisms of melatonin actions.

5.2 MELATONIN METABOLISM

5.2.1 Biosynthesis

Melatonin is synthesized from tryptophan via 5-hydroxylation by tryptophan-5-hydroxylase to 5-hydroxytryptophan, decarboxylation by aromatic amino acid decarboxylase to 5-hydroxytryptamine (serotonin), N-acetylation by *N*-acetyltransferase to *N*-acetylserotonin (NAT), and O-methylation by hydroxyindole-*O*-methyltransferase (to melatonin (*N*-acetyl-5-methoxytryptamine) (Figure 5.1). The cardinal feature of this synthetic pathway is its rhythmicity. The activity of the enzyme NAT in particular increases from 30- to 70-fold at night and, in most circumstances, is rate-limiting in melatonin synthesis.[19] The synthesis of melatonin is initiated by the binding of norepinephrine to adrenergic β1 receptors, subsequent activation of pineal adenylate cyclase, increase in cyclic AMP (cAMP), binding, and de novo synthesis of NAT or of its activator. The potent cAMP-induced gene transcription repressor (ICER) is activated in conjunction with NAT and represents a mechanism that limits the nocturnal production of melatonin.[20] The β1 adrenergic receptor stimulus is enhanced by α1-adrenoceptors, via calcium (Ca_{2+})-phospholipid-dependent protein kinase C (PKC) and by prostaglandins, whose synthesis is activated by the influx of Ca_{2+} into the pinealocyte that follows α1-adrenergic action.[21] Additional stimuli to melatonin synthesis derive from vasoactive intestinal peptide-ergic neurons that reach the pineal gland through the pineal stalk[22] by opioids that bind to σ receptors[23] and by pituitary adenylate cyclase–activating polypeptide.[24] By contrast, γ-aminobutyric acid, dopamine, glutamate, and delta-sleep-inducing peptide seem to inhibit melatonin production.[21] As in animals, in humans, melatonin synthesis also depends on tryptophan availability and is reduced by acute tryptophan depletion. Evidence indicated that, also in humans, the adrenergic stimulus is important for melatonin secretion. β1-adrenergic "blockers suppress the nocturnal secretion of melatonin, with an effect that seems to be inversely related to nocturnal levels of the hormone.[25] Similarly, a reduction of nocturnal melatonin secretion can be obtained with the administration of either clonidine, which reduces the endogenous adrenergic tonus,[26] or *α*-methyl-

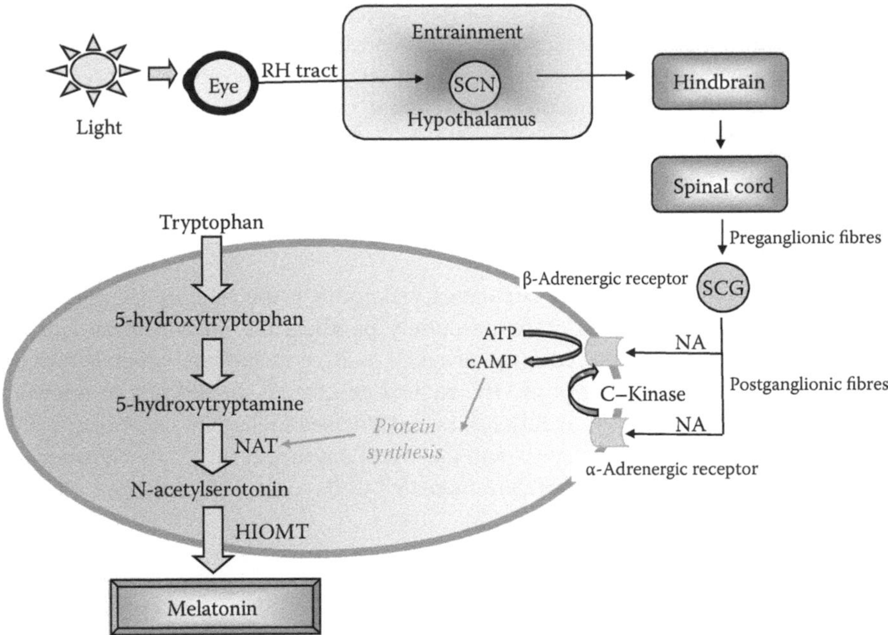

FIGURE 5.1 Mechanisms of melatonin synthesis. The rhythm is generated in the SCN, stimulated by light via the retino-hypothalamic pathway (RH tract). The signal passes across to hindbrain, spinal cord, superior cervical ganglion (SCG) arriving to pineal noradrenergic (NA) receptors. Serotonin *N*-acetyltransferase (NAT) increases 30- to 70-fold during the dark phase through noradrenergic stimulation. HIOMT, hydroxyindole-*O*-methyltransferase. (Modified from Arendt, J., *Rev. Reprod.* 1998;3:13–22.)

para-tyrosine, which reduces presynaptic catecholamine synthesis.[27] Conversely, melatonin secretion is increased by the administration of drugs capable of augmenting catecholamine availability, such as monoamine oxidase inhibitors or tricyclic antidepressants.[28] The importance of intracellular calcium is supported, although not conclusively, by the capability of dihydropyridine calcium antagonists to markedly reduce nocturnal melatonin levels in baboons,[29] whereas the stimulatory effect of prostaglandins is apparent from the decrease in melatonin production that follows the administration of prostaglandin inhibitors.[30] Opiate administration enhances melatonin production, but opioid receptor blocking agents, such as naloxone or naltrexone, do not reduce melatonin levels.[31] Activation of γ-aminobutyric acid receptors by benzodiazepines reduces melatonin at night,[32] whereas manipulation of dopaminergic receptors, with either agonists[33] or antagonists,[20,31] is not capable of markedly modifying melatonin levels.

5.2.2 Secretion

Melatonin displays high lipid and water solubility, which facilitates passage across cell membranes.[2] After release in the circulation, it is present in several fluids, tissues, and cellular compartments (saliva, urine, cerebrospinal fluid, preovulatory follicle, seminal fluid, amniotic fluid, and milk). As no pineal storage of melatonin is available, the plasma hormone profile faithfully reflects the pineal activity.[13] The secretion occurs at night, with maximum plasma levels around 0300–0400 h, varying with chronotype, whereas diurnal levels are undetectable or low in rested subjects. This nycthohemeral rhythm displays the most marked amplitude observed for a hormone, more marked than that of cortisol.[34] Nocturnal melatonin production rates, as estimated by deconvolution analysis applied to plasma melatonin concentration time series, are between 10 and 80 μg per night, the lowest values for a hormone secretion.[35]

The plasma melatonin profile displays a great intersubject heterogeneity. Nonetheless, it is very reproducible from day to day in a same subject and represents one of the most robust circadian rhythms. It provides a good evaluation of the melatonin secretion in the absence of renal or hepatic abnormality.[36] In some subjects, the nocturnal secretion is extremely low or even absent. The consequences of a low melatonin secretion on vulnerability to rhythmic organization and morbidity are again under evaluation.

5.2.3 Catabolism

The liver, which clears more than 90% of circulating melatonin, is the primary site for metabolism. Urine 6-sulfatoxymelatonin (aMT6S) excretion closely parallels the plasma melatonin profile.[37] About 1% melatonin remains unchanged in the urine. 3-Hydroxymelatonin, which is also detected in urine, could represent as a biomarker of OH^- radical generation. In addition to a lower pineal secretory activity, patients with liver cirrhosis show a decreased melatonin clearance, with consequent delayed rise of plasma melatonin peak and increased daytime levels of this hormone.[38] Also, in patients with chronic renal failure, there are increases of daytime melatonin and aMT6S levels and blunted melatonin rhythmicity.[39]

5.2.4 Mechanism of Action

Four mechanisms of melatonin's action in mammalian species have been described so far.[40] These include:

1. Binding to intracellular proteins such as calmodulin;
2. Antioxidative effects;
3. Binding to nuclear receptors of the orphan family;
4. Binding to plasma membrane localized melatonin receptors.

A few reports showed that melatonin can interact with calmodulin, an intracellular protein that is involved in second messenger signal transduction. The antioxidative and beneficial effects of melatonin have been extensively presented in various pathological conditions associated with free radicals and related reactants, such as ischemia/reperfusion (I/R), inflammation, ionizing radiation, and mitochondrial toxins. Melatonin appears to be a natural ligand for the retinoid-related orphan nuclear hormone receptor family (RZR/ROR). However, after identification of this nuclear binding site about 10 years ago, the research has declined and has only continued in recent years.

Melatonin has a variety of means by which it influences the physiology of the organism; some of these actions are receptor-mediated, whereas others are receptor-independent. Besides its classic endocrine effects, melatonin has autocrine and paracrine actions. It has a receptor indirect antioxidant function, whereas has a receptor direct scavenging effect.[41]

To date, three mammalian melatonin receptors have been described: MT1, MT2, and MT3. MT1 and MT2 are G-protein-coupled receptors, and their activations modulate a wide range of intracellular messengers, for example, cAMP, cyclic guanosine monophosphate (cGMP), or $[Ca_{2+}]_i$. Moreover, in mammals, both MT1 and MT2 receptor subtypes are expressed in a wide variety of tissues.[42] The MT3-binding site has been identified as quinone reductase protein, and its physiological significance remains to be clarified.

The cloning of melatonin receptor cDNA resulted in the development of cell lines in which MT1 or MT2 recombinant receptors were expressed. When the human melatonin receptors (hMT1 and hMT2) were cloned and expressed in a variety of cells, they were found to inhibit forskolin-stimulated cAMP. Activation of recombinant hMT1 receptors induces a variety of cellular responses that are mediated by both pertussis (PTX)-sensitive and PTX-insensitive G proteins. The recombinant hMT2 receptor is also coupled to inhibition of adenylyl cyclase activity via a PTX-sensitive

G protein. The significant pharmacology of the membrane melatonin receptors is under intense investigation.[41]

5.3 THE REGULATING SYSTEM OF THE MELATONIN SECRETION

The melatonin rhythm is generated by an endogenous clock located in the suprachiasmatic nucleus (SCN) of the hypothalamus, like other circadian rhythms in mammals (drinking and feeding, sleep/wake cycle, temperature, cortisol or corticosterone, etc.). Results have been reported in animals, mainly in rodents and monkeys, and extended to humans.[43]

The light/dark cycle is the main *zeitgeber* of the regulating system of melatonin secretion. The melatonin rhythm is entrained to the dark period. The photic information is transmitted to the central pacemaker via retino-hypothalamic fibers: during the day, in the presence of light, the output from the retino-hypothalamic tract inhibits melatonin synthesis. Light at night has two major physiological actions, that is, it disrupts circadian rhythms and suppresses the production of melatonin by the pineal gland.[10] In addition, after exposure to light for several consecutive nights, the melatonin secretion escapes the inhibitory effect and progressively shifts (phase delay) to the morning. Full-spectrum bright light is routinely used, but the most effective wavelengths are in the range of 446–477 nm (blue). Because the action spectrum derived from irradiance response curves does not correspond to either scotopic or photopic action spectra, possible new photoreceptors have been hypothesized.[44]

Recently, retinal ganglion cells innervating the SCN were shown to intrinsically respond to light. These melanopsin-containing cells are candidate photoreceptors for the photic entrainment of circadian rhythms because the sensitivity and slow kinctics of the light response are compatible with those of the photic entrainment mechanism.[45] Furthermore, this system appears to send photic information not only to the endogenous clock in the SCN but also to other brain areas involved in irradiance detection, such as light-activated pupil response.

The suppression of melatonin by exposure to low-frequency electromagnetic fields has been considered as a possible mechanism through which exposure to these fields may result in an increased incidence of cancer.[46]

The neural pathway from the SCN to the pineal gland passes first through the upper part of the cervical spinal cord, where synaptic connections are made with preganglionic cell bodies of the superior cervical ganglia of the sympathetic chains (Figure 5.2). Then, neural cells in the superior cervical ganglia send projections to the pineal gland.[47]

5.4 FUNCTIONS OF MELATONIN

Melatonin directly scavenges the highly toxic hydroxyl radical and other oxygen-centered radicals. Also, melatonin displays antioxidative properties: it increases the levels of several antioxidative enzymes including superoxide dismutase, glutathione peroxidase (GPx), and glutathione reductase.[15,48] Evidence exists supporting the idea that oxidative stress is a significant component of specific brain diseases, and melatonin has a clinical potential for the treatment of neurodegenerative disorders in the central as well as in the peripheral nervous system.[49] It is well documented that melatonin and its metabolites have both direct scavenging actions against free radicals and related products[50] as well as indirect antioxidative actions via its ability to stimulate antioxidant enzymes, to inhibit the prooxidative enzyme nitric oxide synthase (NOS),[51] to promote the synthesis of another important intracellular antioxidant, glutathione (GSH),[52] and to diminish free radical formation at the mitochondrial level by reducing the leakage of electrons from the electron transport chain.[53] In addition, melatonin synergizes with other antioxidants to protect against oxidative stress. This combination of actions makes melatonin an important agent in combating some signs of aging and/or the initiation of age-related diseases.[50] In chronic hemodialysis patients, the oxidative stress induced by iron and erythropoietin given for treatment of anemia was prevented by

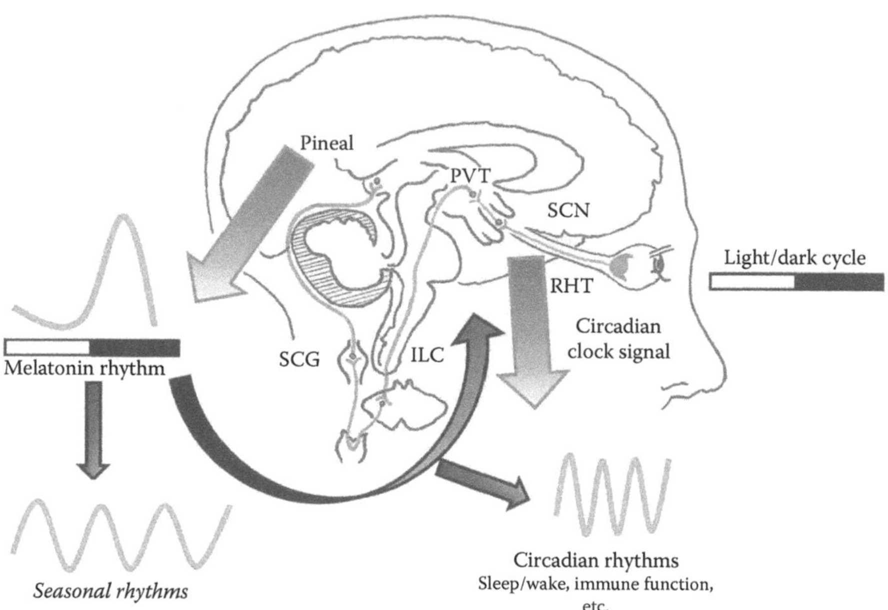

FIGURE 5.2 Control of melatonin secretion. Photic information is conveyed to the SCN. Neuronal efferent pathways from the SCN directly distribute circadian information to different brain areas, including the pineal gland, that generates the melatonin rhythm. The neural route for environmental lighting control of melatonin secretion, after relay in the paraventricular nuclei (PVT), includes the intermediolateral column of the thoracic chord grey (ILC) and the superior cervical ganglion (SCG). The generated melatonin rhythm might be used by the SCN to distribute its rhythmic information. Melatonin can feed back at the level of the SCN, as well as the retina itself. (Modified from *Physiol. Rev*, 9, 11, 2005. American Physiological Society.)

oral administration of melatonin (0.3 mg/kg).[54] Preliminary results in septic newborns showed that high melatonin doses (20 mg per subject) significantly reduced serum levels of lipid peroxidation products and inflammation markers and increased the survival rate and improved the clinical outcome of patients.[55] Similarly, increased blood levels of malondialdehyde (MDA) and nitrite/nitrate observed in asphyxiated newborns were reduced by melatonin treatment (a total dose of 80 mg per infant). Three of the 10 asphyxiated newborns not given melatonin died within 72 hours after birth, whereas none of the 10 who received melatonin died.[56] It has been also demonstrated that melatonin inhibits tumor growth in a variety of clinical situations and prevents the side effects of cancer chemotherapy.[57,58] In particular, melatonin, via activation of its MT1 receptor, suppresses the development and growth of breast cancer by regulation of growth factors, regulation of gene expression, regulation of clock genes, inhibition of tumor cell invasion and metastasis, and even regulation of mammary gland development.[59]

Figure 5.3 summarizes the multiple actions of melatonin above reported.

5.5 MELATONIN AND LIFE

Maternal melatonin, which crosses the placenta, is one of the maternal rhythmic signals capable of synchronizing the fetal biological clock. The pronounced daily melatonin rhythm in the milk could take over in the newborn. After maturation, rhythmic melatonin production reaches the highest levels at the age of 3–6 years. Then, the nocturnal peak drops progressively by 80% until adult levels are reached. This alteration is temporally linked with the appearance of sexual maturity and is not simply the consequence of both increasing body size and constant melatonin production due

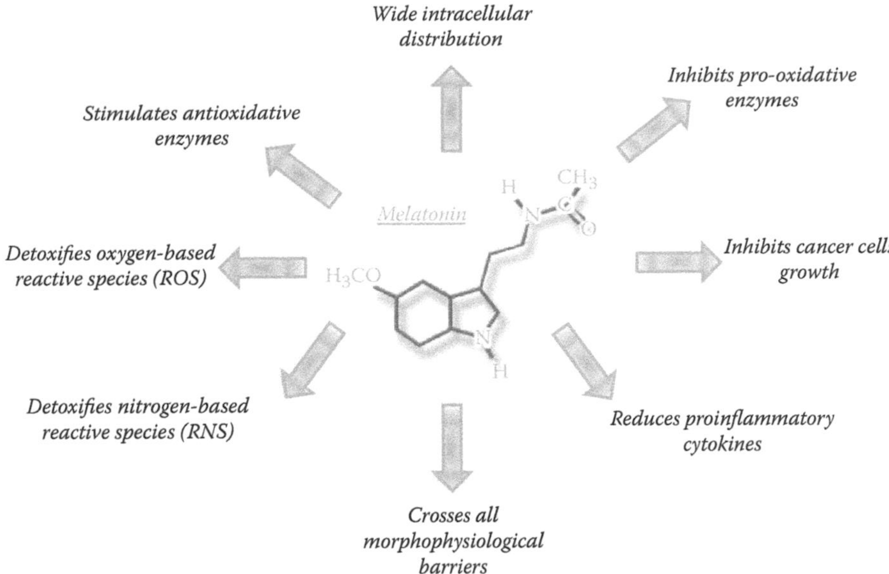

FIGURE 5.3 Some of the actions of melatonin that contribute to its ability to limit tissue damage that is a consequence of injury in the brain as well as in other tissue. Besides scavenging both oxygen- and nitrogen-based reactants, melatonin stimulates (or preserves) the activities of a variety of antioxidant enzymes, such as superoxide dismutase, glutathione peroxidase, glutathione reductase, and catalase. (Modified from Reiter, R.J., et al., *Exp. Biol. Med.* 2005;230:104–17. © Society for Experimental Biology and Medicine.)

to lack of pineal growth during childhood. Data concerning normal precocious puberty treated by gonadotropin-releasing hormone analog suggest that the reduction of melatonin with normal puberty is not likely to be dependent on pubertal gonadotropin or sex steroid influence.[60] During the ovarian cycle, although melatonin may modulate steroidogenesis, especially progesterone production, no clear consensus has emerged as to the melatonin changes that may occur; no preovulatory decrease of melatonin is observed, which could facilitate the ovulation.[61] The transient elevated melatonin secretion during menopause could be related to the dramatic decrease of the estrogen environment.[62] Rather, with aging, the melatonin rhythm progressively dampens, with a tendency to the phase advance, and can be completely abolished in advanced age.[63] The discovery of melatonin and its derivatives as antioxidants has stimulated a large number of studies that have, virtually uniformly, documented the ability of these molecules to detoxify harmful reactants and reduce molecular damage. These observations have clear clinical implications given that numerous age-related diseases in humans have an important free radical component. Moreover, a major theory to explain the processes of aging considers radicals and their derivatives as causative agents. These conditions, coupled with the loss of melatonin as organisms age, suggest that some diseases and some aspects of aging may be aggravated by the diminished melatonin levels in advanced age. Another corollary of this is that the administration of melatonin, which has an uncommonly low toxicity profile, could theoretically defer the progression of some diseases and possibly forestall signs of aging. It is important to remember that increasing life span will not necessarily be a goal of these studies, but improving health and the quality of life in the aged is an aim of all researchers.[1]

5.6 PHYSIOLOGICAL EFFECTS OF MELATONIN IN CARDIOVASCULAR SYSTEM

The evidence from the last 15 years documents that melatonin influences the cardiovascular system,[64,65] but the effects of melatonin on this system are still not definitely proven. Similarly to other organs, the cardiovascular system exhibits diurnal and seasonal rhythms, including the heart

TABLE 5.1
Melatonin Receptors in the Human Cardiovascular System

Localization	Receptor Subtype	Functions
Cardiac ventricular wall	MT1–MT2	Modulate physiological contraction
Coronary arteries and cerebral arteries	MT1–MT2	Vasoconstriction Vasodilatation
Aorta	MT1–MT2	Vasodilatation
Systemic	?	Reduction of peripheral resistance Reduction of blood pressure in human Reduction in core body temperature Sleep promoting

rate, cardiac output, and blood pressure.[66] The SCN of hypothalamus and, possibly, the melatoninergic system modulate the cardiovascular rhythms. Decreases in nocturnal serum melatonin concentration or in urinary aMT6S levels have been reported in patients with coronary heart disease[67] or cardiac failure.[68] Melatonin, which is secreted almost exclusively at night,[13] influences several endocrine and biologic functions. A possible link between melatonin and circulation is suggested by two pieces of evidence. First, the nocturnal increase of melatonin seems to show an inverse temporal relation with the decrease of cardiovascular activity.[20] Second, in rats, melatonin and the pineal gland are able to prevent ischemia and/or reperfusion-induced heart arrhythmias,[69,70] influence the control of blood pressure,[71] and regulate blood flow to the brain.[72]

Moreover, an interesting involvement of melatonin in the cardiovascular regulation of animal models was suggested by pinealectomy experiments that resulted in a temporary hypertension. This hypertension was reversed by the addition of melatonin to drinking water.[73] In addiction, melatonin is effective at reducing blood pressure in hypertensive patients. In a double-blind, placebo-controlled study conducted on 14 normal healthy men, it was noted that the administration of 1 mg of melatonin reduced systolic, diastolic, and mean blood pressure; norepinephrine levels also decreased after administration.[71] Recently, Scheer et al.[74] demonstrated that melatonin given orally (2.5 mg/day) for 3 weeks to patients with essential hypertension reduced significantly both systolic and diastolic blood pressure. The hypotensive action of melatonin may involve either peripheral or central mechanisms.

Melatonin's vasodilatating action is supported by a decrease of the internal artery pulsatile index, which reflects the downstream vasomotor state and resistance.[71] In fact, vasoregulatory actions of melatonin are complex insofar as vasodilatation is mediated via MT2 receptors, whereas MT1-dependent signaling leads to vasoconstriction.[75] The normalization of circadian pacemaker function in the regulation of blood pressure by melatonin treatment has been proposed as a potential strategy for the treatment of essential hypertension.[76]

In the following paragraphs, we summarize the main data on receptor-mediated actions of melatonin in the blood vascular system (Table 5.1).

5.6.1 Heart

The role of melatonin on the heart is unclear at the moment. Mounting evidence indicates an important role of melatonin in its metabolism and physiology. In isolated rat papillary muscle, melatonin has antiadrenergic effects inducing reduction of contractility increase.[77] In particular, the first goal of this study has been to investigate the role of melatonin on myocardial contractility using dose–response curves to melatonin, to isoproterenol, and to calcium either in the presence or in the absence of melatonin (0.3 nM). They found that melatonin has antiadrenergic effects on these muscles and that this phenomenon is abolished in the presence of its receptor antagonist *N*-acetyl-tryptamine.

This suggested that melatonin operates through the specific cardiac receptors. The reduction of contractility increase, induced by forskolin-stimulated adenylate cyclase, shows that melatonin may act through a reduction of cAMP accumulation.

Successively, Ekmekcioglu et al.[78,79] were the first researchers to demonstrate the expression of MT1 and MT2 receptors in left human ventricle specimens. In left ventricle specimens, the authors showed an expression of the MT2 receptor suggesting that melatonin mediates physiological contractile or metabolic functions in human ventricles via receptor subtypes. The presence of melatonin receptors in cardiomyocytes were also suggested by binding studies[80] and also by immunostaining[81] in chick hearts. In the latter study, it was also demonstrated that the MT1-receptor subtype in myocytes is prominent during embryogenesis and declined considerably after hatching. Putative receptor-mediated effects of melatonin on cardiomyocytes may result, according to these studies, in a modulation of calcium homeostasis. Melatonin was shown to stimulate the rat sarcolemma Ca_{2+} pump[82] and to increase the high-voltage activated calcium currents in chick embryonic heart cells.[83] In contrast to possible receptor-mediated effects, several previous studies demonstrated that melatonin has protective effects on the heart through its potent antioxidative properties.[84,85] Therefore, cardiac effects of melatonin are likely to be receptor- and non-receptor–mediated.

Recently, Bojková et al.[86] evaluated the effect of prolonged melatonin administration on chosen metabolic and hormonal variables in male and female Sprague Dawley rats. They found that the relative heart muscle weight in females was increased after melatonin administration. Moreover, melatonin decreased glycemia, heart muscle glycogen concentration in females, and liver glycogen concentration in both sexes. Serum triacylglycerol and heart muscle cholesterol concentrations in females were decreased; however in males, serum and heart muscle cholesterol and phospholipid concentrations were increased. Melatonin increased MDA concentrations in the heart muscle in males and in the liver in both sexes. So, they suggested that melatonin induced prominent sex-dependent changes in both carbohydrate and lipid metabolism.

5.6.2 Blood Vessels

Accumulating evidence indicates that the hormone melatonin regulates vascular tone; however, the nature of the response remains controversial. Both vasoconstrictor and vasodilator responses have been reported; however, data supporting the presence of melatonin receptors are found in some, but not all, vascular beds.[87] In isolated rat caudal arteries, nanomolar concentrations of melatonin potentiate contraction induced by either endogenous or exogenous vasoconstrictors.[88] In rat cerebral arteries and arterioles, melatonin is a direct vasoconstrictor.[89] Melatonin-mediated contraction in caudal and cerebral arteries is blocked by melatonin receptor antagonists.[88,91,92]

Melatonin also dilates rat and rabbit aorta, iliac, renal, and basilar arteries.[93] The lack of specific 2-[^{125}I]iodomelatonin binding in rat aorta[94] suggests either that the melatonin-mediated vasodilatation is not mediated by high-affinity melatonin receptors or that the sensitivity of the binding assay was not sufficient for detection of all melatonin receptor types.[95] In porcine pulmonary, coronary, and marginal colon arteries, high concentrations of melatonin and melatonin analogs may induce vasodilatation by a novel mechanism.[96]

The MT1 and MT2 melatonin receptors are possible mediators of the physiological effects of melatonin.[97] They exhibit distinct structural, chromosomal, and pharmacological differences.[98–100]

It is now well accepted that activation of MT1 melatonin receptors in caudal arteries facilitates adrenergic vasoconstriction.[101,102] However, definitive demonstration of vascular MT2 receptors has been hampered by technical difficulties and discrepancies in technical approaches, rat strains and gender, drug types, and concentrations. Results from our laboratory suggest that the contractile responses to melatonin in male Fischer rat caudal arteries are mediated through activation of at least two distinct receptors.[103,104]

To address these discrepancies, Masana et al.[105] determined the expression of MT1 and MT2 melatonin receptor mRNA using highly sensitive reverse transcription-polymerase chain reaction and in situ hybridization techniques in caudal arteries of three rat strains. Furthermore, they studied the effects of selective MT2 melatonin receptor antagonists on melatonin-mediated potentiation of arterial contraction. They demonstrate that the MT2 melatonin receptor is indeed present in caudal artery and acts to attenuate MT1 melatonin receptor–mediated contraction.

The recent studies by Ekmekcioglu et al.[78,79] showed MT1 and MT2 receptors in human coronary arteries from pathological samples and also from healthy controls. In porcine coronary arteries, melatonin induced vasoconstriction via inhibition of NO effects and potentiation of serotonin effects. There are several potential mechanisms by which melatonin could interfere with the NO pathway and thus potentiate serotonin-induced contractions in coronary arteries. One possibility is that melatonin may inhibit NOS. Although an effect of melatonin on NOS in coronary arteries cannot be ruled out under the present experimental conditions, the inhibitory effect of melatonin on relaxations to sodium nitroprusside, which serves as an exogenous NO donor and is not dependent on NOS, suggests a site of action other than or in addition to inhibition of NOS. Alternatively, melatonin could act by attenuating the action of NO at the level of the vascular smooth muscle. NO relaxes vascular smooth muscle by increasing intracellular cGMP levels and by activating potassium channels in the cell membrane. Recent evidence suggests that melatonin prevents increased cGMP accumulation in several cell types and that the hormone has potassium channel-blocking properties. Thus, it is likely that melatonin may potentiate serotonin-induced vasoconstriction by inhibiting the action of NO on coronary vascular smooth muscle cells rather than by inhibiting the release of NO from endothelial cells.[106]

Regarding the role of melatonin in aorta, Ekmekcioglu[40] showed that both types of MT receptors are present in the human aorta. They assume that melatonin has vasodilatory effects, since studies in aortic rings from rat and rabbits showed that melatonin induces vasodilatation.[107] This effect is endothelium dependent, and probably mediated by the elevation of NO, potentiation of acetylcholine, and/or inhibition of noradrenaline effects as previously demonstrated by Weekley.[108]

The physiological meaning of melatonin on peripheral arteries needs to be clarified. Human studies showed that administration of melatonin during the day decreases core body temperature via selective vasodilatation in distal body regions and induction of sleepiness. Furthermore, intravenous administration of melatonin leads to an increase in peripheral blood flow. These studies confirmed the hypothesis that melatonin in humans is involved in the circadian variation of body temperature and induction of sleep. Several studies showed that melatonin can reduce blood pressure in humans. The mechanisms of these effects are not yet well defined. It is possible that these mechanisms can be due to a reduction in peripheral resistance inducing vasodilatation (NO potentiation, anti-noradrenergic mechanisms, inhibition of vasopressin release). However, since cardiac ventricles also express MT receptors, a negative inotropic effect may also be one reason for the hypotensive effects of melatonin.[40]

5.7 CARDIOVASCULAR DISEASES: CLASSIFICATION AND DEFINITION

Remarkable progress has been made in the past few decades in the field of cardiovascular medicine, as a result of the improved understanding of physiological and pathological pathways that contribute to health and disease. Unfortunately, CVDs (coronary artery disease, hypertension, atherosclerosis, stroke, cerebrovascular disease, congestive heart failure, heart attack, peripheral vascular disease) remain the major cause of death in most developed countries.

The clinical importance of circadian biological rhythms has been strengthened by a number of studies showing a circadian distribution of cardiovascular events such as myocardial infarction, stroke, complex arrhythmia, or sudden cardiac death. Incidence of cardiovascular events showed a maximum level during the early morning hours after awakening from sleep. In addition, a number of pathophysiological mechanisms have been identified to coincide with this peak including blood pressure and heart rate surges, decreased endothelial dilatory capacity of peripheral and coronary arteries, enhanced sympathetic activity, decreased cardiac electrical stability, and increased platelet aggregation. Moreover, the inclusion of other dependent and independent risk factors that may contribute to the apparent multifactorial nature of the CVDs, such as oxidative stress and aging, has been considered. This time window of high risk for the incidence of cardiovascular events has been identified as a target for new treatment and prevention strategies including new release forms of antihypertensive and anti-ischemic drugs.

5.7.1 Cardiovascular Disease and Oxidative Stress

CVDs are some of the most important disease processes in which free radicals impact cardiac physiology.[109,110] Oxidative stress is caused by an imbalance between the oxidant and antioxidant system in favor of the oxidants. Oxidative stress increases the formation of reactive oxygen species (ROS) or free radicals and reactive nitrogen species, which are harmful to cells.[111] ROS are generated constantly in vivo; may cause oxidative damage to nucleic acids, lipids, and proteins; and may affect cell membrane functions. Thus, their accumulation may lead to the oxidative destruction of cells.[112]

ROS also play central roles in cardiac physiology and pathophysiology,[113] and they can directly damage both vascular cells and cardiac myocytes directly. Some studies demonstrated the association of ROS with etiopathogenesis of atherosclerosis and cardiomyopathy in humans.[114] Moreover, ROS are involved in the pathogenesis of cardiac I/R injury through a faltering electron transport chain in mitochondria.[65]

The mechanism for the enhanced ROS generation as well as cellular and subcellular targets of ROS attack is not totally known.

5.7.2 Cardiovascular Disease and Aging

The oxidative stress theory of aging has a long history and has been first formulated by Harman[115] in 1956. Based on this theory, organismal deterioration that occurs as a result of increasing longevity is specifically a consequence of the persistent accumulation of free radical—mediated damage to essential molecules that gradually compromise the function of cells, tissues, and eventually of the organism itself. Since it has been proposed, the free radical theory of aging has been repeatedly modified and redefined.[50]

Aging is defined as a progressive, intrinsic, and irreversible organism change, leading to an increased risk of vulnerability, loss of vigor, diseases, and death. It is a multifactorial process characterized by physiological, metabolic, endocrine, and immune disturbances associated with decline in the bodies' responsiveness against stress. As a result, there is an increase in homeostatic abnormalities, as well as in the incidence of a variety of diseases associated with senescence. Aging is an important risk factor for CVDs not only because there is a process of vascular aging per se but also because aging increases the time of exposure to other cardiovascular risk factors[116]; so the incidence and prevalence of CVDs increase steeply with advancing age. CVDs increase dramatically with aging, not only clinically but also subclinically (occult diseases), such as silent coronary atherosclerosis. The clinical manifestations and prognosis of these diseases and resultant heart failure also worsen with increasing age.[117]

5.8 CARDIOVASCULAR DISEASE AND MELATONIN

Decreased melatonin production was found in several CVDs.[66] The use of melatonin as an antihypertensive, antioxidant, and anti-ischemic drug has been explored and opens new opportunities for the management of cardiovascular dysfunction and disease from a circadian perspective.[118] It is important to note that there is an inverse relationship between plasma melatonin concentrations and acrophase of the blood pressure rhythm in man, as high melatonin level coincides with lower blood pressure values.

A role of melatonin in the control of CVDs is supported by animal and human studies that will be reported in the next paragraphs.

5.8.1 Melatonin and Animal Models in CVD

Since melatonin functions as a free radical scavenger and antioxidant, the ability of this molecule to influence and protect CVDs has been experimentally investigated for a long time.

Tan et al.[119] observed that melatonin protected against arrhythmia induced by I/R reducing the incidence and severity of arrhythmias induced by I/R due to ligation of the anterior descending coronary artery in isolated rat hearts. Presumably, melatonin's beneficial effects in reducing cardiac arrhythmias were due in part to its free radical scavenging activity, which is greatly assisted by the rapidity with which it is taken up into cells. Moreover, melatonin may also reduce cardiac arrhythmias regulating intracellular calcium levels, that is, by preventing calcium overloading, or suppressing sympathetic nerve function and reducing adrenergic receptor function in the myocardium.

Myocardial I/R represents a clinically relevant problem associated with thrombolysis, angioplasty, and coronary bypass surgery. I/R injury is believed to be a consequence of free radical generation in the heart especially during the period of reperfusion.[85,120] In this case, rats were surgically pinealectomized to reduce endogenous levels of melatonin and, 2 months later, they, along with pineal-intact controls, were used in studies of cardiac I/R injury. When the left coronary artery was occluded for 7 minutes followed by 7 minutes of reperfusion, the degree of cardiac arrhythmia was significantly greater in the pinealectomized rats compared with the controls. Even more importantly, the incidence of mortality was 63% in rats lacking their pineal gland compared with only 25% in the pineal-intact rats after I/R induction. These findings suggested that endogenous melatonin levels are protective of the heart during episodes of hypoxia and reoxygenation. Moreover, the same authors demonstrated that melatonin administration immediately before reperfusion still had a protective effect on I/R-induced tissue damage in pinealectomized rats. As most drugs used to prevent I/R injury are known to be effective when they are given before ischemia, it would seem valuable to test melatonin in clinical trials for prevention of possible I/R-induced damage associated with thrombolysis, angioplasty, or coronary bypass surgery.

On the basis of these data, Sahna et al.[121] showed that the cardiac infarct size resulting from I/R was significantly reduced by melatonin administration. I/R increased MDA levels compared with control, and melatonin administration significantly reduced the increased MDA values. I/R leads to lower GSH levels, and melatonin administration significantly increased the GSH levels. These results suggest that melatonin might reduce I/R-induced damage assuming that some of melatonin's antioxidant actions promoting also the activity of glutathione reductase, thereby helping to maintain high levels of reduced GSH. In addition, it has been demonstrated that since melatonin is an effective free radical scavenger, it also decreases intracellular calcium concentrations.[65]

The administration of melatonin reduces blood pressure in spontaneously hypertensive rats (SHR),[122] whereas pinealectomy induces hypertension in rats.[123] K-Laflamme et al.[124] suggested that melatonin may act as the main antihypertensive agent by stimulating the central inhibitory adrenergic pathways, thereby diminishing the basal tone of the peripheral sympathetic nervous system. The hypotensive action of melatonin appears to be, at least partly, associated with the inhibition of basal sympathoadrenal tone and, finally, it could be mediated by blocking the postsynaptic α1-adrenergic receptor-induced inositol phosphate formation. On the other hand, a group of authors from Canada[125] concluded that the hypotensive effect of melatonin in rats was not mediated either by melatonin receptors or by α-adrenoceptors.

Nava et al.[126] demonstrated that, in SHR, melatonin treatment for 6 weeks reduced oxidative stress. SHR exhibit a progressive rise in systolic blood pressure over the same 6-week period. Systolic blood pressure was gradually reduced after treatment of SHR with melatonin. Both intracellular $O_2^{\bullet}$ production and MDA levels were drastically reduced in SHR given melatonin. The melatonin-treated animals exhibited a significant reduction in the expression of nuclear factor κB (NF-κB), an effect that may indirectly contribute to melatonin's role as an antioxidant. In a similar study, Simko and Paulis[64] demonstrated that, in SHR, blood pressure decreased after 6 weeks of melatonin treatment showing also a reduction in interstitial renal tissue inflammation, a decrease of oxidative stress, and an attenuation of kidney NF-κB expression. Moreover, they found that long-term treatment with melatonin increased the antioxidant reserve by normalizing the depressed glutathione peroxidase activity in SHR.

Girouard et al.[127] tested the effect of melatonin on the heart of SHR with left ventricular hypertrophy. The antihypertensive effect of melatonin was not accompanied by a reduction of left ventricular relative weight in these animals. Myocyte hypertrophy and myocardial fibrosis, especially reactive fibrosis that expands from the perivascular space to the intermuscular space, are typical features of hypertensive cardiac remodeling.[128]

There are only few studies testing the ability of melatonin to protect the heart from morphologic changes. Weekley[93] found that melatonin relaxes the smooth muscles lining the aorta in rats. The vascular endothelium may contribute to the regulation of vascular smooth muscle tone by producing such vasoconstrictors as endothelin-1 and thromboxane, as well as vasodilators, such as prostacyclin and nitric oxide (NO). NO was originally identified as a principal endothelium-derived vascular relaxation factor. Okatani et al.[129] demonstrated that a pretreatment with L-N^G-monomethyl arginine, a NOS inhibitor, suppressed the potentiating effect of hydrogen peroxide (H_2O_2) on the vascular tension in umbilical artery segments, suggesting that H_2O_2 may exert its vasospastic effect by inhibiting NOS in the endothelium. Melatonin modulates NOS activity and, thereby, influences NO production. The results of the study of Wakatsuki et al.[130] indicate that H_2O_2 may impair NO synthesis in the endothelium of human umbilical arteries. Melatonin significantly suppresses the H_2O_2-induced inhibition effect of NO production, most likely through its ability to scavenge hydroxyl radicals.

Melatonin reduces the damage induced by chemical hypoxia and reoxygenation in rat cardiomyocytes. Also, Morishima et al.[131] reported that melatonin protected against adriamycin (doxorubicin hydrochloride)–induced cardiomyopathy, the pathogenesis of which may involve free radical and lipid peroxidation. In that study, melatonin has been shown to affect zinc turnover, the element that acts as an antioxidant. Similar results were obtained by Agapito et al.[132] and Xu et al.[84] in an experiment with adriamycin; they found that melatonin was an effective antioxidant against cardiotoxicity of myocardium generated by this antibiotic.

Recently, our team[15] investigated the effects of melatonin on cyclosporine A–induced cardiotoxicity. Histological changes in the heart of cyclosporine A–treated animals included a massive increase in the number of infiltrated cells and disorganization of myocardial fibers with interstitial fibrosis, all of which disappeared after melatonin administration. Moreover, we showed that the cardiac expression of heat shock protein 70, the central component of the cellular network of molecular chaperons and folding catalyst, was significantly increased in the heart of cyclosporine A–treated animals compared with that in the control rats. Melatonin coadministration decreased cyclosporine A–induced heat shock protein 70 expression with respect to cyclosporine A-only-treated rats (Figure 5.4). On the basis of our results, we presumed, in the heart, a mechanism similar to that proposed by the previous authors is operative.[133] The binding of melatonin to membrane receptors (MT1, MT2), via G inhibitory protein, activates the PKC pathway. The consequential increase in intracellular Ca_{2+} concentrations phosphorylates PKC, which activates the protein/activation transcription factor (CREB/ATF). This pathway modulates immediate early gene (IEG) transcription and consequently gene transcription regulation and antioxidant enzyme activities (Figure 5.5).

Although the actions of melatonin are clearly diverse, collectively, both melatonin's receptor signal transduction pathways and its scavenging or antioxidant receptor–independent properties are likely involved in the protective actions of the indole. In the past decade, melatonin as an agent to prevent apoptosis has been a major field of interest.[134] The role that melatonin exerts on apoptosis in different tissues as well as the mechanisms whereby melatonin alters this process is not always

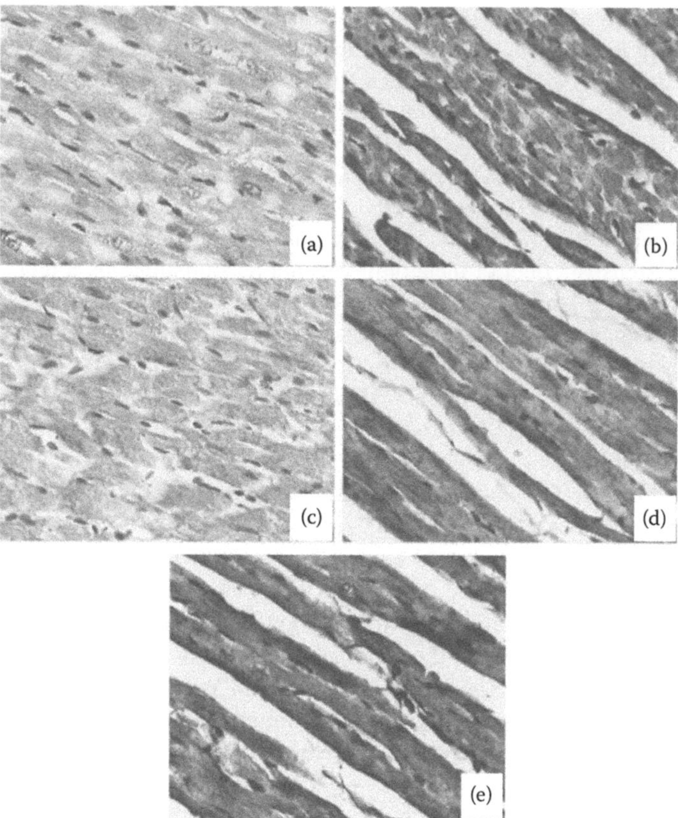

FIGURE 5.4 Photomicrographs of rat heart with heat shock protein 70 immunohistochemistry, respectively, in (a) control, (b) cyclosporine A–treated, (c) cyclosporine A + melatonin, (d) cyclosporine A + melatonin + luzindole, and (e) luzindole alone (original magnification ×400). (Rezzani, R. et al.: *J. Pineal Res.* 2006. 41. 288–95. Copyright Wiley-VCH Verlag GmbH & Co. KGaA. Reproduced with permission.)

clear.[135] To address this point, we evaluated whether melatonin is a useful tool for counteracting cyclosporine A–induced apoptosis and if the antiapoptotic effects of melatonin derive from its ability to engage specific membrane receptors or to its radical scavenging activities. This latter issue particularly requires resolution. Our data and that of others[15,136] underlined that the dominant antioxidant effect of melatonin requires receptors on cell membranes and that only a small portion of the protection is provided by the direct scavenging action of the indole amine. Using nanoparticles as an effective melatonin delivery system, we showed that melatonin may interfere with the apoptotic signaling by scavenging free radicals or by any of the signal transduction events triggered by its multiple direct targets (receptors) within the cells. As melatonin alone is less effective on the apoptotic process, we concluded that the signal transduction elicited by interaction with MT1/MT2 is not enough for such an effect. After administration of nanoparticles, we observed a very significant reduction of myocyte cell death. This could be justified considering the ability of cells to rapidly absorb macromolecules, such as nanoparticles, through endocytosis. This mechanism, common to all cells in the body, internalizes macromolecules and retains them in transport vesicles. The endosomes release drug molecules, such as melatonin, for determining their successful delivery without involving MT1/MT2 receptors. Moreover, these findings suggest that, when melatonin is

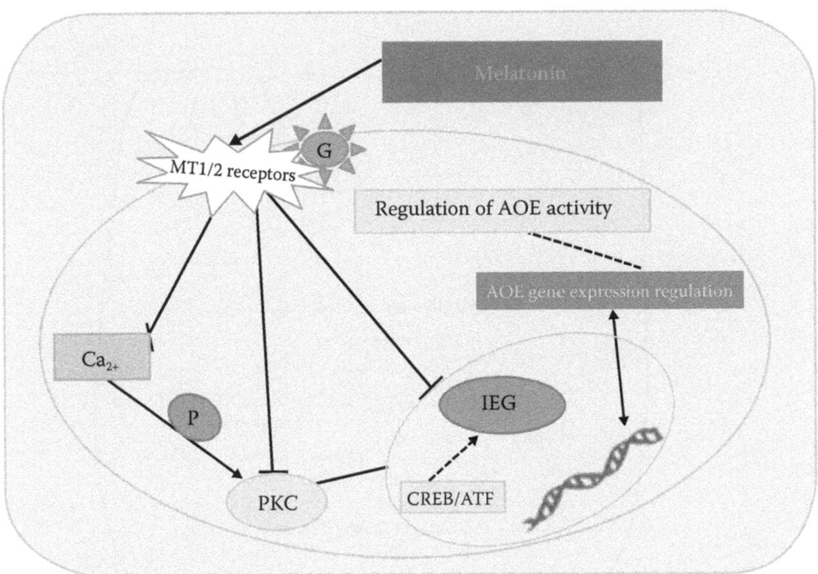

FIGURE 5.5 Hypothetical pathway involved in melatonin regulation of antioxidant enzyme (AOE) gene expression and activity. Melatonin activation of MT1/2 receptors, via G inhibitory protein (G), activates the PKC pathway. The consequential increase in Ca_{2+} concentrations PKC, which activates CREB/ATF thereby increasing the transcription of immediate early gene and, consequently, gene transcription regulation and antioxidant enzyme activity (Rezzani, R. et al.: *J. Pineal Res.* 2006. 41. 288–95. Copyright Wiley-VCH Verlag GmbH & Co. KGaA. Reproduced with permission.)

administered alone, the MT1/MT2 pathway might be necessary but not completely sufficient for apoptosis antagonism and an additional intracellular effect may be required. We have also indicated a hypothetical apoptotic pathway used from internalization of melatonin by nanoparticles (Figure 5.6).

The last paper published by our team regards the beneficial effects of melatonin on nicotine-induced vasculopathy. Among the components of cigarette smoke, nicotine is known to exert proatherosclerotic, prothrombotic, and proangiogenic effects on vascular endothelial cells. This experimental study was designed to investigate the mechanisms by which nicotine induces endothelial dysfunction and further to examine whether melatonin protects against nicotine-induced vasculopathy. Our results show that nicotine induces marked structural and functional alterations in the aorta. Nicotine receptor binding results in activation and phosphorylation of extracellular signal-regulated kinase 1/2. This enzyme, in turn, activates both TGF-β1 and NF-κB; they stimulate, respectively, the synthesis of type I collagen, responsible for fibrosis, and, moreover, intercellular adhesion molecule-1 and vascular cellular adhesion molecule-1 (Figure 5.7). Based on these findings, melatonin is able to minimize the negative effects of nicotine by blocking the activation of extracellular signal-regulated kinase and the other signaling pathways in which this enzyme is involved.

5.8.2 Clinical Trials of Melatonin in CVDs

The effects of melatonin on blood pressure in hypertensive patients are less studied with respect to those observed in animal models. Recently, there are some data pointing to a role of melatonin in cardiovascular homeostasis. Escames et al.[137] investigated the changes in macrophage iNOS activity, oxidative stress, and melatonin levels in human essential hypertension, before and after 6 months

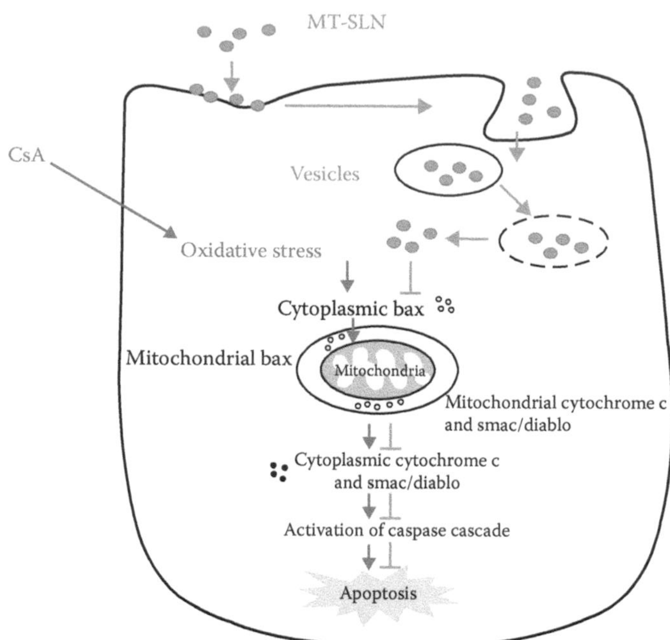

FIGURE 5.6 Hypothetical pathway through which nanosphere and melatonin (MT-SLN) interferes with the intrinsic pathway of cyclosporine A (CsA)–induced apoptosis. CsA induces apoptotic mechanism determining oxidative stress; MT-SLN is internalized into the myocytes by vesicles and, successively, melatonin (MT) is released into the cytoplasm of these cells. Melatonin is able to block the translocation of Bax into the mitochondria and the activation of caspase cascade, which induce apoptotic mechanism. (Rezzani, R. et al.: *J. Pineal Res.* 2009. 46. 255–61. Copyright Wiley-VCH Verlag GmbH & Co. KGaA. Reproduced with permission.)

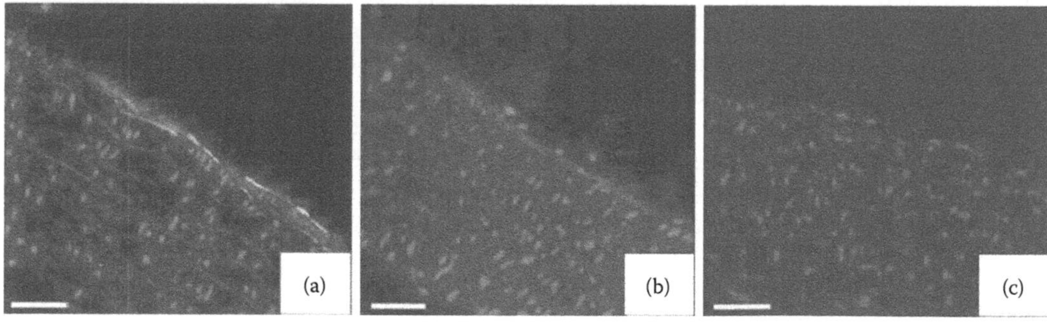

FIGURE 5.7 Immunofluorescence of ICAM-1 (white) and VCAM-1 (gray) expression on the surface of endothelial cells in (a) nicotine-treated animals, (b) control, and (c) nicotine + melatonin groups. Nuclei were stained with DAPI (light gray) (bar = 50 μm). (Rodella, L.F. et al.: *J. Pineal Res.* 2010. 48. 126–32. Copyright Wiley-VCH Verlag GmbH & Co. KGaA. Reproduced with permission.)

of treatment with lacidipine, a Ca_{2+}-channel antagonist. Taken together, lacidipine and melatonin improve endothelial dysfunction by restoring vascular NOS pathway activity and NO availability, through a mechanism probably related to an antioxidant effect. Thus, the use of melatonin as a therapeutic agent in combination with lacidipine may be of interest in the treatment of hypertension.

Another point of interest reported by Lusardi et al.[138] showed that evening administration of 5 mg melatonin increased blood pressure in hypertensive patients who were treated with nifedipine GITS 30 to 60 mg daily. In fact, these authors showed that the chronic evening ingestion of melatonin in hypertensive patients well controlled by nifedipine GITS induces a blood pressure increase and a heart rate acceleration. Kinetic or pharmacodynamic interaction between melatonin and nifedipine is able to impair the antihypertensive efficacy of the calcium-channel blocker. These findings raise the possibility that melatonin may interfere with the blood pressure–lowering effect of antihypertensive agents.

Paskaloglu et al.[139] showed that melatonin or insulin alone can provide limited protection against hyperglycemia-induced oxidative damage in diabetes. Combined treatment with insulin and melatonin can suppress hyperglycemia, prevent oxidative damage, and can restore endothelial function completely, implying that treatment of diabetes mellitus with this combination would be beneficial.

Another interesting point is that melatonin has significant protective actions against the cardiac damage and altered physiology that occurs during I/R injury. Sahna et al.[85,120] showed that physiological concentrations of melatonin were important in preventing I/R-induced cardiac infarct size. The results showing increased I/R-induced cardiac injury after reduction in physiological levels of melatonin have implications for elderly people because in old individuals, endogenous levels of melatonin are significantly lower than in young individuals. Several studies have reported that humans with CVDs have noticeably lower circulating melatonin levels than do age-matched subjects without significant cardiovascular deterioration.[140] Similarly, patients suffering from cardiac syndrome X have an attenuated nocturnal peak in serum melatonin levels relative to those of age-matched individuals with no cardiac pathology.[141] It remains unknown, however, whether the reduced endogenous melatonin levels in patients with CVD is a cause, an effect, or even related to the compromised cardiovascular function.

Zaslavskaya et al.[142] showed the melatonin effects on contractile myocardial function in patients with postmyocardial infarction and heart failure, assessed as stage II–III by the New York Heart Association. They found melatonin associated anti-anginal and anti-ischemic effects, indicating an improvement of contractile function and a normalization of influence on the balance in the oxidant/antioxidant system. Thus, O'Rourke[143] demonstrates that nanomolar concentrations of melatonin inhibit the development of nitrate tolerance in coronary arteries. It should be noted that nitroglycerin is widely used in the treatment of ischemic heart disease, but its long-term clinical usefulness is limited by the development of tolerance.[144] The effect of melatonin appears to be mediated via MT1 or MT2 melatonin receptors; and it is mediated, in part, by inhibition of NO signaling pathways and by protection against oxidative stress,[106,145] properties that may be beneficial in preventing nitrate tolerance and requires the presence of endothelial cells. At the end, melatonin may prove to be a useful pharmacological tool in unraveling mechanisms of nitrate tolerance in blood vessels with intact endothelium vs. those in which the endothelium is absent or dysfunctional.

Scheer et al.[146] reported in hypertensive patients that repeated melatonin intake 1 hour before sleep reduced nighttime systolic and diastolic blood pressure by 6 and 4 mm Hg, respectively.

The trial of Grossman et al.[147] was the first randomized, double-blind, placebo-controlled study showing clearly the benefit from melatonin in treated patients with nocturnal hypertension. The best response was observed in patients treated with an angiotensin-converting enzyme inhibitor and diuretic. There is also evidence that single exogenous melatonin intake can lower blood pressure, but only when melatonin is taken during the daytime, when general SCN neuronal activity is high and endogenous melatonin levels are low. On the contrary, repeated nighttime melatonin intake supports the endogenous melatonin rhythm, improving only the circadian rhythmicity.[148]

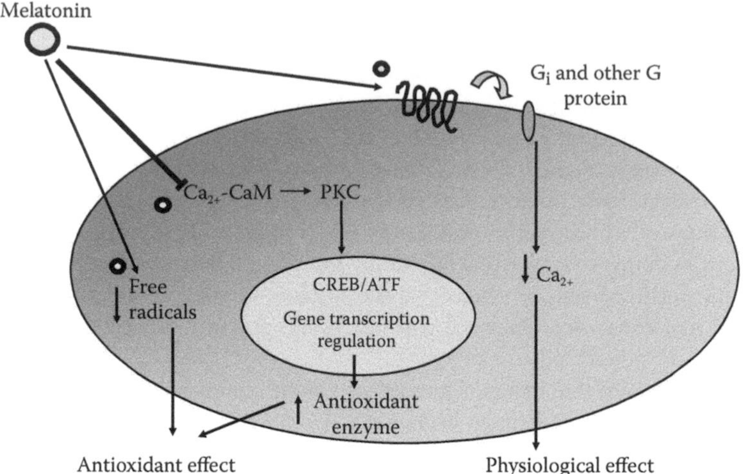

FIGURE 5.8 Hypothetical pathways involved in melatonin regulation of antioxidant enzymes and physiological activity in blood vascular system. Melatonin actions are due to their direct free radical scavenging activity, their indirect actions on anti- and prooxidative enzymes, and also due to receptor-mediated actions on physiological activity.

5.9 SUMMARY AND CONCLUSION

The author reviewed the actions of an endogenously produced molecule, melatonin, in normal and pathological cardiovascular physiology. Furthermore, the evidence presented herein suggests that the protective actions of melatonin and its metabolites are due to their direct free radical scavenging activity, their indirect actions on anti- and prooxidative enzymes, and also due to receptor-mediated actions on physiological activity (Figure 5.8). In particular, the physiological effects of melatonin on the heart are still unclear, but accumulating evidence suggests that melatonin mediates physiological contractile or metabolic functions in human ventricles via receptor subtypes (Figure 5.9a).

The physiological action of melatonin on blood vessels is not clearly defined, and the nature of the response remains controversial even if its action is receptor- and non-receptor–mediated.

Regarding the receptor-mediated action, it is possible to propose, first, a receptor-mediated action stimulating the increase of NOS in intima vascular layer, a decrease of Ca_{2+} and, second, an increase of cGMP inducing vascular relaxation in media vascular layer and an antioxidant activity (Figure 5.9b).

The last but not the least important action of exogenous melatonin is in CVDs. CVDs (coronary artery disease, hypertension, atherosclerosis, stroke, cerebrovascular disease, congestive heart failure, heart attack, peripheral vascular disease) remain the major cause of death in most developed countries. Decreased melatonin production was found in several CVDs and the use of melatonin as an antihypertensive, antioxidant, and anti-ischemic drug has been explored and opens new opportunities for the management of these pathologies. The schematic protective effects of melatonin (increase of antioxidant enzymes, decrease of lipid peroxidation and of blood pressure, etc.) are summarized in Figure 5.10.

In conclusion, given the complexity of melatonin interactions with blood vascular system in normal and pathological cardiovascular physiology, via receptor- and non-receptor–mediated, it will take a lot of more work before a clear picture emerges of how melatonin influences cardiovascular function.

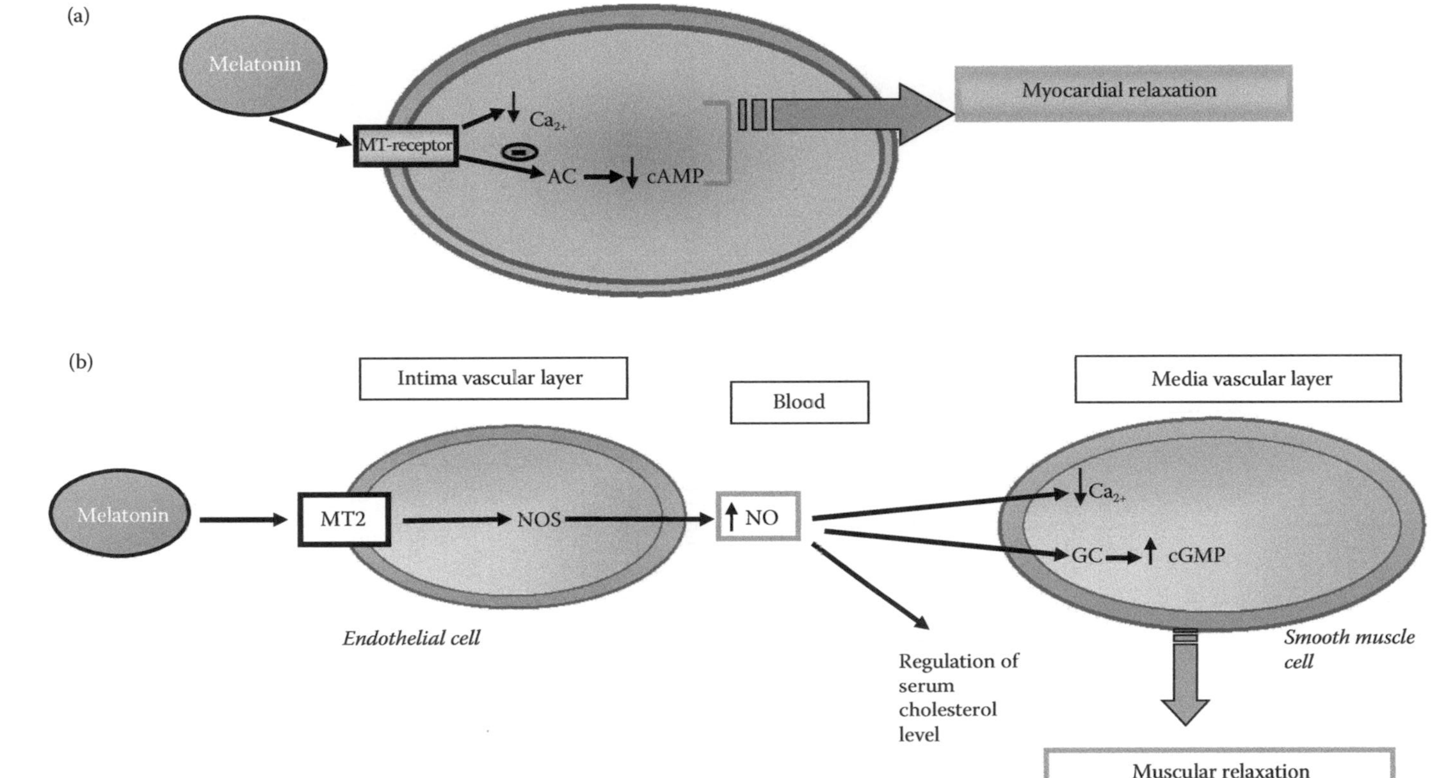

FIGURE 5.9 (a) Receptor- and non-receptor–mediated effects of melatonin in the heart. Melatonin stimulates the sarcolemma Ca_{2+} pump and increases the high-voltage activated calcium currents by MT- receptors. (b) Vascular effects of melatonin are controversial, but it is possible to propose a receptor-mediated action. Melatonin determines an increase of and NOS in intima vascular layer and also, in media vascular layer; a decrease of Ca_{2+}; and an increase of cGMP inducing vascular relaxation.

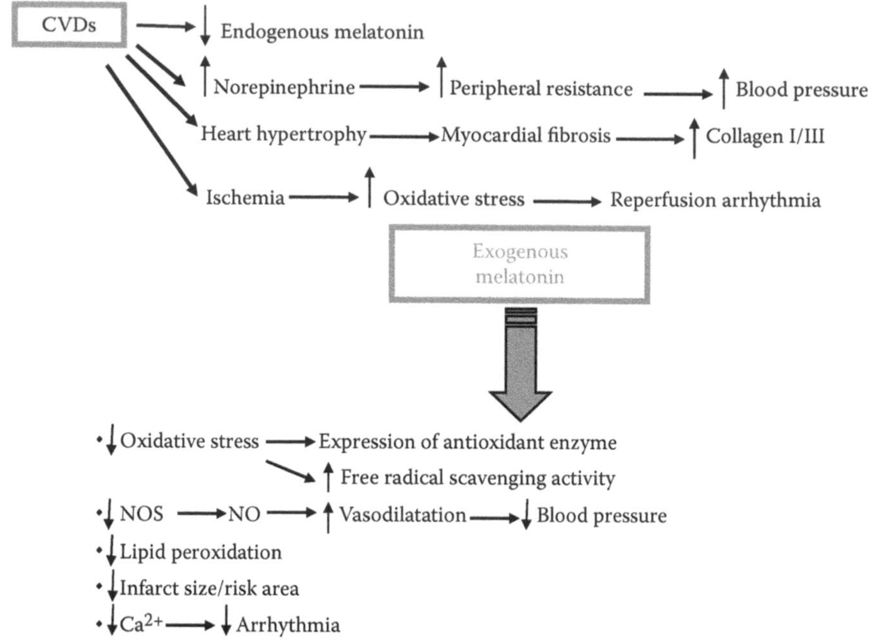

FIGURE 5.10 Damages induced by CVDs and protective effects of melatonin.

ACKNOWLEDGMENTS

The author thanks Dr. Gaia Favero, Dr. Claudia Rossini, and Dr. Foglio Eleonora for their excellent work in writing and improving the chapter.

This review was stimulated by research supported by a grant from the Nathura Srl, Reggio Emilia (Italy), and also by a grant (ex-60% 2009) from the University of Brescia.

REFERENCES

1. Reiter, RJ, Paredes, SD, Manchester, LC, and DX Tan. 2009. Reducing oxidative/nitrosative stress: A newly-discovered genre for melatonin. *Crit. Rev. Biochem. Mol. Biol.* 44:175–200.
2. Claustrat, B, Brun, J, and G Chazot. 2005. The basic physiology and pathophysiology of melatonin. *Sleep. Med. Rev.* 9:11–24.
3. Zrenner, C. 1985. Theories of pineal function from classical antiquity to 1900: A history, in: R.J. Reiter (Ed.), *Pineal Research Reviews* III, Alan R. Liss, New York, 1–40.
4. Adam, C, and P Tannery. 1974. *Oeuvres de Descartes*, vol. XI, Librairie Philosophique J. Vrinn, Paris.
5. Studnicka, FK. 1905. Die Parietalorgane In oppel A (Ed) lehrbuch der vergleichenden mikroskopischen anatomie der worbettiere, Part 5. Gustav Fischer: Jena.
6. Lerner, AB, Case, JD, Takahashi, Y, and W Mori. 1958. Isolation of melatonin, the pineal gland factor that lightens melanocytes. *J. Am. Chem. Soc.* 80:2587.
7. Lerner, AB, Case, JD, and RV Heinzelmann. 1959. Structure of melatonin. *J. Am. Chem. Soc.* 81: 6084–6085.
8. Wurtman, RJ, Axelrod, J, and LS Phillips. 1963. Melatonin synthesis in the pineal gland: Control by light. *Science*. 142:1071–3.
9. Reiter, RJ, and RJ Hester. 1965. Interrelationships of the pineal gland, the superior cervical ganglia and the photoperiod in the regulation of the endocrine systems of hamsters. *Endocrinol.* 79:1168–70.
10. Reiter, RJ, Tan, DX, Korkmaz, A, Erren, TC, Piekarski, C, Tamura, H, and LC 2007. Manchester. Light at night, chronodisruption, melatonin suppression, and cancer risk: A review. *Crit. Rev. Oncog.* 13:303–28.

11. Reiter, RJ. 1993. The melatonin rhythm: Both a clock and a calendar. *Experientia.* 49:654–64.
12. Reiter, RJ. 1980. The pineal and its hormones in the control of reproduction in mammals. *Endocrine. Rev.* 1:109–31.
13. Reiter, RJ. 1991. Pineal melatonin: Cell biology of its synthesis and of its physiological interactions. *Endocrine. Rev.* 12:151–80.
14. Maestroni, GJ. 1993. The immunoneuroendocrine role of melatonin. *J. Pineal. Res.* 14:1–10.
15. Rezzani, R, Rodella, LF, Bonomini, F, Tengattini, S, Bianchi, R, and RJ Reiter. 2006. Beneficial effects of melatonin in protecting against cyclosporine A–induced cardiotoxicity are receptor mediated. *J. Pineal. Res.* 41:288–95.
16. Rezzani, R, Rodella, LF, Fraschini, F, Gasco, MR, Demartini, G, Musicanti, C, and RJ Reiter. 2009. Melatonin delivery in solid lipid nanoparticles: Prevention of cyclosporine A induced cardiac damage. *J. Pineal. Res.* 46:255–61.
17. Rodella, LF, Filippini, F, Bonomini, F, Bresciani, R, Reiter, RJ, and R Rezzani. 2010. Beneficial effects of melatonin on nicotine-induced vasculopathy. *J. Pineal. Res.* 48:126–32.
18. Paulis, L, and F Simko. 2007. Blood pressure modulation and cardiovascular protection by melatonin: Potential mechanisms behind. *Physio.l Res.* 56:671–84.
19. Arendt, J. 1998. Melatonin and the pineal gland: Influence on mammalian seasonal and circadian physiology. *Rev. Reprod.* 3:13–22.
20. Cagnacci, A. 1996. Melatonin in relation to physiology in adult humans. *J Pineal Res.* 21:200–13.
21. Krause, DN, and ML Dubocovich. 1990. Regulatory sites in the melatonin system of mammals. *Trends. Neurosci.* 13:464–70.
22. Cardinali, DP, and MI Vacas. 1987. Cellular and molecular mechanisms controlling melatonin release by mammalian pineal glands. *Cell. Mol. Neurobiol.* 7:323–37.
23. Jansen, KL, Dragunow, M, and RL Faull. 1990. Sigma receptors are highly concentrated in the rat pineal gland. *Brain. Res.* 507:158–60.
24. Yuwiler, A, Brammer, GL, and BL Bennett. 1995. Interaction between adrenergic and peptide stimulation in the rat pineal: Pituitary adenylate cyclase–activating peptide. *J. Neurochem.* 64:2273–80.
25. Cagnacci, A, Soldani, R, Romagnolo, C, and SS Yen. 1994. Melatonin-induced decrease of body temperature in women: A threshold event. *Neuroendocrinology.* 60:549–52.
26. Lewy, AJ, Siever, LJ, Uhde, TW, and SP Markey. 1986. Clonidine reduces plasma melatonin levels. *J. Pharm. Pharmacol.* 38:555–6.
27. Zimmermann, RC, Krahn, L, Klee, G, Delgado, P, Ory, SJ, and SC Lin. 1994. Inhibition of presynaptic catecholamine synthesis with alpha-methyl-para-tyrosine attenuates nocturnal melatonin secretion in humans. *J. Clin. Endocrinol. Metab.* 79:1110–4.
28. Skene, DJ, Bojkowski, CJ, and J Arendt. 1994. Comparison of the effects of acute fluvoxamine and desipramine administration on melatonin and cortisol production in humans. *Br. J. Clin. Pharmacol.* 37:181–6.
29. Meyer, AC, Nieuwenhuis, JJ, Kociszewska, VJ, Joubert, WS, and BJ Meyer. 1986. Dihydropyridine calcium antagonists depress the amplitude of the plasma melatonin cycle in baboons. *Life Sci.* 39:1563–9.
30. Murphy, PJ, Myers, BL, and P Badia. 1996. Nonsteroidal anti-inflammatory drugs alter body temperature and suppress melatonin in humans. *Physiol. Behav.* 59:133–9.
31. Laughlin, GA, Loucks, AB, and SS Yen. 1991. Marked augmentation of nocturnal melatonin secretion in amenorrheic athletes, but not in cycling athletes: Unaltered by opioidergic or dopaminergic blockade. *J. Clin. Endocrinol. Metab.* 73:1321–6.
32. McIntyre, IM, Norman, TR, Burrows, GD, and SM Armstrong. 1993. Alterations to plasma melatonin and cortisol after evening alprazolam administration in humans. *Chronobiol. Int.* 10:205–13.
33. Lal, S, Isaac, I, Pilapil, C, Nair, NP, Hariharasubramanian, N, Guyda, H, and R Quirion. 1987. Effect of apomorphine on melatonin secretion in normal subjects. *Prog. Neuropsychopharmacol. Biol. Psychiatry.* 11:229–33.
34. Follenius, M, Weibel, L, and G Brandenberger. 1995. Distinct modes of melatonin secretion in normal men. *J. Pineal. Res.* 18:135–40.
35. Geoffriau, M, Claustrat, B, and J Veldhuis. 1999. Estimation of frequently sampled nocturnal melatonin production in humans by deconvolution analysis: Evidence for episodic or ultradian secretion. *J. Pineal. Res.* 27:139–44.
36. Grof, E, Grof, P, Brown, GM, Arato, M, and J Lane. 1985. Investigations of melatonin secretion in man. *Prog. Neuropsychopharmacol. Biol. Psychiatry.* 9:609–12.
37. Arendt, J, Bojkowski, C, Franey, C, Wright, J, and V Marks. 1985. Immunoassay of 6-hydroxymelatonin sulfate in human plasma and urine: Abolition of the urinary 24-hour rhythm with atenolol. *J. Clin. Endocrinol. Metab.* 60:1166–73.

38. Iguchi, H, Kato, KI, and H Ibayashi. 1982. Melatonin serum levels and metabolic clearance rate in patients with liver cirrhosis. *J. Clin. Endocrinol. Metab.* 54:1025–7.
39. Lüdemann, P, Zwernemann, S, and A Lerchl. 2001. Clearance of melatonin and 6-sulfatoxymelatonin by hemodialysis in patients with end-stage renal disease. *J. Pineal. Res.* 31:222–7.
40. Ekmekcioglu, C. 2006. Melatonin receptors in humans: Biological role and clinical relevance. *Biomed. Pharmacother.* 60:97–108.
41. Reiter, RJ. 2003. Melatonin: Clinical relevance. *Best. Pract. Res. Clin. Endocrinol. Metab.* 17:273–85.
42. Altun, A, and B Ugur-Altun. 2007. Melatonin: Therapeutic and clinical utilization. *Int. J. Clin. Pract.* 61:835–45.
43. Edgar, DM, Dement, WC, and CA Fuller. 1993. Effect of SCN lesions on sleep in squirrel monkeys: Evidence for opponent processes in sleep-wake regulation. *J. Neurosci.* 13:1065–79.
44. Thapan, K, Arendt, J, and DJ Skene. 2001. An action spectrum for melatonin suppression: Evidence for a novel non-rod, non-cone photoreceptor system in humans. *J. Physiol.* 535:261–7.
45. Berson, DM, Dunn, FA, and M Takao. 2002. Phototransduction by retinal ganglion cells that set the circadian clock. *Science.* 295:1070–3.
46. Warman, GR, Tripp, HM, Warman, VL, and J Arendt. 2003. Circadian neuroendocrine physiology and electromagnetic field studies: Precautions and complexities. *Radiat. Prot. Dosimetry.* 106:369–73.
47. Møller, M, and FM Baeres. 2002. The anatomy and innervation of the mammalian pineal gland. *Cell. Tissue. Res.* 309:139–50.
48. Rodriguez, C, Mayo, JC, Sainz, RM, Antolín, I, Herrera, F, Martín, V, and RJ Reiter. 2004. Regulation of antioxidant enzymes: A significant role for melatonin. *J. Pineal. Res.* 36:1–9.
49. Ortiz, GG, Benítez-King, GA, Rosales-Corral, SA, Pacheco-Moisés, FP, and IE Velázquez-Brizuela. 2008. Cellular and biochemical actions of melatonin which protect against free radicals: Role in neurodegenerative disorders. *Curr. Neuropharmacol.* 6:203–214.
50. Reiter, RJ, Paredes, SD, Korkmaz, A, Manchester, LC, and DX Tan. 2008. Melatonin in relation to the "strong" and "weak" versions of the free radical theory of aging. *Adv. Med. Sci.* 53:119–29.
51. León, J, Escames, G, Rodríguez, MI, López, LC, Tapias, V, Entrena, A, Camacho, E, Carrión, MD, Gallo, MA, Espinosa, A, Tan, DX, Reiter, RJ, and D Acuña-Castroviejo. 2006. Inhibition of neuronal nitric oxide synthase activity by *N*1-acetyl-5-methoxykynuramine, a brain metabolite of melatonin. *J. Neurochem.* 98:2023–33.
52. Winiarska, K, Fraczyk, T, Malinska, D, Drozak, J, and J Bryla. 2006. Melatonin attenuates diabetes-induced oxidative stress in rabbits. *J. Pineal. Res.* 40:168–76.
53. León, J, Acuña-Castroviejo, D, Escames, G, Tan, DX, and RJ Reiter. 2005. Melatonin mitigates mitochondrial malfunction. *J. Pineal. Res.* 38:1–9.
54. Herrera, J, Nava, M, Romero, F, and B Rodríguez-Iturbe. 2001. Melatonin prevents oxidative stress resulting from iron and erythropoietin administration. *Am. J. Kidney. Dis.* 37:750–7.
55. Gitto, E, Karbownik, M, Reiter, RJ, Tan, X, Cuzzocrea, S, Chiurazzi, P, Cordaro, S, Corona, G, Trimarchi, G, and I Barberi. 2001. Effects of melatonin treatment in septic newborns. *Pediatr. Res.* 50:756–60.
56. Fulia, F, Gitto, E, Cuzzocrea, S, Reiter, RJ, Dugo, L, Gitto, P, Barberi, S, Cordaro, S, and I Barberi. 2001. Increased levels of malondialdehyde and nitrite/nitrate in the blood of asphyxiated newborns: Reduction by melatonin. *J. Pineal. Res.* 31:343–9.
57. Neri, B, de Leonardis, V, Gemelli, MT, di Loro, F, Mottola, A, Ponchietti, R, Raugei, A, and G Cini. 1998. Melatonin as biological response modifier in cancer patients. *Anticancer. Res.* 18:1329–32.
58. Guven, A, Yavuz, O, Cam, M, Ercan, F, Bukan, N, and C Comunoglu. 2007. Melatonin protects against epirubicin-induced cardiotoxicity. *Acta. Histochem.* 109:52–60.
59. Hill, SM, Frasch, T, Xiang, S, Yuan, L, Duplessis, T, and L Mao. 2009. Molecular mechanisms of melatonin anticancer effects. *Integr. Cancer. Ther.* 8:337–46.
60. Waldhauser, F, Boepple, PA, Schemper, M, Mansfield, MJ, and WF Jr. Crowley. 1991. Serum melatonin in central precocious puberty is lower than in age-matched prepubertal children. *J. Clin. Endocrinol. Metab.* 73:793–6.
61. Berga, SL, and SS Yen. 1990. Circadian pattern of plasma melatonin concentrations during four phases of the human menstrual cycle. *Neuroendocrinology.* 51:606–12.
62. Okatani, Y, Morioka, N, and A Wakatsuki. 2000. Changes in nocturnal melatonin secretion in perimenopausal women: Correlation with endogenous estrogen concentrations. *J. Pineal. Res.* 28:111–8.
63. Iguchi, H, Kato, KI, and H Ibayashi. 1982. Age-dependent reduction in serum melatonin concentration in healthy human subjects. *J. Clin. Endocrinol. Metab.* 55:27–9.
64. Simko, F, and L Paulis. 2007. Melatonin as a potential antihypertensive treatment. *J. Pineal. Res.* 42:319–22.

65. Tengattini, S, Reiter, RJ, Tan, DX, Terron, MP, Rodella, LF, and R Rezzani. 2008. Cardiovascular diseases: Protective effects of melatonin. *J. Pineal. Res.* 44:16–25.
66. Dominguez-Rodriguez, A, Abreu-Gonzalez, P, and RJ Reiter. 2009. Clinical aspects of melatonin in the acute coronary syndrome. *Curr. Vasc. Pharmacol.* 7:367–73.
67. Yaprak, M, Altun, A, Vardar, A, Aktoz, M, Ciftci, S, and G Ozbay. 2003. Decreased nocturnal synthesis of melatonin in patients with coronary artery disease. *Int. J. Cardiol.* 89:103–7.
68. Girotti, L, Lago, M, Ianovsky, O, Elizari, MV, Dini, A, Lloret, SP, Albornoz, LE, and DP Cardinali. 2003. Low urinary 6-sulfatoxymelatonin levels in patients with severe congestive heart failure. *Endocrine.* 22:245–8.
69. Sallinen, P, Mänttäri, S, Leskinen, H, Ilves, M, Vakkuri, O, Ruskoaho, H, and S Saarela. 2007. The effect of myocardial infarction on the synthesis, concentration and receptor expression of endogenous melatonin. *J. Pineal. Res.* 42:254–60.
70. Reiter, RJ, and DX Tan. 2003. Melatonin: A novel protective agent against oxidative injury of the ischemic/reperfused heart. *Cardiovasc. Res.* 58:10–9.
71. Arangino, S, Cagnacci, A, Angiolucci, M, Vacca, AM, Longu, G, Volpe, A, and GB Melis. 1999. Effects of melatonin on vascular reactivity, catecholamine levels, and blood pressure in healthy men. *Am. J. Cardiol.* 83:1417–9.
72. Dupuis, F, Régrigny, O, Atkinson, J, Limiñana, P, Delagrange, P, Scalbert, E, and JM Chillon. 2004. Impact of treatment with melatonin on cerebral circulation in old rats. *Br. J. Pharmacol.* 141:399–406.
73. Kurcer, Z, Sahna, E, and E Olmez. 2006. Vascular reactivity to various vasoconstrictor agents and endothelium-dependent relaxations of rat thoracic aorta in the long-term period of pinealectomy. *J. Pharmacol. Sci.* 101:329–34.
74. Scheer, FA, Van Montfrans, GA, van Someren, EJ, Mairuhu, G, and RM Buijs. 2004. Daily nighttime melatonin reduces blood pressure in male patients with essential hypertension. *Hypertension.* 43:192–7.
75. Dubocovich, ML, and M Markowska. 2005. Functional MT1 and MT2 melatonin receptors in mammals. *Endocrine.* 27:101–10.
76. Scheer, FA. 2005. Potential use of melatonin as adjunct antihypertensive therapy. *Am. J. Hypertens.* 18:1619–20.
77. Abete, P, Bianco, S, Calabrese, C, Napoli, C, Cacciatore, F, Ferrara, N, and F Rengo. 1997. Effects of melatonin in isolated rat papillary muscle. *FEBS Lett.* 412:79–85.
78. Ekmekcioglu, C, Haslmayer, P, Philipp, C, Mehrabi, MR, Glogar, HD, Grimm, M, Thalhammer, T, and W Marktl. 2001. 24h variation in the expression of the mt1 melatonin receptor subtype in coronary arteries derived from patients with coronary heart disease. *Chronobiol. Int.* 18:973–85.
79. Ekmekcioglu, C, Thalhammer, T, Humpeler, S, Mehrabi, MR, Glogar, HD, Hölzenbein, T, Markovic, O, Leibetseder, VJ, Strauss-Blasche, G, and W Marktl. 2003. The melatonin receptor subtype MT2 is present in the human cardiovascular system. *J. Pineal. Res.* 35:40–4.
80. Pang, CS, Brown, GM, Tang, PL, Cheng, KM, and SF Pang. 1993. 2-[125I]Iodomelatonin binding sites in the lung and heart: A link between the photoperiodic signal, melatonin, and the cardiopulmonary system. *Biol. Signals.* 2:228–36.
81. Pang, CS, Xi, SC, Brown, GM, Pang, SF, and SY Shiu. 2002. 2[125I]Iodomelatonin binding and interaction with beta-adrenergic signaling in chick heart/coronary artery physiology. *J. Pineal. Res.* 32:243–52.
82. Chen, LD, Tan, DX, Reiter, RJ, Yaga, K, Poeggeler, B, Kumar, P, Manchester, LC, and JP Chambers. 1993. In vivo and in vitro effects of the pineal gland and melatonin on [Ca(2+) + Mg2+]-dependent ATPase in cardiac sarcolemma. *J. Pineal. Res.* 14:178–83.
83. Mei, YA, Lee, PP, Wei, H, Zhang, ZH, and SF Pang. 2001. Melatonin and its analogs potentiate the nifedipine-sensitive high-voltage-activated calcium current in the chick embryonic heart cells. *J. Pineal. Res.* 30:13–21.
84. Xu, MF, Tang, PL, Qian, ZM, and M Ashraf. 2001. Effects by doxorubicin on the myocardium are mediated by oxygen free radicals. *Life Sci.* 68:889–901.
85. Sahna, E, Olmez, E, and A Acet. 2002. Effects of physiological and pharmacological concentrations of melatonin on ischemia-reperfusion arrhythmias in rats: Can the incidence of sudden cardiac death be reduced? *J. Pineal. Res.* 32:194–8.
86. Bojková, B, Orendás, P, Friedmanová, L, Kassayová, M, Datelinka, I, Ahlersová, E, and I Ahlers. 2008. Prolonged melatonin administration in 6-month-old Sprague-Dawley rats: Metabolic alterations. *Acta Physiol Hung.* 95:65–76.
87. Mahle, CD, Goggins, GD, Agarwal, P, Ryan, E, and AJ Watson. 1997. Melatonin modulates vascular smooth muscle tone. *J. Biol. Rhythms.* 12:690–6.

88. Geary, GG, Duckles, SP, and DN Krause. 1998. Effect of melatonin in the rat tail artery: Role of K+ channels and endothelial factors. *Br. J. Pharmacol.* 123:1533–40.
89. Geary, GG, Krause, DN, and SP Duckles. 1997. Melatonin directly constricts rat cerebral arteries through modulation of potassium channels. *Am. J. Physiol.* 273:1530–6.
90. Viswanathan, M, Scalbert, E, Delagrange, P, Guardiola-Lemaître, B, and JM Saavedra. 1997. Melatonin receptors mediate contraction of a rat cerebral artery. *Neuroreport.* 8:3847–9.
91. Ting, KN, Dunn, WR, Davies, DJ, Sugden, D, Delagrange, P, Guardiola-Lemaître, B, Scalbert, E, and VG Wilson. 1997. Studies on the vasoconstrictor action of melatonin and putative melatonin receptor ligands in the tail artery of juvenile Wistar rats. *Br. J. Pharmacol.* 122:1299–306.
92. Ting, KN, Blaylock, NA, Sugden, D, Delagrange, P, Scalbert, E, and VG Wilson. 1999. Molecular and pharmacological evidence for MT1 melatonin receptor subtype in the tail artery of juvenile Wistar rats. *Br. J. Pharmacol.* 127:987–95.
93. Weekley, LB. 1991. Melatonin-induced relaxation of rat aorta: Interaction with adrenergic agonists. *J. Pineal. Res.* 11:28–34.
94. Viswanathan, M, Laitinen, JT, and JM Saavedra. 1990. Expression of melatonin receptors in arteries involved in thermoregulation. *Proc. Natl. Acad. Sci. U S A.* 87:6200–3.
95. Dubocovich, ML, Yun, K, Al-Ghoul, WM, Benloucif, S, and MI Masana. 1998. Selective MT2 melatonin receptor antagonists block melatonin-mediated phase advances of circadian rhythms. *FASEB J.* 12:1211–20.
96. Ting, N, Thambyraja, A, Sugden, D, Scalbert, E, Delagrange, P, and VG Wilson. 2000. Pharmacological studies on the inhibitory action of melatonin and putative melatonin analogues on porcine vascular smooth muscle. *Naunyn. Schmiedebergs. Arch. Pharmacol.* 361:327–33.
97. Dubocovich, ML, Masana, MI, and S Benloucif. 1999. Molecular pharmacology and function of melatonin receptor subtypes. *Adv. Exp. Med. Biol.* 460:181–90.
98. Reppert, SM, Godson, C, Mahle, CD, Weaver, DR, Slaugenhaupt, SA, and JF Gusella. 1995. Molecular characterization of a second melatonin receptor expressed in human retina and brain: The Mel1b melatonin receptor. *Proc. Natl. Acad. Sci. U S A.* 92:8734–8.
99. Reppert, SM, Weaver, DR, and C Godson. 1996. Melatonin receptors step into the light: Cloning and classification of subtypes. *Trends. Pharmacol. Sci.* 17:100–2.
100. Slaugenhaupt, SA, Roca, AL, Liebert, CB, Altherr, MR, Gusella, JF, and SM Reppert. 1995. Mapping of the gene for the Mel1a-melatonin receptor to human chromosome 4 (MTNR1A) and mouse chromosome 8 (Mtnr1a). *Genomics.* 27:355–7.
101. Bucher, B, Gauer, F, Pévet, P, and M Masson-Pévet. 1999. Vasoconstrictor effects of various melatonin analogs on the rat tail artery in the presence of phenylephrine. *J. Cardiovasc. Pharmacol.* 33:316–322.
102. Lew, MJ, and S Flanders. 1999. Mechanisms of melatonin-induced vasoconstriction in the rat tail artery: A paradigm of weak vasoconstriction. *Br. J. Pharmacol.* 126:1408–18.
103. Doolen, S, Krause, DN, Dubocovich, ML, and SP Duckles. 1998. Melatonin mediates two distinct responses in vascular smooth muscle. *Eur. J. Pharmacol.* 345:67–9.
104. Doolen, S, Krause, DN, SP. Duckles. 1999. Estradiol modulates vascular response to melatonin in rat caudal artery. *Am. J. Physiol.* 276:1281–8.
105. Masana, MI, Doolen, S, Ersahin, C, Al-Ghoul, WM, Duckles, SP, Dubocovich, ML, and DN Krause. 2002. MT(2) melatonin receptors are present and functional in rat caudal artery. *J. Pharmacol. Exp. Ther.* 302:1295–302.
106. Yang, Q, Scalbert, E, Delagrange, P, Vanhoutte, PM, and ST O'Rourke. 2001. Melatonin potentiates contractile responses to serotonin in isolated porcine coronary arteries. *Am. J. Physiol. Heart. Circ. Physiol.* 280:76–82.
107. Monroe, KK, and SW Watts. 1998. The vascular reactivity of melatonin. *Gen. Pharmacol.* 30:31–5.
108. Weekley, LB. 1995. Pharmacologic studies on the mechanism of melatonin-induced vasorelaxation in rat aorta. *J. Pineal. Res.* 19:133–8.
109. Reiter, RJ, Tan, DX, Mayo, JC, Sainz, RM, Leon, J, and Z Czarnocki. 2003b. Melatonin as an antioxidant: Biochemical mechanisms and pathophysiological implications in humans. *Acta. Biochim. Pol.* 50:1129–46.
110. Reiter, RJ, Tan, DX, Gitto, E, Sainz, RM, Mayo, JC, Leon, J, Manchester, LC, Vijayalaxmi, Kilic, E, and U Kilic. 2004. Pharmacological utility of melatonin in reducing oxidative cellular and molecular damage. *Pol. J. Pharmacol.* 56:159–70.
111. Tuteja, N, Singh, MB, Misra, MK, Bhalla, PL, and R Tuteja. 2001. Molecular mechanisms of DNA damage and repair: Progress in plants. *Crit. Rev. Biochem. Mol. Biol.* 36:337–97.

112. Tuteja, N, Ahmad, P, Panda, BB, and R Tuteja. 2009. Genotoxic stress in plants: Shedding light on DNA damage, repair and DNA repair helicases. *Mutat. Res.* 681:134–49.
113. Kevin, LG, Novalija, E, and DF Stowe. 2005. Reactive oxygen species as mediators of cardiac injury and protection: The relevance to anesthesia practice. *Anesth. Analg.* 101:1275–87.
114. Madamanchi, NR, and MS Runge. Mitochondrial dysfunction in atherosclerosis. *Circ. Res.* 100:460–73.
115. Harman, D. 1956. Aging: A theory based on free radical and radiation chemistry. *J. Gerontol.* 11: 298–300.
116. Versari, D, Daghini, E, Virdis, A, Ghiadoni, L, and S Taddei. 2009. The ageing endothelium, cardiovascular risk and disease in man. *Exp. Physiol.* 94:317–21.
117. Lakatta, EG, and D Levy. Arterial and cardiac aging: Major shareholders in cardiovascular disease enterprises: Part I: Aging arteries: A "set up" for vascular disease. *Circulation.* 107:139–46.
118. Altun, A, and B Ugur-Altun. 2007. Melatonin: Therapeutic and clinical utilization. *Int. J. Clin. Pract.* 61:835–45.
119. Tan, DX, Manchester, LC, Reiter, RJ, Qi, W, Kim, SJ, and GH El-Sokkary. 1998. Ischemia/reperfusion-induced arrhythmias in the isolated rat heart: Prevention by melatonin. *J. Pineal. Res.* 25:184–91.
120. Sahna, E, Parlakpinar, H, Ozer, MK, Ozturk, F, Ozugurlu, F, and A Acet. 2003. Melatonin protects against myocardial doxorubicin toxicity in rats: Role of physiological concentrations. *J. Pineal. Res.* 35:257–61.
121. Sahna, E, Parlakpinar, H, Turkoz, Y, and A Acet. 2005. Protective effects of melatonin on myocardial ischemia/reperfusion induced infarct size and oxidative changes. *Physiol. Res.* 54:491–5.
122. Kawashima, K, Miwa, Y, Fujimoto, K, Oohata, H, Nishino, H, and H Koike. 1987. Antihypertensive action of melatonin in the spontaneously hypertensive rat. *Clin. Exp. Hypertens. A.* 9:1121–31.
123. Karppanen, H, Airaksinen, MM, and I Särkimäki. 1973. Effects of rats of pinealectomy and oxypertine on spontaneous locomotor activity and blood pressure during various light schedules. *Ann. Med. Exp. Biol. Fenn.* 51:93–103.
124. K-Laflamme, A, Wu, L, Foucart, S, and J de Champlain. 1998. Impaired basal sympathetic tone and alpha1-adrenergic responsiveness in association with the hypotensive effect of melatonin in spontaneously hypertensive rats. *Am. J. Hypertens.* 11:219–29.
125. Wu, L, Wang, R, and J de Champlain. 1998. Enhanced inhibition by melatonin of alpha-adrenoceptor-induced aortic contraction and inositol phosphate production in vascular smooth muscle cells from spontaneously hypertensive rats. *J. Hypertens.* 16:339–47.
126. Nava, M, Quiroz, Y, Vaziri, N, and B Rodriguez-Iturbe. 2003. Melatonin reduces renal interstitial inflammation and improves hypertension in spontaneously hypertensive rats. *Am. J. Physiol. Renal. Physiol.* 284:F447–54.
127. Girouard, H, Denault, C, Chulak, C, and J de Champlain. 2004. Treatment by n-acetylcysteine and melatonin increases cardiac baroreflex and improves antioxidant reserve. *Am. J. Hypertens.* 17:947–54.
128. Kai, H, Mori, T, Tokuda, K, Takayama, N, Tahara, N, Takemiya, K, Kudo, H, Sugi, Y, Fukui, D, Yasukawa, H, Kuwahara, F, and T Imaizumi. 2006. Pressure overload-induced transient oxidative stress mediates perivascular inflammation and cardiac fibrosis through angiotensin II. *Hypertens. Res.* 29:711–8.
129. Okatani, Y, Watanabe, K, and Y Sagara. 1997. Effect of nitric oxide, prostacyclin, and thromboxane on the vasospastic action of hydrogen peroxide on human umbilical artery. *Acta. Obstet. Gynecol. Scand.* 76:515–20.
130. Wakatsuki, A, Okatani, Y, Ikenoue, N, Izumiya, C, and C Kaneda. 2000. Melatonin inhibits oxidative modification of low-density lipoprotein particles in normolipidemic post-menopausal women. *J. Pineal. Res.* 28:136–42.
131. Morishima, I, Okumura, K, Matsui, H, Kaneko, S, Numaguchi, Y, Kawakami, K, Mokuno, S, Hayakawa, M, Toki, Y, Ito, T, and T Hayakawa. 1999. Zinc accumulation in adriamycin-induced cardiomyopathy in rats: Effects of melatonin, a cardioprotective antioxidant. *J. Pineal. Res.* 26:204–10.
132. Agapito, MT, Antolín, Y, del Brio, MT, López-Burillo, S, Pablos, MI, and JM Recio. 2001. Protective effect of melatonin against adriamycin toxicity in the rat. *J. Pineal. Res.* 31:23–30.
133. Tomás-Zapico, C, and A Coto-Montes. 2005. A proposed mechanism to explain the stimulatory effect of melatonin on antioxidative enzymes. *J. Pineal. Res.* 39:99–104.
134. Manda, K, Ueno, M, and K Anzai. 2008. Melatonin mitigates oxidative damage and apoptosis in mouse cerebellum induced by high-LET 56Fe particle irradiation. *J. Pineal. Res.* 44:189–96.
135. Sainz, RM, Mayo, JC, Rodriguez, C, Tan, DX, Lopez-Burillo, S, and RJ Reiter. 2003. Melatonin and cell death: Differential actions on apoptosis in normal and cancer cells. *Cell. Mol. Life. Sci.* 60:1407–26.

136. Lochner, A, Genade, S, Davids, A, Ytrehus, K, and JA Moolman. 2006. Short- and long-term effects of melatonin on myocardial post-ischemic recovery. *J. Pineal. Res.* 40:56–63.
137. Escames, G, Khaldy, H, León, J, González, L, and D Acuña-Castroviejo. 2004. Changes in iNOS activity, oxidative stress and melatonin levels in hypertensive patients treated with lacidipine. *J. Hypertens.* 22:629–35.
138. Lusardi, P, Piazza, E, and R Fogari. 2000. Cardiovascular effects of melatonin in hypertensive patients well controlled by nifedipine: A 24-hour study. *Br. J. Clin. Pharmacol.* 49:423–7.
139. Paskaloglu, K, Sener, G, and G Ayanğolu-Dülger. 2004. Melatonin treatment protects against diabetes-induced functional and biochemical changes in rat aorta and corpus cavernosum. *Eur. J. Pharmacol.* 499:345–54.
140. Brugger, P, Marktl, W, and M Herold. 1995. Impaired nocturnal secretion of melatonin in coronary heart disease. *Lancet.* 345:1408.
141. Altun, A, Yaprak, M, Aktoz, M, Vardar, A, Betul, UA, and G Ozbay. 2002. Impaired nocturnal synthesis of melatonin in patients with cardiac syndrome X. *Neurosci. Lett.* 327:143–5.
142. Zaslavskaya, RM, Lilitsa, GV, Dilmagambetova, GS, Halberg, F, Cornélissen, G, Otsuka, K, Singh, RB, Stoynev, A, Ikonomov, O, Tarquini, R, Perfetto, F, Schwartzkopff, O, and EE Bakken. 2004. Melatonin, refractory hypertension, myocardial ischemia and other challenges in nightly blood pressure lowering. *Biomed. Pharmacother.* 58:129–34.
143. O'Rourke, ST, Hammad, H, Delagrange, P, Scalbert, E, and PM Vanhoutte. 2003. Melatonin inhibits nitrate tolerance in isolated coronary arteries. *Br. J. Pharmacol.* 139:1326–32.
144. Parker, JD, and JO Parker. 1998. Nitrate therapy for stable angina pectoris. *N. Engl. J. Med.* 338:520–31.
145. Wakatsuki, A, and Y Okatani. 2000. Melatonin protects against the free radical–induced impairment of nitric oxide production in the human umbilical artery. *J. Pineal. Res.* 28:172–8.
146. Scheer, FA, Van Montfrans, GA, van Someren, EJ, Mairuhu, G, and RM Buijs. 2004. Daily nighttime melatonin reduces blood pressure in male patients with essential hypertension. *Hypertension.* 43:192–7.
147. Grossman, E, Laudon, M, Yalcin, R, Zengil, H, Peleg, E, Sharabi, Y, Kamari, Y, Shen-Orr, Z, and N Zisapel. 2006. Melatonin reduces night blood pressure in patients with nocturnal hypertension. *Am. J. Med.* 119:898–902.
148. Sharkey, KM, and CI Eastman. 2002. Melatonin phase shifts human circadian rhythms in a placebo-controlled simulated night-work study. *Am. J. Physiol. Regul. Integr. Comp. Physiol.* 282:454–63.

6 Melatonin Effect on Reproduction

Maria P. Tsantarliotou and Ioannis A. Taitzoglou

CONTENTS

6.1 INTRODUCTION

The objective of this chapter is to provide a general overview of the physiological role of seasonality in reproduction, which allows mammals to confine their breeding activity to a time of the year when it is most likely to be successful. In the first part, information is provided about the environmental factors that control seasonality of reproduction in humans and various animal species, with photoperiod being the main one. Next, the mode of action of photoperiod on seasonal breeding is analyzed, with two main pathways being investigated: a. the transduction of the light/dark cycle into an endocrine signal which is the circadian secretion of melatonin produced by the pineal gland and b. the regulation of the hypothalamic–pituitary–gonadal axis activity by melatonin secretion from puberty to adulthood, in both sexes. Finally, some novel physiological activities of melatonin (antioxidative, myometrium contractility) that could be considered for new therapeutic strategies in the pathophysiology of the reproductive system are discussed.

6.2 SEASONAL RHYTHMS OF REPRODUCTION

Reproductive activity in many mammals shows pronounced seasonal variations in terms of ovulation frequency (presence or absence of ovulation), spermatogenesis (from moderate to complete absence of sperm production), gamete quality (variation of fertilization rates and embryo survival), and sexual behavior.[1] The time of the year, when animals are reproductively active, varies from species to species and depends mainly on the length of gestation, ensuring that births coincide with a favorable season for the offspring when environmental temperatures are becoming warmer and food availability is increasing (i.e., spring and early summer in animals with either a very short gestational period, such as hamsters, or a gestational period of about a year, such as horses). Thus, the actual mating time is less important than the birthing time, and seasonally breeding species use the time-of-year signal as a message to ensure birth of the young in the spring.[2]

Male Syrian hamsters undergo gonadal regression in autumn and remain reproductively quiescent throughout winter while they reside in the burrows; on the contrary, mating occurs in autumn in animals with a gestational period of around 6 months (sheep, goat, deer).[3,4] The Suffolk ewe becomes sexually active from late summer to early autumn, with unmated having repeated 16-day estrous cycles, until late winter when a 6-month anestrous period begins.[3] In Ile-de-France rams daily sperm production is 50%–80% as high in autumn as in spring,[5] while in the subtropical breed of Damascus buck, semen quality is better during summer.[6]

The timing of reproductive mechanisms is under high selection pressures because temporal errors can prove fatal. Various ultimate and proximate factors act on seasonal rhythms,[5,7,8] with the main ultimate factors food availability and temperature exerting selection pressure to restrict breeding activity to a particular time of the year when it is most likely to be successful. Proximate factors provide the necessary cues for the control of annual rhythms. A proximate factor is a reliable predictor for the preparation of the individual for reproduction, migration, or hibernation, if it is consistent and stable year after year. The day length in a light/dark cycle of a 24-hour photoperiod is the major source of environmental information in the control of a variety of seasonal activities.[1,5]

In sheep, conception is restricted to a certain period of the year—the breeding season, while day length is decreasing; during the remaining anestrous season, the female is anovulatory and the animal does not exhibit estrous behavior.[9] Photoperiod also is used to time puberty in this species by timing the decrease in sensitivity to estradiol inhibition of luteinizing hormone (LH) secretion in both sexes.[10] In sexually mature male golden hamsters exposed to photoperiods shorter than 12.5 hours of light per day, blood plasma levels of the LH, follicle-stimulating hormone (FSH), and testosterone are markedly reduced. Within 8–12 weeks, their testes regress and spermatogenic activity ceases.[11] The predictive nature of photoperiodic information is supported by the fact that the above photoperiod-induced changes are expressed after a dormancy of several weeks. Short-day exposure takes about 6 weeks to stimulate ovulation in sheep and about 8 weeks to induce testicular regression in hamsters.[3,11]

On the other hand, in many species of primates, reproduction involves a seasonal breeding pattern. Rhesus monkeys living outdoors provide an example of a seasonal breeding primate that expresses ovulation in females during the short days of autumn and restricts births during spring;[12–14] furthermore, under natural conditions, season influences the timing of puberty so much that the onset of menarche or first ovulation is better predicted by counting timing in breeding seasons after birth than in months.[15]

Humans are not considered to be seasonal breeders, in the sense that conceptions are spread all over the year; however, most studies suggest seasonality in successful conceptions.[16–19] According to a detailed epidemiological study about correlations between conception rates and various environmental factors in different regions of the earth, photoperiod and temperature in a minor role are the main environmental factors contributing to the annual conception rhythm.[16] There is strong evidence that, during spring, there is an increase in the conception rate in many countries of the northern and southern hemispheres, while extreme temperatures decrease the probability of conception. On the contrary, industrialization seems to be a potent factor, which decreases the amplitude of the human conception rhythms; this negative influence on conception rate is probably due to changes in human working conditions from outdoors to indoors and consequently to the reduction of the environmental impact.[5,19] Moreover, there are vast individual variations in photoresponsiveness, which altogether can account for many contradictions observed in the studies of human sensitivity to photoperiod.[18]

The absolute day length provides the immediate photoperiodic information to animals for their reproductive performance, although it is not the only feature that communicates photoperiodic information.[20,21] In ewes, 13 hours of light per day result in LH secretion if animals have been exposed previously to 16 hours of light, whereas the same day length induces the inhibition of LH secretion if animals have been exposed previously to 10 hours of light.[21] However, for the attainment of puberty, the developing lambs must experience long days before the short-day breeding period, during which their first ovulation occurs.[10]

Siberian hamsters show gonadal regression after they are transferred from 16 to 13.5 hours of light or gonadal growth when they are transferred from 10 to 13.5 hours of light.[20] All the above mean is that animals respond differently to a certain day length if it increases or decreases and that makes the preceding history a very important factor in defying photoperiodic responses. In ewes, progressively changing photoperiod throughout the year is also important to determine the length of the breeding season.[5] Ewes submitted to steep (nonconsecutive) decrease in photoperiod from 16 to 8 or 12 hours of light per day show a stimulation of LH secretion that lasts for only 50 to 60 days. On the contrary, if day length decreases first from 16 to 12 hours and then, during the LH increase, to 8 hours of light, the period of elevated LH levels lasts almost twice as long.[22] Because each day length occurs twice a year, once in summer/autumn and once in winter/spring, its ability to integrate photoperiodic history and the change in photoperiod allow animals to determine precisely the time of the year.

6.3 CIRCADIAN SECRETION OF MELATONIN

It is accepted that seasonal fall and revival of the gonads of photoperiodically sensitive mammals, whether they are long- or short-day breeders, are dependent on the annual fluctuations in day and night lengths, which determine the interval of the nocturnal melatonin rise.[23–25] The photoreceptors that mediate these reproductive events are highly specialized retinal ganglion cells that contain a unique photopigment, melanopsin.[26,27] These cells project via the retinohypothalamic tract to the biological clock (the suprachiasmatic nucleus, SCN) in the anterior part of the hypothalamus.[28,29] Then, the information is sent via sympathetic neurons to the pineal gland, where norepinephrine release on a night basis regulates the nocturnal elevation of melatonin synthsesis.[30] In mice lacking melanopsin, light-dependent entrainment is attenuated; bright light can still entrain circadian rhythms but not to the same extent as in mice expressing melanopsin.[31,32] Besides, when the sympathetic innervation to the pineal gland is destroyed, nocturnal melatonin production does not occur and the gland is no longer capable of regulating reproductive physiology; the animals become continuous breeders and that situation can be very dangerous, especially for the animals living under naturally varying environmental conditions.[33,34]

In humans, melatonin is secreted at night as in other mammals; whether the duration of melatonin secretion varies with season is controversial and results have been conflicting. It seems, however, that the duration of melatonin secretion is longer in winter than in summer at high-temperate subpolar and polar latitudes.[35] The exposure of humans to artificial long or short photoperiods leads to a difference in the duration of secretion, indicating that the retina–pineal axis is capable of detecting changes in photoperiod.[36] Together, these suggest that humans may be seasonally photoperiodic.

So far, it is accepted that in all species, regardless whether they are active at night or during the day, melatonin is synthesized and secreted during the dark phase of the day. Furthermore, the daily melatonin secretion profile varies greatly among species, and a classification into three groups has been proposed, with the ultimate output remaining the same: the duration of elevated melatonin increases when the night lengthens.[5,30] In the type A pattern, melatonin levels remain low during the first part of the night, increasing only during the second half of the night and decreasing to low daytime levels before light onset. This pattern is rare and is observed in the Syrian hamster, the Mongolian gerbil, and the mouse. In the type B pattern, melatonin levels soon after the onset of the night increase slowly, reaching a peak at mid-darkness, while during the second part of the night, melatonin falls to reach daytime levels near the time of light onset; this pattern has been observed among other species, including rats and humans. In type C, melatonin levels reach a plateau soon after the onset of the night (10–30 min in sheep), remaining elevated throughout the entire night and decreasing soon before or around the time of light onset; this profile has been observed in sheep and Siberian hamsters.[37] The lack of storage of melatonin in pinealocytes and its rapid clearance result to very close relationship between the melatonin synthesis and its presence in biological fluids.[5]

6.4 ROLE OF THE PINEAL GLAND

The physiological role of the pineal gland to transmit day-length information was established by accumulating data showing that the effect of photoperiod on seasonal reproduction is intensely altered after the removal or denervation of the pineal gland.[3,38] In humans, pineal tumors that destroy the parenchyma of the gland suppress the release of melatonin, which in turn leads to a premature reactivation of pulsatile gonadotropin-releasing hormone (GnRH) release and results to sexual precocity.[39] Pinealectomy or innervations of the pineal gland by superior cervical ganglionectomy makes rams or ewes insensitive to the inhibitory effects of long days or to the stimulatory effects of short days and unable to display synchronized changes in reproductive activity or in gonadotropin secretion in response to alterations between long and short days.[40–42] During the first trials, pinealectomy failed to show a significant effect of the removal of the pineal gland on the seasonal pattern of ovine reproduction;[43,44] nowadays, it is better understood that this failure was due to the existence of an endogenous rhythm of reproduction in this species, supporting the persistence of alterations between breeding and anestrous even when the external signal is removed (photorefractoriness). On the other hand, this endogenous cycle can be indirectly synchronized in pinealectomized ewes through social signals transmitted by intact males or females.[45]

In male Syrian hamsters, pinealectomy prevents the gonadal regression that is normally provoked by short photoperiod,[46] while the daily administration of melatonin to rats inhibits the estrous phase of their estrous cycle.[47]

6.5 MELATONIN CONTROL OF REPRODUCTION

6.5.1 Melatonin Regulation of the Hypothalamic–Pituitary–Gonadal Axis

Photoperiod induces changes in reproductive activity, in both sexes, through modifications in the secretion of LH and FSH by two mechanisms: one independent of and the other dependent on gonadal steroid.[3,5,11,48–52] Animal studies have demonstrated androgen and estrogen receptors in rat pinealocytes.[53]

In the male Syrian hamster, short photoperiod-induced testicular regression is coupled by decreases in pituitary and serum LH and FSH, leading to repression of testicular function and lowered levels of circulating testosterone.[11] Similar changes are observed in rams transferred from short to long days.[48] In humans, there is accumulating evidence that sex steroids and melatonin levels are inversely related. When sex steroids are high, melatonin is inhibited, and when melatonin levels are high, steroid levels are inhibited.[52,54,55] However, the presence of gonadotropin and gonadal steroid receptors has been demonstrated in human pinealocytes from infancy to old age.[56] All the above suggest the existence of a pineal melatonin–gonadotropin–gonadal steroid feedback mechanism.

The steroid-independent effects of photoperiod are observed in gonadectomized animals. In ovariectomized ewes, the secretion of LH is lower during anestrous than during the breeding season, appearing one pulse every hour or every 30 minutes, respectively (2-fold difference).[49–51] The administration of an estradiol implant in ovariectomized ewes, mimicking midfollicular phase levels, resulted in an LH pulse every 12 to 24 hours or every 30 minutes (20-fold difference) depending on whether animals are experiencing long or short days.[49] Apparently, the final action of melatonin at the level of the central nervous system in both sexes is a control of the hypothalamic GnRH secretion mainly through modulation of steroid-negative feedback; that indirect effect of melatonin on GnRH is also indicative of several neurotransmitter systems to be involved in the regulation of LH. Since the main effect of melatonin is a modification of steroid feedback onto GnRH secretion, melatonin- and steroid-dependent pathways seem to be related.[5]

The mapping of melatonin receptors showed that a great number is present in hypothalamic neurons regulating the release of pituitary gonadotropins as well as in the anterior pituitary.[57,58] Recent studies suggest that melatonin receptors are present in both female and male gonads,[59–63] indicating a direct effect of melatonin on the testis and the ovarian cells.[64] Moreover, both melatonin receptors are present on human and rat myometrial cell membranes,[65] and particularly, these receptors isolated from women's myometrium, during labor are markedly up-regulated.[34,66]

6.5.2 Female

Several studies support the correlation between primates' puberty and melatonin concentration; serum melatonin concentrations in prepubertal children and female monkeys are higher than those in adults.[67–70] The determination of 6-hydroxymelatonin, the main metabolite of the pineal hormone in urinary excretion, showed that the production of melatonin during pubertal development was reduced.[71–73] The finding that menarche and first ovulation are advanced in spring-born female monkeys by imposing a short-day pattern of circulating melatonin during the long days of the summer preceding the third breeding season points out the pineal gland as an important part of the mechanism mediating the seasonal influence on the timing of the onset of puberty in this species.[69] In humans, as previously mentioned, pineal tumors that destroy gland parenchyma induce suppression of melatonin synthesis and pulsatile GnRH release, leading to a precocious puberty.[39] However, in some cases, melatonin concentration seems to be independent from the elevated gonadal hormones. In idiopathic precocious gonadarche, melatonin concentrations were lower than the respective ones of the prepubertal age but similar with those of normal pubertal subjects,[54] while treatment with GnRH analogue, which suppressed pituitary–gonadal hormones, was unable to return melatonin to normal levels.[74] At present, there are not enough data to support the idea that the reduced circulating melatonin concentration is the signal for pubertal resurgence of pulsatile GnRH release in human, so it appears that the capacity of puberty attainment is probably independent of season.

Most studies investigating the regulatory mode of action of melatonin in reproduction have focused in the hypothalamus and pituitary as target tissues, with little attention directed to the role this hormone plays in the gonads itself.

Melatonin concentrations either in human or rat ovarian follicular fluid (FF) obtained from Graafian follicles are significantly higher than those in peripheral serum.[75,76] Although the most likely origin of melatonin in the human preovulatory FF is the general circulation,[75] it may also be synthesized in the granulosa ovarian cells.[77] According to Tamura et al.,[78] melatonin in the FF diffuses into the cumulus oophorus and oocytes to protect them from free radical damage. Among the proposed functions of melatonin in the FF stands the possibility that, via its antioxidative actions, melatonin reduces apoptosis of critical cells and allows preovulatory follicles to fully develop and provide mature oocytes for ovulation.[79]

In human ovarian cells, melatonin stimulated steroid synthesis,[59–81] and that effect seems to be influenced by the diverse endocrine environment of the menstrual phases. Melatonin stimulated progesterone production from preovulatory granulosa cells, enhanced basal and human chorionic gonadotropin–stimulated progesterone production from cells of day 18 to 27 corpora lutea, and stimulated androstenedione synthesis from ovarian stroma.[80,81] On the other hand, the administration of melatonin alone or combined with progesterone inhibited estradiol and LH secretion in normal cycling women and the combination is proposed as a promising contraceptive.[82] However, it is believed that melatonin has the ability to stimulate LH release in order to synchronize the preovulatory rise at night time. Particularly, the LH surge showed a circadian pattern with a maximal incidence at late night–early morning.[83–85] The ability of melatonin to stimulate LH release may be due to its specific action on hypothalamic receptors, by modifying a system of neurotransmitters and hormones that may enhance GnRH release.[52,86–90] The presence of specific melatonin receptors on human anterior pituitary supports the direct effect of melatonin on pituitary cells,[91] through which melatonin may exerts its stimulatory effects during the follicular phase.[92] The loss of this stimulatory effect of melatonin during the luteal phase implies either hormone-induced modification in the number of melatonin receptors or interruptions in the mechanisms in force. As mentioned above, melatonin treatment enhanced basal and human chorionic gonadotropin–stimulated progesterone production from cells of day 18 to 27 corpora lutea[81] and inhibited GnRH and GnRH receptor in the ovary. On this account, a physiological role for local GnRH has been suggested, as a paracrine and/or autocrine molecule, for the regression of corpus luteum.[93] Taking the above into consideration, the involvement of melatonin in the maintenance of the corpus luteum during pregnancy in women could be suggested. Finally, a positive correlation seems to exist between melatonin and the rising pulsatile secretion of prolactin (PRL) without significant changes in its temporal pattern.[94] All studies agree that melatonin administration was able to increase PRL secretion in normal women[52] and that is in accordance with its possible role countering to dopamine (PRL inhibitor) release.[95]

In a recent study by Wood et al.[96] in human-assisted reproduction, seasonality is indicated as a key factor for the greater success in vitro fertilization and embryo transfer (IVF–ET). Specifically, there was a significant improvement in assisted conception outcomes in cycles performed in summer (lighter) months, with more efficient ovarian stimulation, a significantly improved implantation rate per embryo transferred, and greater clinical pregnancy rate during summer cycles. Moreover, in a clinical study of IVF–ET, 56 women were treated with 3 mg of melatonin daily from day 5 of the previous menstrual cycle until the oocyte retrieval, while 59 women were left untreated; melatonin-treated women showed double score in fertilization and pregnancy rates compared with women not treated with melatonin.[78] These results probably validate the beneficial antioxidant role of melatonin of protecting the oocytes from oxidative damages. Likewise, in sheep, pretreatment of ovum pick-up donors with melatonin implants was found to improve oocyte developmental competence, as indicated by the higher fertilization and blastocyst rates obtained.[97] There are accumulated data suggesting that melatonin benefits mouse oocytes and oocytes and early embryo development in the buffalo, pig, and cow;[98–101] in contrast, the enrichment of the in vitro maturation medium with melatonin at various concentrations did not show any improvement in bovine fertilization rate and embryo production.[102] More studies should be addressed to evaluate the benefit of melatonin in various steps of the IVF–ET procedure, taking into consideration the low outcome of the latter.

Espey et al.[103] compared normal ovulation with a local inflammatory response in the wall of the follicle, which resulted in the production of reactive oxygen and nitrogen species (ROS and RNS, respectively) by local inflammatory cells. Cells existing near the follicular rupture suffer irreparable damages and undergo apoptosis; as a consequence, the oocyte may be in toxic danger. Given that melatonin effectively mitigates toxic damage,[104,105] the high endogenous concentrations of melatonin in the FF may serve to protect both the oocytes and the granulosa cells from the abundant radical byproducts.[34] These beneficial actions of melatonin may be either the already known receptor-independent free radical scavenging processes or an indirect melatonin receptor–dependent action.[99]

Many authors suggest that, in humans, the amount of melatonin synthesized in the pineal gland is influenced by age,[106] i.e., slowly declining after 40 years.[107,108] Oocytes and granulosa cells—as in other cells—in aged subjects are threatened by increased oxidative damage; thus, it is probable that melatonin supplementation may be useful in cases of women who are near the end of their reproductive age and want to become pregnant. Whether endogenous blood levels of melatonin fall at all in the aged or whether the drop is secondary due to side effects of drugs older persons take is not clear.[109,110] However, in aged drug-free rats and Syrian hamsters, marked reductions in pineal melatonin production have been proposed.[111,112]

Finally, to enforce the antioxidant defense of the reproductive system against free radicals in pathophysiological states such as preeclampsia, ischemia–reperfusion, hyperoxia, toxic drug administration, etc., in which elevated levels of oxidizing agents are generated, pharmacological doses of antioxidants, melatonin among others, will need to be administered. Melatonin has been found to be more efficient than vitamin C in reducing the extent of oxidative stress in an experimental model of Alzheimer's disease[113] or at least as effective as a combination of vitamins C and E in reducing the oxidative stress in rats.[114] Furthermore, melatonin has a very low toxicity profile, even during pregnancy.[115–117]

Aside from the tissues mentioned above, recent studies have shown that human myometrium is also a target for melatonin, as it expresses melatonin receptors that potentially increase during labor.[65,118,119] Given that human births occur more frequently at night, when melatonin levels are increased, researchers suggested a role for melatonin in parturition. Although Ayar et al.[120] claimed that melatonin inhibited spontaneous and oxytocin-induced contractions of rat myometrium in vitro, Sharkey et al.[66] support that, in myometrial cells, the action of melatonin synergizes with that of oxytocin to promote muscle contractions and gap junction activity, which are important for the coordination of myometrial contractions. These observations on cultured uterine cells need to be confirmed on in vivo clinical trials so that they will give new pharmacological strategies for the management of preterm or delayed parturition.

6.5.3 Male

During long-daylight photoperiod, administration of melatonin in rams either orally in daily doses or by slow release implants induced an increase of LH and FSH concentrations as well as a reduction of PRL level in blood plasma; mean testosterone concentration, basal level, and peak number of testosterone in blood plasma were increased.[121–126] This increase has been attributed to an indirect effect of melatonin on the hypothalamus, with a consequent increase of GnRH secretion and the subsequent increase of pituitary LH secretion.[127–128] Other studies have indicated a direct effect of melatonin on pituitary and increase of LH secretion.[124–126,128,129] Moreover, melatonin implants in Chios rams—a Greek breed—during breeding (autumn) and nonbreeding (spring) seasons increased the activity of some acrosomal enzymes, acrosin, and plasminogen activator, which are released during acrosome reaction,[130] indicating an improvement in the spermatozoa's capability to penetrate the zona pelucida during the fertilization process; these effects have been attributed to the direct or indirect (through testosterone) influence of melatonin.[125,126] However, in a more recent study, it is proposed that long-day exposure followed by melatonin treatment successfully increased testosterone level and improved semen characteristics (sperm motility, viability, total sperm output, percentage of abnormalities, etc.) of Damascus male goats during breeding and nonbreeding seasons.[6] The above beneficial effects were more pronounced during the breeding season, a period in which the hypothalamus–pituitary–testis axis is more active.

Melatonin treatment induced regression of the prostate and atrophy of secretory cell organelles in the accessory sex organs, including the prostate, of golden hamsters.[131] That inhibitory effect of melatonin on the prostate may be mediated through other endocrine systems. Alternatively, a direct action of melatonin has also been proposed, as high-affinity–specific and G protein–coupled melatonin receptors have been reported in the cytosol of human prostate glandular epithelial cells. These receptors may be responsible for the significant inhibitory effect of melatonin on human prostatic cell growth in vitro.[132]

In humans, melatonin may be involved in the modulation of reproductive neuroendocrine axis in males.[133] A strong significant negative correlation has been found between gonadotropins and melatonin release.[134] However, there is much controversy regarding the correlation between melatonin and male fertility. According to Luboshitzky et al.,[135] blood melatonin levels were significantly higher than those of the seminal plasma in a normal man, while no correlation existed among sperm count, motility, morphology, and blood or seminal plasma melatonin concentrations. Sperm motility and seminal melatonin concentration showed no correlation in the study of Bomman et al.,[136] while others found a positive correlation of seminal and serum melatonin with sperm motility and serum PRL.[133] Abnormal sperm motility was correlated with low melatonin levels,[137] whereas in oligozoospermic and azoospermic samples, the higher seminal melatonin was negatively correlated with sperm motility progression.[138] Relative to the mechanism of melatonin action, it is suggested that the hormone possibly controls sperm motility by cAMP protein phosphorylation cascade[139] or/and by influencing the microtubular sliding mechanism of the sperm axoneme.[140] Seminal plasma from infertile men had lower antioxidant levels than that of fertile ones, particularly those semen with poor sperm motility.[141] Melatonin is considered as a potent antioxidant in the semen and this might explain the reduced levels of melatonin in infertile subjects. ROS were significantly higher in infertile subjects with varicocele (88.9%) and leucocytospermia (92.6%) compared with normozoospermic men (55%).[142] Significant variation in the ROS-generating capacity of sperm was also established in infertile as well as in fertile men with varicocele compared with normal fertile cases.[143] The decreased antioxidants in semen in infertile cases with varicocele were corrected after varicocelectomy.[144] It seems that the enhanced ROS production might be the determinant responsible for infertility, and melatonin might protect sperm mitochondria from the damage induced by ROS through its antioxidant potential.[145]

However, Gavella and Lipovac[146] suggested that since melatonin in human semen is at the nanomolar level, its antioxidative role in vivo is of minor importance.

Melatonin alters the morphology, the steroidogenesis, or cGMP production of testicular tissues, the Leydig cells.[147–151] The above findings indicate a direct melatonin action on the testis. High-affinity melatonin receptors are localized in the rat corpus epididymis, while testosterone administration reversed the castration-decreased epididymal 2[^{125}] iodomelatonin-binding density in rats.[152,153] On the other hand, melatonin in vitro reduced forskolin increased c-AMP accumulation in rat epididymal cells.[154] These findings imply a direct melatonin action, via the activation of specific Gi protein–coupled receptors on the regulation of corpus epididymal physiology and reproductive functions in rats.[153]

Mammalian spermatozoa, in order to be capable of fertilizing an oocyte, must be capacitated and thereafter undergo acrosome reaction and hyperactivation. Hyperactivation is a specialized movement of the flagellum of the sperm that permits it to penetrate the zona pellucida. As human seminal fluid contains melatonin[136] and spermatozoa reportedly possess membrane melatonin receptors,[155] Fujinoki[156] investigated whether melatonin would influence hyperactivation of hamster sperm and found that physiological melatonin concentrations in the seminal plasma did not correlate with sperm motility. On the other hand, in mammals with seasonality in reproduction during short photoperiod, there are in vitro indications of a stimulating role of melatonin on reproductive capacity of sperm; in particular, there are data demonstrating that melatonin in vitro determines capacitation of buffalo spermatozoa in a dose-dependent manner.[157]

Further studies are needed to clarify the role of melatonin in sperm activation and function in humans and other species.

6.6 CONCLUSION

Despite the evidence accumulated over the years about the rules governing the melatonin regulation of seasonal reproductive events in long- and short-day breeders, basic questions are still unanswered. How does the same melatonin signal produce opposite effects in long- and short-day breeders? How does the same melatonin signal produce opposite effects depending on the prior melatonin exposure of the individual? Considerable progress has been made in identifying sites of action and receptors of melatonin in various tissues, while many aspects of the seasonal breeding are still unclear. Knowledge of the role of clock genes in melatonin signals decoding, cloning of melatonin receptors subtypes, delineation of the neurotransmitter, and hormone network controlled by melatonin should provide answers into the long-term mechanisms underscore the control of GnRH secretion by melatonin.

On the other hand, melatonin is no longer only applicable to the regulation of seasonal reproductive events through the hypothalamus–pituitary–gonadal axis in long- and short-day breeding mammals or as contraceptive in humans. The discovery of melatonin as a direct free radical scavenger and an indirect antioxidant has greatly expanded the mechanisms whereby melatonin preserves reproductive homeostasis. Recent studies have shown melatonin's ability to protect the gametes from oxidative and nitrosative damage, and it could be further tested to determine if it would improve the outcome of IVF–ET procedures or influence sperm preservation in humans and other species. Given the high failure rate and cost of these procedures, the former could be proved as a significant application. Finally, the possible role of melatonin in reinforcing the antioxidative status of the uterus during pregnancy could attenuate serious dangers. Further investigations in this area are of great interest in human and animal reproductive physiology.

REFERENCES

1. Chemineau, P., Guillaume, D., Migaud, M., Thiery, J.C., Pellicer-Rubio, M.T., and Malpaux, B. Seasonality of reproduction in mammals: Intimate regulatory mechanisms and practical implications. *Reprod. Domest. Anim.* 43, 40–47, 2008.
2. Reiter, R.J. The pineal and its hormones in the control of reproduction in mammals. *Endocr. Rev.* 1, 109–131, 1980.
3. Karsch, F.J., Bittman, E.L., Foster, D.L., Goodman, R.L., Legan, S.J., and Robinson, J.E. Neuroendocrine basis of seasonal reproduction. *Rec. Prog. Horm. Res.* 40, 185–232, 1984.
4. Ortavant, R., Pelletier, J., Ravault, J.P., Thimonier, J., and Volland-Nail, P. Photoperiod: Main proximal and distal factor of the circannual cycle of reproduction in farm mammals. *Oxf. Rev. Reprod. Biol.* 7, 305–345, 1985.
5. Malpaux, B. Seasonal regulation of reproduction in mammals. In Neill, J.D. (ed.), *Knobil and Neill's Physiology of Reproduction*, 3rd edn. Elsevier, Amsterdam, pp. 2231–2281, 2006.
6. Ramadan, T.A., Taha, T.A., Samak, M.A., and Hassan, A. Effectiveness of exposure to long day followed by melatonin treatment on semen characteristics of Damascus male goats during breeding and non-breeding seasons. *Theriogenology* 71, 458–468, 2009.
7. Baker, J.R. The evolution of breeding seasons. In de Beer, G.R. (ed.), *Evolution: Essays on Aspects of Evolutionary Biology,* Oxford University Press, Oxford, pp. 161–177, 1938.
8. Bronson, F.H. *Mammalian Reproductive Biology*. University of Chicago Press, London, 1989.
9. Thwaites, C.J. Photoperiodic control of breeding activity in the Southdown ewe with particular reference to the effects of an equatorial light regime. *J. Agric. Sci. Cambridge* 65, 57–65, 1965.
10. Foster, D.L., and Jackson, L.M. Puberty in the sheep. In Neill, J.D. (ed.), *Knobil and Neill's Physiology of Reproduction*, 3rd edn. Elsevier, Amsterdam, pp. 2127–2176, 2006.
11. Steger, R.W., Matt, K., and Bartke, A. Neuroendocrine regulation of seasonal reproductive activity in the male golden hamster. *Neurosci. Biobehav. Rev.* 9, 191–201, 1985.
12. Walker, M.L., Wilson, M.E., and Gordon, T.P. Endocrine control of the seasonal occurrence of ovulation in rhesus monkeys housed outdoors. *Endocrinology* 114, 1074–1081, 1984.
13. Lindburg, D.G. Seasonality of reproduction in primates. In Mitchell, G., and Erwin, J. (eds.), *Comparative Primate Biology, Vol 2B: Behavior, Cognition and Motivation.* Allan R. Liss, New York, pp. 167–218, 1987.
14. Chik, C.L., Almeida, O.F., Libre, E.A., Booth, J.D., Renquist, D., and Merriam, G.R. Photoperiod-driven changes in reproductive functions in male rhesus monkeys. *J. Clin. Endocrinol. Metab.* 74, 1068–1074, 1992.
15. Rowell, T.E. Variation in age at puberty in monkeys. *Folia Primatol.* 27, 284–290, 1977.
16. Roenneberg, T., and Aschoff, J. Annual rhythm of human reproduction. II. Environmental correlations. *J. Biol. Rhythms* 5, 217–239, 1990.
17. Wehr, T.A. Photoperiodism in humans and other primates: Evidence and implications. *J. Biol. Rhythms* 16, 348–364, 2001.
18. Bronson, F.H. Are humans seasonally photoperiodic? *J. Biol. Rhythms* 19, 180–192, 2004.
19. Roenneberg, T. The decline in human seasonality. *J. Biol. Rhythms* 19, 193–195, 2004.
20. Hoffmann, K., Illnerova, H., and Vanecek, J. Change in duration of the night time melatonin peak may be a signal driving photoperiodic responses in the Djungarian hamster (*Phodopus sungorus*). *Neurosci. Lett.* 67, 68–71, 1986.
21. Robinson, J.E., and Karsch, F.J. Photoperiodic history and a changing melatonin pattern can determine the neuroendocrine response of the ewe to day length. *J. Reprod. Fertil.* 80, 159–165, 1987.
22. Malpaux, B., Robinson, J.E, Brown, M.B., and Karsch, F.J. Importance of changing photoperiod and melatonin secretory pattern in determining the length of the breeding season in the Suffolk ewe. *J. Reprod. Fertil.* 83, 461–470, 1988.
23. Barrett, P., Schuster, C., Mercer, J.P., and Morgan, J.P. Sensitization: A mechanism for melatonin action in the pars tuberalis. *J. Neuroendocrinol.* 15, 415–421, 2003.
24. Lincoln, G.A. Decoding the nightly melatonin signal through circadian clock work. *Mol. Cell Endocrinol.* 252, 69–73, 2006.

25. Dupre, S.M., Butt, D.W., Talbot, R., Downing, A., Mouzaki, D., Waddington, D., Malpaux, B., Davis, J.R., Lincoln, G.A., and Loudon, A.S. Identification of melatonin regulated genes in the ovine pars tuberalis, a target site for seasonal hormonal control. *Endocrinology* 149, 5527–5539, 2008.
26. Panda, S., Nayak, S.K., Compo, B., Walker, J.R., Hogenesch, J.B., and Jegla, T. Illumination of the melanopsin signalling pathway. *Science* 307, 600–604, 2005.
27. Qui, X., Kumbalasiri, T., Carlson, S.M., Wong, K.Y., Krishna, V., Provencio, I., and Berson, D.M. Induction of photosensitivity by heterologous expression of melanopsin. *Nature* 433, 745–749, 2005.
28. Moore, R.Y., Speh, J.C., and Card, J.P. The retino-hypothalamic tract originates from a distinct subset of retinal ganglion cells. *J. Comp. Neurol.* 352, 351–366, 1995.
29. Hattar, S., Liao, H.W., Takao, M., Berson, D.M., and Yau, K.W. Melanopsin containing ganglion cells: Architecture, projections, and intrinsic photosensitivity. *Science* 295, 1065–1070, 2002.
30. Reiter, R.J. Melatonin: The chemical expression of darkness. *Mol. Cell. Endocrinol.* 79, C153–158, 1991.
31. Ruby, N.F., Brennan, T.J., Xie, X., Cao, V., Franken, P., Heller, H.C., and O'Hara, B.F. Role of melanopsin in circadian responses to light. *Science* 298, 2211–2213, 2002.
32. Hattar, S., Lucas, R.J., Mrosovsky, N., Thompson, S., Douglas, R.H., Hankins, M.W., Lem, J., Biel, M., Hofmann, F., Foster, R.G., and Yau, K.W. Melanopsin and rod–cone photoreceptive systems account for all major accessory visual functions in mice. *Nature* 424, 76–81, 2003.
33. Reiter, R.J., and Hester, R.J. Interrelationships of the pineal gland, the superior cervical ganglia and the photoperiod in the regulation of the endocrine systems of hamsters. *Endocrinology* 79, 1168–1170, 1966.
34. Reiter, R.J., Tan, D.X., Manchester, L.C., Paredes, S.D., Mayo, J.C., and Sainz, R.M. Melatonin and reproduction revisited. *Biology of Reproduction* 81, 445–456, 2009.
35. Wehr, T.A. Photoperiodism in humans and other primates: Evidence and implications. *J. Biol. Rhythms* 16, 348–364, 2001.
36. Wehr, T.A., Moul, D.E., Barbato, G., Giesen, H.A., Seidel, J.A., Barker, C., and Bender, C. Conservation of photoperiod-responsive mechanisms in humans. *Am. J. Physiol.*, 265, R846–R857, 1993.
37. Ravault, J.P., and Chesneau, D. The onset of increased melatonin secretion after the onset of darkness in sheep depends on the photoperiod. *J. Pineal Res.* 27, 1–8, 1999.
38. Goldman, B.D. Mammalian photoperiodic system: Formal properties and neuroendocrine mechanisms of photoperiodic time measurement. *J. Biol. Rhythms* 16, 283–301, 2001.
39. Aries Kappers, J. A survey of advances in pineal research. In Reiter, R.J. (ed.), *The Pineal Gland, Vol. 1*. CRC Press, Boca Raton, FL, pp. 1–25, 1981.
40. Lincoln, G.A. Photoperiodic control of seasonal breeding in the ram: Participation of the cranial sympathetic nervous system. *J. Endocrinol.* 82, 135–147, 1979.
41. Bittman, E.L., Dempsey, R.J., and Karsch, F.J. Pineal melatonin secretion drives the reproductive response to daylength in the ewe. *Endocrinology* 113, 2276–2283, 1983.
42. Brinklow, B.R., and Forbes, J.M. Effect of pinealectomy on the plasma concentrations of prolactin, cortisol and testosterone in sheep in short and skeleton long photoperiods. *J. Endocrinol.* 100, 287–294, 1984.
43. Seamark, R.F., Kennaway, D.J., Matthews, C.D., Fellenberg, A.J., Phillipou, G., Kotaras, P., McIntosh, J.E., Dustan, E., and Obst, J.M. The role of the pineal gland in seasonality. *J. Reprod. Fertil.* 30, 15–21, 1981.
44. Kennaway, D.J., Dustan, E.A., Gilmore, T.A., and Seamark, R.F. Effects of pinealectomy oestradiol and melatonin on plasma prolactin and LH secretion in ovariectomized sheep. *J. Endocrinol.* 102, 199–207, 1984.
45. Wayne, N.L., Malpaux, B., and Karsch, F.J. Social cues can play role in timing onset of the breeding season of the ewe. *J. Reprod. Fertil.* 87, 707–713, 1989.
46. Hoffmann, R.A., and Reiter, R.J. Pineal gland: Influence on gonads of male hamsters. *Science* 148, 1609–1611, 1965.
47. Chu, E.W., Wurtman, R.J., and Axelrod, J. An inhibitory effect of melatonin on the estrous phase of the estrous cycle of the rodent. *Endocrinology* 75, 238–242, 1964.
48. Lincoln, G.A., and Short, R.V. Seasonal breeding: Nature's contraceptive. *Rec. Prog. Horm. Res.* 36, 1–52, 1980.
49. Goodman, R.L., Bittman, E.L., Foster, D.L., and Karsch, F.J. Alterations in the control of luteinizing hormone pulse frequency underlie the seasonal variation in estradiol negative feedback in the ewe. *Biol. Reprod.* 27, 580–589, 1982.
50. Montgomery, G.W., Martin, G.B., and Pelletier, J. Changes in pulsatile LH secretion after ovariectomy in Ile-de-France ewes in two seasons. *J. Reprod. Fertil.* 73, 173–183, 1985.

51. Robinson, J.E., Radford, H.M., and Karsch, F.J. Seasonal changes in pulsatile luteinizing hormone (LH) secretion in the ewe: Relationship of frequency of LH pulses to day length and response to estradiol negative feedback. *Biol. Reprod.* 33, 324–334, 1985.
52. Solkoff, D., Inserra, P., and Watson, R.R. Melatonin and Reproduction. In Watson, R.R. (ed.), *Melatonin in the Promotion of Health.* CRC Press, Washington, DC, pp. 191–202, 1999.
53. Gupta, D., Halder, C., Coelevald, M., and Roth, J. Ontogeny, circadian rhythm-pattern and hormonal modulation of 5-alpha-dihydrotestosterone receptors in the rat pineal. *Neuroendocrinology* 57, 45–53, 1993.
54. Waldhauser, F., Boepple, P.A., Schemper, M., Mansfield, M.J., and Crowley, Jr. W.F. Serum melatonin in central precocious puberty is lower than in age-matched prepubertal children. *J. Clin. Endocrinol. Metab.* 73, 793–796, 1991.
55. Luboshitzky, R., Tiosano, D., Ben-Harush, M., Thuma, I., Ayash, A., Lavie, P., and Etziono, A. Pseudo-precocious puberty in a male patient and the melatonin–testosterone–relationship. *J. Ped. Endocrinol. Metab.* 8, 295–299, 1995.
56. Luboshitzky, R, Dharan, M., Goldman, D., Hiss, Y., Herer, P., and Lavie, P. Immunohistochemical localization of gonadotropin and gonadal steroid receptors in human pineal gland. *J. Clin. Endocrinol. Metab.* 82, 977–981, 1997.
57. Roy, D., Angelini, N., Fujeda, H., Brown, G.M., and Belsham, D.D. Cyclical regulation of GnRH gene expression in GTI-7 GnRH secreting neurons by melatonin. *Endocrinology* 142, 4711–4720, 2001.
58. Dubocovich, M.L., and Markowska, M. Functional MT1 and MT2 melatonin receptors in mammals. *Endocrine* 27, 101–110, 2005.
59. Yie, S.M., Brown, G.M., Liu, G.Y., Collins, J.A., Daya, S., Hughes, E.G., Foster, W.G., and Younglai, E.V. Melatonin and steroids in human preovulatory follicular fluid: Seasonal variation and granulosa cell steroid production. *Human Reprod.* 10, 50–55, 1995.
60. Shiu, S., Yu, Z., Chow, P., and Pang, S. Putative melatonin receptors in the male reproductive tissues. In Tang, P., Pang, S., and Reiter, R. (eds.), *Melatonin: A universal photoperiodic signal with diverse actions.* Karger, Hong Kong, pp. 90–100, 1996.
61. Sirotkin, A., and Schaeffer, H.J. Direct regulation of mammalian reproductive organs by serotonin and melatonin. *J. Endocrinol.* 154, 1–5, 1997.
62. Woo, M.M., Tai, C.J., Kang, S.K., Nathwani, P.S., Pang, S.F., and Leung, P.C. Direct action of melatonin in human granulose–luteal cells. *J. Clin. Endocrinol. Metab.* 86, 4789–4797, 2001.
63. Frungieri, M.B., Mayerhofer, A., Zitta, K., Pignarato, O.P., Calandra, R.S., and Gonzalez-Calvar, S.I. Direct action of melatonin on Syrian hamster testes. Melatonin subtype 1a receptors, inhibition of androgen production and interaction with local corticotrophin-releasing hormone system. *Endocrinology* 146, 1541–1552, 2005.
64. Reppert, S.M., Weaver, D.R., and Ebisawa, T. Cloning and characterization of a mammalian melatonin receptor that mediates reproductive and circadian responses. *Neuron* 13, 1177–1185, 1997.
65. Schlabritz-Loutsevitch, N., Hellner, N., Middendorf, R., Muller, D., and Olcese, J. The human myometrium as a target for melatonin. *J. Clin. Endocrinol. Metab.* 88, 908–913, 2003.
66. Sharkey, J.T., Puttaramu, R., Ward, R.A., and Olcese, J. Melatonin synergizes with oxytocin to enhance contractility of human myometrial smooth muscle cells. *J. Clin. Endocrinol. Metab.* 94, 421–427, 2009.
67. Silman, R.E., Leone, R.M., Hooper, R.J.L., and Preece, M.A. Melatonin, the pineal gland and human puberty. *Nature* 282, 301–303, 1979.
68. Attanasio, A., Borelli, P., and Gupta, D. Circadian rhythms in serum melatonin from infancy to adolescence. *J. Clin. Endocrinol. Metab.* 61, 388–390, 1985.
69. Wilson, M.E., and Gordon, T.P. Nocturnal changes in serum melatonin during female puberty in rhesus monkeys: A longitudinal study. *J. Endocrinol.* 121, 553–562, 1988.
70. Salti, R., Galluzzi, F., Bindi, G., Perfetto, F., Tarquini, R., Hallberg, F., and Cornelissen, G. Nocturnal melatonin patterns in children. *J. Clin. Endocrinol. Metab.* 85, 2137–2144, 2000.
71. Tetsuo, M., Poth, M., and Markey, S.P. Melatonin metabolite excretion during childhood and puberty. *J. Clin. Endocrinol. Metab.* 55, 311–313, 1982.
72. Young, I.M., Francis, P.L., Leone, A.M., Stovell, P., and Silman, R.E. Constant pineal output and increasing body mass account for declining melatonin levels during human growth and sexual maturation. *J. Pineal Res.* 5, 71–85, 1988.
73. Cavallo, C., and Dolan, L.M. 6-Hydroxymelatonin sulphate excretion in human puberty. *J. Pineal Res.* 21, 225–230, 1996.
74. Berga, S.L., Jones, K.L., Kaufmann, S.and Yen, S.S.C. Nocturnal melatonin levels are unaltered by ovarian suppression in girls with central precocious puberty. *Fertil. Steril.* 52, 936–941, 1989.

75. Brzezinski, A., Seibel, M.M., Lynch, H.J., Deng, M.H., and Wurtman, R.J. Melatonin in human follicular fluid. *J. Clin. Endocrinol. Metab.* 64, 865–867, 1987.
76. Soares, J.M., Masana, M.I., Ersahin, C., and Dubocovich, M.L. Functional melatonin receptors in rat ovaries at various stages of the estrous cycle. *J. Pharmacol. Exp. Ther.* 306, 694–702, 2003.
77. Itoh, M.T., Ishizaka, B., Kuribayashi, Y., Amemiya, A., and Sumi, Y. Melatonin, its precursors, and synthesizing enzyme activities in the human ovary. *Mol. Hum. Reprod.* 5, 402–408, 1999.
78. Tamura, H., Takasaki, A., Miwa, I., Taniguchi, K., Maekawa, R., Asada, H., Taketani, T., Matsuoka, A., Yamagata, Y., Shimamura, K., Morioka, H., Ishikawa, H., Reiter, R.J., and Sugino, N. Oxidative stress impairs oocyte quality and melatonin protects oocytes from free radical damage and improves fertilization rates. *J. Pineal Res.* 44, 280–287, 2008.
79. Tamura, H., Nakamura, Y., Korkmaz, A., Manchester, L.C., Tan, D.X., Sugino, N., and Reiter, R.J. Melatonin and the ovary: Physiological and pathophysiological implications. *Fertil. Steril.* 92, 328–343, 2009.
80. MacPhee, A.A., Cole, F.E., and Rice, B.F. The effect of melatonin on steroido-genesis by the human ovary in vitro. *J. Clin. Endocrinol. Metab.* 40, 688–696, 1975.
81. Webley, G.E., and Luck, M.R. Melatonin directly stimulates the secretion of progesterone and bovine granulosa cells in vitro. *J. Reprod. Fertil.* 78, 711–717, 1986.
82. Voordouw, B.C., Euser, R., Verdonk, R.E., Alberda, B.T., de Jong, F.H., Drogendijk, A.C., Fauser, B.C., and Cohen, M. Melatonin and melatonin–progestin combinations alter pituitary–ovarian function in women and can inhibit ovulation. *J. Clin. Endocrinol. Metab.* 74, 108–117, 1992.
83. Testart, J., Frydman, R., and Roger, M. Seasonal influence of diurnal rhythms in the onset of the plasma luteinizing hormone surge in women. *J. Clin. Endocrinol. Metab.* 55, 374–377, 1982.
84. Brzezinski, A., Lynch, H.J., Wurtman, R.J., and Seibel, M.M. Possible contribution of melatonin to the timing of the luteinizing hormone surge. *N. Engl. J. Med.* 316, 1550–1551, 1987.
85. Zimmermann, R.C., Schroder, S., Baars, S., Schumacher, M., and Weise, H.C. Melatonin and the ovulatory luteinizing hormone surge. *Fertil. Steril.* 54, 612–618 1990.
86. Kao, L.W., and Weisz, J. Release of gonadotropin releasing hormone (GnRH) from isolated perifused medial–basal hypothalamus by melatonin. *Endocrinology* 100, 1723–1726, 1977.
87. Richardson, S.B., Prasad, J.A., and Hollander, C.S. Acetylcholine, melatonin and potassium depolarization stimulate release of luteinizing hormone releasing hormone (LHRH) from rat hypothalamus in vitro. *Proc. Natl. Acad. Sci. USA* 79, 2686–2689, 1982.
88. Glass, J.D. Neuroendocrine regulation of seasonal reproduction by the pineal gland and melatonin. *Pineal Res. Rev.* 6, 219–259, 1988.
89. Morgan, P.J., and Williams, L.M. Central melatonin receptors: Implication for a mode of action. *Experientia* 45, 955–965, 1989.
90. Rasmussen, D.D. Diurnal modulation of rat hypothalamic gonadotropin releasing hormone (GnRH) release by melatonin in vitro. *J. Endocrinol. Invest.* 16, 1–7, 1993.
91. Weaver, D.R., Stehle, J.H., Stopa, E.G., and Reppert, S.M. Melatonin receptors in human hypothalamus and pituitary implications for circadian and reproductive responses to melatonin. *J. Clin. Endocrinol. Metab.* 76, 295–301, 1993.
92. Yen, S.S. The human menstrual cycle: Neuroendocrine regulation. In Yen SS., and Jaffe, R.B. (eds.), *Reproductive Endocrinology*, 3rd edn. Saunders, Philadelphia, pp. 273–308, 1991.
93. Nathwani, P.S., Kang, S.K., Cheng, K.W., Choi, K.C., and Leung, P.C. Regulation of gonadotropin-releasing hormone and its receptor gene expression by 17beta-estradiol in cultured human granulosa–luteal cells. *Endocrinology* 141, 1754–1763, 2000.
94. Terzolo, M. Revelli, A., Guidetti, D., Piovesan, A., Cassoni, P., Paccotti, P., Angeli, A., and Massobrio, M. Evening administration of melatonin enhances the pulsatile secretion of prolactin but not of LH and TSH in normally cycling women. *Clin. Endocrinol.* 39, 185–191, 1993.
95. Iuvone, P.M., and Gan, J. Functional interaction of melatonin receptors and D1 dopamine receptors in cultured chick retinal neurons. *J. Neurosci.* 15, 2179–2185, 1995.
96. Wood, S., Quinn, A., Troupe, S., Kingsland, C., and Lewis-Jones, I. Seasonal variation in assisted conception cycles and the influence of photoperiodism on outcome in in vitro fertilization cycles. *Hum. Fertil.* 4, 223–229, 2006.
97. Valasi, F., Tsiligianni, Th., Papanikolaou, Th., Dimitriadis, I., Vainas, E., Samartzi, F., and Amiridis, G.S. Melatonin improves the developmental competence of sheep oocytes. *Reprod. Dom. Anim.* 41, 341 2006.
98. Voznesenkaya, T., Makogon, M., Bryzgina, T., Sukhina, V., Grushka, N., and Alexeyeva, I. Melatonin protects against experimental immune ovarian failure in mice. *Biol. Reprod.* 7, 207–220, 2007.

99. Manjunatha, B., Devaraj, M., Gupta, P., Ravindra, J., and Nandi, B. Effect of taurine and melatonin in the culture medium on buffalo in vitro embryo development. *Reprod. Domest. Anim.* 44, 12–16, 2009.
100. Kang, J.T., Koo, O.J., Kwon, D.K., Park, H.J., Jang, G., Kong, S.K., and Lee, B.C. Effects of melatonin on in vitro maturation of porcine oocyte and expression of melatonin receptor RNA in cumulus and granulosa cells. *J. Pineal Res.* 46, 22–28, 2009.
101. Papis, K., Poleszczuk, O., Wenta-Muchalska, E., and Modlinski, J.A. Melatonin effect in bovine embryo development in vitro in relation to oxygen concentration. *J. Pineal Res.* 43, 321–326, 2007.
102. Tsantarliotou, M.P., Attanasio, L., De Rosa, A., Boccia, L., Pellerano, G., and Gasparrini, B. The effect of melatonin on bovine in vitro embryo development. *Ital. J. Animal Sci.* 6, 488–489, 2007.
103. Espey, L.L. Current status of the hypothesis that mammalian ovulation is comparable to an inflammatory reaction. *Biol. Reprod.* 50, 233–238, 1994.
104. Tan, D.X., Chen, L.D., Poeggeler, B., Manchester, L.C., and Reiter, R.J. Melatonin: A potent, endogenous hydroxyl radical scavenger. *Endocrine J.* 1, 57–60, 1993.
105. Manda, K., Ueno, M., and Anzai, K. Melatonin mitigates oxidative damage and apoptosis in mouse cerebellum induced by high-LET ^{56}Fe particle irradiation. *J. Pineal Res.* 44, 189–196, 2008.
106. Reiter, R.J. The aging pineal gland and its physiological consequences. *Bioessays* 14, 169–175, 1992.
107. Zhao, Z.Y., Xie, Y., Fu, Y.R., Bogdan, A., and Touitou, Y. Aging and the circadian rhythm of melatonin: A cross-sectional study of Chinese subjects 30–110 years of age. *Chronobiol. Int.* 19, 1171–1182, 2002.
108. Zhou, J.N., Liu, R.Y., Heerikhuize, J., Hofman, M.A., and Swaab, D.F Alterations in the circadian rhythm of salivary melatonin begin during middle-age. *J. Pineal Res.* 34, 11–16, 2003.
109. Zeiter, J.M., Daniels, J.E., Duffy, J.F., Klerman, E.B., Shanahan, T.L., Dijk, D.J., and Cziesler, C.A. Do plasma melatonin concentrations decline with age? *Am. J. Med.* 108, 432–436, 1999.
110. Stoschitzby, K., Satotnik, A., Lercher, P., Zweiker, R., Maier, R., Liebmann, P., and Lindner, W. Influence of beta-blockers on melatonin release. *Eur. J. Clin. Pharmacol.* 55, 111–115, 1999.
111. Reiter, R.J., Richardson, B.A., Johnson, L.Y., Ferguson, B.N., and Dink, D.T. Pineal melatonin rhythm: Reduction in aging Syrian hamsters. *Science* 210, 1372–1373, 1980.
112. Reiter, R.J., Craft, C.M., Johnson, J.E. Jr., King, T.S., Richardson, B.A., Vaughan, G.M., and Vaughn, M.K. Age-associated reduction in nocturnal pineal melatonin levels in female rats. *Endocrinology* 109, 1295–1297, 1981.
113. Montilla-Lopez, P., Munoz-Agueda, M.C., Feijoo Lopez, M., Munoz-Castaneda, J.R., Bujalance-Arenas, I., and Tunez-Finana, I. Comparison of melatonin versus vitamin C on oxidative stress and antioxidant enzyme activity in Alzheimer's disease induced by okadaic acid in neuroblastoma cells. *Eur. J. Pharmacol.* 451, 237–243, 2002.
114. Gultekin, F., Delibas, N., Yasar, S., and Kilinc, I. In vivo changes in antioxidant systems and protective role of melatonin and a combination of vitamin C and vitamin E on oxidative damage in erythrocytes induced by chlorpyrifos-ethyl in rats. *Arch. Toxicol.* 75, 88–96, 2001.
115. Jahnke, G., Marr, M., Myers, C., Wilson, R., Travlos, G., and Price, C. Maternal and developmental toxicity evaluation of melatonin administered orally to pregnant Sprague–Dawley rats. *Toxicol. Sci.* 50, 271–279, 1999.
116. Cheung, R.T., Tipoe, G.L., Tam, S., Ma, E.S., Zou, L.Y., and Chan, P.S. Preclinical evaluation of pharmacokinetics and safety of melatonin in propylene glycol for intravenous administration. *J. Pineal Res.* 41, 337–343, 2006.
117. Jan, J.E., Wasdell, M.B., Freeman, R.D., and Bax, M. Evidence supporting the use of melatonin in short gestation infants. *J. Pineal Res.* 42, 22–27, 2007.
118. Steffens, F., Zhou, X.B., Sausbier, V., Sailer, C., Motejlek, K., Ruth, P., Olcece, J., Korth, M., and Weiland, T. Melatonin receptor signaling in pregnant and non-pregnant rat uterine myocytes as probed by large conductance Ca+ activated K+ channel activity. *Mol. Endocrinol.* 17, 2103–2115, 2003.
119. Sharkey, J., and Olcese, J. Transcriptional inhibition of oxytocin receptor expression in human myometrial cells by melatonin involves protein kinase C signaling. *J. Clin. Endocrinol. Metab.* 92, 4015–4019, 2007.
120. Ayar, A., Kutlu, S., Yilmaz, B., and Kelestimur, H. Melatonin inhibits spontaneous and oxytocin-induced concentrations of rat myometrium in vitro. *Neuroendocrinol. Lett.* 22, 199–207, 2001.
121. Kennaway, D.J., and Gilmore, T.A. Effects of melatonin implants in ram lambs. *J. Reprod. Fertil.* 73, 85–91, 1985.
122. Lincoln, G.A., and Ebling, F.J.P. Effect of constant-release implants of melatonin on seasonal cycles in reproduction, prolactin secretion and moulting in rams. *J. Reprod. Fertil.* 73, 241–253, 1985.
123. Lincoln, G.A., and Kelly, R.W. Test of ML23 as an antagonist to the effects of melatonin in the ram. *J. Reprod. Fertil.* 86, 737–743, 1989.

124. Chemineau, P., Malpaux, B., Delgadillo, J.A., Guérin, Y., Ravault, J.P., Thimonier, J., and Pelletier, J. Control of sheep and goat reproduction: Use of light and melatonin. *Anim. Reprod. Sc.* 30, 157–184, 1992.
125. Kokolis, N., Theodosiadou, E., Tsantarliotou, M., Rekkas, C., Goulas, P., and Smokovitis, A. The effect of melatonin implants on blood testosterone and acrosin activity in spermatozoa of the ram. *Andrologia* 32, 107–114, 2000.
126. Tsantarliotou, M.P., Kokolis, N.A., and Smokovitis, A. Melatonin administration increased plasminogen activator activity in ram spermatozoa. *Theriogenology* 69, 458–465, 2008.
127. Malpaux, B., Daveau, A., Maurice, F., Gayrard, V., and Thiery, J.C. Short-day effects of melatonin on luteinizing hormone secretion in the ewe: Evidence for central sites of action in the mediobasal hypothalamus. *Biol. Reprod.* 48, 752–760, 1993.
128. Arendt, J. Physiology of the pineal: Role in photoperiodic seasonal functions. In Arendt, J. (ed.), *Melatonin and the mammalian pineal gland*. Chapman & Hall, London, pp. 110–158, 1995.
129. De Reviers, M.M., Ravault, J.P., Tillet, Y., and Pelletier, J. Melatonin binding sites in the sheep pars tuberalis. *Neurosci. Lett.* 100, 89–93, 1989.
130. Taitzoglou, I.A., Kokolis, N., and Smokovitis, A. Release of plasminogen activator and plasminogen activator inhibitor from spermatozoa of man, bull, ram and boar during acrosome reaction. *Mol. Androl.* 8, 187–197, 1996.
131. Chow, P.H., and Pang, S.F. The male accessory sex glands, fertility and melatonin. *Adv. Pineal Res.* 3, 221–224, 1989.
132. Gilad, E., Laudon, M., Matzkin, H., Pick, E., Sofer, M., Braf, Z., and Zisapel, N. Functional melatonin receptors in human prostate epithelial cells. *Endocrinology* 137, 1412–1417, 1996.
133. Awad, H., Halawa, F., Mostafa, T., and Atta, H. Melatonin hormone profile in infertile males. *Int. J. Androl.* 29, 409–413, 2005.
134. Kumanov, P., Tomova, A., Isidori, A., and Nordio, M. Altered melatonin secretion in hypogonadal men: Clinical evidence. *Int. J. Androl.* 28, 234–240, 2005.
135. Luboshitzky, R., Shen-Orr, Z., and Herer, P. Seminal plasma melatonin and gonadal steroids concentrations in normal men. *Arch. Androl.* 48, 225–232, 2002.
136. Bomman, M.S., Oosthuizen, J.M.C., Barnard, H.C., Schulenburg, G.W., Boomker, P., and Reif, S. Melatonin and sperm motility. *Andrologia* 21, 483–485, 1989.
137. Van Vuuren, R.J., Du Plessis, D.J., and Theron, J.J. Melatonin in human semen. *S.A.M.J.* 73, 374–375, 1988.
138. Yie, S.M., Daya, S., Brown, G.M., Deys, L., and Younglai, E.V. Melatonin and aromatase stimulating activity or human seminal plasma. *Andrologia* 23, 227–231, 1991.
139. Guraya, S.S., *Biology of spermatogenesis and spermatozoa in mammals*, Springer-Verlag, Berlin, pp. 286–302, 1987.
140. Pitout, M.J., Van Vuuren, R.J., Van Aswegen, C.H., and Theron, J.J. Melatonin and sperm motility. *S.A.M.J.* 79, 683, 1991.
141. Lewis, S.E., Boyle, P.M., McKinney, K.A., Young, I.S., and Thompson, W. Total antioxidant capacity of seminal plasma is different in fertile and infertile men. *Fertil. Steril.* 64, 868–870, 1995.
142. Mazzilli, F., Rossi, T., Marchesini, M., Ronconi, C., and Dondero, F. Superoxide anion in human semen related to seminal parameters and clinical aspects. *Fertil. Steril.* 62, 862–868, 1994.
143. Weese, D.L., Peaster, M.L., Himsl, K.K., Laech, G.E., Lad, P.M., and Zimmern, P.E. Stimulated reactive oxygen species generation in the spermatozoa of infertile men. *J. Urol.* 149, 64–67, 1993.
144. Mostafa, T., Anis, T.H., El-Nashar, A., Imam, H., and Othman, I.A. Varicocelectomy reduces reactive oxygen species levels and inceases antioxidant activity of seminal plasma from infertile men with varicocele. *Int. J. Androl.* 24, 261–265, 2001.
145. Shang, X., Huang, Y., Ye, Z., Yu, X., and Gu, W. Protection of melatonin against damage of sperm mitochondrial function induced by reactive oxygen species. *Zhonghua Nan Ke Xue* 10, 604–607, 2004.
146. Gavella, M., and Lipovac, V. Antioxidative effect of melatonin on human spermatozoa. *Arch. Androl.* 44, 23–27, 2000.
147. Ellis, L.C. Inhibition of rat testicular androgen synthesis in vitro by melatonin and serotonin. *Endocrinology* 90, 17–28, 1972.
148. Ng, T.B., and Lo, L. Inhibitory actions on pineal indoles on steroidogenesis in isolated rat Leydig cells. *J. Pineal Res.* 5, 229–243, 1988.
149. Persengiev, S., and Kehajova, J. Inhibitory action of melatonin and structurally related compounds on testosterone production by mouse Leydig cells in vitro. *Cell Biochem. Funct.* 9, 281–286, 1991.

150. Niedziela, M. Lerchl, A., and Nieschlag, E. Direct effects of the pineal hormone melatonin on testosterone synthesis of Leydig cells in Djungarian hamsters (*Phodopus sungorus*) in vitro. *Neurosci. Lett.* 201, 247–250, 1995.
151. Valenti, S., Giusti, M. Guido, R., and Giordano, G. Melatonin receptors are present in adult rat Leydig cells and are coupled through a pertussis toxin-sensitive G-protein. *Eur. J. Endocrinol.* 136, 633–639, 1997.
152. Shiu, S.Y.W., Chow, P.H., Yu, Z.H., Tang, F., and Pang, S.F. Autoradiographic distribution and physiological regulation of 2-[^{125}I]iodomelatonin binding in rat epididymis. *Life Sci.* 59, 1165–1174, 1996.
153. Shiu, S.Y.W., Li, L., Wong, J.T.Y., and Pang, S.F. Biology of G protein–coupled melatonin receptors in the epididymis and prostate of mammals. *Chinese Med. J.* 110, 648–655, 1997.
154. Li, L., Xu, J.N., Pang, S.F., and Shiu, S.Y.W. Melatonin modulates cAMP signaling in rat epididymal epithelial cells. *FASEB J.* 12, A 686, 1998.
155. Van Vuuren, R.J.J., Pitout, M.J., Van Aswegen, C.H., and Theron, J.J. Putative melatonin receptor in human spermatozoa. *Clin. Biochem.* 25, 125–127, 1992.
156. Fujinoki, M. Melatonin-enhanced hyperactivation of hamster sperm. *Reproduction* 136, 533–541, 2008.
157. Di Fransesco, S., Mariotti, E., Tsantarliotou, M., Sattar, A., Venditto, I., Rubessa, M., Zicarelli, L., and Gasparrini, B. Melatonin promotes in vitro sperm capacitation in buffalo (Bubbalus Bubalis). *Reprod. Fertil. Dev.* 22, 311–312, 2010.

7 Melatonin and the Prevention of Ultraviolet Solar Skin Damage

Tobias W. Fischer

CONTENTS

7.1 INTRODUCTION

While melatonin was initially discovered by Lerner et al. [1] as a hormone produced by the pineal gland that lightens frog skin, the discovery of its strong antioxidative properties by Tan et al. [2] opened a wide field of research activities and applications of melatonin in a great variety of physiology and pathophysiology conditions in universal biology—from unicellular organisms, to animals, and to human being [3–11].

Classical chronobiology considers melatonin exclusively a neurohormone that regulates the circadian day/night rhythm and seasonal biorhythms [12–14]. Independent of that, in the mammalian system, melatonin has been shown to modulate immune defense responses [15,16], body weight, and reproduction [14] and to exert tumor growth–inhibitory and anti–jet lag effects [17–25]. Independent of these mainly melatonin receptor–dependent effects, melatonin exerts direct, receptor-independent activities, e.g., as a potent direct antioxidant [2,8,26,27], as a chemotoxicity-reducing agent [8,28–31], a putative general antiaging substance [4,32,33], and an anticancer agent [34].

Besides the classical multistep regulated intrapineal synthesis of melatonin, a significant body of evidence for multiple extrapineal sites of melatonin synthesis and significant melatonin levels in different organs and body compartments has accumulated during the past 20 years. These include the bile fluid, bone marrow, cerebrospinal fluid, ovary, eye, lymphocytes, gastric mucosa, and last but not least, the skin and hair [15,35–46]. These observations gave ground for the hypothesis and in fact lead to further clear recognition that melatonin plays a significant role as a strong protective agent in many cells and tissues in order to prevent or lower the impact of oxidative stress and its consequences on their respective biological functions. It is now widely accepted that these extrapineal melatonin production sites generate melatonin levels that suit their biological needs and that, importantly, the physiological levels of melatonin are defined tissue-specific [6]. The body liquids, tissues, or organs mentioned above have melatonin levels that may be 10- to 1000-fold higher than the plasma melatonin concentrations formerly considered as the "physiological" concentration, while concentration magnitudes higher than plasma concentrations had been traditionally considered "pharmacological" [6,47].

The presence of melatonin in high concentrations across very different biological organs and organ systems strongly suggests a ubiquitous and biologically highly relevant existence of tissue-specific, local melatoninergic systems that have the biological role of counteracting specific, tissue-related regional stressors exactly at the place where they occur [6,35,44,47,48]. In fact, such a melatoninergic antioxidative system (MAS) has been recently discovered in a highly differentiated manner in the skin where it regulates skin homeostasis and, most importantly, prevents the harmful consequences of ultraviolet (UV) solar skin damage, i.e., skin aging and skin cancer [41–44,49,50].

7.2 MELATONIN AS A MODULATOR OF PHYSIOLOGICAL SKIN FUNCTION

To comprehensively characterize melatonin as a potent agent in the prevention of UV solar skin damage, some general effects of melatonin on skin cells and tissues under physiological and pathological conditions will be described below.

Since changes in the skin and coat phenotype/function represent a major form of mammalian adaptation to the environmental challenges—and UV solar irradiation is one of its major and a ubiquitous one —it is not surprising that melatonin as a major neuroendocrine regulator that couples photoperiod changes to complex endocrine responses [14,51,52] impacts the mammalian skin physiology and pathology.

To start with, melatonin exerts effects on keratinocytes, the major residential skin cell population in the epidermis (90% of epidermal skin cells), and fibroblasts, the connective tissue cells of the dermis, by targeting growth modification of these cell populations [53,54]. Melatonin suppresses apoptosis and stimulates growth in both serum-starving HaCaT keratinocytes and serum-free cultured fibroblasts [54]. In contrast, growth of serum-supplemented HaCaT keratinocytes is inhibited by melatonin at low concentrations of 10^{-11} M and cell cycle arrest in the G0/G1 phase is induced at 10^{-12} M [54], whereas at very high concentrations ($4–20 \times 10^{-6}$ M) melatonin stimulates cell growth under the same serum-supplemented culture condition [53]. Regarding skin thickness, studies with pinealectomized (i.e., melatonin-deficient) rats revealed distinctly reduced back, abdominal, and thoracic skin thickness, along with an increase of lipid peroxidation and a decrease of protective antioxidative enzymes (catalase [CAT] and glutathione peroxidase [GPx]). Melatonin substitution to these rats reportedly restored skin thickness, reduced lipid peroxidation, and enhanced antioxidative enzyme activity [55]. These results, along with lack of melatonin, but under otherwise physiological (i.e., non-UV exposed) conditions, are strong indicators that melatonin may play a role in UV solar damage protection, since these two biological events (lipid damage and reduction of antioxidative enzymes) are crucial in UV-related oxidative damage in the skin [56]. Further investigations in melatonin-deficient rats showed increased cell atypia, increased nuclear irregularity, atypic tonofilament distribution, and disturbed mitochondrial integrity and dermal collagen fiber structure. These events, which are relevant in skin aging as well, were again reversed by melatonin substitution [57].

In another condition of skin damage induced by exogenous physical forces, such as heat and burn, which are principally similar to UV radiation–induced effects on the skin, melatonin reduced skin damage presumably by lowering oxidative damage, an observation that gives support for the use of melatonin as a therapeutic substance in burn patients [58,59].

7.3 ENHANCEMENT OF ANTIOXIDATIVE ENZYMES

A prerequisite for an efficient UV-protective substance is the enhancing effect on antioxidative enzymes, either on a gene expression levels or directly on enzyme activity. For such properties, melatonin qualifies optimally since it has been shown to enhance the activity of antioxidative enzyme systems in various organs and organ systems [60–64]. The activity of GPx, which reduces H_2O_2 to water, is up-regulated by melatonin in rat brain [60] and in several chicken tissues [63]. Of note, not only enzyme activity, but also gene transcription of antioxidant enzymes such as manganese superoxide dismutase (MnSOD), copper–zinc superoxide dismutase (CuZn–SOD), and GPx is up-regulated by melatonin during porphyrin-induced cell damage in rat brain cortex and in neuronal cell lines [61].

Melatonin effectively up-regulates enzyme gene expression at 10^{-9} M, a concentration that corresponds to the physiological nighttime peak of plasma melatonin [12]. Cultured cells incubated with melatonin for 1 hour generate elevated levels of mRNA for both SOD and GPx and maintain their levels for at least 24 hours. This prolonged elevation suggests a possible involvement of membrane and/or nuclear melatonin receptor activation with signal transduction on transcriptional mRNA level to modify the regulation of antioxidant enzymes by melatonin following outer signals to stress [65,66].

SOD and CAT are not only stimulated by melatonin under conditions of oxidative stress, but also under basal (nonstress) conditions—presumably to build a tissue's baseline protection against subsequent stressful conditions that generate free radicals [67,68]. In the context of the age-related free radical–mediated brain deterioration, melatonin acts more efficiently than vitamin E or vitamin C in detoxifying highly reactive hydroxyl and peroxyl radicals and stimulates GPx, the major antioxidant enzyme in the brain [69]. Considering the common neuroectodermal origin of the brain and epidermis, it is quite likely that these brain related findings are also relevant to the skin, especially since the brain and mammalian skin engage in constitutive and inducible melatonin synthesis to build a tissue protective antioxidative system [42,44–46,70].

Melatonin up-regulates mRNA levels for several antioxidative enzymes (Zn–SOD, CuZn–SOD, GPx, and γ-glutamylcysteine synthetase (γ-GCS), the rate-limiting enzyme of glutathione synthesis [61,62,71]. Currently, it is known that melatonin exerts quite a few of its effects via signal transduction ways mediated by membrane, cytosolic, and nuclear receptors [20,43,72–81]. Although the up-regulation of antioxidant enzyme gene expression by mediation through melatonin receptors has not yet conclusively been shown, some authors have proposed that melatonin-induced up-regulation of antioxidative enzymes involves at least both membrane and nuclear melatonin receptors [82]. Evidence for the latter rises from the observation that melatonin itself and a synthetic nuclear melatonin receptor agonist (CGP 52608) stimulate GPx and glutathione reductase activities in mouse brain [83].

7.4 DIRECT PROTECTIVE EFFECTS AGAINST UV SOLAR SKIN DAMAGE

While reduction of free radicals—the key mediators of oxidative damage—by melatonin has been shown earlier in numerous cell-free and biological systems with several free radical–inducing factors [28,84–88], the suppression of reactive oxygen species (ROS) induced by UV radiation has been first shown only in 2001 [89].

Free radicals and oxidative damage are, in fact, main factors in intrinsic and UV-induced skin aging [56,90,91], and therefore, reduction of free radicals by melatonin was then considered to represent an important function in melatonin-mediated protection against UV solar skin damage. This key observation introduced melatonin as a promising candidate in terms of a potent antioxidant and protective substance in skin photobiology [27,92]. In these studies, which were initially performed in leukocytes, which can be easily stimulated to develop a significant oxidative burst, melatonin was shown to exert radical scavenging properties at maximum effective concentrations of 10^{-8} and 10^{-3} M [89] (Figure 7.1). Additionally, melatonin kept free radical formation significantly low, while under non-melatonin–treated conditions, free radical formation significantly and UV dose–dependently increased at doses of 75, 150, and 300 mJ/cm [93] (Figure 7.2). In the same cell system, melatonin was shown to be a stronger antioxidant than vitamin C and trolox, a vitamin E

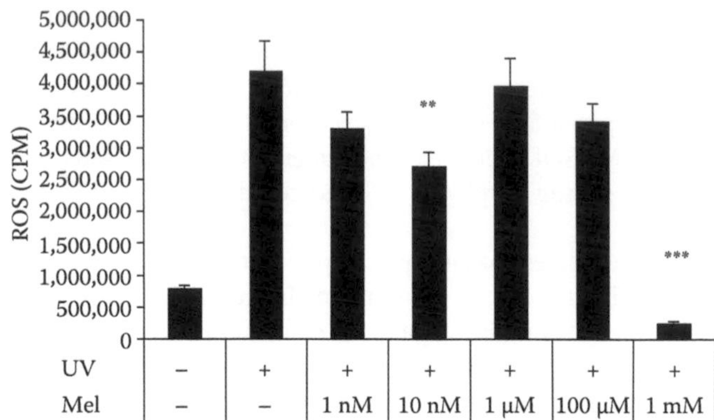

FIGURE 7.1 Melatonin significantly suppresses ROS induced by UV irradiation with UVB/UVA light at a wavelength of 280–360 nm at maximum effective concentrations of 10 nM (** $p < 0.01$) and 1 mM (*** $p < 0.001$) compared to non-melatonin–treated control; CPM, counts per minute as measured by chemiluminescence. (From Fischer, T. W., et al., *Exp. Dermatol.*, 17, 713–730, 2008. With permission.)

analog [94]. This superior potency may be based on the higher reduction potential of melatonin (0.73 V) compared with vitamin C (0.23 V) [8,94]. The lower reduction potential of vitamin C makes the latter even a pro-oxidant leading to the formation of the highly toxic hydroxyl radical, while to-date pro-oxidative properties of melatonin have not been shown [94]. The superiority of melatonin over vitamin E has been shown also in other studies [95]; however, there are also contrary observations in a human lipid bilayer and skin homogenate model, in which vitamin E leads to a higher reduction of peroxidation of liposomes than melatonin [96].

In UV-exposed fibroblasts at the UV dose of 140 mJ/cm^2, melatonin at a concentration of 1 nM leads to a cell survival rate of 92.5%, which was accompanied by significant inhibition of lipid

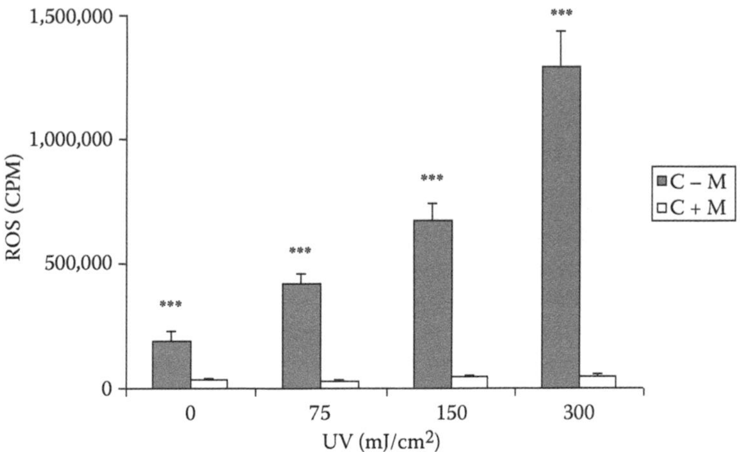

FIGURE 7.2 Formation of ROS in cell solutions (leukocytes) is kept significantly low by melatonin preincubation at 1 mM (white columns) compared with cell solutions that are not treated with melatonin (black columns). Cell solutions were irradiated with increasing doses of UV light (75–300 mJ/cm^2), and differences were highly significant at all applied UV doses (*** $p < 0.001$). (From Fischer, T. W., *J. Pineal Res.*, 37, 107–112, 2004. With permission.)

peroxidation and apoptosis, while fibroblasts not treated with melatonin showed cell survival of only 56% after UV irradiation [97]. A similar study in fibroblasts showed cell protection against UV-induced suppression of cell viability by antiapoptotic effects when they were preincubated with melatonin at a concentration of 100 nM [98].

Referring to human keratinocytes, the main target cell population in UV-induced epidermal skin damage, studies have been performed with UV radiation at increasing doses of 25, 50, 75, and 100 mJ/cm^2, which correspond to minimal erythema dose ranging from very fair, UV-sensible human skin type to darkly pigmented, UV-resistant human skin type and at a wavelength combination of UVB/UVA that mimics the skin's natural UV exposure. The UV-irradiated keratinocytes were investigated for proliferation, colony formation, and apoptotis by [^{3}H]-thymidine-labeled DNA incorporation, clonogeneicity, and terminal deoxynucleotidyl transferase dUTP nick end labeling assay, respectively. Melatonin preincubation with the initially identified maximum effective concentration of 10^{-4} and 10^{-3} M for 30 min led to a significantly increased cell survival and colony formation, which was paralleled by reduced UV-mediated apoptosis [99]. In microarray studies with keratinocytes, the transcription of several classical target genes that are up-regulated after UV exposure and that play an important role in the execution of skin photodamage, namely interstitial collagenase (MMP-1), stromelysin 1 (MMP-3), stromelysin 2 (MMP-10), and aldehyde dehydrogenase 3 type A1 was down-regulated by melatonin pretreatment [43,91,100–103]. Cho et al. [104] performed cDNA microarray analysis from keratinocytes that were pretreated with melatonin at the concentration of 100 nM for 30 min and then exposed to 100 mJ/cm^2. A great variety of genes related to apoptosis (apoptosis-related protein 3), cancer induction, cell cycle (cyclin-dependent kinase 2–interacting protein), enzymes (GPx, ubiquitin-conjugating enzyme E2M), and signal transducer genes (fibroblast growth factor, TGFβ-stimulated protein TSC 22) were down-regulated by melatonin compared with UV-exposed keratinocytes not pretreated with melatonin.

Analysis of mitochondrial (intrinsic) and death receptor–mediated (extrinsic) apoptosis pathways suggests that melatonin inhibits the intrinsic, but not the extrinsic apoptotic pathway and down-regulates its downstream effector caspases, casp-9 and casp-3 [105]. This pathway is induced by reduction of the mitochondrial membrane potential, which is caused by UV-related formation of mitochondrial ROS (mROS). Melatonin has been shown to effectively reduce mROS [106] and therefore is presumably able to significantly normalize mitochondrial membrane potential by reducing mROS also in this condition of UV-induced mitochondrial stress. These mitochondrial protective effects of melatonin have been shown for the concentrations of 10^{-6}, 10^{-4}, and 10^{-3} M in HaCaT keratinocytes [105].

These findings of differential antiapoptotic effects in keratinocyte cell culture give raise to the hypothesis that melatonin may exert effective protection against sunburn cell formation (i.e., intraepidermal keratinocyte apoptosis induced by excessive UV irradiation) in the skin in situ.

However, the antiapoptotic effects of melatonin under UV-induced damage with possible DNA damage would be biologically problematic if DNA damage would not be reduced in parallel. Therefore, the UV-induced activation of poly(ADP-ribose) polymerase (PARP), the key enzyme and direct proportional parameter for DNA damage, was investigated, and melatonin revealed significant inhibition of DNA damage within the first 24 hours after activation [105]. In parallel to molecular investigations, cell morphology analyses showed UV-induced increase of detached apoptotic keratinocytes, formation of dysmorphic cell shape, and nuclear chromatin condensation, which was counteracted by melatonin [105]. Thus, the potent protective effects of melatonin were shown at all relevant molecular and cellular levels of UV-induced apoptosis. With regard to biological relevant aspects on a clinical level, it can be stated that in the condition of diminished rate of DNA damage (as shown indirectly by PARP reduction), the suppressive effects of melatonin on apoptosis would result in the survival of a nonmalignant keratinocyte cell population and therefore may represent an effective strategy for the prevention of UV-induced photocarcinogenesis.

7.5 AUTONOMOUS AND UV-ENHANCED MELATONIN AND METABOLITE PRODUCTION IN SKIN CELLS

The so far described protective effects of melatonin against UV-induced solar skin damage were exclusively shown from investigations with exogenously added melatonin to skin cells. In 2002, Slominski et al. [42] reported that skin cells of multiple types (normal and immortalized skin keratinocytes, hair follicle keratinocytes, fibroblasts from dermis and hair follicle dermal papilla, melanocytes, melanoma cells, and squamous cell carcinoma cell lines) and cutaneous tissue samples from benign as well as malignant skin phenotypes (skin of basal cell carcinoma) express the essential enzymes for melatonin synthesis, namely tryptophan hydroxylase, arylalkylamine *N*-acetyltransferase (AANAT), and hydroxyindole-*O*-methyltransferase (HIOMT), and therefore it seemed very likely that melatonin can be produced in the skin as an extrapineal site of melatonin synthesis. In fact, it was shown already at that time that a product is detectable in HaCaT keratinocyte cell extracts by tandem LC/MS as an adduct ion with the same mass spectrum at *m/z* 233 (calculated mass of 232 Da) and 23-min retention time as melatonin standard. However, this product was detected at a level not very distinct from background, thus suggesting only carefully the presence of melatonin in skin cells [42].

Later, systematic investigations in keratinocytes under different experimental conditions of non-melatonin- and melatonin-supplemented keratinocyte cultures revealed time- and UV-dependent modifications of melatonin production or metabolization to specific melatonin degradants and, of note, definite melatonin detection in keratinocyte cell extracts at defined measurable levels [44]. Specifically, it was shown by high-performance liquid chromatography of keratinocyte cell extracts that naive (i.e., non-melatonin–preincubated) keratinocytes showed intracellular melatonin levels of 146.0 pmol/3 $\times 10^6$ cells, thus indicating autonomous melatonin synthesis by human keratinocytes at a level of approximately 11 fg per single keratinocyte. Given that the cell volume of a HaCaT keratinocyte is approximately 1.43 $\times 10^{-6}$ µl [107], the calculated intracellular melatonin concentration in this cell can be approximated to be 34 µM. Evaluation of melatonin levels after 24 hours of keratinocyte proliferation in culture showed decrease of melatonin down to 65.0 pmol/3 $\times 10^6$ cells, while there was a time-parallel increase of the melatonin metabolites 2-hydroxymelatonin from 7.8 pmol/3 $\times 10^6$ to 20.4 pmol/3 $\times 10^6$ cells and N^1-acetyl-N^2-formyl-5-methoxykynuramine (AFMK) from 17.4 pmol/3 $\times 10^6$ to 33.6 pmol/3 $\times 10^6$ cells, thus indicating a 24-hour consumption of melatonin with metabolism to above-mentioned melatonin metabolites [44]. Interestingly, these two metabolites are strong free radical scavengers themselves, especially AFMK, which is an up to four times stronger antioxidant than melatonin itself [85,108]. AFMK is also known to have anti-inflammatory properties, e.g., reduction of LPS-induced COX-2 up-regulation, decrease of inducible nitric oxide synthase and prostaglandin E2 [109]. Moreover, AFMK inhibits 5-aminolevulinic acid–induced DNA damage [110] and prevents protein destruction [111], therefore representing a potent antioxidative and anti-inflammatory agent against many different types of UV-induced solar damage.

These observations have also been seen in the context of the study setting in which they were generated. While earlier studies had investigated melatonin metabolites only in UV wavelengths that are not essentially related to UV-induced stress in cutaneous biology in naturam (300–575 nm, UV–visible light) [112], the above-mentioned and more recent studies have developed a human skin–related approach using relevant UV wavelengths within UVB/UVA range and also a mixed UV source (UVB 60% and UVA 30%) that is closer to the naturally occurring solar irradiation [44]. More interestingly, increasing UV doses (25, 50, and 100 mJ/cm^2) lead to direct proportional increase of melatonin metabolites, thus defining an UV-enhanced melatonin metabolism.

While earlier studies with detection of melatonin metabolites were carried out in cell-free systems [108,112], the recent studies with melatonin provided the first evidence for UV-enhanced photolytic and/or enzymatic melatonin metabolism in cultured human keratinocytes. Therefore, it can be concluded with almost certainty that human keratinocytes, and likely the skin and its appendages in vivo themselves too, are not only targets for protective exogenous melatonin treatment but also an extrapineal site of melatonin synthesis and of fully functioning local autonomous melatonin metabolism. Since cutaneous local synthesis and metabolism are inducible by UV irradiation, it can be further postulated that the skin provides itself a self-regulated protective system that is switched on by environmental stressors such as UV and ionizing radiation and also by inflammation [27,41–45,54,92,97–99,105,113–117].

7.6 THE MELATONINERGIC ANTIOXIDATIVE SYSTEM (MAS) OF THE SKIN

By identifying the UV-induced melatonin metabolism leading to the generation of antioxidant melatonin metabolites in human keratinocytes that exert strong antioxidative properties themselves, an antioxidative cascade that has been described earlier for chemical or other tissue homogenate systems [85,86,108] had been defined as the MAS of the skin [44] (Figure 7.3). The MAS would protect the skin as an important barrier organ against UV-induced oxidative stress–mediated damaging events on DNA, subcellular, protein, and cell morphology level. Because all metabolites are lipophilic, they would diffuse in every skin compartment, therefore extending the MAS beyond the epidermis, namely to the dermis and the hair follicle [43,46,118], where it represents a defense mechanism against the multifaceted threats of environmental stress, especially UV radiation, to which the skin is life-long exposed [27,41,43,119–125].

ROS, mainly the hydroxyl radical, occurring under UV irradiation in the skin react directly with melatonin [8,119,126,127]. Melatonin is either autonomously produced in epidermal and/or hair follicle keratinocytes where it engages in intracrine signaling/interactions or is released into the extracellular space to regulate autocrine, paracrine, or endocrine signaling [7,44,46]. The reaction of melatonin with hydroxyl radicals induces the formation of 2-OH- and 4-OH-melatonin, which are then further metabolized to AFMK and by arylamine formamidase or CAT to AMK [108,128]. During all steps of this process, hydroxyl radicals are scavenged, and resulting damaging events are either indirectly or directly reduced via decrease of lipid peroxidation, protein oxidation, mitochondrial damage, and DNA damage. This makes the melatoninergic antioxidative cascade very potent in reducing the extensive amounts of free radicals occurring under UV solar radiation and therefore represents a very promising strategy to protect the skin against this main environmental stressor and causative factor for skin aging and tumor promotion.

7.7 EFFECTS OF MELATONIN AGAINST UV-INDUCED SKIN DAMAGE IN CLINICAL DERMATOLOGY

In a clinical study, the lower back of 20 healthy volunteers was treated with 0.6 mg/cm^2 of melatonin or vehicle either 15 min before or 1, 30, or 240 min after UV irradiation. The irradiation was performed with solar spectrum, i.e., UVA and UVB light at a wavelength between 290 and 390 nm, and UV erythema was assessed 24 hours after irradiation by visual score and chromametry. It was shown that melatonin treatment 15 min before irradiation significantly suppressed erythema compared with treatment with vehicle alone, while treatment with melatonin after UV irradiation did not suppress UV erythema, nonrespective to whether treatment was 1, 30, or 240 min after UV exposure [114]. In a dose–response study, the concentration of 0.5% revealed to be the most potent UV erythema–suppressive melatonin concentration [113].

It has to be pointed out that topically applied melatonin reduced UV erythema only when administered before, but not when applied after, UV irradiation. This was confirmed by another group showing that melatonin, and also other antioxidants (vitamins E and C) have no effect on UV erythema when administered after UV irradiation, irrespective of the time-course of application [129]. A parallel can be drawn to immunological skin responses, such as suppression of the Mantoux response by UV irradiation, where the skin response is also only inhibited by melatonin when

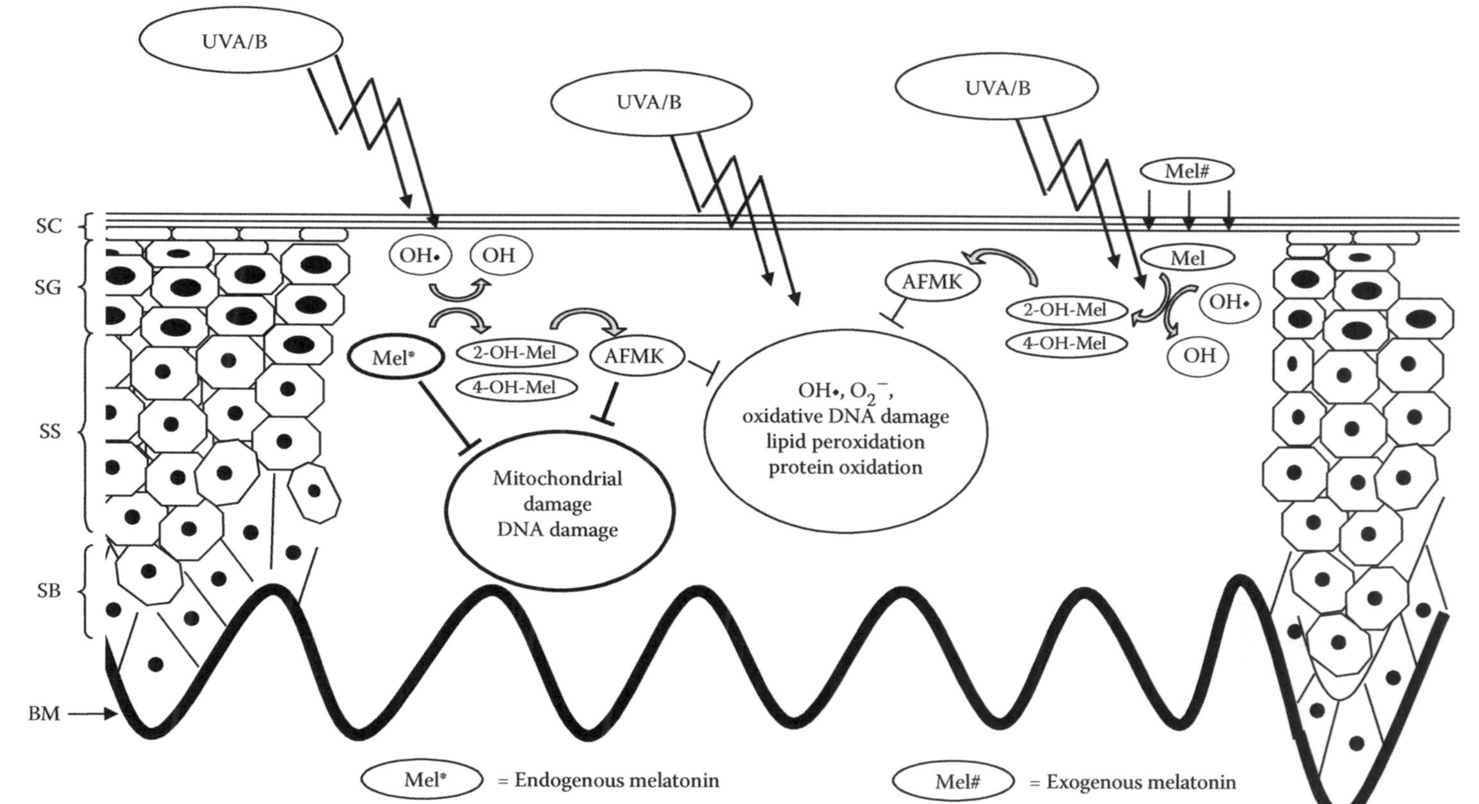

FIGURE 7.3 The MAS of the skin. Parallel to directly scavenging UVB-induced ROS, namely hydroxyl radicals, melatonin is transformed to 2-hydroxymelatonin, 4-hydroxymelatonin, and consecutively to AFMK. All metabolites are strong antioxidants themselves creating a potent antioxidative cascade that reduces lipid peroxidation, protein oxidation, and mitochondrial and DNA damage. Endogenous intracutaneous melatonin production, together with topical application of exogenous melatonin, which penetrates easily through the stratum corneum into deeper layers of the skin, represents the MAS of the skin. SC, stratum corneum; SG, stratum granulosum; SS, stratum spinosum; SB, stratum basale; BM, basement membrane.

applied before UV exposure [130]. Taking into account that the UV-induced free radical formation in the skin is an immediate event upon UV irradiation, the oxidative stress leading to all known consecutive damaging events in the skin can obviously only be antagonized by antioxidants such as melatonin that are already present at the target sites at the time point of UV exposure [99,114,129].

7.8 CONCLUSION AND PERSPECTIVES

Since the discovery of the strong antioxidant properties of melatonin [2], a tremendously wide spectrum of targets and effects of melatonin has evolved, thus showing that melatonin is an important bioregulator as well as pluripotent and essential protective agent in many cells, tissues, and compartments of unicellular organisms, animal, and human body [9,10,12,86,106,131]. The predominant feature of melatonin therein is that of a potent cytoprotective and tissue-protective substance on multiple molecular and cellular damage levels and mechanisms, both in physiological and pharmacological concentrations [6–8,15,19,28,30,35,39,59,63,67,69,86,97,109,132–142].

Within these melatonin "playgrounds," the human skin is an only recently discovered target of protective melatonin effects [27,41,49,50] and at the same time site of extrapineal melatonin synthesis [42,44]. While melatonin exerts many effects on cell growth regulation and tissue homeostasis via melatonin receptors [54], the strong protective effects of melatonin against UV solar skin damage are mainly mediated through its strong direct radical scavenging and antioxidative enzyme stimulating effects [8,50,89,93,98].

The fact that the essential enzymes for melatonin synthesis are expressed in skin cells and cutaneous tissue at a great variety and that skin cells are able to autonomously produce melatonin and develop metabolism with the generation of metabolites with strong antioxidative properties renders the skin a major extrapineal site of melatonin production and activity [42–44,54,108]. The continuous increase of the body of evidence over the past decade supports the important role of melatonin in skin biology and pathology and implicates significant effects of melatonin and its metabolites on skin ulcer formation, heat- and pressure-induced skin injury, melanogenesis, apoptosis, and necrosis as well as tumor growth suppression [20,59,99,143,144].

Moreover, the effects of the main environmental skin stressor, UV radiation, are significantly counteracted or modulated by melatonin in the context of a complex intracutaneous MAS of the skin, with UV radiation–enhanced melatonin metabolism generating even more active agents such as AFMK [41,44,49,99,105].

It therefore seems to be very likely that melatonin is not only a potent UV protective substance in vitro but also in vivo. First, clinical observations indicate that melatonin prevents the manifestation of UV-induced erythema, an event representing the first acute inflammatory skin response that leads by increase of frequency or intensity of UV dose to skin aging processes and direct DNA damage, which is the prerequisite for UV-induced mutation and tumor promotion. However, although melatonin significantly up-regulates the free radical scavenging systems in many body compartments [60–63,69], the evidence that analogous effects are indeed present in the skin remains to be demonstrated in vivo.

The clinical and pharmaceutical key challenge for melatonin in the promotion of skin health and disease is now to explore the most effective and safe approaches to stimulate the skin's endogenous MAS (including its capacity to generate the potent antioxidant melatonin metabolite AFMK) or to additionally or synergistically support the endogenous MAS with externally applied melatonin metabolites or analogues for photodamage prevention and repair.

For application in clinical dermatology, exogenous melatonin should rather be used topically than orally, since orally administered melatonin appears in rather low levels in the blood due to prominent first-pass degradation in the liver [12], thus limiting skin access. Topical administration would circumvent this problem. Also, pharmacodynamically speaking, topical application might be effective because melatonin, with its distinct lipophilic chemical structure, can penetrate and build a depot in the stratum corneum [6,145]. Therefore, endogenous intracutaneous melatonin production, together with topically applied exogenous melatonin or metabolites, can be expected to represent one of the most potent antioxidative defense systems against UV-induced solar damage in the skin [41,43,44,50].

7.9 SUMMARY POINTS

- Melatonin suppresses ROS induced by UV radiation.
- Melatonin down-regulates classical target genes that are up-regulated upon UV exposure (MMP-1, MMP-3, MMP-10, and aldehyde dehydrogenase 3 type A1) and enhances gene expression and enzyme activity of classical antioxidative enzymes (Mn–SOD, CuZn–SOD, CAT, and GPx).
- Melatonin increases survival of keratinocytes and fibroblasts through its antiapoptotic property and protects the mitochondria and DNA.
- Keratinocytes possess an autonomous extrapineal melatonin production, and UV irradiation–enhanced melatonin metabolism generates a cascade of strong antioxidant melatonin metabolites that defines the MAS of the skin.
- Clinically, topical application of melatonin before UV irradiation significantly reduces UV-induced erythema.

REFERENCES

1. Lerner, A. B., Case, J. D., and Takahashi, Y. 1958. Isolation of melatonin, a pineal factor that lightens melanocytes. *J Am Chem Soc* 80: 2587.
2. Tan, D. X., Chen, L. D., Poeggeler, B., Manchester, L. C., and Reiter, R. J. 1993. Melatonin: A potent, endogenous hydroxyl radical scavenger. *Endocr J* 1: 57–60.
3. Reiter, R. J. 2003. Melatonin: Clinical relevance. *Best Pract Res Clin Endocrinol Metab* 17: 273–285.
4. Reiter, R. J., Tan, D., Kim, S. J., et al. 1999. Augmentation of indices of oxidative damage in life-long melatonin-deficient rats. *Mech Ageing Dev* 110: 157–173.
5. Reiter, R. J., and Tan, D. X. 2002. Melatonin: An antioxidant in edible plants. *Ann N Y Acad Sci* 957: 341–344.
6. Reiter, R. J., Tan, D. X., and Maldonado, M. D. 2005. Melatonin as an antioxidant: Physiology versus pharmacology. *J Pineal Res* 39: 215–216.
7. Tan, D. X., Manchester, L. C., Hardeland, R., et al. 2003. Melatonin: A hormone, a tissue factor, an autocoid, a paracoid, and an antioxidant vitamin. *J Pineal Res* 34: 75–78.
8. Tan, D. X., Reiter, R. J., Manchester, L. C., et al. 2002. Chemical and physical properties and potential mechanisms: Melatonin as a broad spectrum antioxidant and free radical scavenger. *Curr Top Med Chem* 2: 181–197.
9. Hardeland R. F. B. 1996. Ubiquitous melatonin—Presence and effects in unicells, plants and animals. *Trends Comp Biochem Physiol* 2: 25–45.
10. Karbownik, M., Lewinski, A., and Reiter, R. J. 2001. Anticarcinogenic actions of melatonin which involve antioxidative processes: Comparison with other antioxidants. *Int J Biochem Cell Biol* 33: 735–753.
11. Lissoni, P., Malugani, F., Malysheva, O., et al. 2002. Neuroimmunotherapy of untreatable metastatic solid tumors with subcutaneous low-dose interleukin-2, melatonin and naltrexone: Modulation of interleukin-2–induced antitumor immunity by blocking the opioid system. *Neuroendocrinol Lett* 23: 341–344.
12. Arendt, J. 1988. Melatonin. *Clin Endocrinol (Oxf)* 29: 205–229.
13. Bubenik, G. A., and Smith, P. S. 1987. Circadian and circannual rhythms of melatonin in plasma of male white-tailed deer and the effect of oral administration of melatonin. *J Exp Zool* 241: 81–89.
14. Lerchl, A., and Schlatt, S. 1993. Influence of photoperiod on pineal melatonin synthesis, fur color, body weight, and reproductive function in the female Djungarian hamster, *Phodopus sungorus*. *Neuroendocrinology* 57: 359–364.
15. Carrillo-Vico, A., Calvo, J. R., Abreu, P., et al. 2004. Evidence of melatonin synthesis by human lymphocytes and its physiological significance: Possible role as intracrine, autocrine, and/or paracrine substance. *FASEB J* 18: 537–539.

16. Guerrero, J. M., and Reiter, R. J. 2002. Melatonin–immune system relationships. *Curr Top Med Chem* 2: 67–79.
17. Herxheimer, A., and Petrie, K. J. 2002. Melatonin for the prevention and treatment of jet lag. *Cochrane Database Syst Rev* CD001520.
18. Waterhouse, J., Reilly, T., Atkinson, G., and Edwards, B. 2007. Jet lag: Trends and coping strategies. *Lancet* 369: 1117–1129.
19. Bartsch, C., Bartsch, H., and Karasek, M. 2002. Melatonin in clinical oncology. *Neuroendocrinol Lett* 23 (Suppl 1): 30–38.
20. Fischer, T. W., Zmijewski, M. A., Zbytek, B., et al. 2006. Oncostatic effects of the indole melatonin and expression of its cytosolic and nuclear receptors in cultured human melanoma cell lines. *Int J Oncol* 29: 665–672.
21. Kumar, C. A., and Das, U. N. 2000. Effect of melatonin on two stage skin carcinogenesis in Swiss mice. *Med Sci Monit* 6: 471–475.
22. Winczyk, K., Pawlikowski, M., Guerrero, J. M., and Karasek, M. 2002. Possible involvement of the nuclear RZR/ROR-alpha receptor in the antitumor action of melatonin on murine Colon 38 cancer. *Tumour Biol* 23: 298–302.
23. Hu, D. N., and Roberts, J. E. 1997. Melatonin inhibits growth of cultured human uveal melanoma cells. *Melanoma Res* 7: 27–31.
24. Helton, R. A., Harrison, W. A., Kelley, K., and Kane, M. A. 1993. Melatonin interactions with cultured murine B16 melanoma cells. *Melanoma Res* 3: 403–413.
25. Bartsch, H., Bartsch, C., and Fleming, B. 1986. Differential effect of melatonin on slow and fast growing passages of a human melanoma cell line. *Neuroendocrinol Lett* 8: 289–293.
26. Reiter, R. J., Tan, D. X., Poeggeler, B., et al. 1994. Melatonin as a free radical scavenger: Implications for aging and age-related diseases. *Ann NY Acad Sci* 719: 1–12.
27. Fischer, T. W., and Elsner, P. 2001. The antioxidative potential of melatonin in the skin. *Curr Probl Dermatol* 29: 165–174.
28. Reiter, R. J., Tan, D. X., Sainz, R. M., Mayo, J. C., and Lopez-Burillo, S. 2002. Melatonin: Reducing the toxicity and increasing the efficacy of drugs. *J Pharm Pharmacol* 54: 1299–1321.
29. Atessahin, A., Sahna, E., Turk, G., et al. 2006. Chemoprotective effect of melatonin against cisplatin-induced testicular toxicity in rats. *J Pineal Res* 41: 21–27.
30. Oz, E., Erbas, D., Surucu, H. S., and Duzgun, E. 2006. Prevention of doxorubicin-induced cardiotoxicity by melatonin. *Mol Cell Biochem* 282: 31–37.
31. Parlakpinar, H., Ozer, M. K., Sahna, E., et al. 2003. Amikacin-induced acute renal injury in rats: Protective role of melatonin. *J Pineal Res* 35: 85–90.
32. Karasek, M., and Reiter, R. J. 2002. Melatonin and aging. *Neuroendocrinol Lett* 23 (Suppl 1): 14–16.
33. Reiter, R. J., Tan, D. X., Manchester, L. C., and El Sawi, M. R. 2002. Melatonin reduces oxidant damage and promotes mitochondrial respiration: Implications for aging. *Ann N Y Acad Sci* 959: 238–250.
34. Karbownik, M. 2002. Potential anticarcinogenic action of melatonin and other antioxidants mediated by antioxidative mechanisms. *Neuroendocrinol Lett* 23 (Suppl 1): 39–44.
35. Tan, D. X., Manchester, L. C., Reiter, R. J., et al. 1999. Identification of highly elevated levels of melatonin in bone marrow: Its origin and significance. *Biochim Biophys Acta* 1472: 206–214.
36. Tan, D. X., Manchester, L. C., Reiter, R. J., et al. 1999. High physiological levels of melatonin in the bile of mammals. *Life Sci* 65: 2523–2529.
37. Skinner, D. C., and Malpaux, B. 1999. High melatonin concentrations in third ventricular cerebrospinal fluid are not due to Galen vein blood recirculating through the choroid plexus. *Endocrinology* 140: 4399–4405.
38. Bubenik, G. A., Hacker, R. R., Brown, G. M., and Bartos, L. 1999. Melatonin concentrations in the luminal fluid, mucosa, and muscularis of the bovine and porcine gastrointestinal tract. *J Pineal Res* 26: 56–63.
39. Cahill, G. M., and Besharse, J. C. 1992. Light-sensitive melatonin synthesis by *Xenopus* photoreceptors after destruction of the inner retina. *Vis Neurosci* 8: 487–490.
40. Itoh, M. T., Ishizuka, B., Kuribayashi, Y., Amemiya, A., and Sumi, Y. 1999. Melatonin, its precursors, and synthesizing enzyme activities in the human ovary. *Mol Hum Reprod* 5: 402–408.
41. Slominski, A., Wortsman, J., and Tobin, D. J. 2005. The cutaneous serotoninergic/melatoninergic system: Securing a place under the sun. *FASEB J* 19: 176–194.
42. Slominski, A., Pisarchik, A., Semak, I., et al. 2002. Serotoninergic and melatoninergic systems are fully expressed in human skin. *FASEB J* 16: 896–898.
43. Slominski, A., Fischer, T. W., Zmijewski, M. A., et al. 2005. On the role of melatonin in skin physiology and pathology. *Endocrine* 27: 137–148.

44. Fischer, T. W., Sweatman, T. W., Semak, I., et al. 2006. Constitutive and UV-induced metabolism of melatonin in keratinocytes and cell-free systems. *FASEB J* 20: 1564–1566.
45. Slominski, A., Baker, J., Rosano, T. G., et al. 1996. Metabolism of serotonin to *N*-acetylserotonin, melatonin, and 5-methoxytryptamine in hamster skin culture. *J Biol Chem* 271: 12281–12286.
46. Kobayashi, H., Kromminga, A., Dunlop, T. W., et al. 2005. A role of melatonin in neuroectodermal–mesodermal interactions: The hair follicle synthesizes melatonin and expresses functional melatonin receptors. *FASEB J* 19: 1710–1712.
47. Reiter, R. J., and Tan, D. X. 2003. What constitutes a physiological concentration of melatonin? *J Pineal Res* 34: 79–80.
48. Tan, D. X., Manchester, L. C., Reiter, R. J., et al. 1999. High physiological levels of melatonin in the bile of mammals. *Life Sci* 65: 2523–2529.
49. Slominski, A., Tobin, D. J., Zmijewski, M. A., Wortsman, J., and Paus, R. 2007. Melatonin in the skin: Synthesis, metabolism and functions. *Trends Exp Dermatol* in press.
50. Fischer, T. W., Slominski, A., Zmijewski, M. A., Reiter, R. J., and Paus, R. 2008. Melatonin as a major skin protectant: From free radical scavenging to DNA damage repair. *Exp Dermatol* 17: 713–730.
51. Paterson, A. M., and Foldes, A. 1994. Melatonin and farm animals: Endogenous rhythms and exogenous applications. *J Pineal Res* 16: 167–177.
52. Cardinali, D. P. 1990. [Regulation of the biologic rhythms in mammals. Function of the pineal gland]. *An R Acad Nac Med (Madr)* 107: 433–442.
53. Hipler, U. C., Fischer, T. W., and Elsner, P. 2003. HaCaT cell proliferation influenced by melatonin. *Skin Pharmacol Appl Skin Physiol* 16: 379–385.
54. Slominski, A., Pisarchik, A., Zbytek, B., et al. 2003. Functional activity of serotoninergic and melatoninergic systems expressed in the skin. *J Cell Physiol* 196: 144–153.
55. Esrefoglu, M., Seyhan, M., Gul, M., et al. 2005. Potent therapeutic effect of melatonin on aging skin in pinealectomized rats. *J Pineal Res* 39: 231–237.
56. Sander, C. S., Chang, H., Salzmann, S., et al. 2002. Photoaging is associated with protein oxidation in human skin in vivo. *J Invest Dermatol* 118: 618–625.
57. Esrefoglu, M., Gul, M., Seyhan, M., and Parlakpinar, H. 2006. Ultrastructural clues for the potent therapeutic effect of melatonin on aging skin in pinealectomized rats. *Fundam Clin Pharmacol* 20: 605–611.
58. Maldonado, M. D., Murillo-Cabezas, F., Calvo, J. R., et al. 2007. Melatonin as pharmacologic support in burn patients: A proposed solution to thermal injury-related lymphocytopenia and oxidative damage. *Crit Care Med* 35: 1177–1185.
59. Tunali, T., Sener, G., Yarat, A., and Emekli, N. 2005. Melatonin reduces oxidative damage to skin and normalizes blood coagulation in a rat model of thermal injury. *Life Sci* 76: 1259–1265.
60. Barlow-Walden, L. R., Reiter, R. J., Abe, M., et al. 1995. Melatonin stimulates brain glutathione peroxidase activity. *Neurochem Int* 26: 497–502.
61. Antolin, I., Rodriguez, C., Sainz, R. M., et al. 1996. Neurohormone melatonin prevents cell damage: Effect on gene expression for antioxidant enzymes. *FASEB J* 10: 882–890.
62. Kotler, M., Rodriguez, C., Sainz, R. M., Antolin, I., and Menendez-Pelaez, A. 1998. Melatonin increases gene expression for antioxidant enzymes in rat brain cortex. *J Pineal Res* 24: 83–89.
63. Pablos, M. I., Agapito, M. T., Gutierrez, R., et al. 1995. Melatonin stimulates the activity of the detoxifying enzyme glutathione peroxidase in several tissues of chicks. *J Pineal Res* 19: 111–115.
64. Reiter, R. J., Melchiorri, D., Sewerynek, E., et al. 1995. A review of the evidence supporting melatonin's role as an antioxidant. *J Pineal Res* 18: 1–11.
65. Rodriguez, C., Mayo, J. C., Sainz, R. M., et al. 2004. Regulation of antioxidant enzymes: A significant role for melatonin. *J Pineal Res* 36: 1–9.
66. Martin, V., Sainz, R. M., Antolin, I., et al. 2002. Several antioxidant pathways are involved in astrocyte protection by melatonin. *J Pineal Res* 33: 204–212.
67. Taskiran, D., Tanyalcin, T., Sozmen, E. Y., et al. 2000. The effects of melatonin on the antioxidant systems in experimental spinal injury. *Int J Neurosci* 104: 63–73.
68. Oner-Iyidogan, Y., Gurdol, F., and Oner, P. 2001. The effects of acute melatonin and ethanol treatment on antioxidant enzyme activities in rat testes. *Pharmacol Res* 44: 89–93.
69. Reiter, R. J. 1995. Oxidative processes and antioxidative defense mechanisms in the aging brain. *FASEB J* 9: 526–533.
70. Slominski, A., Semak, I., Pisarchik, A., et al. 2002. Conversion of L-tryptophan to serotonin and melatonin in human melanoma cells. *FEBS Lett* 511: 102–106.
71. Urata, Y., Honma, S., Goto, S., et al. 1999. Melatonin induces gamma-glutamylcysteine synthetase mediated by activator protein-1 in human vascular endothelial cells. *Free Radic Biol Med* 27: 838–847.

72. Masana, M. I., and Dubocovich, M. L. 2001. Melatonin receptor signaling: Finding the path through the dark. *Sci STKE* 2001: E39.
73. Dillon, D. C., Easley, S. E., Asch, B. B., et al. 2002. Differential expression of high-affinity melatonin receptors (MT1) in normal and malignant human breast tissue. *Am J Clin Pathol* 118: 451–458.
74. Brydon, L., Roka, F., Petit, L., et al. 1999. Dual signaling of human Mel1a melatonin receptors via G(i2), G(i3), and G(q/11) proteins. *Mol Endocrinol* 13: 2025–2038.
75. Chan, A. S., Lai, F. P., Lo, R. K., et al. 2002. Melatonin mt1 and MT2 receptors stimulate c-Jun N-terminal kinase via pertussis toxin-sensitive and -insensitive G proteins. *Cell Signal* 14: 249–257.
76. Kadekaro, A. L., Andrade, L. N. S., Floeter-Winter, L. M., et al. 2004. MT-1 melatonin receptor expression increases the antiproliferative effect of melatonin on S-91 murine melanoma cells. *J Pineal Res* 36: 204–211.
77. Moretti, R. M., Montagnani Marelli, M., Sala, A., Motta, M., and Limonta, P. 2004. Activation of the orphan nuclear receptor RORalpha counteracts the proliferative effect of fatty acids on prostate cancer cells: Crucial role of 5-lipoxygenase. *Int J Cancer* 112: 87–93.
78. Naji, L., Carrillo-Vico, A., Guerrero, J. M., and Calvo, J. R. 2004. Expression of membrane and nuclear melatonin receptors in mouse peripheral organs. *Life Sci* 74: 2227–2236.
79. Nosjean, O., Nicolas, J. P., Klupsch, F., et al. 2001. Comparative pharmacological studies of melatonin receptors: MT1, MT2 and MT3/QR2. Tissue distribution of MT3/QR2. *Biochem Pharmacol* 61: 1369–1379.
80. Wiesenberg, I., Missbach, M., and Carlberg, C. 1998. The potential role of the transcription factor RZR/ROR as a mediator of nuclear melatonin signaling. *Restor Neurol Neurosci* 12: 143–150.
81. Yuan, L., Collins, A. R., Dai, J., Dubocovich, M. L., and Hill, S. M. 2002. MT(1) melatonin receptor overexpression enhances the growth suppressive effect of melatonin in human breast cancer cells. *Mol Cell Endocrinol* 192: 147–156.
82. Tomas-Zapico, C., and Coto-Montes, A. 2005. A proposed mechanism to explain the stimulatory effect of melatonin on antioxidative enzymes. *J Pineal Res* 39: 99–104.
83. Pablos, M., Guerrero, J. M., Ortiz, G. G., Agapito, M. T., and Reiter, R. J. 1997. Both melatonin and putative nuclear melatonin receptor antagonist CGP 52608 stimulate glutathione peroxidase and glutathione reductase activities in mouse brain in vivo. *Neuro Endocrinol Lett* 18: 49–58.
84. Poeggeler, B., Saarela, S., Reiter, R. J., et al. 1994. Melatonin—A highly potent endogenous radical scavenger and electron donor: New aspects of the oxidation chemistry of this indole accessed in vitro. *Ann N Y Acad Sci* 738: 419–420.
85. Tan, D. X., Manchester, L. C., Reiter, R. J., et al. 2000. Significance of melatonin in antioxidative defense system: Reactions and products. *Biol Signals Recept* 9: 137–159.
86. Tan, D. X., Manchester, L. C., Terron, M. P., Flores, L. J., and Reiter, R. J. 2007. One molecule, many derivatives: A never-ending interaction of melatonin with reactive oxygen and nitrogen species? *J Pineal Res* 42: 28–42.
87. Hardeland, R. 2005. Antioxidative protection by melatonin: Multiplicity of mechanisms from radical detoxification to radical avoidance. *Endocrine* 27: 119–130.
88. Livrea, M. A., Tesoriere, L., D'Arpa, D., and Morreale, M. 1997. Reaction of melatonin with lipoperoxyl radicals in phospholipid bilayers. *Free Radic Biol Med* 23: 706–711.
89. Fischer, T. W., Scholz, G., Knoll, B., Hipler, U. C., and Elsner, P. 2001. Melatonin reduces UV-induced reactive oxygen species in a dose-dependent manner in IL-3–stimulated leukocytes. *J Pineal Res* 31: 39–45.
90. Emerit, I. 1992. Free radicals and aging of the skin. *EXS* 62: 328–341.
91. Krutmann, J. 2003. Premature skin aging by ultraviolet radiation and other environmental hazards. The molecular basis. *Hautarzt* 54: 809–817.
92. Fischer, T. W., and Elsner, P. 2005. Melatonin: A hormone, drug, or cosmeceutical. In *Cosmeceuticals and Active Cosmetics* (Elsner, P., and Maibach, H. I., eds.), pp. 413–419, Taylor & Francis, Boca Raton, FL.
93. Fischer, T. W., Scholz, G., Knoll, B., Hipler, U. C., and Elsner, P. 2004. Melatonin suppresses reactive oxygen species induced by UV irradiation in leukocytes. *J Pineal Res* 37: 107–112.
94. Fischer, T. W., Scholz, G., Knoll, B., Hipler, U. C., and Elsner, P. 2002. Melatonin suppresses reactive oxygen species in UV-irradiated leukocytes more than vitamin C and trolox. *Skin Pharmacol Appl Skin Physiol* 15: 367–373.
95. Pieri, C., Marra, M., Moroni, F., Recchioni, R., and Marcheselli, F. 1994. Melatonin: A peroxyl radical scavenger more effective than vitamin E. *Life Sci* 55: L271–L276.
96. Morreale, M., and Livrea, M. A. 1997. Synergistic effect of glycolic acid on the antioxidant activity of alpha-tocopherol and melatonin in lipid bilayers and in human skin homogenates. *Biochem Mol Biol Int* 42: 1093–1102.

97. Ryoo, Y. W., Suh, S. I., Mun, K. C., Kim, B. C., and Lee, K. S. 2001. The effects of the melatonin on ultraviolet-B irradiated cultured dermal fibroblasts. *J Dermatol Sci* 27: 162–169.
98. Lee, K. S., Lee, W. S., Suh, S. I., et al. 2003. Melatonin reduces ultraviolet-B induced cell damages and polyamine levels in human skin fibroblasts in culture. *Best Pract Res Clin Endocrinol Metab* 35: 263–268.
99. Fischer, T. W., Zbytek, B., Sayre, R. M., et al. 2006. Melatonin increases survival of HaCaT keratinocytes by suppressing UV-induced apoptosis. *J Pineal Res* 40: 18–26.
100. Krutmann, J. 2006. The interaction of UVA and UVB wavebands with particular emphasis on signalling. *Prog Biophys Mol Biol* 92: 105–107.
101. Leccia, M. T., Yaar, M., Allen, N., Gleason, M., and Gilchrest, B. A. 2001. Solar simulated irradiation modulates gene expression and activity of antioxidant enzymes in cultured human dermal fibroblasts. *Exp Dermatol* 10: 272–279.
102. Kulms, D., and Schwarz, T. 2002. Mechanisms of UV-induced signal transduction. *J Dermatol* 29: 189–196.
103. Scharffetter-Kochanek, K., Brenneisen, P., Wenk, J., et al. 2000. Photoaging of the skin from phenotype to mechanisms. *Exp Gerontol* 35: 307–316.
104. Cho, J. W., Kim, C. W., and Lee, K. S. 2007. Modification of gene expression by melatonin in UVB-irradiated HaCaT keratinocyte cell lines using a cDNA microarray. *Oncol Rep* 17: 573–577.
105. Fischer, T. W., Zmijewski, M. A., Wortsman, J., and Slominski, A. 2008. Melatonin maintains mitochondrial membrane potential and attenuates activation of initiator (casp-9) and effector caspases (casp-3/casp-7) and PARP in UVR-exposed HaCaT keratinocytes. *J Pineal Res* 44: 397–407.
106. Jou, M. J., Peng, T. I., Hsu, L. F., et al. 2009. Visualization of melatonin's multiple mitochondrial levels of protection against mitochondrial Ca(2+)-mediated permeability transition and beyond in rat brain astrocytes. *J Pineal Res* 48: 20–38.
107. Watt, F. M., Jordan, P. W., and O'Neill, C. H. 1988. Cell shape controls terminal differentiation of human epidermal keratinocytes. *Proc Natl Acad Sci USA* 85: 5576–5580.
108. Tan, D. X., Manchester, L. C., Burkhardt, S., et al. 2001. *N*1-acetyl-*N*2-formyl-5-methoxykynuramine, a biogenic amine and melatonin metabolite, functions as a potent antioxidant. *FASEB J* 15: 2294–2296.
109. Mayo, J. C., Sainz, R. M., Tan, D. X., et al. 2005. Anti-inflammatory actions of melatonin and its metabolites, *N*1-acetyl-*N*2-formyl-5-methoxykynuramine (AFMK) and *N*1-acetyl-5-methoxykynuramine (AMK), in macrophages. *J Neuroimmunol* 165: 139–149.
110. Onuki, J., Almeida, E. A., Medeiros, M. H., and Di Mascio, P. 2005. Inhibition of 5-aminolevulinic acid–induced DNA damage by melatonin, N1-acetyl-N2-formyl-5-methoxykynuramine, quercetin, or resveratrol. *J Pineal Res* 38: 107–115.
111. Ressmeyer, A. R., Mayo, J. C., Zelosko, V., et al. 2003. Antioxidant properties of the melatonin metabolite N1-acetyl-5-methoxykynuramine (AMK): Scavenging of free radicals and prevention of protein destruction. *Redox Rep* 8: 205–213.
112. Maharaj, D. S., Anoopkumar-Dukie, S., Glass, B. D., et al. 2002. The identification of the UV degradants of melatonin and their ability to scavenge free radicals. *J Pineal Res* 32: 257–261.
113. Bangha, E., Elsner, P., and Kistler, G. S. 1996. Suppression of UV-induced erythema by topical treatment with melatonin (*N*-acetyl-5-methoxytryptamine). A dose response study. *Arch Dermatol Res* 288: 522–526.
114. Bangha, E., Elsner, P., and Kistler, G. S. 1997. Suppression of UV-induced erythema by topical treatment with melatonin (*N*-acetyl-5-methoxytryptamine). Influence of the application time point. *Dermatology* 195: 248–252.
115. Dreher, F., Gabard, B., Schwindt, D. A., and Maibach, H. I. 1998. Topical melatonin in combination with vitamins E and C protects skin from ultraviolet-induced erythema: A human study in vivo. *Br J Dermatol* 139: 332–339.
116. Kim, B. C., Shon, B. S., Ryoo, Y. W., Kim, S. P., and Lee, K. S. 2001. Melatonin reduces X-ray irradiation–induced oxidative damages in cultured human skin fibroblasts. *J Dermatol Sci* 26: 194–200.
117. Slominski, A., Chassalevris, N., Mazurkiewicz, J., Maurer, M., and Paus, R. 1994. Murine skin as a target for melatonin bioregulation. *Exp Dermatol* 3: 45–50.
118. Fischer, T. W., Slominski, A., Tobin, D. J., and Paus, R. 2008. Melatonin and the hair follicle. *J Pineal Res* 44: 1–15.
119. Scharffetter-Kochanek, K., Wlaschek, M., Brenneisen, P., et al. 1997. UV-induced reactive oxygen species in photocarcinogenesis and photoaging. *Biol Chem* 378: 1247–1257.
120. Scharffetter-Kochanek, K., Wlaschek, M., Briviba, K., and Sies, H. 1993. Singlet oxygen induces collagenase expression in human skin fibroblasts. *FEBS Lett* 331: 304–306.
121. Schwarz, T. 2005. Mechanisms of UV-induced immunosuppression. *Keio J Med* 54: 165–171.

122. Kulms, D., Zeise, E., Poppelmann, B., and Schwarz, T. 2002. DNA damage, death receptor activation and reactive oxygen species contribute to ultraviolet radiation-induced apoptosis in an essential and independent way. *Oncogene* 21: 5844–5851.
123. Krutmann, J. 2000. Ultraviolet A radiation-induced biological effects in human skin: Relevance for photoaging and photodermatosis. *J Dermatol Sci* 23 Suppl 1: S22–26.
124. Berneburg, M., Plettenberg, H., and Krutmann, J. 2000. Photoaging of human skin. *Photodermatol Photoimmunol Photomed* 16: 239–244.
125. Arck, P. C., Slominski, A., Theoharides, T. C., Peters, E. M. J., and Paus, R. 2006. Neuroimmunology of stress: Skin takes center stage. *J Invest Dermatol* 126: 1697–1704.
126. Krutmann, J., and Grewe, M. 1995. Involvement of cytokines, DNA damage, and reactive oxygen intermediates in ultraviolet radiation-induced modulation of intercellular adhesion molecule-1 expression. *J Invest Dermatol* 105: 67S–70S.
127. Berneburg, M., Grether-Beck, S., Kurten, V., et al. 1999. Singlet oxygen mediates the UVA-induced generation of the photoaging-associated mitochondrial common deletion. *J Biol Chem* 274: 15345–15349.
128. Hardeland, R., Reiter, R. J., Poeggeler, B., and Tan, D. X. 1993. The significance of the metabolism of the neurohormone melatonin: Antioxidative protection and formation of bioactive substances. *Neurosci Biobehav Rev* 17: 347–357.
129. Dreher, F., Denig, N., Gabard, B., Schwindt, D. A., and Maibach, H. I. 1999. Effect of topical antioxidants on UV-induced erythema formation when administered after exposure. *Dermatology* 198: 52–55.
130. Howes, R. A., Halliday, G. M., and Damian, D. L. 2006. Effect of topical melatonin on ultraviolet radiation-induced suppression of Mantoux reactions in humans. *Photodermatol Photoimmunol Photomed* 22: 267–269.
131. Lissoni, P., Vaghi, M., Ardizzoia, A., et al. 2002. A phase II study of chemoneuroimmunotherapy with platinum, subcutaneous low-dose interleukin-2 and the pineal neurohormone melatonin (P.I.M.) as a second-line therapy in metastatic melanoma patients progressing on dacarbazine plus interferon-alpha. *In Vivo* 16: 93–96.
132. Hardeland, R., and Pandi-Perumal, S. R. 2005. Melatonin, a potent agent in antioxidative defense: Actions as a natural food constituent, gastrointestinal factor, drug and prodrug. *Nutr Metab (Lond)* 2: 22.
133. Reiter, R. J., Tan, D. X., and Allegra, M. 2002. Melatonin: Reducing molecular pathology and dysfunction due to free radicals and associated reactants. *Neuroendocrinol Lett* 23 Suppl 1: 3–8.
134. Tunez, I., del Carmen Munoz, M., Feijoo, M., et al. 2003. Melatonin effect on renal oxidative stress under constant light exposure. *Cell Biochem Funct* 21: 35–40.
135. Vijayalaxmi, Reiter, R. J., Herman, T. S., and Meltz, M. L. 1996. Melatonin and radioprotection from genetic damage: In vivo/in vitro studies with human volunteers. *Mutat Res* 371: 221–228.
136. Maestroni, G. J. 2001. The immunotherapeutic potential of melatonin. *Expert Opin Investig Drugs* 10: 467–476.
137. Liu, F., and Ng, T. B. 2000. Effect of pineal indoles on activities of the antioxidant defense enzymes superoxide dismutase, catalase, and glutathione reductase, and levels of reduced and oxidized glutathione in rat tissues. *Biochem Cell Biol* 78: 447–453.
138. Leon, J., Acuna-Castroviejo, D., Escames, G., Tan, D. X., and Reiter, R. J. 2005. Melatonin mitigates mitochondrial malfunction. *J Pineal Res* 38: 1–9.
139. Jou, M. J., Peng, T. I., Yu, P. Z., et al. 2007. Melatonin protects against common deletion of mitochondrial DNA-augmented mitochondrial oxidative stress and apoptosis. *J Pineal Res* 43: 389–403.
140. Bubenik, G. A. 2002. Gastrointestinal melatonin: Localization, function, and clinical relevance. *Dig Dis Sci* 47: 2336–2348.
141. Albarran, M. T., Lopez-Burillo, S., Pablos, M. I., Reiter, R. J., and Agapito, M. T. 2001. Endogenous rhythms of melatonin, total antioxidant status and superoxide dismutase activity in several tissues of chick and their inhibition by light. *J Pineal Res* 30: 227–233.
142. Fischer, T. W., Burmeister, G., Schmidt, H. W., and Elsner, P. 2004. Melatonin increases anagen hair rate in women with androgenetic alopecia, or diffuse alopecia: Results of a pilot randomized controlled trial. *Br J Dermatol* 150: 341–345.
143. Logan, A., and Weatherhead, B. 1980. Post-tyrosinase inhibition of melanogenesis by melatonin in hair follicles in vitro. *J Invest Dermatol* 74: 47–50.
144. Sener, G., Sert, G., Ozer Sehirli, A., et al. 2006. Melatonin protects against pressure ulcer-induced oxidative injury of the skin and remote organs in rats. *J Pineal Res* 40: 280–287.
145. Fischer, T. W., Greif, C., Fluhr, J. W., Wigger-Alberti, W., and Elsner, P. 2004. Percutaneous penetration of topically applied melatonin in a cream and an alcoholic solution. *Skin Pharmacol Physiol* 17: 190–194.

8 Melatonin and Type 2 Diabetes

Andreas Gunter Bach and Elmar Peschke

CONTENTS

8.1 MELATONIN—AN OLD FRIEND

5-Methoxy-*N*-acetyltryptamine, better known as melatonin, is phylogenetically a very old hormone with a large prevalence among vertebrates, invertebrates, fungi, plants, multicellular algae, and unicells. It was isolated from bovine pineal glands by Lerner et al. in 1958 [1]. The biosynthesis of the molecule progresses through a multistage process, starting with the essential amino acid tryptophan. In some unicells, the concentration of melatonin can reach very high values of up to 1 mM [2]. Because of its antioxidant properties, this hormone provides an effective protection against radiation- and chemically induced molecular damage [2].

In mammals, this direct protective function has evolved into a hormonal signal. Not light, but darkness, is the stimulus for secretion in the pineal gland, which is the main organ of melatonin synthesis. The melatonin concentration in the blood oscillates in a circadian manner, with peak concentrations in the dark. In mammals, melatonin is the most important synchronizing signal of circadian and circannual rhythms [2–4].

Melatonin receptors on the cell membrane are coupled to G-proteins. In addition to the MT1 receptor, two further receptor subtypes have been classified. The MT2 receptor is most prevalent in the retina of mammals [4,5], and the MT3 receptor is only detectable in amphibians, fish, and birds. In addition, several cytosolic and nuclear binding sites have been discussed for melatonin [4]. Melatonin is postulated to directly influence the calcium–calmodulin budget [4,6], adenylate cyclase, phosphodiesterase, various protein kinases, and cytoskeletal proteins [4]. In addition, melatonin is thought to regulate gene expression via binding to nuclear receptors of the orphan family [7], to cyclic AMP response element binding protein (CREB), and to mitogen-activated protein kinases (MAPK) [8].

In mammals, melatonin receptors are located in the primary and secondary sexual organs [4,9], in the digestive tract [10], spleen [11], kidney [12], lung [2], retina [4,13], in several types of blood vessels [4], in pancreatic β-cells [14], and in cells of the immune system [2]. All these organs and tissues are subject to the influence of melatonin, which can be of either pineal or local origin.

8.2 TYPE 2 DIABETES AND ANTIDIABETICS

The maintenance of glucose homeostasis in the blood is an essential basic function in all organisms. Due to the glucose dependence, above all, of the central nervous system, but also of the erythrocytes and the renal medulla, the need to closely regulate blood glucose concentrations is of utmost importance. As the primary organ synthesizing and storing blood sugar-regulating hormones, the endocrine pancreas is integral in the control and regulation of glucose homeostasis, and the blood sugar–lowering hormone insulin plays a particularly vital role.

Type 2 diabetes is a chronic disease characterized by hyperglycaemia due to absolute or relative insulin deficiency, and it is associated with disturbances of carbohydrate, protein, and lipid metabolism. A common misunderstanding is that type 2 diabetes is caused exclusively by an insufficiency of insulin; this is an oversimplified and even misleading idea.

Let us look first at the normal regulatory circuit. The human body consumes glucose during normal meals, which subsequently causes the blood sugar level to rise. Blood glucose is transferred via the insulin-dependent glucose transporter 2 by facilitated diffusion into the β-cell. Intracellular glucose is phosphorylated by glucokinase to glucose-6-phosphate and is processed through a series of connected chain reactions: glycolysis, citric acid cycle, and oxidative phosphorylation. This sequence leads to an increase in ATP concentrations. By the strong binding of ATP to ATP-sensitive potassium channels in the cell membrane, the channels are inhibited, which, in turn, impedes the efflux of potassium ions and, thus, depolarizes the cell membrane. This results in the activation of voltage-dependent calcium channels, coupled with the influx of calcium into the cell. As a result, the exocytotic secretion of insulin is initiated; the insulin-containing granules fuse with the plasma membrane and release their contents into the extracellular space.

In addition to lowering the blood glucose concentration by accelerating glucose uptake in muscle and fat cells, insulin acts in an anabolic manner through stimulation of protein, glycogen, and triglyceride synthesis, and in an anticatabolic manner by inhibition of lipolysis, proteolysis, and gluconeogenesis. Insulin also regulates cell growth and proliferation by activating genes that are essential for the control and progression of the cell cycle. The target cells for insulin are liver cells, muscle cells, and adipocytes, which are stimulated to take up glucose from the blood. The blood sugar level then drops again, thus completing the regulatory cycle.

What happens in type 2 diabetes? Overfeeding, genetic predisposition, and other unknown factors decrease the sensitivity of the liver, muscles, and fat tissues toward insulin. The compensatory response of the body is to increase insulin secretion. However, in the long term, this leads to overuse of the insulin-producing pancreatic β-cells and, ultimately, their degeneration [15].

Acute metabolic complications of the disease are often life-threatening metabolic disorders such as ketoacidosis, hyperglycemic–hyperosmolar dehydration, hyperglycemic shock, and lactic acidosis.

Through chronic illness or insufficient control of glucose levels, microangiopathy and macroangiopathy occur due to the deposition of nondegradable sugar compounds. These conditions, in turn, lead to long-term complications such as nephropathy, polyneuropathy, skin diseases, increased susceptibility to infections, retinopathy, and atherosclerosis with the subsequent increased risk of myocardial infarction and cerebral apoplexy.

Type 2 diabetes is colloquially often referred to as "diabetes." In contrast to type 2 diabetes, the much rarer type 1 diabetes is caused primarily by pancreatic β-cell destruction; an autoimmune reaction is presumably the trigger.

It is easy to imagine that evolutionary factors dictated that humans, equipped with adrenaline (epinephrine), noradrenaline (norepinephrine), glucagon, and a vegetative nervous system, possess many means of increasing the blood sugar level, but only one counter regulatory mechanism—insulin.

The present blessing and simultaneous curse of early diabetes research is that it has led to a symptom-oriented treatment of the disease, i.e., with medications to increase the production of or substitute insulin. However, this approach has the potential drawback of exacerbating insulin resistance. Over the past several decades, approaches have been explored to pharmacologically normalize the insulin sensitivity of tissues and intervene in the metabolic processes of hepatic glucose. Unfortunately, the negative side effects and low effectiveness of the available agents have prevented resounding success along this line. Thus, the administration of insulin-enhancing drugs and insulin itself remain the therapy of choice.

8.3 THE DISCOVERY OF MELATONIN AS AN ENDOGENOUS ANTIDIABETIC

In the 1950s, Romanian scientists [16,17] described that an extract of the pineal gland showed effects similar to those of insulin; in other words, it was able to reduce the blood glucose level. A pineal peptide was suspected of being the active agent; this peptide was called pinealin.

The isolation and description of the pineal indoleamine melatonin in 1958 [1] subsequently provided evidence that most of the insulin-like effects attributed to pinealin were actually caused by melatonin [18].

Using different study approaches, it has been repeatedly demonstrated that elimination of the pineal gland causes a metabolic state similar to diabetes [19–22] and that this state is reversible by substitution with melatonin [23–26].

Interestingly, recent genome-wide association studies show that variants of the MT2 receptor gene may be associated with elevated levels of fasting blood glucose and a reduced functionality in β-cells [27]. Furthermore, it has been demonstrated that certain frequently occurring single-nucleotide polymorphisms at this gene locus are associated with an increased risk of type 2 diabetes [27–29].

In some studies, partially contradictory results have been presented; these have stimulated an ongoing and controversial discussion among professionals. The reason for many misunderstandings in the melatonin–insulin debate is that melatonin exerts effects not only on the pancreatic β-cell but also on other cell types. Furthermore, short-term effects are often different from long-term effects. Finally, melatonin synthesis itself is affected by insulin and glucose. In addition, different boundary conditions were often insufficiently considered. For example, the time of day is crucial when it comes to the experimental use of melatonin in trials; this should be familiar to anyone who has ever used melatonin as an antidote to jet lag. Moreover, melatonin can act very differently in different species. This phylogenetically old substance has developed different signaling pathways over the course of evolution [30].

It is not necessary to recapitulate here all of the misunderstandings that have arisen in past decades. Currently, there is broad consensus on the antidiabetic effect of melatonin; the details on how this process functions will be explained in the following.

8.4 TECHNIQUE: THE TYPE 2 DIABETIC RAT MODEL

This chapter focuses on the effect of melatonin in humans. Many far-reaching manipulative studies of this effect are, for obvious reasons, only feasible on animal models of human type 2 diabetes. One of the most frequently used animal models is the type 2 diabetic Goto–Kakizaki (GK) rat. It is therefore sensible to characterize this strain of animal here and to elucidate its differences to humans.

The GK rat is named after its developers, Goto and Kakizaki [31]. It is an inbred strain that originated from a common, healthy strain of Wistar rats, by repeated cross-breeding of organisms with poor glucose tolerance over many generations. Essentially, the "diabetes genes" were selected for those that occur in the natural population. As a result, animals have emerged that, due to their substantial genetic predisposition, always develop type 2 diabetes. These rats show, in contrast to their healthy counterparts, a slightly elevated blood sugar concentration [32]; a reduced amount of insulin-producing pancreatic β-cells [33], which display a weaker response to blood glucose elevations due to disturbed glucose tolerance [32,34]; hepatic glucose overproduction [35]; as well as an increased insulin resistance in the liver, muscles, and fat tissues [31]. All these changes are also typical of human type 2 diabetes. Furthermore, GK rats develop the characteristic long-term complications of diabetes, such as vascular disease, nephropathy, neuropathy, and retinopathy. For these reasons, GK rats are still widely accepted as a polygenetic model for the study of human type 2 diabetes [36,37].

A very important difference between humans and rats is that rats are nocturnal, which means that they also feed primarily at night. The endogenous rhythm of food intake is therefore shifted by 12 hours between rats and humans, and yet despite the shift, the melatonin rhythm peaks (acrophase) in humans, rats, and in almost every other type of mammal at night.

Another important difference between humans and rats lies in the way melatonin synthesis is regulated. The nocturnal rise in melatonin synthesis is mainly due to an accumulation of active arylalkylamine-*N*-acetyltransferase (AA-NAT). In rats, protein synthesis of the enzyme increases at night, so some time passes after the onset of darkness before melatonin levels rise in the blood. In contrast, in humans, a continuously high amount of AA-NAT exists, which is activated post-translationally in the dark. Therefore, humans produce melatonin at night with less delay than do rats [38–40]. Thus, it is clear that the results obtained for rats cannot be transferred indiscriminately to humans.

8.5 TECHNIQUE: FUNCTIONAL ANALYSIS OF PANCREATIC β-CELLS

Detailed studies involving living pancreatic β-cells are for obvious reasons not possible on humans but require animal models. A common technique for such examinations is, first, to surgically remove the pancreas of type 2 diabetic GK rats. Then, the islets of insulin-producing pancreatic β-cells are isolated under the microscope.

Pancreatic β-cells, together with other types of cells, are components of the islet of Langerhans (in short: islets). Depending on the species, hundreds or thousands of these islets make up the endocrine pancreas.

For basic physiological studies on isolated pancreatic β-cells, two cell culture systems are fundamentally available: primary cells freshly isolated from animal or human tissues and permanent cell lines that have been immortalized by genetic modification. The extraction of islets from rats [41] or pigs [42] and the subsequent isolation of native β-cells from the islets [43] lead to primary cell cultures.

The major advantage of a primary cell culture is that these directly derived cells are—at least at the beginning of the culture—very similar in their physiological characteristics to the corresponding cells in vivo. The disadvantages of using primary cells for cellular studies are their limited ability to proliferate and survive, the increased effort required for extraction, the sometimes considerable interindividual differences and the complex demands required for cell culture [44]. On the contrary, permanent, immortal cell lines are readily available and easy to maintain in culture, and they also exhibit a nearly unlimited ability to proliferate and uniform basic physiological characteristics.

An ideal model system for primary pancreatic β-cells meets the following criteria: inducible insulin secretion by different stimuli at physiological concentrations with native kinetics of secretion through the nearly immutable metabolic processes and the preservation of physiological pathways, stability over many cycles of division, and immortality. It is, therefore, evident that both a high degree of differentiation and a good growth potential are needed [45]. This may explain why only a few cell lines meet the required criteria.

Among the currently established cell lines are the mouse MIN6 insulinoma line, the hamster insulinoma line HIT, as well as the rat insulinoma lines RIN and β-TC. From a hybrid culture of lymphocytes and the RIN line, the glucose-responsive, insulin-producing rat insulinoma (INS-1) cell line was derived. To varying degrees, all insulinoma cell lines possess characteristics that distinguish them from native pancreatic β-cells and that, therefore, have to be taken into account.

For example, in both RIN and HIT cells, an insulin content up to 1000-fold lower than that in native pancreatic β-cells can be observed [46–48]. None of the tumor cell lines secreted insulin in response to a glucose stimulus in the same pattern as is seen in native pancreatic β-cells. Some cell lines already respond to low glucose levels with maximum secretion levels [49]. Others, like the INS-1 cell line, secrete insulin within the physiological range of from 5 to 15 mM glucose [48], but compared with basal secretion, the increase is less significant than that seen in native β-cells. More recently, attempts have been made, with varying success, to resolve the problem of insufficient insulin secretion by artificial amplification of cellular glucokinase and/or glucose transporter 2 activity [50].

Among the available cell lines, the INS-1 rat insulinoma line described by Asfari et al. in 1992 [48] fulfils the previously mentioned criteria relatively well. The insulin content is about 20% of the value of native β-cells, and the responsiveness to glucose lies within the physiological range. In addition, immunofluorescence only detected insulin in INS-1 cells; glucagon, somatostatin, pancreatic polypeptide, and other hormones were not detected [48]. This selectivity demonstrates the high degree of differentiation preserved. Furthermore, proliferation of the INS-1 cell line remains stable for years, without significant changes in their traits [48]. Functional tests are carried out with whole islets or the pancreatic β-cells from a cell line. Again, two different techniques are applied. First, the classical batch technique can be used, whereby the cells are kept in a culture dish. At regular intervals the medium must be exchanged. The batch technique is simple and allows a large number of replicates, which is advantageous for the study of many issues. Second, the cells can be examined in a superfusion system, where they are immersed in a temperate, oxygenated nutrient solution maintained at constant flow and pH; this state best simulates the in vivo situation. In enriched culture medium, the concentration of glucose, melatonin, and other substances can be set at will. With the nutrient solution removed, the concentrations of insulin and other cells produced can be measured. The cells and cell groups remain viable and functional in the system for several days. The composition of the medium is controlled and the temporal dynamics involved in the secretion of substances such as insulin can be closely monitored.

8.6 MELATONIN MODULATES INSULIN SECRETION

Early on, it was shown that melatonin inhibits the insulin secretion of the pancreatic β-cell [5,14,51]. However, it remained unclear for some time exactly how this happened. Functional analysis of pancreatic β-cells finally proved that melatonin activates three major intracellular signaling cascades: the 3′–5′-cyclic adenosine monophosphate (cAMP) cascade [52,53], the 3′–5′-cyclic guanosine monophosphate (cGMP) cascade [54,55], and the inositol-1,4,5-triphosphate (IP_3) cascade [56,57]. The hypothesis that melatonin has a regulatory influence on the pancreatic β-cell has been strengthened by the detection of two melatonin receptors, MT1 [14,58] and MT2 [59], in whole-tissue examinations of the pancreas in rats and humans [28,60].

However, the pancreatic islets only represent a small proportion of the pancreas and the insulin-producing pancreatic β-cells, only one of several cell types in each islet. So, the melatonin receptors found could still have been on another type of cell. To specifically locate these receptors, isolated pancreatic β-cells were studied. Here, the INS-1 cell line came into play. Both receptor subtypes have been found in INS-1 cells, although the quantification of messenger ribonucleic acid (mRNA) and the amounts of protein indicated predominance of the MT1 isoform [60]. Both types of receptors may be prerequisites for the three signal cascades.

A schematic illustration of the influence of melatonin on the pancreatic β-cell is given in Figure 8.1. In contrast to the melatonin-induced inhibition of the cAMP and cGMP signaling cascades, which culminates in the inhibition of insulin secretion, the melatonin-mediated activation of the IP_3 cascade promotes insulin secretion.

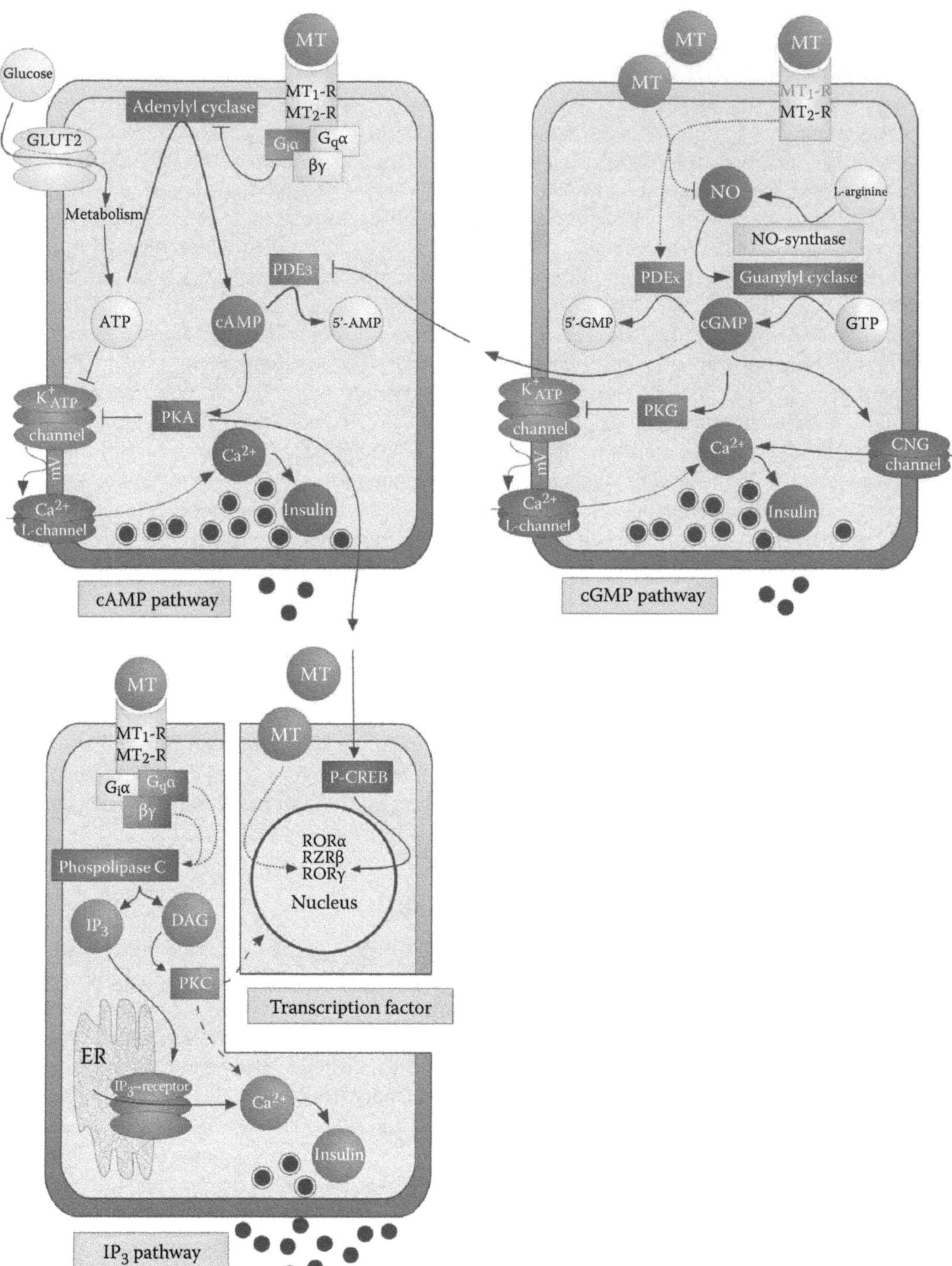

FIGURE 8.1 The signaling pathways of melatonin in the insulin-producing pancreatic β-cell. (Peschke, E.: *J. Pineal Res.* 2008. 44. 26–40. Copyright Wiley-VCH Verlag GmbH & Co. KGaA. Reproduced with permission.)

This phenomenon is by no means unusual. For example, the hormone insulin acts in a similar manner: it reduces cAMP levels through activation of phosphodiesterases and increases IP_3 levels by activating the phospholipase Cγ.

As far as the effect of melatonin is concerned, the temporal differences in the expression of the signaling pathways have to be taken into account. The inhibitory effect on the cAMP signaling cascade occurs only after prolonged incubation with melatonin but is then dominant. The stimulating effect on IP_3 levels is executed almost immediately but is significantly weaker. Precisely this pattern of the insulin secretion has already been described for the hormones of the pineal organ [61].

It should be made clear, however, that melatonin can only exert an effect on insulin secretion in combination with stimulants such as glucose, acetylcholine, or forskolin. Melatonin thus has a modulating influence. Both the active insulin-promoting and insulin-inhibiting signaling pathways are modulated. First, via the IP_3 signaling cascade, the insulin-stimulating effect of substances such as cholecystokinin and the parasympathetic transmitter substance acetylcholine at the muscarinic receptor are enhanced [50]. Then, after a relatively long period in the dark, the cAMP-inhibitory effect of melatonin becomes predominant. All in all, cAMP-mediated insulin secretion is inhibited by enhancement of the effects of cAMP-inhibiting substances such as gastric inhibitory polypeptide (GIP), glucagon-like peptide (GLP), glucagon, and somatostatin as well as by a weakening of the cAMP-stimulatory effects of, for example, sympathetic transmitter substances at the β-receptor [50]. In this sense, a modulation of postprandial insulin secretion is conceivable. After the consumption of food, local intestinal melatonin synthesis could cause a short-term increase in insulin release. In the further course, the cAMP-mediated inhibitory effect may help prevent excessive insulin secretion.

In connection with circadian modulation, pineal melatonin becomes a focal point, although various physiological regulatory mechanisms are still hypothetical. For example, melatonin could mediate, via IP_3, an increased responsiveness of the pancreatic β-cells to cholecystokinin at the beginning of food consumption or, via cAMP, the protection of pancreatic β-cells toward the end of the activity phase. It must be stressed that the evidence gathered to date is applicable to the pancreatic β-cell of the rat; this is physiologically relevant for any interpretation because the rat is a nocturnal animal. Their periods of activity are displaced by 12 hours in comparison to those of humans. The food consumption of rats primarily takes place in the dark [62]. However, in humans, similar mechanisms could form physiologically useful response patterns, e.g., the cAMP-mediated reduction in insulin and accompanying increase in glucose concentration before the start of the activity phase in the morning, in other words, a reinforcement of the so-called dawn phenomenon [63–66].

Unlike many antidiabetics that increase insulin secretion directly, the effect of melatonin on the insulin-producing pancreatic β-cell is, on the whole, inhibitory. This has been demonstrated in both rats [52,67–69] and humans [70]. How is this effect compatible with the "insulin-like" effect of melatonin?

We believe that β-cells are protected by melatonin against long-term overstimulation. The treatment of diabetic rats with melatonin for a relatively long period reduced insulin levels, prevented insulin resistance, and normalized plasma lipid ratios [71]. Studies with type 2 diabetic patients have yielded similar results [72].

However, this indirect, protective effect of melatonin may also be dependent on its discharge at a suitable time. The indirect, long-term effect and the importance of the correctly timed application have probably hindered the commercial use of melatonin as an antidiabetic agent.

8.7 MELATONIN PREVENTS INSULIN RESISTANCE

Insulin resistance is characterized by impairment of the insulin-signaling cascade in such a way that glucose-consuming hepatic glucogen synthesis is reduced, the uptake of glucose in skeletal muscles is inhibited, and the blood circulation in skeletal muscles is diminished. Overall, the glucose-reducing effects of insulin are weakened.

It has been shown that melatonin prevents insulin resistance at all levels. First, liver cells take up more glucose and produce more glycogen under the influence of melatonin [73]. Second, several authors have demonstrated that melatonin increases the activity of the insulin receptor kinase in skeletal muscle, which increases phosphorylation of the insulin receptor substrate 1 (IRS-1), leading in turn to enhanced insulin action in muscle tissue [74,75]. Third, other authors have demonstrated that the lack of MT1 receptors in mice severely disrupts their ability to metabolize glucose [76]. Fourth, in overfed mice, it has been shown that melatonin is important for the flow of blood in skeletal muscles by supporting the insulin-mediated vasodilatation and, in this manner, again increases glucose utilization [77].

In contrast, some studies have described an exacerbation of insulin resistance after melatonin administration [66,78]; this may, however, be due to the fact that only short-term, opposing effects were observed.

8.8 MELATONIN PROTECTS PANCREATIC β-CELLS AGAINST RADICALS

The importance of free radicals in the pathogenesis of malignant and degenerative diseases, as well as in type 2 diabetes, has been emphasized in recent decades. The deleterious effects of free radicals cause alterations in DNA and numerous enzymes, as well as direct membrane damage [79]. Insulin-producing pancreatic β-cells only have weak defenses against radicals [80] and are therefore particularly vulnerable.

Radical donors such as alloxan and streptozotocin accumulate in pancreatic β-cells and can be used to produce a greatly increased burden of free radicals. Both chemicals are "diabetogenic" because they lead to a decline of pancreatic β-cells in animals and, thus, to the development of diabetes [80,81]. In the specific case of primary β-cell failure, we speak of type 1 diabetes.

Interestingly, a high dosage of melatonin can prevent the above response because, as a radical scavenger, melatonin protects pancreatic β-cells against free radicals [18,82,83]. In addition to its direct antioxidant effect, especially against dangerous hydroxyl radicals [84–87], melatonin induces the production of antioxidant enzymes such as superoxide dismutase, catalase, and glutathione peroxidase [88,89].

Furthermore, after surgical removal of the pineal gland, rats show both a reduced density of islets in the pancreas as well as increased degenerative, pathological tissue changes, such as necrosis and/or apoptosis, inflammation, increased interstitial clefts, and deviations in cell differentiation and growth [22].

Both mechanisms, the damage by free radicals and the protection by melatonin, can be applied, within certain limits, to the processes involved in type 2 diabetes. Here, the damage caused by free radicals occurs at a much lower dosage and over a period of several decades. The physiological concentration of melatonin is several orders of magnitude lower than that used in radical scavenging experiments. In real life, many other substances may function as radical scavengers in humans in addition to melatonin.

The antioxidant activity of melatonin is unequivocal. Despite its high efficiency, however, the low physiological concentrations of melatonin of between 200 and 300 pM in rats and humans are hardly sufficient to neutralize unpaired electrons and thus protect the pancreatic β-cell against radicals [85]. The importance of this mechanism in the development or prevention of type 2 diabetes is therefore only speculative.

8.9 RELATIONSHIPS BETWEEN CIRCADIAN RHYTHMS AND GLUCOSE METABOLISM

Since many factors have an influence on the concentration of insulin and glucose, it is difficult to determine the specific strength of the modulatory effect of melatonin. It is undisputed, however, that, in mammals, blood glucose concentration, insulin secretion, and insulin sensitivity are subject to a circadian rhythm [90–93].

Biological rhythms have stabilizing and anticipatory function. The food consumption of a species occurs at relatively fixed times, e.g., during the day for humans, at night for rats, and at dawn for certain predatory animals. Therefore, synchronization of the digestive and metabolic systems with a biological rhythm represents an adaptation to environmental conditions, thus securing a survival advantage in an evolutionary sense.

In addition, there are groups that consider not only the daytime but also seasonal rhythms to be important. Thus, an interesting theory has been postulated, namely, that the long-term metabolic changes in type 2 diabetes correspond in many ways to the short-term weight gain of numerous species in adaptation to winter conditions [94].

The loss or desynchronization of these rhythms is of clinical significance [18]. It has been shown for night-shift workers that insulin, blood sugar, and triglyceride levels are distinctly higher after a meal taken at night than after a meal taken during the day, showing the poorer adaptation of humans to a nocturnal lifestyle [95]. Some authors consider night work to be an independent health risk, in addition to obesity and type 2 diabetes [96].

According to current knowledge, many, perhaps all, cells follow rhythms. A circadian rhythm of insulin secretion is known in decentralized islets of dogs [97], mice [18], rats [98], and humans [70,99]. Pancreatic islets in the superfusion system, i.e., in vitro and without an external timer, show an endogenous rhythm of insulin secretion [92,93,100]. Both humans and rats show different reactions to oral and intravenous glucose tolerance tests depending on the time of day [101,102]. On the one hand, the central rhythm generator in the suprachiasmatic nucleus (SCN) has an influence on food consumption [103] and on the responsiveness of tissues to insulin [90,104]. On the other hand, melatonin can synchronize the endogenous rhythm of pancreatic islets [93]. The intracellular mechanisms behind this synchronization are yet unclear. Presumably however, a mechanism of gene regulation is responsible via CREB, via orphan receptors, or via MAPK [8]. In pancreatic β-cells it has been shown that different time genes are influenced by melatonin [100].

In addition, information exists that increased nocturnal melatonin is needed to ensure regular differentiation of pancreatic islets [105]. The absence of the nocturnal melatonin signal can therefore lead to desynchronization and dysfunction of the pancreatic islets.

In addition to the central rhythm generator in the SCN of mammals, the existence of independent circadian rhythms in individual organs and cell associations has been postulated. These peripheral rhythms are synchronized with the central rhythm as a result of signals from the SCN [103]; this occurs via the autonomic nervous system and melatonin (Figure 8.2, point 1). Certain endocrine organs play a special mediating role in this process. The pineal gland, with its dominant hormone melatonin, is regarded as an extension of the SCN [106]. In addition, the intestine is being discussed as another organ probably involved in melatonin synthesis (Figure 8.2, point 2).

Postprandial glucose influx (Figure 8.2, point 3) is the main stimulus in pancreatic β-cells leading to insulin secretion (Figure 8.2, point 4). Insulin, in turn, exerts its well-known stimulatory effects on certain tissues, e.g., it initiates the storage of glucose as glycogen in the liver, the consumption of glucose in the skeletal muscles, and the storage of glucose as fat in adipose tissue (Figure 8.2, point 5). Overall insulin stimulates the consumption of blood glucose, which leads to the reduction of blood glucose levels and, thus, completes the course of the main feedback loop of glucose homeostasis.

However, there are further feedback loops. The SCN exerts effects via the autonomic nervous system on both the pancreatic β-cell and all the peripheral tissues. The hormone melatonin directly modulates the insulin secretion of the pancreatic β-cell (Figure 8.2, point 6) and prevents insulin resistance (Figure 8.2, point 7). It has been proposed that this is how an organism prepares itself for glucose metabolization in advance to food uptake [90]. The SCN and the pineal gland harbor insulin receptors [107]. Insulin and glucose affect the central rhythm generator and modulate the

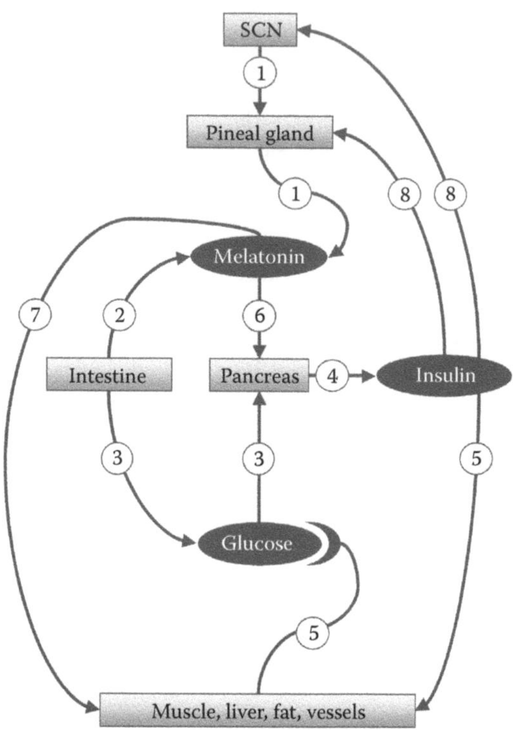

FIGURE 8.2 The postprandial and circadian regulation of glucose metabolism: the interaction of glucose, insulin, and melatonin.

biosynthesis of melatonin [108–110], resulting in a second feedback loop that integrates circadian rhythms.

To preserve clarity in the figure, only the feedback of insulin on the SCN is presented (Figure 8.2, point 8); however, glucose and melatonin effect the SCN in a similar manner. Surprisingly, melatonin actives a receptor tyrosine kinase in the SCN in such a way that, on an intracellular level, both insulin and melatonin signals are intertwined [111].

It is precisely the feedback between the metabolism of glucose and melatonin secretion that casts an interesting light on situations in which the metabolism of glucose is disrupted. Indeed, a disruption in the secretion of melatonin has been demonstrated in type 2 diabetic rats, hamsters [110,112,113], and humans [18,57]. Cause and effect probably cannot be separated in this feedback loop, which can evolve into a vicious circle in type 2 diabetes [114,115].

8.10 THE INTESTINE AS A SOURCE OF MELATONIN

Melatonin receptors exist throughout almost the entire digestive tract of all mammals, including humans [116–118]. The total amount of melatonin in the digestive tract can be up to 400 times higher than that found in the pineal gland [2,119,120].

The key enzymes of melatonin biosynthesis are detectable in the intestines and pancreas [120]. This may explain why melatonin can still be detected in the digestive tract, even after the removal of the pineal gland [121]. This autochthonous production of melatonin, which presumably takes place in the enterochromaffin cells of the gastrointestinal tract [121] is supplemented by a significant uptake of the substance and its precursor tryptophan from food. Melatonin, which enters the duodenum from the stomach, is thought to be a potent stimulus for the secretion of bicarbonate [122]. Further studies have documented that luminal melatonin accelerates intestinal transit [123] and increases the activity of the exocrine pancreas [120]. These observations recognize the hormone as an important mediator of hepatogastrointestinal communication [120,121].

Therefore, with respect to the pancreatic β-cell, both circadian and postprandial modulations by melatonin should be considered.

8.11 REDUCED MELATONIN LEVELS IN TYPE 2 DIABETES

As shown previously, melatonin influences the metabolism of glucose at many different levels. Several authors have emphasized the importance of an intact melatonin signal for glucose homeostasis [124] and shown that an insufficiency of melatonin coincides with type 2 diabetes [57,60].

In turn, insulin itself is able to increase the noradrenaline-stimulated synthesis of pineal melatonin [125]. The significance of this mechanism in humans has not yet been determined. It is, however, known that first a relative and then an absolute insufficiency of insulin in type 2 diabetes is associated with reduced melatonin levels [18,126–129].

Even though some opposing opinions have been voiced [130], most studies describe disruptions in the nocturnal secretion of melatonin already as a consequence of relatively early stages of overnutrition [131], as well as of type 2 diabetes [132].

In type 2 diabetes significantly increased mRNA and protein levels of melatonin receptors can be detected in human pancreatic β-cells [133]. Nuclear receptors of the retinoid orphan receptor and retinoid Z receptor families, which are associated with signaling by melatonin, are increased as well. This increase in receptors is considered an attempt to counteract the decreased melatonin levels in type 2 diabetic organisms.

Type 2 diabetes and an insufficiency of melatonin may not only be associated with one another but may also enhance each other in a vicious circle.

8.12 IMPAIRED INNERVATION OF THE PINEAL GLAND IN TYPE 2 DIABETES

The decisive stimulator of the pineal gland is noradrenaline, which originates in the sympathetic nerve fibers and rises by a factor of 100 during the night [40].

In someone with type 2 diabetes, the total content of noradrenaline in the pineal region is significantly reduced. In response, inhibitory α2-adrenoceptors are significantly more strongly expressed in the pineal glands of type 2 diabetic animals [134]. In this context, functional studies show that the pineal glands of type 2 diabetic rats react to noradrenaline stimulation with weaker pineal melatonin secretion than do pineal glands of nondiabetic rats [135]. One reason for the reduced melatonin synthesis in type 2 diabetes can therefore be seen in a disrupted noradrenergic supply to the pineal, possibly due to diabetic neuropathy [132,136]. Other authors have shown that reduced insulin levels, such as those found in type 2 diabetes after the pancreatic β-cells have been exhausted, are associated with a reduction in the stimulation of noradrenergic in the pineal gland [137].

8.13 DECREASED MELATONIN SYNTHESIS IN TYPE 2 DIABETES

Melatonin synthesis starts with the essential amino acid tryptophan [138]. This amino acid is already found in much smaller amounts in the pineal glands of type 2 diabetic rats. In humans, there are also indications that the availability of tryptophan has a direct influence on melatonin synthesis [139].

All intermediary substances on the way to melatonin, 5-hydroxytryptophan, serotonin, and *N*-acetylserotonin, are also significantly decreased in the pineal gland of type 2 diabetic animals. Notable is the especially large deficit in 5-hydroxytryptophan. The hydroxylation of tryptophan to 5-hydroxytryptophan is catalyzed by tetrahydrobiopteridin (5,6,7,8-tetrahydropteridine) [140,141]. This factor is decreased in type 2 diabetic rats [142,143] and mice [144]. In addition, tetrahydrobiopteridin plays a crucial role in the synthesis of tyrosine hydroxylase [141], a key enzyme of noradrenaline synthesis [145]. Reduced noradrenaline levels in type 2 diabetes have not only been described in rats but also in humans [146,147]. Ultimately, these results point to insufficiencies of tryptophan and tetrahydrobiopteridin as causes of reduced pineal melatonin synthesis in type 2 diabetic organisms [134,135]. In addition, reduced activity of AA-NAT has been documented in type 2 diabetic rats, so that the immediate precursor of melatonin is likewise synthesized more slowly [18].

Last, but not least, it has been shown that cerebral blood flow is impaired in type 2 diabetic humans [148]; this may be another reason why pineal melatonin synthesis is reduced in type 2 diabetic humans.

8.14 SUMMARY

1. Melatonin modulates the insulin secretion of pancreatic β-cells, predominantly in an inhibitory manner, via the cAMP and cGMP signaling pathways. This is putatively a protection mechanism against the exhaustion of β-cells. In addition to the pineal gland, the intestine is another possible site of melatonin synthesis.
2. In supraphysiological concentrations, melatonin acts as a radical scavenger in the pancreatic β-cells.
3. Melatonin prevents insulin resistance in peripheral tissues by increasing the glucose uptake of the liver and skeletal muscles.
4. As a zeitgeber, melatonin mediates the central, endogenous rhythm of the SCN to the pancreatic β-cells. The SCN and the pineal gland are under the influence of both insulin and glucose. The circadian rhythm and the metabolism of glucose are intertwined. A disruption of this interaction has clinical significance.
5. In type 2 diabetes, the nocturnal secretion of pineal melatonin is disrupted. It causes diabetic neuropathy, folic acid insufficiency, reduced cerebral blood flow, and impaired insulin feedback.

REFERENCES

1. Lerner, A. B., J. D. Case, T. H. Lee, and W. Mori. "Isolation of Melatonin, the Pineal Gland Factor That Lightens Melanocytes." *J Am Chem Soc* 80 (1958): 2587–89.
2. Hardeland, R. "New Actions of Melatonin and Their Relevance to Biometeorology." *Int J Biometeorol* 41, no. 2 (1997): 47–57.
3. Reiter, R. J. "The Melatonin Rhythm: Both a Clock and a Calendar." *Experientia* 49, no. 8 (1993): 654–64.
4. Dubocovich, M. L. "Melatonin Receptors: Are There Multiple Subtypes?" *Trends Pharmacol Sci* 16, no. 2 (1995): 50–6.
5. Peschke, E., D. Peschke, T. Hammer, and V. Csernus. "Influence of Melatonin and Serotonin on Glucose-Stimulated Insulin Release from Perifused Rat Pancreatic Islets in Vitro." *J Pineal Res* 23, no. 3 (1997): 156–63.
6. Soto-Vega, E., I. Meza, G. Ramirez-Rodriguez, and G. Benitez-King. "Melatonin Stimulates Calmodulin Phosphorylation by Protein Kinase C." *J Pineal Res* 37, no. 2 (2004): 98–106.
7. Becker-Andre, M., I. Wiesenberg, N. Schaeren-Wiemers, E. Andre, M. Missbach, J. H. Saurat, and C. Carlberg. "Pineal Gland Hormone Melatonin Binds and Activates an Orphan of the Nuclear Receptor Superfamily." *J Biol Chem* 269, no. 46 (1994): 28531–4.
8. Chan, A. S., F. P. Lai, R. K. Lo, T. A. Voyno-Yasenetskaya, E. J. Stanbridge, and Y. H. Wong. "Melatonin MT1 and MT2 Receptors Stimulate C-Jun N-Terminal Kinase Via Pertussis Toxin-Sensitive and -Insensitive G Proteins." *Cell Signal* 14, no. 3 (2002): 249–57.
9. Frungieri, M. B., A. Mayerhofer, K. Zitta, O. P. Pignataro, R. S. Calandra, and S. I. Gonzalez-Calvar. "Direct Effect of Melatonin on Syrian Hamster Testes: Melatonin Subtype 1a Receptors, Inhibition of Androgen Production, and Interaction with the Local Corticotropin-Releasing Hormone System." *Endocrinology* 146, no. 3 (2005): 1541–52.

10. Lee, P. P., and S. F. Pang. "Melatonin and Its Receptors in the Gastrointestinal Tract." *Biol Signals* 2, no. 4 (1993): 181–93.
11. Markowska, M., A. Mrozkowiak, J. Pawlak, and K. Skwarlo-Sonta. "Intracellular Second Messengers Involved in Melatonin Signal Transduction in Chicken Splenocytes in Vitro." *J Pineal Res* 37, no. 3 (2004): 207–12.
12. Song, Y., C. W. Chan, G. M. Brown, S. F. Pang, and M. Silverman. "Studies of the Renal Action of Melatonin: Evidence That the Effects Are Mediated by 37 Kda Receptors of the Mel1a Subtype Localized Primarily to the Basolateral Membrane of the Proximal Tubule." *Faseb J* 11, no. 1 (1997): 93–100.
13. Nash, M. S., and N. N. Osborne. "Pertussis Toxin–Sensitive Melatonin Receptors Negatively Coupled to Adenylate Cyclase Associated with Cultured Human and Rat Retinal Pigment Epithelial Cells." *Invest Ophthalmol Vis Sci* 36, no. 1 (1995): 95–102.
14. Peschke, E., J. D. Fauteck, U. Musshoff, F. Schmidt, A. Beckmann, and D. Peschke. "Evidence for a Melatonin Receptor within Pancreatic Islets of Neonate Rats: Functional, Autoradiographic, and Molecular Investigations." *J Pineal Res* 28, no. 3 (2000): 156–64.
15. Araki, E., S. Oyadomari, and M. Mori. "Impact of Endoplasmic Reticulum Stress Pathway on Pancreatic Beta-Cells and Diabetes Mellitus." *Exp Biol Med (Maywood)* 228, no. 10 (2003): 1213–7.
16. Parhon, C. I., I. Potop, and E. Felix. "Influenta Epifisectomiei Si a Administrarii De Extract Epifisar Asupra Unor Data Metabolice Privind Mineralele (Ca, K, P, Si, Mg), Lipidele, Protidele Si Glucidele, La Sobolanul Alb Adult." *Stud Cercet Endocr* 3, no. 3 (1952): 321–29.
17. Milcou, I., L. Nanu, and R. Marcean. "[Existence of a Hypoglycemic Pineal Hormone Synergistic with Insulin.]." *Ann Endocrinol (Paris)* 18, no. 4 (1957): 612–20.
18. Peschke, E. "Melatonin, Endocrine Pancreas and Diabetes." *J Pineal Res* 44, no. 1 (2008): 26–40.
19. Diaz, B., and E. Blazquez. "Effect of Pinealectomy on Plasma Glucose, Insulin and Glucagon Levels in the Rat." *Horm Metab Res* 18, no. 4 (1986): 225–9.
20. Mellado, C., V. Rodriguez, J. G. de Diego, E. Alvarez, and E. Blazquez. "Effect of Pinealectomy and of Diabetes on Liver Insulin and Glucagon Receptor Concentrations in the Rat." *J Pineal Res* 6, no. 4 (1989): 295–306.
21. Rodriguez, V., C. Mellado, E. Alvarez, J. G. De Diego, and E. Blazquez. "Effect of Pinealectomy on Liver Insulin and Glucagon Receptor Concentrations in the Rat." *J Pineal Res* 6, no. 1 (1989): 77–88.
22. de Lima, L. M., L. C. dos Reis, and M. A. de Lima. "Influence of the Pineal Gland on the Physiology, Morphometry and Morphology of Pancreatic Islets in Rats." *Braz J Biol* 61, no. 2 (2001): 333–40.
23. Shima, T., S. J. Chun, A. Niijima, J. G. Bizot-Espiard, B. Guardiola-Lemaitre, M. Hosokawa, and K. Nagai. "Melatonin Suppresses Hyperglycemia Caused by Intracerebroventricular Injection of 2-Deoxy-D-Glucose in Rats." *Neurosci Lett* 226, no. 2 (1997): 119–22.
24. Nishida, S., T. Segawa, I. Murai, and S. Nakagawa. "Long-Term Melatonin Administration Reduces Hyperinsulinemia and Improves the Altered Fatty-Acid Compositions in Type 2 Diabetic Rats Via the Restoration of Delta-5 Desaturase Activity." *J Pineal Res* 32, no. 1 (2002): 26–33.
25. Hussain, S. A., H. M. Khadim, B. H. Khalaf, S. H. Ismail, K. I. Hussein, and A. S. Sahib. "Effects of Melatonin and Zinc on Glycemic Control in Type 2 Diabetic Patients Poorly Controlled with Metformin." *Saudi Med J* 27, no. 10 (2006): 1483–8.
26. Kadhim, H. M., S. H. Ismail, K. I. Hussein, I. H. Bakir, A. S. Sahib, B. H. Khalaf, and S. A. Hussain. "Effects of Melatonin and Zinc on Lipid Profile and Renal Function in Type 2 Diabetic Patients Poorly Controlled with Metformin." *J Pineal Res* 41, no. 2 (2006): 189–93.
27. Prokopenko, I., C. Langenberg, J. C. Florez, R. Saxena, N. Soranzo, G. Thorleifsson, et al. "Variants in Mtnr1b Influence Fasting Glucose Levels." *Nat Genet* 41, no. 1 (2009): 77–81.
28. Bouatia-Naji, N., A. Bonnefond, C. Cavalcanti-Proenca, T. Sparso, J. Holmkvist, M. Marchand, et al. "A Variant near Mtnr1b Is Associated with Increased Fasting Plasma Glucose Levels and Type 2 Diabetes Risk." *Nat Genet* 41, no. 1 (2009): 89–94.
29. Staiger, H., F. Machicao, S. A. Schafer, K. Kirchhoff, K. Kantartzis, M. Guthoff, G. Silbernagel, N. Stefan, H. U. Haring, and A. Fritsche. "Polymorphisms within the Novel Type 2 Diabetes Risk Locus Mtnr1b Determine Beta-Cell Function." *PLoS One* 3, no. 12 (2008): e3962.
30. Tan, D. X., R. Hardeland, L. C. Manchester, S. D. Paredes, A. Korkmaz, R. M. Sainz, J. C. Mayo, L. Fuentes-Broto, and R. J. Reiter. "The Changing Biological Roles of Melatonin During Evolution: From an Antioxidant to Signals of Darkness, Sexual Selection and Fitness." *Biol Rev Camb Philos Soc* (2009).
31. Goto, Y., K. Suzuki, T. Ono, M. Sasaki, and T. Toyota. "Development of Diabetes in the Non-Obese Niddm Rat (Gk Rat)." *Adv Exp Med Biol* 246 (1988): 29–31.

32. Portha, B., P. Serradas, D. Bailbe, K. Suzuki, Y. Goto, and M. H. Giroix. "Beta-Cell Insensitivity to Glucose in the Gk Rat, a Spontaneous Nonobese Model for Type Ii Diabetes." *Diabetes* 40, no. 4 (1991): 486–91.
33. Movassat, J., C. Saulnier, P. Serradas, and B. Portha. "Impaired Development of Pancreatic Beta-Cell Mass Is a Primary Event During the Progression to Diabetes in the Gk Rat." *Diabetologia* 40, no. 8 (1997): 916–25.
34. Frese, T., I. Bazwinsky, E. Muhlbauer, and E. Peschke. "Circadian and Age-Dependent Expression Patterns of Glut2 and Glucokinase in the Pancreatic Beta-Cell of Diabetic and Nondiabetic Rats." *Horm Metab Res* 39, no. 8 (2007): 567–74.
35. Bisbis, S., D. Bailbe, M. A. Tormo, F. Picarel-Blanchot, M. Derouet, J. Simon, and B. Portha. "Insulin Resistance in the Gk Rat: Decreased Receptor Number but Normal Kinase Activity in Liver." *Am J Physiol* 265, no. 5 Pt 1 (1993): E807–13.
36. Ghanaat-Pour, H., Z. Huang, M. Lehtihet, and A. Sjoholm. "Global Expression Profiling of Glucose-Regulated Genes in Pancreatic Islets of Spontaneously Diabetic Goto-Kakizaki Rats." *J Mol Endocrinol* 39, no. 2 (2007): 135–50.
37. Sena, C. M., C. Barosa, E. Nunes, R. Seica, and J. G. Jones. "Sources of Endogenous Glucose Production in the Goto-Kakizaki Diabetic Rat." *Diabetes Metab* 33, no. 4 (2007): 296–302.
38. Klein, D. C., S. L. Coon, P. H. Roseboom, J. L. Weller, M. Bernard, J. A. Gastel, M. Zatz, P. M. Iuvone, I. R. Rodriguez, V. Begay, J. Falcon, G. M. Cahill, V. M. Cassone, and R. Baler. "The Melatonin Rhythm-Generating Enzyme: Molecular Regulation of Serotonin *N*-Acetyltransferase in the Pineal Gland." *Recent Prog Horm Res* 52 (1997): 307–57; discussion 57–8.
39. Stehle, J. H., C. von Gall, C. Schomerus, and H. W. Korf. "Of Rodents and Ungulates and Melatonin: Creating a Uniform Code for Darkness by Different Signaling Mechanisms." *J Biol Rhythms* 16, no. 4 (2001): 312–25.
40. Simonneaux, V., and C. Ribelayga. "Generation of the Melatonin Endocrine Message in Mammals: A Review of the Complex Regulation of Melatonin Synthesis by Norepinephrine, Peptides, and Other Pineal Transmitters." *Pharmacol Rev* 55, no. 2 (2003): 325–95.
41. Lacy, P. E., and M. Kostianovsky. "Method for the Isolation of Intact Islets of Langerhans from the Rat Pancreas." *Diabetes* 16, no. 1 (1967): 35–9.
42. Ricordi, C., C. Socci, A. M. Davalli, C. Staudacher, P. Baro, A. Vertova, I. Sassi, F. Gavazzi, G. Pozza, and V. Di Carlo. "Isolation of the Elusive Pig Islet." *Surgery* 107, no. 6 (1990): 688–94.
43. Van De Winkel, M., and D. Pipeleers. "Autofluorescence-Activated Cell Sorting of Pancreatic Islet Cells: Purification of Insulin-Containing B-Cells According to Glucose-Induced Changes in Cellular Redox State." *Biochem Biophys Res Commun* 114, no. 2 (1983): 835–42.
44. Kaiser, N., A. P. Corcos, I. Sarel, and E. Cerasi. "Monolayer Culture of Adult Rat Pancreatic Islets on Extracellular Matrix: Modulation of B-Cell Function by Chronic Exposure to High Glucose." *Endocrinology* 129, no. 4 (1991): 2067–76.
45. Wollheim, C. B., P. Meda, and P. A. Halban. "Establishment and Culture of Insulin-Secreting Beta Cell Lines." *Methods Enzymol* 192 (1990): 223–35.
46. Santerre, R. F., R. A. Cook, R. M. Crisel, J. D. Sharp, R. J. Schmidt, D. C. Williams, and C. P. Wilson. "Insulin Synthesis in a Clonal Cell Line of Simian Virus 40–Transformed Hamster Pancreatic Beta Cells." *Proc Natl Acad Sci U S A* 78, no. 7 (1981): 4339–43.
47. Praz, G. A., P. A. Halban, C. B. Wollheim, B. Blondel, A. J. Strauss, and A. E. Renold. "Regulation of Immunoreactive-Insulin Release from a Rat Cell Line (Rinm5f)." *Biochem J* 210, no. 2 (1983): 345–52.
48. Asfari, M., D. Janjic, P. Meda, G. Li, P. A. Halban, and C. B. Wollheim. "Establishment of 2-Mercaptoethanol-Dependent Differentiated Insulin-Secreting Cell Lines." *Endocrinology* 130, no. 1 (1992): 167–78.
49. Poitout, V., L. K. Olson, and R. P. Robertson. "Insulin-Secreting Cell Lines: Classification, Characteristics and Potential Applications." *Diabetes Metab* 22, no. 1 (1996): 7–14.
50. McClenaghan, N. H., and P. R. Flatt. "Physiological and Pharmacological Regulation of Insulin Release: Insights Offered through Exploitation of Insulin-Secreting Cell Lines." *Diabetes Obes Metab* 1, no. 3 (1999): 137–50.
51. Bailey, C. J., T. W. Atkins, and A. J. Matty. "Melatonin Inhibition of Insulin Secretion in the Rat and Mouse." *Horm Res* 5, no. 1 (1974): 21–8.
52. Peschke, E., E. Muhlbauer, U. Musshoff, V. J. Csernus, E. Chankiewitz, and D. Peschke. "Receptor (MT(1)) Mediated Influence of Melatonin on Camp Concentration and Insulin Secretion of Rat Insulinoma Cells INS-1." *J Pineal Res* 33, no. 2 (2002): 63–71.

53. Picinato, M. C., E. P. Haber, J. Cipolla-Neto, R. Curi, C. R. de Oliveira Carvalho, and A. R. Carpinelli. "Melatonin Inhibits Insulin Secretion and Decreases Pka Levels without Interfering with Glucose Metabolism in Rat Pancreatic Islets." *J Pineal Res* 33, no. 3 (2002): 156–60.
54. Stumpf, I., E. Muhlbauer, and E. Peschke. "Involvement of the Cgmp Pathway in Mediating the Insulin-Inhibitory Effect of Melatonin in Pancreatic Beta-Cells." *J Pineal Res* 45, no. 3 (2008): 318–27.
55. Stumpf, I., I. Bazwinsky, and E. Peschke. "Modulation of the Cgmp Signaling Pathway by Melatonin in Pancreatic Beta-Cells." *J Pineal Res* 46, no. 2 (2009): 140–7.
56. Bach, A. G., S. Wolgast, E. Muhlbauer, and E. Peschke. "Melatonin Stimulates Inositol-1,4,5-Trisphosphate and Ca2+ Release from INS1 Insulinoma Cells." *J Pineal Res* 39, no. 3 (2005): 316–23.
57. Peschke, E., T. Frese, E. Chankiewitz, D. Peschke, U. Preiss, U. Schneyer, R. Spessert, and E. Muhlbauer. "Diabetic Goto Kakizaki Rats as Well as Type 2 Diabetic Patients Show a Decreased Diurnal Serum Melatonin Level and an Increased Pancreatic Melatonin-Receptor Status." *J Pineal Res* 40, no. 2 (2006): 135–43.
58. Peschke, E., E. Muhlbauer, U. Musshoff, V. J. Csernus, E. Chankiewitz, and D. Peschke. "Receptor (MT(1)) Mediated Influence of Melatonin on Camp Concentration and Insulin Secretion of Rat Insulinoma Cells INS-1." *J Pineal Res* 33, no. 2 (2002): 63–71.
59. Muhlbauer, E., and E. Peschke. "Evidence for the Expression of Both the MT1- and in Addition, the MT2-Melatonin Receptor, in the Rat Pancreas, Islet and Beta-Cell." *J Pineal Res* 42, no. 1 (2007): 105–6.
60. Peschke, E., I. Stumpf, I. Bazwinsky, L. Litvak, H. Dralle, and E. Muhlbauer. "Melatonin and Type 2 Diabetes—A Possible Link?" *J Pineal Res* 42, no. 4 (2007): 350–8.
61. Neacsu, C. "Pineal–Pancreas Interaction: Pineal Hormone E5 Action on Insulin Activity." *Physiologie* 25, no. 3 (1988): 119–27.
62. Pauly, J. E., and L. E. Scheving. "Circadian Rhythms in Blood Glucose and the Effect of Different Lighting Schedules, Hypophysectomy, Adrenal Medullectomy and Starvation." *Am J Anat* 120, no. 3 (1967): 627–36.
63. Van Cauter, E., K. S. Polonsky, and A. J. Scheen. "Roles of Circadian Rhythmicity and Sleep in Human Glucose Regulation." *Endocr Rev* 18, no. 5 (1997): 716–38.
64. Bolli, G. B., P. De Feo, S. De Cosmo, G. Perriello, M. M. Ventura, F. Calcinaro, C. Lolli, P. Campbell, P. Brunetti, and J. E. Gerich. "Demonstration of a Dawn Phenomenon in Normal Human Volunteers." *Diabetes* 33, no. 12 (1984): 1150–3.
65. Trumper, B. G., K. Reschke, and J. Molling. "Circadian Variation of Insulin Requirement in Insulin Dependent Diabetes Mellitus the Relationship between Circadian Change in Insulin Demand and Diurnal Patterns of Growth Hormone, Cortisol and Glucagon During Euglycemia." *Horm Metab Res* 27, no. 3 (1995): 141–7.
66. Cagnacci, A., S. Arangino, A. Renzi, A. M. Paoletti, G. B. Melis, P. Cagnacci, and A. Volpe. "Influence of Melatonin Administration on Glucose Tolerance and Insulin Sensitivity of Postmenopausal Women." *Clin Endocrinol (Oxf)* 54, no. 3 (2001): 339–46.
67. Wolden-Hanson, T., D. R. Mitton, R. L. McCants, S. M. Yellon, C. W. Wilkinson, A. M. Matsumoto, and D. D. Rasmussen. "Daily Melatonin Administration to Middle-Aged Male Rats Suppresses Body Weight, Intraabdominal Adiposity, and Plasma Leptin and Insulin Independent of Food Intake and Total Body Fat." *Endocrinology* 141, no. 2 (2000): 487–97.
68. Peschke, E., D. Peschke, T. Hammer, and V. Csernus. "Influence of Melatonin and Serotonin on Glucose-Stimulated Insulin Release from Perifused Rat Pancreatic Islets in Vitro." *J Pineal Res* 23, no. 3 (1997): 156–63.
69. Picinato, M. C., E. P. Haber, J. Cipolla-Neto, R. Curi, C. R. de Oliveira Carvalho, and A. R. Carpinelli. "Melatonin Inhibits Insulin Secretion and Decreases Pka Levels without Interfering with Glucose Metabolism in Rat Pancreatic Islets." *J Pineal Res* 33, no. 3 (2002): 156–60.
70. Boden, G., J. Ruiz, J. L. Urbain, and X. Chen. "Evidence for a Circadian Rhythm of Insulin Secretion." *Am J Physiol* 271, no. 2 Pt 1 (1996): E246–52.
71. Nishida, S., T. Segawa, I. Murai, and S. Nakagawa. "Long-Term Melatonin Administration Reduces Hyperinsulinemia and Improves the Altered Fatty-Acid Compositions in Type 2 Diabetic Rats Via the Restoration of Delta-5 Desaturase Activity." *J Pineal Res* 32, no. 1 (2002): 26–33.
72. Kadhim, H. M., S. H. Ismail, K. I. Hussein, I. H. Bakir, A. S. Sahib, B. H. Khalaf, and S. A. Hussain. "Effects of Melatonin and Zinc on Lipid Profile and Renal Function in Type 2 Diabetic Patients Poorly Controlled with Metformin." *J Pineal Res* 41, no. 2 (2006): 189–93.
73. Shieh, J. M., H. T. Wu, K. C. Cheng, and J. T. Cheng. "Melatonin Ameliorates High Fat Diet-Induced Diabetes and Stimulates Glycogen Synthesis Via a Pkczeta-Akt-Gsk3beta Pathway in Hepatic Cells." *J Pineal Res* 47, no. 4 (2009): 339–44.

74. Ha, E., S. V. Yim, J. H. Chung, K. S. Yoon, I. Kang, Y. H. Cho, and H. H. Baik. "Melatonin Stimulates Glucose Transport Via Insulin Receptor Substrate-1/Phosphatidylinositol 3-Kinase Pathway in C2c12 Murine Skeletal Muscle Cells." *J Pineal Res* 41, no. 1 (2006): 67–72.
75. Nishida, S. "Metabolic Effects of Melatonin on Oxidative Stress and Diabetes Mellitus." *Endocrine* 27, no. 2 (2005): 131–6.
76. Contreras-Alcantara, S., K. Baba, and G. Tosini. "Removal of Melatonin Receptor Type 1 Induces Insulin Resistance in the Mouse." *Obesity* (*Silver Spring*) (2010).
77. Sartori, C., P. Dessen, C. Mathieu, A. Monney, J. Bloch, P. Nicod, U. Scherrer, and H. Duplain. "Melatonin Improves Glucose Homeostasis and Endothelial Vascular Function in High-Fat Diet–Fed Insulin-Resistant Mice." *Endocrinology* 150, no. 12 (2009): 5311–7.
78. Dhar, M., S. S. Dayal, C. S. Ramesh Babu, and S. R. Arora. "Effect of Melatonin on Glucose Tolerance and Blood Glucose Circadian Rhythm in Rabbits." *Ind J Physiol Pharmacol* 27, no. 2 (1983): 109–17.
79. Tiedge, M., S. Lortz, R. Munday, and S. Lenzen. "Protection against the Co-Operative Toxicity of Nitric Oxide and Oxygen Free Radicals by Overexpression of Antioxidant Enzymes in Bioengineered Insulin-Producing Rinm5f Cells." *Diabetologia* 42, no. 7 (1999): 849–55.
80. Tiedge, M., S. Lortz, J. Drinkgern, and S. Lenzen. "Relation between Antioxidant Enzyme Gene Expression and Antioxidative Defense Status of Insulin-Producing Cells." *Diabetes* 46, no. 11 (1997): 1733–42.
81. Peschke, E., H. Ebelt, H. J. Bromme, and D. Peschke. " 'Classical' and 'New' Diabetogens—Comparison of Their Effects on Isolated Rat Pancreatic Islets in Vitro." *Cell Mol Life Sci* 57, no. 1 (2000): 158–64.
82. Reiter, R. J., D. X. Tan, and S. Burkhardt. "Reactive Oxygen and Nitrogen Species and Cellular and Organismal Decline: Amelioration with Melatonin." *Mech Ageing Dev* 123, no. 8 (2002): 1007–19.
83. Reiter, R. J., D. Tan, S. J. Kim, L. C. Manchester, W. Qi, J. J. Garcia, J. C. Cabrera, G. El-Sokkary, and V. Rouvier-Garay. "Augmentation of Indices of Oxidative Damage in Life-Long Melatonin-Deficient Rats." *Mech Ageing Dev* 110, no. 3 (1999): 157–73.
84. Bromme, H. J., W. Morke, and E. Peschke. "Transformation of Barbituric Acid into Alloxan by Hydroxyl Radicals: Interaction with Melatonin and with Other Hydroxyl Radical Scavengers." *J Pineal Res* 33, no. 4 (2002): 239–47.
85. Bromme, H. J., W. Morke, D. Peschke, H. Ebelt, and D. Peschke. "Scavenging Effect of Melatonin on Hydroxyl Radicals Generated by Alloxan." *J Pineal Res* 29, no. 4 (2000): 201–8.
86. Ebelt, H., D. Peschke, H. J. Bromme, W. Morke, R. Blume, and E. Peschke. "Influence of Melatonin on Free Radical-Induced Changes in Rat Pancreatic Beta-Cells in Vitro." *J Pineal Res* 28, no. 2 (2000): 65–72.
87. Bromme, H. J., H. Ebelt, D. Peschke, and E. Peschke. "Alloxan Acts as a Prooxidant Only under Reducing Conditions: Influence of Melatonin." *Cell Mol Life Sci* 55, no. 3 (1999): 487–93.
88. Reiter, R. J., D. X. Tan, C. Osuna, and E. Gitto. "Actions of Melatonin in the Reduction of Oxidative Stress. A Review." *J Biomed Sci* 7, no. 6 (2000): 444–58.
89. Rodriguez, C., J. C. Mayo, R. M. Sainz, I. Antolin, F. Herrera, V. Martin, and R. J. Reiter. "Regulation of Antioxidant Enzymes: A Significant Role for Melatonin." *J Pineal Res* 36, no. 1 (2004): 1–9.
90. La Fleur, S. E. "Daily Rhythms in Glucose Metabolism: Suprachiasmatic Nucleus Output to Peripheral Tissue." *J Neuroendocrinol* 15, no. 3 (2003): 315–22.
91. Zawalich, W. S., K. C. Zawalich, G. J. Tesz, J. A. Sterpka, and W. M. Philbrick. "Insulin Secretion and Ip Levels in Two Distant Lineages of the Genus Mus: Comparisons with Rat Islets." *Am J Physiol Endocrinol Metab* 280, no. 5 (2001): E720–8.
92. Picinato, M. C., E. P. Haber, A. R. Carpinelli, and J. Cipolla-Neto. "Daily Rhythm of Glucose-Induced Insulin Secretion by Isolated Islets from Intact and Pinealectomized Rat." *J Pineal Res* 33, no. 3 (2002): 172–7.
93. Peschke, E., and D. Peschke. "Evidence for a Circadian Rhythm of Insulin Release from Perifused Rat Pancreatic Islets." *Diabetologia* 41, no. 9 (1998): 1085–92.
94. Scott, E. M., and P. J. Grant. "Neel Revisited: The Adipocyte, Seasonality and Type 2 Diabetes." *Diabetologia* 49, no. 7 (2006): 1462–6.
95. Morgan, L., S. Hampton, M. Gibbs, and J. Arendt. "Circadian Aspects of Postprandial Metabolism." *Chronobiol Int* 20, no. 5 (2003): 795–808.
96. Qin, L. Q., J. Li, Y. Wang, J. Wang, J. Y. Xu, and T. Kaneko. "The Effects of Nocturnal Life on Endocrine Circadian Patterns in Healthy Adults." *Life Sci* 73, no. 19 (2003): 2467–75.
97. Stagner, J. I., E. Samols, and G. C. Weir. "Sustained Oscillations of Insulin, Glucagon, and Somatostatin from the Isolated Canine Pancreas During Exposure to a Constant Glucose Concentration." *J Clin Invest* 65, no. 4 (1980): 939–42.

98. Chou, H. F., N. Berman, and E. Ipp. "Evidence for Pancreatic Pacemaker for Insulin Oscillations in Low-Frequency Range." *Am J Physiol* 266, no. 6 Pt 2 (1994): R1786–91.
99. Marchetti, P., D. W. Scharp, M. McLear, R. Gingerich, E. Finke, B. Olack, C. Swanson, R. Giannarelli, R. Navalesi, and P. E. Lacy. "Pulsatile Insulin Secretion from Isolated Human Pancreatic Islets." *Diabetes* 43, no. 6 (1994): 827–30.
100. Muhlbauer, E., S. Wolgast, U. Finckh, D. Peschke, and E. Peschke. "Indication of Circadian Oscillations in the Rat Pancreas." *FEBS Lett* 564, no. 1–2 (2004): 91–6.
101. Ben-Dyke, R. "Diurnal Variation of Oral Glucose Tolerance in Volunteers and Laboratory Animals." *Diabetologia* 7, no. 3 (1971): 156–9.
102. Gibson, T., L. Stimmler, R. J. Jarrett, P. Rutland, and M. Shiu. "Diurnal Variation in the Effects of Insulin on Blood Glucose, Plasma Non-Esterified Fatty Acids and Growth Hormone." *Diabetologia* 11, no. 1 (1975): 83–8.
103. Schibler, U., J. Ripperger, and S. A. Brown. "Peripheral Circadian Oscillators in Mammals: Time and Food." *J Biol Rhythms* 18, no. 3 (2003): 250–60.
104. Bizot-Espiard, J. G., A. Double, B. Guardiola-Lemaitre, P. Delagrange, A. Ktorza, and L. Penicaud. "Diurnal Rhythms in Plasma Glucose, Insulin, Growth Hormone and Melatonin Levels in Fasted and Hyperglycaemic Rats." *Diabetes Metab* 24, no. 3 (1998): 235–40.
105. Picinato, M. C., A. E. Hirata, J. Cipolla-Neto, R. Curi, C. R. Carvalho, G. F. Anhe, and A. R. Carpinelli. "Activation of Insulin and IGF-1 Signaling Pathways by Melatonin through MT1 Receptor in Isolated Rat Pancreatic Islets." *J Pineal Res* 44, no. 1 (2008): 88–94.
106. Gastel, J. A., P. H. Roseboom, P. A. Rinaldi, J. L. Weller, and D. C. Klein. "Melatonin Production: Proteasomal Proteolysis in Serotonin *N*-Acetyltransferase Regulation." *Science* 279, no. 5355 (1998): 1358–60.
107. Bruning, J. C., D. Gautam, D. J. Burks, J. Gillette, M. Schubert, P. C. Orban, R. Klein, W. Krone, D. Muller-Wieland, and C. R. Kahn. "Role of Brain Insulin Receptor in Control of Body Weight and Reproduction." *Science* 289, no. 5487 (2000): 2122–5.
108. Lynch, H. J., M. Ho, and R. J. Wurtman. "The Adrenal Medulla May Mediate the Increase in Pineal Melatonin Synthesis Induced by Stress, but Not That Caused by Exposure to Darkness." *J Neural Transm* 40, no. 2 (1977): 87–97.
109. Champney, T. H., R. W. Steger, D. S. Christie, and R. J. Reiter. "Alterations in Components of the Pineal Melatonin Synthetic Pathway by Acute Insulin Stress in the Rat and Syrian Hamster." *Brain Res* 338, no. 1 (1985): 25–32.
110. Champney, T. H., A. P. Holtorf, C. M. Craft, and R. J. Reiter. "Hormonal Modulation of Pineal Melatonin Synthesis in Rats and Syrian Hamsters: Effects of Streptozotocin-Induced Diabetes and Insulin Injections." *Comp Biochem Physiol A* 83, no. 2 (1986): 391–5.
111. Anhe, G. F., L. C. Caperuto, M. Pereira-Da-Silva, L. C. Souza, A. E. Hirata, L. A. Velloso, J. Cipolla-Neto, and C. R. Carvalho. "In Vivo Activation of Insulin Receptor Tyrosine Kinase by Melatonin in the Rat Hypothalamus." *J Neurochem* 90, no. 3 (2004): 559–66.
112. Conti, A., and G. J. Maestroni. "Melatonin Rhythms in Mice: Role in Autoimmune and Lymphoproliferative Diseases." *Ann N Y Acad Sci* 840 (1998): 395–410.
113. Champney, T. H., G. C. Brainard, B. A. Richardson, and R. J. Reiter. "Experimentally-Induced Diabetes Reduces Nocturnal Pineal Melatonin Content in the Syrian Hamster." *Comp Biochem Physiol A* 76, no. 1 (1983): 199–201.
114. Radziuk, J., and S. Pye. "Diurnal Rhythm in Endogenous Glucose Production Is a Major Contributor to Fasting Hyperglycaemia in Type 2 Diabetes. Suprachiasmatic Deficit or Limit Cycle Behaviour?" *Diabetologia* 49, no. 7 (2006): 1619–28.
115. Van Cauter, E. "Putative Roles of Melatonin in Glucose Regulation." *Therapie* 53, no. 5 (1998): 467–72.
116. Bubenik, G. A., and S. F. Pang. "Melatonin Levels in the Gastrointestinal Tissues of Fish, Amphibians, and a Reptile." *Gen Comp Endocrinol* 106, no. 3 (1997): 415–9.
117. Bubenik, G. A., R. R. Hacker, G. M. Brown, and L. Bartos. "Melatonin Concentrations in the Luminal Fluid, Mucosa, and Muscularis of the Bovine and Porcine Gastrointestinal Tract." *J Pineal Res* 26, no. 1 (1999): 56–63.
118. Messner, M., G. Huether, T. Lorf, G. Ramadori, and H. Schworer. "Presence of Melatonin in the Human Hepatobiliary–astrointestinal Tract." *Life Sci* 69, no. 5 (2001): 543–51.
119. Huether, G., B. Poeggeler, A. Reimer, and A. George. "Effect of Tryptophan Administration on Circulating Melatonin Levels in Chicks and Rats: Evidence for Stimulation of Melatonin Synthesis and Release in the Gastrointestinal Tract." *Life Sci* 51, no. 12 (1992): 945–53.

120. Leja-Szpak, A., J. Jaworek, K. Nawrot-Porabka, M. Palonek, M. Mitis-Musiol, A. Dembinski, S. J. Konturek, and W. W. Pawlik. "Modulation of Pancreatic Enzyme Secretion by Melatonin and Its Precursor; L-Tryptophan. Role of Cck and Afferent Nerves." *J Physiol Pharmacol* 55 Suppl 2 (2004): 33–46.
121. Jaworek, J., T. Brzozowski, and S. J. Konturek. "Melatonin as an Organoprotector in the Stomach and the Pancreas." *J Pineal Res* 38, no. 2 (2005): 73–83.
122. Sjoblom, M., and G. Flemstrom. "Melatonin in the Duodenal Lumen Is a Potent Stimulant of Mucosal Bicarbonate Secretion." *J Pineal Res* 34, no. 4 (2003): 288–93.
123. Drago, F., S. Macauda, and S. Salehi. "Small Doses of Melatonin Increase Intestinal Motility in Rats." *Dig Dis Sci* 47, no. 9 (2002): 1969–74.
124. Claustrat, B., J. Brun, and G. Chazot. "The Basic Physiology and Pathophysiology of Melatonin." *Sleep Med Rev* 9, no. 1 (2005): 11–24.
125. Garcia, R. A., S. C. Afeche, J. H. Scialfa, F. G. do Amaral, S. H. dos Santos, F. B. Lima, M. E. Young, and J. Cipolla-Neto. "Insulin Modulates Norepinephrine-Mediated Melatonin Synthesis in Cultured Rat Pineal Gland." *Life Sci* 82, no. 1–2 (2008): 108–14.
126. O'Brien, I. A., I. G. Lewin, J. P. O'Hare, J. Arendt, and R. J. Corrall. "Abnormal Circadian Rhythm of Melatonin in Diabetic Autonomic Neuropathy." *Clin Endocrinol (Oxf)* 24, no. 4 (1986): 359–64.
127. Tutuncu, N. B., M. K. Batur, A. Yildirir, T. Tutuncu, A. Deger, Z. Koray, B. Erbas, G. Kabakci, S. Aksoyek, and T. Erbas. "Melatonin Levels Decrease in Type 2 Diabetic Patients with Cardiac Autonomic Neuropathy." *J Pineal Res* 39, no. 1 (2005): 43–9.
128. Peschke, E., T. Frese, E. Chankiewitz, D. Peschke, U. Preiss, U. Schneyer, R. Spessert, and E. Muhlbauer. "Diabetic Goto Kakizaki Rats as Well as Type 2 Diabetic Patients Show a Decreased Diurnal Serum Melatonin Level and an Increased Pancreatic Melatonin-Receptor Status." *J Pineal Res* 40, no. 2 (2006): 135–43.
129. Peschke, E., I. Stumpf, I. Bazwinsky, L. Litvak, H. Dralle, and E. Muhlbauer. "Melatonin and Type 2 Diabetes—A Possible Link?" *J Pineal Res* 42, no. 4 (2007): 350–8.
130. Robeva, R., G. Kirilov, A. Tomova, and P. Kumanov. "Low Testosterone Levels and Unimpaired Melatonin Secretion in Young Males with Metabolic Syndrome." *Andrologia* 38, no. 6 (2006): 216–20.
131. Cano, P., V. Jimenez-Ortega, A. Larrad, C. F. Reyes Toso, D. P. Cardinali, and A. I. Esquifino. "Effect of a High-Fat Diet on 24-H Pattern of Circulating Levels of Prolactin, Luteinizing Hormone, Testosterone, Corticosterone, Thyroid-Stimulating Hormone and Glucose, and Pineal Melatonin Content, in Rats." *Endocrine* 33, no. 2 (2008): 118–25.
132. Tutuncu, N. B., M. K. Batur, A. Yildirir, T. Tutuncu, A. Deger, Z. Koray, B. Erbas, G. Kabakci, S. Aksoyek, and T. Erbas. "Melatonin Levels Decrease in Type 2 Diabetic Patients with Cardiac Autonomic Neuropathy." *J Pineal Res* 39, no. 1 (2005): 43–9.
133. Godson, C., and S. M. Reppert. "The Mel1a Melatonin Receptor Is Coupled to Parallel Signal Transduction Pathways." *Endocrinology* 138, no. 1 (1997): 397–404.
134. Bach, A. G., E. Muhlbauer, and E. Peschke. "Adrenoceptor Expression and Diurnal Rhythms of Melatonin and Its Precursors in the Pineal Gland of Type 2 Diabetic Goto-Kakizaki Rats." *Endocrinology* 151, no. 6 (2010): 2483–93.
135. Frese, T., A. G. Bach, E. Muhlbauer, K. Ponicke, H. J. Bromme, A. Welp, and E. Peschke. "Pineal Melatonin Synthesis Is Decreased in Type 2 Diabetic Goto-Kakizaki Rats." *Life Sci* 1, no. 13–14 (2009): 526–33.
136. O'Brien, I. A., I. G. Lewin, J. P. O'Hare, J. Arendt, and R. J. Corrall. "Abnormal Circadian Rhythm of Melatonin in Diabetic Autonomic Neuropathy." *Clin Endocrinol (Oxf)* 24, no. 4 (1986): 359–64.
137. Garcia, R. A., S. C. Afeche, J. H. Scialfa, F. G. do Amaral, S. H. dos Santos, F. B. Lima, M. E. Young, and J. Cipolla-Neto. "Insulin Modulates Norepinephrine-Mediated Melatonin Synthesis in Cultured Rat Pineal Gland." *Life Sci* 82, no. 1–2 (2008): 108–14.
138. Wurtman, R. J., F. Larin, J. Axelrod, H. M. Shein, and K. Rosasco. "Formation of Melatonin and 5-Hydroxyindole Acetic Acid from 14c-Tryptophan by Rat Pineal Glands in Organ Culture." *Nature* 217, no. 5132 (1968): 953–4.
139. Harada, T., M. Hirotani, M. Maeda, H. Nomura, and H. Takeuchi. "Correlation between Breakfast Tryptophan Content and Morning–Evening in Japanese Infants and Students Aged 0–15 Yrs." *J Physiol Anthropol* 26, no. 2 (2007): 201–7.
140. Noguchi, T., M. Nishino, and R. Kido. "Tryptophan 5-Hydroxylase in Rat Intestine." *Biochem J* 131, no. 2 (1973): 375–80.
141. Fitzpatrick, P. F. "Tetrahydropterin-Dependent Amino Acid Hydroxylases." *Annu Rev Biochem* 68 (1999): 355–81.

142. Okumura, M., M. Masada, Y. Yoshida, H. Shintaku, M. Hosoi, N. Okada, Y. Konishi, T. Morikawa, K. Miura, and M. Imanishi. "Decrease in Tetrahydrobiopterin as a Possible Cause of Nephropathy in Type II Diabetic Rats." *Kidney Int* 70, no. 3 (2006): 471–6.
143. Hamon, C. G., P. Cutler, and J. A. Blair. "Tetrahydrobiopterin Metabolism in the Streptozotocin Induced Diabetic State in Rats." *Clin Chim Acta* 181, no. 3 (1989): 249–53.
144. Cai, S., J. Khoo, S. Mussa, N. J. Alp, and K. M. Channon. "Endothelial Nitric Oxide Synthase Dysfunction in Diabetic Mice: Importance of Tetrahydrobiopterin in Enos Dimerisation." *Diabetologia* 48, no. 9 (2005): 1933–40.
145. Flatmark, T. "Catecholamine Biosynthesis and Physiological Regulation in Neuroendocrine Cells." *Acta Physiol Scand* 168, no. 1 (2000): 1–17.
146. Pietraszek, M. H., Y. Takada, A. Takada, M. Fujita, I. Watanabe, A. Taminato, and T. Yoshimi. "Blood Serotonergic Mechanisms in Type 2 (Non-Insulin-Dependent) Diabetes Mellitus." *Thromb Res* 66, no. 6 (1992): 765–74.
147. Vakov, L. "[Basal Blood Level of Serotonin in Diabetes Mellitus Patients]." *Vutr Boles* 23, no. 1 (1984): 79–84.
148. Kaplar, M., G. Paragh, A. Erdei, E. Csongradi, E. Varga, I. Garai, L. Szabados, L. Galuska, and J. Varga. "Changes in Cerebral Blood Flow Detected by Spect in Type 1 and Type 2 Diabetic Patients." *J Nucl Med* 50, no. 12 (2009): 1993–8.

9 Melatonin, Sleep, and Immune Modulation: Role in Health and Disease

Daniel P. Cardinali

CONTENTS

9.1 INTRODUCTION

Sleep and the immune system share regulatory molecules [1]. These molecules, mostly cytokines, are involved in both physiological sleep and the disturbed sleep observed during infection. It is feasible that sleep influences the immune system through the action of centrally produced cytokines that are regulated during sleep (see, for example, ref. [2]). In humans, both sleep and the neuroendocrine–immune system are controlled by a double-command system given by predictive and reactive homeostasis processes [3,4]. Predictive homeostasis is the primary role of the circadian system.

Pineal melatonin is a major circadian signal released to circulation daily at night. In all mammals, circulating melatonin is synthesized primarily in the pineal gland [5] and constitutes the "chemical code of night." Thus, many of the reported effects of melatonin on the immune system may depend on melatonin's role in sleep. In addition, melatonin is also locally found in various cells, tissues, and organs including lymphocytes [6], human and murine bone marrow [7,8], the thymus [9], the gastrointestinal tract [10], skin [11], and the eyes [12], where it plays either an autocrine or paracrine role [13].

Melatonin is a powerful antioxidant that scavenges superoxide radicals as well as other radical oxygen and nitrogen species (ROS and RNS, respectively) and gives rise to a cascade of metabolites sharing its antioxidant properties [14]. The antioxidant effect of melatonin is also exerted indirectly via promotion of gene expression of antioxidant enzymes and inhibition of gene expression of pro-oxidant enzymes [15]. The objective of the review is to summarize some of the mechanisms implicated in the mutual interaction among sleep, melatonin, and the immune system.

9.2 REACTIVE AND PREDICTIVE HOMEOSTASIS

The term *homeostasis* was introduced more than 80 years ago by Walter Cannon [16] to define the physiological factors that maintain the equilibrium status of the organism. Following Claude Bernard, Cannon improved the concept of constancy of the internal milieu. As Cannon stated, the prefix *homeo* [alike] was selected rather than *homo* [the same] to include explicitly the normal oscillation detectable in physiological variables. The first time the term *homeostasis* was used was in reference to the mechanisms regulating blood glucose levels. Cannon used the term to describe how blood glucose was controlled with normal values oscillating between a minimum and a maximum. When these limits were trespassed, mechanisms become activated to compensate for them. Then, these processes only function in the face of disturbances rather than anticipating them ("reactive" homeostasis) [16].

It must be noted that most regulatory mechanisms have a latency that can be inappropriately long for the expected response. For example, if a new protein is needed, latency may be as long as 1–2 hours, a time that can increase if there is a need to synthesize a hormone. A significant contribution of the circadian organization is that it allows the physiological response to be ready in advance to the expected perturbations of the internal milieu, provided the perturbation occurs at approximately the same hour every day ("predictive homeostasis" [16]).

In humans, such a predictive activity can be demonstrable. Body temperature and ACTH and cortisol rhythms increase some hours in advance to the major stress of morning awakening; the digestive system anticipates meal time; the cardiovascular system starts in advance during sleep the major changes in cardiovascular control to overcome the change in position during awakening. What evolution has selected is the development of a precise "biological clock," flexible enough to be resynchronized readily to new temporal situations.

Therefore, because of the seminal influence of Cannon and Moore-Ede, the term *homeostasis* is used today not only for describing the biological strategies to cope with changes in environment (reactive homeostasis) but also the time-related mechanisms that allow the organisms to predict an expected environmental modification by preparing to do it in advance (predictive homeostasis).

As a consequence of the development of the concept of homeostasis, disease can be analyzed both as the alteration of the internal environment it provokes as well as the result of the compensatory mechanisms triggered by the body to protect itself from the disease. As first defined by Hans Selye, the stress response implies a number of processes that are the consequence, not of the original noxious agent, but of the body itself in the course of the defense reaction [17]. Lately, McEwen introduced the concept of allostasis to define the price everyone pays for the stress response [18,19]. Even a moderate stimulus leaves its mark if repeatedly administered. In follow-up studies on urban populations, the allostatic charge was found to be proportional to sleep disturbance. In addition, the following factors also relate directly to the allostatic debt: (a) arterial systolic pressure, (b) nocturnal excretion of cortisol and catecholamines, (c) body mass index, (d) glycosylated hemoglobin, and (e) high-density lipoprotein/cholesterol ratio. Levels of hormones such as melatonin [20,21] appears to be inversely linked to the allostatic charge. Therefore, at least, a part of the allostatic process includes modification of the circadian organization (sleep/wake cycle, melatonin secretion).

9.3 SLEEP IS A COMPLEX PHENOMENON COMPRISING TWO SUBSTATES

Sleep is an essential process in life. It is a behavioral state defined by (a) characteristic relaxation of posture, (b) raised sensory thresholds, (c) distinctive electroencephalographic (EEG) pattern, and (d) ready reversibility. Sleep is not a unitary state, but it is composed of two substates. Based on polysomnographic measures, sleep has been divided into categories of rapid eye movement (REM) sleep and non-REM (NREM) sleep (also called slow-wave sleep) [22].

NREM sleep comprises four stages (stages 1–4), with stages 3 and 4 being characterized by slow, high-amplitude EEG waves in the frequency range below 4 Hz (delta rhythm). Sleep alternates between NREM stages 1–4 and REM sleep approximately every 90–120 minutes [23]. Periods of NREM sleep constitute about 75% of the total sleep time, and NREM reaches its greatest depth during the first half of the night. After completion of the fourth stage, the next stage does not begin immediately. Instead, the first four stages reverse quickly and are then immediately followed by a period of REM sleep.

REM sleep is defined by a faster EEG activity, rapid horizontal eye movements on electrooculography, vital sign instability, and the occurrence of skeletal muscle hypotonia and dysautonomia [24]. The tone in most voluntary muscles is minimal, but the diaphragm and the eye muscles are phasically active, giving REM sleep some resemblance to the wake state, for which reason it is sometimes referred to as "paradoxical sleep."

The length of the NREM and REM stages is not static. The first REM sleep will occur 90–120 minutes after falling asleep and will last approximately 10 minutes. As night proceeds, the length of stages 3 and 4 of NREM (delta or deep sleep) begins to wane and the length of REM sleep increases up to about 0.5 hour in length after a number of cycles. After a prolonged period of wake activity (as in humans), the first cycles are characterized by a preponderance of high-voltage, slow-wave activity (i.e., the NREM phase is enhanced), whereas the last cycles show more low-voltage, fast-wave activity (i.e., the REM phase is enhanced) [25–27].

The recurrent cycles of NREM and REM sleep are accompanied by major changes in the body's physiology. Indeed, it can be said that we live sequentially in three different physiological states (or "bodies"): that of wakefulness, that of NREM sleep, and that of REM sleep. For an average of 8 hours of sleep per day, a 76-year-old adult has lived about 50 years in wakefulness, 20 years in NREM sleep, and 6 years in REM sleep. NREM sleep duration readily decreases (about 30 minutes per decade), and stages 3 and 4 of NREM sleep represent less than 10% of total sleep after 40–50 years of age. This decrease is compensated by increases in stages 1 and 2 of NREM, while REM sleep or total duration of sleep remains more stable.

Since most epidemiological data indicate that, in our modern society, we only sleep for about 6 hours per day, for a 76-year-old adult, approximately 55 years are lived in wakefulness, 15 years in NREM sleep, and 6 years in REM sleep [25,26]. There is increasing evidence that obesity, metabolic syndrome, and possibly neurodegenerative diseases can be related to the prevalence of wakefulness in face of sleep loss in our contemporary, 24/7 society [27–29].

As shown in Table 9.1, significant physiological differences exist among the three physiological stages discussed above. Wakefulness is a catabolic, sympathotonic stage as reflected in every physiological system examined with a predominant activity of the hypothalamic–pituitary axis and high cortisol and norepinephrine levels (and none or very few melatonin in circulation), whereas NREM sleep is an anabolic stage characterized by a parasympathetic predominance, with decreases in blood pressure, heart rate, and respiratory rate and occurrence of a pulsatile release of anabolic hormones like growth hormone (GH), insulin, and prolactin and the secretory period of pineal melatonin. Indeed, NREM sleep is functionally associated with several cytoprotective processes, and in the brain, several neurotrophic factors are synthesized during this period [30–32].

In contrast, REM sleep is typically an "antihomeostatic" stage (Table 9.1). The regulatory mechanisms controlling cardiovascular, respiratory, and thermoregulatory functions become grossly inefficient, leaving functional the spinal, metameric responses only. Heart rate and blood pressure as well as their variability increase and the respiratory rate becomes irregular in REM sleep [26]. Awakening from REM sleep yields reports of hallucinoid dreaming, even in subjects who rarely or never recall dreams spontaneously. This indicates that the brain activation of this phase of sleep is sufficiently intense and organized to support complex mental processes and again argues against a rest function for REM sleep. Indeed, several areas of the brain, e.g., the limbic system, are more active in REM than during wakefulness [33]. The evolutionary logic of somatic and autonomic disconnection during REM is that if acted, this period of sleep could be damaging for an individual's survival.

TABLE 9.1
Three Physiological States ("Bodies") of Our Life

	Wakefulness	NREM Sleep	REM Sleep
	"Active brain in an active body"	"Inactive brain in an active body"	"Hallucinating brain in a paralyzed body"
Neurochemical "microclimate"	Tonic firing of neurons in the locus ceruleus (noradrenergic) and raphe nuclei (serotonergic) driven by orexinergic hypothalamic neurons Phasic discharge of the pedunculopontine nucleus of the pontine tegmentum (PPT, cholinergic)	Inhibition by VLPO area of the arousal systems Decreased aminergic activity in face of progressive increase of cholinergic activity (tonic firing of PPT neurons) Both responsible for decreased consciousness	Prevalent cholinergic activity (PPT nucleus) concomitant with extreme reduction of aminergic activity REM sleep and wakefulness are states of cortical activation with different neuromodulating pattern (cholinergic vs. noradrenergic) and different contents of consciousness
Afferent	Actively functioning Thalamocortical circuit in "open-gate fashion" so that sensory information can reach the cerebral cortex Activated dorsolateral prefrontal cortex (working memory)	Thalamocortical circuit in "gate-closed fashion" (which prevents sensory information from reaching the cerebral cortex) 25% Decrease in cerebral blood flow and oxygen consumption Synthesis of neurotrophins	Thalamic activity changes to operation "open-gate fashion" as during wakefulness
Efferent	Actively functioning	Episodic muscle activity, hypotonia	Skeletal muscle paralysis as a protective mechanism to prevent the locomotor correlates of a highly activated brain
Content awareness	Attention, logical thinking, memory	Disconnection, episodic memory, amnesia	Dream activity characterized by vivid hallucinations, illogical thinking, and intense emotion
Perception	Externally generated	Absent	Generated internally, preferential activation of the pons and limbic system with deactivation of dorsolateral prefrontal cortex
Physiological pattern in organs and systems	Predominance of sympathetic activity in organs and systems, e.g., Th2 responses Augmented plasma norepinephrine and cortisol	Parasympathetic hyperfunction in organs and systems GH, prolactin, and insulin secretion Th1 responses	Generalized disconnection of autonomic regulatory system (this prevents expression of dreaming's emotions) Antihomeostatic physiology

Two interacting processes regulate the timing, duration, and depth (intensity) of sleep: a homeostatic process that keeps the duration and intensity of sleep within certain boundaries and a circadian rhythm that determines the timing of sleep (Figure 9.1). The homeostatic process depends on immediate history: the interval since the previous sleep episode and the intensity of sleep in that episode. This drive to enter sleep increases, possibly exponentially, with the duration since the end of the previous sleep episode. It declines exponentially once sleep has been initiated. This reinforces the cyclical nature of sleep and wakefulness and equates sleep with other physiological needs such as hunger or thirst. The homeostatic sleep drive controls NREM sleep rather than REM sleep [25].

In contrast, the phase and amplitude of the circadian rhythm are independent of the history of previous sleep but are generated by the major pacemaker, the hypothalamic suprachiasmatic nuclei (SCN) (Figure 9.2). The circadian variation of human sleep propensity is roughly the inverse of the core body temperature rhythm: maximum propensity for sleep and the highest continuity of sleep occur in proximity to the minimum of temperature. Reactive homeostatic mechanisms link the depth of sleep with duration of preceding wakefulness while the circadian mechanisms play a fundamental role to determine initiation of sleep and relative duration of REM and NREM sleep phases.

Studies in humans under constant routine conditions have led to the definition of the so-called biological night as the period during which melatonin is produced and secreted into the bloodstream (Figures 9.1 and 9.2). The beginning of the biological night is characterized by onset of the melatonin surge, an accompanying increase in sleep propensity (Figure 9.1) as well as a decrease in core body temperature; the opposite occurs as the biological night and sleep end [34]. Rising nocturnal levels of endogenous melatonin contribute significantly to the nocturnal decline in core body temperature. The inability to fall asleep during the "wake maintenance zone" or "sleep forbidden zone" occurs just prior to the opening of the "sleep gate" [35] (Figure 9.1, arrow). The sleep gate is represented by the steep rise in sleepiness that occurs during the late evening and that begins a period characterized by a consistently high degree of sleep propensity. The nocturnal onset of melatonin secretion predictably precedes the opening of the sleep gate by about 2 hours, and it is believed to initiate at the SCN and via MT_1 receptors (Figure 9.2) a cascade of events culminating 1–2 hours later in the "opening of the sleep gate" [36]. Taken together, current findings suggest that

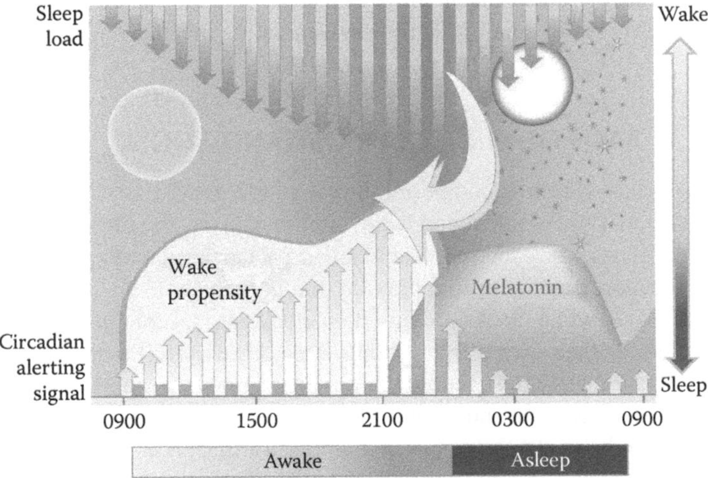

FIGURE 9.1 A two-process model has been proposed for the sleep/wake cycle that posits opposing homeostatic (sleep-dependent) and circadian (sleep-independent) influences. The circadian cycle promotes arousal, while the homeostatic system is driven by the need for sleep. In this model, an alerting signal is dominant during the wake period, during which time a sleep load increases as the wake period progresses. During the evening, the alerting signal is thought to be attenuated via melatonin allowing sleep to occur.

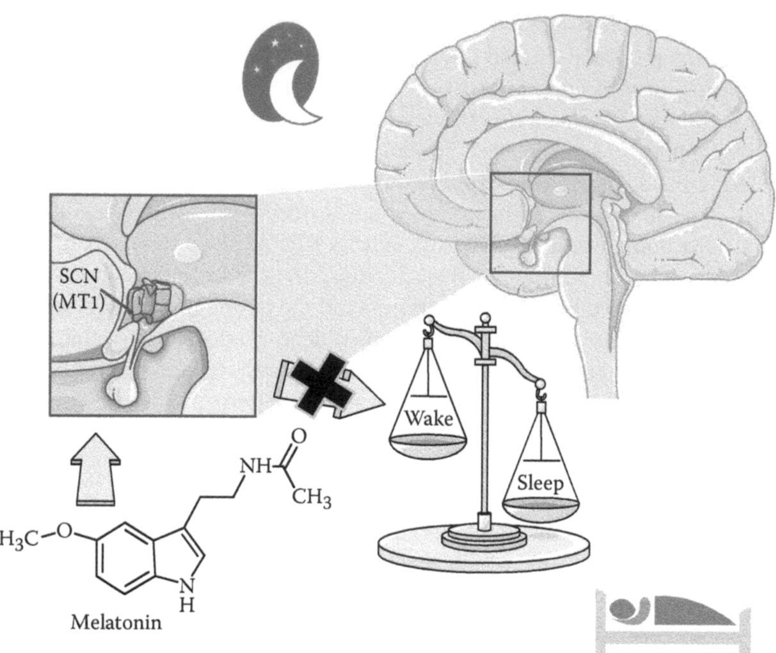

FIGURE 9.2 In mammals, there is evidence that a region in the anterior hypothalamus, the SCN, is the central pacemaker for the circadian rhythms. These nuclei, which contain a few thousand neurons in humans, have the property to generate circadian rhythms even in isolation from other brain structures. SCN integrity is required for generation and maintenance of 24-hour rhythms, as well as for their synchronization by the environmental light/dark cycle. SCN are also essential to promote wakefulness. Information generated in the SCN neurons is conveyed to specific areas in the basal hypothalamus that control the two major communicating systems in the body, the endocrine and the autonomic nervous systems. Melatonin secreted at night suppresses activity of SCN wake-promoting neurons via MT_1 receptors.

the endogenous nocturnal circadian melatonin signal is involved in the circadian rhythm of sleep propensity by turning off the circadian wakefulness-generating mechanism rather than by actively inducing sleep.

9.4 BIOLOGICAL BASIS OF CIRCADIAN ORGANIZATION

In mammals, the circadian system is composed of many individual, tissue-specific cellular clocks [37]. To generate coherent physiological and behavioral responses, the phases of this multitude of cellular clocks are orchestrated by the master circadian pacemaker residing in the SCN [38]. The sleep/wake cycle is the most prominent circadian rhythm in humans.

At a molecular level, circadian clocks are based on clock genes, some of which encode proteins able to feedback and inhibit their own transcription. These cellular oscillators consist of interlocked transcriptional and post-translational feedback loops that involve a small number of core clock genes (about 12 genes identified currently) [39]. The positive drive to the daily clock is constituted by two, basic helix–loop–helix, PAS domain containing transcription factor genes, called *Clock* and *Bmal1*. The protein products of these genes form heterodimeric complexes that control the transcription of other clock genes, notably three period (*Per1/Per2/Per3*) genes and two cryptochrome (*Cry1/Cry2*) genes, which in turn provide the negative feedback signal that shuts down the *Clock/Bmal* drive to complete the circadian cycle [40].

Per and Cry messenger RNAs peak in the SCN in mid-to-late circadian day, regardless of whether an animal is nocturnal or diurnal. Other clock genes provide additional negative and positive transcriptional/translational feedback loops to form the rest of the core clockwork, which has been characterized in rodents by a transgenic gene deletion methodology. Clock gene expression oscillates because of the delay in the feedback loops, regulated in part by the phosphorylation of the clock proteins that control their stability, nuclear reentry, and transcription complex formation [41,42].

9.5 THE NEUROENDOCRINE–IMMUNE RHYTHMS

Like sleep, the neuroendocrine–immune system is controlled in humans by a double-command system given by the predictive and the reactive homeostasis processes, i.e., the interaction of the circadian clock with the sleep homeostat [3,4,43]. In the case of pituitary hormones, pulsatile ultradian components of about 90–120 minutes (which is the time elapsed between every NREM and REM) are also found. Hormonal rhythms depend mostly on the sleep homeostat (e.g., GH, prolactin, insulin, leptin), on the circadian clock (e.g., cortisol, melatonin), or on both (e.g., TSH) [43–46].

In the case of the cytokine rhythms, although less examined, their dependence on the sleep homeostat seems to be prevalent. The 24-hour sleep/wake rhythm correlates with specific circadian patterns of immune responses [47,48]. NREM sleep is associated with T helper (Th) 1 responses, whereas during wakefulness Th2 responses are predominant. Th1 cells release mainly interferon γ (IFN-γ), aside from other cytokines including interleukin (IL) 2 and tumor necrosis factor (TNF) α; they become activated in response to intracellular viral and bacterial challenges supporting cellular (type 1) responses, such as macrophage activation and antigen presentation. Wakefulness is associated with predominance of cytokines characteristic of Th2 immunity, e.g., IL-4, IL-5, IL-10, and IL-13, that mediate humoral (type 2) defense via stimulating mast cells, eosinophils, and B cells against extracellular pathogens [48–50]. Types 1 and 2 cytokine balance is crucial for the control of immune function, with type 1 cytokines overall supporting cellular aspects of immune responses and type 2 cytokines moderating the type 1 response [51,52].

An excessive production of either cytokine type leads to inflammation and tissue damage on the one hand and to susceptibility to infection and allergy on the other. To prevent overactivity, the types 1 and 2 cytokine balance is tightly regulated by mutual inhibition and via a complex neuroendocrine control. The clinical relevance of the balancing function of sleep is indicated by the findings of an increased type 2–mediated allergic skin reaction after sleep deprivation in patients with atopic dermatitis [53]. Also, sleep deprivation after inoculation suppresses antibody responses to hepatitis A virus and influenza vaccinations [53–55].

Several reports indicate that the shift toward Th1-mediated immune defense occurring in NREM sleep is driven by the neuroendocrine environment (see, for example, refs. [1,50,56]). The circadian peak of the ratio of IFN-γ/IL-10 in whole blood samples during nocturnal sleep is abolished by administering glucocorticoids the preceding evening. Thus, the suppression of endogenous cortisol release and the increase in melatonin secretion, both driven by the SCN during early sleep, seems to play a promoting role for Th1 shift. In addition, NREM sleep that is dominant during the early part of nocturnal sleep promotes the release of GH and prolactin (Table 9.1), which supports Th1 cell–mediated immunity. In summary, GH, prolactin, and melatonin are known to shift the types 1 and 2 balance toward type 1, whereas cortisol and norepinephrine can shift it toward type 2 [49,50].

Many studies have described circadian variations in immune parameters such as lymphocyte subpopulations, proliferation, antigen presentation, and cytokine gene expression [39,57]. The number of lymphocytes and monocytes in the human blood reach maximal values during the night and are lowest after waking. Natural killer (NK) cells, by contrast, reach their highest level in the afternoon, with a normal decrease in number and activity around midnight [58–60]. Changes in lymphocyte subset populations can depend on time-of-day–associated changes in cell proliferation of immunocompetent organs and/or on diurnal modifications in lymphocyte release and traffic among lymphoid organs. In our laboratory, we examined the regulation of circadian rhythmicity of lymph cell proliferation in a number of experimental models in rats using the submaxillary lymph nodes. The bilateral anatomical location of submaxillary lymph nodes and their easily manipulable autonomic innervation allowed us to dissect the humoral and neural mechanisms regulating the lymphoid organs and their interaction. A significant diurnal variation of rat submaxillary lymph node cell proliferation was uncovered, displaying maximal activity at early afternoon [61]. Such a maximum coincided with peak mitotic responses. A purely neural pathway including the autonomic nervous system innervating the lymph nodes as a motor leg was identified [62]. The combined sympathetic–parasympathetic denervation of the lymph node suppressed circadian variation in lymph cell proliferation. In addition, a hormonal pathway involving the circadian secretion of melatonin also plays a role to induce rhythmicity [63].

In view of their significant circadian changes, immune cells have been tested for the presence of clock genes [57,64–68]. In a study aimed to investigate whether circadian clock genes function in human peripheral blood mononuclear cells, clock genes *Perl*, *Per2*, and *Per3* were found to be expressed in a circadian manner in human peripheral blood mononuclear cells, with a peak level occurring during the second part of the active phase [69,70]. The presence of molecular clock mechanisms in NK cells conjointly with the circadian expression of critical factors involved in NK cell function were verified by demonstrating the 24-hour expression of clock genes (*Perl*, *Per2*, *Bmall*, *Clock*), *Dbp* (a clock-controlled output gene), *CREB* (involved in clock signaling), cytolytic factors (granzyme B and perforin), and cytokines IFN-γ and TNF-α in NK cells enriched from the rat spleen [71]. Thus, the existence of a molecular clock machinery seems to be conserved across different lymphocyte subsets and peripheral blood cells. Moreover, they may share common entrainment signals.

Rhythms in the number of circulating T cells persisted in rats with disrupted circadian output [72] and SCN ablation did not affect the 24-hour rhythms in cell cycle phase distribution in bone marrow cells [73]. These observations suggest that some rhythms in the immune system are SCN-independent. Entrainment signals other than light can be coordinating the rhythm in NK cell function and other immunological parameters. For example, feeding is an important synchronizer for peripheral clock gene expression [72], and the internal desynchronization produced by restricted feeding during the light period can slow tumor progression in mice [74]. Daily locomotor activity rhythms are also considered to act as entrainment cues for peripheral tissues [75] and may as well influence the molecular clock in lymphocyte cells. In addition, intrinsic immunological outputs such as cytokine secretion could function as entrainment factors for immune cells. Indeed, IL-6 has been shown to induce *Perl* expression in vitro [76].

Several studies have investigated the changes in cytokine levels that occur during the 24-hour sleep/wake cycle in humans (see refs. [2,50]). Plasma TNF-α levels peak during the dark phase of cycle, and this circadian rhythm of TNF-α release is disrupted by sleep pathology, e.g., obstructive sleep apnea. Plasma IL-1β levels also have a diurnal variation, being highest at the onset of NREM sleep. Both intrahypothalamic IL-1 and TNF-α regulate sleep.

The levels of other cytokines (including IL-2, IL-6, IL-10, and IL-12) and the proliferation of T cells in response to mitogens also change during the 24-hour cycle. The production of macrophage-related cytokines (such as TNF-α) increases during sleep (in response to in vitro stimulation) in parallel with the rise in monocyte numbers in the blood. The production of T-cell–related cytokines (such as IL-2) increases during sleep, independent of migratory changes in T-cell distribution [2,50].

Sleep deprivation is associated with a shift of the types 1 and 2 cytokine balance toward type 2 activity, as found in healthy subjects acutely deprived of sleep and in chronic sleep deficits occurring in insomnia, alcoholism, stress, and during the course of aging [50]. A consistent finding is that proinflammatory cytokines are elevated in all these groups [77–79]. People with sleep apnea and narcolepsy have higher TNF-α levels compared with controls, whereas abstinent alcoholics and people partially deprived of sleep show elevations of both TNF-α and IL-6. Together with increased levels of inflammatory cytokines, people with insomnia show decreased T-helper ($CD3^+$, $CD4^+$) and T-cytotoxic ($CD8^+$) cells and decreased NK cell activity [77,80]. Experimentally induced sleep deprivation has been found to alter the diurnal pattern of cellular and humoral immune functions [81,82] and to decrease overall immune function [83] in normal adults.

IL-6 is one of the cytokines whose levels fluctuate in response to partial sleep deprivation. IL-6 has a circadian rhythm, peaking at night, with lower levels during the day. In healthy men, the levels of IL-6 increased with peak values occurring 2.5 hours after sleep onset [83]. During partial sleep deprivation, the nocturnal increase of IL-6 was delayed and did not occur until sleep was allowed. Hence, like GH, prolactin, or leptin secretion, sleep, rather than a circadian pacemaker, influences nocturnal IL-6 secretion [83].

To study the role of nocturnal sleep on normal immune regulation in a design to assess acute sleep loss rather than excessive sleep loss, normal volunteers slept two consecutive regular sleep/wake cycles or remained awake for 24 hours followed by recovery sleep [84,85]. No alteration in the absolute production of IL-1β and TNF-α between the two experimental conditions was found; however, the expected decrease of IL-1β and TNF-α during sleep was blocked when subjects were kept awake. Hence, there was an increase in the nocturnal production of both cytokines during the sleep deprivation period. Other studies evaluating sleep restriction found a delayed nocturnal release of sleep-associated cytokines, IL-1, IL-6, and TNF-α, with subsequent recuperation of normal levels on recovery nights [83,86,87]. This suggests that cytokines depend more on the activity of the sleep homeostat than on the circadian oscillator.

Several reports indicate a possible immune feedback regulation of the circadian clock (for example, see ref. [88]). For example, immunosuppressant drugs such as cyclosporine affect the phase of locomotor activity [89] and hormone secretion [90,91]. Moreover, immune-related transcription factors are present and active in the SCN, and its activity is partially necessary for light-induced phase shifts [89].

9.6 IMMUNOMODULATION BY MELATONIN

9.6.1 Basic Biology of Melatonin

Circulating melatonin binds to albumin and is metabolized mainly in the liver where it is hydroxylated in the C6 position by cytochrome P450 monooxygenases (CYPA2 and CYP1A). Melatonin is then conjugated with sulfate to form 6-sulfatoxymelatonin, the main melatonin metabolite found in urine. Melatonin is also metabolized in tissues by oxidative pyrrole-ring cleavage into kynuramine derivatives. The primary cleavage product is N^1-acetyl-N^2-formyl-5-methoxykynuramine (AFMK), which is deformylated, either by arylamine formamidase or hemoperoxidase, to N^1-acetyl-5-methoxykynuramine (AMK) [92]. It has been proposed that AFMK is the primitive and primary active metabolite of melatonin [93]. Melatonin is also converted into cyclic 3-hydroxymelatonin in a process that directly scavenges two hydroxyl radicals [93].

Orally administered melatonin exhibits extensive first-pass metabolism and its absolute bioavailability is reported to be around 15% with a wide range of variability [94,95]. The wide variations in melatonin's bioavailability is attributed to interindividual variations in the expression of and activity of CYPA2 and CYP1A [96].

Melatonin exerts many physiological actions by acting on membrane and nuclear receptors although other actions are receptor-independent (e.g., scavenging of free radicals or interaction with cytoplasmic proteins) [14,36]. The two melatonin receptors cloned so far (MT_1 and MT_2) are membrane receptors that have seven membrane domains and belong to the superfamily of G-protein–coupled receptors [97]. Melatonin receptor activation induces a variety of responses that are mediated both by pertussis-sensitive and pertussis-insensitive G_i proteins. In the cytoplasm, melatonin interacts with proteins such as calmodulin and tubulin. Nuclear receptors of retinoic acid receptor superfamily (RZR/ROR-α) have been identified in several cells, among them in human lymphocytes and monocytes [98].

The immunomodulatory role of melatonin is related in part to its action on specific melatonin receptors located in immunocompetent cells. In a study on two human lymphocytic (Jurkat) and monocytic (U937) cell lines, the addition of melatonin was found to enhance IL-2 and IL-6 production by acting primarily through nuclear ROR-α receptors [99]. Melatonin synthesized by human lymphocyte may play a crucial role in modulating the IL-2/IL-2 receptor system, as indicated by studies showing that when melatonin biosynthesis is blocked by the tryptophan hydroxylase inhibitor parachlorophenylalanine, both IL-2 and IL-2 receptor levels fall, an effect counteracted by the addition of exogenous melatonin [98]. Similarly, prostaglandin (PG) E_2–induced inhibition on IL-2 production increased when melatonin membrane receptors were blocked by the MT_1/MT_2 blocker luzindole. Taken together, these data indicate that melatonin synthesized in human lymphocytes is involved in the physiological regulation of the IL-2/IL-2R expression through a mechanism comprising both membrane and nuclear melatonin receptors [98].

The contribution of MT_1 and MT_2 receptors in mediating the melatonin-induced enhancement of cellular and humoral immune function was explored in mice [100]. Melatonin enhanced splenocyte proliferation in both wild typ, and MT_1 –/– mice, an effect that was blocked by luzindole, indicating that the melatonin-induced enhancement of immune function is mediated via MT_2 receptors [100].

Repeated stimulation of Th cells in the presence of IL-12 causes Th cells to differentiate into Th1 cells, which produce IL-2 and IFN-γ and are particularly effective in enhancing immune responses that involve macrophages and other phagocytes. Melatonin augments IFN-γ production by Th1 cells. The enhancement of NK cell activity by melatonin is attributed to the increased production of IL-2 and IL-12 [98].

9.6.2 Innate Immunity

A number of studies support the immunoregulatory action of melatonin on the body's innate immunity. Melatonin stimulates the production of progenitor cells for granulocytes and macrophages (GM-CFU) and has a general stimulatory action on hemopoiesis [98]. Melatonin receptors are detectable in monocyte/macrophage lineage and melatonin binding to both membrane and nuclear receptors stimulates the production of GM-CFU cells [98]. Exogenous melatonin augments NK cells and monocytes in both the bone marrow and the spleen with a latency of 7 to 14 days. The action of melatonin on monocyte production can be partly due to its direct action on melatonin receptors or may be due to an increase of monocyte sensitivity to stimulants like IL-3, IL-4, IL-6, or GM colony-stimulating factor (GM-CSF) [101]. As stromal cells contain receptors for κ-opioid cytokine peptides, the melatonin-induced release of opioid peptides from these stromal cells in bone marrow could be involved in the regulation of hemopoietic cell proliferation [102].

Melatonin increases the actual production of GM-CSF cell lineage and not the interorgan trafficking of myeloid precursors [101]. An increased activation of monocytes/macrophages by melatonin has been reported in yet another study in rodents [103]. As both macrophage cells and neutrophils form important components of the innate immune system, the stimulatory action of melatonin reflects a significant immunoenhancing property.

Macrophages have been shown to form large amounts of nitric oxide (NO) upon activation by reactive ROS that mediate their microbiocidal properties. Melatonin decreased NO concentration in macrophages by suppressing inducible NO synthase (iNOS) expression [104]. When melatonin's effects on phagocytic activity of macrophages were tested at different concentrations, the greatest phagocytic stimulation was obtained at melatonin concentrations resembling the unstressed situation [105]. Hence, pharmacological amounts of melatonin may well decrease the optimal phagocytic activity of macrophages.

The time course of the innate immunological response involves a proinflammatory phase followed by an anti-inflammatory phase. Proinflammatory responses serve as a defense against several stressor conditions and sequential processes that shut down these responses are necessary to avoid exacerbation or the development of chronic diseases. It has been proposed that melatonin can play a role in both phases of the inflammatory response, both after release from the pineal gland as well as by the release from activated mononuclear and polymorphonuclear cells in a paracrine manner at the site of injury [106].

Not only melatonin but also its oxidation product AFMK is very effective in acting on neutrophils [107]. Both melatonin and AFMK have been shown to inhibit IL-8 release from neutrophils and AFMK has been found to be more active than melatonin in this aspect. The production of TNF-α by neutrophils is also inhibited by melatonin and AFMK. Since TNF-α and IL-8 contribute to the severity of inflammatory conditions, the finding of melatonin inhibiting the release of IL-8 and TNF-α assumes significance for it may help to reduce acute and chronic inflammation. Neutrophils are more responsive than monocytes to AFMK, suggesting that melatonin biosynthesis and metabolism participate in the chemical communication among leukocytes. Melatonin may be effective in optimizing intrinsic immune responses rather than acting simply as an antioxidant [108]. Melatonin is recognized to increase the production of Th1 type and inflammatory cytokines and to enhance both cell mediated and humoral responses.

9.6.3 Acquired Immunity

Orally administered melatonin can substantially promote the survival (antiapoptosis) of precursor B lymphocytes (responsible for humoral immunity) in the B lymphocyte generating site, i.e., the bone marrow [109]. This indicates that melatonin treatment can boost the survival of mature B cells, which are the functional elements in humoral immunity.

The immunostimulatory role of melatonin is exerted mainly on Th cells and on T-lymphocyte precursors, and melatonin could act as an autacoid in bone marrow as shown by the demonstration of melatonin synthesis in bone marrow cells of mice and humans [8]. Melatonin augments $CD4^+$ lymphocytes and decreases $CD8^+$ lymphocytes in rat submaxillary lymph nodes [110]. Collectively, published studies indicate that melatonin possesses important immunoenhancing properties and suggest that melatonin may favor a Th1 response, for example, during the natural history of human immunodeficiency virus type I infection [111].

It must be noted, however, that besides the release of proinflammatory Th1 cytokines, such as IFN-γ and IL-2, administration of melatonin to antigen-primed mice increased the production of IL-10, indicating that melatonin can also activate anti-inflammatory Th2-like immune responses under certain circumstances [112]. Therefore, it is not yet clear whether melatonin acts only on Th1 cells or also affects Th2 cells. This is an important subject since, as discussed above, the Th1/Th2 balance is significant for the immune response. Relevant to this, melatonin treatment augmented the subsequent in vitro stimulation by the mitogenic agents lipopolysaccharide (LPS, which stimulates B cells) and concanavalin A (which stimulates T cells) in submaxillary lymph nodes [110]. In addition, an inhibitory influence of melatonin on parameters of the immune function has also been demonstrated, i.e., in human NK cell activity, DNA synthesis, IFN-γ and TNF-α synthesis, as well as the proliferation of T lymphocytes and lymphoblastoid cell lines were depressed by melatonin.

9.7 MELATONIN AS AN ANTI-INFLAMMATORY DRUG

Inflammation is a complex phenomenon that involves numerous mediators triggering physiological defense effects against pathogenic microorganisms or stress. Most of the proinflammatory stimuli in inflamed tissues and migratory cells activate both cyclooxygenase 2 (COX-2) and iNOS enzymes [113]. This overproduction of prostaglandins (PGs) and NO plays important roles in inflammation, being responsible for blood vessel dilatation as well as for local and systemic symptoms of fever, pain, and edema [114]. Therefore, since both COX-2 and iNOS are inducible forms up-regulated in response to inflammatory responses, they have been the focus of interest for understanding melatonin's role in the pathophysiology of inflammation.

Data accumulated in the past decade strongly indicate that melatonin plays an important role in antioxidant defense [14]. The regulation of enzymes involved in the redox pathway is one of the ways by which melatonin exerts its antioxidant effects. This action is complementary to the nonenzymatic, radical scavenger effect that melatonin and some of its metabolites (notably AFMK and

AMK) have to scavenge ROS, RNS, and organic radicals [92]. Other antioxidant effects could be mediated by binding to quinone reductase 2, which had previously been assumed to represent a new melatonin receptor.

More recently, mitochondrial effects of melatonin have come into focus, including safeguarding of respiratory electron flux, reduction of oxidant formation by lowering electron leakage, and inhibition of opening of the mitochondrial permeability transition pore [115]. These effects of melatonin and its metabolites are rather unique. For example, the MT_1/MT_2 melatonergic agonist ramelteon displays no relevant antioxidant activity [116].

In one of the earliest studies on melatonin role in inflammation, zymosan-activated plasma was locally injected to induce paw inflammation [117]. Zymosan-activated plasma or complement trigger the production of ROS and RNS [118]. Injection of zymosan-activated plasma in rat's paws readily evokes an inflammatory reaction as evidenced by the presence of edema within 30 minutes that reached a maximum at 3 hours [117]. Nitrite/nitrate levels were found to be elevated at 3 hours after injection. Local melatonin administration significantly reduced zymosan-activated plasma-induced edema in a dose-dependent manner. Melatonin treatment also reduced nitrite/nitrate ratio, myeloperoxidase (MPO) activity, and malonaldehyde levels [117].

Early data pointed out to an inhibitory effect of melatonin on COX [119]. Indeed, melatonin readily inhibits COX-2 [120] and iNOS [118,121]. Other possible mechanisms for melatonin's anti-inflammatory effects included activation of nuclear factor κB [122] and inhibition of neutrophil infiltration [118].

The anti-inflammatory actions of melatonin and its metabolites AFMK and AMK were evaluated in LPS-activated RAW 264.7 macrophages [123]. In LPS-stimulated RAW 264.7 macrophages, melatonin addition at millimolar concentrations significantly inhibited COX-2 and iNOS activity and thus the increase of PGE_2. Melatonin also inhibited LPS-induced increase of COX-2 protein expression in a dose-dependent manner [123]. Both AFMK and AMK shared the effect of melatonin to prevent the increase in COX-2 induced by LPS in macrophages. COX-2 inhibition by melatonin and its analogs resulted in apoptosis in RAW 264.7 macrophages. From this study, the authors concluded that melatonin and its metabolites AFMK or AMK have the potential to be a new class of anti-inflammatory agents [123].

The hypothesis that melatonin suppresses the expression of the proinflammatory genes COX-2 and iNOS by a common transcriptional mechanism was also tested. Melatonin, but not tryptophan or serotonin, inhibited COX-2 and iNOS transcriptional activation by inhibiting p300 histone acetyltransferase activity, thereby suppressing p52 acetylation, binding, and transactivation [124]. Another study aimed to define the effect of melatonin on inflammation-related gene expression in LPS-stimulated human peripheral blood mononuclear cells. Melatonin inhibits LPS-induced CC chemokine subfamily gene expression in human peripheral blood mononuclear cells in a microarray analysis [125].

The formation of potent oxidants catalyzed by MPO has been implicated in the pathogenesis of various diseases including atherosclerosis, asthma, arthritis, and cancer [126–128], and so far, no effective inhibitors have been identified for MPO. Galijasevic et al. [129] recently demonstrated that melatonin serves as a potent inhibitor of MPO under physiological-like conditions. In the presence of chloride, melatonin inactivated MPO at two points in the peroxidase cycle through binding to MPO to form an inactive complex, melatonin–MPO–Cl, and accelerating MPO compound II formation, an inactive form of MPO [129]. This dual regulation by melatonin is unique and may represent a new means through which melatonin can control MPO and its downstream inflammatory pathways.

9.8 MELATONIN IN INFECTIOUS DISEASE: SEPTIC SHOCK, MALARIA, CHAGAS DISEASE

Melatonin has been identified to protect organisms against bacterial, viral, and parasitic infections [130–137], presumably by acting through a variety of mechanisms, like immunomodulation or direct or indirect antioxidant activity. Melatonin's therapeutic efficacy has been advocated in septic shock, a lethal condition caused by a pathogen-induced sequential intracellular event occurring in immune cells, epithelium, endothelium, and the neuroendocrine system [138,139]. The lethal effects of septic shock are associated with the production and release of numerous proinflammatory biochemical mediators such as cytokines, NO, ROS, and RNS radicals, together with development of massive apoptosis.

Melatonin has been shown to be beneficial for reversing symptoms of septic shock in experimental animals [140,141] as well as it reduced oxidative stress in human newborns with sepsis, distress, or other conditions where there is excessive ROS production (see, for example, ref. [142]). Although understanding the melatonin's action in the pathogenesis of septic shock is yet to be achieved, studies so far point out that melatonin through its immunomodulatory, antioxidant, and antiapoptotic actions exert beneficial effects in septic shock and multiorgan failure. Melatonin also acts specifically at the mitochondrial level, protecting the electron leakage and respiratory chain failure, thereby augmenting the respiratory efficiency [115].

Malaria, a disease caused by the protozoan species *Plasmodium*, infects more than 300 million people and results in the death of more than 1 million people annually. It is known that malaria affects several organs including kidney, heart, spleen, heart, and cerebral tissue [143]. Malaria has been shown to increase the generation of ROS in tissues and decreases the level of critical antioxidant enzymes. Malarial infection activates immune effector and regulatory cells, thereby causing intravascular lesions in target organs, lungs, kidney, and brain, thus accounting for the broad systemic complications that inevitably accompany progression of the disease [144,145].

Melatonin administration may have both enhancing and inhibitory effects on malaria development (for example, see ref. [146]). Via its receptors, melatonin increases the ability of *Plasmodium* to invade erythrocytes, a process that involves phospholipase C activation and release of calcium from the intracellular storage sites. On the other hand, melatonin inhibits free radical-mediated mitochondrial-dependent hepatocyte apoptosis and liver damage induced by malarial infection, indicating that appropriate antioxidant doses of melatonin could be particularly useful to limit ROS production and ROS-induced hepatocyte apoptosis and hence protect liver from apoptosis and dysfunction [147].

A major argument in favor of the promoting effect of *Plasmodium* infection via melatonin receptors was provided by the inhibition of this melatonin action in vivo and in vitro by the MT_1/MT_2 receptor antagonist luzindole [148,149]. Since melatonin effects on ROS production under these circumstances may not be receptor-mediated the association of melatonin antagonists (to impair the synchronizing effect of melatonin on *Plasmodia*) with pharmacological doses of melatonin (to impair ROS and RNS production) might have therapeutic significance in the treatment of malaria. Future investigations should consider two-tiered or multimodal approaches to the use of melatonin, melatonin agonists, and melatonin antagonists as new therapeutic strategies in combating malarial infection [146].

Chagas disease is a severe health problem in Latin America, causing approximately 50,000 deaths a year, with approximately 18 million infected people. About 25%–30% of the patients infected with *Trypanosoma cruzi* develop the chronic form of the disease, with progressive myocardial damage and, often, sudden death [150]. No curative treatment for Chagas disease is presently available. The protective response against *T. cruzi* depends on both innate and acquired immunity involving macrophages, NK cells, T and B lymphocytes, and the production of proinflammatory Th1 cytokines. In addition, an increased NO production in macrophages leading to effective microbicidal action is needed to control parasitemia [151,152]. Melatonin is detectable in *T. cruzi* [153] and may play a role in promoting infection, whereas when administered in high doses during the acute phase of *T. cruzi* infection, it can decrease parasitemia while reducing NO production [154–156]. During chronic disease progression, the sustained oxidative stress concomitant to myocardial damage could be reduced by administering melatonin. It is hypothesized that the coordinated administration of a melatonin agonist such as the MT_1/MT_2 agonist ramelteon, which lacks antioxidant activity and may not affect

NO production during the acute phase and of melatonin in doses high enough to decrease oxidative damage, preserve mitochondria, and to prevent cardiomyopathy during the chronic phase, could be a novel add-on treatment of Chagas disease.

ACKNOWLEDGMENTS

Studies in the author's laboratory were supported by grants from Agencia Nacional de Promoción Científica y Tecnológica, Argentina (PICT 2007-01045) and the University of Buenos Aires (M 006). D.P.C. is a Superior Investigator, Argentine Research Council (CONICET), and Professor Emeritus, University of Buenos Aires.

REFERENCES

1. Krueger, J. M. 2008. The role of cytokines in sleep regulation. *Curr. Pharm. Des.* 14: 3408–16.
2. Pandi-Perumal, S. R., D. P. Cardinali, and G. P. Chrousos, eds. 2007. *Neuroimmunology of Sleep.* New York: Springer Science + Business Media, LLC.
3. Copinschi, G., K. Spiegel, R. Leproult, et al. 2000. Pathophysiology of human circadian rhythms. *Novartis Found. Symp.* 227: 143–57.
4. Pace-Schott, E. F., and J. A. Hobson. 2002. The neurobiology of sleep: Genetics, cellular physiology and subcortical networks. *Nat. Rev. Neurosci.* 3: 591–605.
5. Claustrat, B., J. Brun, and G. Chazot. 2005. The basic physiology and pathophysiology of melatonin. *Sleep Med. Rev.* 9: 11–24.
6. Carrillo-Vico, A., J. R. Calvo, P. Abreu, et al. 2004. Evidence of melatonin synthesis by human lymphocytes and its physiological significance: Possible role as intracrine, autocrine, and/or paracrine substance. *FASEB J.* 18: 537–9.
7. Tan, D. X., L. C. Manchester, R. J. Reiter, et al. 1999. Identification of highly elevated levels of melatonin in bone marrow: Its origin and significance. *Biochim. Biophys. Acta* 1472: 206–14.
8. Conti, A., S. Conconi, E. Hertens, et al. 2000. Evidence for melatonin synthesis in mouse and human bone marrow cells. *J. Pineal Res.* 28: 193–202.
9. Naranjo, M. C., J. M. Guerrero, A. Rubio, et al. 2007. Melatonin biosynthesis in the thymus of humans and rats. *Cell Mol. Life Sci.* 64: 781–90.
10. Raikhlin, N. T., and I. M. Kvetnoy. 1976. Melatonin and enterochromaffine cells. *Acta Histochem.* 55: 19–24.
11. Slominski, A., T. W. Fischer, M. A. Zmijewski, et al. 2005. On the role of melatonin in skin physiology and pathology. *Endocrine.* 27: 137–48.
12. Lundmark, P. O., S. R. Pandi-Perumal, V. Srinivasan, et al. 2006. Role of melatonin in the eye and ocular dysfunctions. *Vis. Neurosci.* 23: 853–62.
13. Tan, D. X., L. C. Manchester, R. Hardeland, et al. 2003. Melatonin: A hormone, a tissue factor, an autocoid, a paracoid and an antioxidant vitamin. *J. Pineal Res.* 34: 75–8.
14. Reiter, R. J., S. D. Paredes, L. C. Manchester, et al. 2009. Reducing oxidative/nitrosative stress: A newly-discovered genre for melatonin. *Crit. Rev. Biochem. Mol. Biol.* 44: 175–200.
15. Jimenez-Ortega, V., P. Cano, D. P. Cardinali, et al. 2009. 24-Hour variation in gene expression of redox pathway enzymes in rat hypothalamus: Effect of melatonin treatment. *Redox Rep.* 14: 132–8.
16. Moore-Ede M. C., F. M. Sulzmanand C. A. Fuller. 1982. *The Clock that Times Us: Physiology of the Circadian System.* Cambridge: Harvard University Press.
17. Selye, H. 1936. Syndrome produced by diverse nocuous agents. *Nature* 138: 32–8.
18. McEwen, B. 1998. Protective and damaging effects of stress mediators. *N. Engl. J. Med.* 338: 171–9.
19. McEwen, B. S. 2006. Sleep deprivation as a neurobiologic and physiologic stressor: Allostasis and allostatic load. *Metabolism* 55: S20–S23.
20. Girotti, L., M. Lago, O. Ianovsky, et al. 2000. Low urinary 6-sulphatoxymelatonin levels in patients with coronary artery disease. *J. Pineal Res.* 29: 138–42.
21. Girotti, L., M. Lago, O. Ianovsky, et al. 2003. Low urinary 6-sulphatoxymelatonin levels in patients with severe congestive heart failure. *Endocrine* 22: 245–8.
22. Rechtschaffen A.and A. Kales. 1968. *A Manual of Standardized Terminology, Techniques and Scoring System for Sleep Stages of Human Subjects.* Bethesda, MD: US Department of Health, Education and Welfare Public Health Service-NIH/NIND.

23. Beersma, D. G. M. 1998. Models of human sleep regulation. *Sleep Med. Rev.* 2: 31–43.
24. Vigo, D. E., J. Domínguez, M. Scaramal, et al. 2010. Nonlinear analysis of heart rate variability within independent frequency components during the sleep–wake cycle. *Auton. Neurosci. Basic Clin.* 154: 84–8.
25. Pace-Schott, E. F., and J. A. Hobson. 2002. The neurobiology of sleep: Genetics, cellular physiology and subcortical networks. *Nat. Neurosci. Rev* 3: 591–605.
26. Parmeggiani, P. L., and R. Velluti, eds. 2005. *The Physiological Nature of Sleep*. London: Imperial College Press.
27. Dijk, D. J. 2009. Regulation and functional correlates of slow wave sleep. *J. Clin. Sleep Med.* 5: S6–15.
28. Gangwisch, J. E. 2009. Epidemiological evidence for the links between sleep, circadian rhythms and metabolism. *Obes. Rev.* 10 Suppl. 2: 37–45.
29. Gimble, J. M., M. S. Bray, and A. Young. 2009. Circadian biology and sleep: Missing links in obesity and metabolism? *Obes. Rev.* 10 Suppl. 2: 1–5.
30. Gorgulu, Y., and O. Caliyurt. 2009. Rapid antidepressant effects of sleep deprivation therapy correlates with serum BDNF changes in major depression. *Brain Res. Bull.* 80: 158–62.
31. Lee, K. S., T. A. Alvarenga, C. Guindalini, et al. 2009. Validation of commonly used reference genes for sleep-related gene expression studies. *BMC Mol. Biol* 10: 45.
32. Faraguna, U., V. V. Vyazovskiy, A. B. Nelson, et al. 2008. A causal role for brain-derived neurotrophic factor in the homeostatic regulation of sleep. *J. Neurosci.* 28: 4088–95.
33. Hobson, J. A. 2009. REM sleep and dreaming: Towards a theory of protoconsciousness. *Nat. Rev. Neurosci.* 10: 803–13.
34. Lewy, A. J., J. Emens, A. Jackman, et al. 2006. Circadian uses of melatonin in humans. *Chronobiol. Int.* 23: 403–12.
35. Lavie, P. 2001. Sleep–wake as a biological rhythm. *Annu. Rev. Psychol.* 52: 277–303.
36. Pandi-Perumal, S. R., I. Trakht, V. Srinivasan, et al. 2008. Physiological effects of melatonin: Role of melatonin receptors and signal transduction pathways. *Prog. Neurobiol.* 185: 335–53.
37. Reddy, A. B., G. K. Wong, J. O'Neill, et al. 2005. Circadian clocks: Neural and peripheral pacemakers that impact upon the cell division cycle. *Mutat. Res.* 574: 76–91.
38. Morin, L. P., and C. N. Allen. 2006. The circadian visual system, 2005. *Brain Res. Brain Res. Rev.* 51: 1–60.
39. Bonnefont, X. 2010. Circadian timekeeping and multiple timescale neuroendocrine rhythms. *J. Neuroendocrinol.* 22: 209–16.
40. Okamura, H. 2003. Integration of mammalian circadian clock signals: From molecule to behavior. *J. Endocrinol.* 177: 3–6.
41. Collins, B., and J. Blau. 2006. Keeping time without a clock. *Neuron* 50: 348–50.
42. Lakin-Thomas, P. L. 2006. Transcriptional feedback oscillators: Maybe, maybe not. *J. Biol. Rhythms* 21: 83–92.
43. Cardinali, D. P., and Pandi-Perumal, S. R. 2006. *Neuroendocrine Correlates of Sleep/Wakefulness*. New York: Springer.
44. Van Cauter, E., and G. Copinschi. 2000. Interrelationships between growth hormone and sleep. *Growth Horm. IGF. Res.* 10 Suppl. B: S57–S62.
45. Touitou, Y., and E. Haus. 2000. Alterations with aging of the endocrine and neuroendocrine circadian system in humans. *Chronobiol. Int.* 17: 369–90.
46. Penev, P., K. Spiegel, M. L'Hermite-Baleriaux, et al. 2003. Relationship between REM sleep and testosterone secretion in older men. *Ann. Endocrinol. (Paris)* 64: 157.
47. Dimitrov, S., T. Lange, S. Tieken, et al. 2004. Sleep associated regulation of T helper 1/T helper 2 cytokine balance in humans. *Brain Behav. Immun.* 18: 341–8.
48. Berger, J. 2008. A two-clock model of circadian timing in the immune system of mammals. *Pathol. Biol (Paris)* 56: 286–91.
49. Chrousos, G. P. 2009. Stress and disorders of the stress system. *Nat. Rev. Endocrinol.* 5: 374–81.
50. Opp, M. R. 2009. Sleep and psychoneuroimmunology. *Immunol. Allergy Clin. North Am.* 29: 295–307.
51. Kidd, P. 2003. Th1/Th2 balance: The hypothesis, its limitations and implications for health and disease. *Altern. Med. Rev.* 8: 223–46.
52. Corthay, A. 2009. How do regulatory T cells work? *Scand. J. Immunol.* 70: 326–36.
53. Williams, H. C., and D. J. Grindlay. 2010. What's new in atopic eczema? An analysis of systematic reviews published in 2007 and 2008. Part 1. Definitions, causes and consequences of eczema. *Clin. Exp. Dermatol.* 35: 12–5.
54. Miller, G. E., S. Cohen, S. Pressman, et al. 2004. Psychological stress and antibody response to influenza vaccination: When is the critical period for stress and how does it get inside the body? *Psychosom. Med.* 66: 215–23.

55. Dopp, J. M., N. A. Wiegert, J. J. Moran, et al. 2007. Humoral immune responses to influenza vaccination in patients with obstructive sleep apnea. *Pharmacotherapy* 27: 1483–9.
56. Rector, D. M., J. L. Schei, H. P. Van Dongen, et al. 2009. Physiological markers of local sleep. *Eur. J. Neurosci.* 29: 1771–8.
57. Bollinger, T., A. Bollinger, H. Oster, et al. 2010. Sleep, immunity and circadian clocks: A mechanistic model. *Gerontology* 56: 574–80.
58. Petrovsky, N., and L. C. Harrison. 1998. The chronobiology of human cytokine production. *Int. Rev. Immunol.* 16: 635–49.
59. Buijs, R. M., F. A. Scheer, F. Kreier, et al. 2006. Chapter 20: Organization of circadian functions: Interaction with the body. *Prog. Brain Res.* 153: 341–60.
60. Cutolo, M., A. Sulli, C. Pizzorni, et al. 2006. Circadian rhythms: Glucocorticoids and arthritis. *Ann. N. Y. Acad. Sci.* 1069: 289–99.
61. Cardinali, D. P., R. Cutrera, P. Castrillon, et al. 1996. Diurnal rhythms in ornithine decarboxylase activity and norepinephrine and acetylcholine synthesis and acetylcholine synthesis of rat submaxillary lymph nodes: Effect of pinealectomy, superior cervical ganglionectomy and melatonin replacement. *Neuroimmunomodulation* 3: 102–11.
62. Cardinali, D. P., and A. I. Esquifino. 1998. Neuroimmunoendocrinology of the cervical autonomic nervous system. *Biomed. Rev.* 9: 47–59.
63. Cardinali, D. P., A. P. Garcia, P. Cano, et al. 2004. Melatonin role in experimental arthritis. *Curr. Drug Targets. Immune Endocr. Metabol. Disord.* 4: 1–10.
64. Hayashi, M., S. Shimba, and M. Tezuka. 2007. Characterization of the molecular clock in mouse peritoneal macrophages. *Biol. Pharm. Bull.* 30: 621–6.
65. Murphy, B. A., M. M. Vick, D. R. Sessions, et al. 2007. Acute systemic inflammation transiently synchronizes clock gene expression in equine peripheral blood. *Brain Behav. Immun.* 21: 467–76.
66. Zhu, Y., D. Leaderer, C. Guss, et al. 2007. Ala394Thr polymorphism in the clock gene NPAS2: A circadian modifier for the risk of non-Hodgkin's lymphoma. *Int. J. Cancer* 120: 432–5.
67. Liu, J., G. Mankani, X. Shi, et al. 2006. The circadian clock Period 2 gene regulates gamma interferon production of NK cells in host response to lipopolysaccharide-induced endotoxic shock. *Infect. Immun.* 74: 4750–6.
68. Arjona, A., and D. K. Sarkar. 2006. Evidence supporting a circadian control of natural killer cell function. *Brain Behav. Immun.* 20: 469–76.
69. Boivin, D. B., F. O. James, A. Wu, et al. 2003. Circadian clock genes oscillate in human peripheral blood mononuclear cells. *Blood* 102: 4143–5.
70. Kusanagi, H., K. Mishima, K. Satoh, et al. 2004. Similar profiles in human period1 gene expression in peripheral mononuclear and polymorphonuclear cells. *Neurosci. Lett.* 365: 124–7.
71. Arjona, A., and D. K. Sarkar. 2005. Circadian oscillations of clock genes, cytolytic factors and cytokines in rat NK cells. *J. Immunol.* 174: 7618–24.
72. Kobayashi, H., K. Oishi, S. Hanai, et al. 2004. Effect of feeding on peripheral circadian rhythms and behaviour in mammals. *Genes Cells* 9: 857–64.
73. Filipski, E., V. M. King, M. C. Etienne, et al. 2004. Persistent twenty-four hour changes in liver and bone marrow despite suprachiasmatic nuclei ablation in mice. *Am. J. Physiol. Regul. Integr. Comp. Physiol.* 287: R844-R851.
74. Wu, M. W., X. M. Li, L. J. Xian, et al. 2004. Effects of meal timing on tumor progression in mice. *Life Sci.* 75: 1181–93.
75. Schibler, U., J. Ripperger, and S. A. Brown. 2003. Peripheral circadian oscillators in mammals: Time and food. *J. Biol. Rhythms* 18: 250–60.
76. Motzkus, D., U. Albrecht, and E. Maronde. 2002. The human *Per1* gene is inducible by interleukin-6. *J. Mol. Neurosci* 18: 105–9.
77. Irwin, M., C. Clark, B. Kennedy, et al. 2003. Nocturnal catecholamines and immune function in insomniacs, depressed patients and control subjects. *Brain Behav. Immun.* 17: 365–72.
78. Okun, M. L., S. Giese, L. Lin, et al. 2004. Exploring the cytokine and endocrine involvement in narcolepsy. *Brain Behav. Immun.* 18: 326–32.
79. Vgontzas, A. N., E. Zoumakis, E. O. Bixler, et al. 2004. Adverse effects of modest sleep restriction on sleepiness, performance and inflammatory cytokines. *J. Clin. Endocrinol. Metab.* 89: 2119–26.
80. Savard, J., L. Laroche, S. Simard, et al. 2003. Chronic insomnia and immune functioning. *Psychosom. Med.* 65: 211–21.
81. Dinges, D. F., S. D. Douglas, S. Hamarman, et al. 1995. Sleep deprivation and human immune function. *Adv. Neuroimmunol.* 5: 97–110.

82. Heiser, P., B. Dickhaus, W. Schreiber, et al. 2000. White blood cells and cortisol after sleep deprivation and recovery sleep in humans. *Eur. Arch. Psychiatry Clin. Neurosci.* 250: 16–23.
83. Redwine, L., R. L. Hauger, J. C. Gillin, et al. 2000. Effects of sleep and sleep deprivation on interleukin-6, growth hormone, cortisol and melatonin levels in humans. *J. Clin. Endocrinol. Metab.* 85: 3597–603.
84. Marshall, L., and J. Born. 2002. Brain-immune interactions in sleep. *Int. Rev. Neurobiol.* 52: 93–131.
85. Born, J., T. Lange, K. Hansen, et al. 1997. Effects of sleep and circadian rhythm on human circulating immune cells. *J. Immunol.* 158: 4454–64.
86. Vgontzas, A. N., E. O. Bixler, H. M. Lin, et al. 2005. IL-6 and its circadian secretion in humans. *Neuroimmunomodulation.* 12: 131–40.
87. Moldofsky, H., and J. B. Dickstein. 1999. Sleep and cytokine-immune functions in medical, psychiatric and primary sleep disorders. *Sleep Med. Rev.* 3: 325–37.
88. Coogan, A. N., and C. A. Wyse. 2008. Neuroimmunology of the circadian clock. *Brain Res.* 1232: 104–12.
89. Marpegan, L., T. A. Bekinschtein, R. Freudenthal, et al. 2004. Participation of transcription factors from the Rel/NF-[kappa]B family in the circadian system in hamsters. *Neurosci. Lett.* 358: 9–12.
90. Selgas, L., D. Pazo, A. Arce, et al. 1998. Circadian rhythms in adenohypophysial hormone levels and hypothalamic monoamine turnover in mycobacterial adjuvant-injected rats. *Biol. Signals Recept.* 7: 15–24.
91. Esquifino, A. I., L. Selgas, E. Vara, et al. 1999. Twenty-four rhythms of hypothalamic corticotropin-releasing hormone, thyrotropin-releasing hormone, growth hormone-releasing hormone and somatostatin in rats injected with Freund's adjuvant. *Biol. Signals Recept.* 8: 178–90.
92. Hardeland, R., D. X. Tan, and R. J. Reiter. 2009. Kynuramines, metabolites of melatonin and other indoles: The resurrection of an almost forgotten class of biogenic amines. *J. Pineal Res.* 47: 109–16.
93. Tan, D. X., L. C. Manchester, M. P. Terron, et al. 2007. One molecule, many derivatives: A never-ending interaction of melatonin with reactive oxygen and nitrogen species? *J. Pineal Res.* 42: 28–42.
94. Di, W. L., A. Kadva, A. Johnston, et al. 1997. Variable bioavailability of oral melatonin. *N. Engl. J. Med.* 336: 1028–9.
95. DeMuro, R. L., A. N. Nafziger, D. E. Blask, et al. 2000. The absolute bioavailability of oral melatonin. *J. Clin. Pharmacol* 40: 781–4.
96. Hartter, S., C. Ursing, S. Morita, et al. 2001. Orally given melatonin may serve as a probe drug for cytochrome P450 1A2 activity in vivo: A pilot study. *Clin. Pharmacol. Ther.* 70: 10–6.
97. Dubocovich, M. L. 2007. Melatonin receptors: Role on sleep and circadian rhythm regulation. *Sleep Med.* 8 Suppl. 3: 34–42.
98. Carrillo-Vico, A., R. J. Reiter, P. J. Lardone, et al. 2006. The modulatory role of melatonin on immune responsiveness. *Curr. Opin. Investig. Drugs* 7: 423–31.
99. Garcia-Maurino, S., D. Pozo, J. R. Calvo, et al. 2000. Correlation between nuclear melatonin receptor expression and enhanced cytokine production in human lymphocytic and monocytic cell lines. *J. Pineal Res.* 29: 129–37.
100. Drazen, D. L., and R. J. Nelson. 2001. Melatonin receptor subtype MT2 (Mel 1b) and not mt1 (Mel 1a) is associated with melatonin-induced enhancement of cell-mediated and humoral immunity. *Neuroendocrinology* 74: 178–84.
101. Currier, N. L., L. Z. Sun, and S. C. Miller. 2000. Exogenous melatonin: Quantitative enhancement in vivo of cells mediating non-specific immunity. *J. Neuroimmunol.* 104: 101–8.
102. Maestroni, G. J. 2001. The immunotherapeutic potential of melatonin. *Expert. Opin. Investig. Drugs* 10: 467–76.
103. Kaur, C., and E. A. Ling. 1999. Effects of melatonin on macrophages/microglia in postnatal rat brain. *J. Pineal Res.* 26: 158–68.
104. Zhang, S., W. Li, Q. Gao, et al. 2004. Effect of melatonin on the generation of nitric oxide in murine macrophages. *Eur. J. Pharmacol.* 501: 25–30.
105. Barriga, C., M. I. Martin, E. Ortega, et al. 2002. Physiological concentrations of melatonin and corticosterone in stress and their relationship with phagocytic activity. *J. Neuroendocrinol.* 14: 691–5.
106. Markus, R. P., Z. S. Ferreira, P. A. Fernandes, et al. 2007. The immune-pineal axis: A shuttle between endocrine and paracrine melatonin sources. *Neuroimmunomodulation* 14: 126–33.
107. Silva, S. O., M. R. Rodrigues, S. R. Carvalho, et al. 2004. Oxidation of melatonin and its catabolites, *N*1-acetyl-*N*2 -formyl-5-methoxykynuramine and *N*1-acetyl-5-methoxykynuramine, by activated leukocytes. *J. Pineal Res.* 37: 171–5.
108. Bondy, S. C., D. K. Lahiri, V. M. Perreau, et al. 2004. Retardation of brain aging by chronic treatment with melatonin. *Ann. N. Y. Acad. Sci.* 1035: 197–215.

109. Yu, Q., S. C. Miller, and D. G. Osmond. 2000. Melatonin inhibits apoptosis during early B-cell development in mouse bone marrow. *J. Pineal Res.* 29: 86–93.
110. Castrillón, P., D. P. Cardinali, D. Pazo, et al. 2001. Effect of superior cervical ganglionectomy on 24-h variations in hormone secretion from anterior hypophysis and in hypothalamic monoamine turnover, during the preclinical phase of Freund's adjuvant arthritis in rats. *J. Neuroendocrinol.* 13: 288–95.
111. Nunnari, G., L. Nigro, F. Palermo, et al. 2003. Reduction of serum melatonin levels in HIV-1-infected individuals' parallel disease progression: Correlation with serum interleukin-12 levels. *Infection* 31: 379–82.
112. Raghavendra, V., V. Singh, S. K. Kulkarni, et al. 2001. Melatonin enhances Th2 cell mediated immune responses: Lack of sensitivity to reversal by naltrexone or benzodiazepine receptor antagonists. *Mol. Cell Biochem.* 221: 57–62.
113. Vane, J. R., and R. M. Botting. 1998. Anti-inflammatory drugs and their mechanism of action. *Inflamm. Res.* 47 Suppl. 2: S78–S87.
114. Kiefer, W., and G. Dannhardt. 2002. COX-2 inhibition and the control of pain. *Curr. Opin. Investig. Drugs* 3: 1348–58.
115. Acuna-Castroviejo, D., G. Escames, M. I. Rodriguez, et al. 2007. Melatonin role in the mitochondrial function. *Front. Biosci.* 12: 947–63.
116. Mathes, A., D. Kubuls, L. Waibel, et al. 2008. Selective activation of melatonin receptors with ramelteon improves liver function and hepatic perfusion after hemorrhagic shock in rat. *Crit. Care Med.* 36: 2863–70.
117. Costantino, G., S. Cuzzocrea, E. Mazzon, et al. 1998. Protective effects of melatonin in zymosan-activated plasma-induced paw inflammation. *Eur. J. Pharmacol.* 363: 57–63.
118. Cuzzocrea, S., B. Zingarelli, E. Gilad, et al. 1997. Protective effect of melatonin in carrageenan-induced models of local inflammation: Relationship to its inhibitory effect on nitric oxide production and its peroxynitrite scavenging activity. *J. Pineal Res.* 23: 106–16.
119. Cardinali, D. P., M. N. Ritta, A. M. Fuentes, et al. 1980. Prostaglandin E release by rat medial basal hypothalamus in vitro. Inhibition by melatonin at submicromolar concentrations. *Eur. J. Pharmacol.* 67: 151–3.
120. Cuzzocrea, S., G. Costantino, E. Mazzon, et al. 1999. Regulation of prostaglandin production in carrageenan-induced pleurisy by melatonin. *J. Pineal Res.* 27: 9–14.
121. Pozo, D., R. J. Reiter, J. R. Calvo, et al. 1994. Physiological concentrations of melatonin inhibit nitric oxide synthase in rat cerebellum. *Life Sci.* 55: L455-L460.
122. Mohan, N., K. Sadeghi, R. J. Reiter, et al. 1995. The neurohormone melatonin inhibits cytokine, mitogen and ionizing radiation induced NF-kappa B. *Biochem. Mol. Biol. Int.* 37: 1063–70.
123. Mayo, J. C., R. M. Sainz, D. X. Tan, et al. 2005. Anti-inflammatory actions of melatonin and its metabolites, *N*1-acetyl-*N*2-formyl-5-methoxykynuramine (AFMK) and *N*1-acetyl-5-methoxykynuramine (AMK), in macrophages. *J. Neuroimmunol.* 165: 139–49.
124. Deng, W. G., S. T. Tang, H. P. Tseng, et al. 2006. Melatonin suppresses macrophage cyclooxygenase-2 and inducible nitric oxide synthase expression by inhibiting p52 acetylation and binding. *Blood* 108: 518–24.
125. Park, H. J., H. J. Kim, J. Ra, et al. 2007. Melatonin inhibits lipopolysaccharide-induced CC chemokine subfamily gene expression in human peripheral blood mononuclear cells in a microarray analysis. *J. Pineal Res.* 43: 121–9.
126. Podrez, E. A., H. M. Abu-Soud, and S. L. Hazen. 2000. Myeloperoxidase-generated oxidants and atherosclerosis. *Free Radic. Biol. Med.* 28: 1717–25.
127. Nicholls, S. J., and S. L. Hazen. 2005. Myeloperoxidase and cardiovascular disease. *Arterioscler. Thromb. Vasc. Biol* 25: 1102–11.
128. Pattison, D. I., and M. J. Davies. 2006. Reactions of myeloperoxidase-derived oxidants with biological substrates: Gaining chemical insight into human inflammatory diseases. *Curr. Med. Chem.* 13: 3271–90.
129. Galijasevic, S., I. Abdulhamid, and H. M. Abu-Soud. 2008. Melatonin is a potent inhibitor for myeloperoxidase. *Biochemistry* 47: 2668–77.
130. Ben Nathan, D., G. J. Maestroni, S. Lustig, et al. 1995. Protective effects of melatonin in mice infected with encephalitis viruses. *Arch. Virol.* 140: 223–30.
131. Wiid, I., E. Hoal-van Helden, D. Hon, et al. 1999. Potentiation of isoniazid activity against Mycobacterium tuberculosis by melatonin. *Antimicrob. Agents Chemother.* 43: 975–7.
132. Bonilla, E., N. Valero, L. Chacin-Bonilla, et al. 2004. Melatonin and viral infections. *J. Pineal Res.* 36: 73–9.

133. Baltaci, A. K., C. S. Bediz, R. Mogulkoc, et al. 2003. Effect of zinc and melatonin supplementation on cellular immunity in rats with toxoplasmosis. *Biol. Trace Elem. Res.* 96: 237–45.
134. Baltaci, A. K., R. Mogulkoc, Y. Turkoz, et al. 2004. The effect of pinealectomy and zinc deficiency on nitric oxide levels in rats with induced Toxoplasma gondii infection. *Swiss. Med. Wkly.* 134: 359–63.
135. El Sokkary, G. H., H. M. Omar, A. F. Hassanein, et al. 2002. Melatonin reduces oxidative damage and increases survival of mice infected with Schistosoma mansoni. *Free Radic. Biol. Med.* 32: 319–32.
136. Budu, A., R. Peres, V. B. Bueno, et al. 2007. *N*1-Acetyl-*N*2-formyl-5-methoxykynuramine modulates the cell cycle of malaria parasites. *J. Pineal Res.* 42: 261–6.
137. Beraldo, F. H., and C. R. Garcia. 2005. Products of tryptophan catabolism induce Ca2+ release and modulate the cell cycle of *Plasmodium falciparum* malaria parasites. *J. Pineal Res.* 39: 224–30.
138. Mongardon, N., A. Dyson, and M. Singer. 2009. Is MOF an outcome parameter or a transient, adaptive state in critical illness? *Curr. Opin. Crit. Care* 15: 431–6.
139. O'Brien, J. M., Jr., N. A. Ali, and E. Abraham. 2008. Year in review 2007: Critical care—Multiple organ failure and sepsis. *Crit. Care* 12: 228.
140. Escames, G., D. Acuna-Castroviejo, L. C. Lopez, et al. 2006. Pharmacological utility of melatonin in the treatment of septic shock: Experimental and clinical evidence. *J. Pharm. Pharmacol.* 58: 1153–65.
141. Shang, Y., S. P. Xu, Y. Wu, et al. 2009. Melatonin reduces acute lung injury in endotoxemic rats. *Chin. Med. J. (Engl.)* 122: 1388–93.
142. Gitto, E., S. Pellegrino, P. Gitto, et al. 2009. Oxidative stress of the newborn in the pre- and postnatal period and the clinical utility of melatonin. *J. Pineal Res.* 46: 128–39.
143. D'Alessandro, U. 2009. Existing antimalarial agents and malaria—Treatment strategies. *Expert Opin. Pharmacother.* 10: 1291–306.
144. Schofield, L. 2007. Intravascular infiltrates and organ-specific inflammation in malaria pathogenesis. *Immunol. Cell Biol.* 85: 130–7.
145. Schofield, L., and G. E. Grau. 2005. Immunological processes in malaria pathogenesis. *Nat. Rev. Immunol.* 5: 722–35.
146. Srinivasan, V., D. W. Spence, A. Moscovitch, et al. 2010. Malaria: Therapeutic implications of melatonin. *J. Pineal Res.* 48: 1–8.
147. Guha, M., P. Maity, V. Choubey, et al. 2007. Melatonin inhibits free radical-mediated mitochondrial-dependent hepatocyte apoptosis and liver damage induced during malarial infection. *J. Pineal Res.* 43: 372–81.
148. Hotta, C. T., M. L. Gazarini, F. H. Beraldo, et al. 2000. Calcium-dependent modulation by melatonin of the circadian rhythm in malarial parasites. *Nat. Cell Biol.* 2: 466–8.
149. Hotta, C. T., R. P. Markus, and C. R. Garcia. 2003. Melatonin and *N*-acetyl-serotonin cross the red blood cell membrane and evoke calcium mobilization in malarial parasites. *Braz. J. Med. Biol. Res.* 36: 1583–7.
150. Coura, J. R., and J. C. Dias. 2009. Epidemiology, control and surveillance of Chagas disease: 100 years after its discovery. *Mem. Inst. Oswaldo Cruz* 104 Suppl. 1: 31–40.
151. Sathler-Avelar, R., D. M. Vitelli-Avelar, A. Teixeira-Carvalho, et al. 2009. Innate immunity and regulatory T-cells in human Chagas disease: What must be understood? *Mem. Inst. Oswaldo Cruz* 104 Suppl. 1: 246–51.
152. Cunha-Neto, E., L. G. Nogueira, P. C. Teixeira, et al. 2009. Immunological and non-immunological effects of cytokines and chemokines in the pathogenesis of chronic Chagas disease cardiomyopathy. *Mem. Inst. Oswaldo Cruz* 104 Suppl. 1: 252–8.
153. Macias, M., M. N. Rodriguez-Cabezas, R. J. Reiter, et al. 1999. Presence and effects of melatonin in *Trypanosoma cruzi*. *J. Pineal Res.* 27: 86–94.
154. Santello, F. H., E. O. Frare, C. D. Dos Santos, et al. 2007. Melatonin treatment reduces the severity of experimental *Trypanosoma cruzi* infection. *J. Pineal Res.* 42: 359–63.
155. Santello, F. H., E. O. Frare, L. C. Caetano, et al. 2008. Melatonin enhances pro-inflammatory cytokine levels and protects against Chagas disease. *J. Pineal Res.* 45: 79–85.
156. Santello, F. H., E. O. Frare, C. D. Dos Santos, et al. 2008. Suppressive action of melatonin on the TH-2 immune response in rats infected with *Trypanosoma cruzi*. *J. Pineal Res.* 45: 291–6.

10 Melatonin as a Treatment for Uveitis

Ruth E. Rosenstein, Pablo H. Sande, Diego C. Fernandez, Mónica Chianelli, and Daniel A. Sáenz

CONTENTS

10.1 BACKGROUND

Melatonin is a ubiquitous natural substance that is widely distributed in nature, being found in both plants and animals [1–3]. Melatonin is probably one of the first biologically significant compounds that appeared in living organisms. Although in all mammals including humans, melatonin is primarily synthesized in the pineal gland, its synthesis also occurs in other tissues, such as bone marrow, gut, gastrointestinal tract, lymphocytes, and in various parts of the eye in most mammals, i.e., the retina [4–6], the ciliary body [7], and the lachrymal gland [8].

In the eye, melatonin, which is locally synthesized or enters from the circulation, may contribute to the regulation of retinomotor movements, rod outer segment disc shedding, dopamine synthesis and release, and intraocular pressure (IOP). Moreover, melatonin is an effective antioxidant and free radical scavenger [9–12], which protects the photoreceptor outer segment and other ocular tissues from oxidative damage induced by light [13–18].

Uveitis is a common ophthalmic disorder characterized by an acute, recurrent, or persistent ocular inflammation. Uveitis is associated with the disruption of the blood–ocular barrier (BOB) as well as protein leakage and leukocyte infiltration into the aqueous humor. Several lines of evidence support the view that uveitis results from damage generated by infiltrated leukocytes, which release cytokines and other inflammatory chemical mediators [19], including arachidonic acid (AA) metabolites [20], reactive oxygen species (ROS) [21], NO [22], and superoxide anion [23], among many others. At present, the therapy for uveitis generally based on the use of corticoids is essentially directed toward pain reduction and avoidance of ocular tissue lesions [24,25]. However, the immunosuppressive effect of corticoids may contribute to the development of systemic disease. Moreover, this strategy carries with it the attendant risk of cortisonic glaucoma induction that usually follows its chronic use

[26,27]. Thus, despite the fact that uveitis is a highly prevalent cause of blindness, there are currently no optimal treatments for these ocular diseases. In recent years, melatonin has been identified as a neuroprotector in experimental animal models of various neurological and neurodegenerative disorders [28–30]. In this context, we will consider evidence supporting that melatonin should be regarded as an important ophthalmic therapeutic resource, particularly for the management of uveitis.

10.2 MELATONIN BIOSYNTHESIS IN THE EYE

Melatonin is synthesized intraocularly through the same pathway that occurs in the pineal gland [31]. Tryptophan taken up from the blood is converted into serotonin, which is subsequently metabolized to *N*-acetyl serotonin by the enzyme arylalkylamine *N*-acetyltransferase (AA-NAT). *N*-Acetyl serotonin is then converted into melatonin by the enzyme hydroxyindole-*O*-methyltransferase (HIOMT). The earliest finding supporting melatonin's biosynthetic pathway in the mammalian retina was the description of HIOMT activity [4] and the demonstration that labeled serotonin is converted into melatonin in the rat retina [5]. The presence of HIOMT in the chicken retina at both the protein and mRNA level has been confirmed [32,33]. The gene encoding HIOMT is selectively expressed in retinal photoreceptors. In a recent study, the promoter of the HIOMT gene Otx2 was detected both in the chicken retina and pineal gland [34]. These findings are significant in view of the fact that Otx2 protein is present at "the right place and at the right time" to play a role in the onset of HIOMT gene expression in retinal photoreceptors and pineal gland [34]. AA-NAT levels show a circadian rhythm, peaking at night in the chicken and rat retina [35,36]. The presence of AA-NAT in the human eye has been well documented [37]. In the rhesus monkey, AA-NAT activity in pineal and retina shows more than a fourfold increase at night [38].

Melatonin biosynthesis in the retina is regulated by the light/dark cycle [39]. In addition, the finding that isolated *Xenopus* photoreceptor cells rhythmically secrete melatonin suggests that photoreceptors contain an endogenous circadian clock that regulates melatonin biosynthesis [40]. This hypothesis has been confirmed in the golden hamster and mouse retinas [6,41]. In fact, several genes identified as components of the core oscillator in the suprachiasmatic nuclei (SCN) have also been localized in the retina [42–44]. At present, it is not known whether the circadian rhythms in mammalian photoreceptors are driven by inner retinal clocks through synaptic ribbons or by paracrine outputs. Experiments with the rodless mouse have shown that melatonin synthesis is not abolished by the complete loss of photoreceptors, but that its circadian expression disappears [6,45]. This finding suggests that rods are necessary for the rhythmic synthesis of melatonin. However, new evidences indicate that chick retinal ganglion cells are able to rhythmically synthesize melatonin, even in isolated conditions [46].

Regulated by the interaction between a circadian clock and the photic information, retinal melatonin levels rise rapidly after the onset of darkness and decrease after light exposure in the golden hamster and rat [47,48]. The entire sequence of events has been elegantly studied in chicken photoreceptor cells. The depolarization of photoreceptors that occurs during darkness induces AA-NAT activity by a Ca^{2+} and cAMP dependent mechanism [49]. Depolarization of the photoreceptor membrane opens dihydropyridine-sensitive voltage-gated Ca^{2+} channels, resulting in sustained increases in intracellular Ca^{2+} concentrations in the inner segments of photoreceptors, which, in turn, stimulate cAMP formation through the activation of calmodulin-dependent adenyl cyclase [50]. Increased levels of cAMP induce AA-NAT gene transcription and increase its activity causing an augmented production of melatonin [51,52]. Stability of AA-NAT is regulated by cAMP, and light; a decrease in cAMP levels in photoreceptor cells results in rapid degradation of AA-NAT protein by proteasomal proteolysis [53].

As for the regulation of melatonin biosynthesis by a circadian clock, the gating process involves an E box–mediated transcriptional activation of the adenyl cyclase gene. This regulates melatonin synthesis by regulating the expression of type 1 adenyl cyclase and the synthesis of cAMP in photoreceptors [54]. Cyclic AMP signaling may play a key role in the input and output components of the central circadian axis, the retina, the SCN, and the pineal gland [54]. In addition to cAMP, binding of AA-NAT to 14-3-3 proteins in retinal photoreceptors appears to be important in the response to light and darkness [55]. During darkness, retinal AA-NAT is phosphorylated and forms a complex with 14-3-3 proteins, which protects it from dephosphorylation and degradation. Binding of AA-NAT to 14-3-3 proteins is disrupted by light in photoreceptors, which allows AA-NAT degradation. Although the studies cited above have been conducted in the chicken, several in vivo and in vitro studies have established that there is a circadian clock system in the mammalian eye independent from the SCN [56]. Besides the retina, it has been reported that both AA-NAT and HIOMT are present in other ocular structures such as rabbit and rat lens [57,58].

10.3 MELATONIN RECEPTORS IN THE EYE

Since most of melatonin functions are attributed to its interaction with specific receptors, the study of the distribution of melatonin receptor subtypes in the eye assumes functional significance [16]. Immunocytochemical analysis of ocular tissues obtained from various species, including chickens, rats, and humans, shows that melatonin receptors MT_1 and MT_2 are localized in the cornea, choroid, sclera, retina, and retinal blood vessels [59–65]. In *Xenopus* eyes, MT_1 melatonin receptors have been described in the corneal epithelium, stroma, sclera, and endothelium [66], suggesting melatonin's involvement in the differential regulation of growth and remodeling of the fibrous and cartilaginous scleral layers that affect eye size and refraction. On the other hand, the localization of melatonin receptors in the iris and ciliary processes could indicate that they may be involved in regulating IOP [67]. The presence of melatonin receptor Mel_{1c} in the nonpigmented epithelium of the chicken [68] suggests that melatonin may affect the rate of aqueous humor secretion by the ciliary epithelium and the circadian rhythm of IOP. The Mel_{1c} receptor subtype was first cloned in the chicken [69] but has never been identified in mammals [70]. The three identified melatonin receptors, namely MT_1, MT_2, and Mel_{1c}, show different daily rhythms of protein expression in the retinal pigment epithelium (RPE) and choroid, with peak levels of MT_1 and MT_2 occurring during the night and peak levels of Mel_{1c} occurring during the day in the chick [65].

The presence of MT_2 in *Xenopus* apical microvillar cell membrane but not on the basement membrane of the RPE supports the hypothesis that melatonin is involved in photoreceptor outer segment disc shedding and phagocytosis [66,70]. MT_1 receptors have been identified in retinal ganglion cells (RGCs) and amacrine cells in rat and guinea pig [61,71]. In humans, MT_1 immunoreactivity was found in cell bodies along the inner border of the inner nuclear layer, and in its outer border almost exclusively in horizontal cells, in cell bodies within the ganglion cell layer, and in the inner segments of rod photoreceptors [61]. In addition, about two thirds of CA1 and CA2 dopaminergic neurons exhibited MT_1 immunolabeling. MT_1 receptors were also identified in human and macaque AII amacrine cells, which are critical neurons in the rod pathway of the mammalian retina.

The MT_2 receptor is expressed in the sclera, lens, RPE, and neural retina of *Xenopus* eye [64]. In older humans, MT_2 has recently been localized to ganglion and bipolar cells in the inner nuclear layer, to the inner segments of photoreceptors, and to cellular processes in inner and outer plexiform layers [72]. The presence of melatonin receptors in multiple cell types suggests that melatonin could have multiple physiological functions in the retina. In human retinal RGCs, MT_1 receptors represent nearly 90% of the total number of melatonin receptors [73]. The MT_1 receptor has been identified in the adventitial cells of retinal vessels, suggesting that melatonin could have an indirect action on vascular smooth muscle [62].

10.4 OCULAR FUNCTIONS OF MELATONIN

Systemic administration of melatonin has been found to produce significant changes in anterior and vitreous chamber depth, suggesting that melatonin may play a role in ocular growth and development [65]. Retinal melatonin acts as a neuromodulator that mediates dark adaptive regulation of retinomotor movements [74]. The expression of MT_1 receptors in most dopaminergic amacrine cells in human retina implicates melatonin in the modulation of dopaminergic function [63]. Both dopamine and melatonin are key signaling agents in the regulation of retinal rhythmicity. These two substances are mutually inhibitory, acting as signals for day and night, respectively. It was demonstrated that picomolar concentrations of melatonin selectively inhibit the calcium-dependent release of dopamine from rabbit retina [75]. Moreover, experimental evidence that supports the model of mutual signaling between melatonin and dopamine has been provided by Doyle et al. [76], who demonstrated that in C3H+/+ mice, which lack melatonin and show no circadian rhythmicity of dopamine content, the deficiency could be corrected by cyclical administration of melatonin. The action of melatonin on the rod pathway at the level of horizontal and amacrine cells has been proposed as a unique mechanism by which the retina adapts to low light intensities [61]. A correlation between melatonin levels and the electroretinographic response has been shown in human studies, which suggest that daily melatonin and electroretinogram (ERG) cycling are associated [77]. On the other hand, melatonin decreases retinal cAMP accumulation [39] and regulates the activity of the retinal glutamate/glutamine cycle activity [78].

10.4.1 Melatonin as a Retinal Antioxidant

The possibility that melatonin could detoxify highly ROS was originally suggested by Ianas et al. [79]. Shortly thereafter, Poeggeler et al. [9] and Reiter et al. [80], using spin trapping and electron resonance spectroscopy, demonstrated melatonin's capacity to directly scavenge highly reactive hydroxyl radicals. Since then, several reports have shown that melatonin acts as a free radical scavenger and an efficient antioxidant [2,81–84]. Not only melatonin but also several of its metabolites generated during its free radical scavenging action act as antioxidants [85]. The kynurenic pathway of melatonin metabolism includes a series of radical scavengers with the possible sequence: melatonin → cyclic 3-hydroxymelatonin → N^1-acetyl-N^2-formyl-5-methoxykynuramine (AFMK) → N^1-acetyl-5-methoxykynuramine (AMK). In the metabolic step from melatonin to AFMK, up to four free radicals can be consumed [85–88]. Because of this pathway, melatonin's efficacy as an antioxidant is greatly increased. Melatonin has been shown to protect against oxidative stress in various, highly divergent experimental systems. Melatonin's functions as an antioxidant include (a) direct free radical scavenging, (b) stimulation of antioxidative enzymes, (c) increasing the efficiency of mitochondrial oxidative phosphorylation and reducing electron leakage (thereby lowering free radical generation), and (d) augmenting the efficiency of other antioxidants [89]. Melatonin has been shown to scavenge free radicals generated in mitochondria, reduce electron leakage from the respiratory complexes, and improve ATP synthesis [90,91]. Moreover, melatonin preserves mitochondrial glutathione levels, thereby enhancing the antioxidant potential [92]. It was recently demonstrated that the low-affinity MT3 melatonin receptor binding site is identical with quinone reductase 2 (QR2) [93] and that melatonin inhibits the activity of this enzyme [94,95], and there is evidence that, contrary to previous belief [96], QR2 is an activating enzyme [97,98] since its deletion from living organisms leads to increased toxicity of quinines [97]. Thus, inhibition of the enzyme could have antioxidant effects. Moreover, *N*-acetylserotonin interacts with QR2 and, in fact, has an affinity for this enzyme that is higher than that of melatonin [95,99,100]. Therefore, endogenous levels of *N*-acetylserotonin are even more inhibitory to QR2 in producing an antioxidant action and may well be the endogenous ligand for this enzyme.

The retina is a particularly susceptible tissue to oxidative stress because of its high consumption of oxygen, its high proportion of polyunsaturated fatty acids, and its direct exposure to light. It was demonstrated that melatonin decreases lipid peroxidation of polyunsaturated fatty acids located in rod outer segment membranes [101], it may protect retinal pigment epithelial cells from oxidative stress [102], and it prevents retinal oxidative damage from ischemia–reperfusion injury [103]. In cultures of human retinal neuronal cells subjected to experimental hypoxanthine/xanthine oxidase–induced injury, melatonin is able to rescue retinal neurons [104]. Furthermore, in dark-adapted, single photoreceptors isolated from the frog retina after illumination with saturating light, melatonin at picomolar and low-nanomolar concentrations was shown to be 100 times more potent in inhibiting the light-induced oxidative processes than vitamin E [18]. Recently, we have shown that melatonin increases superoxide dismutase activity and reduced glutathione levels, whereas it decreases lipid peroxidation in the rat retina [105]. Taken together, these results strongly support the role of melatonin as an effective retinal antioxidant.

10.4.2 Melatonin and the Retinal Nitridergic Pathway

NO, a highly reactive short-lived radical species, plays an important role as an intercellular and intracellular messenger in the central nervous system. NO is generated by a family of enzymes called NO synthases (NOS) that oxidate L-arginine to L-citrulline producing NO. NO acts as an endogenous activator of a soluble guanylyl cyclase, thereby increasing cGMP levels. There is evidence from different studies supporting that NO is involved in the regulation of several retinal processes. NO activates a retinal soluble guanylyl cyclase and modulates a Ca^{2+} channel and a voltage-independent conductance in the inner segment of photoreceptors [106]. Effects of NO were also recorded on hemigap junction channels in horizontal cells of the catfish retina [107], on cGMP-gated channels in retinal ganglion cells [108], and ON-bipolar cells [109]. Intracellular application of L-arginine prevents the prolongation of the light responses in frog isolated rods [110], and it blocks gap junctions between horizontal cells in the turtle retina [111]. Besides these physiological actions, NO can react with superoxide producing peroxynitrite, a powerful and deleterious oxidant. We have shown that in isolated conditions, melatonin may directly react with NO yielding at least one stable product, *N*-nitrosomelatonin, which was characterized by NMR and x-ray spectroscopy [112,113]. In addition to a direct scavenging of NO, low concentrations of melatonin significantly decrease hamster retinal NOS activity. Melatonin behaves as a noncompetitive inhibitor of this enzyme, since it decreases the V_{max}, with no changes on the K_m [114]. This result agrees with the previously described effect of melatonin on NOS from other neural structures such as hypothalamus [115], cerebellum [116], striatum, and cerebral frontal cortex [117]. However, while the inhibitory effect of melatonin in those tissues was evident up to 1 nM, in the retina, a much higher sensitivity to the methoxyindole was evident, as it was effective even at 1 pM. In addition, while in other systems melatonin was active when added to crude homogenates, in the hamster retina, it was only effective when the whole tissues were preincubated in the presence of the methoxyindole. The high sensitivity of this melatonin inhibitory effect and the fact that the tissue integrity seems to be necessary suggest that, in the retina, melatonin modulates NOS activity through a receptor-mediated mechanism but not through its binding to calmodulin. The reasons of this discrepancy are not clear. It should be noted that the retina, unlike the cerebellum, the hypothalamus, or the striatum, is able to synthesize melatonin. Being a highly lipophilic molecule, melatonin has the capability of crossing all physiological barriers. However, these results suggest that the effect of melatonin on NOS activity could be restricted to those cell types that coexpress melatonin receptors and NOS.

Besides NOS, another limiting step in NO synthesis is the availability of its precursor, L-arginine, which depends on the presence and activity of a specific uptake system. Physiological concentrations of melatonin significantly decrease retinal L-arginine influx [114]. The lower V_{max} of this mechanism observed in the presence of the methoxyindole suggests that melatonin decreases the number of active transporter molecules, without changing the affinity. Since melatonin decreases both L-arginine influx and its conversion to NO, a decrease in L-arginine–induced response is expectable in the presence of the methoxyindole. Indeed, the increase in cGMP accumulation induced by L-arginine is significantly reduced by melatonin [114]. Despite the fact that NO donors, such as sodium nitroprusside (SNP) releases NO in a NOS-independent way, we showed that melatonin also decreases its effect on cGMP accumulation, probably through its capacity to directly scavenge NO. In agreement with these results, it was shown that uncontrolled NO elevation causes morphological and nuclear changes in the retina and that melatonin significantly suppresses the NO-induced increase in mean

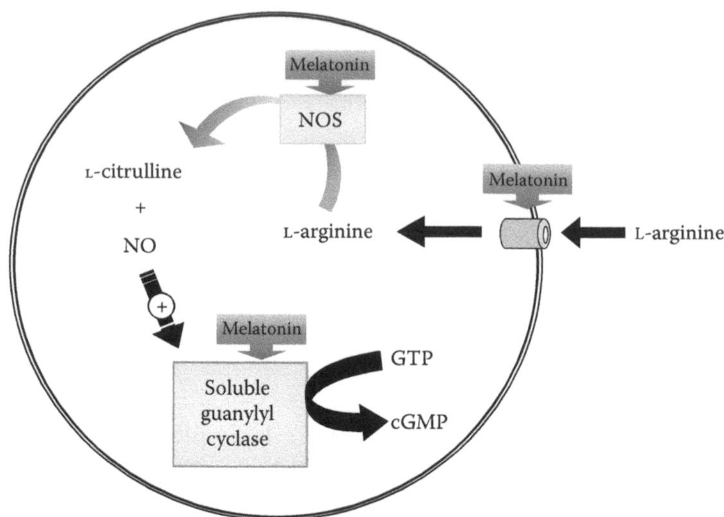

FIGURE 10.1 Schematic representation of the retinal nitridergic pathway and its modulation by melatonin. As shown, melatonin decreases NOS activity and L-arginine uptake as well as the increase in cGMP levels induced by L-arginine and SNP.

inner retinal layer thickness, nuclei in the inner nuclear layer, as well as the number of retinas expressing hyperchromatic expression, and apoptotic ganglion cells [118]. In addition, it was demonstrated that melatonin reduces NO-induced lipid peroxidation in rat retinal homogenates [119]. Peroxynitrite is a toxic oxidant formed from the reaction of superoxide and NO under conditions of inflammation and oxidant stress, and it was shown that melatonin is a scavenger of peroxynitrite [120]. Furthermore, it was demonstrated that melatonin is protective against oxidative damage in situations where NO is known to account for molecular destruction [121]. The effects of melatonin on the retinal nitridergic pathway are summarized in Figure 10.1.

10.5 UVEITIS

Uveitis is the term used to describe many forms of intraocular inflammation involving the uveal tract (iris, ciliary body, and choroid) and adjacent ocular structures (retina, vitreous, and optic nerve). Uveitis is derived from the Latin *uva*, or "grape"; a peeled blue grape has a bluish vein structure that resembles the middle, vascular layer of the eye, the uvea. Uveitis is the most common form of intraocular inflammation and remains a significant cause of visual loss. Inflammation of the anterior uvea is termed *anterior uveitis* or *iridocyclitis*. If only the iris is involved, the condition is called *iritis*. Inflammation of the ciliary body is *cyclitis*, and choroidal inflammation is termed *choroiditis*. In clinical usage, uveitis has come to describe most forms of intraocular inflammation. If a layer contiguous with the uvea is predominantly involved in an inflammatory process, the term used for the intraocular inflammation is modified accordingly, that is, *retinochoroiditis*, *retinitis*, or *vitritis* [122]. Hogan et al. [123] have used the classification anterior, posterior, and diffuse uveitis (or panuveitis). Anterior uveitis consists of either *iritis* or *iridocyclitis*, whereas uveitis involving the middle portion of the eye is termed either *cyclitis* or *intermediate uveitis* (Figure 10.2). The classification of posterior uveitis depends on which intraocular layer is predominantly involved. It is termed *choroiditis* or *retinitis* when just the choroid or the retina is involved, whereas *retinochoroiditis* or *chorioretinitis* is used when both layers are involved; in the latter situation, the first portion of the term denotes the most intensely involved layer of the eye. *Panuveitis* is a generalized inflammation of not only the whole of the uveal tract, but also involves the retina and vitreous humor.

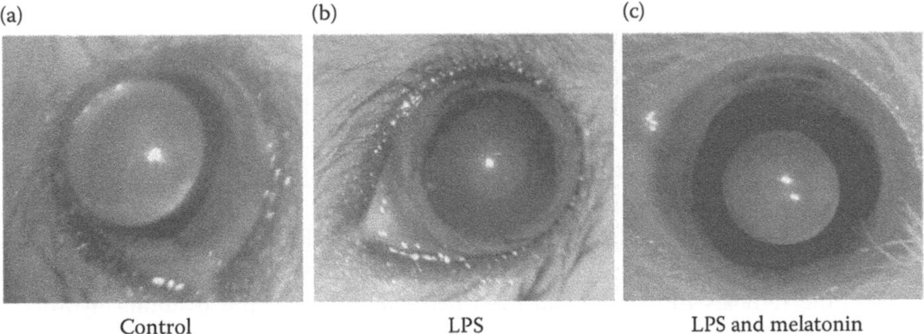

FIGURE 10.2 Representative photographs of eyes injected with (a) vehicle and LPS (b) in the absence and (c) in the presence of melatonin. In eyes injected with LPS in the absence of melatonin, episcleral hyperemia, miosis, synechiae, and distorted fundus reflection were observed. In the presence of melatonin, a decrease in the inflammatory process was evident, with only a mild conjunctival congestion and lens opacity.

In anterior uveitis, there is often vascular congestion of the conjunctiva and the sclera (ciliary flush). Inflammation of the anterior uvea (iris and ciliary body) results in increased vascular permeability; cells and protein are detectable on slit-lamp biomicroscopy of the anterior chamber (aqueous humor). Inflammatory cells may be deposited on the posterior corneal surface, anterior chamber angle, or on either the anterior surface or pupillary border of the iris. These depositions may result in an adhesion between the papillary margin of the iris and the lens, which are termed *posterior synechiae*. Peripheral anterior synechiae may occur between the anterior iris and the cornea; if these peripheral anterior synechiae occur for 360 degrees, the anterior chamber angle is closed and IOP increases (resulting in glaucoma). Alternatively, as a result of uveitis, IOP may decrease and aqueous humor production by the inflamed ciliary body be diminished. Chronic or recurrent anterior uveitis often leads to opacification of the lens with visually significant cataract formation.

Vision often decreases as a result of posterior segment inflammation, due to opacities in the vitreous, or from inflammation or vascular occlusions of the macular area (fovea) or the optic nerve. Inflammatory single cells or aggregates in the vitreous cavity are perceived by a patient as "floaters" and may be detected either by a slit-lamp examination or with an ophthalmoscope. The retina, which is normally transparent, appears cloudy or white when inflamed. Inflammation involving only the choroid appears as yellow, white, or gray patches with well-defined borders.

Retinal vasculitis may occur with vascular cuffing, arterial or venous occlusions, or hemorrhages. Histologically, there are lymphocytes cuffing the inflamed retinal vessels. Increased vascular permeability of retinal vessels in either the macula or the optic nerve leads to edema and diminution of vision. Persistent macular edema results in permanent visual disability due to the formation of macular cysts. Optic atrophy may occur as a consequence of chronic inflammation of the optic nerve (revised in ref. [124]). In children, the most common causes of uveitis are juvenile rheumatoid arthritis, ankylosing spondylitis, Behcet's syndrome, sarcoidosis, toxocariasis, toxoplasmosis, and chronic cyclitis. In adults with anterior uveitis, the differential diagnoses include ankylosing spondylitis, Reiter's syndrome, inflammatory bowel disease, sarcoidosis, and those of infectious causes. Posterior uveitis syndromes are usually due to toxoplasmosis, syphilis, cytomegalovirus, and *Candida*. Diffuse forms of uveitis in adults are usually due tochronic cyclitis, sarcoidosis, Behcet's disease, Vogt–Koyanagi–Harada's syndrome, and masquerade syndromes (revised by Lowder and Char [124]).

10.5.1 Mechanisms Involved in Uveitis

Uveitis is characterized by a disruption of the BOB, accompanied by protein leakage and leukocyte infiltration into the aqueous humor. Resident cells are activated and inflammatory cells are recruited. Despite that uveitis is one of the main causes of eye morbidity and loss of visual functions, the complexity of the biochemical and immune mechanisms involved in its generation and development remain unknown. In this sense, several animal models such as interleukin (IL)-1–induced uveitis, experimental autoimmune uveitis (EAU), and endotoxin induced uveitis (EIU), among others, were developed for understanding disease pathogenesis and testing new therapies for ocular inflammatory diseases [125].

Several lines of evidence support that uveitis is due to damage generated by infiltrated leukocytes, which release cytokines [19,126] and other inflammatory chemical mediators, such as AA metabolites [20], ROS [127], NO [23], and superoxide anion (O_2^-) [22], among many others. Oxygen-derived free radicals have been implicated in the inflammation associated with EIU in experimental animals [128]. Free radicals initiate retinal lipid peroxidation, and the resultant hydroperoxides serve as amplification factors, such as chemotaxis of inflammatory cells [129,130]. The presence of oxidative stress in the photoreceptor mitochondria appears to be an early event in the development of uveitis, which initiates the subsequent irreversible retinal damage in experimental uveitis by attracting phagocytic cells to this initial site of injury [131]. In fact, there is evidence that free radical scavengers and antioxidants can act as anti-inflammatory agents, thus protecting the eye from inflammation-mediated tissue damage [132].

Prostaglandins (PGs) can be synthesized through the activities of two cyclooxygenase (COX) isoforms. COX-1 is constitutively expressed in most tissues and its activity provides for the relative small amounts of PGs required for the mediation and modulation of normal physiological functions. In inflammatory conditions, COX-2 is rapidly induced by cytokines, growth factors, and bacterial endotoxin, and its enzymatic activity accounts for the large amounts of PGs produced during inflammation [133]. PGs in small doses administered topically or intraocularly produce some of the responses of injury and inflammation, such as hyperemia, miosis, breakdown of the blood–aqueous barrier, and rise in IOP. Also, E-type PGs administered topically together with histamine (but not the individual components) cause cellular infiltration and produce edema in conjunctival tissues [134]. Moreover, it was shown that AA metabolites regulate vascular permeability, chemotaxis, and contribute to uveitis amplification [134,135].

Studies from animal models of uveitis and human patients with uveitis implicate reactive oxygen/nitrogen radicals in the inflammatory process. Parks et al. [136] demonstrated that multiple intraperitoneal injections of L-NAME, a well-known NOS inhibitor, reduced clinical signs of uveitis in EIU, suggesting that NO could participate to the pathogenesis of experimental uveitis as a proinflammatory mediator. Furthermore, it has been shown that the hemodynamic and vascular permeability changes associated with EIU in the rat are in part due to increased production of NO. High levels of nitrite in the aqueous humor and vitreous of rats at the time of maximal ocular inflammation following injection with lipopolysaccharide (LPS) as well as the presence of a calcium-independent NOS activity in the anterior segment during endotoxin-induced uveitis [137] have been demonstrated. Furthermore, reverse transcriptase–polymerase chain reaction assays show an increased expression of inducible isoform of NO synthase (iNOS) mRNA in the iris–ciliary body and in the retina of rats with EIU [138]. In situ hybridization revealed that epithelial cells of the iris–ciliary body and cells infiltrating (macrophages, polymorphonuclear leukocytes) the anterior segment and in the retina are the major source of NO [22]. Moreover, a significant correlation was obtained between the nitrite level in aqueous humor and clinical signs of EIU. The efficacy of treatment with NOS inhibitors in EIU in rat or in rabbit suggests that treatments that reduce NO production or NO action would be beneficial and would provide new prospects for treatment of human uveitis [139]. Activated phagocytes synthesize large amounts of nitric oxide (NO) through a reaction catalyzed by the iNOS [138,140].

10.5.2 Current Treatment for Uveitis

The treatment of uveitis has three main goals: to prevent vision-threatening complications, to relieve the patient's complaints, and, when feasible, to treat the underlying disease [141]. Current treatment for uveitis employs systemic medications that have severe side effects and are globally immunosuppressive. Clinically, chronic progressive or relapsing forms of noninfectious uveitis are treated with topical and/or systemic corticosteroids. In addition to steroids, macrolides such as cyclosporine and rapamycin are used, and in some cases, cytotoxic agents such as cyclophosphamide and chlorambucil and antimetabolites such as azathioprine, methotrexate, and lefunomide. While often effective, these drugs have potential serious side effects, and they compromise protective immunity to pathogens [142].

The increased knowledge in immunology and the progresses of pharmacology have improved our treatment of autoimmune diseases. The main anti-inflammatory effects of corticosteroids are an attenuation of the hypersensibility reactions, a sequestration of intravascular lymphocytes and an inhibition of the production of cytokines and eicosanoids. The nonsteroidal anti-inflammatory drugs (NSAIDs) form another group of medications particularly useful for the treatment of chronic uveitis. Several COX-2 inhibitory medications are under clinical investigation and some are commercially available. One of their characteristics is to present less of the most undesirable side effects seen with conventional NSAIDs, such as irritation of the gastrointestinal tract and platelets aggregation inhibition. Agents such as cyclophosphamide, leukeran, imuran, methotrexate, and cyclosporin have been used extensively for the treatment of severe uveitis. Because of its efficacy and safety, methotrexate is the best immunosuppressive agent to be tried for the treatment of chronic uveitis. However, immunosuppressive treatments and corticosteroids have many side effects and are not very selective [125].

A more specific approach to therapy that will target primarily the cells involved in pathogenesis and leave the rest of the immune system alone is urgently needed. Thus, there is urgent need to develop effective immunotherapeutic strategies that are nontoxic and that specially target the pathogenic cell population.

10.6 MELATONIN AND UVEITIS

As already mentioned, current treatments for uveitis have limited effectiveness and a considerable range of side effects. Kukner et al. [143] have investigated the effect of melatonin on autoimmune uveitis. In this study, intravitreal injections of bovine serum albumin were used to induce uveitis in the guinea pig. Melatonin, vitamin E, or aprotinin were intraperitoneally administered 3 days after albumin injection. A significant increase in leptin expression occurs in the retina, choroid, sclera, and episclera; RGCs were edematous and inner plexiform layer thickness increased in uveitic eyes. In animals treated with melatonin, vitamin E, or aprotinin, leptin expression was similar to the control group and edema and histopathological changes were reduced.

More recently, we have studied the effect of melatonin on EIU, another established experimental model for uveitis, giving a single intravitreal injection of LPS in the golden hamster [144]. LPS, a component of Gram-negative bacterial outer membranes, enhances the expression of various inflammatory mediators including tumor necrosis factor (TNF) α, interleukin (IL) 6 [19], PGE_2 [20], and NO [22,23]. In this study, a pellet of melatonin was implanted subcutaneously 2 hours before the intravitreal injection of LPS. As described in other species [135,145], the intravitreal injection of LPS in the golden hamster induces several signs of uveitis such as disruption of the BOB, dilatation of conjunctival vessels, iridial hyperemia, and flare in the anterior chamber, as shown in Figure 10.3. In addition to these anterior segment (anterior chamber, iris, and ciliary body) alterations, the examination of the posterior segment showed retinal vasculitis, hemorrhagic exudates, focal destruction of photoreceptor cells, and retinal infiltration (Figure 10.4). Clinical and histopathological abnormalities were evident at 24 hours postinjection, and the hamsters mostly recovered by 8 days. The presence of melatonin significantly reduces clinical symptoms induced by LPS, as shown in Figure 10.4. This effect is unspecific for particular signs, since a reduction of all of them was evident in the presence of melatonin. Moreover, melatonin reduces cell infiltration in the iris, ciliary body, and limbus, as well as in the retina and vitreous (Figure 10.4) and it decreases

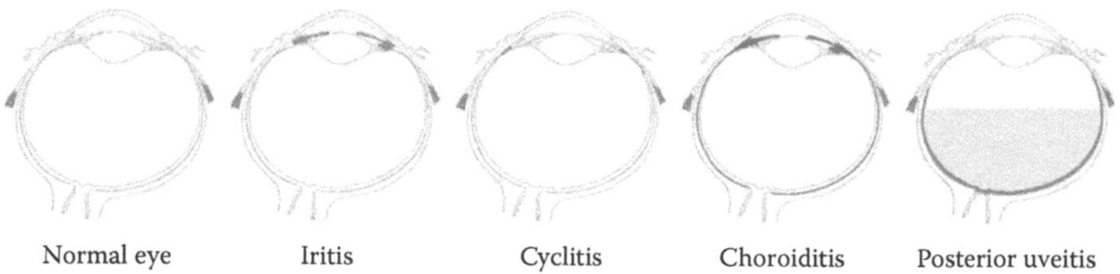

FIGURE 10.3 Schematic representations of different forms of clinical and experimental uveitis.

the leakage of proteins and cells in the anterior segment of LPS-injected eyes and protects the ultrastructure of BOBs. In animals injected with LPS, a remarkable disorganization of rod outer segment membranous disks was observed, whereas no morphological changes in photoreceptor outer segments were observed in animals treated with LPS plus melatonin (Figure 10.4). To assess retinal function in experimental uveitis, scotopic flash ERGs were registered in eyes from animals injected with vehicle or LPS, since the hamster has a predominantly rod–retina. A significant reduction of a- and b-wave amplitude, but not their latencies, was observed after 8 days of intravitreal injection of LPS. The fact that ERG alterations are evident at a period in which most of the clinical and histological changes are not evident (8 days), suggests that LPS provokes retinal sequels that are also prevented by melatonin.

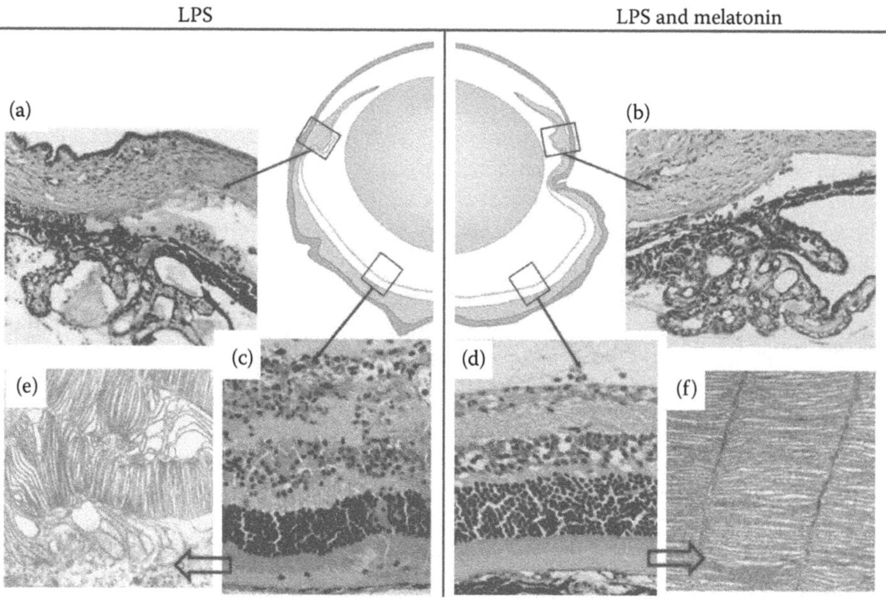

FIGURE 10.4 Micrographs of hematoxylin and eosin–stained sections of anterior chamber angle and retina, 24 hours after vehicle or LPS injection in the absence or presence of melatonin. (a) An intense inflammatory cell infiltration was observed in anterior chamber structures after LPS injection, (b) whereas the treatment with melatonin decreased cell infiltration. As for retinal morphology, note (c) the altered thickness of retinal layers, focal hemorrhages, and cellular infiltration induced by LPS injection and (d) the apparently normal morphology in retinas from eyes injected with LPS in the presence of melatonin. Ultrastructural analysis of photoreceptors from retinas obtained 8 days after LPS injection in the (e) absence and (f) presence of melatonin. LPS injection provoked a high disorganization of photoreceptor outer segments, whereas an ultrastructural preservation of photoreceptor outer segments was observed in the presence of melatonin.

As for the mechanism/s involved in the protection induced by melatonin, it is well established that LPS induces iNOS expression as well as a cascade of cytokine synthesis in different systems (for a review, see ref. [146]). Melatonin decreases the effect of LPS on two key signals involved in inflammatory processes, such as retinal NOS activity and TNF-α levels. NFκB is one of the most important transcription factors in transcriptional regulation of inflammatory proteins [147,148]. Activated NFκB translocates to the nucleus, where it binds to kB binding sites in the promoter regions of target genes, and induces the transcription of proinflammatory mediators, e.g., iNOS, TNF-α, COX-2, and IL-1b, IL-6, and IL-8 [149]. The fact that melatonin prevents the LPS-induced increase in nuclear levels of p50 and p65 could account for the decrease in NOS activity and TNF-α levels. These results point at NFκB as a key target for the anti-inflammatory effect of melatonin in EIU. In agreement, it was shown that melatonin inhibits iNOS expression by inhibiting the activation of NFκB in immunostimulated murine macrophages [150] and rat skeletal muscle [151]. Furthermore, it was shown that melatonin reduces colonic inflammatory injury [152] by down-regulating proinflammatory molecules such as TNF-α mediated by NFκB inhibition [152].

Besides the already mentioned effects, several other mechanisms could be involved in the anti-inflammatory effect of melatonin, such as inhibition of activity and expression of COX [153] and PG release [154], inhibition of the rolling and adherence of leukocytes to endothelial layers, limiting cell migration [155], reduction of proinflammatory [156] and increase in anti-inflamatory cytokines (such as IL-1, IL-6, and IL-12], [157], decrease in vascular endothelial growth factor [158] and chemokines levels [159], and reduction of Fas ligand-mediated apoptosis, among many others, but up to now most of them were not confirmed at ocular level. Further investigations of the mechanisms by which melatonin affects its ocular target tissues may unveil new concepts of ocular therapeutic.

10.7 CONCLUDING REMARKS

Uveitis, a disease with potentially blinding sequels (synequiae, cataracts, macular and optic nerve edema, with loss of vision and loss of the eye), remains a challenging field to ophthalmologists as the disease causes significant morbidity, and the use of traditional forms of treatment is restricted by limited effectiveness and considerable side effects. Thus, it represents a significant public health concern. Several lines of evidence support the involvement of oxidative damage and increased NO production as ethiopathogenic mechanisms of uveitis, while melatonin by itself exhibits both antioxidant and antinitridergic properties, among many other anti-inflammatory effects. As mentioned before, ocular inflammation is mainly treated with topical and/or systemic application of corticosteroids. During long-term treatment with corticosteroids, however, care must be taken to guard against both ocular and systemic complications such as cataract, glaucoma, diabetes, hypertension, and osteoporosis. Therefore, the establishment of additive anti-inflammatory approaches is desirable to decrease the rate and degree of these complications. The present results suggest that melatonin, which lacks adverse collateral effects even at high doses, could be a promissory resource in the management of uveitis. Alone or combined with corticosteroid therapy, the anti-inflammatory effects of melatonin may benefit patients with chronic uveitis and decrease the rate and degree of corticosteroid-induced complications. Although in the mentioned study only the preventive effect of melatonin in experimental uveitis was demonstrated, this "relative weakness" does not preclude its clinical relevance. Indeed, uveitis is a common consequence of ocular surgery (cataract surgery and vitrectomy, among others). Thus, even as preventive strategy, the present results suggest that melatonin, a very safe compound for human use, should be included in the ophthalmic therapeutic resources. Moreover, we have recently shown that melatonin is an effective anti-inflammatory even when administered 12 or 24 hours after the intravitreal injection of LPS. In summary, melatonin appears as a potentially useful anti-inflammatory drug, particularly in ophthalmology, and as an alternative or eventually as a complement to glucocorticoids, since it resulted to be highly effective and it does not present the side effects of these steroids.

REFERENCES

1. Hardeland, R., and Poeggeler, B. (2003). Non-vertebrate melatonin. *Journal of Pineal Research* 34 (4): 233–241.
2. Pandi-Perumal, S.R., Srinivasan, V., Maestroni, G.J., Cardinali, D.P., Poeggeler, B., and Hardeland, R. (2006). Melatonin: Nature's most versatile biological signal? *FEBS Journal* 273(13): 2813–2838.
3. Paredes, S.D., Korkmaz, A., Manchester, L.C., Tan, D.X., and Reiter, R.J. (2009). Phytomelatonin: A review. *Journal of Experimental Botany* 60(1): 57–69.
4. Cardinali, D.P., and Rosner, J.M. (1971). Metabolism of serotonin by the rat retina *in vitro*. *Journal of Neurochemistry* 18(9): 1769–1770.
5. Cardinali, D.P., and Rosner, J.M. (1971). Retinal localization of the hydroxyindole-*O*-methyl transferase (HIOMT) in the rat. *Endocrinology* 89(1): 301–303.
6. Tosini, G., and Menaker, M. (1998). The clock in the mouse retina: Melatonin synthesis and photoreceptor degeneration. *Brain Research* 789(2): 221–228.
7. Martin, X.D., Malina, H.Z., Brennan, M.C., Hendrickson, P.H., and Lichter, P.R. (1992). The ciliary body—The third organ found to synthesize indoleamines in humans. *European Journal of Ophthalmology* 2(2): 67–72.
8. Mhatre, M.C., Van Jaarsveld, A.S., and Reiter, R.J. (1988). Melatonin in the lacrimal gland: First demonstration and experimental manipulation. *Biochemical and Biophysical Research Communications* 153(3): 1186–1192.
9. Poeggeler, B., Reiter, R.J., Tan, D.X., Chen, L.D., and Manchester, L.C. (1993). Melatonin, hydroxyl radical-mediated oxidative damage, and aging: A hypothesis. *Journal of Pineal Research* 14(4): 151–168.
10. Hardeland, R., Tan, D.X., and Reiter, R.J. (2009). Kynuramines, metabolites of melatonin and other indoles: The resurrection of an almost forgotten class of biogenic amines. *Journal of Pineal Research* 47(2): 109–126.
11. Peyrot, F., and Ducrocq, C. (2008). Potential role of tryptophan derivatives in stress responses characterized by the generation of reactive oxygen and nitrogen species. *Journal of Pineal Research* 45(3): 235–246.
12. Reiter, R.J., Paredes, S.D., Manchester, L.C., and Tan, D.X. (2009). Reducing oxidative/nitrosative stress: A newly-discovered genre for melatonin. *Critical Reviews in Biochemistry and Molecular Biology* 44(4): 175–200.
13. Siu, A.W., Maldonado, M., Sanchez-Hidalgo, M., Tan, D.X., and Reiter, R.J. (2006). Protective effects of melatonin in experimental free radical–related ocular diseases. *Journal of Pineal Research* 40(2): 101–109.
14. Lundmark, P.O., Pandi-Perumal, S.R., Srinivasan, V., and Cardinali, D.P. (2006). Role of melatonin in the eye and ocular dysfunctions. *Visual Neuroscience* 23(6): 853–862.
15. Lundmark, P.O., Pandi-Perumal, S.R., Srinivasan, V., Cardinali, D.P., and Rosenstein, R.E. (2007). Melatonin in the eye: Implications for glaucoma. *Experimental Eye Research* 84(6): 1021–1030.
16. Alarma-Estrany, P., and Pintor, J. (2007). Melatonin receptors in the eye: Location, second messengers and role in ocular physiology. *Pharmacology & Therapeutics* 113(3): 507–522.
17. Siu, A.W., Reiter, R.J., and To, C.H. (1999). Pineal indoleamines and vitamin E reduce nitric oxide–induced lipid peroxidation in rat retinal homogenates. *Journal of Pineal Research* 27(2): 122–128.
18. Marchiafava, P.L., and Longoni, B. (1999). Melatonin as an antioxidant in retinal photoreceptors. *Journal of Pineal Research* 26(3): 184–189.
19. de Vos, A.F, Klaren, V.N., and Kijlstra, A. (1994). Expression of multiple cytokines and IL-1RA in the uvea and retina during endotoxin-induced uveitis in the rat. *Investigative Ophthalmology & Visual Science* 35(11): 3873–3883.
20. Bellot, J.L., Palmero, M., García-Cabanes, C., Espí, R., Hariton, C., and Orts, A. (1996). Additive effect of nitric oxide and prostaglandin-E2 synthesis inhibitors in endotoxin-induced uveitis in the rabbit. *Inflammation Research* 45(4): 203–208.
21. Sasaki, M., Ozawa, Y., Kurihara, T., Noda, K., Imamura, Y., Kobayashi, S., et al. (2009). Neuroprotective effect of an antioxidant, lutein, during retinal inflammation. *Investigative Ophthalmology & Visual Science* 50(3): 1433–1439.
22. Jacquemin, E., De Kozak, Y., Thillaye, B., Courtois, Y., and Goureau, O. (1996). Expression of inducible nitric oxide synthase in the eye from endotoxin-induced uveitis rats. *Investigative Ophthalmology & Visual Science* 37(6): 1187–1196.
23. Hashida, M., Fukushima, A., Zhang, J., Kodama, H., and Ueno, H. (2000). Involvement of superoxide generated by polymorphonuclear leukocytes in endotoxin-induced uveitis. *Graefe's Archive for Clinical and Experimental Ophthalmology* 238(4): 359–365.

24. McCluskey, P.J., Towler, H.M., and Lightman, S. (2000). Management of chronic uveitis. *British Medical Journal (Clinical Research Edition)* 320(7234): 555–558.
25. Gaudio, P.A. (2004). A review of evidence guiding the use of corticosteroids in the treatment of intraocular inflammation. *Ocular Immunology and Inflammation* 12(3): 169–192.
26. McGhee, C.N., Dean, S., and Danesh-Meyer, H. (2002). Locally administered ocular corticosteroids: Benefits and risks. *Drug Safety* 25(1): 33–55.
27. El Afrit, M.A., Mazlout, H., Trojet, S., Larguech, L., Megaieth, K., Belhaj, S., et al. (2007). Cortisone glaucoma: Epidemiological, clinical, and therapeutic study. *Journal Français d'Ophtalmologie* 30(1): 49–52.
28. Reiter, R.J., Cabrera, J., Sainz, R.M., Mayo, J.C., Manchester, L.C., and Tan, D.X. (1999). Melatonin as a pharmacological agent against neuronal loss in experimental models of Huntington's disease, Alzheimer's disease and parkinsonism. *Annals of the New York Academy of Sciences* 890: 471–485.
29. Srinivasan, V., Pandi-Perumal, S.R., Maestroni, G.J., Esquifito, A.I., Hardeland, R., and Cardinali, D.P. (2005). Role of melatonin in neurodegenerative diseases. *Neurotoxicity Research* 7(4): 293–318.
30. Srinivasan, V., Pandi-Perumal, S.R., Cardinali, D.P., Poeggeler, B., and Hardeland, R. (2006). Melatonin in Alzheimer's disease and other neurodegenerative disorders. *Behavioral and Brain Functions* 2: 15.
31. Axelrod, J. (1974). The pineal gland: A neurochemical transducer. *Science* 184(144): 1341–1348.
32. Bernard, M., Guerlotte, J., Greve, P., Gréchez-Cassiau, A., Iuvone, M.P., and Zatz, M. (1999). Melatonin synthesis pathway: Circadian regulation of the genes encoding the key enzymes in the chicken pineal gland and retina. *Reproduction Nutrition Development* 39(3): 325–334.
33. Liu, C., Fukuhara, C., Wessel, J.H., 3rd, Iuvone, P.M., and Tosini, G. (2004). Localization of Aa-Nat mRNA in the rat retina by fluorescence in situ hybridization and laser capture microdissection. *Cell and Tissue Research* 315(2): 197–201.
34. Dinet, V., Girard-Naud, N., Voisin, P., and Bernard, M. (2006). Melatoninergic differentiation of retinal photoreceptors: Activation of the chicken hydroxyindole-*O*-methyltransferase promoter requires a homeodomain-binding element that interacts with Otx2. *Experimental Eye Research* 83(2): 276–290.
35. Niki, T., Hamada, T., Ohtomi, M., Sakamoto, K., Suzuki, S., Kako, K., et al. (1998). The localization of the site of arylalkylamine *N*-acetyltransferase circadian expression in the photoreceptor cells of mammalian retina. *Biochemical and Biophysical Research Communications* 248(1): 115–120.
36. Iuvone, P.M., Brown, A.D., Haque, R., Weller, J., Zawilska, J.B., Chaurasia, S.S., et al. (2002). Retinal melatonin production: Role of proteasomal proteolysis in circadian and photic control of arylalkylamine *N*-acetyltransferase. *Investigative Ophthalmology & Visual Science* 43(2): 564–572.
37. Coon, S.L., Mazuruk, K., Bernard, M., Roseboom, P.H., Klein, D.C., and Rodriguez, I.R. (1996). The human serotonin *N*-acetyltransferase (EC 2.3.1.87) gene (AANAT): Structure, chromosomal localization, and tissue expression. *Genomics* 34(1): 76–84.
38. Coon, S.L., Del, OE, Young, W.S. 3rd, and Klein, D.C. (2002). Melatonin synthesis enzymes in Macaca mulatta: Focus on arylalkylamine *N*-acetyltransferase (EC 2.3.1.87). *Journal of Clinical Endocrinology & Metabolism* 87(10): 4699–4706.
39. Faillace, M.P., Sarmiento, M.I., Siri, L.N., and Rosenstein, R.E. (1994). Diurnal variations in cyclic AMP and melatonin content of golden hamster retina. *Journal of Neurochemistry* 62(5): 1995–2000.
40. Cahill, G.M., and Besharse, J.C. (1993). Circadian clock functions localized in *Xenopus* retinal photoreceptors. *Neuron* 10(4): 573–577.
41. Tosini, G., and Menaker, M. (1996). Circadian rhythms in cultured mammalian retina. *Science* 272(5260): 419–421.
42. Haque, R., Chaurasia, S.S., Wessel, J.H. 3rd., and Iuvone, P.M. (2002). Dual regulation of cryptochrome 1 mRNA expression in chicken retina by light and circadian oscillators. *Neuroreport* 13(17): 2247–2251.
43. Bailey, M.J., Chong, N.W., Xiong, J., and Cassone, V.M. (2002). Chickens' Cry2: Molecular analysis of an avian cryptochrome in retinal and pineal photoreceptors. *FEBS Letters* 513(2–3): 169–174.
44. Namihira, M., Honma, S., Abe, H., Masubuchi, S., Ikeda, M., and Honmaca, K. (2001). Circadian pattern, light responsiveness and localization of rPer1 and rPer2 gene expression in the rat retina. *Neuroreport* 12(3): 471–475.
45. Tosini, G. Melatonin circadian rhythm in the retina of mammals. (2000). *Chronobiology International* 17(5): 599–612.
46. Garbarino-Pico, E., Carpentieri, A.R., Contin, M.A., Sarmiento, M.I., Brocco, M.A., Panzetta, P., et al. (2004). Retinal ganglion cells are autonomous circadian oscillators synthesizing *N*-acetylserotonin during the day. *Journal of Biological Chemistry* 279(49): 51172–51181.
47. Fukuhara, C., Dirden, J.C., and Tosini, G. (2001). Photic regulation of melatonin in rat retina and the role of proteasomal proteolysis. *Neuroreport* 12(17): 3833–3837.

48. Faillace, M.P., Cutrera, R., Sarmiento, M.I., and Rosenstein, R.E. (1995). Evidence for local synthesis of melatonin in golden hamster retina. *Neuroreport* 6(15): 2093–2095.
49. Ivanova, T.N., and Iuvone, P.M. (2003). Melatonin synthesis in retina: Circadian regulation of arylalkylamine *N*-acetyltransferase activity in cultured photoreceptor cells of embryonic chicken retina. *Brain Research* 973(1): 56–63.
50. Gan, J., Alonso-Gomez, A.L., Avendano, G., Johnson, B., and Iuvone, P.M. (1995). Melatonin biosynthesis in photoreceptor-enriched chick retinal cell cultures: Role of cyclic AMP in the K(+)-evoked, Ca(2+)-dependent induction of serotonin *N*-acetyltransferase activity. *Neurochemistry International* 27(2): 147–155.
51. Alonso-Gomez, A.L., and Iuvone, P.M. (1995). Melatonin biosynthesis in cultured chick retinal photoreceptor cells: Calcium and cyclic AMP protect serotonin *N*-acetyltransferase from inactivation in cycloheximide-treated cells. *Journal of Neurochemistry* 65(3): 1054–1060.
52. Grève, P., Alonso-Gómez, A., Bernard, M., Ma, M., Haque, R., Klein, D.C., et al. (1999). Serotonin *N*-acetyltransferase mRNA levels in photoreceptor-enriched chicken retinal cell cultures: Elevation by cyclic AMP. *Journal of Neurochemistry* 73(5): 1894–1900.
53. Tosini, G., Chaurasia, S.S., and Michael, I.P. (2006). Regulation of arylalkylamine *N*-acetyltransferase (AANAT) in the retina. *Chronobiology International* 23(1–2): 381–391.
54. Fukuhara, C., Liu, C., Ivanova, T.N., Chan, G.C., Storm, D.R., Iuvone, P.M., et al. (2004). Gating of the cAMP signaling cascade and melatonin synthesis by the circadian clock in mammalian retina. *Journal of Neuroscience* 24(8): 1803–1811.
55. Pozdeyev, N., Taylor, C., Haque, R., Chaurasia, S.S., Visser, A., Thazyeen, A., et al. (2006). Photic regulation of arylalkylamine *N*-acetyltransferase binding to 14–3–3 proteins in retinal photoreceptor cells. *Journal of Neuroscience* 26(36): 9153–9161.
56. Tosini, G., Pozdeyev, N., Sakamoto, K., and Iuvone, P.M. (2008). The circadian clock system in the mammalian retina. *Bioessays* 30(7): 624–633.
57. Abe, M., Itoh, M.T., Miyata, M., Ishikawa, S., and Sumi, Y. (1999). Detection of melatonin, its precursors and related enzyme activities in rabbit lens. *Experimental Eye Research* 68(2): 255–262.
58. Itoh, M.T., Takahashi, N., Abe, M., and Shimizu, K. (2007). Expression and cellular localization of melatonin-synthesizing enzymes in the rat lens. *Journal of Pineal Research* 42(1): 92–96.
59. Ascher, J.A., Cole, J.O., Colin, J.N., Feighner, J.P., Ferris, R.M., Fibiger, H.C., et al. (1995). Bupropion: A review of its mechanism of antidepressant activity. *Journal of Clinical Psychiatry* 56(9): 395–401.
60. Fujieda, H., Hamadanizadeh, S.A., Wankiewicz, E., Pang, S.F., and Brown, G.M. (1999). Expression of mt1 melatonin receptor in rat retina: Evidence for multiple cell targets for melatonin. Neuroscience 93(2): 793–799.
61. Scher, J., Wankiewicz, E., Brown, G.M., and Fujieda, H. (2002). MT(1) melatonin receptor in the human retina: Expression and localization. *Investigative Ophthalmology & Visual Science* 43(3): 889–897.
62. Savaskan, E., Wirz-Justice, A., Olivieri, G., Pache, M., Kräuchi, K., Brydon, L., et al. (2002). Distribution of melatonin MT1 receptor immunoreactivity in human retina. *Journal of Histochemistry and Cytochemistry* 50(4): 519–526.
63. Scher, J., Wankiewicz, E., Brown, G.M., and Fujieda, H. (2003). AII amacrine cells express the MT1 melatonin receptor in human and macaque retina. *Experimental Eye Research* 77(3): 375–382.
64. Wiechmann, A.F., Udin, S.B., and Summers Rada, J.A. (2004). Localization of Mel1b melatonin receptor-like immunoreactivity in ocular tissues of *Xenopus laevis*. *Experimental Eye Research* 79(4): 585–594.
65. Rada, J.A., and Wiechmann, A.F. (2006). Melatonin receptors in chick ocular tissues: Implications for a role of melatonin in ocular growth regulation. *Investigative Ophthalmology & Visual Science* 47(1): 25–33.
66. Wiechmann, A.F., and Rada, J.A. (2003). Melatonin receptor expression in the cornea and sclera. *Experimental Eye Research* 77(2): 219–225.
67. Osborne, N.N., Nash, M.S., and Wood, J.P. (1998). Melatonin counteracts ischemia-induced apoptosis in human retinal pigment epithelial cells. *Investigative Ophthalmology & Visual Science* 39(12): 2374–2383.
68. Wiechmann, A.F., and Wirsig-Wiechmann, C.R. (2001). Multiple cell targets for melatonin action in *Xenopus laevis* retina: Distribution of melatonin receptor immunoreactivity. *Visual Neuroscience* 18(5): 695–702.
69. Liu, F., Yuan, H., Sugamori, K.S., Hamadanizadeh, A., Lee, F.J., Pang, S.F., et al. (1995). Molecular and functional characterization of a partial cDNA encoding a novel chicken brain melatonin receptor. *FEBS Letters* 374(2): 273–278.
70. Wiechmann, A.F., and Summers, J.A. (2008). Circadian rhythms in the eye: The physiological significance of melatonin receptors in ocular tissues. *Progress in Retinal and Eye Research* 27(2): 137–160.

71. Fujieda, H., Scher, J., Hamadanizadeh, S.A., Wankiewicz, E., Pang, S.F., and Brown, G.M. (2000). Dopaminergic and GABAergic amacrine cells are direct targets of melatonin: Immunocytochemical study of mt1 melatonin receptor in guinea pig retina. *Visual Neuroscience* 17(1): 63–70.
72. Savaskan, E., Jockers, R., Ayoub, M., Angeloni, D., Fraschini, F., Flammer, J., et al. (2007). The MT2 melatonin receptor subtype is present in human retina and decreases in Alzheimer's disease. *Current Alzheimer Research* 4(1): 47–51.
73. Meyer, P., Pache, M., Loeffler, K.U., Brydon, L., Jockers R., Flammer J., et al. (2002). Melatonin MT-1-receptor immunoreactivity in the human eye. *British Journal of Ophthalmology* 86(9): 1053–1057.
74. Pierce, M.E., and Besharse, J.C. (1985). Circadian regulation of retinomotor movements. I. Interaction of melatonin and dopamine in the control of cone length. *Journal of General Physiology* 86(5): 671–689.
75. Dubocovich, M.L. (1983). Melatonin is a potent modulator of dopamine release in the retina. *Nature (London)* 306(5945): 782–784.
76. Doyle, S.E., Grace, M.S., Mcivor, W., and Menaker, M. (2002). Circadian rhythms of dopamine in mouse retina: The role of melatonin. *Visual Neuroscience* 19(5): 593–601.
77. Rufiange, M., Dumont, M., and Lachapelle, P. (2002). Correlating retinal function with melatonin secretion in subjects with an early or late circadian phase. *Investigative Ophthalmology & Visual Science* 43(7): 2491–2499.
78. Sáenz, D.A., Goldin, A.P., Minces, L., Chianelli, M., Sarmiento, M.I., and Rosenstein, R.E. (2004). Effect of melatonin on the retinal glutamate/glutamine cycle in the golden hamster retina. *FASEB Journal* 18(15): 1912–1913.
79. Ianas, O., Olinescu, R., and Badescu, I. (1991). Melatonin involvement in oxidative processes. *Endocrinologie* 29(3–4): 147–153.
80. Reiter, R.J., Tan, D.X., Poeggeler, B., Menendez-Pelaez, A., Chen, L.D., and Saarela, S. (1994). Melatonin as a free radical scavenger: Implications for aging and age-related diseases. *Annals of the New York Academy of Sciences* 719: 1–12.
81. Hardeland, R., Balzer, I., Poeggeler, B., Fuhrberg, B., Uría, H., Behrmann, G., et al. (1995). On the primary functions of melatonin in evolution: Mediation of photoperiodic signals in a unicell, photooxidation, and scavenging of free radicals. *Journal of Pineal Research* 18(2): 104–111.
82. Reiter, R.J., Guerrero, J.M., Escames, G., Pappolla, M.A., and Acuña-Castroviejo, D. (1997). Prophylactic actions of melatonin in oxidative neurotoxicity. *Annals of the New York Academy of Sciences* 825: 70–78.
83. Reiter, R.J., Garcia, J.J., and Pie J. (1998). Oxidative toxicity in models of neurodegeneration: Responses to melatonin. *Restorative Neurology and Neuroscience* 12(2–3): 135–142.
84. Reiter, R.J., Tan, D.X., Osuna, C., and Gitto, E. (2000). Actions of melatonin in the reduction of oxidative stress. A review. *Journal of Biomedical Science* 7(6): 444–458.
85. Tan, D.X., Manchester, L.C., Terron, M.P., Flores, L.J., and Reiter, R.J. (2007). One molecule, many derivatives: A never-ending interaction of melatonin with reactive oxygen and nitrogen species? *Journal of Pineal Research* 42(1): 28–42.
86. Adler, L.J., Gyulai, F.E., Diehl, D.J., Mintun, M.A., Winter, P.M., and Firestone, L.L. (1997). Regional brain activity changes associated with fentanyl analgesia elucidated by positron emission tomography. *Anesthesia & Analgesia* 84(1): 120–126.
87. Guenther, A.L., Schmidt, S.I., Laatsch, H., Fotso, S., Ness, H., Ressmeyer, A.R., et al. (2005). Reactions of the melatonin metabolite AMK (*N*1-acetyl-5-methoxykynuramine) with reactive nitrogen species: Formation of novel compounds, 3-acetamidomethyl-6-methoxycinnolinone and 3-nitro-AMK. *Journal of Pineal Research* 39(3): 251–260.
88. Hardeland, R. (2005). Antioxidative protection by melatonin: Multiplicity of mechanisms from radical detoxification to radical avoidance. *Endocrine* 27(2): 119–130.
89. Reiter, R.J., Tan, D.X., Mayo, J.C., Sainz, R.M., Leon, J., and Czarnocki, Z. (2003). Melatonin as an antioxidant: Biochemical mechanisms and pathophysiological implications in humans. *Acta Biochimica Polonica* 50(4): 1129–1146.
90. Acuña-Castroviejo, D., Escames, G., León, J., Carazo, A., and Khaldy, H. (2003). Mitochondrial regulation by melatonin and its metabolites. *Advances in Experimental Medicine and Biology* 527: 549–557.
91. León, J., Acuña-Castroviejo, D., Escames, G., Tan, D.X., and Reiter, R.J. (2005). Melatonin mitigates mitochondrial malfunction. *Journal of Pineal Research* 38(1): 1–9.
92. Leon, J., Acuña-Castroviejo, D., Sainz, R.M., Mayo, J.C., Tan, D.X., and Reiter, R.J. (2004). Melatonin and mitochondrial function. *Life Sciences* 75(7): 765–790.
93. Nosjean, O., Ferro, M., Coge, F., Beauverger, P., Henlin, J.M., Lefoulon, F., et al. (2000). Identification of the melatonin-binding site MT3 as the quinone reductase 2. *Journal of Biological Chemistry* 275(40): 31311–31317.

94. Boutin, J.A., Marcheteau, E., Hennig, P., Moulharat, N., Berger, S., Delagrange, P., et al. (2008). MT3/QR2 melatonin binding site does not use melatonin as a substrate or a co-substrate. *Journal of Pineal Research* 45(4): 524–531.
95. Calamini, B., Santarsiero, B.D., Boutin, J.A., and Mesecar, A.D. (2008). Kinetic, thermodynamic and X-ray structural insights into the interaction of melatonin and analogues with quinone reductase 2. *Biochemical Journal* 413(1): 81–91.
96. Tan, D.X., Manchester, L.C., Terron, M.P., Flores, L.J., Tamura, H., and Reiter, R.J. (2007). Melatonin as a naturally occurring co-substrate of quinone reductase-2, the putative MT3 melatonin membrane receptor: Hypothesis and significance. *Journal of Pineal Research* 43(4): 317–320.
97. Long, D.J. 2nd, Iskander, K., Gaikwad, A., Arin, M., Roop, D.R., Knox, R., et al. (2002). Disruption of dihydronicotinamide riboside: quinone oxidoreductase 2 (NQO2) leads to myeloid hyperplasia of bone marrow and decreased sensitivity to menadione toxicity. *Journal of Biological Chemistry* 277(48): 46131–46139.
98. Celli, C.M., Tran. N., Knox, R., Jaiswal, A.K. (2006). NRH: quinone oxidoreductase 2 (NQO2) catalyzes metabolic activation of quinones and anti-tumor drugs. *Biochemical Pharmacology* 72(3): 366–376.
99. Molinari, E.J., North, P.C., and Dubocovich, M.L. (1996). 2-[125I]iodo-5-methoxycarbonylamino-*N*-acetyltryptamine: A selective radioligand for the characterization of melatonin ML2 binding sites. *European Journal of Pharmacology* 301(1–3): 159–168.
100. Mailliet, F., Ferry, G., Vella, F., Berger, S., Cogé, F., Chomarat, P., et al. (2005). Characterization of the melatoninergic MT3 binding site on the NRH: quinone oxidoreductase 2 enzyme. *Biochemical Pharmacology* 71(1–2): 74–88.
101. Guajardo, M.H., Terrasa, A.M., and Catala, A. (2003). Protective effect of indoleamines on *in vitro* ascorbate-Fe2+ dependent lipid peroxidation of rod outer segment membranes of bovine retina. *Journal of Pineal Research* 35(4): 276–282.
102. Liang, F.Q., Green, L., Wang, C., Alssadi, R., and Godley, B.F. (2004). Melatonin protects human retinal pigment epithelial (RPE) cells against oxidative stress. *Experimental Eye Research* 78(6): 1069–1075.
103. Celebi, S., Dilsiz, N., Yilmaz, T., and Kukner, A.S. (2002). Effects of melatonin, vitamin E and octreotide on lipid peroxidation during ischemia–reperfusion in the guinea pig retina. *European Journal of Ophthalmology* 12(2): 77–83.
104. Lee, M.C., Chung, Y.T., Lee, J.H., Jung, J.J., Kim, H.S., and Kim, S.U. (2001). Antioxidant effect of melatonin in human retinal neuron cultures. *Experimental Neurology* 172(2): 407–415.
105. Belforte, N.A., Moreno, M.C., de Zavalía, N., Sande, P.H., Chianelli, M.S., Keller Sarmiento, M.I., et al. (2010). Melatonin: A novel neuroprotectant for the treatment of glaucoma. *Journal of Pineal Research* 48(4): 353–364.
106. Kurenny, D.E., Moroz, L.L., Turner, R.W., Sharkey, K.A., and Barnes, S. (1994). Modulation of ion channels in rod photoreceptors by nitric oxide. *Neuron* 13(2): 315–324.
107. DeVries, S.H., and Schwartz, E.A. (1992). Hemi-gap junction channels in solitary cells of the catfish retina. *Journal of Physiology* 445: 201–230.
108. Ahmad, I., Leinders-Zufall, T., Kocsis, J.D., Shepherd, G.M., Zufall, F., and Barnstable, C.J. (1994). Retinal ganglion cells express a cGMP-gated cation conductance activatable by nitric oxide donors. *Neuron* 12(1): 155–165.
109. Nawy, S., and Jahr C.E. (1990). Suppression by glutamate of cGMP-activated conductance in retinal bipolar cells. *Nature* 346(6281): 269–271.
110. Tsuyama, Y., Noll, G.N., and Schmidt, K.F. (1993). L-Arginine and nicotinamide adenine dinucleotide phosphate alter dark voltage and accelerate light response recovery in isolated retinal rods of the frog (*Rana temporaria*). *Neuroscience Letters* 149(1): 95–98.
111. Miyachi, E., Murakami, M., and Nakaki, T. (1990). Arginine blocks gap junctions between retinal horizontal cells. *Neuroreport* 1(2): 107–110.
112. Turjanski, A.G., Chaia, Z., Doctorovich, F., Estrin, D.A., Rosenstein, R.E., and Piro, O. (2000). *N*-Nitrosomelatonin. *Acta Crystallographica Section C* 56(Pt 6): 682–683.
113. Turjanski, A.G.,Leonik, F., Estrin, D.A., Rosenstein, R.E., Doctorovich F.A. (2000). Scavenging of NO by melatonin. *Journal of the American Chemical Society* 122(42): 10468–10469.
114. Saenz, D.A,, Turjanski, A.G., Sacca, G.B., Marti, M., Doctorovich, F., Sarmiento M.I., et al. (2002). Physiological concentrations of melatonin inhibit the nitridergic pathway in the Syrian hamster retina. *Journal of Pineal Research* 33(1): 31–36.
115. Bettahi, I., Pozo, D., Osuna, C., Reiter, R.J., Acuña-Castroviejo, D., and Guerrero, J.M. (1996). Melatonin reduces nitric oxide synthase activity in rat hypothalamus. *Journal of Pineal Research* 20(4): 205–210.

116. Pozo, D., Reiter, R.J., Calvo, J.R., and Guerrero, J.M. (1997). Inhibition of cerebellar nitric oxide synthase and cyclic GMP production by melatonin via complex formation with calmodulin. *Journal of Cellular Biochemistry* 65(3): 430–442.
117. León, J., Vives, F., Crespo, E., Camacho, E., Espinosa, A., Gallo, M.A., et al. (1998). Modification of nitric oxide synthase activity and neuronal response in rat striatum by melatonin and kynurenine derivatives. *Journal of Neuroendocrinology* 10(4): 297–302.
118. Siu, A.W., Ortiz, G.G., Benitez-King, G., To, C.H., and Reiter, R.J. (2004). Effects of melatonin on the nitric oxide treated retina. *British Journal of Ophthalmology* 88(8): 1078–1081.
119. Siu, A.W., Reiter, R.J., and To, C.H. (1999). Pineal indoleamines and vitamin E reduce nitric oxide–induced lipid peroxidation in rat retinal homogenates. *Journal of Pineal Research* 27(2): 122–128.
120. Gilad, E., Cuzzocrea, S., Zingarelli, B., Salzman, A.L., and Szabó, C. (1997). Melatonin is a scavenger of peroxynitrite. *Life Sciences* 60(10): 169–174.
121. Cuzzocrea, S., Costantino, G., Gitto, E., Mazzon, E., Fulia, F., Serraino, I., et al. (2000). Protective effects of melatonin in ischemic brain injury. *Journal of Pineal Research* 29(4): 217–227.
122. Char, D.H., and Schlaegel, T.F. Jr. (1982). General factors in uveitis, Chap 39. In: Duane, T.D. (ed.), *Clinical Ophthalmology*, Vol. 4. Philadelphia: Harper & Row, pp. 1–7.
123. Hogan, M.J., Kimura, S.J., and Thygeson, P. (1959). Signs and symptoms of uveitis—I. Anterior uveitis. American Journal of Ophthalmology 47(5, Part 2): 155–176.
124. Lowder, C.Y., and Char, D.H. (1984). Uveitis. A review. *Western Journal of Medicine.* 140(3): 421–432.
125. Srivastava, A., Rajappa, M., and Kaur, J. (2010). Uveitis: Mechanisms and recent advances in therapy. *Clinica Chimica Acta.* 411(17–18): 1165–1171.
126. Planck, S.R., Huang, X.N., Robertson, J.E., and Rosenbaum, J.T. (1994.) Cytokine mRNA levels in rat ocular tissues after systemic endotoxin treatment. *Investigative Ophthalmology & Visual Science* 35(3): 924–930.
127. Rao, N. (1990). Role of oxygen free radicals in retinal damage associated with experimental uveitis. *Transaction of the American Ophthalmological Society* 88: 797–850.
128. Satici, A., Guzey, M., Gurler, B., Vural H, and Gurkan, T. (2003). Malondialdehyde and antioxidant enzyme levels in the aqueous humor of rabbits in endotoxin-induced uveitis. *European Journal of Ophthalmology* 13(9–10): 779–783.
129. Goto, H., Wu, G.S., Gritz, D.C., Atalla, L.R., and Rao N.A. (1991). Chemotactic activity of the peroxidized retinal membrane lipids in experimental autoimmune uveitis. *Current Eye Research* 10(11): 1009–1014.
130. Wu, G.S., Sevanian, A., and Rao, N.A (1992). Detection of retinal lipid hydroperoxides in experimental uveitis. *Free Radical Biology and Medicine* 12(1): 19–27.
131. Saraswathy, S., and Rao, N.A. (2008). Photoreceptor mitochondrial oxidative stress in experimental autoimmune uveitis. *Ophthalmic Research* 40(3–4): 160–164.
132. Bosch-Morell, F., Romá, J., Marín, N., Romero, B., Rodriguez-Galietero, A., Johnsen-Soriano, S., et al. (2002). Role of oxygen and nitrogen species in experimental uveitis: Anti-inflammatory activity of the synthetic antioxidant ebselen. *Free Radical Biology and Medicine* 33(5): 669–675.
133. Masferrer, J.L., and Kulkarni, P.S. (1997). Cyclooxygenase-2 inhibitors: A new approach to the therapy of ocular inflammation. *Survey of Ophthalmology* 41(Suppl. 2): S35–40.
134. Bhattacherjee, P. (1980). Prostaglandins and inflammatory reactions in the eye. *Methods & Findings in Experimental & Clinical Pharmacology* 2(1): 17–31.
135. Howes, E.L. Jr, and McKay, D.G. (1976). The effects of aspirin and indomethacin on the ocular response to circulating bacterial endotoxin in the rabbit. *Investigative Ophthalmology & Visual Science* 15(8): 648–651.
136. Parks, D.J., Cheung, M.K., Chan, C.C., and Roberge, F.G. (1994). The role of nitric oxide in uveitis. *Archives of Ophthalmology* 112(4): 544–546.
137. Mandai, M., Mittag, T.W., Kogishi, J., Iwaki, M., Hangai, M., and Yoshimura, N. (1994). The role of nitric oxide synthase in endotoxin-induced uveitis: Effect of N^{G}-nitro L-arginine. *Investigative Ophthalmology & Visual Science* 35(10): 3673–3681.
138. Goureau, O., Bellot, J., Thillaye, B., Courtois, Y., and de Kozak, Y. (1995). Increased nitric oxide production in endotoxin-induced uveitis: Reduction of uveitis by an inhibitor of nitric oxide synthase. *Journal of Immunology* 154(12): 6518–6523.
139. Becquet. F., Courtois, Y., and Goureau, O. (1997). Nitric oxide in the eye: Multifaceted roles and diverse outcomes. *Survey of Ophthalmology* 42(1): 71–82.

140. Sonoki, T., Nagasaki, A., Gotoh, T., Takiguchi, M., Takeya, M., Matsuzaki, H., et al. (1997). Coinduction of nitric-oxide synthase and arginase I in cultured rat peritoneal macrophages and rat tissues *in vivo* by lipopolysaccharide. *Journal of Biological Chemistry* 272(6): 3689–3693.
141. Biswas, J., Rao, N.A. (1989). Management of intraocular inflammation. In: Ryan, S.J. (ed.). *Retina*, Vol. 2. St. Louis, MO: CV Mosby, pp. 139–146.
142. Nussenblatt, R.B., Whitcup S.M., and Palestine, A.G. (1996). *Uveitis: Fundamentals and Clinical Practice*, 2nd ed. St. Louis, MO: Mosby Year Book.
143. Kükner, A., Colakoğlu, N., Serin, D., Alagöz, G., Celebi, S., and Kükner, A.S. (2006). Effects of intraperitoneal vitamin E, melatonin and aprotinin on leptin expression in the guinea pig eye during experimental uveitis. *Acta Ophthalmologica Scandinavica* 84(1): 54–61.
144. Sande, P.H., Fernandez, D.C., Aldana Marcos, H.J., Chianelli, M.S., Aisemberg. J., Silberman, D.M., et al. (2008). Therapeutic effect of melatonin in experimental uveitis. *American Journal of Pathology* 173(6): 1702–1713.
145. Koga, T., Koshiyama, Y., Gotoh, T., Yonemura, N., Hirata, A., Tanihara, H., et al. (2002). Coinduction of nitric oxide synthase and arginine metabolic enzymes in endotoxin-induced uveitis rats. *Experimental Eye Research* 75(6): 659–667.
146. Murphy, K., Haudek, S.B., Thompson, M., and Giroir, B.P. (1998). Molecular biology of septic shock. *New Horizons (Baltimore, Md.)* 6(2): 181–193.
147. Xie, Q.W., Kashiwabara, Y., and Nathan, C. (1994). Role of transcription factor NF-κB/Rel in induction of nitric oxide synthase. *Journal of Biological Chemistry* 269(45): 4705–4708.
148. Ghosh, S., May, M.J., and Kopp, E.B. (1998). NF-kappa B and Rel proteins: Evolutionarily conserved mediators of immune responses. *Annual Review of Immunology* 16: 225–260.
149. Griscavage, J.M., Wilk, S., and Ignarro, L.J. (1996). Inhibitors of the proteasome pathway interfere with induction of nitric oxide synthase in macrophages by blocking activation of transcription factor NF-κB. *Proceedings of the National Academy of Sciences USA* 93(8): 3308–3312.
150. Gilad, E., Wong, H.R., Zingarelli, B., Virág, L., O'Connor, M., Salzman, A.L., et al. (1998). Melatonin inhibits expression of the inducible isoform of nitric oxide synthase in murine macrophages: Role of inhibition of NFkappaB activation. *FASEB Journal* 12(9): 685–693.
151. Alonso, M., Collado, P.S., and González-Gallego, J. (2006). Melatonin inhibits the expression of the inducible isoform of nitric oxide synthase and nuclear factor kappa B activation in rat skeletal muscle. *Journal of Pineal Research* 41(1): 8–14.
152. Li, J.H., Yu, J.P., Yu, H.G., Xu, X.M., Yu, L.L., Liu, J., et al. (2005). Melatonin reduces inflammatory injury through inhibiting NF-kappaB activation in rats with colitis. *Mediators of Inflammation* 2005(4): 185–193.
153. Martínez-Campa, C., González, A., Mediavilla, M.D., Alonso-González, C., Alvarez-García, V., Sánchez-Barceló, E.J., et al. (2009). Melatonin inhibits aromatase promoter expression by regulating cyclooxygenases expression and activity in breast cancer cells. *British Journal of Cancer* 101(9): 1613–1619.
154. Pawlikowski, M., Juszczak, M., Karasek, E., Muszynska, B., and Karasek, M. (1984). Melatonin inhibits prostaglandin E release from the medial basal hypothalamus of pinealectomized rats. *Journal of Pineal Research* 1(4): 317–321.
155. Markus, R.P., Ferreira, Z.S., Fernandes, P.A., and Cecon, E. (2007). The immune–pineal axis: A shuttle between endocrine and paracrine melatonin sources. *Neuroimmunomodulation* 14(3–4): 126–133.
156. Escames, G., Acuña-Castroviejo, D., López, L.C., Tan, D.X., Maldonado, M.D., Sánchez-Hidalgo, M., et al. (2006). Pharmacological utility of melatonin in the treatment of septic shock: Experimental and clinical evidence. *Journal of Pharmacy and Pharmacology* 58(9): 1153–1165.
157. Maestroni, G.J. (2001).The immunotherapeutic potential of melatonin. *Expert Opinion on Investigational Drugs* 10(3): 467–476.
158. Kaur, C., Sivakumar, V., Yong, Z., Lu, J., Foulds, W.S., and Ling, E.A. (2007). Blood–retinal barrier disruption and ultrastructural changes in the hypoxic retina in adult rats: The beneficial effect of melatonin administration. *Journal of Pathology* 212(4): 429–439.
159. Park, H.J., Kim, H.J., Ra, J., Hong, S.J., Baik, H.H., Park, H.K., et al. (2007). Melatonin inhibits lipopolysaccharide-induced chemokine subfamily gene expression in human peripheral blood mononuclear cells in a microarray analysis. *Journal of Pineal Research* 43(2): 121–129.

11 Role of Melatonin in Regulating Gut Motility

Jennie Wong and Khek-Yu Ho

CONTENTS

11.1 INTRODUCTION

Melatonin is primarily synthesized and released from the pineal gland and is known for its multiple neurohormonal functions, exerting its action centrally within the nervous system, as well as peripherally, in many tissues.[1–3] Melatonin exhibits both receptor-dependent and receptor-independent effects. In the gastrointestinal tract, melatonin is released from the serotonin-rich enteroendocrine cells and is reported to exert endocrine, autocrine, paracrine, as well as luminal functions.[4–6] Concentration of melatonin in the gastrointestinal tract, which is derived from both the pineal gland and local de novo synthesis, is reported to be as much as 100 times that found in blood and 400 times that found in the pineal gland.[5–7] While melatonin's central role on the maintenance of the circadian rhythm and sleep–wake cycle is well known, its roles in the modulation of gastrointestinal functions are less well characterized, and the associated regulatory pathways remain largely unclear. Gastrointestinal motility follows a circadian rhythm with reduced nocturnal activity, but circadian rhythms are frequently found disrupted in patients with gastrointestinal motility disorders such as irritable bowel syndrome (IBS), and subjects with upset day/night cycle such as those working on night shifts and subjects traveling over time zones. These subjects often experience exacerbations of abdominal symptoms as well as episodes of diarrhea or constipation.[8–15]

11.2 CLINICAL STUDIES

In the early 2000s, we conducted a double-blind cross-over study to determine the effect of melatonin on IBS patients and healthy subjects. In the study, we showed that, compared with controls ($n = 17$), colonic transit time (mean ± SD) in constipation-predominant IBS patients ($n = 7$) was prolonged (65.2 ± 33.3 vs. 25.2 ± 7.7 hours in controls; $p < 0.01$). In healthy control patients, treatment with 3 mg/day melatonin at bedtime for 8 weeks significantly increased the colonic transit time from 27.4 ± 10.5 to 37.4 ± 23.8 hours ($p = 0.04$). However, melatonin treatment did not significantly change the colonic transit time of IBS patients.[15] The findings pointed to the possibility of melatonin's inhibitory role on normal human gut transit. In another similar study we conducted on 17 female IBS patients, we demonstrated that an 8-week course of oral melatonin at a dose of 3 mg/day was effective in improving bowel symptoms in these patients.[16] Using validated questionnaires—the GI symptom, the sleep questionnaires, and the Hospital Anxiety and Depression Scale—to assess symptom severity and to compute the IBS, sleep, and anxiety/depression scores, respectively, we showed that improvements in mean IBS scores were significantly greater after treatment with melatonin (3.9 ± 2.6) than with placebo (1.3 ± 4.0) ($p = 0.037$). Percent response rate, defined as percentage of subjects achieving mild-to-excellent improvement in IBS symptoms, was also higher in the melatonin-treated arm (88% vs. 47% in placebo controls, $p = 0.04$). However, changes in mean sleep, anxiety, and depression scores were similar in melatonin and placebo treatment, suggesting that melatonin's therapeutic effect in IBS is independent of these factors. These findings have since been confirmed in a study by Saha et al.[17] in which they randomly assigned 18 IBS patients to receive either melatonin 3 mg ($n = 9$) or matching placebo ($n = 9$) at bedtime for 8 weeks. The study showed that melatonin significantly improved IBS score in IBS patients (45% vs. 16.66% in placebo controls, $p < 0.05$). Overall extracolonic IBS score was also significantly lower in melatonin-treated patients (49.16% to 13.88%, $p < 0.05$), as compared with that of patients treated with placebo.

Melatonin's mechanism of action in the gastrointestinal tract is not entirely known. Studies in rats have shown that melatonin is physiologically involved in the preprandial and postprandial changes of gastrointestinal motility and that it exerts both excitatory and inhibitory effects on the smooth musculature of the gut.[18–19] Melatonin is also believed to act as an antagonist of serotonin and has been shown to reduce the tone but not amplitude or frequency of gastrointestinal contraction.[20–21] A recent study using a rodent model demonstrated that melatonin administration could reverse lipopolysaccharide-induced gastrointestinal motility disturbances via its inhibition of oxidative stress.[22] In human studies, Wisniewska-Jarosinska et al.[23] had shown that, compared with healthy individuals, women with both diarrhea and constipation form of IBS had significantly higher urinary excretion of 6-hydroxymelatonin sulfate, while Radwan et al.[4] showed that compared with healthy controls, patients with IBS had significantly lower 6-sulfatoxymelatonin/creatinine ratio in their urine. These findings suggested that disturbances in melatonin metabolism and secretion might be involved in the pathogenesis of IBS and potentially other motility-related gastrointestinal disorders. Two studies conducted in animal models suggest that this may be attributed to the blockade of nicotinic channels by melatonin and/or the interaction between melatonin and Ca^{2+}-activated K^+ channels.[24–25] Yet, another study showed that pharmacological doses of melatonin delay gastric emptying via mechanisms that involve CCK2 and 5-HT3 receptors.[26]

The precise mechanism through which melatonin regulates gastrointestinal motility is still uncertain. One common setback in the evaluation of the cause–effect relationship between melatonin and gastrointestinal motility related diseases is the subjectivity of common determinants such as self-reported sleep disturbances and associated psychological distress scores used to assess the severity of the gastrointestinal disorders and patient's psychological factors that could have a bearing on the disease manifestations. Due to the nonobjective nature of the assessment parameters/methods commonly used, meaningful interpretation of study results is difficult and might result in inconclusive inferences or deductions that are conflicting. To overcome that in our subsequent investigation, our research team attempted approaching the issue in a more objective manner—by manipulation of pertinent IBS-determining parameters with melatonin, a modulator of sleep and gastrointestinal sensitivity and motility, and then measuring the effects.[27] We conducted a randomized, double-blind, placebo-controlled trial in which we randomized 40 IBS patients with sleep disturbances to receive either melatonin 3 mg ($n = 20$) or matching placebo ($n = 20$) at bedtime for 2 weeks. Before and after the treatment, all patients were assessed with validated IBS symptoms evaluation score questionnaire, hospital anxiety and depression scale, PSQI, and the Epworth sleepiness scale for evaluation of their bowel symptoms, psychological status, sleep disturbance, and level of daytime sleepiness, respectively. In addition, rectal manometry and overnight polysomnography were conducted on all subjects before and after treatment. Polysomnography included electroencephalogram, electrooculogram, nasal airflow pressure transducer and oronasal thermistor, electromyogram, microphone for snoring detection, electrocardiogram, thoracic and abdominal pietzo belts for movement detection, and bilateral leg electromyogram. Rectal manometry evaluated rectal sensory thresholds, resting pressure, push pressure, and maximal voluntary squeeze pressure. In the 2-week study, we showed that in IBS patients with concomitant sleep disturbances, gastrointestinal visceral sensitivity, as determined by feelings of abdominal pain and rectal sensitivity, was significantly attenuated after 2 weeks of treatment with 3 mg melatonin. In comparison with placebo treatment, 3 mg/day melatonin taken for 2 weeks significantly decreased mean abdominal pain score (2.35 vs. 0.70 in placebo controls; $p < 0.001$) and increased mean rectal pain threshold (8.9 vs. −1.2 mm Hg in placebo controls; $p < 0.01$). The therapeutic effect of melatonin in the IBS patients was associated with heightened pressure and volume thresholds for both rectal urgency and pain sensations. Melatonin's effect on gastrointestinal visceral sensitivity occurred in the absence of any observable change to biophysiological sleep parameters as determined by polysomnography and the anxiety/depression profiles of patients, suggesting that melatonin's modulation of gastrointestinal visceral sensitivity could be independent of its better known action on sleep and psychological factors. These findings reaffirm our earlier observations that melatonin effect on IBS symptoms occurred independently of patient's sleep, anxiety, and depression scores.[15–16]

It is still not clear exactly how melatonin affects gastrointestinal visceral sensitivity in IBS patients. In IBS, alterations to autonomic function, gastrointestinal visceral sensitivity, and motility are all known to contribute to the symptoms. Based on evidence of impaired autonomic function found in IBS and the reduced sympathetic responses in these patients,[28–31] it is tempting to speculate that melatonin might exert its therapeutic effects through the brain–gut axis with a key modulatory action on autonomic functions. In this regard, exogenously administered melatonin might have a potential role in the treatment of certain IBS patients whose symptoms are principally due to altered gastrointestinal visceral sensitivity arising from autonomic dysfunction rather than other etiologic factors. Well-designed clinical trials with sufficient sample size would, however, be needed for proper evaluation of melatonin's efficacy and safety in the treatment of these patients.

11.3 SUMMARY

The role of melatonin in gastrointestinal physiology is as complex as it is intriguing. Aberrant sleep pattern is commonly reported by patients with gastrointestinal motility disorders, such as IBS. Sleep disturbances have been associated with perceived intensification of abdominal symptoms in IBS. Central to the physiology of sleep is the role of melatonin, which is also widely believed to modulate gastrointestinal symptoms. Although melatonin-mediated neurohumoral modulation of gastrointestinal motility is a plausible explanation to abdominal symptoms especially prominent in night shift workers, the actual pathophysiologic pathways involved in the regulation of these disorders remain to be clearly elucidated. Numerous recent studies have sought to demonstrate the cause–effect relationship, but the subjectivity of common determinants of sleep disturbances and the often associated psychological distress makes interpretation of study results difficult, resulting in inconclusive inferences or deductions that are often conflicting. Our study team had recently attempted approaching the issue in a more objective manner by manipulation of pertinent IBS-determining parameters with melatonin, a known modulator of sleep and gastrointestinal sensitivity and motility, and then measuring the effects. We were able to show in a randomized, double-blind, placebo-controlled trial that, in IBS patients with concomitant sleep disturbances, gastrointestinal visceral sensitivity, as determined by feelings of abdominal pain and rectal sensitivity, was significantly attenuated after 2 weeks of treatment with 3 mg melatonin. This occurred in the absence of observable change to biophysiological sleep parameters as determined by polysomnography and to the anxiety/depression profiles of patients, suggesting that melatonin's modulation of gastrointestinal visceral sensitivity could be independent of its better known action on sleep and psychological factors. The finding is intriguing and opens the way to investigating the potential use of exogenous melatonin in the treatment of IBS patients whose symptoms are principally due to increased gastrointestinal visceral sensitivity.

REFERENCES

1. Brown GM. Light, melatonin and the sleep–wake cycle. *J Psychiatry Neurosci*. 1994 Nov;19(5):345–353.
2. Pandi-Perumal SR, Srinivasan V, Maestroni GJ, Cardinali DP, Poeggeler B, Hardeland R. Melatonin: Nature's most versatile biological signal? *FEBS J*. 2006 Jul;273(13):2813–2838.

3. Konturek SJ, Konturek PC, Brzozowska I, et al. Localization and biological activities of melatonin in intact and diseased gastrointestinal tract (GIT). *J Physiol Pharmacol.* 2007 Sep;58(3):381–405.
4. Radwan P, Skrzydlo-Radomanska B, Radwan-Kwiatek K, Burak-Czapiuk B, Strzemecka J. Is melatonin involved in the irritable bowel syndrome? *J Physiol Pharmacol.* 2009 Oct;60 Suppl 3:67–70.
5. Bubenik GA. Gastrointestinal melatonin: Localization, function, and clinical relevance. *Dig Dis Sci.* 2002;47:2336–2348.
6. Bubenik GA, Hacker RR, Brown GM, Bartos L. Melatonin concentration in luminal fluid, mucosa and muscularis of the bovine and porcine gastrointestinal tract. *J Pineal Res.* 1999;26:56–63.
7. Huether G. The contribution of extrapineal sites of melatonin to circulating melatonin levels in higher vertebrates. *Experientia.* 1994;49:665–670.
8. Kumar D, Idzikowski C, Wingate DL, et al. Relationship between enteric migrating motor complex and the sleep cycle. *Am J Physiol.* 1990;259:G983–G990.
9. Hoogerwerf WA. Role of clock genes in gastrointestinal motility. *Am J Physiol Gastrointest Liver Physiol.* 2010 Sep;299(3):G549–G555.
10. Fass R, Fullerton S, Tung S, et al. Sleep disturbances in clinic patients with functional bowel disorders. *Am J Gastroenterol.* 2000;95:1195–1200.
11. Elsenbruch S, Thompson JJ, Hamish MJ, et al. Behavioral and physiological sleep characteristics in women with irritable bowel syndrome. *Am J Gastroenterol.* 2002;97:2306–2314.
12. Merle A, Delagrange P, Renard P, et al. Effect of melatonin on motility pattern of small intestine in rats and its inhibition by melatonin receptor antagonist S. 22153. *J Pineal Res.* 2000 Sep;29(2):116–124.
13. Rotem AY, Sperber AD, Krugliak P, et al. Polysomnographic and actigraphic evidence of sleep fragmentation in patients with irritable bowel syndrome. *Sleep.* 2003;26:747–752.
14. Jarrett M, Heitkemper M, Cain KC, et al. Sleep disturbance influences gastrointestinal symptoms in women with irritable bowel syndrome. *Dig Dis Sci.* 2000;45:952–959.
15. Lu WZ, Song GH, Gwee KA, Ho KY. The effects of melatonin on colonic transit time in normal controls and IBS patients. *Dig Dis Sci.* 2009 May;54(5):1087–1093.
16. Lu WZ, Gwee KA, Moochhalla S, Ho KY. Melatonin improves bowel symptoms in female patients with irritable bowel syndrome: A double-blind placebo-controlled study. *Aliment Pharmacol Ther.* 2005 Nov 15;22(10):927–934.
17. Saha L, Malhotra S, Rana S, Bhasin D, Pandhi P. A preliminary study of melatonin in irritable bowel syndrome. *J Clin Gastroenterol.* 2007 Jan;41(1):29–32.
18. Storr M, Koppitz P, Sibaev A, et al. Melatonin reduces non-adrenergic, non-cholinergic relaxant neurotransmission by inhibition of nitric oxide synthase activity in the gastrointestinal tract of rodents in vitro. *J Pineal Res.* 2002;33:101–108.
19. Harlow HJ, Weekley BL. Effect of melatonin on the force of spontaneous contractions of in vitro rat small and large intestine. *J Pineal Res.* 1986;3:277–284.
20. Bubenik GA, Dhanvantari S. Influence of serotonin and melatonin on some parameters of gastrointestinal activity. *J Pineal Res.* 1989;7:333–344.
21. Lee PP and Pang SF. Melatonin and its receptors in the gastrointestinal tract. *Biol Signals.* 1993;2: 181–193.
22. De Filippis D, Iuvone T, Esposito G, et al. Melatonin reverses lipopolysaccharide-induced gastrointestinal motility disturbances through the inhibition of oxidative stress. *J Pineal Res.* 2008;44: 45–51.
23. Wisniewska-Jarosinska M, Chojnacki J, Konturek S, Brzozowski T, Smigielski J, Chojnacki C. Evaluation of urinary 6-hydroxymelatonin sulphate excretion in women at different age with irritable bowel syndrome. *J Physiol Pharmacol.* 2010 Jun;61(3):295–300.
24. Barajas-Lopez C, Peres AL, Espinosa-Luna R, et al. Melatonin modulates cholinergic transmission by blocking nicotinic channels in the guinea-pig submucous plexus. *Eur J Pharmacol.* 1996;312:319–325.
25. Storr M, Schusdziarra V, Allescher HD. Inhibition of small conductance K+-channels attenuated melatonin-induced relaxation of serotonin-contracted rat gastric fundus. *Can J Physiol Pharmacol.* 2000;78:799–806.
26. Kasimay O, Cakir B, Devseren E, Yegen BC. Exogenous melatonin delays gastric emptying rate in rats: Role of CCK2 and 5-HT3 receptors. *J Physiol Pharmacol.* 2005 Dec;56(4):543–353.
27. Song GH, Leng PH, Gwee KA, Moochhala SM, Ho KY. Melatonin improves abdominal pain in irritable bowel syndrome patients who have sleep disturbances: A randomised, double blind, placebo controlled study. *Gut.* 2005 Oct;54(10):1402–1407.
28. Orr WC, Elsenbruch S, Harnish MJ. Autonomic regulation of cardiac function during sleep in patients with irritable bowel syndrome. *Am J Gastroenterol.* 2000;95:2865–2871.

29. Nishiyama K, Yasue H, Moriyama Y, et al. Acute effects of melatonin administration on cardiovascular autonomic regulation in healthy men. *Am Heart J.* 2001;141:E9.
30. Ray CA. Melatonin attenuates the sympathetic nerve responses to orthostatic stress in humans. *J Physiol.* 2003;551(Pt 3):1043–1048.
31. Manabe N, Tanaka T, Hata J, Kusunoki H, Haruma K. Pathophysiology underlying irritable bowel syndrome—From the viewpoint of dysfunction of autonomic nervous system activity. *J Smooth Muscle Res.* 2009 Feb;45(1):15–23.

12 Melatonin and Food Safety: Investigating a Possible Role in the Seasonality of the Bacterial Pathogen *Escherichia coli* O157:H7 in Cattle

Tom S. Edrington and David J. Nisbet

CONTENTS

12.1 INTRODUCTION

Seasonal shedding of *Escherichia coli* O157:H7 in cattle is typically higher in the summer months and very low to nonexistent during the winter months. Interestingly, while this phenomenon is well documented and generally consistent, viable explanations are lacking. Ambient temperature is most often presented as the explanation for the seasonality of this pathogen and at first appearance would appear reasonable and logical. However, upon further examination of cattle prevalence and human outbreak data and consideration of our own research experience with *E. coli* O157:H7, we felt there must be a better explanation. Herein we discuss our own hypothesis regarding the seasonality of *E. coli* O157:H7 in feedlot cattle.

12.2 UNDERSTANDING *E. Coli* O157:H7

E. coli O157:H7 was first identified as a human pathogen following an outbreak linked to hamburger in 1982 [1]. Since that time, this pathogen has become one of the most important foodborne pathogens in the United States having been responsible for numerous illnesses and deaths. In humans, *E. coli* O157:H7 causes a range of symptoms, primarily in children and older persons, including bloody diarrhea, vomiting, hemorrhagic colitis, and hemolytic uremic syndrome characterized by acute renal failure [2].

Recently, it was estimated that the health-related costs of foodborne illness in the United States is \$152 billion a year, of which \$993 million is attributed to *E. coli* O157:H7 [3]. Even though numerous routes of transmission have been identified (water, vegetables, contact at petting zoos, apple cider), a link to cattle or exposure to products that have been contaminated with cattle manure are most often implicated. Cattle are considered the primary reservoir for *E. coli* O157:H7 with ground beef linked to more human outbreaks than any other source [2,4]. Accordingly, the beef industry in the United States has been severely affected by this pathogen, incurring added costs of approximately $2.7 billion over 10 years (1990s) due to loss of demand, impact on beef prices, product recalls, and cost of implementing intervention strategies [5]. The good news is that intervention strategies utilized during the slaughter and processing are highly effective in reducing the prevalence of *E. coli* O157:H7 in beef products. However, as evidenced by multiple large-scale ground beef recalls in the past few years, these techniques are not 100% effective.

Anyone who has spent any appreciable amount of time researching *E. coli* O157:H7 in cattle likely found the above subheading humorous. Cattle are asymptomatic shedders of *E. coli* O157:H7 with no visible signs that can be used as indicators of colonization. Fecal prevalence is unpredictable as well. Some cattle may shed detectable quantities consistently, some sporadically, some only once in a while. Cattle may shed high concentrations in the feces ("supershedders") but as above, do so with no rhyme or reason. These variations in individual shedding are compounded when pen prevalence is examined in a feedlot. The one thing that is predictable about the prevalence of this pathogen in cattle is that it is typically unpredictable. In general, fecal shedding of this bacterium is low in the winter, increases throughout the spring to peak levels in late summer and early fall, and then decreases again throughout the late fall and early winter [6–8]. Human outbreaks, not surprisingly, occur predominantly in the summer months and mirror the seasonal shedding patterns in cattle [9,10] and the prevalence of *E. coli* O157:H7 in ground beef [11]. Please note that the seasonality mentioned above and in the remainder of the chapter is in relation to cattle and *E. coli* O157:H7 prevalence in North America. While this pathogen is of concern in countries throughout the world and seasonality has been reported [12], differences in cattle management and housing can confound interpretation of the results. Beyond seasonality, and not even season is absolutely consistent, finding anything that is reliably and repeatedly correlated to *E. coli* O157:H7 prevalence remains a daunting task.

Based on how well-documented and generally accepted seasonality is, it was surprising to find how little research has been conducted investigating this phenomenon. The simple explanation, and the most plausible initially, is ambient temperature. Elevated ambient temperatures in the summer months could provide for a more suitable environment for *E. coli* O157:H7 outside of the animal host (i.e., soil, water, feed, etc.) and thereby produce a more constant source of infection or reinfection for cattle. However, if this was the case, you would expect to see a higher prevalence in cattle in the southern latitudes of the United States and potentially more human cases as well. Published reports suggest just the opposite with Canada and the northern regions of the United States responsible for a greater number of human outbreaks than the southern states [2,13,14]. Additionally, in research conducted at our laboratory in College Station, TX, with beef and dairy cattle naturally colonized with *E. coli* O157:H7, we observed on multiple occasions a significant seasonal decrease in fecal prevalence during the fall compared with summer months, even though ambient temperatures were comparable to summer temperatures in the northern latitudes of the United States. What about other livestock species with relatively low to nonexistent prevalence of *E. coli* O157:H7 such as swine and poultry? Could the fact that most are raised indoors under strictly controlled lighting regimes that do not vary with season explain, at least in part, the relative low prevalence of *E. coli* O157:H7 in these species?

12.2.1 So What Does All of This Have to Do with Melatonin?

Based on these observations, we compared ambient temperatures in two distinct geographic locations within North America (Calgary, Alberta, Canada, and Amarillo, TX), both of which have a significant number of feedlot cattle [15]. The monthly average temperature in Amarillo exceeds the average monthly high temperature in Calgary every month of the year. Yet, as we mentioned above, there are more reported cases of human infections in the northern compared with southern latitudes and no consistent regional differences in cattle prevalence. So in our minds, the ambient temperature argument was fallible and we began the search for more plausible explanations. We asked the question, "What is relatively consistent year in and year out beyond ambient temperature?" The answer: day length. Going back to our comparison of Calgary and Amarillo and looking at average day length each month, we found that in Calgary, day length is longer in the summer months when *E. coli* O157:H7 is most prevalent. Could this, at least in part, explain the similar animal prevalence in the colder as opposed to warmer regions of North America?

We know that the effects of changing day length on animals are numerous. For instance, many mammals breed seasonally as decreasing day length in the fall of the year influences various hormones involved in reproduction [16]. Additionally, seasonal changes in immune system function are affected by photoperiod [17,18]. Essentially, decreasing day length stimulates a "dormant" immune system to prepare the animal for the stress and demands of winter, thereby creating a survival advantage. These changes, in part, are thought to be mediated by hormones produced by the pineal and thyroid glands [19]. Perhaps hormone production in response to changing day length stimulates the immune system and thereby the animal's own defense system exerts a control on *E. coli* O157:H7 populations within the gastrointestinal tract (GIT). Plausible, but cattle are typically asymptomatic carriers of *E. coli* O157:H7 and do not suffer any apparent ill effects from this bacterium. That being the case, it does not stand to reason that an "activated" immune system would seek out a "nonthreatening" bacteria species.

So hormones, known to be influenced by changing day length, affect physiological processes within animals, but do these same hormones have any effect on bacteria within the animal's gastrointestinal system? *In vitro* and *in vivo* research indicates that hormones do play a role in the regulation of bacterial populations. The catecholamines are reportedly involved in the quorum sensing system that *E. coli* O157:H7 utilizes to stimulate growth and regulate virulence gene expression [20,21]. Quorum sensing has been dubbed "the language that bacteria use to communicate with host cells" [20] and is a regulatory mechanism for basic physiological functions of *E. coli* O157:H7 such as growth and division, protein biosynthesis, metabolism, and pathogenesis.

12.3 LET THE RESEARCH BEGIN

Based on our own observations with *E. coli* O157:H7 shedding in cattle, coupled with the well-documented seasonality of this pathogen, the geographic distribution of outbreaks (human) and prevalence (cattle), and the evidence that hormones do influence bacteria, we developed a new hypothesis regarding the seasonality of this pathogen in cattle: seasonal shedding of *E. coli* O157:H7 in cattle is influenced, at least partially, by physiological changes within the host animal in response to changing day length.

Our first experiment was conducted in a commercial feedlot in which cattle were exposed to artificial lighting in the fall of the year when natural daylight was decreasing. Our thought was that maintaining a level of light exposure (duration) similar to summer time levels would support fecal shedding whereas the decreasing day length experienced by the control cattle would result in a lower fecal prevalence. This was largely what we observed: fecal prevalence of *E. coli* O157:H7 in the lighted pens remained constant while the nonlighted control pens decreased. Upon removal of the lighting from the treated pens, fecal prevalence returned to levels comparable to control cattle [15]. As cattle type, days on feed, cattle sex, and pen conditions including ambient temperature were all similar among treatments, these data support our hypothesis that day length may be the key contributing factor to the seasonality of *E. coli* O157:H7.

Numerous hormones are affected by day length (increasing or decreasing) that may result in the initiation or cessation of hormone production/release. Melatonin is one such hormone with diurnal as well as seasonal patterns of production/secretion. Pineal production of melatonin increases in the fall and peaks during the winter months when day length is the shortest, decreasing to low levels during the long days of summer [22,23]. Could this potentially explain the seasonality of *E. coli* O157:H7 prevalence in cattle? Do the elevated winter melatonin concentrations reach a threshold that exerts an inhibitory effect on *E. coli* O157:H7 in the gastrointestinal tract of cattle that subsequently diminishes as melatonin levels recede in the summer months?

A second experiment sought to answer these questions and determine if exogenous melatonin would influence fecal prevalence of *E. coli* O157:H7 in feedlot cattle [24]. Cattle in a commercial feedlot were identified as naturally colonized with *E. coli* O157:H7 and transported to our laboratory facilities where they were maintained on a high-concentrate ration. One half of the steers received an oral bolus of melatonin (0.5 mg/kg BW) for seven consecutive days. Following a 5-day period of no treatment, these same steers received a second melatonin dose [5.0 mg/kg BW) for four consecutive days followed by a 10-day period of no treatment. Control steers received an empty gelatin capsule and were handled identically to the melatonin-treated cattle. Fecal shedding of *E. coli* O157:H7 was monitored daily throughout the entire course of the experimental period. No statistically significant differences were observed in fecal prevalence when the low melatonin dose was administered or during the period of no treatment prior to administration of the high melatonin dose. However, during the 4-day period of administering the high melatonin dose, the percentage of fecal samples positive for *E. coli* O157:H7 was decreased ($p = 0.05$) in the melatonin treatment-compared with the control. This difference was not observed during the following 10-day period of no treatment. Serum concentrations of melatonin were determined throughout the course of the experiment as well but are somewhat confounding. As expected, serum concentrations were increased ($p < 0.05$) during the period of the low melatonin dose administration; however, concentrations, although substantially elevated compared with previous concentrations, were not different among treatments when cattle received the high melatonin dose. However, as melatonin concentrations in all cattle were significantly higher in the 10-day period of no treatment at the conclusion of the experiment when compared with levels at the initiation of the study, we feel that decreasing day length and naturally increasing melatonin concentrations may have masked the effect of the high dose of melatonin. Additionally, the large variation in serum melatonin concentrations observed for each animal from one collection to the next likely influenced the serum melatonin results. Even so, the results of the experiment, in particular, that a low dose of melatonin had no effect whereas a high dose did significantly influence fecal shedding of *E. coli* O157:H7, are intriguing. Possibly, the low dose of melatonin was digested in the rumen and, while enough to alter serum melatonin concentrations, did not reach the lower GIT where *E. coli* O157:H7 primarily resides, whereas the high dose of melatonin was enough to provide for some melatonin to escape rumen degradation/absorption, reach the lower GIT, and thereby influence fecal prevalence of *E. coli* O157:H7. Or is there a threshold of GIT melatonin concentration that once exceeded will produce a subsequent effect on *E. coli* O157:H7 prevalence? This would seem a more viable explanation especially when considering melatonin production by the GIT.

12.4 GASTROINTESTINAL MELATONIN

Originally, it was thought that the pineal gland was the sole source of melatonin; however, more recently, melatonin-producing cells have been discovered in the GIT, pancreas, suprarenal glands, thyroid gland, thymus, airway epithelium, placenta, Harderian glands, and others [25,26]. Of these, the highest concentrations are found in the GIT, where levels may exceed pineal gland production by 400-fold [27]. While the production of melatonin in the gut is significant, it is unclear what impact this has on circulating levels of melatonin. Some have speculated that the overall contribution is relatively low [26] while others reported melatonin produced by the lower porcine GIT contributed significantly to a short-term increase in circulating melatonin following refeeding [28]. Our data would support this latter research, as we observed an increase in serum concentrations of melatonin following both low and high doses, an effect that was quickly diminished when melatonin treatments were stopped [24].

Melatonin is synthesized in the enterochromaffin cells of the GIT [27,29] and is dependent on the precursor amino acid, tryptophan [30]. Research demonstrated that administration of melatonin or the melatonin precursor tryptophan resulted in accumulation of melatonin in the GIT [31–35] and subsequent increases in circulating melatonin [30,31,36]. When tryptophan was administered to pinealectomized chicks and rats, an increase in serum melatonin was observed that was suggested as being derived from an extrapineal organ [36]. Taken together, this supports our conclusion that the oral melatonin administered to cattle increased the gastrointestinal melatonin concentration and subsequently the serum concentrations as well. The lack of effect on serum concentrations when the high melatonin dose was administered was discussed above and is likely a factor of natural variation and sampling protocol and not a failure of the treatment itself to increase serum melatonin concentrations.

Our results coupled with previous research indicate that administration of melatonin or a melatonin precursor increases GIT melatonin. Therefore, we conducted a third experiment [24], very similar to the second, in which cattle were administered tryptophan orally instead of melatonin. If our treatment was successful in increasing GIT melatonin and subsequently decreasing fecal prevalence of *E. coli* O157:H7 as observed previously, we may be able to develop a cost-effective preharvest intervention strategy. Supplementation of melatonin at the levels tested would be cost-prohibitive in cattle production; however, supplementation with tryptophan offers some intriguing possibilities. Similar to the melatonin study, we dosed cattle naturally colonized with *E. coli* O157:H7 with a low and a high tryptophan dose and monitored fecal shedding daily.

No differences in the percentage of fecal samples positive for *E. coli* O157:H7 were observed during administration of the low or high tryptophan dose, although significant increases in serum tryptophan concentrations were observed in tryptophan-treated compared with control cattle [24]. Serum melatonin concentrations, however, were not different. In cattle, amino acids including tryptophan are rapidly degraded by rumen microbes. Therefore, we needed a dose large enough so that some tryptophan would escape ruminal digestion and reach the lower intestine but low enough to avoid overdosing the cattle and causing pulmonary edema [37]. The serum data suggested tryptophan was absorbed either from the rumen or small intestine into the serum but was not sufficient enough to increase GIT melatonin concentrations as might be indicated by a concomitant increase in serum melatonin concentrations [24]. The increase in serum melatonin reported by others following tryptophan administration [30,36,38] but not observed in our study may be due to species differences and/or tryptophan dose, as their dose was considerably higher than what we used in our cattle experiment. If we assume the differences in fecal shedding of *E. coli* O157:H7 observed in the melatonin experiment were a result of increased GIT melatonin as indicated by increased serum melatonin, then the lack of differences in serum melatonin in the tryptophan experiment would suggest that our dose was not sufficient to elevate GIT melatonin concentrations.

Results of these first three experiments support our hypothesis that decreasing day length and physiological responses to changing day length, in particular, the hormone melatonin, are responsible at least in part for the seasonal prevalence of *E. coli* O157:H7. Data from our melatonin and tryptophan experiments and from others' research suggest that GIT melatonin should be our primary focus. The question then arises, is GIT melatonin produced/secreted seasonally, similar to pineal melatonin, or are other factors involved?

Some researchers have reported diurnal differences in GIT melatonin concentrations [39–42] while others have reported no differences [34,43,44]. We have not found any research reporting circadian, or more importantly to our research efforts with *E. coli* O157:H7, annual rhythms of GIT melatonin secretion in ruminants. Research is currently underway in our laboratory to determine if GIT melatonin in feedlot cattle is secreted seasonally in response to changing day length and to determine if concentrations are correlated to *E. coli* O157:H7 prevalence.

Other factors may be involved in the initiation of GIT melatonin synthesis and release, such as response to food intake and composition, which has been demonstrated in several studies [26,45]. With this relationship between food intake and GIT melatonin, it has been suggested that the enterochromaffin cells are where nutritional information is received and translated into a chemical messenger, plasma melatonin level [27]. If this is in fact the case, it offers intriguing possibilities for impacting *E. coli* O157:H7 populations in cattle preharvest. Let us assume that high GIT melatonin concentrations decrease GIT *E. coli* O157:H7 as our melatonin experiment suggests and that there is a seasonal increase in GIT concentrations of melatonin that influence the seasonality of this pathogen. Let us also assume that GIT melatonin in ruminants is secreted as has been reported in other species, not diurnally, but in response to food intake. Taken together, this suggests that modifying food intake in cattle prior to slaughter in the summertime, when GIT melatonin concentrations are low, could possibly trigger a "flushing" effect with GIT melatonin increasing to wintertime levels and thereby reduce *E. coli* O157:H7 populations.

More recently, it has been reported [26,45] that GIT melatonin exerts a protective effect on GIT tissues in a number of ways including enhancing submucosal blood flow, stimulating production of gastroprotective hormones, protecting gastrointestinal mucosa from ulceration, stimulating the immune system, decreasing secretion of hydrochloric acid, and fostering epithelial regeneration. Quite possibly, the mechanism in which melatonin decreased fecal prevalence in our melatonin study is related to one or more of these protective functions exerted in the GIT. Melatonin treatment may have prevented or reduced binding of *E. coli* O157:H7 to the GIT mucosa, resulting in the decreased incidence of shedding we observed in melatonin-treated steers compared with control animals.

In addition to melatonin, we have also investigated the influence of other hormones and hormone-like compounds known to respond to changing day length (thyroid hormones, prolactin, vitamin D) on *E. coli* O157:H7 populations in cattle. Initial research examining the thyroid gland found that a hyperthyroid state following chemical inhibition of the thyroid tended to increase fecal shedding of *E. coli* O157:H7 in cattle [46]. Subsequent research in which cattle were administered triiodothyronine to achieve a hyperthyroid status decreased fecal prevalence of *E. coli* O157:H7 [47]. The influence of prolactin was recently investigated in our laboratory and found to have minimal, if any, impact on *E. coli* O157:H7 (Edrington, unpublished results). Vitamin D, the "sunshine vitamin" and a compound considered by many to be more hormone-like in its actions, was also investigated by our laboratory. Initial research found that a high dose of vitamin D tended to increase fecal shedding of *E. coli* O157:H7 (Edrington, unpublished results). Research is currently underway in our laboratory to determine if a correlation exists between the *E. coli* O157:H7 prevalence and serum concentrations of vitamin D in feedlot cattle in the winter and summer. While these results are not as interesting as the melatonin research, they do indicate that other hormones may play a role in the population dynamics of this pathogen and the seasonality observed in cattle is likely due to a cascade of events involving these hormones and possibly others yet to be identified.

12.5 SUMMARY

The seasonality of *E. coli* O157:H7 prevalence in feedlot cattle in the United States has been well documented but poorly understood. Herein, we present our hypothesis, that this phenomenon is related to hormonal changes within the animal in response to changing day length, as well as data that support our hypothesis. Our data suggest that melatonin, and in particular gastrointestinal melatonin, is likely involved in the seasonal population dynamics of *E. coli* O157:H7 in cattle and that further research in this area is warranted. Understanding the seasonality of this pathogen could potentially lead to preharvest intervention strategies to reduce *E. coli* O157:H7 in cattle and subsequently infections in humans when they are most prevalent.

REFERENCES

1. Riley, L.W., R.S. Remis, S.D. Helgerson, H.B. McGee, J.G. Wells, B.R. Davis, R.J. Hebert, E.S. Olcott, L.M. Johnson, N.T. Hargrett, P.A. Blake, and M.L. Cohen. 1983. Hemorrhagic colitis associated with a rare *E. coli* serotype. *N. Engl. J. Med.* 308:681–685.

2. Griffin, P.M., and R.V. Tauxe. 1991. The epidemiology of infections casued by *E. coli* O157:H7, other enterohemorrhagic *E. coli* and the associated hemolytic uremic syndrome. *Epidemiol. Rev.* 13:60–98.
3. Scharff, R.L. 2010. Health-related costs from foodborne illness in the United States. Georgetown University. Available at http://www.producesafetyproject.org/admin/assests/files/Health-Related-Foodborne-Illness-Costs-Report.pdf-1.pdf (accessed May 3, 2010).
4. Capriola, A., S. Morabito, H. Brugere, and E. Oswald. 2005. Enterohaemorrhagic *Escherichia coli*: Emerging issues on virulence and modes of transmission. *Vet. Res.* 36:289–311.
5. Kay, S. 2003. The cost of *E. coli* O157:H7. *Meat Poult.* 2:26–34.
6. VanDonkersgoed, J., T. Graham, and V. Gannon. 1999. The prevalence of verotoxins, *Escherichia coli* O157:H7 and *Salmonella* in the feces and rumen of cattle at processing. *Can. Vet. J.* 40:332–338.
7. Chapman, P.A., C.A. Siddons, A.T. Cerdan Malo, and M.A. Harkin. 1997. A 1-year study of *Escherichia coli* O157 in cattle, sheep, pigs and poultry. *Epidemiol. Infect.* 119:245–250.
8. Hancock, D.D., T.E. Besser, D.H. Rice, D.E. Herriott, and P.I. Tarr. 1997. A longitudinal study of *Escherichia coli* O157 in fourteen cattle herds. *Epidemiol. Infect.* 118:193–195.
9. Rangel, J.M., P.H. Sparling, C. Crowe, P.M. Griffin, and D.L. Swerdlow. 2005. Epidemiology of *Escherichia coli* O157:H7 outbreaks, United States, 1982–2002. *Emerg. Inf. Dis.* 11:603–609.
10. Besser, R.E., P.M. Griffin, and L. Slutsker. 1999. *Escherichia coli* O157:H7 gastroenteritis and the hemolytic uremic syndrome, an emerging infectious disease. *Annu. Rev. Med.* 50:355–367.
11. Chapman, P.A., A.T. Cerdan Malo, M. Ellin, R. Ashton, and M.A. Harkin. 2001. *Escherichia coli* O157 in cattle and sheep at slaughter, on beef and lamb carcasses and in raw beef and lamb products in South Yorkshire, UK. *Int. J. Food Microbiol.* 64:139–150.
12. Ogden, I.D., M. MacRae, and N.J.C. Strachan. 2004. Is the prevalence and shedding concentrations of *E. coli* O157:H7 in beef cattle in Scotland seasonal? *FEMS Microbiol. Lett.* 233:297–300.
13. Hancock, D., T. Besser, J. LeJeune, M. Davis, and D. Rice. 2001. The control of VTEC in the animal reservoir. *Int. J. Food Microbiol.* 66:71–78.
14. Meyer-Broseta, S., S.N. Bastian, P.D. Arne, O. Cerf, and M. Sanaa. 2001. Review of epidemiological surveys on the prevalence of contamination of healthy cattle with *Escherichia coli* serogroup O157:H7. *Int. J. Environ. Hyg.* 203:347–361.
15. Edrington, T.S., T.R. Callaway, S.E. Ives, M.J. Engler, M.L. Looper, R.C. Anderson, and D.J. Nisbet. 2006. Seasonal shedding of *Escherichia coli* O157:H7 in ruminants: A new hypothesis. *Foodborne Pathol. Dis.* 3:413–421.
16. Legan, S.J., and F.J. Karsch. 1979. Neuroendocrine regulation of the estrous cycle and seasonal breeding in the ewe. *Biol. Reprod.* 20:74–85.
17. Drazen, D.L, L.J. Kriegsfeld, J.E. Schneider, and R.J. Nelson. 2000. Leptin, but not immune function, is linked to reproductive responsiveness to photoperiod. *Am. J. Physiol.* 278:R1401–R1407.
18. Nelson, R.J., and J.M.C. Blom. 1994. Photoperiodic effects on tumor development and immune function. J. Biol. Rhythms 9:233–249.
19. Nelson, R.J., and D.L. Drazen. 1999. Melatonin mediates seasonal adjustments in immune function. *Reprod. Nutr. Dev.* 39:383–398.
20. Sperandio, V., A.G. Torres, B. Jarvis, J.P. Nataro, and J.B. Kaper. 2003. Bacteria–host communication: The language of hormones. *Proc. Natl. Acad. Sci. USA* 100:8951–8956.
21. Lyte, M., C.D. Frank, and B.T. Green. 1996. Production of an autoinducer of growth by norepinephrine cultured *Escherichia coli* O157:H7. *FEMS Microbiol. Lett.* 139:155–159.
22. Pevet, P. 2003. Melatonin: From seasonal to circadian signal. *J. Neuroendocrinol.* 15:422–426.
23. Alila-Johansson, A., L. Eriksson, T. Soveri, and M.L. Laakso. 2001. Seasonal variation in endogenous serum melatonin profiles in goats: A difference between spring and fall? *J. Biol. Rhythms* 16:254–263.
24. Edrington, T.S., T.R. Callaway, D.M. Hallford, L. Chen, R.C. Anderson, and D.J. Nisbet. 2008. Effects of exogenous melatonin and tryptophan on fecal shedding of *E. coli* O157:H7 in cattle. *Microb. Ecol.* 55:553–560.
25. Jawaorek, J., K. Nawrot, S.J. Konturek, A. Leja-Szpak, P. Thor, and W.W. Pawlik. 2004. Melatonin and its precursor, L-tryptophan: Influence on pancreatic amylase secretion *in vivo* and *in vitro*. *J. Pineal Res.* 36:155–164.
26. Kvetnoy, I.M., I.E. Ingel, T.V. Kvetnaia, N.K. Malinovskaya, S.I. Rapoport, N.T. Raikhlin, A.V. Trofimov, and V.V. Yuzhakov. 2002. Gastrointestinal melatonin: Cellular identification and biological role. *Neuroendocrinol. Lett.* 23:121–132.
27. Huether, G. 1993. The contribution of extrapineal sites of melatonin synthesis to circulating melatonin levels in higher vertebrates. *Experientia* 49:665–670.

28. Bubenik, G.A., S.F. Pang, R.R. Hacker, and P.S. Smith. 1996. Melatonin concentrations in serum and tissues of porcine gastrointestinal tract and their relationship to the intake and passage of food. *J. Pineal Res.* 21:251–256.
29. Quay, W.B., and Y.H. Ma. 1976. Demonstration of gastrointestinal hydroxyindole-*O*-methyl transferase. *IRCS Med. Sci.* 4:563.
30. Huether, G., B. Poeggeler, A. Reimer, and A. George. 1992a. Effect of tryptophan administration on circulating melatonin levels in chicks and rats: Evidence for stimulation of melatonin synthesis and release in the gastrointestinal tract. *Life Sci.* 51:945–953.
31. Huether, G., G. Hajak, A. Reimer, R. Poeggeler, M. Blomer, A. Rodenbeck, and E. Ruther. 1992b. The metabolic fate of infused L-tryptophan in men: Possible clinical implications of the accumulation of circulating tryptophan and tryptophan metabolites. *Psychopharmacology* 106:422–432.
32. Bubenik, G.A., H.L. Ayles, R.O. Ball, R.M. Friendship, and G.M. Brown. 1998. Relationship between melatonin levels in plasma and gastrointestinal tissues and the incidence and severity of gastric ulcers in pigs. *J. Pineal Res.* 24:62–66.
33. DeBoer, H. 1988. The influence of photoperiod and melatonin on hormone levels and operand light demand in the pig. PhD thesis. University of Guelph, Ontario, Canada, 1988.
34. Bubenik, G.A. 1980. Localization of melatonin in the digestive tract of the rat: Effect of maturation, diurnal variation, melatonin treatment, and pinealectomy. *Horm. Res.* 12:313–323.
35. Kopin, I.J., C.M.B. Pare, J. Axelrod, and H. Weissbach. 1961. The fate of melatonin in animals. *J. Biol. Chem.* 236:3072–3075.
36. Yaga, K., R.J. Reiter, and B.A. Richardson. 1993. Tryptophan loading increases daytime serum melatonin levels in intact and pinealectomized rats. *Life Sci.* 52:1231–1238.
37. Carlson, J.R., M.T. Yokoyama, and E.O. Dickinson. 1972. Induction of pulmonary edema and emphysema in cattle and goats with 3-methylindole. *Science* 176:298.
38. Hajak, G., A. Rodenbeck, H.D. Ehrenthal, S. Leonard, D. Wedekind, G. Sengos, D. Zhou, and G. Huether. 1997. No evidence for a physiological coupling between melatonin and glucocorticoids. *Psychopharmacology* 133:313–322.
39. Lee, P.P., S.Y. Shiu, P.H. Chow, and S.F. Pang. 1995. Regional and diurnal studies of melatonin and melatonin binding sites in the duck gastro-intestinal tract. *Biol. Signals* 4:212–224.
40. Bubenik, G.A., L.P. Niles, S.F. Pang, and P.J. Pentney. 1993. Diurnal variation and binding characteristics of melatonin in the mouse brain and gastrointestinal tissues. *Comp. Biochem. Physiol. C.* 104:221–224.
41. Lee, P.P., and S.F. Pang. 1993. Melatonin and its receptors in the gastrointestinal tract. *Biol. Signals* 2:181–193.
42. Vakkuri, O., H. Rintamaki, and J. Leppaluoto. 1985. Presence of immunoreactive melatonin in different tissues of the pigeon (*Columba livia*). *Gen. Comp. Endo.* 58:69–75.
43. Kennaway, D.J., R.G. Firth, G. Philipou, C.D. Mathews, and R.F. Seamark. 1977. A specific radioimmunoassay for melatonin in biological tissue and fluids and its validation by gas chromatography–mass spectrometry. *Endocrinology* 101:119–127.
44. Ozaki, Y., and H.J. Lynch. 1976. Presence of melatonin in plasma and urine of pinealectomized rats. *Endocrinology* 99:641–644.
45. Bubenik, G.A. 2002. Gastrointestinal melatonin. Localization, function, and clinical relevance. *Dig. Dis. Sci.* 47:2336–2348.
46. Schultz, C.L., T.S. Edrington, S.B. Schroeder, D.M. Hallford, K.J. Genovese, T.R. Callaway, R.C. Anderson, and D.J. Nisbet. 2005. Effect of the thyroid on faecal shedding of *E. coli* O157:H7 and *Escherichia coli* in naturally infected yearling cattle. *J. Appl. Microbiol.* 99:1176–1180.
47. Edrington, T.S., T.R. Callaway, D.M. Hallford, R.C. Anderson, and D.J. Nisbet. 2007. Influence of exogenous triiodothyronine (T_3) on fecal shedding of *Escherichia coli* O157 in cattle. *Microb. Ecol.* 53:664–669.

13 Melatonin in Dentistry

Luigi F. Rodella, Mauro Labanca, and Eleonora Foglio

CONTENTS

13.1 MELATONIN

Melatonin is an indolamine hormone (*N*-acetyl-5-methoxytryptamine) synthesized from the essential amino acid tryptophan in a series of four enzymatic steps.[1,2] It was originally discovered in 1958 by the American dermatologist Aaron Lerner and his coworkers at the Yale University School of Medicine as an amphibian skin-lighting factor present in extracts of bovine pineal glands. Lerner named the molecule "melatonin" because it induces contraction of stellate amphibian melanophores.[3] The fact that melatonin is an evolutionarily highly conserved molecule, ubiquitously distributed in living systems, seems to demonstrate that it has important physiological roles.[4]

13.1.1 Biosynthesis, Secretion, and Metabolism

In vertebrates, melatonin is primarily secreted by the pineal gland, a neuroendocrine transducer considered until the first half of the 20th century as an epithalamic appendage of brain with enigmatic functions;[5,6] therefore, there are also extrapineal sites of melatonin production, on which it exerts a local action. However, with the exception of the retina and the GI tract (in which melatonin is stored)[7], the physiological significance of these extrapineal sites is still a matter of debate. In the pineal gland, melatonin is synthesized by pinealocytes, whereas in the retina, it is produced by photoreceptor cells.[8–10] Melatonin produced by the pineal gland is immediately released into the blood vascular system and cerebrospinal fluid of the third ventricle where exerts various biological actions upon reaching melatonin receptor-rich target tissues; melatonin secreted by the retina instead is not released into the circulation and so exerts a paracrine function.[11] Once melatonin is released into the circulation (where 50%–75% of melatonin is bound reversibly to albumin and glycoproteins), it has a short half-life:[4] most of the circulating melatonin (95%) is primarily metabolized in the liver by cytochrome P450 enzymes; alternatively, it is metabolized by oxidative pyrrole-ring cleavage[12] in a number of extrahepatic tissues by both enzymatic and nonenzymatic mechanisms.[13]

13.1.2 Mechanism of Action

Although the mechanisms by which melatonin modulates the pathways in which it is involved are currently not completely understood, it has been demonstrated that it acts on its target cells/tissue through transmembrane G-protein–coupled receptors MT1, MT2, and MT3 or through orphan nuclear receptors of the retinoic acid receptor family.[14] However, in other particular biological contexts, no specific receptors appear to be required for melatonin's actions;[15,16] being a lipophilic molecule, it has the capacity to pass freely in and out of all cellular and fluid compartments of the body having free access to all cells of the body and thereby offers an additional receptor-independent nonhormonal role of free radical scavenger in reducing the oxidative stress.[13]

13.1.3 Main Biological Functions

Studies in various animals, especially in mammals, have shown that, at either physiological or pharmacological concentrations, melatonin appears to be involved in numerous physiological and pathophysiological processes including the control of sleep, circadian rhythms, retinal physiology, seasonal reproductive cycles, cancer development and growth (melatonin has oncostatic potentials), regulation of the immune response,[17,18] antioxidation, and free radical scavenging (up-regulating several antioxidative enzymes and down-regulating pro-oxidant enzymes),[19] mitochondrial respiration, cardiovascular function and blood pressure control,[20,21] bone metabolism, and gastrointestinal physiology.[13,22] Other actions of this hormone include the inhibition of dopamine (DA) release in the hypothalamus and in the retina,[23] and it is also involved in pubertal development[24,25] and the aging process.[26,27] On this purpose, it has been remembered that the amount of melatonin produced during the night appears to be greatest around the time just before puberty, with a steady decrease thereafter through middle and old age. For this reason, the decrease in melatonin production has implications for various diseases, including age-associated neurodegenerative diseases and cancer initiation.[28]

13.2 MELATONIN IN THE ORAL CAVITY

In the following pages, we will report the specific roles that melatonin exerts at the oral cavity level, both in physiological and in pathological conditions. In particular, the purpose of this review is to explain the potential utility of melatonin in the treatment of the most relevant pathologies affecting the oral cavity: tooth decay, periodontal diseases (PDs), and oral cavity cancer–associated inflammation.

13.2.1 Melatonin in the Oral Cavity of Healthy Subjects

Saliva may be described as a heterogeneous fluid composed of proteins, glycoproteins, electrolytes, and small organic molecules, as well as compounds transported from the blood.[29] It represents a combination of gingival crevicular fluid (similar to serum for its composition) and other fluids released from salivary glands, of which the parotid, submandibular, and sublingual are the three major sources.[30] The secretion of saliva has been shown to be affected by different forms of stimulation: time of day, diet, age, sex, a variety of disease states, and several pharmacological agents.[31]

Once in the blood, melatonin gets to the saliva by passive diffusion. The ratio between salivary and plasmatic melatonin in a (24-hour) cycle is relatively stable and varies from 0.24 to 0.33: it means that the salivary melatonin concentration is equivalent to 24%–33% of the plasma levels.[32,33] As reported above, the amount of melatonin in saliva is lower when compared with that of blood probably due to the fact that the major part of the plasma melatonin is bound to albumin (nearly 70%) and so it is not free to diffuse into saliva. Thus, salivary melatonin reflects in appreciable extent the portion of circulating melatonin not bound to proteins (the free-circulating melatonin).[34] It is possible that melatonin is also produced and released locally by the mucosal lining of the oral cavity, but this still requires direct experimental evidence. Salivary melatonin can be reliably assayed. By measuring salivary melatonin, oral pathologies can be studied in relation to plasma and salivary melatonin behavior. A significant positive correlation between salivary and plasma melatonin exists: according to Konturek et al.,[35] the concentration of salivary melatonin under basal conditions is negligible, but following local oral application of indoleamine, its plasma level dose-dependently increases, and this is consequently accompanied by an increase of salivary melatonin.

Melatonin has several specific functions in the oral cavity, so its effects on oral health warrant further investigations. It acts as a potent antioxidant and free radical scavenger, immunomodulatory agent, strong promoter of bone formation, and anti-inflammatory factor in PDs.[36] Recently, it has been claimed that the imbalances in levels of free radicals and reactive oxygen species (ROS) with antioxidants may play an important role in the onset and development of several inflammatory oral pathologies.[37] On this purpose, current evidences for oxidative damage in the most prevalent oral cavity diseases and the possible therapeutic effects of antioxidants like melatonin[38] have been extensively reviewed in the last years.

13.3 MELATONIN AND ORAL CAVITY DISEASES

13.3.1 Tooth Decay

Dental caries, also known as tooth decay, is the localized destruction of susceptible dental hard tissues by acidic by-products from bacterial fermentation of dietary carbohydrates.[39,40] Tooth decay can affect the enamel (the outer covering of the crown), cementum (the outermost layer of the root), and dentine (the tissue beneath both the enamel and the cementum). As partially reported above, dental caries results from interactions over time between the products of bacteria metabolism and many host factors that include teeth and saliva. So, even if dental caries is a multifactorial disease (related, for instance, to high numbers of cariogenic bacteria, insufficient fluoride exposure, gingival recession, immunological components, need for special health care, and genetic factors)[39,41] resulting from an ecological imbalance in the physiological equilibrium between tooth minerals and oral microbial biofilms,[42] it is greatly affected by salivary flow and composition and also by dietary habits.[43]

Given the presence of melatonin in the oral cavity because of its release in saliva[11] and given its beneficial properties, it has been hypothesized that this hormone could have a cariostatic potential. On this purpose, with the strong influence of diet on cariogenesis, Mechin and Toury[44] suggested that, melatonin, being abundantly available in the foodstuffs, may diminish the caries development with its antioxidant activity. In their study, Mechin and Toury[44] tested the effects of melatonin administration on caries development in rats receiving a standard or a modified cariogenic diet 2000M: a large increase in the caries score was induced by the cariogenic diet as compared with the control group. Moreover, in groups receiving melatonin, a highly significant decrease in the caries score was obtained. However, the explanation of these results can only be speculative. In fact, no antibacterial action was attributed to melatonin, and there are no evidences about the possible action of melatonin on calcium metabolism and on the mineralization/demineralization equilibrium. Nevertheless, the hypothesis of the possible action of melatonin on various salivary components that can modify the cariostatic potential of saliva is more intriguing and needs further investigation.

13.3.2 Periodontal Disease

PD is an oral inflammatory disorder of the periodontium that affects the supporting tissues of the teeth (alveolar bone, gums, and periodontal ligament), leading to progressive destruction of connective tissue attachment and alveolar bone. A consequence is the severe loss of supporting periodontal tissues and teeth, seen prevalently among adults and older people. Current information indicates that bacterial infection and accumulations on the teeth may be the primary causative agent of PD.[45,46] Nowadays, PD represents one of the most commonly reported chronic inflammatory adult conditions. Approximately 48% of U.S. adults have chronic PD, and similar or higher rates (up to 70%) have been reported in other populations.[47] PD incidence is increased by several risk factors; in general, all those conditions that provide the anaerobes ample time to survive in periodontal tissue or any medical conditions (e.g., HIV infections) that trigger host antibacterial defense mechanisms will likely promote PDs.[48]

The severity of periodontitis is characterized by the degree of marginal bone loss, depth of periodontal pockets, degree of attachment loss, and number of teeth with furcation development.[49] In diagnosing PD, the probing depth is a good indicator of the advance of the disease. In a healthy periodontium, there is no loss of epithelial attachment or pocket formation and the periodontal pocket is less than 2 mm deep.[50] The disease state ranges from gingivitis to periodontitis and advanced periodontitis.

Gingivitis, the most prevalent and mild form of PD, is characterized by the inflammation of the gums caused by plaque deposits, with possible bleeding when brushed or probed.[49]

Periodontitis can be identified by the hardening of plaque to form calculus, causing gum recession. This results in the formation of pockets between 3.5 and 5.5 mm between the tooth surface and the gum.[51] The symptoms are similar to those of gingivitis but are more severe due to higher accumulation of bacteria and stronger inflammatory responses.

Advanced forms of periodontitis are also prevalent, affecting approximately 10%–30% of the adult population in the United States.[52] Advanced periodontitis is distinguished by excessive tissue loss of gingiva and alveolar bone and pockets greater than 5.5 mm in depth. This condition often leads to tooth exfoliation due to the destruction of the tooth connective ligaments.[53]

The etiology and pathogenesis of PD are not completely clear. Human gingivitis and periodontitis are the results of an imbalance in the bacterial species that colonize the oral cavity and are characterized by complex interactions between pathogenic bacteria and the host's immunoinflammatory responses.[55,56] In the past three decades, marked advances have occurred in our understanding of the infectious agents of PD. There are more than 300 distinct species of bacteria present in the gingival area of the mouth, most of which exist in a commensal relationship with the host. However, three Gram-negative, anaerobic, or microaerophilic bacteria species, known as periodontal pathogens (*Actinobacillus actinomycetemcomitans*, *Bacteroides forsythus*, and *Porphyromonas gingivalis*), have been identified as being ubiquitous in periodontal plaque formations.[53,54,56] Moreover, within the past years, various herpes viruses, such as human cytomegalovirus and Epstein–Barr virus, have also emerged as pathogens in the destructive PD.[57]

As reported above, the damage of periodontal tissues results both from a direct effect of the toxic products released by the bacteria and from the action of the immune system that, if stimulated by bacterial infection, produces and releases mediators that induce the effectors of connective tissue breakdown.[58,59] Numerous studies have showed that the destruction of periodontal tissue in PD is mainly due to host-derived mediators and free radicals.[60,61] Different mechanisms, including DNA damage, lipid peroxidation, protein damage, oxidation of important enzymes, and stimulation of proinflammatory cytokine release, have been implicated as causes of tissue damage by an increase in both ROS and reactive nitrogen species (RNS).[62,63] An inverse relationship between peroxidation products and antioxidant molecules or enzymes in spontaneous or in experimental PD has been stressed.[64–66] Chapple et al.[53] reported that total antioxidant activity is reduced in saliva of patients with periodontitis relative to that in nonperiodontitis subjects. The imbalance between oxidative stress induced by ROS and the concentrations (or activity) of the antioxidants may lead to a further oxidative attack and substantial deterioration of the periodontal tissues,[67,68] resulting in tissue damage.[69,70]

Microbial components, especially lipopolysaccharide (LPS), have the capacity to induce an initial infiltrate of inflammatory cells. Activated macrophages synthesize and secrete a variety of proinflammatory molecules, including some interleukins (IL-1α, IL-β, IL-6, and IL-8), tumor necrosis factor α (TNF-α), prostaglandins (PGE2), and hydrolytic enzymes.[71] These cytokines recruit polymorphonuclear leukocytes (PMN) to the site of infection.[54] PMN play a relevant role in the etiology of PD, as they are the predominant host immune response to oral bacterial infection. Upon stimulation by bacterial antigens, cytokines promote the PMN to express adhesion molecules and move out of the circulation to the site of infection.[72] When PMN arrive here, they can induce an autoamplification effect producing IL-8 to attract more PMN into the infection site. This is exacerbated by the ability of *P. gingivalis* to modulate the mobility and function of PMN within the site of infection:[54] a reduction of IL-8 secretion in epithelial cells, mediated by the bacterium, inhibits the recruitment of PMN to the infected area. At the site of infection, PMN produce proteolytic enzymes (e.g., elastase), but also ROS. Indeed, PMN in periodontal patients display an increased number, adhesion, and oxidative activity.[73] As the release of ROS is not target-specific, damage to host tissue also occurs. Gingival epithelial cells are highly susceptible to attack by PMN-derived oxidants;[74] human PMN produce in vitro desquamation (as a consequence of the digestion of extracellular matrix constituents by PMN neutral proteases) and lysis of gingival epithelial cells (caused by PMN oxidants generated by myeloperoxidase).[38]

In PD, a number of proteases that degrade collagen and extracellular matrix (ECM) play key roles in periodontal tissue breakdown.[75] A particular subgroup of matrix metalloproteinases (MMPs), called collagenases, is the major group of enzymes responsible for degradation of ECM and for collagen destruction in periodontitis. These latent collagenolytic enzymes are activated by ROS in the inflammatory environment, giving rise to elevated levels of interstitial collagenase in inflamed gingival tissue.[76] The attachment loss deepens the sulcus, creating a periodontal pocket. This pocket provides a microbial niche that can harbor on the order of 100 bacterial cells.[77] This event marks the transition from gingivitis to periodontitis.

PD is clearly an important and potentially life-threatening condition, often underestimated by health professionals and the general population. The available evidence implicating inflammatory mediators and cells in the disease process suggests that local antioxidant status may be of importance in determining susceptibility to the disease and its progression following initial bacterial colonization.

13.3.2.1 Gold Standard Therapies in PD

Due the minimal symptoms of gingival bleeding and attachment loss, many individuals neglect to treat their disease. Left untreated, gingivitis may progress to irreversible periodontitis, resulting in tooth loss.

Periodontal research has provided sufficient evidence indicating that, once diagnosed, chronic PD is successfully treatable.[78] The first therapeutic goal in treatment of PD is to alter or eliminate the origin of the microbes as well as the contributing risk factors. The majority of periodontal treatment modalities, however, attempt to arrest the progression of periodontal destruction in order to avoid tooth loss and preserve the healthy state of the periodontium.[79] Furthermore, in severe cases, regeneration of the periodontal attachments must be attempted.[80] The first nonsurgical step of PD treatment involves special cleaning called scaling and root planing. Supplemental treatment may include antiseptic mouth medications, either to aid the healing process or to further control the bacterial infection. Often, antibiotics may be administered, which may offer an effective alternative. Doxycycline, a wide-spectrum antibiotic, and other tetracyclines are frequently used in dental treatments for soft tissue and bone regeneration after PD because of their strong activity against periodontal pathogens; they are able to inhibit the activity of human MMPs and reduce the severity and progression of PDs in animal models and humans.[81] Along with antibiotic therapy, if the periodontal pockets are not reduced or further loss of alveolar bone is observed, surgical treatment may therefore be beneficial to PD patients to prevent bone loss. If the PD has caused excessive loss of gum tissue or bone, then soft-tissue grafts or bone grafts may be performed to reduce further gum recession and bone loss.

13.3.2.2 New Perspectives in PD Treatment: Melatonin Supplementation

In recent years, the role of ROS, lipid peroxidation products, and antioxidant systems in the pathology of PD have been well clarified. It is now of importance to determine the possible contribution of diet to salivary antioxidant status because the use of antioxidant supplementation in the treatment or prevention of these chronic diseases of the oral cavity can be an excellent chance for preventing them. Recent medical and dental research in this area is geared toward the prevention of free radical–mediated diseases by using specific nutrient antioxidants supplementation.[38] Melatonin was found to be released with saliva into the oral cavity and to be implicated in various dental and PDs: for this reason, it is one of the more prominent antioxidants used for this purpose. In particular, melatonin possesses two functions of great interest to dental professionals: first of all, its capacity to scavenge free radicals, thereby exerting antioxidative action,[82,83] and second, the cell protective effect exerted by melatonin in situations of inflammation.[37,84]

Nowadays, it is well known that melatonin not only would stimulate the immune system through the plasma fraction of the hormone but would also afford local protection though the salivary melatonin fraction[85] to better protect the cell populations affected by the periodontal process from the ROS generated by the inflammatory process. Saliva antioxidant capacity was significantly lower in diseased patients compared with controls. In addition, the ratio between saliva and serum antioxidants was also significantly lower in the diseased patients. It was proposed that the reduction in antioxidant capacity was either a direct causal factor in the PD patients or that the reduction was due to a reduction in scavenging antioxidants mediated through an increase in oxidative stress due to the pathogenesis of the disease. Cutando et al.[85] emphasized the physiological impact of melatonin in saliva: this little amine displays noticeable antioxidant activity in saliva[86] and helps protect the oral cavity from tissue damage due to oxidative stress. In a recent study, it was indirectly shown that nitric oxide (NO) production was elevated in the diseased periodontium. In ligature-induced periodontitis in rats, inducible nitric oxide synthase (iNOS) was expressed at higher concentrations at the ligated sites than at the nonligated sites.[87] The diseased tissue biopsies from periodontitis patients demonstrated a greater level of iNOS expression than the healthy tissue biopsies from the clinically nonperiodontitis patients. In particular, the basal layers of epithelium and macrophages, lymphocytes, and neutrophils in the connective tissue were found to stain positively for iNOS, only in diseased patients.[88] Recent evidence suggests that the pineal hormone melatonin, acting as a potent free radical scavenger, plays an important acute and chronic role in reducing or eliminating the oxidant damage produced by NO.[89,13] Based on a number of studies, it is estimated that melatonin inhibits the activity of NOS,[90,91] in particular iNOS, which produces excessive amounts of NO, thus contributing to the pathophysiology of inflammation and increasing the oxidative stress.[92]

Furthermore, in PDs, the increase in free radical production coexists with a decrease in antioxidant defense. Besides its direct action as a free radical scavenger, melatonin influences the oxidative stress status indirectly by stabilizing the inner mitochondrial membrane and improving the electron transport chain located there.[93] It has been demonstrated that melatonin is a broad-spectrum antioxidant:[94,95] in pharmacological and physiological doses, it increases gene expression and activity of endogenous antioxidants, which are important in maintaining the integrity of vasculature and other tissues.[96,97] These antioxidant properties of melatonin could turn out very beneficial for treatment of the local inflammatory lesions and for accelerating the healing process (e.g., after tooth extration and other surgical procedures in the oral cavity). Recently, Cutando et al.[98] have shown the favorable effects of the local melatonin administration to the alveolar sockets after molar or premolar extraction in dogs. The animals without melatonin regimen showed an increase in lipid peroxidation, nitrite plus nitrate levels in plasma, and glutathione disulfide/glutathione ratio. Dogs who were administered 2 mg melatonin to the extration socket just after extraction did not show this increase.[98] This suggests that locally applied melatonin to the oral cavity lining may be useful in the treatment of oral lesions.[99] Czesnikiewicz-Guzik et al.[99] attempted to measure the concentrations of melatonin in the saliva and plasma of patients after application of melatonin to restricted areas of oral mucosa, such as the palate. It was found that melatonin is quickly and in a time-dependent fashion absorbed into the circulation from the mucosa of the oral cavity as documented by the increment of plasma immunoreactive melatonin levels that was paralleled by the increase in salivary concentrations of this indole. These results may have important clinical implications because melatonin could be applied directly on oral mucosa in a variety of infectious and noninfectious oxidative stress diseases of the oral cavity including denture-induced stomatitis, gingivitis, healing of lesions, and ulcerations caused by tooth extration (alveolitis). Moreover, these studies indicate that topically applied melatonin to the oral mucosa in the area of damage or inflammation is effective in combating the inflammatory processes and acceleration of the healing of erosions and ulcerations in the oral cavity.

Furthermore, melatonin seems to also have a direct effect above the cell populations of the immune system. It is known, for instance, that the metabolic products of periodontopathic bacteria decrease cytokine production including IL-2.[100,101] IL-2 regulates a series of processes in different cells of the immune system. A relationship between IL-2 and melatonin was described when it was found that melatonin stimulates the production of IL-2 by T lymphocytes.[102] On the other end, IL-2 can modulate the synthesis of melatonin at the level of the pineal gland.[103] Without doubt, this reciprocal modulation has important consequences at the time of treatment of periodontal patients who have, in one way or another, an altered immunological system. Thus, it was of interest to study the changes in the relationship between melatonin and IL-2 during periodontal pathologies. Moreover, earlier studies[104,105] showed that an increase in salivary and plasma melatonin resulted in stimulation of the CD4+ T cells, which possess membrane and nuclear receptors for the hormone.[102] This would stimulate the other immune cell populations via cytokine secretion (e.g., CD3+, CD19+, CD8+ cells), thereby facilitating the host reaction to an existing oral infection.[106]

Such beneficial effects of melatonin could open new perspectives for the treatment of oral inflammatory processes,[85,86] suggesting that this indole hormone could have a protective function in fighting periodontal infection. However, the relationship between PDs and melatonin level remains to be better understood.

13.3.3 Oral Cavity Cancer

Oral cavity cancer, predominantly oral squamous cell carcinoma (OSCC), is an important cancer, globally affecting 270,000 people worldwide each year.[107] Despite of the recent progress in the diagnosis and therapy of OSCC, the 5-year survival rate has not improved in more than two decades.[108] Therefore, a more comprehensive understanding of the molecular pathogenesis of OSCC is urgently needed to identify new targets for the effective therapy and to recognize the early state of OSCC or, when it is possible, premalignant lesions. The development of OSCC has been reported as one of the most important complications of a chronic inflammatory disease of the oral mucosa,[109] called oral lichen planus (OLP),[110,111] even if in OLP patients the underlying mechanisms of malignant transformation have not been clearly established.

The association of chronic inflammation with a variety of cancers, including OSCC, has been amply addressed.[112–114] ROS and RNS are considered to play a key role in inflammation-mediated carcinogenesis. ROS can generate DNA base alterations, strand breaks, damage to tumor suppressor genes, and enhanced expression of proto-oncogenes.[115] ROS-induced mutation could also arise from protein damage and attack on lipids, which then initiate lipid peroxidation,[116] resulting in the transformation of normal cells into malignant cells.[117] Any changes in enzymatic and nonenzymatic antioxidant defense systems may break cellular equilibrium and cause damages and ultimately malignant transformation. In addition, overproduction of NO leads to generation of various RNS.[118] Excess of NO is produced from inflammatory cells via the expression of iNOS.[119,120] Chronic inflammation induced iNOS-dependent DNA damage in not only inflammatory cells but also epithelial cells, which could potentially develop into cancer.[121,122] Therefore, this DNA damage could possibly imply an association between the existence of OLP and development into oral cancer. Moreover, the magnitude of the inflammation damage associated to carcinogenesis depends not only on ROS/RNS levels but also on the body's defense mechanisms, mediated by various cellular antioxidants. Disruption of this delicate oxidant/antioxidant balance in the body seems to play a causative role in carcinogenesis.[123] Therefore, melatonin, which is a potent scavenger of the hydroxyl radical and peroxynitrate, may be useful in treating oxygen radical pathophysiology.[124] Parallel to that, melatonin stimulates the activity of antioxidative enzymes and inhibits pro-oxidative enzymes, thus physiologically synergizing with its direct free radical scavenging properties. For all these reasons, an inverse interaction between melatonin and carcinogenic processes is of focal importance.[125]

Generally, OSCC is considered to arise through the progressive accumulation of multiple genetic abnormalities that impair the functions of oncogenes or tumor-suppressor genes.[126] Besides genetic alterations, evidence has emerged that the DNA methylation of 5′-CpG islands has been shown to be a major cause of inactivation of tumor-suppressor genes in human OSCC.[127] Melatonin receptor 1A (*MTNR1A*), which encodes for one of two high affinity forms of a melatonin receptor, seems to be a candidate target involved in the etiopathogenesis of OSCC. Interestingly, expression of this gene was frequently silenced in OSCC cell lines without its homozygous loss, although it was present in normal oral mucosa, suggesting that *MTNR1A* might be inactivated epigenetically in OSCC and contribute to oral carcinogenesis. In several cancers, indeed, it has been reported that melatonin treatment or ectopic expression of MTNR1A has a growth suppressive effect on cancer cells in vitro and in vivo,[128,129] even though the intracellular mechanisms behind the antiproliferative actions of melatonin remain unclear.

13.3.3.1 Melatonin in Treatment of Oral Mucositis, a Complication of Chemotherapy

Oral mucositis is a consequence of the toxic effects of chemotherapeutic agents and irradiation on oral mucosa cells.[130–132] It is estimated that oral mucositis is a complication in 40% of patients receiving chemotherapy, more than 90% of those irradiated for head and neck cancer. This condition is frequently associated with severe pain and inflammation and can cause malnutrition, systemic infections, and low quality of life, as well as limiting chemotherapy doses. The clinical appearance of oral mucositis may range from mild discomfort and erythema to painful erythema and edema and/or ulcerations.[133]

The pathophysiology of mucositis is not known in detail. A complex hypothesis has been proposed to elucidate the mechanism by which mucositis develops and resolves. According to this, mucositis is a complex process, divided into four phases: an initial inflammatory/vascular phase, an epithelial phase, an ulcerative/bacteriological phase, and a healing phase.[130] The hypothesis speculates on the importance of the inflammatory response induced in the involved tissues by chemotherapy and ionizing radiation that occurs through the activation of intracellular and intercellular signaling pathways, regulating gene expression of specific proteins involved in immune and inflammatory processes (e.g., cytokines, adhesion molecules).[134,135] Of the many drugs and methods used to treat mucositis, none has been shown to be uniformly effective. Trials investigating locally and systemically applied treatments of mucositis include immunomodulatory drugs, anticholinergic drugs, cytokines, antiviral drugs, glutamine, and antioxidants.

Among the antioxidants currently under investigation, the pineal hormone melatonin could be added, as it has been claimed to have activity in the prevention of mucositis.[136,137] Locally and systemically applied melatonin has been shown to prevent and treat mucositis in patients with cancer.[138] The pineal hormone melatonin inhibits the production of free radicals that mediate the toxicity of chemotherapy. Nevertheless, experimental data are still controversial: chemotherapy-induced stomatitis was not reduced in a study with the use of melatonin, although other toxic effects were decreased.[139–141] Additional basic and clinical researches are needed to determine whether melatonin can be used to treat chemotherapy-induced mucositis.

13.4 ROLE OF MELATONIN IN BONE METABOLISM

It is known that melatonin is involved in skeletal development: in particular, increasing evidences from in vitro and in vivo experiments using rodent and chicken have suggested the possible role of melatonin on bone metabolism.[142,143] The structural integrity of mammalian bone is dependent upon a balance between the activity of osteoclasts (the bone-resorptive cells) and osteoblasts (the bone-formative cells).[144,145] The aim of this remodeling process is the renewing of the skeleton while maintaining its anatomical and structural integrity.[146] Under normal conditions, bone is constantly degraded and replaced with new bone in cycles in which osteoclasts adhere to bone and subsequently remove it by acidification and proteolytic digestion. After the osteoclasts have left the resorption site, osteoblasts invade the area, and begin the process of forming new bone by secreting osteoid (a matrix of collagen and other proteins), which is eventually mineralized. After bone formation has ceased, the surface of the bone is covered by lining cells, a distinct type of terminally differentiated osteoblasts.[146]

Several reports indicate that melatonin is involved in the regulation of calcium homeostasis. The effects of melatonin on calcium metabolism were first studied by Csaba et al.,[147,148] who proposed that this hormone could influence the secretion of calcitonin[149] and parathyroid hormone.[147] Indeed, it was demonstrated that suppression of melatonin secretion by white light (at the intensity used to treat hyperbilirubinemia in human infants) in newborn rats or synthesis in adult rats (by administration of the beta-adrenoceptor blocker propranolol) lowered serum calcium concentration.[150] Moreover, in both studies, treatment of rats with melatonin prevented serum calcium decrease.[150–152]

The in vitro effect of melatonin on cellular proliferation and differentiation has stimulated interest in its role in bone regeneration. Therefore, the effect of melatonin on bone metabolism was recently examined using different kinds of osteoblastic cell lines.[153,154] Roth et al.,[26] for instance, examined the direct effect of melatonin on osteoblasts using MC3T3-El preosteoblasts and rat osteoblast-like osteosarcoma 17/2.8 cells.[142] Both cell lines in the presence of nanomolar concentrations of melatonin augmented gene expression of bone sialoprotein (an extracellular bone matrix protein that is expressed during osteoblastic cell differentiation and is required for mineralization), as well as several other essential bone marker proteins including alkaline phosphatase, osteocalcin, and osteopontin, and stimulated both osteoblast differentiation and mineralization.[142] This relationship is supported by the fact that the genes of a large portion of bone matrix contain the sequence of bases (RGGTCA) necessary for the nuclear receptor of melatonin to bind with its promoting zone.[155] In these preosteoblastic cell lines, melatonin seems to reduce the period of differentiation into osteoblasts, and this reaction seems to be mediated by the membrane receptors for the indole.[156]

Previous studies have shown that melatonin stimulates the synthesis and proliferation of collagen type I fibers in human osteoblasts in vitro.[153] Similar results were reported in clinically relevant human bone cells, in which micromolar concentrations of melatonin significantly increase procollagen type Ic peptide production (a measure of type I collagen synthesis) in a concentration-dependent manner.[153] Some authors reported that the mitogen-activated protein kinase (MAP-K) signal transduction pathway may be responsible for melatonin's effects on osteoblasts differentiation,[157–159] even if further studies are needed. In another study, melatonin acted directly on human bone cells (HOB-M) and human osteoblastic cell line (SV-HFO) and dose-dependently increased the proliferation in both cell types by twofolds.[153] Type I collagen synthesis was also elevated in both cell types, but neither alkaline phosphatase activity nor osteocalcin secretion was influenced by melatonin.[153]

Furthermore, seems that these effects on osteoblasts are mediated through melatonin transmembrane receptors.[160] Two genes have been isolated for membrane melatonin receptors in mammals including humans: one is the melatonin 1a receptor[161] and the other is the 1b receptor.[162] In a recent study, reverse transcription–polymerase chain reaction and Western blot analysis showed that human osteoblasts express the melatonin 1a receptor and that its expression levels decrease gradually with age.[163] In this study, Satomura et al. confirm a possible role of melatonin in human bone formation, showing that at pharmacological doses, it is able to enhance proliferation and differentiation of normal human osteoblasts, even if its mechanisms of action remain unclear. Moreover, to demonstrate the possible utility of melatonin as a pharmaceutical agent to shorten the period of bone regeneration, the effects of this hormone on bone formation in vivo were also tested; in mice, intraperitoneally administered melatonin to mice induced a significant increase in the ratio of new to old bone mass in the cortex of the femur.[162] Collectively, all these findings indicate that melatonin has a promotional action on osteoblasts.

The bone complex, therefore, includes osteoblasts, osteoclasts, and the bone matrix. An interaction between osteoclasts and osteoblasts has been recently noted in mammals, and it is necessary to consider both their actions.[146,164] On the whole, osteoclasts are under the control of local modulator factors produced, among other cells, by the osteoblasts. The receptor activator of nuclear factor j B (RANK) and the receptor activator of the nuclear factor j B ligand (RANKL) have been identified in osteoclasts and osteoblasts, respectively.[165] Exposure of osteoblasts to substances such as parathyroid hormone stimulated the expression of osteoclast differentiating factors: in particular, it was found that the bound RANKL to RANK induces multinucleated osteoclasts (active type of osteoclasts)[165] and then can activate bone resorption.[166] Another osteoblastic protein, osteoprotegerin (a soluble member of the superfamily of tumor necrosis factor receptors), on the contrary, can inhibit the differentiation of osteoclasts by binding to osteoclast differentiation factor as a decoy.[166] The effect of melatonin on the expression of RANK and osteoprotegerin was investigated in mouse MC3T3-E1 osteoblastic cells.[154] In this study, melatonin at pharmacological doses causes an inhibition of bone resorption and an increase in bone mass by down-regulating RANK-mediated osteoclast formation and activation:[154] the authors observed a significant dose-dependent decrease of RANK mRNA and an increase in both mRNA and protein levels of osteoprotegerin in MC3T3-E1 cells. On the other hand, melatonin is capable of influencing the RANKL system, suppressing its activity[36,154] and favoring the formation of new bone: this indicates that melatonin may bring about a reduction in bone resorption and an increase in bone mass because of its repression of osteoclast activation by means of RANK.[167] Moreover, in in vivo studies on intact mice, pharmacological doses of melatonin elevated the bone mineral density[154] aside from the trabecular thickness of the vertebra and the cortical thickness of the femur already showed in ovariectomized mice.[168] This treatment significantly reduced the bone resorption parameters (osteoclastic surface and osteoclastic number) but did not increase the histomorphometric bone formation parameters (bone formation rate, mineral apposition rate, and osteoid volume).[154] So the skeletal effects of melatonin are, presumably, a result of the inhibition of osteoclast activity.

In a recent study, the effects of melatonin on osteoclastic and osteoblastic cells were examined using a culture system of the teleost scale.[169] The teleost scale is a calcified tissue that contains osteoclasts, osteoblasts,[170] and also components of the bone matrix;[171,172] hydroxyapatite also exists in the scale.[173] The scales of teleosts contain as much as 20% of the total body calcium and are a functional internal calcium reservoir during periods of increased calcium demand.[169,174,175] Thus, there are many similarities between the teleost scale and mammalian membrane bone. In this "in vitro assay system," melatonin directly suppressed both tartrate-resistant acid phosphatase and alkaline phosphatase activities, markers of osteoclastic and osteoblastic activity, respectively, by suppressing their growth and differentiation.[169] This was the first report related to the function of melatonin in osteoclasts and on the inhibitory effect of melatonin in osteoblasts when incubated in the presence of osteoclastic cells. Indeed, the authors argued that the previously reported effects of melatonin to stimulate proliferation of mammalian osteoblasts[142] were artifacts because the experiments were conducted with isolated osteoblasts, while in bone formation and metabolism, cell-to-cell contacts between osteoblasts and osteoclasts occur.[146]

Moreover, melatonin acts directly on osteoclasts, which use a variety of chemical agents and different mechanisms to resorb the extracellular matrix and degrade bone, including the production of free radicals. Osteoclasts generate high levels of free radicals, superoxide anions, in particular, during bone resorption, which contribute to the degradative process.[176] Thus, melatonin, being an antioxidant and a free radical scavenger at both physiological and pharmacological concentrations[177] may interfere in this function of the osteoclast detoxifying free radicals, which are produced during osteoclastogenesis,[178] leading to an inhibition of reabsorption of the bone.[167] Therefore, the effect of melatonin in preventing osteoclast activity in the bone may depend in part on its free radical scavenging properties. These data point toward an osteogenic effect of melatonin, which may be of clinical importance because it could be used as a therapeutic agent in situations when bone formation would be advantageous, such as in occlusal reconstruction using dental implants.

13.4.1 Melatonin Promotes Bone Regeneration around Dental Implants

All the actions of melatonin on bone metabolism described above are of interest, as it may possible to apply melatonin during endo-osseous dental implant surgery as biomimetic agent.[179] Occlusal reconstruction using dental implants is of importance from the point of view of the quality of life of patients: for this reason, osseointegration should be promptly completed and it should be maintained for as long as possible. So, in order to obtain functional bone as soon as possible, it is critical to enhance at the same time both the proliferation and differentiation of osteogenic cells.

The long-term success of many dental implants depends on their ability to become well integrated in bone. Titanium (Ti) is the implant material of choice for use in dental applications, even if the surface properties of this material are not well suited for bonding to bone. Modifications of both surface topography and chemistry have led to significant improvements in the integration of such materials in bone. Several measures have been proposed to improve and accelerate osseous healing using topical treatments. They include the application of platelet-rich plasma, bone morphogenetic proteins, and growth factors (e.g., melatonin).[180] Tacheki et al. focused on the possibility that melatonin may be an effective hormone in the treatment of bone changes around dental implants; its efficiency has been shown when melatonin acts synergistically with fibroblast growth factor 2 (FGF-2) to promote bone formation around titanium implants placed in the tibia of rat by enhancing both the proliferation and differentiation of osteogenic cells.[181] The results of Tacheki et al. strongly suggest that these two molecules have the potential to promote osteointegration of titanium implants, even if their exact roles during osteogenesis are not completely understood; FGF-2 is typically thought to control osteoprogenitor cell proliferation, whereas melatonin is more important in osteoblast differentiation. Moreover, in a recent study, it has been stated that topical application of melatonin successfully activated osteogenesis around titanium implants in a canine mandibular model. Considering a possible future application of melatonin in dentistry, the authors of this study thought that it was beneficial to introduce the effects of melatonin in implant treatment and showed that when applied topically, melatonin promotes peri-implant bone formation. A study with experimental beagle dogs was carried out to evaluate the effect of the topical application of melatonin mixed with a very biocompatible collagenized bone substitutes of porcine origin[182,183] on the osteointegration of dental implants. Bone grafts have been usually placed in bone defects or into extraction sockets to facilitate healing, used, for instance, in order to increase the width of the crest or for augmentation of the maxillary sinus floor to enable implant placement.[184] The results of Calvo-Guirado et al. showed that melatonin, combined with collagenized porcine bone substitutes, reveals more bone-to-implant contact and less crestal bone resorption than control implants, suggesting a positive role of melatonin in osteointegration around dental implants.[185]

As emerged from all these studies, melatonin, with its capacity to induce bone cell proliferation and differentiation, could facilitate the process of healing of bone tissue in dental implant surgery, reducing the period of osteointegration and settling of the implant, and therefore, the quality of life of the patient may be improved.

13.5 MELATONIN USE IN SURGERY AS AN ANESTHETIC ADJUVANT

13.5.1 Potential Anesthetic Effects of Exogenously Administered Melatonin

General anesthesia is a pharmacologically induced state that entails amnesia, analgesia, hypnosis (unconsciousness), immobility, and blunted autonomic responsiveness.[186] Experimental literature in animals[187] and anecdotal observations in humans[188] have shown that melatonin has hypnotic actions.[189] Anton-Tay et al.[190] were the first to demonstrate clearly that exogenously administered melatonin has hypnotic properties in human subjects and that the loss of consciousness is accompanied by a pattern of electroencephalographic activity similar to that seen during intravenous and volatile anesthesia.[191] At the molecular level, general anesthetics enhance the function of inhibitory gamma-aminobutyric acid type A ($GABA_A$): positive modulation of $GABA_A$ receptor function has been recognized as an important component of the central depressant effects of many intravenous anesthetics, including propofol.[192] There is evidence to suggest that the central effects of melatonin, at least in part, involve facilitation of GABA-ergic transmission by modulating the GABA receptor.[193,194] Also, significant dose-dependent increases in GABA concentrations were noted in the central nervous system after the administration of melatonin.[195]

In rats, intravenous administration of large doses of melatonin induced a profound dose-dependent hypnotic state that was characterized by a rapid loss of righting reflex and antinociceptive effects against thermal, chemical, and electrical stimuli (resulted from the release of b-endorphin[196]), less potent, but similar to that observed with equipotent doses of thiopental and propofol;[197] moreover, orally administered melatonin has been shown to potentiate the anesthetic effects of thiopental and ketamine.[198] Furthermore, in a study using melatonin pretreatment associated with thiopental (a hyperalgesic molecule), the latter did not increase paw withdrawal threshold;[199] these findings underlie the anesthetic adjuvant properties of melatonin. However, even if melatonin exhibited antinociceptive effects, it was not as effective as other anesthetic agents in abolishing the response to tail clamping. Loss of righting reflex (hypnosis) and abolition of purposeful movement response to tail clamp (immobilization) are used for determination of anesthetic potencies of volatile anesthetics.[200] Thus, melatonin on its own does not seem to possess sufficient efficacy to warrant consideration as a general anesthetic.

The above observations raised the question whether melatonin might be suitable at least as an anesthetic adjuvant in preoperative treatments. Orally administered melatonin (5 mg) is used as a preoperative medication in both paediatric[201] and adult surgical patients.[202,203] The management of anxiety in children undergoing dental procedures, for instance, has developed considerably in the past decades. The approach with behavior management techniques combined with relative analgesia (inhaled nitrous oxide and oxygen) is unsuccessful in some children. In such cases, control of pain and anxiety poses a significant barrier to dental care, and sedation or general anesthesia is seen as the only option. Clinical trials with melatonin as a premedication agent in anxious children under N_2O/O_2 sedation for dental treatment have shown good results, but so far, only limited data are available.[189] Naguib et al.[202,203] noted that premedication with 0.05, 0.1, or 0.2 mg/kg sublingual/oral melatonin is associated with preoperative anxiolysis and sedation in adults and children without impairment of psychomotor skills or impact on the quality of recovery; oral melatonin is often used to enhance both the onset and quality of sleep for premedication of adult patients.[204,205] Furthermore, it should be mentioned that melatonin has been effective in preventing postsurgical adhesions,[206] delirium,[207] and sleep disturbances.[208]

A number of melatonin analogues of greater potency and efficacy (e.g., 2-bromomelatonin, phenylmelatonin) are currently being studied to determine their effects on the induction of general anesthesia. In contrast to melatonin, 2-bromomelatonin was effective in abolishing the response to a supramaximal stimulus, as tail clamping, even in some animals that did not lose their righting reflex. Substitution with a lipophilic substituent, bromine, at the 2-indole position of *N*-acetyl-5-methoxytryptamine increases the hypnotic and antinociceptive, as well as the melatonergic properties of this molecule.[209] The profile of the hypnotic properties of this melatonin analogue is similar to that induced by propofol, which has a rapid onset and a short duration of action, but unlike propofol, the reduced nocifensive behavior persisted for a longer period. Those data support the notion that 2-bromomelatonin might find use as an anesthetic agent.

13.5.2 Effect of Anesthesia and Surgery on Melatonin Homeostasis

The effects of surgery and anesthesia on melatonin secretion and endocrine function have not been thoroughly evaluated, even if many factors, such as sleep disturbances, pain, drugs, and stress, associated with surgical procedures and anesthesia are all potentially capable of interaction with melatonin production.[210,211] A possible explanation for the change in melatonin and melatonin metabolites levels around surgery can be related to anesthesia, and in particular, the administration of benzodiazepines was found to partially suppress melatonin secretion.[212] It is also possible that the same influence is exercised by other anesthetic drugs. Reber et al.[210] reported that isoflurane and propofol anesthesia elicited elevated plasma melatonin levels. In contrast, Karkela et al.[211] reported that both spinal and general anesthesia significantly decreased melatonin secretion during the first postoperative period, noticing a postanesthesia phase delay in melatonin secretion. The conflicting results on melatonin secretion in the perioperative period in these studies could be due to the differences in the methodology of melatonin concentration measurement and in the variables of surgical procedures and preoperative preparation. Further studies are needed to better understand the short- and long-term changing levels of melatonin around surgical intervention.

13.6 CONCLUSIONS

From an accurate analysis of scientific literature, it seems that melatonin, either systemically or locally administered, has some interesting properties that both protect the oral cavity from inflammatory processes or infections and modulate the activity of cells involved in bone metabolism. Nowadays, experimental and clinical evidences are still inconsistent, so further studies are needed to clarify melatonin role in the homeostasis of oral tissues and enable the use of this hormone in the therapy of oral pathologies. Nevertheless, the scientific community believes that assumptions exist to look at this molecule with attention.

REFERENCES

1. Wiechmann, A.F., and Summers, J.A. 2008. Circadian rhythms in the eye: The physiological significance of melatonin receptors in ocular tissues. *Prog. Retin. Eye Res.* 27(2):137–60.
2. Malhotra, S., Sawhney, G., and Pandhi, P. 2004. The therapeutic potential of melatonin: A review of the science. *Med. Gen. Med.* 6(2):46.
3. Lerner, A.B., Case, J.D., Takahashi, Y., Lee, T.H., and Mori, W. 1960. Isolation of melatonin and 5-methoxyindole-3-acetic acid from bovine pineal glands. *J. Biol. Chem.* 235:1992–7.
4. Claustrat, B., Brun, J., and Chazot, G. 2005. The basic physiology and pathophysiology of melatonin. *Sleep Med. Rev.* 9(1):11–24.
5. Korf, H.W., Schomerus, C., and Stehle, J.H. 1998. The pineal organ, its hormone melatonin, and the photoneuroendocrine system. *Adv. Anat. Embryol. Cell. Biol.* 146:1–100.
6. Reiter, R.J. 1991. Pineal melatonin: Cell biology of its synthesis and of its physiological interactions. *Endocr. Rev.* 12(2):151–80.
7. Bubenik, G.A. 2002. Gastrointestinal melatonin: Localization, function, and clinical relevance. *Dig. Dis. Sci.* 47(10):2336–48.
8. Arendt, J. 1995. *Melatonin and the Mammalian Pineal Gland.* Chapman & Hall, London.

9. Takahashi, J.S., Murakami, N., Nikaido, S.S., Pratt, B.L., and Robertson, L.M. 1989. The avian pineal, a vertebrate model system of the circadian oscillator: Cellular regulation of circadian rhythms by light, second messengers, and macromolecular synthesis. *Recent Prog. Horm. Res.* 45:279–348.
10. Zawilska, J.B., and Iuvone, P.M. 1992. Melatonin synthesis in chicken retina: Effect of kainic acid–induced lesions on the diurnal rhythm and D2-dopamine receptor–mediated regulation of serotonin *N*-acetyltransferase activity. *Neurosci. Lett.* 135(1):71–4.
11. Vakkuri, O., Leppäluoto, J., and Kauppila, A. 1985. Oral administration and distribution of melatonin in human serum, saliva and urine. *Life Sci.* 37(5):489–95.
12. Wurtman, R.J., and Moskowitz, M.A. 1977. The pineal organ (second of two parts). *N. Engl. J. Med.* 296(24):1383–6.
13. Reiter, R.J. 1991. Melatonin: The chemical expression of darkness. *Mol. Cell. Endocrinol.* 79(1–3):153–8.
14. Ekmekcioglu, C. 2006. Melatonin receptors in humans: Biological role and clinical relevance. *Biomed. Pharmacother.* 60(3):97–108.
15. Pandi-Perumal, S.R., Srinivasan, V., Maestroni, G.J., Cardinali, D.P., Poeggeler, B., and Hardeland, R. 2006. Melatonin: Nature's most versatile biological signal? *FEBS J.* 273(13):2813–38.
16. Blask, D.E. 2007. Melatonin. In: *McGraw-Hill Yearbook of Science and Technology*. 142–4. McGraw-Hill, New York.
17. Srinivasan, V., Maestroni, G.J., Cardinali, D.P., Esquifino, A.I., Perumal, S.R., and Miller, S.C. 2005. Melatonin, immune function and aging. *Immun. Ageing.* 2:17.
18. Carrillo-Vico, A., Calvo, J.R., Abreu, P., Lardone, P.J., García-Mauriño, S., Reiter, R.J., and Guerrero, J.M. 2004. Evidence of melatonin synthesis by human lymphocytes and its physiological significance: Possible role as intracrine, autocrine, and/or paracrine substance. *FASEB J.* 18(3):537–9.
19. Tan, D.X., Manchester, L.C., Terron, M.P., Flores, L.J., and Reiter, R.J. 2007. One molecule, many derivatives: A never-ending interaction of melatonin with reactive oxygen and nitrogen species? *J. Pineal Res.* 42(1):28–42.
20. Cagnacci, A., Arangino, S., Angiolucci, M., Melis, G.B., Facchinetti, F., Malmusi, S., and Volpe, A. 2001. Effect of exogenous melatonin on vascular reactivity and nitric oxide in postmenopausal women: Role of hormone replacement therapy. *Clin. Endocrinol. (Oxf.).* 54(2):261–6.
21. Cavallo, A., Daniels, S.R., Dolan, L.M., Khoury, J.C., and Bean, J.A. 2004. Blood pressure response to melatonin in type 1 diabetes. *Pediatr. Diabetes.* 5(1):26–31.
22. Arendt, J. 2006. Melatonin and human rhythms. *Chronobiol. Int.* 23(1–2):21–37.
23. Zisapel, N. 2001. Melatonin–dopamine interactions: From basic neurochemistry to a clinical setting. *Cell. Mol. Neurobiol.* 21(6):605–16.
24. Commentz, J.C., Uhlig, H., Henke, A., Hellwege, H.H., and Willig, R.P. 1997. Melatonin and 6-hydroxymelatonin sulfate excretion is inversely correlated with gonadal development in children. *Horm. Res.* 47(3):97–101.
25. Salti, R., Galluzzi, F., Bindi, G., Perfetto, F., Tarquini, R., Halberg, F., and Cornélissen, G. 2000. Nocturnal melatonin patterns in children. *J. Clin. Endocrinol. Metab.* 85(6):2137–44.
26. Reiter, R.J., Guerrero, J.M., Garcia, J.J., and Acuña-Castroviejo, D. 1998. Reactive oxygen intermediates, molecular damage, and aging. Relation to melatonin. *Ann. N.Y. Acad. Sci.* 854:410–24.
27. Karasek, M. 2004. Melatonin, human aging, and age-related diseases. *Exp. Gerontol.* 39(11–12):1723–9.
28. Karasek, M., and Winczyk, K. 2006. Melatonin in humans. *J. Physiol. Pharmacol.* 57(S5):19–39.
29. FDI Working Group 10, CORE. 1992. Saliva: Its role in health and disease. *Int. Dent. J.* 42:291–304.
30. Navazesh, M. 1993. Methods for collecting saliva. *Ann. N.Y. Acad. Sci.* 694:72–7.
31. Mandel, I.D. 1974. Relation of saliva and plaque to caries. *J. Dent. Res.* 53(2):246–66.
32. Laakso, M.L., Porkka-Heiskanen, T., Alila, A., Stenberg, D., and Johansson, G. 1990. Correlation between salivary and serum melatonin: Dependence on serum melatonin levels. *J. Pineal Res.* 9(1):39–50.
33. McIntyre, I.M., Norman, T.R., Burrows, G.D., and Armstrong, S.M. 1987. Melatonin rhythm in human plasma and saliva. *J. Pineal Res.* 4(2):177–83.
34. Voultsios, A., Kennaway, D.J., and Dawson, D. 1997. Salivary melatonin as a circadian phase marker: Validation and comparison to plasma melatonin. *J. Biol. Rhythms.* 12(5):457–66.
35. Konturek, S.J., Konturek, P.C., Brzozowski, T., and Bubenik, G.A. 2007. Role of melatonin in upper gastrointestinal tract. *J. Physiol. Pharmacol.* 58(S6):23–52.
36. Cutando, A., Gómez-Moreno, G., Arana, C., Acuña-Castroviejo, D., and Reiter, R.J. 2007. Melatonin: Potential functions in the oral cavity. *J. Periodontol.* 78(6):1094–102.
37. Chapple, I.L. 1997. Reactive oxygen species and antioxidants in inflammatory diseases. *J. Clin. Periodontol.* 24(5):287–96.

38. Battino, M., Bullon, P., Wilson, M., and Newman, H. 1999. Oxidative injury and inflammatory periodontal diseases: The challenge of anti-oxidants to free radicals and reactive oxygen species. *Crit. Rev. Oral Biol. Med.* 10(4):458–76.
39. Fejerskov, O., and Kidd, E.A. 2003. *Dental Caries: The Disease and Its Clinical Management.* Blackwell Monksgaard, Copenhagen, Denmark.
40. Marsh, P., and Martin, M.V. 1999. *Oral Microbiology*, 4th ed. Wright, Oxford.
41. Hassell, T.M., and Harris, E.L. 1995. Genetic influences in caries and periodontal diseases. *Crit. Rev. Oral Biol. Med.* 6(4):319–42.
42. Fejerskov, O. 2004. Changing paradigms in concepts on dental caries: Consequences for oral health care. *Caries Res.* 38(3):182–91.
43. Selwitz, R.H., Ismail, A.I., and Pitts, N.B. 2007. Dental caries. *Lancet.* 369(9555):51–9.
44. Mechin, J.A., and Toury, C. 1976. Action of melatonin on caries development in rats. *J. Dent. Res.* 55(3):555.
45. Löe, H. 1983. Principles of aetiology and pathogenesis governing the treatment of periodontal disease. *Int. Dent. J.* 33(2):119–26.
46. Olsen, I. 2008. Update on bacteraemia related to dental procedures. *Transfus. Apher. Sci.* 39(2):173–8.
47. Albandar, J.M. 2005. Epidemiology and risk factors of periodontal diseases. *Dent. Clin. North Am.* 49(3):517–32.
48. Loesche, W.J., and Grossman, N.S. 2001. Periodontal disease as a specific, albeit chronic, infection: Diagnosis and treatment. *Clin. Microbiol. Rev.* 14(4):727–52.
49. Ridgeway, E.E. 2000. Periodontal disease: Diagnosis and management. *J. Am. Acad. Nurse Pract.* 12(3):79–84.
50. Angeli, F., Verdecchia, P., Pellegrino, C., Pellegrino, R.G., Pellegrino, G., Prosciutti, L., Giannoni, C., Cianetti, S., and Bentivoglio, M. 2003. Association between periodontal disease and left ventricle mass in essential hypertension. *Hypertension.* 41(3):488–92.
51. Nuttall, N.M., Steele, J.G., Pine, C.M., White, D., and Pitts, N.B. 2001. The impact of oral health on people in the UK in 1998. *Br. Dent. J.* 190(3):121–6.
52. Fuster, V., Badimon, L., Badimon, J.J., and Chesebro, J.H. 1992. The pathogenesis of coronary artery disease and the acute coronary syndromes (1). *N. Engl. J. Med.* 326(4):242–50.
53. Chapple, I.L., Mason, G.I., Garner, I., Matthews, J.B., Thorpe, G.H., Maxwell, S.R., and Whitehead, T.P. 1997. Enhanced chemiluminescent assay for measuring the total antioxidant capacity of serum, saliva and crevicular fluid. *Ann. Clin. Biochem.* 34 (Pt 4):412–21.
54. Lamont, R.J., and Jenkinson, H.F. 1998. Life below the gum line: Pathogenic mechanisms of Porphyromonas gingivalis. *Microbiol. Mol. Biol. Rev.* 62(4):1244–63.
55. Page, R.C. 1999. Milestones in periodontal research and the remaining critical issues. *J. Periodontal Res.* 34(7):331–9.
56. Jenkinson, H.F., and Dymock, D. 1999. The microbiology of periodontal disease. *Dent. Update.* 26(5):191–7.
57. Slots, J., Kamma, J.J., and Sugar, C. 2003. The herpesvirus–*Porphyromonas gingivalis*–periodontitis axis. *J. Periodontal Res.* 38(3):318–23.
58. Zambon, J.J., Reynolds, H., Fisher, J.G., Shlossman, M., Dunford, R., and Genco, R.J. 1988. Microbiological and immunological studies of adult periodontitis in patients with noninsulin-dependent diabetes mellitus. *J. Periodontol.* 59(1):23–31.
59. Gustafsson, A., and Asman, B. 1996. Increased release of free oxygen radicals from peripheral neutrophils in adult periodontitis after Fc delta-receptor stimulation. *J. Clin. Periodontol.* 23(1):38–44.
60. Meikle, M.C., Atkinson, S.J., Ward, R.V., Murphy, G., and Reynolds, J.J. 1989. Gingival fibroblasts degrade type I collagen films when stimulated with tumor necrosis factor and interleukin 1: Evidence that breakdown is mediated by metalloproteinases. *J. Periodontal Res.* 24(3):207–13.
61. Séguier, S., Gogly, B., Bodineau, A., Godeau, G., and Brousse, N. 2001. Is collagen breakdown during periodontitis linked to inflammatory cells and expression of matrix metalloproteinases and tissue inhibitors of metalloproteinases in human gingival tissue? *J. Periodontol.* 72(10):1398–406.
62. Bartold, P.M., Wiebkin, O.W., and Thonard, J.C. 1984. The effect of oxygen-derived free radicals on gingival proteoglycans and hyaluronic acid. *J. Periodontal Res.* 19(4):390–400.
63. Finkel, T. 2001. Reactive oxygen species and signal transduction. *IUBMB Life.* 52(1–2):3–6.
64. Mishchenko, V.P., Silenko, I.u.I., Khavinson, V.K., and Tokar', D.L. 1991. The effect of periodontal cytomedin onlipid peroxidation and hemostasis in spontaneous periodontitis in rats. *Stomatologiia.* (5):12–4.

65. Silenko, I.u.I., Vesnina, L.E., and Mishchenko, V.P. 1994. Effect of paradentium polypeptide on the lipid peroxidation of the membranes and coagulation of erythrocytes in rats with spontaneous paradentitis. *Fiziol. Zh.* 40(2):88–91.
66. Bobyrev, V.N., Kovalev, E.V., Rozkolupa, N.V., Eremina, N.F., and Voskresenskiĭ, O.N. 1994. Biochemical and ultrastructural changes in the periodontium during the chronic administration of pro-oxidant xenobiotics. *Stomatologiia.* 73(4):57–61.
67. Halliwell, B. 1994. Free radicals, antioxidants, and human disease: Curiosity, cause, or consequence? *Lancet.* 344(8924):721–4.
68. Sies, H. 1997. Oxidative stress: Oxidants and antioxidants. *Exp. Physiol.* 82(2):291–5.
69. Sies, H. 1991. Oxidative stress: From basic research to clinical application. *Am. J. Med.* 91(3C):31S–38S.
70. Moslen, M.T. 1994. In: Armstrong, D. *Free Radicals in Diagnostic Medicine.* Eds. Plenum Press, New York.
71. Kim, J., and Amar, S. 2000. Periodontal disease and systemic conditions: A bidirectional relationship. *Odontology.* 94(1):10–21.
72. Gainet, J., Chollet-Martin, S., Brion, M., Hakim, J., Gougerot-Pocidalo, M.A., and Elbim, C. 1998. Interleukin-8 production by polymorphonuclear neutrophils in patients with rapidly progressive periodontitis: An amplifying loop of polymorphonuclear neutrophil activation. *Lab. Invest.* 78(6):755–62.
73. Asman, B. 1988. Peripheral PMN cells in juvenile periodontitis. Increased release of elastase and of oxygen radicals after stimulation with opsonized bacteria. *J. Clin. Periodontol.* 15(6):360–4.
74. Altman, L.C., Baker, C., Fleckman, P., Luchtel, D., and Oda, D. 1992. Neutrophil-mediated damage to human gingival epithelial cells. *J. Periodontal Res.* 27(1):70–9.
75. Sorsa, T., Ingman, T., Suomalainen, K., Haapasalo, M., Konttinen, Y.T., Lindy, O., Saari, H., and Uitto, V.J. 1992. Identification of proteases from periodontopathogenic bacteria as activators of latent human neutrophil and fibroblast-type interstitial collagenases. *Infect Immun.* 60(11):4491–5.
76. Lee, W., Aitken, S., Sodek, J., and McCulloch, C.A. 1995. Evidence of a direct relationship between neutrophil collagenase activity and periodontal tissue destruction in vivo: Role of active enzyme in human periodontitis. *J. Periodontal Res.* 30(1):23–33.
77. Geerts, S.O., Legrand, V., Charpentier, J., Albert, A., and Rompen, E.H. 2004. Further evidence of the association between periodontal conditions and coronary artery disease. *J. Periodontol.* 75(9):1274–80.
78. American Academy of Periodontology (AAP). 1998. Guidelines for periodontal therapy. *J. Periodontol.* 69:405–8.
79. Becker, W., Berg, L., and Becker, B.E. 1979. Untreated periodontal disease: A longitudinal study. *J. Periodontol.* 50(5):234–44.
80. Ebersole, J.L., Capelli, D., and Steffen, M.J. 1995. Longitudinal dynamics of infection and serum antibody in *A. actinomycetemcomitans* periodontitis. *Oral Dis.* 1:129–38.
81. Ramamurthy, N.S., Rifkin, B.R., Greenwald, R.A., Xu, J.W., Liu, Y., Turner, G., Golub, L.M., and Vernillo, A.T. 2002. Inhibition of matrix metalloproteinase–mediated periodontal bone loss in rats: A comparison of 6 chemically modified tetracyclines. *J. Periodontol.* 73(7):726–34.
82. Baydas, G., Canatan, H., and Turkoglu, A. 2002. Comparative analysis of the protective effects of melatonin and vitamin E on streptozocin-induced diabetes mellitus. *J. Pineal Res.* 32(4):225–30.
83. Zhang, Z., Araghi-Niknam, M., Liang, B., Inserra, P., Ardestani, S.K., Jiang, S., Chow, S., and Watson, R.R. 1999. Prevention of immune dysfunction and vitamin E loss by dehydroepiandrosterone and melatonin supplementation during murine retrovirus infection. *Immunology.* 96(2):291–7.
84. Packer, L. Nutrition and biochemistry of the lipophilic antioxidants vitamin E and carotenoids. In: Ong, A.S.H., Niki, E., and Packer, L. 1995. *Nutrition, Lipids, Health and Disease.* AOCS Press, Champaign, IL.
85. Cutando, A., Gómez-Moreno, G., Villalba, J., Ferrera, M.J., Escames, G., and Acuña-Castroviejo, D. 2003. Relationship between salivary melatonin levels and periodontal status in diabetic patients. *J. Pineal Res.* 35(4):239–44.
86. Moore, S., Calder, K.A., Miller, N.J., and Rice-Evans, C.A. 1994. Antioxidant activity of saliva and periodontal disease. *Free Radic. Res.* 21(6):417–25.
87. Lohinai, Z., Benedek, P., Fehér, E., Györfi, A., Rosivall, L., Fazekas, A., Salzman, A.L., and Szabó, C. 1998. Protective effects of mercaptoethylguanidine, a selective inhibitor of inducible nitric oxide synthase, in ligature-induced periodontitis in the rat. *Br. J. Pharmacol.*123(3):353–60.
88. Lappin, D.F., Kjeldsen, M., Sander, L., and Kinane, D.F. 2000. Inducible nitric oxide synthase expression in periodontitis. *J. Periodontal Res.* 35(6):369–73.

89. Yerer, M.B., Yapislar, H., Aydogan, S., Yalcin, O., and Baskurt, O. 2004. Lipid peroxidation and deformability of red blood cells in experimental sepsis in rats: The protective effects of melatonin. *Clin. Hemorheol. Microcirc.* 30(2):77–82.
90. Pozo, D., Reiter, R.J., Calvo, J.R., and Guerrero, J.M. 1994. Physiological concentrations of melatonin inhibit nitric oxide synthase in rat cerebellum. *Life Sci.* 55(24):455–60.
91. Storr, M., Koppitz, P., Sibaev, A., Saur, D., Kurjak, M., Franck, H., Schusdziarra, V., and Allescher, H.D. 2002. Melatonin reduces non-adrenergic, non-cholinergic relaxant neurotransmission by inhibition of nitric oxide synthase activity in the gastrointestinal tract of rodents in vitro. *J. Pineal Res.* 33(2):101–8.
92. Aydogan, S., Yerer, M.B., and Goktas, A. 2006. Melatonin and nitric oxide. *J. Endocrinol. Invest.* 29(3):281–7.
93. Bongiorno, D., Ceraulo, L., Ferrugia, M., Filizzola, F., Ruggirello, A., and Liveri, V.T. 2005. Localization and interactions of melatonin in dry cholesterol/lecithin mixed reversed micelles used as cell membrane models. *J. Pineal Res.* 38(4):292–8.
94. Tan, D.X., Manchester, L.C., Reiter, R.J., Qi, W.B., Karbownik, M., and Calvo, J.R. 2000. Significance of melatonin in antioxidative defense system: Reactions and products. *Biol. Signals Recept.* 9(3–4):137–59.
95. Allegra, M., Reiter, R.J., Tan, D.X., Gentile, C., Tesoriere, L., and Livrea, M.A. 2003. The chemistry of melatonin's interaction with reactive species. *J. Pineal Res.* 34(1):1–10.
96. Guzik, T.J., Olszanecki, R., Sadowski, J., Kapelak, B., Rudziński, P., Jopek, A., Kawczynska, A., Ryszawa, N., Loster, J., Jawien, J., Czesnikiewicz-Guzik, M., Channon, K.M., and Korbut, R. 2005. Superoxide dismutase activity and expression in human venous and arterial bypass graft vessels. *J. Physiol. Pharmacol.* 56(2):313–23.
97. Tomás-Zapico, C., and Coto-Montes, A. 2005. A proposed mechanism to explain the stimulatory effect of melatonin on antioxidative enzymes. *J. Pineal Res.* 39(2):99–104.
98. Cutando, A., Arana, C., Gómez-Moreno, G., Escames, G., López, A., Ferrera, M.J., Reiter, R.J., and Acuña-Castroviejo, D. 2007. Local application of melatonin into alveolar sockets of beagle dogs reduces tooth removal-induced oxidative stress. *J. Periodontol.* 78(3):576–83.
99. Czesnikiewicz-Guzik, M., Konturek, S.J., Loster, B., Wisniewska, G., and Majewski, S. 2007. Melatonin and its role in oxidative stress related diseases of oral cavity. *J. Physiol. Pharmacol.* 58(S3):5–19.
100. Kurita-Ochiai, T., Fukushima, K., and Ochiai, K. 1995. Volatile fatty acids, metabolic by-products of periodontopathic bacteria, inhibit lymphocyte proliferation and cytokine production. *J. Dent. Res.* 74(7):1367–73.
101. Yamamoto, M., Fujihashi, K., Hiroi, T., McGhee, J.R., Van Dyke, T.E., and Kiyono, H. 1997. Molecular and cellular mechanisms for periodontal diseases: Role of Th1 and Th2 type cytokines in induction of mucosal inflammation. *J. Periodontal Res.* 32:115–9.
102. Garcia-Mauriño, S., Gonzalez-Haba, M.G., Calvo, J.R., Goberna, R., and Guerrero, J.M. 1998. Involvement of nuclear binding sites for melatonin in the regulation of IL-2 and IL-6 production by human blood mononuclear cells. *J. Neuroimmunol.* 92(1–2):76–84.
103. Cutando, A., and Silvestre, F.J. 1995. Melatonin: Implications at the oral level. *Bull. Group Int. Rech. Sci. Stomatol. Odontol.* 38(3–4):81–6.
104. Maestroni, G.J., and Conti, A. 1990. The pineal neurohormone melatonin stimulates activated CD4+, Thy-1+ cells to release opioid agonist(s) with immunoenhancing and anti-stress properties. *J. Neuroimmunol.* 28(2):167–76.
105. Maestroni, G.J. 2001. The immunotherapeutic potential of melatonin. *Expert Opin. Invest Drugs.* 10(3):467–76.
106. Gómez-Moreno, G., Cutando-Soriano, A., Arana, C., Galindo, P., Bolaños, J., Acuña-Castroviejo, D., and Wang, H.L. 2007. Melatonin expression in periodontal disease. *J. Periodontal Res.* 42(6):536–40.
107. Parkin, D.M., Bray, F., Ferlay, J., and Pisani, P. 2005. Global cancer statistics, 2002. *CA Cancer J. Clin.* 55(2):74–108.
108. Lippman, S.M., and Hong, W.K. 2001. Molecular markers of the risk of oral cancer. *N Engl J Med.* 344(17):1323–6.
109. Scully, C., Beyli, M., Ferreiro, M.C., Ficarra, G., Gill, Y., Griffiths, M., Holmstrup, P., Mutlu, S., Porter, S., and Wray, D. 1998. Update on oral lichen planus: Etiopathogenesis and management. *Crit. Rev. Oral Biol. Med.* 9(1):86–122.
110. Rajentheran, R., McLean, N.R., Kelly, C.G., Reed, M.F., and Nolan, A. 1999. Malignant transformation of oral lichen planus. *Eur. J. Surg. Oncol.* 25(5):520–3.

111. Mignogna, M.D., Fedele, S., Lo Russo, L., Lo Muzio, L., and Bucci, E. 2004. Immune activation and chronic inflammation as the cause of malignancy in oral lichen planus: Is there any evidence? *Oral Oncol.* 40(2):120–30.
112. Coussens, L.M., and Werb, Z. 2002. Inflammation and cancer. *Nature.* 420(6917):860–7.
113. Clevers, H. 2004. At the crossroads of inflammation and cancer. *Cell.* 118(6):671–4.
114. Philip, M., Rowley, D.A., and Schreiber, H. 2004. Inflammation as a tumour promoter in cancer induction. *Semin. Cancer Biol.* 14(6):433–9.
115. Cerutti, P.A. 1994. Oxy-radicals and cancer. *Lancet.* 344(8926):862–3.
116. Burdon, R.H. 1995. Superoxide and hydrogen peroxide in relation to mammalian cell proliferation. *Free Radic. Biol. Med.* 18(4):775–94.
117. Guyton, K.Z., and Kensler, T.W. 1993. Oxidative mechanisms in carcinogenesis. *Br. Med. Bull.* 49(3):523–44.
118. Halliwell, B. 1999. Oxygen and nitrogen are pro-carcinogens. Damage to DNA by reactive oxygen, chlorine and nitrogen species: Measurement, mechanism and the effects of nutrition. *Mutat. Res.* 443(1–2):37–52.
119. Ohshima, H., Tatemichi, M., and Sawa, T. 2003. Chemical basis of inflammation-induced carcinogenesis. *Arch. Biochem. Biophys.* 417(1):3–11.
120. Hussain, S.P., Hofseth, L.J., and Harris, C.C. 2003. Radical causes of cancer. *Nat. Rev. Cancer.* 3(4):276–85.
121. Pinlaor, S., Hiraku, Y., Ma, N., Yongvanit, P., Semba, R., Oikawa, S., Murata, M., Sripa, B., Sithithaworn, P., and Kawanishi, S. 2004. Mechanism of NO-mediated oxidative and nitrative DNA damage in hamsters infected with *Opisthorchis viverrini*: A model of inflammation-mediated carcinogenesis. *Nitric Oxide.* 11(2):175–83.
122. Rasheed, M.H., Beevi, S.S., Rajaraman, R., and Bose, S.J. 2007. Alleviation of oxidative and nitrosative stress following curative resection in patient with oral cavity cancer. *J. Surg. Oncol.* 96(3):194–9.
123. Beevi, S.S., Rasheed, M.H., and Geetha, A. 2007. Evidence of oxidative and nitrosative stress in patients with cervical squamous cell carcinoma. *Clin. Chim. Acta.* 375(1–2):119–23.
124. Reiter, R.J., Tang, L., Garcia, J.J., and Munoz, H.A. 1997. Pharmacological actions of melatonin in oxygen radical pathophysiology. *Life Sci.* 60:2255–71.
125. Bartsch, C., and Bartsch, H. 2006. The anti-tumour activity of pineal melatonin and cancer enhancing life styles in industrialized societies. *Cancer Causes Control.* 17(4):559–71.
126. Scully, C., Field, J.K., and Tanzawa, H. 2000. Genetic aberrations in oral or head and neck squamous cell carcinoma (SCCHN): 1. Carcinogen metabolism, DNA repair and cell cycle control. *Oral Oncol.* 36(3):256–63.
127. Ha, P.K., and Califano, J.A. 2006. Promoter methylation and inactivation of tumour-suppressor genes in oral squamous-cell carcinoma. *Lancet Oncol.* 7(1):77–82.
128. Tamarkin, L., Cohen, M., Roselle, D., Reichert, C., Lippman, M., and Chabner, B. 1981. Melatonin inhibition and pinealectomy enhancement of 7,12-dimethylbenz(*a*)anthracene-induced mammary tumours in the rat. *Cancer Res.* 41:4432–6.
129. Jung, B., and Ahmad, N. 2006. Melatonin in cancer management: Progress and promise. *Cancer Res.* 66(20):9789–93.
130. Sonis, S.T. 1993. Oral complications of cancer therapy. In: DeVita, V.T., Hellma, S., and Rosenberg, S.A. *Cancer: Principles and Practice of Oncology*, 5th ed. JB Lippincott, Philadelphia.
131. Gallagher, J.G. Mucositis. In: Klastersky, J., Schimp, S.C., and Lenn, H.J. 1995. *Handbook of Supportive Care in Cancer.* Marcel Dekker, New York.
132. Sonis, S.T. 2009. Mucositis: The impact, biology and therapeutic opportunities of oral mucositis. *Oral Oncol.* 45(12):1015–20.
133. Martin, M.V. 1993. Irradiation mucositis: A reappraisal. *Eur. J. Cancer B. Oral Oncol.* 29B(1):1–2.
134. Hallahan, D.E., Haimovitz-Friedman, A., Kufe, D.W., Fuks, Z., and Weichselbaum, R.R. 1993. The role of cytokines in radiation oncology. *Important Adv. Oncol.* 71–80.
135. Koj, A. 1996. Initiation of acute phase response and synthesis of cytokines. *Biochim. Biophys. Acta.* 1317(2):84–94.
136. Plevová, P. 1999. Prevention and treatment of chemotherapy- and radiotherapy-induced oral mucositis: A review. *Oral Oncol.* 35(5):453–70.
137. Sharma, R., Tobin, P., and Clarke, S.J. 2005. Management of chemotherapy-induced nausea, vomiting, oral mucositis, and diarrhoea. *Lancet Oncol.* 6(2):93–102.
138. Büntzel, J., Küttner, K., Fröhlich, D., and Glatzel, M. 1998. Selective cytoprotection with amifostine in concurrent radiochemotherapy for head and neck cancer. *Ann. Oncol.* 9(5):505–9.

139. Lissoni, P., Barni, S., Mandalà, M., Ardizzoia, A., Paolorossi, F., Vaghi, M., Longarini, R., Malugani, F., and Tancini, G. 1999. Decreased toxicity and increased efficacy of cancer chemotherapy using the pineal hormone melatonin in metastatic solid tumor patients with poor clinical status. *Eur. J. Cancer*. 35(12):1688–92.
140. Herrstedt, J. 2000. Prevention and management of mucositis in patients with cancer. *Int. J. Antimicrob. Agents*. 16(2):161–3.
141. Lissoni, P., Paolorossi, F., Ardizzoia, A., Barni, S., Chilelli, M., Mancuso, M., Tancini, G., Conti, A., and Maestroni, G.J. 1997. A randomized study of chemotherapy with cisplatin plus etoposide versus chemo-endocrine therapy with cisplatin, etoposide and the pineal hormone melatonin as a first-line treatment of advanced non-small cell lung cancer patients in a poor clinical state. *J. Pineal Res*. 23(1):15–9.
142. Roth, J.A., Kim, B.G., Lin, W.L., and Cho, M.I. 1999. Melatonin promotes osteoblast differentiation and bone formation. *J. Biol. Chem*. 274(31):22041–7.
143. Machida, M., Dubousset, J., Yamada, T., Kimura, J., Saito, M., Shiraishi, T., and Yamagishi, M. 2006. Experimental scoliosis in melatonin-deficient C57BL/6J mice without pinealectomy. *J. Pineal Res*. 41(1):1–7.
144. Simmons, D.J., and Grynpass, M.D. 1990. *Mechanisms of Bone Formation In Vivo*. Telford Press, Caldwell.
145. Ducy, P., Schinke, T., and Karsenty, G. 2000. The osteoblast: A sophisticated fibroblast under central surveillance. *Science*. 289(5484):1501–4.
146. Manolagas, S.C. 2000. Birth and death of bone cells: Basic regulatory mechanisms and implications for the pathogenesis and treatment of osteoporosis. *Endocr. Rev*. 21(2):115–37.
147. Csaba, G., and Baráth, P. 1974. The effect of pinealectomy on the parafollicular cells of the rat thyroid gland. *Acta Anat. (Basel)*. 88(1):137–46.
148. Csaba, G., and Bókay, J. 1977. The effect of melatonin and corpus pineal extract on serum electrolytes in the rat. *Acta Biol. Acad. Sci. Hung*. 28(1):143–4.
149. Kiss, J., Bánhegyi, D., and Csaba, G. 1969. Endocrine regulation of blood calcium level. II. Relationship between the pineal body and the parathyroid glands. *Acta Med. Acad. Sci. Hung*. 26(4):363–70.
150. Hakanson, D.O., and Bergstrom, W.H. 1981. Phototherapy-induced hypocalcemia in newborn rats: Prevention by melatonin. *Science*. 214(4522):807–9.
151. Hakanson, D.O., Penny, R., and Bergstrom, W.H. 1987. Calcemic responses to photic and pharmacologic manipulation of serum melatonin. *Pediatr. Res*. 22(4):414–6.
152. Hakanson, D.O., and Bergstrom, W.H. 1990. Pineal and adrenal effects on calcium homeostasis in the rat. *Pediatr. Res*. 27(6):571–3.
153. Nakade, O., Koyama, H., Ariji, H., Yajima, A., and Kaku, T. 1999. Melatonin stimulates proliferation and type I collagen synthesis in human bone cells in vitro. *J. Pineal Res*. 27(2):106–10.
154. Koyama, H., Nakade, O., Takada, Y., Kaku, T., Lau, K.H. 2002. Melatonin at pharmacologic doses increases bone mass by suppressing resorption through down-regulation of the RANKL-mediated osteoclast formation and activation. *J. Bone Miner. Res*. 17(7):1219–29.
155. Guardia, J., Gómez-Moreno, G., Ferrera, M.J., and Cutando, A. 2009. Evaluation of Effects of Topic Melatonin on Implant Surface at 5 and 8 Weeks in Beagle Dogs. *Clin. Implant. Dent. Relat. Res*. ([Epub ahead of print] PubMed PMID: 19681939).
156. Jockers, R., Maurice, P., Boutin, J.A., and Delagrange, P. 2008. Melatonin receptors, heterodimerization, signal transduction and binding sites: What's new? *Br. J. Pharmacol*. 154(6):1182–95.
157. Suzuki, A., Guicheux, J., Palmer, G., Miura, Y., Oiso, Y., Bonjour, J.P., and Caverzasio, J. 2002. Evidence for a role of p38 MAP kinase in expression of alkaline phosphatase during osteoblastic cell differentiation. *Bone*. 30(1):91–8.
158. Bordt, S.L., McKeon, R.M., Li, P.K., Witt-Enderby, P.A., and Melan, M.A. 2001. N1E-115 mouse neuroblastoma cells express MT1 melatonin receptors and produce neurites in response to melatonin. *Biochim. Biophys. Acta*. 1499(3):257–64.
159. Witt-Enderby, P.A., MacKenzie, R.S., McKeon, R.M., Carroll, E.A., Bordt, S.L., and Melan, M.A. 2000. Melatonin induction of filamentous structures in non-neuronal cells that is dependent on expression of the human mt1 melatonin receptor. *Cell. Motil. Cytoskeleton*. 46(1):28–42.
160. Radio, N.M., Doctor, J.S., and Witt-Enderby, P.A. 2006. Melatonin enhances alkaline phosphatase activity in differentiating human adult mesenchymal stem cells grown in osteogenic medium via MT2 melatonin receptors and the MEK/ERK (1/2) signalling cascade. *J. Pineal Res*. 40(4):332–42.
161. Reppert, S.M., Godson, C., Mahle, C.D., Weaver, D.R., Slaugenhaupt, S.A., and Gusella, J.F. 1995. Molecular characterization of a second melatonin receptor expressed in human retina and brain: The Mel1b melatonin receptor. *Proc. Natl. Acad. Sci. USA*. 92(19):8734–8.

162. Satomura, K., Tobiume, S., Tokuyama, R., Yamasaki, Y., Kudoh, K., Maeda, E., and Nagayama, M. 2007. Melatonin at pharmacological doses enhances human osteoblastic differentiation in vitro and promotes mouse cortical bone formation in vivo. *J. Pineal Res.* 42(3):231–9.
163. Suzuki, N., Somei, M., Seki, A., Reiter, R.J., and Hattori, A. 2008. Novel bromomelatonin derivatives as potentially effective drugs to treat bone diseases. *J. Pineal Res.* 45(3):229–34.
164. Suda, T., Takahashi, N., Udagawa, N., Jimi, E., Gillespie, M.T., and Martin, T.J. 1999. Modulation of osteoclast differentiation and function by the new members of the tumor necrosis factor receptor and ligand families. *Endocr. Rev.* 20(3):345–57.
165. Teitelbaum, S.L. 2000. Bone resorption by osteoclasts. *Science.* 289(5484):1504–8.
166. Krane, S.M. 2002. Genetic control of bone remodelling—Insights from a rare disease. *N. Engl. J. Med.* 347(3):210–2.
167. Cardinali, D.P., Ladizesky, M.G., Boggio, V., Cutrera, R.A., and Mautalen, C. 2003. Melatonin effects on bone: Experimental facts and clinical perspectives. *J. Pineal Res.* 34(2):81–7.
168. Uslu, S., Uysal, A., Oktem, G., Yurtseven, M., Tanyalçin, T., and Başdemir, G. 2007. Constructive effect of exogenous melatonin against osteoporosis after ovariectomy in rats. *Anal. Quant. Cytol. Histol.* 29(5):317–25.
169. Suzuki, N., and Hattori, A. 2002. Melatonin suppresses osteoclastic and osteoblastic activities in the scales of goldfish. *J. Pineal Res.* 33(4):253–8.
170. Yamada, J. 1961. Studies on the structure and growth of the scales in the goldfish. *Mem. Fac. Fish Hokkaido Univ.* 9:181–226.
171. Nishimoto, S.K., Araki, N., Robinson, F.D., and Waite, J.H. 1992. Discovery of bone gamma-carboxyglutamic acid protein in mineralized scales. The abundance and structure of *Lepomis macrochirus* bone gamma-carboxyglutamic acid protein. *J. Biol. Chem.* 267(16):11600–5.
172. Lehane, D.B., McKie, N., Russell, R.G., and Henderson, I.W. 1999. Cloning of a fragment of the osteonectin gene from goldfish, *Carassius auratus*: Its expression and potential regulation by estrogen. *Gen. Comp. Endocrinol.* 114(1):80–7.
173. Onozato, H., and Watabe, N. 1979. Studies on fish scale formation and resorption. III. Fine structure and calcification of the fibrillary plates of the scales in *Carassius auratus* (Cypriniformes: Cyprinidae). *Cell Tissue Res.* 201(3):409–22.
174. Berg, A. 1968. Studies on the metabolism of calcium and strontium in freshwater fish. I. Relative contribution of direct and intestinal absorption. *Mem. Ist. Ital. Idrobiol.* 23:161–196.
175. Persson, P., Sundell, K., Bjornsson, B.T., and Lundqvist, H. 1998. Calcium metabolism and osmoregulation during sexual maturation of river running Atlantic salmon. *J. Fish Biol.* 52:334–349.
176. Fraser, J.H., Helfrich, M.H., Wallace, H.M., and Ralston, S.H. 1996. Hydrogen peroxide, but not superoxide, stimulates bone resorption in mouse calvariae. *Bone.* 19(3):223–6.
177. Okatani, Y., Wakatsuki, A., Reiter, R.J., and Miyahara, Y. 2002. Melatonin reduces oxidative damage of neural lipids and proteins in senescence-accelerated mouse. *Neurobiol. Aging.* 23(4):639–44.
178. Maldonado, M.D., Murillo-Cabezas, F., Terron, M.P., Flores, L.J., Tan, D.X., Manchester, L.C., and Reiter, R.J. 2007. The potential of melatonin in reducing morbidity–mortality after craniocerebral trauma. *J. Pineal Res.* 42(1):1–11.
179. Simon, Z., and Watson, P.A. 2002. Biomimetic dental implants—New ways to enhance osseointegration. *J. Can. Dent. Assoc.* 68(5):286–8.
180. Zechner, W., Tangl, S., Tepper, G., Fürst, G., Bernhart, T., Haas, R., Mailat, G., and Watzek, G. 2003. Influence of platelet-rich plasma on osseous healing of dental implants: A histologic and histomorphometric study in minipigs. *Int. J. Oral Maxillofac. Implants.* 18(1):15–22.
181. Takechi, M., Tatehara, S., Satomura, K., Fujisawa, K., and Nagayama, M. 2008. Effect of FGF-2 and melatonin on implant bone healing: A histomorphometric study. *J. Mater. Sci. Mater. Med.* 19(8):2949–52.
182. Muñoz, F., López-Peña, M., Miño, N., Gómez-Moreno, G., Guardia, J., and Cutando, A. 2009. Topical application of melatonin and growth hormone accelerates bone healing around dental implants in dogs. *Clin. Implant. Dent. Relat. Res.*
183. Orsini, G., Scarano, A., Piattelli, M., Piccirilli, M., Caputi, S., and Piattelli, A. 2006. Histologic and ultrastructural analysis of regenerated bone in maxillary sinus augmentation using a porcine bone–derived biomaterial. *J. Periodontol.* 77(12):1984–90.
184. McAllister, B.S., and Haghighat, K. 2007. Bone augmentation techniques. *J. Periodontol.* 78(3):377–96.
185. Calvo-Guirado, J.L., Gómez-Moreno, G., Barone, A., Cutando, A., Alcaraz-Baños, M., Chiva, F., López-Marí, L., and Guardia, J. 2009. Melatonin plus porcine bone on discrete calcium deposit implant surface stimulates osteointegration in dental implants. *J. Pineal Res.* 47(2):164–72.

186. Naguib, M., Gottumukkala, V., and Goldstein, P.A. 2007. Melatonin and anesthesia: A clinical perspective. *J. Pineal Res.* 42(1):12–21.
187. Marczynski, T.J., Yamaguchi, N., Ling, G.M., and Grodzinska, L. 1964. Sleep induced by the administration of melatonin (5-methoxyn-acetyltryptamine) to the hypothalamus in unrestrained cats. *Experientia.* 20(8):435–7.
188. Lerner, A.B., and Case, J.D. 1960. Melatonin. *Fed. Proc.* 19:590–2.
189. Isik, B., Baygin, O., and Bodur, H. 2008. Premedication with melatonin vs midazolam in anxious children. *Paediatr. Anaesth.* 18(7):635–41.
190. Antón-Tay, F., Díaz, J.L., and Fernández-Guardiola, A. 1971. On the effect of melatonin upon human brain. Its possible therapeutic implications. *Life Sci.* 10(15):841–50.
191. Clark, D.L., and Rosner, B.S. 1973. Neurophysiologic effects of general anesthetics. The electroencephalogram and sensory evoked responses in man. *Anesthesiology.* 38(6):564–82.
192. Naguib, M., Baker, M.T., Spadoni, G., and Gregerson, M. 2003. The hypnotic and analgesic effects of 2-bromomelatonin. *Anesth. Analg.* 97(3):763–8.
193. Coloma, F.M., and Niles, L.P. 1988. Melatonin enhancement of [3H]-gamma-aminobutyric acid and [3H]muscimol binding in rat brain. *Biochem. Pharmacol.* 37(7):1271–4.
194. Niles, L.P., Pickering, D.S., and Arciszewski, M.A. 1987. Effects of chronic melatonin administration on GABA and diazepam binding in rat brain. *J. Neural Transm.* 70(1–2):117–24.
195. Rosenstein, R.E., and Cardinali, D.P. 1986. Melatonin increases in vivo GABA accumulation in rat hypothalamus, cerebellum, cerebral cortex and pineal gland. *Brain Res.* 398(2):403–6.
196. Shavali, S., Ho, B., Govitrapong, P., Sawlom, S., Ajjimaporn, A., Klongpanichapak, S., and Ebadi, M. 2005. Melatonin exerts its analgesic actions not by binding to opioid receptor subtypes but by increasing the release of beta-endorphin an endogenous opioid. *Brain Res. Bull.* 64(6):471–9.
197. Naguib, M., Hammond, D.L., Schmid, P.G., Baker, M.T., Cutkomp, J., Queral, L., and Smith, T. 2003. Pharmacological effects of intravenous melatonin: Comparative studies with thiopental and propofol. *Br. J. Anaesth.* 90(4):504–7.
198. Budhiraja, S., and Singh, J. 2005. Adjuvant effect of melatonin on anesthesia induced by thiopental sodium, ketamine, and ether in rats. *Methods Find. Exp. Clin. Pharmacol.* 27(10):697–9.
199. Kitahata, L.M., and Saberski, L. 1992. Are barbiturates hyperalgesic? *Anesthesiology.* 77(6):1059–61.
200. Deady, J.E., Koblin, D.D., Eger, E.I. 2nd, Heavner, J.E., and D'Aoust, B. 1981. Anesthetic potencies and the unitary theory of narcosis. *Anesth. Analg.* 60(6):380–4.
201. Samarkandi, A., Naguib, M., Riad, W., Thalaj, A., Alotibi, W., Aldammas, F., and Albassam, A. 2005. Melatonin vs. midazolam premedication in children: A double-blind, placebo-controlled study. *Eur. J. Anaesthesiol.* 22(3):189–96.
202. Naguib, M., and Samarkandi, A.H. 2000. The comparative dose–response effects of melatonin and midazolam for premedication of adult patients: A double-blinded, placebo-controlled study. *Anesth. Analg.* 91(2):473–9.
203. Naguib, M., and Samarkandi, A.H. 1999. Premedication with melatonin: A double-blind, placebo-controlled comparison with midazolam. *Br. J. Anaesth.* 82(6):875–80.
204. Owens, J.A., Rosen, C.L., and Mindell, J.A. 2003. Medication use in the treatment of pediatric insomnia: Results of a survey of community-based pediatricians. *Pediatrics.* 111:628–35.
205. Sweis. D. 2005. The uses of melatonin. *Arch. Dis. Child. Educ. Pract. Ed.* 90: 74–77.
206. Ozçelik, B., Serin, I.S., Basbug, M., Uludag, S., Narin, F., and Tayyar, M. 2003. Effect of melatonin in the prevention of post-operative adhesion formation in a rat uterine horn adhesion model. *Hum. Reprod.* 18(8):1703–6.
207. Hanania, M., and Kitain, E. 2002. Melatonin for treatment and prevention of postoperative delirium. *Anesth. Analg.* 94(2):338–9.
208. Cronin, A.J., Keifer, J.C., Davies, M.F., King, T.S., and Bixler, E.O. 2000. Melatonin secretion after surgery. *Lancet.* 356(9237):1244–5.
209. Naguib, M., Baker, M.T., Spadoni, G., and Gregerson, M. 2003. The hypnotic and analgesic effects of 2-bromomelatonin. *Anesth. Analg.* 97(3):763–8.
210. Reber, A., Huber, P.R., Ummenhofer, W., Gürtler, C.M., Zurschmiede, C., Drewe, J., and Schneider, M. 1998. General anaesthesia for surgery can influence circulating melatonin during daylight hours. *Acta Anaesthesiol. Scand.* 42(9):1050–6.
211. Kärkelä, J., Vakkuri, O., Kaukinen, S., Huang, W.Q., and Pasanen, M. 2002. The influence of anaesthesia and surgery on the circadian rhythm of melatonin. *Acta Anaesthesiol. Scand.* 46(1):30–6.
212. McIntyre, I.M., Norman, T.R., Burrows, G.D., and Armstrong, S.M. 1993. Alterations to plasma melatonin and cortisol after evening alprazolam administration in humans. *Chronobiol. Int.* 10(3):205–13.

14 Melatonin as a Potential Treatment of Gastrointestinal Diseases

George A. Bubenik

CONTENTS

14.1 INTRODUCTION

It has been more than 10 years since the publication of the first edition of the book *Melatonin in the Promotion of Health.* The research performed since that time led to a great expansion of our knowledge about utilization of melatonin in treatment as well as prevention of various gastrointestinal (GIT) and hepatobiliary (HB) diseases. Because of the increase in the amount of new data, I have concentrated my review mostly on the literature published in the past 5 to 10 years.

Melatonin was first detected in the bovine pineal gland [1] but was later identified in the entire GIT system [2]. The research elucidating the role of this indolalkylamine in the function of the GIT and the physiology and pathology of the HB system indicated that it is prevalently GIT melatonin and not pineal melatonin that is participating in these functions [3–5]. It has been calculated by Huether [6] that at any time of the day, the GIT contains around 400 times more melatonin than the pineal gland. Furthermore, concentrations of melatonin in the GIT and the HB tissues exceed those in plasma by 10 to 100 times [3,7–9]. In addition to being produced in the enterochromaffin cells of the gut [10], melatonin may also be produced by the intestinal flora [11,12], and its concentration in the intestinal segments is modulated by food intake [7,13]. Therefore, GIT melatonin can act not only as an endocrine but also as a paracrine, autocrine, and luminal hormone [14]. Melatonin increases mucosal blood flow by relieving the spastic actions of the melatonin precursor serotonin [15]. Melatonin also stimulates the function of the immune system and fosters re-epithelization of mucous membranes. Finally, as an effective scavenger of free radicals [16,17], melatonin may alleviate numerous pathological conditions of the alimentary tract. Because of these properties melatonin was effective in animal and human experiments as a preventive or therapeutic remedy in numerous pathological conditions of the GIT and HB systems [18], such as the oral cavity, esophagus, stomach, pancreas, liver, gall bladder, ulcerative colitis (UC), irritable bowel syndrome (IBS), children's colic, and GI cancer. The following chapter presents the results of those investigations.

14.2 ORAL CAVITY

As an increase of melatonin in plasma and saliva was found in diabetic patients, it was speculated that this elevation is connected with melatonin function as a scavenger of free radicals [16,19]. Furthermore, it has been suggested, that an increase of melatonin in the saliva may have a protective periodontal function. Finally, because of its strong antioxidant, immunomodulatory, and anticancer properties, melatonin has been proposed to be used for the treatment of the mechanical damage, bacterial, fungal and viral infections of the oral mucosa and periodontal diseases, oral cancer, and alveolar wound caused by tooth extraction [17,20,21].

14.3 ESOPHAGUS

Mucosal injury to esophagus by a hydrochloric acid or pepsin reflux from the stomach (gastroesophageal reflux disease, or GERD), of which the most prominent symptom is "heartburn," is a common disease affecting up to 44% of the adult U.S. population [22]. The dangerous complications of GERD are esophageal ulcer, esophageal hemorrhage, esophageal stricture, Barrett's esophagus, and esophageal adenocarcinoma. The cause of GERD is a lack of resistance to corrosive and proteolytic action of gastric acid/pepsin and biliary secretion as well as a malfunction of lower esophageal and pyloric sphincters. The esophageal defense mechanisms include an increase of mucous and salivary secretion as well as an increase in the production of epidermal growth factor and prostaglandins [23]. It has been established that cyclooxygenase and nitric oxide synthase are a part of the paracrine system protecting the mucosal membrane, but the entire defense mechanism of the esophageal protection has not yet been fully elucidated. Particularly little is know about the role of melatonin, a strong antioxidant protecting the mucosa of the entire alimentary tract [24]. In the study of Konturek et al. [24] acute esophageal lesions were induced by perfusion with an acid pepsin solution using a tube inserted via oral cavity into mid-esophagus. Such perfusion caused substantial injury as compared with the infusion of saline. Pretreatment with melatonin significantly reduced the extent of injury, increased mucosal blood flow, elevated mucosal content of PGE_2, while decreasing the levels of TNF-α. Recent research study in humans revealed that the night-time melatonin serum concentration was highest in healthy subjects (34.7 ± 4.8 pg/ml). In patients with GERD and with recurrent duodenal ulcer, the serum melatonin concentration was only 27.2 ± 8.5 and 25.5 ± 6.2 pg/ml, respectively. The authors concluded that a high concentration of melatonin in serum is needed to prevent peptic changes in esophageal and duodenal mucosa [25]. In a human study, a dietary supplementation containing 2.5 mg of melatonin, L-tryptophan (TRP), vitamin B12, methionine, and betaine given to a group of patients lead to a complete regression of GERD symptoms in 100% of subjects. On the other hand, patients treated with omeprazole (a proton pump inhibitor, or PPI) reported a decrease of GERD symptoms in only 65.7%. In addition, whereas melatonin has virtually no significant side effects, PPIs have potentially serious side effects. In rats, the complete suppression of hydrochloric acid secretion by PPI led to carcinogenesis detected in enterochromaffin-like cells [26]. The effectiveness of melatonin as a remedy for GERD has been ascribed to their capacity to inhibit a secretion of gastric acid, promote healing of ulcers as well as inhibit nitric oxide synthesis [26]. A formula, known under the commercial name Protexid and containing melatonin, vitamin B12, and several amino acids, is produced and sold for treatment of GERD by the U.S. firm Eades Nutritional (Ricardo de Souza Pereira, personal communication).

In rats, experimental pretreatment with melatonin significantly reduced hemorrhagic lesions and decreased esophageal lipid peroxidation, which were aggravated by reflux esophagitis (RE). In addition, melatonin replenished levels of superoxide dismutase and glutathione, which was detected in RE rats; this indicates that melatonin exhibits free radical scavenging properties. Furthermore, whereas melatonin suppressed the up-regulated levels of expression of proinflammatory cytokines such as TNF-α, interleukin (IL) 1β, and IL-10, it also increased levels of an anti-inflammatory cytokine IL-10. The failure of the MT_2 receptor antagonist luzindole to block the protective effect of melatonin indicates that melatonin is acting in a receptor-independent fashion [27].

The experimental as well as clinical studies indicate the potential capacity of melatonin in the prevention or treatment of GERD or other RE diseases.

14.4 STOMACH

Melatonin was successful in preventing damage on the gastric mucosa in many studies in which a variety of models (such as overcrowding, ethanol, acetic acid, water immersion and restraint stress, nonsteroidal anti-inflammatory drugs [NSAIDs], or alendronate) were used. One of the first investigations of the role of melatonin in the prevention and treatment of gastric ulcers was done in young pigs, in which ulcers occurred spontaneously, probably due to overcrowding. In this study, the lowest concentrations of melatonin in the plasma and stomach tissues were found in pigs that exhibited the most severe ulceration. On the other hand, a 4-week administration of melatonin in the diet (5 mg/kg food) significantly reduced the incidence and severity of gastric ulcers. It was concluded that a development of ulcers may be due to the deficiency of melatonin concentration in the plasma and in the gastric tissue itself [28]. In experiments with human patients, 5 mg melatonin or placebo was given daily for 12 weeks to 60 patients. Dyspepsic symptoms completely disappeared in 17 patients and partially improved in 9 subjects. Statistical analysis revealed that melatonin significantly improved the ulcer-like dyspepsia [29]. Furthermore, exposure to continuous darkness (which elevates plasma levels of melatonin) significantly reduced gastric inflammation caused by ethanol [30]. Similarly, Konturek et al. [24] reported that stress-induced gastric lesions are showing circadian variations with an increase during the day and decrease during the night. These changes are inversely related to the circadian variation of melatonin. As these changes occurred also after pinealectomy, it was concluded that the prevention of ulceration is mediated by changes in local gastric melatonin. In the recent study by Brzozowski et al. [31], gastric bleeding in rats was induced by water immersion and restrained stress (WRS). In intact animals, the nighttime increase of endogenous melatonin prevented mucosal damage by increased mucosal blood flow, inhibition of gastric secretion of hydrochloric acid, and by scavenging of free radicals. On the other hand, pinealectomy, which reduced melatonin levels, augmented the WRS-induced gastric mucosal lesions. Furthermore, parenteral administration of melatonin to rats prevented ethanol-induced gastric ulceration, depletion of total glutathione, infiltration of polymorphonuclear leukocytes, and a decrease of activity of glutathione reductase. These data indicate that the protection provided by melatonin is presumably due to its antioxidant capacity [32]. Melatonin capacity to prevent ethanol-induced ulceration of the stomach in mice is related to the reduction of matrix metalloproteinases (MMPs), which play an important role in degradation of gastric extracellular matrix protein [33]. The formation of stomach ulcers is connected with the remodeling of extracellular matrix by various MMPs. However, how MMPs are regulated during NSAID-induced gastric ulceration has not been elucidated yet. Melatonin, given to mice at the dose of 60 mg/kg of body weight, was successful in the prevention or healing of acute gastric ulcers, which are characterized by infiltration of inflammatory cells and disruption of gastric mucosa [34]. Alendromate (used for the treatment of osteoporosis under the name of Fosamax) causes serious GIT adverse effects. In the experimental study done on rats, a significant impairment of the stomach function (such as increased acidity, increased lipid peroxidation, elevation of glutathione levels, substantial tissue damage) was induced by a chronic oral administration of alendromate. Conversely, treatments with omeprazole or melatonin prevented such alendromate-induced gastric damage [35]. Treatments with omeprazole or melatonin prevented these damages, with melatonin being more efficient in protecting the mucosa than omeprazole. Conversely, intraperitoneal injections of alendronate did not induce much gastric irritation [35]. Finally, serosal application of acetic acid caused mucosal ulceration accompanied by a reduction of mucosal microcirculation. Daily intragastric treatment with melatonin (25 mg/kg/day) or melatonin precursor TRP (100 mg/kg) accelerated ulcer healing by affecting cyclooxygenase 2 (COX-2)–prostaglandin system, with an accelerated production of protective prostaglandins and an increased mucosal blood flow. After intragastric treatment with the melatonin receptor blocker luzindol (25 mg/kg/day), the acceleration of ulcer healing by melatonin slowed down significantly. Melatonin induced an acceleration of mucosal cell proliferation by releasing gastrin and ghrelin [36]. It can be concluded that experimental studies on animals as well as on humans indicate that melatonin might be effective as a primary or secondary remedy for the treatment of gastritis or gastric ulcers.

14.5 PANCREAS

An exogenous melatonin or TRP, given intraperitonealy, attenuates pancreatitis induced by cerulein or by ischemia/reperfusion. These effects were ascribed to the reduction of lipid peroxidation and the decrease of TNF-α, combined with an increase of plasma IL-10 [37]. Furthermore, melatonin or TRP given intraperitonealy induced a dose-dependent increase of pancreatic amylase secretion as well as a dose-dependent increase of cholecystokinin. The stimulation of pancreatic secretion by melatonin was completely abolished by vagotomy [38]. Moreover, melatonin or TRP induced a dose-dependent elevation of pancreatic protein secretion after a diversion of pancreatobiliary juice. This was accompanied by a dose-dependent increase of plasma levels of cholecystokinin [38]. Melatonin secreted into the gut lumen appears to be involved not only in the acceleration of the healing of chronic gastric ulcers but also in the postprandial secretion of pancreatic enzymes [39]. Experimental pancreatitis (induced by continuous infusion of cerulein at a rate of 15 mg/kg/h) was alleviated by melatonin delivered by intraperitoneal route at doses of 2 or 10 mg/kg, 30 minutes after the cerulein administration. Melatonin reduced the local prostaglandin production toward the control levels. Higher doses of melatonin were somewhat more effective in preventing pancreatitis than lower ones [40]. In the most recent experiment, an acute pancreatitis was induced by intraperitoneal injections of L-arginine. A subsequent administration of melatonin significantly improved the nucleic acid content, rate of DNA synthesis, pancreatic protein, and amylase contents. Histopathological examination demonstrated that melatonin treatment promotes spontaneous regeneration of pancreatic tissues [41]. Finally, Jaworek et al. [42] reported that melatonin strongly stimulated secretion of pancreatic amylase when applied intraperitonealy or injected into gut lumen. Using immunohistology, melatonin receptors MT_2 were localized not only in the pancreatic tissues but also in the duodenum, stomach, and colon. The highest concentrations of MT_2 melatonin receptors were observed in *Muscularis mucosae* and *Muscularis externa.* The highest density of MT_2 receptors was detected in the colon. Nighttime levels of melatonin were higher than the daytime levels in the stomach, duodenum, and pancreas, but no circadian variation was observed in the colon [43].

14.6 LIVER

Melatonin reduced the damage caused to the liver by the administration of carbon tetrachloride. Hepatic damage such as a lipid dystrophy, massive necrosis of hepatocytes, an increase of free and conjugated bilirubin, elevation of many hepatic enzymes, as well as NO accumulation in the liver and in the blood were all significantly ameliorated by melatonin [44]. In another study, melatonin prevented liver cirrhosis in rats induced by a long-term administration of thioacetamide [45]. Fasting plasma level of melatonin is five time higher in patients with liver cirrhosis (LC), as compared with healthy controls. This difference is probably due to impaired degradation in the liver and the shunting of portal blood around the liver due to formation of portosystemic collaterals [46].

Finally, in one in vitro study, melatonin prevented in a dose- and time-dependent manner the loss of viability, leakage of lactate dehydrogenase, depletion of intracellular glutathione, and malonedealdehyde accumulation, which was caused by the herbicide paraquat [47].

14.7 BILIARY PASSAGES

Gallstones are one of the most common gastroenterological problems requiring surgery. They affect around 10%–15% of the adult U.S. population, which leads to approximately 700,000 cholecystectomies a year. Free radicals can cause damage to the gallbladder epithelium and predispose it to gallstone formation. Melatonin, a potent antioxidant, reduces gall bladder inflammation and gallstone by decreasing the biliary levels of cholesterol. A cholesterol reduction occurs either via a decrease of its absorption across the intestinal epithelium or by an increase of the conversion of cholesterol to bile acids [48]. Melatonin, which passes through the liver on the way from the intestine, concentrates in the bile and reaches an extreme concentration of melatonin (up to a thousand times higher than levels in the gut). It was proposed that those high levels in the bile prevent oxidative damage to the gut mucosa caused by the bile acids [9].

14.8 ULCERATIVE COLITIS

UC is an inflammatory bowel disease affecting around 1 million people in the United States alone. It usually starts between the ages of 15 and 30 years. The etiology and pathogenesis have not been elucidated yet, but it is suspected that they are of autoimmune origin with some contributing genetic factors. Unfortunately, the treatments for this condition are nonspecific, not always effective, and often have serious side effects. Therefore, there is an increasing effort to find an alternative, more tolerable, and less expensive treatment for this disease [49]. In humans, symptoms of UC are chronic abdominal pain, diarrhea, rectal bleeding, loss of appetite, fatigue, and weight loss. The condition is aggravated by stress, spicy food, raw fruits and vegetable, caffeinated drinks, alcohol, and NSAIDs [50]. Since the first study in mice reporting a successful treatment of UC (induced by dextran sodium sulfate) with melatonin [51], there were 14 other studies performed that repeated such experiments. In these animal models, UC was induced by dextran sodium sulfate [51], dinitrobenzene sulfonic acid [52], trinitrobenzene sulfonic acid [53], acetic acid [54,55], and methotrexate [56]. The results of these studies (using four different models of UC) were recently summarized in the exhaustive review of Terry et al. [49]. Thirteen of these studies have demonstrated an alleviation of colitis symptoms after melatonin treatment. Only one of these results showed a worsening of colitis, and it is the one with the highest dose used long-term. Conversely, all short-term administrations of various doses of melatonin used in this study were beneficial [53]. These results may indicate that the effectiveness of melatonin may depend on the sensitivity of the individual subject or on the animal species used. The alleviation of UC symptoms by melatonin were ascribed to a variety of mechanisms: (1) an inhibition of nitric oxide production, (2) an inhibition of COX-2 expression [54], (3) an inhibition of NF-κ activation, (4) the reduction of immunological damage via regulation of macrophage activity, (5) the reduction of proinflammatory cytokines, (6) the reduction of MMP-2 and MMP-9 activity [57], and (7) modulation of signal transduction pathway and apoptosis [58]. In addition, melatonin influences the regulation of gut motility [59]. Finally, melatonin was also proposed as a physiological inhibitor of serotonin [4,60]. In the most recent rodent model, melatonin reversed lipopolysaccharide-induced GIT motility through inhibition of oxidative stress [49].

In addition to animal experiments, there are data from several human studies that indicate that melatonin can reduce inflammation and other pathological symptoms of UC. Jan and Freeman [61] reported that treating children with sleep disorders with melatonin significantly improved their GIT disorders. Furthermore, a German businessman with UC intermittently took melatonin to alleviate symptoms of jet lag when flying to the United States and he reported to his physician that his UC symptoms disappeared each time he used melatonin [62]. Finally, researchers in India reported unpublished data showing some improvement in patients with refractory colitis when treated with melatonin [63]. Conversely, in one case, UC symptoms reappeared in a patient 2 months after he started to take melatonin daily for sleep initiation [64]. These results indicate that the effectiveness of melatonin as a prophylactic or therapeutic remedy may depend on the dose, length of administration, and sensitivity of the subject to melatonin.

14.9 IRRITABLE BOWEL SYNDROME

IBS affects the function of the colon in as many as 20% of the American, British, and Chinese population and is more prevalent in women than men. The characteristic symptoms are abdominal discomfort, cramps and pain, bloating from intestinal gas, impaired motility, and water reabsorption from the intestine causing either diarrhea or constipation. The causes of these conditions are not known, but IBS is aggravated by certain food (such as rye, barley, milk), caffeinated drinks, stress, and menstruation [65]. Unfortunately, none of the drugs used for the treatment of irritable bowel disease (IBD), such as antispasmodics, antidiarrheals, osmotics, cathartics, bulking agents, tranquilizers, or sedatives, is always safe or effective [66]. Melatonin can function as a natural antagonist of serotonin [60], which may predestine it as an effective remedy for the treatment of IBS [14]. In vitro, melatonin relieved spasm caused by serotonin and was effective in the restoration of intestinal motility [15], and in vivo, melatonin improved food transit time in mice [59]. Melatonin in 3-mg dose given for 2–8 weeks was more effective than placebo in improving IBD symptoms and abdominal pain scores, without affecting sleep [67]. Recently, three studies were performed investigating the effect of melatonin on IBD symptoms in human subjects. These studies showed a dramatic, statistically significant decrease of IBD symptoms in the treatment groups. Melatonin, but not placebo, reduced the pain score, the abdominal distention score, the abnormal defecation scores, and the quality of life score (summarized by Terry et al. [49]). The improvement of overall symptoms among IBD symptoms and the quality of life observed in those experiments [68] warrants further adequately designed clinical trials [67].

14.10 COLON CANCER

Colon cancer is the second most common cancer in the Western world. Most colon cancers develop from the precancerous polyps. Fortunately, it takes several years to transform polyps into cancers; thus, a screening test, such as colonoscopy may detect polyps or cancers in time for the treatment. Melatonin exhibits strong immunomodulatory [69], apoptotic [70], and oncostatic properties [8,71] and so may play a role in the diagnosis and treatment of colon cancer. In an in vitro study, melatonin inhibited the proliferation of human colon cancer cells (CaCo-2 line) [72], and in higher doses, melatonin inhibited the growth of the colon adenocarcinoma line [73]. In another study, melatonin decreased the incidence of colon cancer induced by dimethylhydrazine [69]. Several recent reviews summarized the anticarcinogenic effects of melatonin [8,74–76]. A rapid progress has been made in the past decade regarding the role of melatonin as an oncostatic agent, but as some contradictory effects were reported, more research is needed to elucidate its role in the treatment of colon cancer.

14.11 INFANT COLIC

Infant colic is characterized by prolonged crying of an otherwise healthy child. About 20% of children of both sexes experience this condition, which is characterized by the accumulation of gas in their intestines. In breastfeeding mothers, avoidance of certain foods, such as cruciferous vegetable, beans, onions, coffee, and alcohol may reduce the symptoms. The physiological cause of the colic is not known, but it has been hypothesized that it results from the lack of balance between serotonin and melatonin concentrations in the GIT. Melatonin is a natural antagonist of serotonin [59], which in excess causes intestinal spasms [14]. In human children, melatonin levels decline precipitously after birth, but they rebound at about 3 months of life [77], the time when colic usually stops. Because melatonin relieves intestinal spasms, promotes regular motility [59], and initiates sleep [78], this indole was suggested as a treatment for infant colic [79].

14.12 CONCLUSION

Most research studies on the physiological role of melatonin in the GIT indicate that this indolealkylamine is an integral part of the digestive function and has an important role in GIT physiology. Despite the overwhelming evidence derived from hundreds of research studies indicating beneficial effects of melatonin in the prevention and treatment of GIT and HB diseases, only a few clinical investigations were performed up to date. Perhaps, it is now time to "adopt" melatonin as an "orphan drug" and test its effectiveness in humans in large-scale clinical studies. Millions of people are taking melatonin daily without major side effects, which may demonstrate that melatonin is a safe and effective drug against a variety of GIT conditions. However, several studies indicate that the effectiveness of melatonin as a prophylactic or therapeutic remedy may depend on the dose used in the treatment, the length of administration, and the sensitivity of the subject to this remarkable indole [80].

REFERENCES

1. Lerner AA, Case JD, Takahashi Y, Lee TH, Mori W. Isolation of melatonin, the pineal factor that lightens melanocytes. *J Am Chem Soc* 1958; 80: 33.
2. Bubenik GA, Brown GM, Grota LJ. Immunohistological localization of melatonin in the rat digestive tract. *Experientia* 1977; 49: 662–663.
3. Bubenik GA, Brown GM. Pinealectomy reduces melatonin levels in serum but not in the gastrointestinal tract of the rat. *Biol Signals* 1997; 6: 40–44.
4. Bubenik GA. Gastrointestinal melatonin: Localization, function and clinical relevance. *Dig Dis Sci* 2002; 47: 2336–2348.
5. Martin MT, Azpiroz F, Malagelada JR. Melatonin and the gastrointestinal tract. *Therapie* 1998; 53: 453–458.
6. Huether G. The contribution of extrapineal sites of melatonin to circulating melatonin levels in higher vertebrates. *Experientia* 1993; 49: 665–670.
7. Bubenik GA, Hacker RR, Pang SF, Smith PS. Melatonin concentrations in serum and tissues of porcine gastrointestinal tract and their relationship to the intake and passage of food. *J Pineal Res* 1996; 21: 251–256.
8. Reiter RJ. Mechanisms of cancer inhibition by melatonin. *J Pineal Res* 2004; 37: 213–214.
9. Tan DX, Manchester LC, Reiter RJ, Qi W, Hanes M, Farley NJ. High physiological levels of melatonin in the bile of mammals. *Life Sci* 1999; 65: 2523–2529.
10. Raikhlin NT, Kvetnoy AM, Tolkachev VN. Melatonin may be synthetized in enterochromaffine cells. *Nature* 1975; 255: 334–345.
11. Bubenik GA, Hacker RR, Brown GM, Bartos L. Melatonin concentrations in luminal fluid, mucosa and muscularis of the bovine and porcine gastrointestinal tract. *J Pineal Res* 1996; 29: 56–63.
12. Saps M. Ecology of functional gastrointestinal disorders. *J Pediatr Gastroenterol Nutr* 2008; 47: 684–687.
13. Bubenik GA, Pang SF, Cockshut J, Smith PS, Grovum LW, Friendship RM. Circadian variation of portal, arterial and venous blood levels of melatonin in pigs and its relationship to food intake and sleep. *J Pineal Res* 2000; 28: 9–15.
14. Bubenik GA. Therapeutic perspectives of gastrointestinal melatonin. In: *Melatonin: From Molecules to Therapy*. Eds. SR Pandi-Perumal & DP Cardinali. Nova Science Publishing, New York, 2007; pp. 529–524.
15. Bubenik GA. The effect of serotonin, *N*-acetylserotonin and melatonin of spontaneous contraction of isolated rat intestine. *J Pineal Res* 1986; 3: 41–54.
16. Hardeland R, Pandi-Perumal SR. Melatonin, a potent agent in antioxidative defense: Actions as a natural food constituent, gastrointestinal factor, drug and prodrug. *Nutr Metab* 2005; 2: 2–35.

17. Cutando A, Arana C, Gomez-Moreno G, Ferrera MJ, Hardeland R, Pandi-Perumal SR. Local application of melatonin into alveolar sockets of beagle dogs reduces tooth removal-induced oxidative stress. *J Periodontol* 2007; 78: 576–583.
18. Bubenik GA. Treatment of gastrointestinal diseases with melatonin. In: *Contemporary Perspectives in Clinical Pharmacotherapeutics*. Eds, K Kohli, M Gupta, and SJ Thejwany. Elsevier, India, 2006; pp. 356–365.
19. Huether G. Melatonin synthesis in the gastrointestinal tract and the impact of nutritional factors on circulating melatonin. *Ann N Y Acad Sci* 1994; 719: 146–158.
20. Cutando A, Gomez-Moreno G, Ferrera MJ, Vilalba J, Escamez G, Acuna- Castroviejo D. Relationship between salivary melatonin levels and periodontal status in diabetic patients. *J Pineal Res* 2003; 35: 239–244.
21. Czesnikiewicz-Guzik SJ, Konturek SJ, Loster B, Wisniewska G, Majewski S. Melatonin and its role in oxidative stress related diseases of oral cavity. *J Physiol Pharmacol* 2007; 58: Suppl. 3, 5–19.
22. Pereira RS. Regression of gastroesophageal reflux disease symptoms using supplementation with melatonin, vitamins and aminoacids: Comparison with omeprazole. *J Pineal Res* 2006; 41: 195–200.
23. Konturek SJ, Zayachkivska O, Havriluk XO, Brzozowski T, Sliwowski Z, Pawlik. M, Konturek PC, Czesniekiewicz-Guzik M, Gzhegotsky MR, Pawlik WW. Protective influence of melatonin against acute esophageal lesions involves prostaglandins, nitric oxide and sensory nerves. *J Physiol Pharmacol.* 2007; 58: 361–377.
24. Konturek SJ, Brzozowski T, Konturek PC, Zwirska-Korczala K, Reiter RJ. Day/night differences in stress-induced gastric lesions in rats with an intact pineal gland or after pinealectomy. *J Pineal Res* 2007; 44: 408–415.
25. Klupinska G, Wisniewska-Jarosinska M, Harasiuk A, Chojnacki C, Stech-Michalska K, Blasiak J, Reiter RJ, Chojnacki J. Nocturnal secretion of melatonin in patients with upper digestive tract disorders. *J Physiol Pharmacol* 2006; 57: Suppl 5, 41–50.
26. Pereira RS. Regression of esophageal ulcer using a dietary supplement containing melatonin. *J Pineal Res* 2006; 40: 355–356.
27. Lahiri S, Singh P, Singh S, Rasheed N, Palit G, Pant KK. Melatonin protects against experimental reflux esophagitis. *J Pineal Res* 2009; 46: 207–313.
28. Bubenik GA, Ayles HL, Ball RO, Friendship R, Brown GM. Relationship between melatonin levels in plasma and gastrointestinal tissues and the incidence and severity of gastric ulcers in pigs. *J Pineal Res* 1998; 24: 62–66.
29. Klupinska G, Poplawski T, Drzewoski J, Reiter RJ, Blasiak J, Chojnacki J. Therapeutic effect of melatonin in patients with functional dyspepsia. *J Clin Gastroenterol* 2007; 41: 270–274.
30. Cevik H, Erkanli G, Ercan F, Isman CA, Yegen BC. Exposure to continuous darkness ameliorates gastric and colonic inflammation in the rat: Both receptor and non-receptor–mediated processes. *J Gastroenterol Hepatol* 2005; 20: 294–303.
31. Brzozowski T, Zwirska-Korczala K, Konturek PC, Konturek SJ, Sliwowski Z, Pawlik M, Kwiecien S, Drozdowicz D, Mazurkiewicz-Janik M, Bielanski W, Pawlik WW. Role of circadian rhythm and endogenous melatonin in pathogenesis of acute gastric bleeding erosion induced by stress. *J Physiol Pharmacol.* 2007; 58: Suppl. 6, 53–64.
32. Bilici D, Suleyman H, Banoglu ZN, Kiziltunc A, Afci B, Cificioglu A. Melatonin prevents enthanol-induced gastric mucosal damage possibly due to its antioxidant effect. *Digest Dis Sci* 2002; 47: 856–861.
33. Swarnakar S, Mishra A, Ganguly K, Sharma V. Matrix metalloproteinase-9 activity and expression is reduced by melatonin during prevention of ethanol-induced gastric ulcer in mice. *J Pineal Res* 2007; 43: 56–64.
34. Ganguly K, Swarnakar S. Induction of matrix metalloproteinase-9 and -3 in nosteroidal anti-inflammatory drug-induced acute gastric ulcers in mice: Regulation by melatonin. *J Pineal Res* 2009; 47: 43–55.
35. Sener G, Goren FO, Ulusoy NB, Ersoy Y, Arbak S, Dulger GA. Protective effect of melatonin and omeprazol against alendronat-induced gastric damage. *Digest Dis Sci* 2005; 50: 1506–1512.
36. Konturek PC, Konturek SJ, Burnat G, Brzozowski T, Brzozowska I, Reiter RJ. Dynamic physiological and molecular gastric ulcer healing achieved by melatonin and its precursor L-tryptophan in rats. *J Pineal Res* 2008; 45: 180–190.
37. Jaworek J, Leja-Szpak A, Bonior J, Nawrot K, Tomaszewska R, Stachura J, Sendur A, Pawlik W, Brzozowski T, Konturek S. Protective effect of melatonin and its precursor L-tryptophan on acute pancreatitis induced by caerulein overstimulation or ischemia/reperfusion. *J Pineal Res* 2003; 34: 34–40.

38. Jaworek J, Brzozowski T, Konturek SJ. Mini review: Melatonin and its precursor, L-tryptophan: Influence on pancreatic amylase secretion *in vivo* and *in vitro*. *J Pineal Res* 2004; 36: 155–164.
39. Jaworek J, Nawrot K, Konturek SJ, Leja-Szpak A, Thor P, Pawlik W. Mini review: Melatonin as an organoprotector in the stomach and the pancreas. *J Pineal Res* 2005; 38: 73–83.
40. Chen H-M, Chen J-C, Ng C-J, Chiu D-F, Chen M-F. Melatonin reduces pancreatic prostaglandins production and protects against caerulein-induced pancreatitis in rats. *J Pineal Res* 2006; 40: 34–39.
41. Sidhu S, Pandhi P, Malhotra S, Vaiphei K, Khanduja KL. Melatonin treatment is beneficial in pancreatic repair process after experimental acute pancreatitis. *Eur J Pharmacol* 2010; 628: 282–289.
42. Jaworek J, Nawrot-Porabka K, Leja-Szpak A, Bonior J, Szklarczyk J, Kot M, Konturek SJ and Pawlik WW. Melatonin as a modulator of pancreatic enzyme secretion and pancreatoprotector. *J Physiol Pharmacol* 2007; 59, Suppl 6, 65–80.
43. Stebelova K, Antilla K, Manttari S, Saarela S, Zeman M. Immunohistochemical definition of MT_2 receptors and melatonin in the gastrointestinal tissues of rat. *Acta Histochem* 2010; 112: 26–33.
44. Zavodnik LB, Zavodnik IB, Lapshina EA, Belonovskaya EB, Martinchik MDI, Kravchuk RI, Bryszewska M, Reiter RJ. Protective effects of melatonin against carbon tetrachloride hepatotoxicity in rats. *Cell Biochem Funct* 2005; 23: 353–359.
45. Cruz A, Padillo FJ, Torres E, Navarrete CM, Munoz-Castaneda RJ, Caballero FJ, Briceno J, Marchal T, Tunez I, Montilla P, Pera C, Muntane J. Melatonin prevents experimental liver cirrhosis induced by thioacetamide in rats. *J Pineal Res* 2005; 39: 143–150.
46. Celinski K, Konturek PC, Slomka M, Cichoz-Lach H, Gonciarz M, Bielanski W, Reiter RJ, Konturek PC. Altered basal and postprandial plasma melatonin, gastrin, ghrelin, leptin and insulin in patients with liver cirrhosis and portal hypertension without and with oral administration of melatonin or tryptophan. *J Pineal Res* 2009; 46: 408–414.
47. Garcia-Rubio L, Matas P, Miguez MP. Protective effect of melatonin in paraquat-induced toxicity in isolated rat hepatocytes. *Hum Exp Toxicol* 2005; 24: 475–480.
48. Koppisetti S, Jenigiri B, Terron MP, Tengatinni S, Tamura H, Flores LJ, Tan DX, Reiter RJ. Reactive oxygen species and the hypomotility of the gall bladder as targets for treatment of gallstones with melatonin: A review. *Dig Dis Sci* 2008; 53: 2592–2603.
49. Terry PD, Villinger F, Bubenik GA, Sitaraman SV. Melatonin and ulcerative colitis: Evidence, biological mechanisms and future research. *Inflamm Bowel Dis* 2009; 15: 134–140.
50. Hanauer SB. Inflammatory bowel diseases. *New England J Med* 1996; 334, 841–848.
51. Pentney P, Bubenik GA. Melatonin reduces the severity of dextran-induced colitis in mice. *J Pineal Res* 1995; 19: 31–39.
52. Cuzzocrea S, Mazzon E, Serraino I, Lepore W, Terranova M, Ciccolo A, Caputi A. Melatonin reduces dinitrobenzene sulfonic acid–induced colitis. *J Pineal Res* 2001; 30: 1–12.
53. Marquez S, Sanchez-Fidalgo S, Calvo J, Alarcon de la Lastra C, Motilva V. Acutely administered melatonin is beneficial while chronic melatonin treatment aggravates the evolution of TNBS-induced colitis. *J Pineal Res* 2006; 40: 48–55.
54. Dong W-G, Mei Q, Yu JP, Xu J-M, Xiang L, Xu Y. Effects of melatonin in the expression of iNOS and COX-2 in rats model of colitis. *World J Gastroenterol* 2003; 9: 1307–1311.
55. Nosalova V, Zeman M, Cerna S, Navarova J, Zakalova M. Protective effect of melatonin in acetic acid induced colitis in rats. *J Pineal Res* 2007; 42: 364–370.
56. Jahovic N, Sener G, Cevic H, Ersoy Y, Arbak S, Yegen BC. Amelioration of methotrexate-induced enteritis by melatonin in rats. *Cell Biochem Funct* 2004; 22: 169–178.
57. Esposito E, Mazzon E, Riccardi L, Rocco C, Meli R, Cuzzocrea S. Matrix metalloproteinase-9 and metalloproteinase-2 activity and expression is reduced by melatonin during experimental colitis. *J Pineal Res* 2008; 45: 166–173.
58. Mazzon E, Esposito E, Crisafulli LR, Muia C, DiBella P, Meli R, Cuzzocrea S. Melatonin modulates signal transaction pathways and apoptosis in experimental colitis. *J Pineal Res* 2006; 41: 3363–373.
59. Bubenik GA, Dhanvantari S. The influence of melatonin on some parameters of gastrointestinal activity. *J Pineal Res* 1989; 7: 333–344.
60. Bubenik GA, Pang SF. The role of serotonin and melatonin in the gastrointestinal physiology: Ontogeny, regulation of food intake and mutual 5-HT, melatonin feedback. *J Pineal Res* 1994; 16: 91–99.
61. Jan JE, Freeman RD. Re: Mann—Melatonin for ulcerative colitis? *Am J Gastroenterol* 2003; 98: 1446.
62. Mann S. Melatonin for ulcerative colitis? *Am J Gastroenterol* 2003; 98: 1446.
63. Malhotra S, Bhasin D, Shafig N, Pandi P. Drug treatment of ulcerative colitis: Unfractionated heparin, low molecular weight heparin and beyond. *Expert Opin Pharmacother* 2004; 4: 329–334.

64. Maldonado MD, Calvo RL. Melatonin usage in ulcerative colitis: Case report. *J Pineal Res* 2008; 45: 339–340.
65. Song HG, Gwee KA, Moochhala SM, Ho KY. Melatonin improves abdominal pain in irritable bowel syndrome patients, who have sleep disturbances: A randomized double blind placebo controlled study. *GUT* 2005; 54: 1402–1407.
66. Chang F-Y, Lu C-L. Treatment of irritable bowel syndrome using complementary and alternative medicine. *J Clin Med Assoc* 2009; 72: 294–300.
67. Saad RJ, Chey WD. Recent developments in the therapy of irritable bowel syndrome. *Expert Opinion Invest Drugs* 2008; 17: 117–130.
68. Saha L, Malhotra S, Rana S, Basin D, Pandhi PA. A preliminary study on melatonin in irritable bowel syndrome. *J Clin Gastroenterol* 2007; 41: 29–32.
69. Hotchkiss AK, Nelson RJ. Melatonin and the immune function: hype or hypothesis? *Critical Rev Immunol* 20020; 22: 351–371.
70. Anisimov VN, Popovich IG, Zabezhinski MA, Anisimov SV, Gurevich P, Vesnushkin GM, Vinogradova LA. Melatonin as antioxidant, gyroprotector and anticarcinogen. *Biochem Biophys Acta* 2006; 1757: 573–589.
71. Anisimov V, Popovich I, Shtylik A, Zabezhinski M, Ben-Huh H, Gurevich P, Berman V, Tendler Y, Zusman I. Melatonin and colon carcinogenesis. III. Effects of melatonin on proliferative activity and apoptosis in colon mucosa and colon tumours induced by 1,2-dimethylhydrazine in rats. *Exp Toxicol Pathol* 2000; 52: 71–76.
72. Pentney P. An investigation of melatonin in the gastrointestinal tract. Ch. 4. In vitro inhibition of CaCO-2 human colorectal cancer cells by melatonin, melatonin analogues and benzodiazepines. MSc thesis, University of Guelph, Ontario, 1995; pp. 114–169.
73. Fariol M, Venerco Y, Orta X, Castellaos J, Segovia-Silvestre T. *In vitro* effect of melatonin upon cell proliferation in colon adenocarcinoma line. *J Appl Toxicol* 2000; 21: 21–24.
74. Mills E, Wu P, Seeley D, Guyatt G. Melatonin in the treatment of cancer: A systemic review of randomized controls trials and meta-analysis. *J Pineal Res* 2006; 39: 360–366.
75. Wenzel U, Nickel A, Daniel H. Melatonin potentiates flavone-induced apoptosis in human colon cancer cells by increasing the level of glyconic end products. *Int J Cancer* 2005; 116: 236–242.
76. Hoang BX, Shaw DG, Pham PT, Levine SA. Neurobiological effects of melatonin as related to cancer. *Eur J Cancer Prevent* 2007; 16: 511–516.
77. Waldhauser F, Weiszenbacher G, Tatzer E, Gisinger B, Waldhouser M, Schemper M, Frisch H. Alteration in nocturnal serum melatonin levels in human with growth and aging. *J Clin Endocrinol Metabol* 1988; 66: 648–652.
78. Reiter RJ. Pineal melatonin: Cell biology of its synthesis and of its physiological interactions. *Endocrine Rev* 1991; 12: 151–180.
79. Weissbluth L, Weissbluth M. Infant colic: The effect of serotonin and melatonin circadian rhythm on the intestinal smooth muscles. *Med Hypotheses* 2005; 40: 158–164.
80. Reiter RJ, Tan D-X. What constitutes a physiological concentrations of melatonin. *J Pineal Res* 2003; 34: 79–80.

15 The Uses of Melatonin in Anesthesia and Surgery

Hany A. Mowafi and Salah A. Ismail

CONTENTS

15.1 INTRODUCTION

Melatonin is a hormone secreted by the pineal gland. It is available as a dietary supplement, taken primarily for the relief of insomnia. Increasing evidence from human and animal studies suggests that melatonin may be efficacious as a preoperative anxiolytic, a postoperative analgesic, and a preventative for postoperative delirium. It has also been reported to decrease intraocular pressure. Melatonin's high efficacy, wide safety profile in terms of dose, and virtual lack of toxicity make it of interest in anesthetic and surgical practice. This chapter reviews clinical trial data describing the efficacy and safety of melatonin in the perioperative anesthetic and surgical setting. We shall also focus our attention on animal and human experimental studies that concern these issues.

15.2 EFFECT OF ANESTHESIA AND SURGERY ON MELATONIN HOMEOSTASIS

Many studies have demonstrated that general anesthesia, alone or in conjunction with surgery, disturbs the circadian rhythm of melatonin secretion in humans and experimental animals [1–14]. In turn, this disruption in melatonin levels may be the cause of postoperative sleep disorders occurring in patients following anesthesia and surgery [2]. However, the reports of the extent of these alterations in perioperative melatonin homeostasis are inconsistent and contradictory.

General anesthesia administered for hysterectomy operations reduced the nocturnal plasma concentrations of melatonin on the first postoperative night [2]. In another study of patients undergoing orthopedic surgery, the total urinary sulfatoxymelatonin (a major metabolite of melatonin) decreased on the first postoperative evening following thiopental and isoflurane anesthesia [3]. In addition, a reduction in the night/day ratio of urinary sulfatoxymelatonin level was found on the fourth postoperative day after major abdominal surgical procedures. This contradiction may be explained by a phase delay of the sulfatoxymelatonin rhythm [15]. Thus, general anesthesia may influence either the timing or amplitude of postoperative melatonin secretion.

Additionally, the plasma melatonin concentration has been shown to decrease under general anesthesia and surgery [6] and appeared to be unaffected during the immediate postoperative hours [9]. Other studies contradict these findings. For example, general intravenous anesthesia (fentanyl and thiopental or propofol) increased plasma melatonin levels during anesthesia [10] and also during the first 8 hours following propofol and isoflurane anesthesia [1].

There is some evidence that the choice of anesthetic administered, intravenous or inhalational, may influence the plasma melatonin levels, intraoperatively and postoperatively. For example, during the recovery period, the elevation in plasma melatonin levels persisted in patients who had received inhalational isoflurane anesthesia but gradually decreased in those who received intravenous propofol. (In the same study, it appeared that altered melatonin levels following isoflurane and propofol anesthesia may also explain the differences in postoperative sedation scores in those patients.) [1]. According to another report, the type of inhalational anesthetic may influence melatonin homeostasis differently where isoflurane increased the intraoperative plasma level of melatonin, whereas sevoflurane reduced it [5]. It has been also reported that melatonin concentration did not change in the immediate postoperative hours in the children who received intravenous thiopental or midazolam anesthesia for ambulatory surgery [4].

In a further study, no significant effects after extracorporeal artificial circulation using a heart–lung machine for open heart surgery were found on either perioperative circadian melatonin profile or on postoperative mood changes [12]. However, there was a disruption in perioperative melatonin and cortisol secretions in the patients who underwent coronary artery bypass grafting surgery with cardiopulmonary bypass. For that study, a circadian secretion pattern for melatonin, but not for cortisol, was present on the second postoperative day in most patients [16]. There was also severe disturbance in the circadian activity parameters and sleep after both laparoscopic cholecystectomy and major abdominal surgery, with the greater disruption following the latter [13].

Recently, it was found that propofol anesthesia per se decreased the plasma melatonin concentration during the immediate 3 hours and increased it at 20 hours following awakening from anesthesia in rats exposed to normal light conditions [14]. As we can see, the data are growing and somewhat contradictory. Such conflicting findings could be clarified through diverse times of sampling and methods of melatonin level assessment, differences in the duration and/or complexity of surgeries performed, variability in anesthetic techniques, and perioperative treatment. Since most anesthetic drugs and regimens were used in conjunction with surgery and premedication, it is hard to differentiate the effects of general anesthesia from those of surgery and other perioperative medications [11]. Further studies are required to definitely recognize the immediate and late effects of anesthesia and/or surgery on melatonin secretion and its perioperative implications.

15.3 HYPNOTIC EFFECTS OF MELATONIN ADMINISTRATION

Large intravenous melatonin administration induced unconsciousness and produced an electroencephalographic (EEG) pattern similar to that caused by intravenous thiopental and propofol-induced loss of consciousness in rats [17,18]. Moreover, it has been demonstrated that melatonin markedly reduces the mean latency of sleep onset time in young and older subjects [19–21]. Oral melatonin was used as a preoperative medication in both pediatric [22] and adult surgical patients [23,24]. In older patients who were premedicated with oral melatonin 10 mg, preoperative anxiety decreased by 33% compared with a 21% reduction in the placebo group [25].

Naguib et al. [22–24] demonstrated that premedication with sublingual/oral melatonin, unlike midazolam, was associated with preoperative anxiolysis and sedation in adults and children, which did not impair psychomotor skills or impact the quality of recovery. A preoperative melatonin supplement was accompanied with a tendency toward faster recovery and a lower incidence of postoperative excitement than midazolam. Additionally, administration of a single low dose of melatonin (0.3 or 1 mg) did not blunt rapid eye movement (REM) sleep [19]. Furthermore, unlike benzodiazepines, melatonin had no "hangover" effects [19].

In a meta-analysis of randomized controlled studies on the effects of exogenous melatonin on sleep, it was reported that melatonin treatment significantly reduced sleep onset latency, increased sleep efficiency, and increased total sleep duration [26]. Variability in the activity of exogenously administered melatonin could be attributed to differences in the dose/preparation, subject profiles, and the time of administration.

Oral premedication with 0.2 mg/kg melatonin significantly reduced intravenous propofol and thiopental doses required for loss of responses to verbal commands and eyelash stimulation [27]. At the ED_{50} values reflecting loss of responses to verbal command and eyelash reflex, the relative potency of propofol after melatonin premedication was 1.7–1.8 times greater than that of propofol after placebo [27]. Similarly, the relative potency of thiopental following melatonin premedication was 1.3–1.4 times greater than that of thiopental after placebo [27]. In rats, it has been shown that orally administered melatonin potentiated the anesthetic effects of thiopental and ketamine [28]. Furthermore, intraperitoneal injection of 100 mg/kg melatonin significantly reduced the minimum anesthetic concentration of isoflurane in rats by 24%, when compared with controls [29].

Melatonin might be promising as an anesthetic induction agent. Data from in vivo rat models have revealed that melatonin and its analogs, 2-bromomelatonin and phenylmelatonin, have anesthetic properties [17,18,30,31]. Anesthetic doses of melatonin produced effects on processed electroencephalographic variables similar to those of thiopental and propofol in rats [17,18]. The profile of the hypnotic properties of 2-bromomelatonin and phenylmelatonin was similar to that induced by propofol, and the similarity lies on the rapid onset and a short duration of action of these compounds. Unlike propofol and thiopental, melatonin and its analogs have potent antinociceptive effects [17,18]. Evidence suggests that melatonin-induced analgesia could be attributed to the release of β-endorphin [32]. These data support the concept that melatonin, or one of its analogs, might be used as an anesthetic agent. However, in a recent study, melatonin premedication did not enhance sevoflurane induction of anesthesia in women undergoing hysteroscopy as assessed by bispectral index [33].

15.3.1 Melatonin Analgesic Effects

Melatonin has a promising role as an analgesic drug that could be used for alleviating pain associated with surgical procedures.

Several animal studies have shown that systemic melatonin provided dose-dependent antinociception and enhanced morphine analgesia [34]. Moreover, in a further clinical study of female patients undergoing abdominal hysterectomy under epidural anesthesia, Caumo et al. [35] proved that melatonin premedication enhanced postoperative analgesia. In addition, it was demonstrated that melatonin improved tourniquet tolerance and enhanced postoperative analgesia in patients receiving intravenous regional anesthesia [36]. Moreover, after melatonin premedication in patients undergoing cataract surgery under topical anesthesia, the study group had lower pain scores and the fewer subjects who needed fentanyl, with a reduction in the intraoperative fentanyl consumption [37]. In another study, the preoperative melatonin has anxiolytic and postoperative analgesic effects similar to that of clonidine, albeit greater than placebo, in patients undergoing abdominal hysterectomy [38].

In a recent study, oral administration of melatonin the night before and 1 hour before surgery was effective in decreasing both postoperative pain and patient-controlled analgesia with tramadol. It also improved sleep quality and subjective analgesic efficacy in patients undergoing prostatectomy [39]. The precise mechanism and site of action of melatonin antinociception are not completely obvious. However, the mechanism of analgesic effects of melatonin could be through controlling the release of proinflammatory mediators, suppressing the activation of nociceptors and pain perception in the brain and promoting sleep, which is extremely essential for modifying pain perception. Glutamate, γ-aminobutyric acid, opioid neurotransmission, or melatonin receptors may be involved in melatonin's analgesia. Other alternative mechanisms may be through scavenging free radicals or nitric oxide synthase inhibition [40].

15.3.2 Melatonin Anxiolytic Effects

Several studies reported that melatonin was useful for reducing anxiety prior to surgery, presumably due to its sedative effects [23,24,27,37]. The anxiolytic effects of melatonin may be mediated via γ-aminobutyric acid system activation. However, other researchers have been unable to confirm these results. Melatonin did not significantly reduce anxiety in older patients undergoing elective surgery [25]. Similarly, in anxious children, oral 0.5 mg/kg melatonin premedication was similar to placebo for sedation during dental treatment [41]. In a more recent study, it was shown that oral melatonin given to children before surgery in doses up to 0.4 mg/kg was less effective than oral midazolam in reducing preoperative anxiety [42]. However, methodological concerns may have limited the validity of these studies. These include discrepancies in the time of day in which the studies were performed, the lack of valid evaluative tools for anxiety, and variability in the bioavailability of the formulations used could explain this debate.

15.3.3 Melatonin and Postoperative Delirium

Postoperative delirium is a common problem and can be a result of sleep/wake cycle disruptions that occurs in the hospital environment. Plasma melatonin levels, essential in regulation of the sleep/wake rhythm, are decreased after surgery and in hospitalized patients. The reduction in postoperative melatonin secretion triggers sleep disturbances in the older patients, which in turn causes delirium [43]. Profound sleep disturbance in postoperative patients could be prevented by exogenous melatonin supplementation [2]. It may be useful to use melatonin as a treatment or prophylaxis for postoperative delirium in patients with a history of postoperative confusion.

15.3.4 Melatonin and Postoperative Cognitive Dysfunction

It was found that patients with postoperative cognitive dysfunction had poorer sleep but without significant differences in 6-sulfatoxymelatonin levels compared with the control patients who were free from cognitive dysfunction [7,8]. The 6-sulfatoxymelatonin rhythm was disturbed after surgery with a significantly reduced night/day ratio and higher daytime excretion. Further studies are required for more comprehensive analysis of the melatonin rhythm.

15.3.5 Melatonin and Regional Anesthesia

Melatonin is an effective premedication before intravenous regional anesthesia since it reduces patient anxiety, decreases tourniquet-related pain, and improves perioperative analgesia [36]. Although still under trial, melatonin seems to be effective in the relief of postdural puncture headache in humans (Ismail and Mowafi, ongoing study).

15.3.6 Melatonin and Ophthalmologic Surgery

Oral melatonin premedication for patients undergoing cataract surgery under topical anesthesia provided anxiolytic effects, enhanced analgesia, and decreased intraocular pressure, resulting in better operating conditions [37].

15.3.7 Melatonin and Surgical Oxidative Stress

Both experimental and human studies suggest that modulation of oxidative stress that results from surgical intervention can improve organ function and probably reduce morbidity and mortality. Melatonin has potent antioxidant properties. As proven experimentally, it is more effective than the classical antioxidants with minimal toxicity. Studies showed that melatonin reduced the oxidative damage related to surgical insults and ischemia/reperfusion and improved morbidity and mortality [44].

The effect of melatonin as an antioxidant in relation to surgery on humans has only been tested in newborns. The drug was safe and reduced oxidative stress caused by surgery. Melatonin reduced cytokines levels and modified serum inflammatory parameters in neonates undergoing major operation with a significant improvement in clinical parameters [45]. Similar beneficial effects of melatonin in the adult population remain to be documented.

15.3.8 Melatonin and Organ Transplantation

Melatonin is a versatile preparation that has immunostimulatory, antioxidative, antiapoptotic, antibiotic, and antiviral properties that could modulate several pathological and physiological processes associated with organ transplantation. It could protect against ischemia–reperfusion injury and prolong graft survival following transplantation, as demonstrated in animal models [46]. However, more studies are required to evaluate melatonin's beneficial effects for transplantation of different organs and to assess it as a potential adjuvant therapeutic drug in humans.

15.3.9 Melatonin and Wound Healing

In 2003, Soybir et al. demonstrated that the administration of melatonin in rats significantly improved angiogenesis and wound healing, probably secondary to release of growth factors [47]. However, further randomized clinical trials are required before final confirmation of its beneficial effects especially in patients with disturbed healing.

15.3.10 Melatonin and Bone Healing

It has been shown that both fibroblast growth factor 2 and melatonin have similar stimulatory effects on osteogenesis. Together, they synergistically enhanced new bone formation around titanium implants in rats [48]. However, further clinical trials in humans may be performed to confirm this effect.

15.3.11 Melatonin and Postpinealectomy Syndrome

It had been reported that the tumors of the pineal gland distinctly decreased the circadian rhythm of melatonin before surgery. The lack of melatonin rhythm in these tumors may help in the diagnosis of this condition. Moreover, postoperative melatonin deficiency could justify melatonin supplementation to prevent a sleep/wake cycle disturbance occurring following surgery and the probable post-pinealectomy syndrome in patients with resected pineal gland [49].

15.3.12 Melatonin and Intra-Abdominal Adhesions

Melatonin may be a valuable agent in preventing peritoneal adhesions in rats [50]. Intra-abdominal adhesions following abdominal surgery could induce intestinal obstruction or infertility. However, randomized clinical studies are required in humans to evaluate its potential clinical benefits.

15.3.13 Melatonin and Major Vascular Surgery

Treatment of patients undergoing major aortic surgery with intravenous melatonin in a dose up to 60 mg intraoperatively was demonstrated to be safe and lacks adverse effects [51]. Melatonin may decrease oxidative damage resulting from this surgery, but randomized clinical trials are required before definitive conclusions can be drawn regarding its clinical benefit.

15.3.14 Melatonin and Cardiac Surgery

It has been found that melatonin may have a protective effect against ischemic–reperfusion injury during coronary artery bypass grafting, as high plasma levels of melatonin may be associated with low levels of reperfusion injury markers [52]. However, additional studies may be required for the preoperative administration of melatonin in cardiac surgery patients with cardiopulmonary bypass to improve myocardial protection. Melatonin administration effectively reduced postoperative pericardial adhesions in dogs [53]. The use of melatonin for the prophylaxis of pericardial adhesions following cardiac operations in human subjects warrants further investigations.

15.3.15 Melatonin and Hemorrhagic Shock

Treatment with melatonin suppresses the release of the proinflammatory cytokines, tumor necrosis factor (TNF)-α and interleukin (IL)-6. The levels of markers of organ injury associated with hemorrhagic shock are decreased; therefore, ameliorating hemorrhagic shock–induced organ damage in rats [54]. However, further studies are required to elucidate these effects in patients with hemorrhagic shock.

15.3.16 Melatonin and Sedation during Diagnostic Procedures

Clinically, it has been used to induce sleep to facilitate performing electroencephalography (EEG) in children [55]. Melatonin may also be useful for magnetic resonance imaging (MRI) examination and has been reported to be successful in 55%–76% of children [56]. However, this study included series of cases, lacking control group for comparison.

In a further study, melatonin tablets of 3 or 6 mg doses given 10 minutes before MRI were not valuable for sedation of children. Children tended to be sedated more quickly after melatonin and were slower to recover, although statistically insignificant. These findings may denote that there was wide variation in the onset of sedation following melatonin premedication. Additionally, interindividual variations in children who need MRI and contrasting criteria for sedation could explain some of the differences in sedation times [57].

15.3.17 Melatonin and Thermal Injury

There is good evidence that melatonin therapy possesses potential advantage in reducing the morbidity and mortality in patients with thermal injury [58]. It is a powerful free radical scavenger and antioxidant, particularly in the skin. It has some influence on intracellular organelles that improve the cells' ability to resist damage associated with burn. Melatonin has also immunomodulatory and inhibitory effects on proinflammatory cytokines. Therefore, it ameliorates the immune disorders that often result following thermal injury. Finally, melatonin triggers sleep mechanisms that are disturbed in patients with burn.

15.3.18 Melatonin and Liver Resection

Experimental data suggest that preoperative melatonin, as a potent immunomodulator and antioxidant, would decrease postoperative infectious and noninfectious complications induced by major abdominal surgery. Therefore, a clinical trial is going to determine if melatonin can improve the general outcome after liver resection [59].

Because of melatonin's antioxidant effects and its capacity to cross physiological barriers, it may be administered therapeutically against surgically induced oxidative stress. In the work of Ochoa et al., who studied the effects of melatonin during cardiopulmonary bypass surgery, their findings provided grounds for the use of melatonin for preventive and therapeutic purposes in open heart surgery [60].

15.3.19 Melatonin and Thyroid Surgery

In an interesting study, diurnal serum melatonin profiles in patients with a very large goiter were assessed before and after the surgery. The authors found that nocturnal serum melatonin concentrations were significantly higher after the surgery than before the operation. They concluded that the manipulations of very large goiters during its surgical resection may compress the superior cervical ganglia, indirectly altering melatonin synthesis, although other mechanisms cannot be excluded [61].

15.4 CONCLUSIONS

Based on the available evidence in clinical and experimental studies, with melatonin's beneficial effects in anesthetic and surgical settings, it is highly likely that its dietary supplementation will be a safe and inexpensive option for perioperative clinical practice. Melatonin has significant potential for clinical uses as a premedication in adults and children for several perioperative settings. However, further studies are required to definitely identify the short- and long-term effects of anesthesia, alone and combined with surgery, on melatonin secretion. Moreover, clinical trials are needed to verify the clinical usefulness of melatonin in humans for the different experimental surgical models.

REFERENCES

1. Reber A, Huber PR, Ummenhofer W, Gurtler CM, Zurschmiede C, Drewe J, et al. (1998). General anaesthesia for surgery can influence circulating melatonin during daylight hours. *Acta Anaesthesiologica Scandinavica* 42:1050–6.
2. Cronin AJ, Keifer JC, Davies MF, King TS, Bixler EO. (2000). Melatonin secretion after surgery. *Lancet* 356:1244–5.
3. Karkela J, Vakkuri O, Kaukinen S, Huang WQ, Pasanen M. (2002). The influence of anaesthesia and surgery on the circadian rhythm of melatonin. *Acta Anaesthesiologica Scandinavica* 46:30–6.

4. Munoz-Hoyos A, Heredia F, Moreno F, Molina-Carballo A, Escames G, Acuna-Castroviejo D. (2002). Evaluation of plasma levels of melatonin after midazolam or sodium thiopental anesthesia in children. *Journal of Pineal Research* 32:253–6.
5. Arai YP, Ueda W, Okatani Y, Fukaya T, Manabe M. (2004). Isoflurane increases, but sevoflurane decreases blood concentrations of melatonin in women. *Journal of Anesthesia* 18:228–31.
6. Ram E, Vishne TH, Weinstein T, Beilin B, Dreznik Z. (2005). General anesthesia for surgery influences melatonin and cortisol levels. *World Journal of Surgery* 29:826 –9.
7. Gögenur I, Middleton B, Burgdorf S, Rasmussen LS, Skene DJ, Rosenberg J. (2007). Impact of sleep and circadian disturbances in urinary 6-sulphatoxymelatonin levels, on cognitive function after major surgery. *Journal of Pineal Research* 43:179–84.
8. Gögenur I, Middleton B, Kristiansen VB, Skene DJ, Rosenberg J. (2007). Disturbances in melatonin and core body temperature circadian rhythms after minimal invasive surgery. *Acta Anaesthesiologica Scandinavica* 51(8):1099–106.
9. Fassoulaki A, Kostopanagiotou G, Meletiou P, Chasiakos D, Markantonis S. (2007). No change in serum melatonin or plasma beta-endorphin levels after sevoflurane anesthesia. *Journal of Clinical Anesthesia* 19:120–4.
10. Castro MR, Pastor AB, Alcantud JF, Salvan JH, Osado IR, Roca AP. (2007). [Altered plasma melatonin concentrations after administration of propofol in continuous infusion]. *Revista Española de Anestesiología y Reanimación* 54:469–74.
11. Dispersyn G, Pain L, Challet E, Touitou Y. (2008). General anesthetics effects on circadian temporal structure: An update. *Chronobiology International* 25:835–50.
12. Chenevard R, Suter Y, Erne P. (2008). Effects of the heart–lung machine on melatonin metabolism and mood disturbances. *European Journal of Cardio-Thoracic Surgery* 34:338–43.
13. Gögenur I, Bisgaard T, Burgdorf S, van Someren E, Rosenberg J. (2009). Disturbances in the circadian pattern of activity and sleep after laparoscopic versus open abdominal surgery. *Surgical Endoscopy* 23(5):1026–31.
14. Dispersyn G, Pain L, Touitou Y. (2010). Propofol anesthesia significantly alters plasma blood levels of melatonin in rats. *Anesthesiology* 112(2):333–7.
15. Gögenur I, Ocak U, Altunpinar O, Middleton B, Skene DJ, Rosenberg J. (2007). Disturbances in melatonin, cortisol and core body temperature rhythms after major surgery. *World Journal of Surgery* 31:290–8.
16. Guo X, Kuzumi E, Charman SC, Vuylsteke A. (2002). Perioperative melatonin secretion in patients undergoing coronary artery bypass grafting. *Anesthesia and Analgesia* 94:1085–91.
17. Naguib M, Hammond DL, Schmid PG 3rd, Baker MT, Cutkomp J, Queral L, et al. (2003). Pharmacological effects of intravenous melatonin: Comparative studies with thiopental and propofol. *British Journal of Anaesthesia* 90:504–7.
18. Naguib M, Schmid PG III, Baker MT. (2003). The electroencephalographic effects of IV anesthetic doses of melatonin: Comparative studies with thiopental and propofol. *Anesthesia and Analgesia* 97:238–43.
19. Zhdanova IV, Wurtman RJ, Lynch HJ, Ives JR, Dollins AB, Morabito C, et al. (1995). Sleep-inducing effects of low doses of melatonin ingested in the evening. *Clinical Pharmacology and Therapeutics* 57:552–8.
20. Wade AG, Ford I, Crawford G, McMahon AD, Nir T, Laudon M, Zisapel N. (2007). Efficacy of prolonged release melatonin in insomnia patients aged 55–80 years: Quality of sleep and next-day alertness outcomes. *Current Medical Research Opinion* 23(10):2597–605.
21. Wang-Weigand S, McCue M, Ogrinc F, Mini L. (2009). Effects of ramelteon 8 mg on objective sleep latency in adults with chronic insomnia on nights 1 and 2: Pooled analysis. *Current Medical Research Opinion* 25(5):1209–13.
22. Samarkandi A, Naguib M, Riad W, Thalaj A, Alotibi W, Aldammas F, et al. (2005). Melatonin vs. midazolam premedication in children: A double-blind, placebo-controlled study. *European Journal of Anaesthesiology* 22:189–96.
23. Naguib M, Samarkandi AH. (1999). Premedication with melatonin: A double-blind, placebo-controlled comparison with midazolam. *British Journal of Anaesthesia* 82:875–80.
24. Naguib M, Samarkandi AH. (2000). The comparative dose response effects of melatonin and midazolam for premedication of adult patients: A double-blinded, placebo-controlled study. *Anesthesia and Analgesia* 91:473–9.
25. Capuzzo M, Zanardi B, Schiffino E, Buccoliero C, Gragnaniello D, Bianchi S, et al. (2006). Melatonin does not reduce anxiety more than placebo in the elderly undergoing surgery. *Anesthesia and Analgesia* 103:121–3.

26. Brzezinski A, Vangel MG, Wurtman RJ, Norrie G, Zhdanova I, Ben-Shushan A, et al. (2005). Effects of exogenous melatonin on sleep: A meta-analysis. *Sleep Medicine Reviews* 9:41–50.
27. Naguib M, Samarkandi AH, Moniem MA, Mansour Eel-D, Alshaer AA, Al-Ayyaf HA, et al. (2006). Effects of melatonin premedication on propofol and thiopental induction dose–response curves: A prospective, randomized, double blind study. *Anesthesia and Analgesia* 103(6):1448–52.
28. Budhiraja S, Singh J. (2005). Adjuvant effect of melatonin on anesthesia induced by thiopental sodium, ketamine, and ether in rats. *Methods and Findings in Experimental and Clinical Pharmacology* 27:697–9.
29. Miyoshi H, Ono T, Sumikawa K. (2001). Melatonin reduces minimum alveolar concentration for isoflurane in rats. *Anesthesiology* 95:A–113.
30. Duranti E, Stankov B, Spadoni G, Duranti A, Lucini V, Capsoni S, et al. (1992). 2-Bromomelatonin: Synthesis and characterization of a potent melatonin agonist. *Life Sciences* 51:479–85.
31. Naguib M, Baker MT, Flood P et al. (2004). Melatonin and its analogs do not induce general anesthesia by potentiating the responsiveness of postsynaptic GABA receptors. *American Society of Anesthesiologists* 101:A817.
32. Shavali S, Ho B, Govitrapong P, Sawlom S, Ajjimaporn A, Klongpanichapak S, et al. (2005). Melatonin exerts its analgesic actions not by binding to opioid receptor subtypes but by increasing the release of beta-endorphin an endogenous opioid. *Brain Research Bulletin* 64:471–9.
33. Evagelidis P, Paraskeva A, Petropoulos G, Staikou C, Fassoulaki A. (2009). Melatonin premedication does not enhance induction of anaesthesia with sevoflurane as assessed by bispectral index monitoring. *Singapore Medical Journal* 50(1):78–81.
34. Yu CX, Zhu B, Xu SF, Cao XD, Wu GC. (2000). The analgesic effects of peripheral and central administration of melatonin in rats. *European Journal of Pharmacology* 403:49–53.
35. Caumo W, Torres F, Moreira NL Jr, Auzani JA, Monteiro CA, Londero G, Ribeiro DF, Hidalgo MP. (2007). The clinical impact of preoperative melatonin on postoperative outcomes in patients undergoing abdominal hysterectomy. *Anesthesia and Analgesia* 105:1263–71.
36. Mowafi HA, Ismail SA. (2008). Melatonin improves tourniquet tolerance and enhances postoperative analgesia in patients receiving intravenous regional anesthesia. *Anesthesia and Analgesia* 107:1422–6.
37. Ismail SA, Mowafi HA. (2009). Melatonin provides anxiolysis, enhances analgesia, decreases intraocular pressure, and promotes better operating conditions during cataract surgery under topical anesthesia. *Anesthesia and Analgesia* 108:1146–51.
38. Caumo W, Levandovski R, Hidalgo MP. (2009). Preoperative anxiolytic effect of melatonin and clonidine on postoperative pain and morphine consumption in patients undergoing abdominal hysterectomy: A double-blind, randomized, placebo-controlled study. *Journal of Pain* 10(1):100–8.
39. Borazan H, Tuncer S, Yalcin N, Erol A, Otelcioglu S. (2010). Effects of preoperative oral melatonin medication on postoperative analgesia, sleep quality, and sedation in patients undergoing elective prostatectomy: A randomized clinical trial. *Journal of Anesthesia* 24(2):155–60.
40. Srinivasan V, Pandi-Perumal SR, Spence DW, Moscovitch A, Trakht I, Brown GM, et al. (2010). Potential use of melatonergic drugs in analgesia: Mechanisms of action. *Brain Research Bulletin* 81:362–71.
41. Isik B, Baygin O, Bodur H. (2008). Premedication with melatonin vs midazolam in anxious children. *Paediatric Anaesthesia* 18(7):635–41.
42. Kain ZN, MacLaren JE, Herrmann L, Mayes L, Rosenbaum A, Hata J, et al. (2009). Preoperative melatonin and its effects on induction and emergence in children undergoing anesthesia and surgery. *Anesthesiology* 111:44–9.
43. Shigeta H, Yasui A, Nimura Y, Machida N, Kageyama M, Miura M, Menjo M, Ikeda K. (2001). Postoperative delirium and melatonin levels in elderly patients. *American Journal of Surgery* 182(5):449–54.
44. Kücükakin B, Gögenur I, Reiter RJ, Rosenberg J. (2009). Oxidative stress in relation to surgery: Is there a role for the antioxidant melatonin? *Journal of Surgical Research* 152(2):338–47.
45. Gitto E, Romeo C, Reiter RJ, Impellizzeri P, Pesce S, Basile M, et al. (2004). Melatonin reduces oxidative stress in surgical neonates. *Journal of Pediatric Surgery* 39(2):184–9.
46. Fildes J, Yonan N, Keevil B. (2009). Melatonin — a pleiotropic molecule involved in pathophysiological processes following organ transplantation. *Immunology* 127:443–9.
47. Soybir G, Topuzlu C, Odabas Ö, Dolay K, Bilir A, Köksoy F. (2003). The effects of melatonin on angiogenesis and wound healing. *Surgery Today* 33:896–901.
48. Takechi M, Tatehara S, Satomura K, Fujisawa K, Nagayama M. (2008). Effect of FGF-2 and melatonin on implant bone healing: A histomorphometric study. *Journal of Materials Science: Materials in Medicine* 19:2949–52.
49. Leston J, Mottolese C, Champier J, Jouvet A, Brun J, Sindou M, et al. (2009). Contribution of the daily melatonin profile to diagnosis of tumors of the pineal region. *Journal of Neurooncology* 93:387–94.

50. Ersoz N, Ozler M, Altinel O, Sadir S, Ozerhan IH, Uysal B, et al. (2009). Melatonin prevents peritoneal adhesions in rats. *Journal of Gastroenterology and Hepatolology* 24(11):1763–7.
51. Kücükakin B, Lykkesfeldt J, Nielsen HJ, Reiter RJ, Rosenberg J, Gögenur I. (2008). Utility of melatonin to treat surgical stress after major vascular surgery — a safety study. *Journal of Pineal Research* 44(4):426–31.
52. Sokullu O, Sanioğlu S, Kurç E, Sargin M, Deniz H, Tartan Z, Aka SA, Bilgen F. (2009). Does the circadian rhythm of melatonin affect ischemia–reperfusion injury after coronary artery bypass grafting? *Heart Surg Forum* 12(2):E95–9.
53. Saeidi M, Sobhani R, Movahedi M, Alsaeidi S, Samani RE. (2009). Effect of melatonin in the prevention of postoperative pericardial adhesion formation. *Interactive Cardiovascular and Thoracic Surgery* 9(1):26–8.
54. Yang FL, Subeq YM, Lee CJ, Lee RP, Peng TC, Hsu BG. (2009). Melatonin ameliorates hemorrhagic shock–induced organ damage in rats. *Journal of Surgical Research.* In press, available online 15 August 2009.
55. Wassmer E, Carter PF, Quinn E, McLean N, Welsh G, Seri S, et al. (2001). Melatonin is useful for recording sleep EEGs: A prospective audit of outcome. *Developmental Medicine and Child Neurology* 43:735–8.
56. Johnson K, Page A, Williams H, Wassemer E, Whitehouse W. (2002). The use of melatonin as an alternative to sedation in uncooperative children undergoing an MRI examination. *Clinical Radiology* 57:502–6.
57. Sury MR, Fairweather K. (2006). The effect of melatonin on sedation of children undergoing magnetic resonance imaging. *British Journal of Anaesthesia* 97(2):220–5.
58. Maldonado MD, Murillo-Cabezas F, Calvo JR, Lardone PJ, Tan DX, Guerrero JM, et al. (2007). Melatonin as pharmacologic support in burn patients: A proposed solution to thermal injury–related lymphocytopenia and oxidative damage. *Critical Care Medicine* 35(4):1177–85.
59. Schemmer P, Nickkholgh A, Schneider H, Sobirey M, Weigand M, Koch M, et al. (2008). PORTAL: Pilot study on the safety and tolerance of preoperative melatonin application in patients undergoing major liver resection: A double-blind randomized placebo-controlled trial. *BMC Surgery* 8:2.
60. Ochoa JJ, Vílchez MJ, Palacios MA, García JJ, Reiter RJ, Muñoz-Hoyos A. (2003). Melatonin protects against lipid peroxidation and membrane rigidity in erythrocytes from patients undergoing cardiopulmonary bypass surgery. *Journal of Pineal Research* 35:104–8.
61. Karasek M, Stankiewicz A, Bandurska-Stankiewicz E, Zylinska K, Pawlikowski M, Kuzdak K. (2000). Melatonin concentrations in patients with large goiter before and after surgery. *Neuro-Endocrinolology Letters* 21(6):437–9.

16 Melatonin in Bone Health

Paula A. Witt-Enderby, William P. Clafshenkel, Mary P. Kotlarczyk, and Shalini Sethi

CONTENTS

The prevalence of osteoporosis-related fractures is predicted to increase from about 10 million to greater than 14 million by 2020 [1]. The prevalence of osteoporosis is greater among women than men, and women comprise the majority of hip and wrist fractures associated with osteoporosis [1]. As estimated for 2005, women 65 years and older account for nearly 74% of all fractures, while men 65 years or older account for 61% [1]. The majority of fractures occur in Caucasian women, with a smaller percentage of these fractures estimated for African Americans and Hispanics. However, women of all ethnicities are considered at risk for developing osteoporosis. After 50 years old, 10% of Hispanic women, 5% of non-Hispanic black women, and 20% of non-Hispanic white and Asian women are estimated to have osteoporosis [2]. Approximately 50% of women in these ethnicities are estimated to have low bone mass [2]. These figures highlight the importance of taking proper preventive measures, including timely screening and diagnosis of osteoporosis, obtaining accurate patient histories, and examining and discussing risk factors associated with its development.

Risk factors for osteoporosis range from lifestyle habits, to disease states, to the use of certain medications. Physical conditions such as low body weight, small body frame, increasing age, low bone mineral density, low peak bone mass at maturity, surgically-induced menopause, and estrogen deficiency are all contributors to osteoporosis risk [2,3]. Several disease states can increase osteoporosis risk, including diabetes type 1, adrenal insufficiency, inflammatory bowel disease, rheumatoid arthritis, multiple sclerosis, epilepsy, and congestive heart failure. Likewise, the medications used to treat these conditions such as oral glucocorticoids, anticoagulants, barbiturates, and lithium can further increase the risk of developing osteoporosis [2]. Lifestyle habits that contribute to osteoporosis and osteoporosis-related fractures include cigarette smoking, immobility, low physical activity, alcohol consumption, poor diet, particularly a diet low in calcium and vitamin D, and, more recently discovered, night shift work [4]. Shift work is a risk factor for breast cancer in women as reviewed [5], and it has been hypothesized that the light-induced suppression of the natural nocturnal surge in melatonin in the body is what predisposes one to breast cancer or bone disease [5,6].

16.1 CURRENT OSTEOPOROSIS THERAPIES

Many women will seek traditional osteoporosis therapies to counter the bone loss resulting from imbalances in bone remodeling. Current therapies used to prevent or treat osteoporosis or build bone in bone grafting procedures include calcitonin, bisphosphonates, selective estrogen receptor modulators (SERMs), parathyroid hormone (PTH) analogs (teriparatide, FORTEO), calcium and vitamin D supplements, and, more recently, a RANK ligand inhibitor, denosumab (PROLIA), and recombinant human bone morphogenetic protein 2 (BMP-2; INFUSE). All of these therapies work through unique mechanisms to inhibit bone resorption or enhance bone deposition; their mechanisms of action will be discussed in later sections.

Bisphosphonates such as alendronate (FOSAMAX), risedronate (ACTONEL), ibandronate (BONIVA), and zoledronic acid (RECLAST) are indicated for the prevention and treatment of osteoporosis or the treatment of glucocorticoid-induced osteoporosis in both men and women. These drugs have a high affinity for sites of active bone remodeling and inhibit osteoclast activity to limit the resorption of bone. The results of clinical trials have shown bisphosphonate therapy reduces the risk of vertebral fractures by 40%–50% and nonvertebral fractures including fractures of the hip by 20%–40% [7], but their efficacy, particularly alendronate use, over time has been questioned especially with respect to the formation of atypical fractures [8]. While these therapies may offer some protection against bone loss, they are not without untoward effects. Most of these therapies focus on decreasing the activity of osteoclasts or act as antiresorptive agents, and these include bisphosphonates, calcitonin, raloxifene, denosumab, and estrogen-based hormone replacement therapies. As such, they minimize further bone loss, which is problematic in cases of severe osteoporosis, which requires new bone to be formed. There are few bone-forming drugs on the market and the one most widely used in severe cases of osteoporosis is the PTH analog, teriparatide (FORTEO). Teriparatide is effective at increasing bone mass by stimulating the formation of new bone, particularly by increasing bone density, improving the microarchitecture of the bone, and reducing risk of vertebral and nonvertebral fractures [9]. While PTH therapy is effective, patient compliance can be affected by the need for daily subcutaneous injections. Also, this therapy is usually limited to a 2-year duration, at which time antiresorptive therapy is often necessary to maintain bone mass developed while on PTH [9]. Calcitonin, another antiresorptive therapy, is approved for the treatment of postmenopausal osteoporosis 5 years after menopause; however, the development of newer drugs has led to a decline in its usage [10].

Estrogen replacement therapy can protect against bone loss associated with menopause; however, there are health concerns with long-term hormone replacement therapy, including increased risk of breast cancer and adverse cardiovascular events [11]. As such, SERMs, such as raloxifene, have been developed and approved in the United States for both the prevention and treatment of postmenopausal osteoporosis. SERMs possess both agonist and antagonist activity with responses being tissue-specific. While they maintain the beneficial effects of estrogen on bone and breast, unwanted side effects with SERM therapy include hot flashes, vaginal dryness, and increased risk of venous thromboembolism [12]. Side effects such as these can affect patient compliance and may limit the duration of treatment.

16.2 MELATONIN AS A POTENTIAL OSTEOPOROTIC THERAPY

The use of melatonin clinically to maintain good bone health in women should be considered, bearing in mind the growing body of evidence of melatonin's efficacy to induce osteoblast formation, inhibit osteoclast activity, and scavenge free radicals as reviewed [6,13,14]. Supplementation with melatonin during the hours of darkness may serve as a preventive agent to reduce the loss of bone associated with aging, delay or reduce the need for therapies like bisphosphonates or SERMs, treat bone loss due to disease or drug therapy, or prevent the untoward effects of existing antiresorptive therapies (Figure 16.1).

Levels of melatonin, similar to estrogen, decrease with age and after menopause [14]. A combination of these factors along with genetics, diet, and lack of exercise could increase the risk of osteoporosis. Melatonin may be an important factor in maintaining bone density, and, as such, a lack of melatonin may be involved in the development of postmenopausal osteoporosis in women [15–18] and other bone-related disorders such as adolescent idiopathic scoliosis (AIS) [6]. While one study found no change in circulating melatonin levels in AIS patients [19], other researchers have found altered

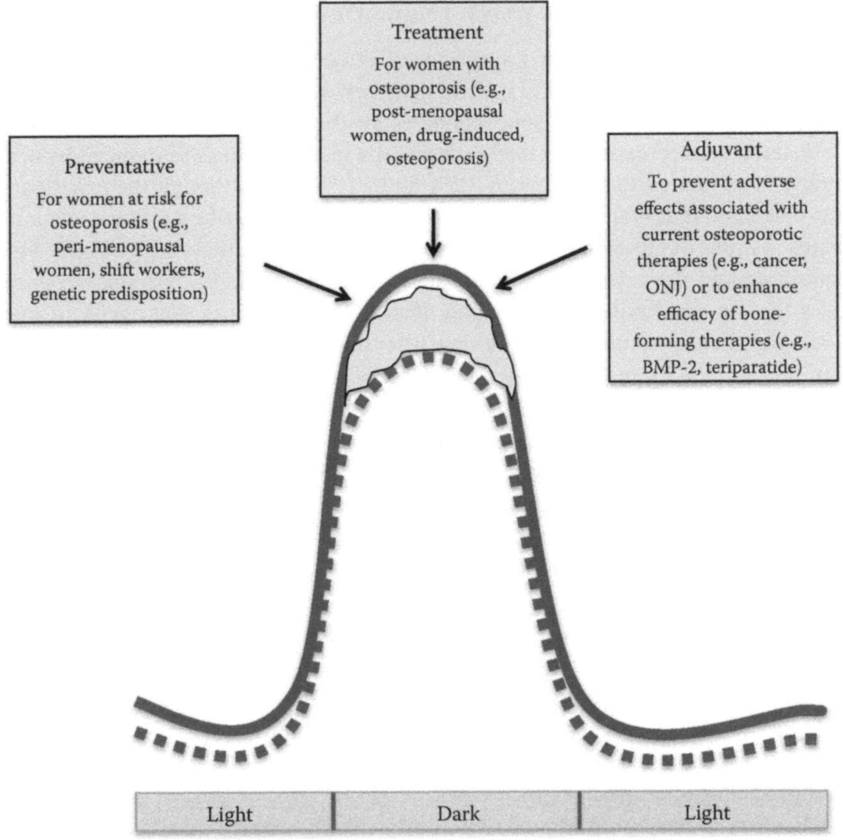

FIGURE 16.1 Use of melatonin to maintain bone health. Melatonin levels fluctuate throughout the light/dark cycle with levels of melatonin being highest during the hours of darkness. Factors that suppress the endogenous nocturnal surge in melatonin (dotted line; e.g., light exposure at night, age) could predispose one to osteoporosis. Supplementing one's diet with melatonin, particularly during the hours of darkness, could restore the daily rhythm of melatonin and prevent bone disease. Besides preventing bone disease, melatonin supplementation could act as a potential treatment for osteoporosis either due to menopause or induced following drug therapy (e.g., glucocorticoid therapy) or can be used in combination with existing osteoporotic therapies to minimize their adverse effects (e.g., osteonecrosis of the jaw (ONJ)).

melatonin signaling in osteoblasts from AIS patients compared with cells from healthy individuals [20,21], suggesting an important role for melatonin and melatonin receptors in this disease [6].

The rhythm of melatonin fluctuates throughout the light/dark cycle with levels being the highest during the hours of darkness [22]. Like melatonin, bone metabolism has a diurnal rhythm, which may be attributed to the rhythmic release of melatonin throughout the light/dark cycle ascribing a role for melatonin in osteogenesis [23–26]. Decreases in melatonin levels are associated with increases in biochemical markers of bone resorption, suggesting that melatonin may be an endogenous inhibitor of osteoclast activity [27]. Exposure to artificial light at night decreases plasma melatonin levels in the body [28], and these decreases in nocturnal levels of melatonin may predispose one to the development of osteoporosis. This is supported in a 2009 study where an increase in the risk of wrist and hip fractures occurred in women who worked 20 or more years of night shift work compared with women who never worked night shifts. Also, it was found that the risk for these fractures increased in women with a lower body mass index and who never used hormone replacement therapy [4].

16.3 MELATONIN AS AN ADJUVANT THERAPY

Melatonin has the potential to prevent the untoward effects of existing antiresorptive therapies including osteonecrosis of the jaw (ONJ). Clinicians report the incidence of ONJ is increasing among menopausal patients utilizing bisphosphonates for the prevention and treatment of osteoporosis [29,30]. Based on cases reported in the literature, the incidence of ONJ induced by oral bisphosphonate therapy is estimated to be between 2.5% and 27.3% [7]. Although the exact pathology is unknown, it is theorized that oral bisphosphonate–induced ONJ is attributed to the accumulation of bisphosphonates in areas of elevated bone remodeling due, in part, to their high affinity for calcium, limited metabolism, and their down-regulation of bone turnover [7,29]. Osteonecrosis of the jaw further reduces the already limited quantity and quality of bone in the oral cavity of menopausal females and can significantly prolong healing time after oral surgery. The limited quality and quantity of bone in the oral cavity may be attributed to decreases in salivary flow that accompany the transition through menopause and, over time, decreases in oral bone mineral density can lead to marked atrophy of dentoalveolar bone along the mandibular and maxillary ridges causing the early loss of posterior molar teeth [29,31,32]. Symptoms of ONJ include pain, swelling, exposed bone, and purulent secretions [7]. These events can substantially affect the utility and results of oral implant procedures and corrective surgeries sought to repair and/or replace jaw bone and missing teeth. If implant procedures are undertaken in these conditions, they often are unsuccessful [31].

Melatonin is released into the saliva and may have protective roles in periodontal disease [33]. Periodontal disease is known to be aggravated by free radicals and by alterations in the immune response to microorganisms that are in plaque. Melatonin, through its receptors, by direct interaction with cytosolic proteins, or through its free radical scavenging, can reduce factors known to be involved in the inflammatory process [6]. Melatonin has been shown to mitigate the proinflammatory cytokines tumor necrosis factor α (TNF-α), interleukin 12 (IL-12), and interferon γ (INF-γ), while increasing the anti-inflammatory mediator IL-10 [34].

Topical application of melatonin around dental implants in beagle dogs facilitates osteointegration and results in a greater quantity and density of newly formed bone [35–37]. When melatonin is combined with fibroblast growth factor 2, the enhancement in bone formation facilitated the osteointegration of titanium tibia implants in female Wistar rats [38]. Melatonin also has synergistic effects on bone regeneration when combined with growth hormone [39]. These studies substantiate claims that melatonin may accelerate the synthesis and mineralization of the osteoid matrix and aid in bone formation and, if used in combination with other drugs, for example, recombinant human bone morphogenetic protein 2, may improve health outcomes in bone grafting procedures. To date, there have been no studies on the ability of melatonin to regenerate bone in human subjects. Therefore, melatonin alone or in combination with other therapies may be an attractive option for re-establishing local bone loss in the jaws of women with ONJ.

16.4 MECHANISMS UNDERLYING BONE CELL ACTIVITY AND THEIR MODULATION BY MELATONIN

Preclinical and in vitro cell culture studies are beginning to reveal the mechanisms underlying melatonin's effects on bone cells [13,14]. As shown in Figure 16.2, melatonin's actions on bone remodeling involve both osteoclasts and osteoblasts. Melatonin has been reported to increase osteoblast differentiation [40,41] or proliferation [42,43] and inhibit osteoclast activity [44,45]. Melatonin can also scavenge free radicals produced by excessive bone resorption protecting osteoblasts and bone in general from their destruction [6].

The main trigger for osteogenesis is the formation of osteoblasts from mesenchymal stem cells. Melatonin can enhance osteoblast formation via activation of MT_2 melatonin receptors expressed on mesenchymal stem cells [40,46] (Figure 16.2). This process is regulated by complex signal transduction mechanisms and gene expression described below and depicted in Figure 16.3. The initial

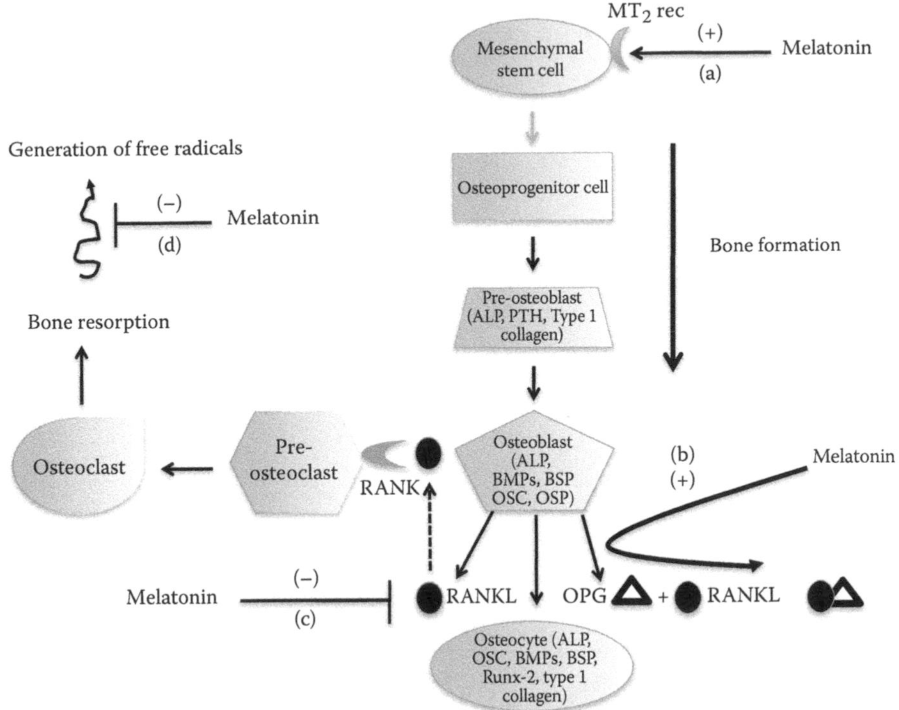

FIGURE 16.2 Mechanisms of melatonin action on osteoblasts and osteoclasts. As shown, melatonin acts at many levels to modulate bone. (a) Melatonin, acting through MT_2 melatonin receptors (MT_2 recs) expressed on mesenchymal stem cells, induces their differentiation into osteoblasts. (b) Melatonin induces the expression of osteoprotegerin (OPG) in osteoblasts, which binds to the receptor activator of NF-κB ligand (RANKL) acting as a decoy to prevent RANKL binding to its receptor (RANK) expressed on osteoclasts. (c) Melatonin-induced formation of OPG–RANKL complexes prevents osteoclastogenesis, osteoclast activity and ultimately bone resorption. (d) Melatonin, through its potent free radical scavenging properties, can prevent radical-induced destruction of osteoblasts and osteoclasts to prevent bone loss. ALP, alkaline phosphatase, PTH, parathyroid hormone, BMPs, bone morphogenetic proteins, BSP, bone sialoprotein, OSC, osteocalcin, OSP, osteopontin, Runx-2, runt-related transcription factor.

process of differentiation of stem cells involves self-renewal, which maintains the stem cell population by giving rise to another stem cell. This stem cell can then divide to form a preosteoblast, an intermediate stage of osteoblast differentiation, which begins to express certain bone marker proteins like alkaline phosphatase, PTH, and type I collagen. Mature osteoblasts, formed by the differentiation of preosteoblasts, express proteins like alkaline phosphatase, osteopontin, bone morphogenetic proteins, bone sialoprotein, and osteocalcin [47]. Osteocyte formation is the last stage of osteogenesis, and these cells express multiple proteins including alkaline phosphatase, osteocalcin, bone morphogenetic proteins, runt-related transcription factor 2 (Runx-2), bone sialoprotein, and type I collagen.

Besides inducing osteoblast formation from mesenchymal stem cells [40,46], melatonin can inhibit osteoclast activity via stimulation of osteoblasts directly as shown in Figure 16.2. Melatonin has been shown to increase osteoprotegerin levels in mouse MC3T3-E1 osteoblastic cells [45]. Osteoprotegerin (OPG) can bind receptor activator of NF-κB ligand, RANKL, another protein released from osteoblasts and act as a decoy to prevent RANKL's interaction with RANK receptors expressed on osteoclasts. In the normal process of bone remodeling, RANKL, released from

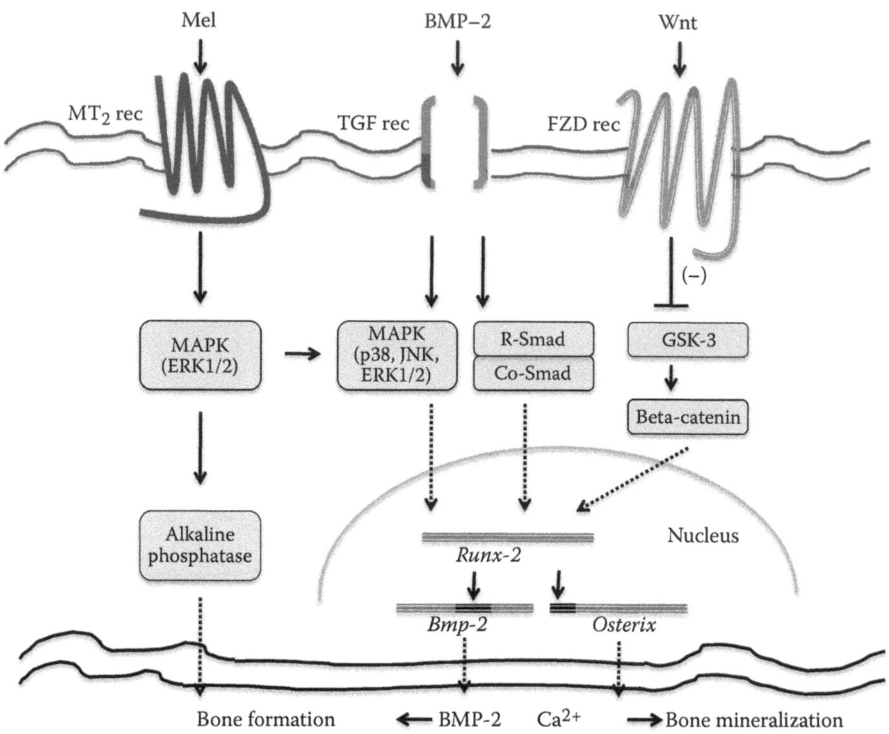

FIGURE 16.3 Mechanisms of melatonin action in osteoblasts. As shown, multiple signaling cascades are involved in osteoblast function and formation and include melatonin, bone morphogenetic proteins (BMPs), and Wnt proteins. As shown, activation of TGF receptors by BMP-2 leads to the phosphorylation of R-Smads, which complex with Co-Smads, leading to their translocation into the nucleus and activation of osteogenic genes like *Runx-2*, *BMP-2*, and *osterix*. BMPs can also act independently of Smads and activate the mitogen activated protein kinase (MAPK) pathway; proteins belonging to the MAPK family include ERK, JNK, and p38 [52,67]. ERK1/2, activated by BMPs [68] or melatonin [46], increases the transcription of the osteogenic genes, *Runx-2* and *osteocalcin*, and the activity of ALP [40,67,69] to induce the differentiation of osteoblasts. Another signaling mechanism in osteoblast differentiation is the Wnt/β-catenin pathway. Wnts are glycoproteins that are ligands for seven membrane-spanning frizzled receptors (FZDs) [56]. The activation of FZD receptors by Wnts cause a down regulation of glycogen synthase kinase 3 (GSK-3) and hypophosphorylation of its substrate β-catenin. β-Catenin then translocates to the nucleus and activates osteogenic genes like *Runx-2* and *osteocalcin* [57].

osteoblasts, induces osteoclastogenesis by binding to its receptor, RANK, expressed on the surface of osteoclasts. Activation of RANK by RANKL induces the differentiation of preosteoclasts to form mature osteoclasts enhancing bone resorption [48,49]. RANKL inhibitors such as denosumab (PROLIA) are currently being developed to treat women with osteoporosis and their use in combination with melatonin may enhance their efficacy to reduce bone resorption.

As shown in Figure 16.2, throughout the process of osteogenesis, specific proteins are expressed. One set of proteins called bone morphogenetic proteins (BMPs) play a particularly vital role in osteoblast formation and bone development. Drugs such as recombinant human bone morphogenetic protein 2 (BMP-2; INFUSE) are being introduced clinically for bone grafting procedures [50]. As shown in Figure 16.3, BMPs belong to the TGF-β superfamily of proteins [51] because they bind to TGF-β receptors located in the plasma membrane of osteoblasts, and after their activation, transmit intracellular signals via downstream signal transducers of TGF-β receptors called Smad proteins [52]. BMP-2–mediated activation of TGF-β receptors leads to phosphorylation of Smads resulting in their interaction with common-partner Smads called Co-Smads (Figure 16.3). These R-Smad/Co-Smad complexes translocate into the nucleus where they regulate transcription of osteogenic genes like *Runx-2*, *BMP-2*, and *osterix* [53–55] to name a few. The expression of *BMP-2* mRNA leads to the secretion of BMP-2 protein from the osteoblast to further bone formation in an autocrine or paracrine manner. The expression of *osterix* mRNA leads to bone mineralization. Another signaling mechanism involved in osteoblast differentiation is the Wnt/β-catenin pathway. Wnts are glycoproteins that are ligands for seven membrane-spanning frizzled receptors (FZD) [56]. The activation of FZD receptors by Wnts causes an increase in β-catenin (unphosphorylated) via an inhibition/down regulation of glycogen synthase kinase 3. β-Catenin then translocates to the nucleus and activates osteogenic genes like *Runx-2* [57]. Many other signaling mechanisms are involved in osteogenesis (i.e., fibroblast growth factors, Notch receptors, PTH, and molecules like Indian hedgehog) [56,58,59] making osteogenesis a complex and incompletely understood process.

Melatonin-mediated activation of MT_2 receptors expressed on mesenchymal stem cells results in osteoblast formation via stimulation of ERK1/2, one of the members of the mitogen-activated protein kinase (MAPK) family through a complicated process involving MT_2 receptor/Gi protein/β-arrestin/MEK/ERK1/2 complex formation [40,46]. Melatonin, acting through MT_2 melatonin receptors, also induces the expression of genes involved in osteogenesis including *Runx-2* and *BMP-2* [46], and this may occur through a cross-talk with other MAPKs such as p38 and ERK1/2, proteins reported to promote the differentiation of osteoblasts [40,60–62].

In keeping then, melatonin, given in combination with other drugs utilizing common signaling pathways, for example, human recombinant BMP-2 drugs, may further increase osteoblast function and levels leading to greater bone formation through intracellular cross-talk mechanisms involving MAPKs. In another scenario, melatonin may be used in combination with RANKL inhibitors to further attenuate osteoclast activity. Making melatonin an even more attractive candidate for use in the clinic to prevent or treat osteoporosis is its ability to scavenge free radicals; free radicals accumulate with age, in response to oxidative stress and through excessive bone resorption [63]. This accumulation in free radicals may lead to poor bone health via destruction of osteoblasts [64]. Because melatonin and its radicals are a potent free radical scavengers [6], then supplementing one's diet with melatonin at night to enhance the protective endogenous nocturnal surge may reduce radical-induced damage to the bone.

16.5 CONCLUSION

With more of the U.S. population approaching the age range that puts individuals at higher risk for developing osteoporosis, there is a public health concern regarding osteoporosis, particularly in its prevention and treatment. In 2005, bone fractures accounted for $17 billion of direct medical costs; this number is estimated to exceed $20 billion by 2025 [1]. Melatonin may be a useful alternative therapy for preventing or treating osteoporosis. If given as a combination therapy, it may either maximize the efficacy of existing osteoporotic drug therapies or minimize their adverse effects. Combination therapies using drugs targeting different cellular mechanisms is commonly used in the treatment of other diseases like diabetes mellitus type 2 to improve health outcomes and should be a strategy used for preventing or treating osteoporosis. Melatonin should be considered as one of the drugs to be used in combination with other osteoporotic agents like bisphosphonates, SERMS, denosumab (PROLIA), BMP-2, or teriparatide to prevent or treat bone disease. Melatonin is inexpensive and free of side effects. As such, the economic savings to the taxpayer may be great and its use in an aged population feasible. Aside from its potential bone protective effects, melatonin may also improve quality of life through improvements in sleep. Disturbances in sleep are a common symptom reported by women during menopause [65] as well as in the elderly population. Because melatonin alleviates insomnia and improves sleep quality in middle-aged to older patients without harmful side effects [66], this may be an added benefit to its use in this population.

REFERENCES

1. Burge, R, Dawson-Hughes, B, Solomon, DH, Wong, JB, King, A, Tosteson, A. 2007. Incidence and economic burden of osteoporosis-related fractures in the United States, 2005–2025. *J Bone Miner Res* 22: 465–475.
2. Nochowitz, B, Siegert, S, Wasik, M. 2009. An update on osteoporosis. *Am J Ther* 16: 437–445.
3. Kalu, DU. 1995. Evolution of the pathogenesis of postmenopausal bone loss. *Bone* 17: 135S–144S.
4. Feskanich, D, Hankinson, SE, Schernhammer, ES. 2009. Nightshift work and fracture risk: The Nurses' Health Study. *Osteoporos Int* 20: 537–542.
5. Grant, SG, Melan, MA, Latimer, JJ, Witt-Enderby, PA. 2009. Melatonin and breast cancer: Cellular mechanisms, clinical studies and future perspectives. *Expert Rev Mol Med* 11: e5.
6. Sanchez-Barcelo, EJ, Mediavilla, M.D., Reiter, R.J. 2010. Scientific basis for the potential use of melatonin in bone diseases: Osteoporosis and adolescent idiopathic scoliosis. *J Osteoporosis*. doi: 10.4061/2010/830231.
7. Yarom, N, Yahalom, R, Shoshani, Y, Hamed, W, Regev, E, Elad, S. 2007. Osteonecrosis of the jaw induced by orally administered bisphosphonates: Incidence, clinical features, predisposing factors and treatment outcome. *Osteoporos Int* 18: 1363–1370.
8. Abrahamsen, B, Eiken, P, Eastell, R. 2009. Subtrochanteric and diaphyseal femur fractures in patients treated with alendronate: A register-based national cohort study. *J Bone Miner Res* 24: 1095–1102.
9. Bilezikian, JP. 2008. Combination anabolic and antiresorptive therapy for osteoporosis: Opening the anabolic window. *Curr Osteoporos Rep* 6: 24–30.
10. Yasothan, U, Kar, S. 2008. Osteoporosis: Overview and pipeline. *Nat Rev Drug Discov* 7: 725–726.
11. Shifren, JL, Schiff, I. 2010. Role of hormone therapy in the management of menopause. *Obstet Gynecol* 115: 839–855.
12. Gennari, L, Merlotti, D, Nuti, R. 2010. Selective estrogen receptor modulator (SERM) for the treatment of osteoporosis in postmenopausal women: Focus on lasofoxifene. *Clin Interv Aging* 5: 19–29.
13. Cardinali, DP, Ladizesky, MG, Boggio, V, Cutrera, RA, Mautalen, C. 2003. Melatonin effects on bone: Experimental facts and clinical perspectives. *J Pineal Res* 34: 81–87.
14. Witt-Enderby, PA, Radio, NM, Doctor, JS, Davis, VL. 2006. Therapeutic treatments potentially mediated by melatonin receptors: Potential clinical uses in the prevention of osteoporosis, cancer and as an adjuvant therapy. *J Pineal Res* 41: 297–305.
15. Sack, RL, Lewy, AJ, Erb, DL, Vollmer, WM, Singer, CM. 1986. Human melatonin production decreases with age. *J Pineal Res* 3: 379–388.
16. Waldhauser, F, Weiszenbacher, G, Frisch, H, Zeitlhuber, U, Waldhauser, M, Wurtman, RJ. 1984. Fall in nocturnal serum melatonin during prepuberty and pubescence. *Lancet* 1: 362–365.
17. Ladizesky, MG, Cutrera, RA, Boggio, V et al. 2001. Effect of melatonin on bone metabolism in ovariectomized rats. *Life Sci* 70: 557–565.
18. Uslu, S, Uysal, A, Oktem, G, Yurtseven, M, Tanyalcin, T, Basdemir, G. 2007. Constructive effect of exogenous melatonin against osteoporosis after ovariectomy in rats. *Anal Quant Cytol Histol* 29: 317–325.
19. Brodner, W, Krepler, P, Nicolakis, M et al. 2000. Melatonin and adolescent idiopathic scoliosis. *J Bone Joint Surg Br* 82: 399–403.
20. Moreau, A, Wang DA, S, Forget, S et al. 2004. Melatonin signaling dysfunction in adolescent idiopathic scoliosis. *Spine* 29: 1772–1781.
21. Azeddine, B, Letellier, K, Wang DA, S, Moldovan, F, Moreau, A. 2007. Molecular determinants of melatonin signaling dysfunction in adolescent idiopathic scoliosis. *Clin Orthop Relat Res* 462: 45–52.
22. Zawilska, JB, Skene, DJ, Arendt, J. 2009. Physiology and pharmacology of melatonin in relation to biological rhythms. *Pharmacol Rep* 61: 383–410.
23. Greenspan, SL, Dresner-Pollak, R, Parker, RA, London, D, Ferguson, L. 1997. Diurnal variation of bone mineral turnover in elderly men and women. *Calcif Tissue Int* 60: 419–423.
24. Heshmati, HM, Riggs, BL, Burritt, MF, Mcalister, CA, Wollan, PC, Khosla, S. 1998. Effects of the circadian variation in serum cortisol on markers of bone turnover and calcium homeostasis in normal postmenopausal women. *J Clin Endocrinol Metab* 83: 751–756.
25. Hassager, C, Risteli, J, Risteli, L, Jensen, SB, Christiansen, C. 1992. Diurnal variation in serum markers of type I collagen synthesis and degradation in healthy premenopausal women. *J Bone Miner Res* 7: 1307–1311.
26. Ostrowska, Z, Kos-Kudla, B, Marek, B, Kajdaniuk, D. 2003. Influence of lighting conditions on daily rhythm of bone metabolism in rats and possible involvement of melatonin and other hormones in this process. *Endocr Regul* 37: 163–174.

27. Ostrowska, Z, Kos-Kudla, B, Marek, B, Swietochowska, E, Gorski, J. 2001. Assessment of the relationship between circadian variations of salivary melatonin levels and type I collagen metabolism in postmenopausal obese women. *Neuro Endocrinol Lett* 22: 121–127.
28. Graham, C, Cook, MR, Gerkovich, MM, Sastre, A. 2001. Examination of the melatonin hypothesis in women exposed at night to EMF, or bright light. *Environ Health Perspect* 109: 501–507.
29. Torres, J, Tamimi, F, Garcia, I, Cebrian, JL, Lopez-Cabarcos, E, Lopez, A. 2008. Management of atrophic maxilla in severe osteoporosis treated with bisphosphonates: A case report. *Oral Surg Oral Med Oral Pathol Oral Radiol Endod* 106: 668–672.
30. Ruggiero, SL, Mehrotra, B, Rosenberg, TJ, Engroff, SL. 2004. Osteonecrosis of the jaws associated with the use of bisphosphonates: A review of 63 cases. *J Oral Maxillofac Surg* 62: 527–534.
31. Friedlander, AH. 2002. The physiology, medical management and oral implications of menopause. *J Am Dent Assoc* 133: 73–81.
32. Von Wowern, N. 2001. General and oral aspects of osteoporosis: A review. *Clin Oral Investig* 5: 71–82.
33. Cutando, A, Gomez-Moreno, G, Arana, C, Acuna-Castroviejo, D, Reiter, RJ. 2007. Melatonin: Potential functions in the oral cavity. *J Periodontolog* 78: 1094–1102.
34. Carrillo-Vico, A, Lardone, PJ, Naji, L et al. 2005. Beneficial pleiotropic actions of melatonin in an experimental model of septic shock in mice: Regulation of pro-/anti-inflammatory cytokine network, protection against oxidative damage and anti-apoptotic effects. *J Pineal Res* 39: 400–408.
35. Guardia, J, Gomez-Moreno, G, Ferrera, MJ, Cutando, A. 2009. Evaluation of effects of topical melatonin on implant surface at 5 and 8 weeks in beagle dogs. *Clin Implant Dent Relat Res.* doi: 0.1111/j.1708-8208.2009.00211.x.
36. Cutando, A, Gomez-Moreno, G, Arana, C et al. 2008. Melatonin stimulates osteointegration of dental implants. *J Pineal Res* 45: 174–179.
37. Calvo-Guirado, JL, Gomez-Moreno, G, Barone, A et al. 2009. Melatonin plus porcine bone on discrete calcium deposit implant surface stimulates osteointegration in dental implants. *J Pineal Res* 47: 164–172.
38. Takechi, M, Tatehara, S, Satomura, K, Fujisawa, K, Nagayama, M. 2008. Effect of FGF-2 and melatonin on implant bone healing: A histomorphometric study. *J Mater Sci Mater Med* 19: 2949–2952.
39. Munoz, F, Lopez-Pena, M, Mino, N, Gomez-Moreno, G, Guardia, J, Cutando, A. 2009. Topical application of melatonin and growth hormone accelerates bone healing around dental implants in dogs. *Clin Implant Dent Relat Res.* doi: 10.1111/j.1708–8208.2009.00242.x.
40. Radio, NM, Doctor, JS, Witt-Enderby, PA. 2006. Melatonin enhances alkaline phosphatase activity in differentiating human adult mesenchymal stem cells grown in osteogenic medium via MT2 melatonin receptors and the MEK/ERK (1/2) signaling cascade. *J Pineal Res* 40: 332–342.
41. Roth, JA, Kim, BG, Lin, WL, Cho, MI. 1999. Melatonin promotes osteoblast differentiation and bone formation. *J Biol Chem* 274: 22041–22047.
42. Satomura, K, Tobiume, S, Tokuyama, R et al. 2007. Melatonin at pharmacological doses enhances human osteoblastic differentiation in vitro and promotes mouse cortical bone formation in vivo. *J Pineal Res* 42: 231–239.
43. Nakade, O, Koyama, H, Ariji, H, Yajima, A, Kaku, T. 1999. Melatonin stimulates proliferation and type I collagen synthesis in human bone cells in vitro. *J Pineal Res* 27: 106–110.
44. Suzuki, N, Hattori, A 2002. Melatonin suppresses osteoclastic and osteoblastic activities in the scales of goldfish. *J Pineal Res* 33: 253–258.
45. Koyama, H, Nakade, O, Takada, Y, Kaku, T, Lau, KH. 2002. Melatonin at pharmacologic doses increases bone mass by suppressing resorption through down-regulation of the RANKL-mediated osteoclast formation and activation. *J Bone Miner Res* 17: 1219–1229.
46. Sethi, S, Radio, NM, Kotlarczyk, MP et al. 2010. Determination of the minimal melatonin exposure required to induce osteoblast differentiation from human mesenchymal stem cells and these effects on downstream signaling pathways. *J Pineal Res.* doi: 10.1111/j.1600-079X.2010.00784.x.
47. Thomas, D, Kansara, M. 2006. Epigenetic modifications in osteogenic differentiation and transformation. *J Cell Biochem* 98: 757–769.
48. Wada, T, Nakashima, T, Hiroshi, N, Penninger, JM. 2006. RANKL–RANK signaling in osteoclastogenesis and bone disease. *Trends Mol Med* 12: 17–25.
49. Boyce, BF, Xing, L. 2007. The RANKL/RANK/OPG pathway. *Curr Osteoporos Rep* 5: 98–104.
50. Mckay, WF, Peckham, SM, Badura, JM. 2007. A comprehensive clinical review of recombinant human bone morphogenetic protein-2 (INFUSE Bone Graft). *Int Orthop* 31: 729–734.
51. Chen, D, Zhao, M, Mundy, GR. 2004. Bone morphogenetic proteins. *Growth Factors* 22: 233–241.
52. Derynck, R, Zhang, YE. 2003. Smad-dependent and Smad-independent pathways in TGF-beta family signalling. *Nature* 425: 577–584.

53. Miyazono, K, Maeda, S, Imamura, T. 2005. BMP receptor signaling: Transcriptional targets, regulation of signals, and signaling cross-talk. *Cytokine Growth Factor Rev* 16: 251–263.
54. Lee, MH, Kim, YJ, Kim, HJ et al. 2003. BMP-2–induced Runx2 expression is mediated by Dlx5, and TGF-beta 1 opposes the BMP-2-induced osteoblast differentiation by suppression of Dlx5 expression. *J Biol Chem* 278: 34387–34394.
55. Nakashima, K, Zhou, X, Kunkel, G et al. 2002. The novel zinc finger-containing transcription factor osterix is required for osteoblast differentiation and bone formation. *Cell* 108: 17–29.
56. Huang, W, Yang, S, Shao, J, Li, YP 2007. Signaling and transcriptional regulation in osteoblast commitment and differentiation. *Front Biosci* 12: 3068–3092.
57. Day, TF, Guo, X, Garrett-Beal, L, Yang, Y. 2005. Wnt/beta-catenin signaling in mesenchymal progenitors controls osteoblast and chondrocyte differentiation during vertebrate skeletogenesis. *Dev Cell* 8: 739–750.
58. Chau, JF, Leong, WF, Li, B. 2009. Signaling pathways governing osteoblast proliferation, differentiation and function. *Histol Histopathol* 24: 1593–1606.
59. Guo, X, Wang, XF. 2009. Signaling cross-talk between TGF-beta/BMP and other pathways. *Cell Res* 19: 71–88.
60. Rawadi, G, Ferrer, C, Spinella-Jaegle, S, Roman-Roman, S, Bouali, Y, Baron, R. 2001. 1-(5-Oxohexyl)-3,7-Dimethylxanthine, a phosphodiesterase inhibitor, activates MAPK cascades and promotes osteoblast differentiation by a mechanism independent of PKA activation (pentoxifylline promotes osteoblast differentiation). *Endocrinology* 142: 4673–4682.
61. Suzuki, A, Palmer, G, Bonjour, JP, Caverzasio, J. 1999. Regulation of alkaline phosphatase activity by p38 MAP kinase in response to activation of Gi protein-coupled receptors by epinephrine in osteoblast-like cells. *Endocrinology* 140: 3177–3182.
62. Matsushita, T, Chan, YY, Kawanami, A, Balmes, G, Landreth, GE, Murakami, S. 2009. Extracellular signal-regulated kinase 1 (ERK1) and ERK2 play essential roles in osteoblast differentiation and in supporting osteoclastogenesis. *Mol Cell Biol* 29: 5843–5857.
63. Fraser, JH, Helfrich, MH, Wallace, HM, Ralston, SH. 1996. Hydrogen peroxide, but not superoxide, stimulates bone resorption in mouse calvariae. *Bone* 19: 223–226.
64. Sanchez-Rodriguez, MA, Ruiz-Ramos, M, Correa-Munoz, E, Mendoza-Nunez, VM. 2007. Oxidative stress as a risk factor for osteoporosis in elderly Mexicans as characterized by antioxidant enzymes. *BMC Musculoskelet Disord* 8: 124.
65. Woods, NF, Mitchell, ES. 2005. Symptoms during the perimenopause: Prevalence, severity, trajectory, and significance in women's lives. *Am J Med* 118 Suppl 12B: 14–24.
66. Wade, A, Downie, S. 2008. Prolonged-release melatonin for the treatment of insomnia in patients over 55 years. *Expert Opin Invest Drugs* 17: 1567–1572.
67. Guicheux, J, Lemonnier, J, Ghayor, C, Suzuki, A, Palmer, G, Caverzasio, J. 2003. Activation of p38 mitogen-activated protein kinase and c-Jun-NH2-terminal kinase by BMP-2 and their implication in the stimulation of osteoblastic cell differentiation. *J Bone Miner Res* 18: 2060–2068.
68. Ge, C, Xiao, G, Jiang, D, Franceschi, RT. 2007. Critical role of the extracellular signal-regulated kinase-MAPK pathway in osteoblast differentiation and skeletal development. *J Cell Biol* 176: 709–718.
69. Ahmed, I, Gesty-Palmer, D, Drezner, MK, Luttrell, LM. 2003. Transactivation of the epidermal growth factor receptor mediates parathyroid hormone and prostaglandin F2 alpha-stimulated mitogen-activated protein kinase activation in cultured transgenic murine osteoblasts. *Mol Endocrinol* 17: 1607–1621.

17 Prevention and Treatment of Breast Cancer Using Melatonin

Vicki L. Davis, Balasunder R. Dodda, and Paula A. Witt-Enderby

CONTENTS

Breast cancer is the most prevalent cancer among American women, excluding skin cancers, and it is the second leading cause of cancer-related deaths next to lung cancer [1]. Several novel strategies are under investigation for their effectiveness in preventing and treating breast cancer. Chemoprevention is one such strategy that involves administration of drugs to prevent, suppress, or reverse the carcinogenesis process. In breast cancer management, chemoprevention is aimed at preventing mammary cancer progression to invasive cancer [2]. In a breast cancer prevention trial using tamoxifen, its use resulted in a 49% reduction in the incidence of estrogen receptor (ER)–positive breast cancers in high-risk women [3]. Tamoxifen is approved by the U.S. Food and Drug Administration for use in high-risk women to prevent breast cancer. Widespread use of tamoxifen for breast cancer prevention, however, is limited by its lack of efficacy in ER-negative tumors and the increased risk of endometrial cancer and thromboembolic events associated with its long-term use [4]. Hence, there remains a need to develop other agents for chemoprevention of breast cancer without increasing uterine cancer risk. The potential for melatonin to protect those at risk for cancer, treat those with cancer, and prevent the recurrence of breast cancer is great. Considering that most preclinical and clinical studies show melatonin use to be protective against mammary cancer, more studies in women should be conducted to move it from the bench to the bedside.

17.1 MELATONIN AND BREAST CANCER IN HUMANS

Physiological aging is associated with decreases in endogenous melatonin levels with lower nocturnal peaks in older people [5]. Decreases in melatonin output in older people have been consistently linked to insomnia and a higher prevalence of cancer [6,7]. The therapeutic significance of melatonin has been proven in circadian rhythm disorders such as insomnia, jet lag, sleep/wake cycle disturbances in shift work, and blind people [8]. For these therapeutic uses, melatonin is currently available as an over-the-counter drug or food supplement in Argentina, China, Poland, and the United States [9].

The relationship linking melatonin and breast cancer was first proposed by Cohen et al. [10] in 1978 who hypothesized that decreases in melatonin secretion could cause hyperestrogenism, which in turn promotes breast carcinogenesis. Supporting this hypothesis, an inverse relationship between melatonin and estrogen is seen in vivo [11,12] and in breast cancer where low nocturnal serum melatonin concentrations and urinary 6-sulfatoxymelatonin (urinary metabolite of melatonin) levels are found in women with ER-positive breast cancer patients [13,14]. In 1987, Stevens [15] hypothesized that the increased incidence of breast cancer in industrial societies is related to greater exposure to high levels of light at night. Epidemiological studies in women who frequently work during nights for long periods show an increase in breast cancer risk [16,17]. Coleman and Reiter in 1992 advanced a hypothesis that blindness from an early age reduces breast cancer risk by increasing melatonin secretion from the pineal gland [18]. This hypothesis is partly supported by the results of the cohort study in blind women that showed an inverse relationship between level of visual blindness and breast cancer risk [19]. These observations have led to the hypothesis that conditions that suppress nocturnal melatonin levels, like working the night shift, may increase breast cancer risk. In fact, shift work was recently classified as a potential carcinogen by the International Agency for Research on Cancer and the World Health Organization as reviewed in [20].

The existing clinical and epidemiological data demonstrate a causal relationship between low melatonin levels and breast cancer development. Levels of melatonin during the night or in breast cyst fluids [21] in cancer patients may be prognostic in nature, thus affecting treatment or therapeutic outcome [20]. For example, low nocturnal levels of melatonin are associated with poor prognosis in breast cancer based on measures of tumor "aggressiveness" or proliferative status [22], its level of differentiation or nuclear grade [23], and its invasive potential due to loss of ER or progesterone receptor (PR) expression [24].

A meta-analysis of the human trials using melatonin alone as a chemotherapy agent or in combination with other therapies was conducted as reviewed [25]. All studies were performed on advanced cancer patients using melatonin alone or in combination with other chemotherapies, including cisplatin. Three studies were conducted on patients with lung cancer (one alone and two in conjunction with cisplatin chemotherapy). One study each on breast cancer, renal cell cancer, glioblastoma, and malignant melanoma was conducted. Two studies of patients with either advanced or metastatic solid tumors and one study specifically of brain metastases from assorted solid tumors was also performed. The average number of subjects in these studies was 75 and they were single-arm, unblinded studies. The results from the meta-analysis conclude that melatonin significantly reduced the risk of death in cancer patients at 1 year [26] and suggest that administration of relatively high doses of melatonin (10–50 mg daily), either alone or in combination therapies, favorably influence the course of advanced malignant diseases including breast cancer [6,27]. Hence, supplementation with melatonin is thought to benefit women who are at risk of developing breast cancer or with an established diagnosis of breast cancer. Melatonin could also be used to protect one against radical-induced damage associated with certain chemotherapeutic regimens through its ability to scavenge free radicals (discussed in detail in later sections). It is known that melatonin is protective against chemical mimics of oxidative stress, like tobacco smoke [28], or in individuals who were exposed to ionizing radiation [29]. Melatonin may also be working through melatonin receptors to produce these protective actions. Melatonin receptors type 1 (MT_1R) were detected in luminal and myoepithelial cells in milk ducts in both cancerous (39/42 specimens) and noncancerous (40/42 specimens) tissue independent of HER2, PR, and ER status [30].

In endocrine-dependent breast cancer, the antiestrogenic effects of melatonin may interfere with one's susceptibility to carcinogenesis, estrogen-induced cell proliferation, and tumor progression [31] through a variety of mechanisms (Figure 17.1). Breast tumor cells are often hormone-dependent, making them high responders to therapies designed to lower endogenous hormone levels. Other

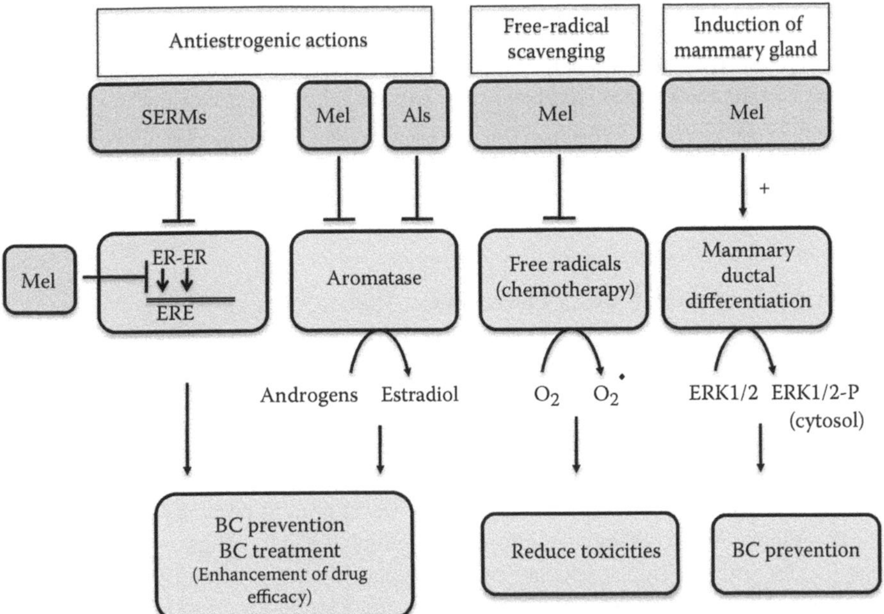

FIGURE 17.1 Therapeutic considerations for use of melatonin in the clinical setting for breast cancer. Melatonin (Mel) has multiple modes of action and these attributes of melatonin, in addition to its cost and safety profile, make it an ideal drug candidate to use in combination with other therapies to enhance the efficacy and reduce side effects (e.g., vaginal dryness) of drugs like selective estrogen receptor modulators (SERMs; tamoxifen, raloxifene) or aromatase inhibitors (AIs; letrozole, anastrozole) to increase therapeutic outcomes. Melatonin can be added in combination with AIs to enhance the attenuation in local estrogen levels in the breast. Also, melatonin can be added with SERMs to enhance their efficacy by working through two different mechanisms to reduce estrogen-mediated signaling in the breast. SERMs function as estrogen receptor antagonists in breast tissue blocking the interaction of estrogen with estrogen receptors (ERs) preventing ER dimerization and reducing ER-mediated gene activation. Melatonin acts to block ER interaction with estrogen response elements (EREs) on genes also reducing ER-mediated gene activation. The use of melatonin in combination with more toxic chemotherapeutic drugs may protect normal cells from free radical damage through its antioxidant properties. Also, chronic melatonin therapy could be used to induce breast tissue differentiation by increasing cytosolic compartmentalization of the mitogen activated protein kinase, ERK1/2, protecting against breast cancer development, growth, and progression.

characteristics of hormone-dependent breast cancers are that they create a tumor environment conducive to hormone-induced growth, for example, by overexpressing hormone receptors similar to what occurs in HER2-type breast cancer as well as in estrogen- (ER+) or progesterone-dependent (PR+) breast cancers [32], by expressing altered ratios of these receptors [33], or by overexpressing accessory proteins that aid in receptor function [34]. Therefore, the therapies used commonly in the clinical setting include those targeted to reduce endogenous levels of hormones (e.g., estrogen using anastrozole or letrozole) or to block hormone/receptor interactions (e.g., raloxifene or tamoxifen to block estrogen's interactions with ERs) or combinations thereof to reduce hormone receptor-mediated signaling through hormone response elements. Recently, it was shown that combination anastrozole (1 mg, noon dose) and melatonin (20 mg evening dose) therapy improved therapeutic outcomes in patients with metastatic breast cancer. Specifically, 57% of patients given this combination therapy showed either complete (2/14 patients) or partial response (6/14 patients) with tumor regression for 26 months [27]. Melatonin may be working through aromatases to inhibit their activity, thereby decreasing the production of biologically active estrogens. Melatonin's effects on these pathways will be discussed in greater detail in later sections.

17.2 MELATONIN AND MAMMARY CANCER IN PRECLINICAL MODELS

Preclinical studies are routinely used to investigate the potential of agents to prevent, treat, or increase the risk of human diseases, such as breast cancer. Although no animal model can exactly replicate the human systems, rodent models are valuable for predicting the beneficial or adverse outcomes of chemicals in women. The effects of melatonin deficiency and supplementation have been studied in multiple model systems to demonstrate the ability of melatonin to inhibit mammary cancer development or to treat existing tumors.

17.2.1 Light on Mammary Cancer Development (Latency)

Melatonin deficiencies can be induced in rodents primarily by light exposure (loss of darkness) or by pinealectomy to remove the main source of circulating levels of melatonin (although local production of melatonin in some organs can still occur). In chemically-induced mammary cancer, constant light exposure (LL or 24:0) results in a higher incidence and shorter latency in mammary tumor formation compared to light/dark cycles (LD) with 12 to 14 hours of darkness [35]. Pinealectomy has similar effects on mammary tumor development compared with sham controls [36]. In classic replacement experiments, administering melatonin to compensate for the deficiency induced by pinealectomy or light exposure reversed the effects by extending the latency and/or decreasing the incidence of tumors compared to the vehicle-treated animals as reviewed in [37]. However, in some studies, melatonin treatment is less effective or does not reverse the increased mammary tumor incidence in pinealectomy, unlike with light exposure [38,39]. These findings suggest that light exposure may be a more specific means to decrease melatonin. In addition, light exposure is correlative with melatonin deficiency in women due to light pollution [40]. In contrast to reducing melatonin levels, enhancing pineal secretion of melatonin by exposing animals to constant darkness (light deprivation) or by other means, such as using anosmic or blinded animals or low environmental temperatures, decreases mammary tumor incidence and lengthens the latency [36,37]. These experiments verify that the risk of mammary cancer is modified by inhibiting the normal nocturnal secretion of melatonin (increases risk) and by increasing melatonin levels either by stimulating endogenous secretion or by exogenous supplementation (decreases risk). This was also demonstrated using human breast tumor xenografts grown in rats and perfused with human blood exposed to light at night (melatonin-deficient) or not exposed to light at night (melatonin-rich) [41]. The results from this study show that human breast tumor xenografts perfused with human blood taken from women who were exposed to a light pulse during the night showed an increase in tumor growth compared with tumors perfused with human blood taken at night with no light exposure. The tumor growth suppressive effects of the melatonin-rich blood were blocked when a melatonin receptor antagonist was added. These data demonstrate two important findings: (1) that light exposure at night was modifying melatonin levels to impact on tumor growth rates and (2) that melatonin's effects on tumor growth suppression were being mediated by melatonin receptors [41]. The results of such animal studies demonstrate excellent correlation with epidemiological studies in night-shift workers (dark deficiency) and blind women (light deficiency), indicating that rodent models can be used as good predictors of melatonin's influence on human breast cancer.

17.2.2 Melatonin on Mammary Cancer Development (Latency)

The protective effects of melatonin on mammary tumor development have been tested in multiple animal models. Most studies have been performed in rats with chemically-induced mammary cancer, either with dimethylbenz[*a*]anthracene (DMBA) [42] or methylnitrosourea (MNU) (see the review in ref. [37]); however, spontaneous and transgenic mammary cancer mouse models [43–45] have also been examined. The preventative actions of melatonin have been supported in these multiple models, suggesting melatonin may have antitumor actions against multiple types of breast cancer.

Melatonin has been reported to decrease the incidence, increase the latency, and decrease multiplicity (number of tumors/animal) [46,47] of mammary cancer. These anticancer actions suggest melatonin may act to inhibit both tumor initiation and promotion. By beginning melatonin treatment at different times relative to the cancer-inducing agent, its effects on mammary tumor initiation and promotion were examined in several studies. In rats with MNU-induced mammary cancer, melatonin administered (subcutaneously) for 2 weeks prior and up to the day of the second MNU injection did not alter tumor development, but when melatonin was started 4 weeks after the MNU treatments, tumor incidence was reduced [48]. These results suggest that melatonin only influenced tumor promotion and not initiation in this model. However, in DMBA-treated rats, if melatonin was provided in the initiation phase (prior to and up to 1 week following DMBA), it effectively reduced the incidence of mammary tumors [42,49] as it did when started 1 week after DMBA administration [42]. Therefore, in the DMBA model, melatonin could prevent both the initiation and promotion of mammary tumors. If similar effects occur in human breast cancer, supplementing melatonin levels naturally (getting sufficient sleep in the dark) or exogenously may be important at any stage in a woman's life when she is prone to developing breast cancer.

17.2.3 Melatonin on Mammary Cancer Growth

Although most studies have investigated the preventative actions of melatonin for mammary cancer, some have focused on its potential as a treatment for preexisting mammary cancer. Because melatonin levels can be modified based on lighting conditions, adjustments in lighting duration (i.e., constant light, LL, or constant dark, DD) are often used to assess light-induced suppression of endogenous melatonin levels on mammary cancer growth. One study with DMBA-induced mammary adenocarcinomas discovered that exposure to light during the dark cycle (LL), especially dim lighting, increased the growth and decreased survival of the rats and was associated with lower nocturnal secretion of the metabolite of melatonin (6-sulfatoxymelatonin) and higher concentrations of serum estradiol [50]. In other studies, the growth of the primary tumors and the incidence of lung metastases were suppressed in MMTV-*neu* mice with nighttime exposure to darkness (LD, 12:12) [43,44]. These findings suggest that not getting sufficient exposure to darkness can have an adverse effect on breast cancer patients by lowering endogenous nocturnal melatonin levels.

Melatonin supplementation also reduced tumor growth [51,52]. It also slowed tumor growth and the incidence of palpable tumors overexpressing the MT_1R in MCF-7 cells, which were implanted into nude mice exposed to darkness at night (LD 12:12) [53]. These data suggest that the protective effects of melatonin on tumor growth are mediated through the MT_1R. As melatonin receptors are detected in the normal mammary gland of mice [54], the preventative actions of melatonin may also be imparted, at least in part, by its receptor-mediated actions. This was also demonstrated in rats implanted with human breast tumor xenografts, which showed a reversal in tumor suppression in the melatonin-rich blood in the presence of a melatonin receptor antagonist [41].

17.2.4 Melatonin on Mammary Cancer Metastases (Progression)

In addition to inhibiting primary tumor growth, the incidence of lung metastases was suppressed in MMTV-*neu* mice with nighttime exposure to darkness (LD, 12:12) [43,44]. Other studies also suggest melatonin inhibits the invasive and metastatic properties using MCF-7 breast cancer cells and clones expressing HER2, which have high metatastic potential [55,56]. As metastatic progression of breast cancer is intimately linked to patient survival, the ability of melatonin to inhibit this phase of tumorigenesis is of critical importance to women with existing breast cancer and needs to be investigated in clinical trials. Recently, melatonin receptors, particularly MT_1Rs have been associated with metastatic tumors. Using human dermal tumors (melanoma malignum), it was observed that MT_1Rs were expressed in all 38 primary tumor specimens and 10 metastatic lymph nodes examined and that the levels of MT_1R expression was more pronounced in primary tumors than in the lymph nodes [57]. These data suggest that a loss of MT_1R expression may increase invasive potential.

17.3 MELATONIN'S MECHANISMS OF ACTION

A number of mechanisms have been attributed to melatonin's cancer protective actions. Melatonin can lower estrogen levels via aromatases and can inhibit estrogen-responsive genes [31,58]. Melatonin and estrogen have been shown to accumulate in breast cyst fluids and their accumulation is shown to be predictive of growth inhibition and stimulation, respectively. [21]. Melatonin is a lipophilic molecule that produces cellular effects through melatonin receptors or independent of melatonin receptors. The receptor-independent actions of melatonin can be further subdivided into effects targeted at intracellular cytosolic proteins (e.g., calmodulin, aromatase) or effects carried out on its own and through its radicals. Research is showing that melatonin acts through a variety of intracellular mechanisms to produce its cancer protective actions, particularly on delaying tumor onset (latency), inhibiting tumor growth, and reducing tumor progression (metastases). The cancer protective effects of melatonin could be attributed to its ability to scavenge free radicals to reduce the initiating effects of mutations on genes particularly protooncogenes. The tumor promotion and growth inhibitory properties of melatonin may be attributed to its effects on proliferative processes via its antiestrogenic actions and cell differentiating properties while its antimetastatic properties may be attributed to its cell differentiating properties as well as its effects on matrix/cell adhesion proteins (Figure 17.1).

17.3.1 Tumor Development

There are many mechanisms by which melatonin acts to prevent mammary cancer but a reduction in oxidative damage due to melatonin and its radicals' ability to scavenge free radicals may be a significant one. Melatonin is a known free radical scavenger more potent than glutathione [59]. Melatonin decreases stress-induced mitochondrial damage due to radical formation [60,61]. Melatonin's potency is attributed to the findings that both melatonin and its radicals are capable of scavenging free radicals. When melatonin takes on two radicals, it produces cyclic 3-hydroxymelatoin (c3-OHM), which can take on another free radical thus forming *N*1-acetyl-*N*2-formyl-5-methoxykynuramine (AFMK), which, too, can take on another radical to produce *N*1-acetyl-5-methoxykynuramine (AMK) [59]. This radical-on-radical property of melatonin explains the potent free radical scavenging properties of melatonin to reduce oxidative stress to the organism. It is shown that melatonin-deficient (pinealectomized) rats suffer increased oxidative damage over their lifetime [62], whereas lifelong melatonin administration decreases both DNA damage in the brain [63] and the spontaneous incidence of tumors in mice [64]. It is also shown that melatonin can reduce toxicities of chemotherapeutic regimens known to produce free radicals [65].

17.3.2 Growth

The majority of in vitro experiments of melatonin effects on human breast cancer cells were performed on ERα-positive MCF-7, T47D, and ZR-75-1 cells and ERα-negative MDA-MB 231 and BT-20 cells. Most of the studies done in MCF-7 cells demonstrated melatonin's oncostatic effects through its direct antiestrogenic effects on breast cancer cells [66]. The antiproliferative effects of melatonin are also related to the melatonin's ability to prolong the cell cycle by suppressing the progression of MCF-7 cells from the G_0 or G_1 phase to the S phase [67]. The growth inhibitory effects of melatonin in breast cancer cells are mediated, in part, by MT_1Rs, and MT_2Rs demonstrated using melatonin receptor antagonists and recombinant cell models expressing each of the melatonin receptor subtypes [53,68]. Melatonin, acting through MT_1Rs, and Gi proteins, can inhibit the cAMP-dependent signaling pathway and contribute to the inhibition of estrogen responsive genes like *BRCA-1*, *p53*, *p21*, and *c-myc* [69] by preventing ER interaction with estrogen response elements (EREs) located on these genes.

Melatonin may also be suppressing tumor proliferation by acting independently of receptors. Melatonin can traverse cell membranes, enter cells, and inhibit intracellular proteins like calmodulin [70] or aromatase [12,58,71]. The inhibitory actions of melatonin on calmodulin can decrease the activation of calmodulin-dependent adenylyl cyclases located in the plasma membrane to decrease cAMP levels. This decrease in cAMP prevents ER binding to EREs to inhibit the expression of estrogen-responsive genes [12,47,72–74]. (Please refer to the review in ref. [20] for greater detail with respect to molecular mechanisms). The inhibitory actions of melatonin on aromatases can reduce local levels of estrogen in mammary tissue and thus reduce estrogen-responsive gene regulation. Melatonin has been shown to modulate the synthesis and transformation of biologically active estrogens in MCF-7 cells by down-regulating sulfatase and 17-β-hydroxysteroid dehydrogenase and inducing estone sulfotransferase [71]. Melatonin inhibits aromatase activity by down-regulating its expression through an interaction with the promoter regions, pII, pI.3, and pI.4, of aromatase [75]. Decreases in estrogen-responsive genes in mammary tissue, as described above, may also contribute to the melatonin-induced reduction in breast cancer growth and metastases described in the preclinical and clinical studies. These actions of melatonin would make it a useful adjuvant to treat estrogen-dependent breast cancers, along with tamoxifen, raloxifene, or fulvestrant [12,47,76] as shown in Figure 17.1.

Melatonin coadministration with other treatments, such as tamoxifen, aromatase inhibitors, retinoic acid, and lycopene has shown enhanced effects on tumor prevention [46,51,52,56,77–81]. For example, with melatonin plus tamoxifen, the effectiveness of a low dose of tamoxifen for prevention of MNU-induced mammary cancer was significantly enhanced with the addition of melatonin to that equivalent of 3 times the dose of tamoxifen alone [77]. This augmented effect in the combined treatment may be linked to melatonin's known antiestrogenic actions [31], which could supplement the antiestrogenic properties of tamoxifen. These data suggest that a lower dose of tamoxifen may be able to be tested in women to provide sufficient breast cancer prevention with fewer sides effects and possible other benefits of melatonin therapy, such as on mood, bone, and sleep. This may hold true for other classes of cancer therapies like aromatase inhibitors. Therefore, more preclinical and clinical studies investigating how melatonin influences the efficacy of other preventative or therapeutic drugs need to be designed and tested to take advantage of the beneficial effects of melatonin on cancer and other body systems, especially due to its lack of toxicity [20].

The extent of mammary ductal differentiation to increase the number of tertiary branching and lobular structures are associated with a reduction in mammary cancer [82]. This is further supported in human studies, which show that multiple pregnancies and breast-feeding, which induce mammary ductal differentiation, also provide protection in women against breast cancer [82]. Cellular differentiation and proliferation are interconnected; that is, a cell undergoing cellular differentiation will have lower proliferative capacity compared to a cell not undergoing differentiation. Therefore, hormones like melatonin may be protective against breast cancer through its actions on differentiation processes to slow the growth of cells. This would protect against mammary cancer induced by mutations since the mutation would not be propagated. If this occurred in the nontumor mammary tissue, then this could make it more difficult for the tumor to grow and metastasize.

The mechanism by which melatonin induces cellular differentiation probably occurs through many mechanisms, but an important emerging mechanism is one involving the mitogen-activated protein kinase (MAPK), ERK1/2. The MAPKs are protein kinases known to be involved in both cellular differentiation and proliferation. Recent studies show that the cellular compartmentalization of ERK1/2 (cytosolic or nuclear) determines whether a cell will proceed down a path of cellular differentiation (cytosolic localization) or proliferation (nuclear localization) [83]. Therefore, hormones like melatonin may be protective against breast cancer by regulating the compartmentalization patterns of ERK1/2 to reduce nuclear compartmentalization and increase cytosolic compartmentalization to induce cellular differentiation and slow the growth of cells, respectively.

Melatonin induces the differentiation of numerous cell types [84–92], and compartmentalization of ERK1/2 to the cytosol has been shown to occur in human mesenchymal stem cells induced by melatonin to form osteoblasts [93]. In addition to the studies in cells, the slowing effect of the melatonin on the human breast cancer xenografts probably involves these MAPKs because it was shown that melatonin-rich blood (i.e., no light exposure at night) suppresses MAPK (ERK1/2) levels in the breast cancer xenografts, and this effect was blocked in the presence of a melatonin receptor antagonist [41]. As stated previously, melatonin-induced differentiation in nontumor adjacent mammary tissue could reduce the potential for tumor growth and metastases. Melatonin's effects on matrix adhesion proteins may also prevent the spread of breast cancer into other organs. This is supported in studies that show melatonin increases β1-integrin and E-cadherin expression (matrix adhesion proteins) in human (MCF-7) breast cancer tumor cells and promotes their differentiation, thus lowering their invasive status [55].

17.3.3 Therapeutic Considerations for Using Melatonin as Breast Cancer Therapy

The available in vitro and in vivo studies data support the critical role of the time of melatonin administration for the antitumor effects of melatonin. The most effective protocol of melatonin dosing is the simulation of the physiological rhythm of melatonin secretion by administering the melatonin during the night [94]. Melatonin exerts its chemopreventative and therapeutic role in wide range of neoplasms including breast cancer due to its multiple antitumor effects [95]. In addition to its beneficial effects when supplementing animals with a melatonin deficiency, supplementing melatonin levels in animals exposed to normal daily light/dark cycles (10:14 or 12:12), thus with normal melatonin nocturnal peaks and diurnal rhythms, also reduces mammary tumor development [35,39,42–44]. These studies suggest that women without a melatonin deficiency would also benefit from taking supplements at night. In addition, since nocturnal melatonin peaks decrease in women as they age [7], these findings suggest that even without excessive light exposure, women would benefit by using supplements to replace these diminishing levels.

Melatonin prevention preclinical studies administer melatonin only at night, even in the animals not exposed to darkness, to recreate the normal timing for peak levels in the blood. This treatment schedule is designed to mimic the natural peak in melatonin levels that occur during exposure to darkness. Continuous treatments throughout the day or those provided during the light cycle are not expected to provide same level of protection against tumor formation. In addition, one study in MMTV-*neu* transgenic mice, expressing the HER2/*neu* oncogene, demonstrated that only continuous treatment was able to reduce the incidence mammary adenocarcinomas and metastases as well as decrease the size of the mammary tumors compared with animals only treated five times monthly [43]. These findings suggest that women who would take melatonin to reduce their risk of developing breast cancer should take it daily prior to bedtime. The fact that melatonin is normally synthesized and secreted each night in response to darkness suggests that the body's response to daily melatonin replacement over one's lifetime should remain responsive (Figure 17.2).

If sleep patterns are normal and not out of sync with the light/dark cycle, then bedtime dosing rather than evening dosing (6–8 PM) may be recommended so to not to phase shift the individual and make them awake earlier in the morning, as is known to occur [7]. If, however, the individual has sleep disruption (e.g., due to light at night shift work, sleeping condition at home, menopause), timing of the melatonin dose should be considered with the goal being to resynchronize the rhythms back to coincide with the light/dark cycle (Figure 17.2). In combination therapies and depending on the drug and the goal of therapy, melatonin may need to be added concurrently or staggered from the other drugs being given. For example, melatonin should be given separately from drug treatments known to be activated through cytochrome P_{450} enzymes, such as tamoxifen, to avoid any drug–drug interactions [96]. However, if the goal of therapy is to reduce local levels of estrogen in the breast, then the dosing may want to be given concurrently with melatonin to maximize the effect of both drugs [95].

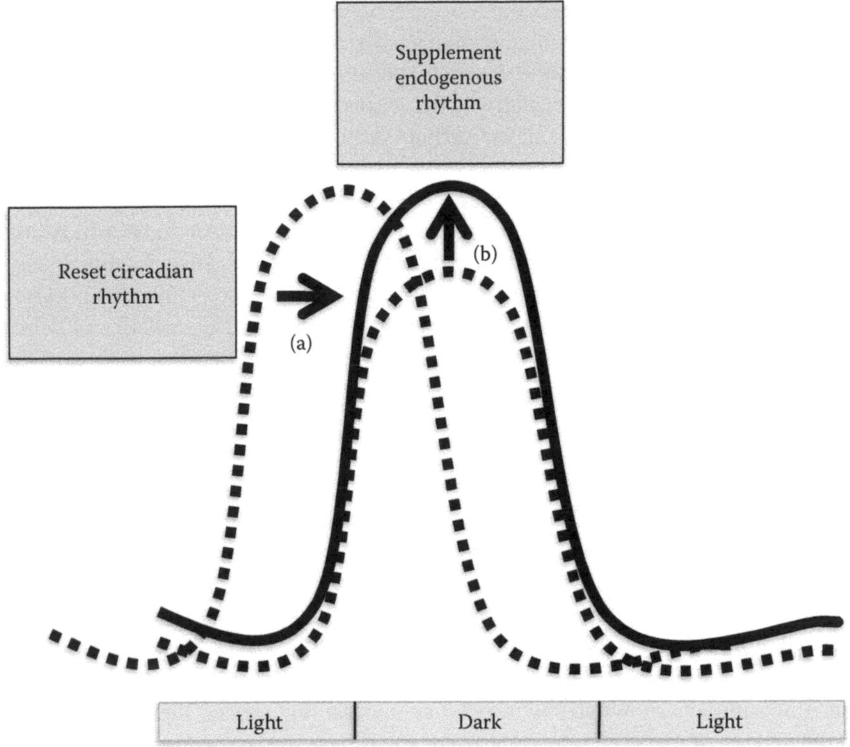

FIGURE 17.2 Levels of melatonin through the 24-hour cycle and the impact of aging and light on its levels. As shown in the graph (solid line), levels of melatonin fluctuate throughout the 24-hour cycle and peak during the hours of darkness. The dotted curves depicted in (a) and (b) show how these curves are affected throughout a woman's life. For example, as shown in (b), factors such as light at night (e.g., shift work) and/or aging (e.g., perimenopausal or postmenopausal women) decrease the nocturnal peak levels to predispose a woman to developing breast cancer. Therefore, supplementing nocturnal melatonin levels may be protective against cancer. Also, it has been shown that the rhythm of melatonin secretion changes during a woman's lifetime in response to fluctuations in her estrogen levels (i.e., pregnancy, menopause, HRT usage). Also, others are showing that clock protein expression in mammary tissue taken from women with breast cancer shows altered patterns of *PER-2* mRNA expression. Because PER-2 is a "clock" protein regulated by light and also a possible tumor suppressor, then resynchronization as shown in (a) melatonin levels and clock proteins to align with the light/dark cycle may provide protection against breast cancer.

Based on the evidence, chronic (i.e., daily bedtime dosing) rather than short-term melatonin dosing produces the greatest benefits on cancer. Melatonin's effects on intracellular mechanisms require constant, persistent exposures to perhaps (1) maintain attenuated levels of aromatases and downstream estrogen responses in the mammary tissue, (2) maintain high enough levels of melatonin to scavenge free radicals to protect the tissue from radical-induced damage, and (3) keep the melatonin receptor in a desensitized stated to modulate ERK1/2 translocation patterns (i.e., maintain cytosolic compartmentalization) that protect the mammary tissue against cancer formation and progression to metastatic disease.

Most over-the-counter melatonin supplements are in tablets with 3 or 5 mg as the recommended nighttime dose. However, if one compares rodent doses to humans only by adjusting for body weight, such as using a microgram per kilogram dose, doses testing mammary tumor prevention in rats or mice are high. That is, if an average woman weighs 70 kg and a mouse weighing 0.04 kg is administered a 50-μg dose or 1.25 mg/kg, the human equivalent would be greater than 87 mg/day. However, mice and rats have a considerably higher metabolism than humans, which should be considered when comparing doses. To account for metabolic rates, if an oral dose is adjusted considering caloric intake for the mouse versus a woman's (such as <18 kcal/day for a mouse versus 1800 kcal/day for an average woman), this same dose may be comparable to a 5-mg melatonin tablet for a woman. This oral dose (50 μg/mouse) effectively decreases the incidence of spontaneous mammary tumors in the C3H/Jax mouse model [42], indicating that tumor prevention can occur at reasonable dosages for women.

When examining the results of animal studies to assess the potential benefits of melatonin, the method of administration as well as the dose needs to be considered. As melatonin is taken orally by women, this delivery method may be more representative than injection (subcutaneously or intraperitoneally). In addition, as melatonin is poorly absorbed in the gut (~15%) [97], bioavailability would be considerably higher for the same dose injected versus given by mouth. As women would be averse to the idea of nightly injections of melatonin, preclinical studies with oral delivery of melatonin may be more correlative for clinical outcomes, especially for comparing effective doses. Several studies using oral administration of melatonin have reported melatonin to be preventative for mammary cancer using doses that are within the range of human consumption, if the metabolic rates of the rats and mice are used for correlating the dose [35,42–44,49].

Due to the strong protective effects of melatonin on breast cancer, conditions that influence its levels should not be ignored for developing preclinical mammary cancer studies. Most cancer studies are investigating melatonin use over a 12-hour or similar dark cycle, yet this level of dark exposure may not be representative of an average woman in an industrialized nation, such as the United States. Since melatonin provides protection against cancer, the use of a long dark cycle may not be accurately reflecting the potential of another therapy or chemical to influence carcinogenesis in women. That is, if a therapy shows strong protection in an animal model, these results could be partially due to the actions of melatonin due to its high levels peaking in the night. However, in women sleeping for 6 hours at night with some light exposure or frequent interruptions, lower nocturnal melatonin levels may not augment the therapy and a reduced efficacy may be observed. Similarly, when investigating risk factors, such as environmental chemicals, the adverse effects may be underestimated due to a beneficial abatement by the nocturnal melatonin peaks in the tested rodents. Therefore, for developing animal studies to assess breast cancer risk or the therapeutic potential of drug, the length of the dark cycle or level of darkness may need to be adjusted to be more representative of women in this country, even for studies not specifically evaluating melatonin.

Even though light-induced decreases in melatonin production probably play very significant roles in increasing breast cancer risk, light effects on clock genes located in the breast tissue may also play a role. The mechanisms underlying light-induced breast cancer are not clear but may involve a key clock protein, PER2. PER2 is a tumor suppressor [98] and mutations in *PER-2* and *PER-3* clock genes result in greater spontaneous tumor formation in mice [99] and an increased risk for pre-menopausal breast cancer [100]. PER-2 activity throughout the light/dark cycle is disrupted in women with breast cancer [101]. PER-2 inhibits the proliferation of several cancers that are epithelial in nature including breast cancer [102] and its down-regulation accelerates breast cancer growth in a circadian-dependent manner [103,104]. PER-2 may also be connected to ER expression, particularly ERα, in a reciprocal manner. High levels of PER2 are associated with low ERα expression and low PER2 is associated with high ERα in [98]. The regulation of PER-2 is poorly understood, but may involve epigenetic regulation through methylation of *PER-2* gene promoters [102] as reviewed in [98]. In addition to the light influences on melatonin levels, light-mediated effects on clock proteins should also be studied concurrently to get the full, yet complicated, picture regarding melatonin's effects as an anticancer agent. Light influences on clock proteins as well as on melatonin levels may explain the differences in melatonin's efficacy to reverse mammary tumor incidence in pinealectomized animals compared to those exposed to light at night [38,39]. Because light exposure at night is more correlative with melatonin deficiency in women due to light pollution [40] other than a natural aging process, then light influences on clock genes as well as on the mechanisms discussed above should be considered when using melatonin as a chemotherapeutic agent. Because light inhibits the synthesis and secretion of melatonin from the pineal gland and that light is a powerful inducer of breast cancer, especially when the exposure occurs during the night [41], then the recommendation would be to reduce light exposure at night by closing blinds, avoid use of nightlights, turn off computers, and wear an eye mask to maximize and maintain the surge in melatonin that occurs during darkness.

The potential for melatonin in improving breast cancer chemotherapeutic outcomes as well as patient-reported outcomes is great. The lack of melatonin use in the clinic is puzzling to those in the melatonin field, especially as a complementary alternative medicine (CAM). Melatonin should be used as a CAM with mainstay chemotherapies to enhance their efficacy and reduce adverse effects or toxicities including sleep disturbances, anxiety, depression, hypotension [105], thrombocytopenia [106,107], and cachexia [108]. Melatonin supplementation has been successful at restoring sleep quality and circadian rhythmicity in older persons [109,110], suggesting that such supplementation could also ameliorate these effects of melatonin disruption as well as the increased cancer incidence. Also, melatonin seems to promote general well-being in cancer patients [111]. This positive effect of melatonin on mood as well as its low toxicity and free radical scavenging property [65] might allow cancer patients to tolerate higher doses of toxic compounds or be more likely to complete the course of standard chemotherapy regimens. These beneficial properties of coadministration of melatonin on making the patient more tolerant to the chemotherapy treatment should be exploited for greater overall treatment benefits in any study.

REFERENCES

1. Jemal, A, Siegel, R, Ward, E, et al. 2008. Cancer statistics, 2008. *CA Cancer J Clin* 58: 71–96.
2. Tsao, AS, Kim, ES, Hong, WK. 2004. Chemoprevention of cancer. *CA Cancer J Clin* 54: 150–180.
3. Fisher, B, Costantino, JP, Wickerham, DL, et al. 1998. Tamoxifen for prevention of breast cancer: Report of the National Surgical Adjuvant Breast and Bowel Project P-1 Study. *J Natl Cancer Inst* 90: 1371–1388.
4. Wolmark, N, Dunn, BK. 2001. The role of tamoxifen in breast cancer prevention: Issues sparked by the NSABP Breast Cancer Prevention Trial (P-1). *Ann N Y Acad Sci* 949: 99–108.
5. Zhdanova, IV, Wurtman, RJ, Balcioglu, A, Kartashov, AI Lynch, HJ. 1998. Endogenous melatonin levels and the fate of exogenous melatonin: Age effects. *J Gerontol A Biol Sci Med Sci* 53: B293–B298.
6. Bartsch, C, Bartsch, H, Karasek, M. 2002. Melatonin in clinical oncology. *Neuro Endocrinol Lett* 23 Suppl 1: 30–38.
7. Zawilska, JB, Skene, DJ, Arendt, J. 2009. Physiology and pharmacology of melatonin in relation to biological rhythms. *Pharmacol Rep* 61: 383–410.
8. Leger, D, Laudon, M, Zisapel, N. 2004. Nocturnal 6-sulfatoxymelatonin excretion in insomnia and its relation to the response to melatonin replacement therapy. *Am J Med* 116: 91–95.
9. Karasek, M, Winczyk, K. 2006. Melatonin in humans. *J Physiol Pharmacol* 57 Suppl 5: 19–39.
10. Cohen, M, Lippman, M, Chabner, B. 1978. Role of pineal gland in aetiology and treatment of breast cancer. *Lancet* 2: 814–816.
11. Kos-Kudla, B, Ostrowska, Z, Marek, B, et al. 2002. Circadian rhythm of melatonin in postmenopausal asthmatic women with hormone replacement therapy. *Neuro Endocrinol Lett* 23: 243–248.
12. Sanchez-Barcelo, EJ, Cos, S, Mediavilla, D, Martinez-Campa, C, Gonzalez, A, Alonso-Gonzalez, C. 2005. Melatonin–estrogen interactions in breast cancer. *J Pineal Res* 38: 217–222.
13. Tamarkin, L, Danforth, D, Lichter, A, et al. 1982. Decreased nocturnal plasma melatonin peak in patients with estrogen receptor positive breast cancer. *Science* 216: 1003–1005.
14. Schernhammer, ES, Hankinson, SE. 2009. Urinary melatonin levels and postmenopausal breast cancer risk in the Nurses' Health Study cohort. *Cancer Epidemiol Biomarkers Prev* 18: 74–79.
15. Stevens, RG. 1987. Electric power use and breast cancer: A hypothesis. *Am J Epidemiology* 125.4: 556–561.
16. Davis, S, Mirick, DK, Stevens, RG. 2001. Night shift work, light at night, and risk of breast cancer. *J Natl Cancer Inst* 93: 1557–1562.
17. Davis, S, Mirick, DK. 2006. Circadian disruption, shift work and the risk of cancer: A summary of the evidence and studies in Seattle. *Cancer Causes Control* 17: 539–545.
18. Coleman, MP, Reiter, RJ. 1992. Breast cancer, blindness and melatonin. *Eur J Cancer* 28: 501–503.

19. Flynn-Evans, EE, Stevens, RG, Tabandeh, H, Schernhammer, ES, Lockley, SW. 2009. Total visual blindness is protective against breast cancer. *Cancer Causes and Control* 20: 1753–1756.
20. Grant, SG, Melan, MA, Latimer, JJ, Witt-Enderby, PA. 2009. Melatonin and breast cancer: Cellular mechanisms, clinical studies and future perspectives. *Expert Rev Mol Med* 11: e5.
21. Burch, JB, Walling, M, Rush, A, et al. 2007. Melatonin and estrogen in breast cyst fluids. *Breast Cancer Res Treat* 103: 331–341.
22. Bartsch, C, Kvetnoy, I, Kvetnaia, T, et al. 1997. Nocturnal urinary 6-sulfatoxymelatonin and proliferating cell nuclear antigen–immunopositive tumor cells show strong positive correlations in patients with gastrointestinal and lung cancer. *J Pineal Res* 23: 90–96.
23. Maestroni, GJ, Conti, A. 1996. Melatonin in human breast cancer tissue: Association with nuclear grade and estrogen receptor status. *Lab Invest* 75: 557–561.
24. Blask, DE. 1997. The melatonin rhythm in cancer patients, Washington, D.C., American Psychiatric Press.
25. Panzer, A, Viljoen, M. 1997. The validity of melatonin as an oncostatic agent. *J Pineal Res* 22: 184–202.
26. Mills, E, Wu, P, Seely, D, Guyatt, G. 2005. Melatonin in the treatment of cancer: A systematic review of randomized controlled trials and meta-analysis. *J Pineal Res* 39: 360–366.
27. Lissoni, P, Di Fede, G, Battista, A, et al. 2009. A phase II study of anastrozole plus the pineal anticancer hormone melatonin in the metastatic breast cancer women with poor clinical status. *Cancer Ther* 7: 302–304.
28. Vesnushkin, GM, Plotnikova, NA, Semenchenko, AI, Anisimov, VN. 2006. Dose-dependent inhibitory effect of melatonin on carcinogenesis induced by benzo[a]pyrene in mice. *J Exp Clin Cancer Res* 25: 507–513.
29. Viii, B. 2006. *Health Risks from Exposure to Low Levels of Ionizing Radiation*, National Academies Press, Washington, DC.
30. Rogelsperger, O, Ekmekcioglu, C, Jager, W, et al. 2009. Coexpression of the melatonin receptor 1 and nestin in human breast cancer specimens. *J Pineal Res* 46: 422–432.
31. Cos, S, Gonzalez, A, Martinez-Campa, C, Mediavilla, MD, Alonso-Gonzalez, C Sanchez-Barcelo, EJ. 2006. Estrogen-signaling pathway: A link between breast cancer and melatonin oncostatic actions. *Cancer Detect Prev* 30: 118–128.
32. Treilleux, Peloux, N, Brown, M Sergeant, A. 1997. Human estrogen receptor (ER) gene promoter-P1: Estradiol-independent activity and estradiol inducibility in ER+ and ER- cells. *Mol Endocrinol* 11: 1319–1331.
33. Cunat, S, Hoffmann, P, Pujol, P. 2004. Estrogens and epithelial ovarian cancer. *Gynecol Oncol* 94: 25–32.
34. Naderi, A, Teschendorff, AE, Beigel, J, et al. 2007. BEX2 is overexpressed in a subset of primary breast cancers and mediates nerve growth factor/nuclear factor-kappaB inhibition of apoptosis in breast cancer cell lines. *Cancer Res* 67: 6725–6736.
35. Kothari, LS. 1987. Influence of chronic melatonin on 9,10-dimethyl-1,2-benzanthracene–induced mammary tumors in female Holtzman rats exposed to continuous light. *Oncology* 44: 64–66.
36. Anisimov, VN. 2006. Light pollution, reproductive function and cancer risk. *Neuro Endocrinol Lett* 27: 35–52.
37. Cos, S Sanchez-Barcelo, EJ. 2000. Melatonin, experimental basis for a possible application in breast cancer prevention and treatment. *Histol Histopathol* 15: 637–647.
38. Shah, PN, Mhatre, MC, Kothari, LS. 1984. Effect of melatonin on mammary carcinogenesis in intact and pinealectomized rats in varying photoperiods. *Cancer Res* 44: 3403–3407.
39. Tamarkin, L, Cohen, M, Roselle, D, Reichert, C, Lippman, M, Chabner, B. 1981. Melatonin inhibition and pinealectomy enhancement of 7,12-dimethylbenz(*a*)anthracene-induced mammary tumors in the rat. *Cancer Res* 41: 4432–4436.
40. Graham, C, Cook, Mr, Gerkovich, MM, Sastre, A. 2001. Examination of the melatonin hypothesis in women exposed at night to EMF or bright light. *Environ Health Perspect* 109: 501–507.
41. Blask, DE, Brainard, GC, Dauchy, RT, et al. 2005. Melatonin-depleted blood from premenopausal women exposed to light at night stimulates growth of human breast cancer xenografts in nude rats. *Cancer Res* 65: 11174–11184.
42. Subramanian, A, Kothari, L. 1991. Suppressive effect by melatonin on different phases of 9,10-dimethyl-1, 2-benzanthracene (DMBA–)induced rat mammary gland carcinogenesis. *Anticancer Drugs* 2: 297–303.
43. Anisimov, VN, Alimova, IN, Baturin, DA, et al. 2003. The effect of melatonin treatment regimen on mammary adenocarcinoma development in HER-2/neu transgenic mice. *Int J Cancer* 103: 300–305.

44. Baturin, DA, Alimova, IN, Anisimov, VN, et al. 2001. The effect of light regimen and melatonin on the development of spontaneous mammary tumors in HER-2/neu transgenic mice is related to a downregulation of HER-2/neu gene expression. *Neuro Endocrinol Lett* 22: 441–447.
45. Mediavilla, MD, Guezmez, A, Ramos, S, Kothari, L, Garijo, F, Sanchez Barcelo, EJ. 1997. Effects of melatonin on mammary gland lesions in transgenic mice overexpressing N-ras proto-oncogene. *J Pineal Res* 22: 86–94.
46. Rao, GN, Ney, E, Herbert, RA. 2000. Effect of melatonin and linolenic acid on mammary cancer in transgenic mice with c-neu breast cancer oncogene. *Breast Cancer Res Treat* 64: 287–296.
47. Witt-Enderby, PA, Radio, NM, Doctor, JS, Davis, VL. 2006. Therapeutic treatments potentially mediated by melatonin receptors: Potential clinical uses in the prevention of osteoporosis, cancer and as an adjuvant therapy. *J Pineal Res* 41: 297–305.
48. Blask, DE, Pelletier, DB, Hill, SM, et al. 1991. Pineal melatonin inhibition of tumor promotion in the *N*-nitroso-*N*- methylurea model of mammary carcinogenesis: Potential involvement of antiestrogenic mechanisms in vivo. *J Cancer Res Clin Oncol* 117: 526–532.
49. Lenoir, V, De Jonage-Canonico, MB, Perrin, MH, Martin, A, Scholler, R, Kerdelhue, B. 2005. Preventive and curative effect of melatonin on mammary carcinogenesis induced by dimethylbenz[a]anthracene in the female Sprague–Dawley rat. *Breast Cancer Res* 7: R470–476.
50. Cos, S, Mediavilla, D, Martinez-Campa, C, Gonzalez, A, Alonso-Gonzalez, C, Sanchez-Barcelo, EJ. 2006. Exposure to light-at-night increases the growth of DMBA-induced mammary adenocarcinomas in rats. *Cancer Lett* 235: 266–271.
51. Kothari, A, Borges, A, Kothari, L. 1995. Chemoprevention by melatonin and combined melatonin–tamoxifen therapy of second generation nitroso-methylurea–induced mammary tumours in rats. *Eur J Cancer Prev* 4: 497–500.
52. Kubatka, P, Bojkova, B, K, Mc-K, et al. 2001. Effects of tamoxifen and melatonin on mammary gland cancer induced by *N*-methyl-*N*-nitrosourea and by 7,12-dimethylbenz(a)anthracene, respectively, in female Sprague–Dawley rats. *Folia Biol (Praha)* 47: 5–10.
53. Collins, A, Yuan, L, Kiefer, TL, Cheng, Q, Lai, L, Hill, SM. 2003. Overexpression of the MT1 melatonin receptor in MCF-7 human breast cancer cells inhibits mammary tumor formation in nude mice. *Cancer Lett* 189: 49–57.
54. Recio, J, Cardinali, DP, Sanchez-Barcelo, EJ. 1994. 2-[125I]iodomelatonin binding sites in murine mammary tissue. *Biol Signals* 3: 85–90.
55. Cos, S, Fernandez, R, Guezmes, A, Sanchez-Barcelo, EJ. 1998. Influence of melatonin on invasive and metastatic properties of MCF-7 human breast cancer cells. *Cancer Res* 58: 4383–4390.
56. Hill, SM, Frasch, T, Xiang, S, Yuan, L, Duplessis, T, Mao, L. 2009. Molecular mechanisms of melatonin anticancer effects. *Integr Cancer Ther* 8: 337–346.
57. Danielczyk, K, Dziegiel, P. 2009. The expression of MT1 melatonin receptor and Ki-67 antigen in melanoma malignum. *Anticancer Res* 29: 3887–3895.
58. Martinez-Campa, C, Alonso-Gonzalez, C, Mediavilla, MD, et al. 2006. Melatonin inhibits both ER alpha activation and breast cancer cell proliferation induced by a metalloestrogen, cadmium. *J Pineal Res* 40: 291–296.
59. Reiter, RJ, Paredes, SD, Manchester, LC, Tan, DX. 2009. Reducing oxidative/nitrosative stress: A newly-discovered genre for melatonin. *Crit Rev Biochem Mol Biol* 44: 175–200.
60. Luchetti, F, Betti, M, Canonico, B, et al. 2009. ERK MAPK activation mediates the antiapoptotic signaling of melatonin in UVB-stressed U937 cells. *Free Radic Biol Med* 46: 339–351.
61. Acuna-Castroviejo, D, Escames, G, Rodriguez, MI, Lopez, LC. 2007. Melatonin role in the mitochondrial function. *Front Biosci* 12: 947–963.
62. Reiter, RJ, Tan, D, Kim, SJ, et al. 1999. Augmentation of indices of oxidative damage in life-long melatonin-deficient rats. *Mech Ageing Dev* 110: 157–173.
63. Morioka, N, Okatani, Y, Wakatsuki, A. 1999. Melatonin protects against age-related DNA damage in the brains of female senescence-accelerated mice. *J Pineal Res* 27: 202–209.
64. Anisimov, VN, Alimova, IN, Baturin, DA, et al. 2003. Dose-dependent effect of melatonin on life span and spontaneous tumor incidence in female SHR mice. *Exp Gerontol* 38: 449–461.
65. Vijayalaxmi, Reiter, RJ, Tan, DX, Herman, TS, Thomas, CR, Jr. 2004. Melatonin as a radioprotective agent: A review. *Int J Radiat Oncol Biol Phys* 59: 639–653.
66. Sanchez-Barcelo, EJ, Cos, S, Fernandez, R, Mediavilla, MD. 2003. Melatonin and mammary cancer: A short review. *Endocr Relat Cancer* 10: 153–159.
67. Cos, S, Recio, J, Sanchez-Barcelo, EJ. 1996. Modulation of the length of the cell cycle time of MCF-7 human breast cancer cells by melatonin. *Life Sci* 58: 811–816.

68. Jones, MP, Melan, MA, Witt-Enderby, PA. 2000. Melatonin decreases cell proliferation and transformation in a melatonin receptor–dependent manner. *Cancer Lett* 151: 133–143.
69. Girgert, R, Hanf, V, Emons, G, Grundker, C. 2009. Membrane-bound melatonin receptor MT1 downregulates estrogen responsive genes in breast cancer cells. *J Pineal Res* 47: 23–31.
70. Dai, J, Inscho, EW, Yuan, L, Hill, SM. 2002. Modulation of intracellular calcium and calmodulin by melatonin in MCF-7 human breast cancer cells. *J Pineal Res* 32: 112–119.
71. Gonzalez, A, Cos, S, Martinez-Campa, C, et al. 2008. Selective estrogen enzyme modulator actions of melatonin in human breast cancer cells. *J Pineal Res* 45: 86–92.
72. Del Rio, B, Garcia Pedrero, JM, Martinez-Campa, C, Zuazua, P, Lazo, PS, Ramos, S. 2004. Melatonin, an endogenous-specific inhibitor of estrogen receptor alpha via calmodulin. *J Biol Chem* 279: 38294–38302.
73. Kiefer, T, Ram, PT, Yuan, L, Hill, SM. 2002. Melatonin inhibits estrogen receptor transactivation and cAMP levels in breast cancer cells. *Breast Cancer Res Treat* 71: 37–45.
74. Rato, AG, Pedrero, JG, Martinez, MA, Del Rio, B, Lazo, PS, Ramos, S. 1999. Melatonin blocks the activation of estrogen receptor for DNA binding. *FASEB J* 13: 857–868.
75. Martinez-Campa, C, Gonzalez, A, Mediavilla, MD, et al. 2009. Melatonin inhibits aromatase promoter expression by regulating cyclooxygenases expression and activity in breast cancer cells. *Br J Cancer* 101: 1613–1619.
76. Aust, S, Jaeger, W, Klimpfinger, M, et al. 2005. Biotransformation of melatonin in human breast cancer cell lines: Role of sulfotransferase 1A1. *J Pineal Res* 39: 276–282.
77. Kothari, A, Borges, A, Ingle, A, Kothari, L. 1997. Combination of melatonin and tamoxifen as a chemoprophylaxis against *N*-nitroso-*N*-methylurea–induced rat mammary tumors. *Cancer Lett* 111: 59–66.
78. Hill, SM, Teplitzky, S, Ram, PT, et al. 1999. Melatonin synergizes with retinoic acid in the prevention and regression of breast cancer. *Adv Exp Med Biol* 460: 345–362.
79. Cos, S, Gonzalez, A, Guezmes, A, et al. 2006. Melatonin inhibits the growth of DMBA-induced mammary tumors by decreasing the local biosynthesis of estrogens through the modulation of aromatase activity. *Int J Cancer* 118: 274–278.
80. Melancon, K, Cheng, Q, Kiefer, TL, et al. 2005. Regression of NMU-induced mammary tumors with the combination of melatonin and 9-*cis*-retinoic acid. *Cancer Lett* 227: 39–48.
81. Moselhy, SS, Al Mslmani, MA. 2008. Chemopreventive effect of lycopene alone or with melatonin against the genesis of oxidative stress and mammary tumors induced by 7,12 dimethyl(*a*)benzanthracene in sprague dawely female rats. *Mol Cell Biochem* 319: 175–180.
82. Russo, J, Balogh, GA, Heulings, R, et al. 2006. Molecular basis of pregnancy-induced breast cancer protection. *Eur J Cancer Prev* 15: 306–342.
83. Luttrell, LM. 2002. Activation and targeting of mitogen-activated protein kinases by G-protein–coupled receptors. *Can J Physiol Pharmacol* 80: 375–382.
84. Satomura, K, Tobiume, S, Tokuyama, R, et al. 2007. Melatonin at pharmacological doses enhances human osteoblastic differentiation in vitro and promotes mouse cortical bone formation in vivo. *J Pineal Res* 42: 231–239.
85. Sanchez-Hidalgo, M, Lu, Z, Tan, DX, Maldonado, MD, Reiter, RJ, Gregerman, RI. 2007. Melatonin inhibits fatty acid–induced triglyceride accumulation in ROS17/2.8 cells: Implications for osteoblast differentiation and osteoporosis. *Am J Physiol Regul Integr Comp Physiol* 292: R2208–2215.
86. Schuster, C, Williams, LM, Morris, A, Morgan, PJ, Barrett, P. 2005. The human MT1 melatonin receptor stimulates cAMP production in the human neuroblastoma cell line SH-SY5Y cells via a calcium-calmodulin signal transduction pathway. *J Neuroendocrinol* 17: 170–178.
87. Johnston, JD, Klosen, P, Barrett, P, Hazlerigg, DG. 2006. Regulation of MT melatonin receptor expression in the foetal rat pituitary. *J Neuroendocrinol* 18: 50–56.
88. Radio, NM, Doctor, JS, Witt-Enderby, PA. 2006. Melatonin enhances alkaline phosphatase activity in differentiating human adult mesenchymal stem cells grown in osteogenic medium via MT2 melatonin receptors and the MEK/ERK (1/2) signaling cascade. *J Pineal Res* 40: 332–342.
89. Sainz, RM, Mayo, JC, Tan, DX, Leon, J, Manchester, L, Reiter, RJ. 2005. Melatonin reduces prostate cancer cell growth leading to neuroendocrine differentiation via a receptor and PKA independent mechanism. *Prostate* 63: 29–43.
90. Bellon, A, Ortiz-Lopez, L, Ramirez-Rodriguez, G, Anton-Tay, F, Benitez-King, G. 2007. Melatonin induces neuritogenesis at early stages in N1E-115 cells through actin rearrangements via activation of protein kinase C and Rho-associated kinase. *J Pineal Res* 42: 214–221.
91. Moriya, T, Horie, N, Mitome, M, Shinohara, K. 2007. Melatonin influences the proliferative and differentiative activity of neural stem cells. *J Pineal Res* 42: 411–418.

92. Jimenez-Jorge, S, Jimenez-Caliani, AJ, Guerrero, JM, et al. 2005. Melatonin synthesis and melatonin-membrane receptor (MT1) expression during rat thymus development: Role of the pineal gland. *J Pineal Res* 39: 77–83.
93. Sethi, S, Radio, NM, Kotlarczyk, M, et al. 2010. Determination of the minimal melatonin exposure required to induce osteoblast differentitation from human mesenchymal stem cells and these effects on downstream signaling pathways. *J Pineal Res*. doi:10.1111/j.1600-079X.2010.00784.x.
94. 2005. Melatonin. Monograph. *Altern Med Rev* 10: 326–336.
95. Jung, B, Ahmad, N. 2006. Melatonin in cancer management: Progress and promise. *Cancer Res* 66: 9789–9793.
96. Sideras, K, Ingle, JN, Ames, MM, et al. 2010. Coprescription of tamoxifen and medications that inhibit CYP2D6. *J Clin Oncol* 28: 2768–2776.
97. Demuro, RL, Nafziger, AN, Blask, DE, Menhinick, AM, Bertino, JS, Jr. 2000. The absolute bioavailability of oral melatonin. *J Clin Pharmacol* 40: 781–784.
98. Korkmaz, A, Sanchez-Barcelo, EJ, Tan, DX, Reiter, RJ. 2009. Role of melatonin in the epigenetic regulation of breast cancer. *Breast Cancer Res Treat* 115: 13–27.
99. Canaple, L, Kakizawa, T, Laudet, V. 2003. The days and nights of cancer cells. *Cancer Res* 63: 7545–7552.
100. Zhu, Y, Brown, HN, Zhang, Y, Stevens, RG, Zheng, T. 2005. Period3 structural variation: A circadian biomarker associated with breast cancer in young women. *Cancer Epidemiol Biomarkers Prev* 14: 268–270.
101. Chen, ST, Choo, KB, Hou, MF, Yeh, KT, Kuo, SJ, Chang, JG. 2005. Deregulated expression of the PER1, PER2 and PER3 genes in breast cancers. *Carcinogenesis* 26: 1241–1246.
102. Gery, S, Gombart, AF, Yi, WS, Koeffler, C, Hofmann, WK, Koeffler, HP. 2005. Transcription profiling of C/EBP targets identifies Per2 as a gene implicated in myeloid leukemia. *Blood* 106: 2827–2836.
103. Yang, X, Wood, PA, Oh, EY, Du-Quiton, J, Ansell, CM, Hrushesky, WJ. 2009. Down regulation of circadian clock gene Period 2 accelerates breast cancer growth by altering its daily growth rhythm. *Breast Cancer Res Treat* 117: 423–431.
104. Yang, X, Wood, PA, Ansell, C, Hrushesky, WJ. 2009. Circadian time-dependent tumor suppressor function of period genes. *Integr Cancer Ther* 8: 309–316.
105. Lissoni, P, Pittalis, S, Ardizzoia, A, et al. 1996. Prevention of cytokine-induced hypotension in cancer patients by the pineal hormone melatonin. *Support Care Cancer* 4: 313–316.
106. Lissoni, P, Barni, S, Brivio, F, et al. 1995. A biological study on the efficacy of low-dose subcutaneous interleukin-2 plus melatonin in the treatment of cancer-related thrombocytopenia. *Oncology* 52: 360–362.
107. Lissoni, P, Tancini, G, Barni, S, et al. 1996. The pineal hormone melatonin in hematology and its potential efficacy in the treatment of thrombocytopenia. *Recenti Prog Med* 87: 582–585.
108. Lissoni, P, Paolorossi, F, Tancini, G, et al. 1996. Is there a role for melatonin in the treatment of neoplastic cachexia? *Eur J Cancer* 32A: 1340–1343.
109. Valtonen, M, Niskanen, L, Kangas, AP, Koskinen, T. 2005. Effect of melatonin-rich night-time milk on sleep and activity in elderly institutionalized subjects. *Nord J Psychiatry* 59: 217–221.
110. Gubin, DG, Gubin, GD, Waterhouse, J, Weinert, D. 2006. The circadian body temperature rhythm in the elderly: Effect of single daily melatonin dosing. *Chronobiol Int* 23: 639–658.
111. Norsa, A, Martino, V. 2007. Somatostatin, retinoids, melatonin, vitamin D, bromocriptine, and cyclophosphamide in chemotherapy-pretreated patients with advanced lung adenocarcinoma and low performance status. *Cancer Biother Radiopharm* 22: 50–55.

18 Molecular and Epigenetic Effects of Melatonin in Breast Cancer

Sara Proietti, Alessandra Cucina, Simona Dinicola, Alessia Pasqualato, Fabrizio D'Anselmi, and Mariano Bizzarri

CONTENTS

18.1 INTRODUCTION

Three centuries ago, the French philosopher René Descartes [1] described the pineal gland as "the seat of the soul," but it was not until the late 1950s that melatonin, the principal secretory product of the pineal gland was identified [2]. There is now evidence that melatonin may have a role in several biological functions, among which are circadian rhythms, sleep, mood, reproduction, and aging [3–5]. Moreover, as a pharmaceutical drug, melatonin is thought to be beneficial in some pathological conditions [6–8]. Namely, there is now compelling evidence that melatonin may reduce the incidence and the growth of human tumors. However, uncertainties and doubts still surround the physiological mechanisms and the biochemical pathways through which melatonin exerts its antineoplastic effects [9].

Although the first suggestion relating something of pineal gland origin to cancer was made more than 80 years ago [10], only during the past three decades has the role of melatonin in the control of neoplastic growth been specifically investigated [11,12].

In 1978, the seminal paper of Cohen et al. [13] first proposed that the pineal gland and melatonin are likely to play an important role in the pathogenesis of breast cancer. These authors suggested that a decrease in pineal function, whatever its cause, and the consequent reduction in melatonin secretion could induce a state of relative hyperestrogenism, thus leading to a prolonged exposure of breast tissue to estrogens and eventually ending in cancer induction.

Breast cancer is one of the most frequently occurring cancers among women and one of the leading causes of death among women aged 40 to 55 years [14]. Many factors, including hormonal environment, age, dietary and alcohol consumption, or cigarette smoking, have all been hypothesized as contributors to the development of breast cancer [15]. However, a major consequence of a modern lifestyle is the disruption of circadian rhythms, a condition that leads to several pathological conditions, including sleep disturbances and depression [16]. The day and night cycle is indeed an important regulator of a wide variety of physiological biorhythms in living organisms, including humans. In particular, accumulating evidence shows that changes in circadian rhythms might lead to increased susceptibility to cancer in humans. Epidemiological studies have indeed revealed the risk for breast cancer to be significantly higher in industrialized societies and that the risk increases in women who work night shifts or in individuals who spend more hours per week and years working at night [17].

Growing in parallel with industrialization, the use of artificial light–prolonged "day" has permitted employers to extend their work schedules into the night and in many cases throughout the 24-hour period. Because of this temporal coincidence, light at night suppresses the synthesis and release of melatonin; this drop has been incriminated as a plausible contributor to the elevated cancer risk [18]. What this means is that modern humans are rendering themselves relatively melatonin-deficient by shortening their daily dark period and, therefore, the duration of time during which melatonin can be produced. Kerenyi et al. [19] were the first to propose that "light pollution" may be a potentially important etiologic influence on the genesis of other human cancers. Recent epidemiological studies [20,21] showing that women working night shifts have a significantly elevated risk of breast cancer presumably due to their potential increased exposure to light at night provide additional support for this hypothesis. Indeed, in 1981, Bartsch et al. [22] published the first study demonstrating that plasma concentrations are diminished in patients with breast cancer. Since then, many studies have confirmed that patients with established breast cancer have measurably lower levels of melatonin [23,24].

18.2 MELATONIN EFFECTS ON BREAST CANCER: ANIMAL STUDIES AND CLINICAL TRIALS

Further insights into the relationship between melatonin and cancer have been provided by studies performed on chemically induced mammary cancer in animals. Reducing circulating melatonin levels in rats (through pinealectomy or by exposure to continuous light) generally leads to increased spontaneous tumor induction or enhanced growth of implanted cancers. On the other hand, restoring melatonin levels has been proven to prevent or restrain the development of breast cancer [25,26].

Melatonin significantly reduces the incidence and tumor size of rat mammary cancers induced by 7,12-dimethylbenz[*a*]anthracene (DMBA) or *N*-nitrosomethylurea (NMU) [27,28]. In DMBA-exposed rats, long-term daily administration of melatonin inhibited tumorigenesis, whereas pinealectomy increased the incidence of breast tumors [29]. Similar results have been reported by several authors [30]. Moreover, constant light—known to suppress melatonin release—reduces the latency and increases the number of DMBA-induced mammary tumors in rats and increases the incidence of different spontaneous cancers in female CBA mice [31]. Moreover, in NMU-treated rats, melatonin's cytostatic effects are similar to those exerted by tamoxifen, i.e., melatonin increases tumor latency, reduces cancer incidence (% of animals developing tumors) as well as the number and size of tumors. Furthermore, melatonin slows the rate of tumor growth and enhances spontaneous tumor regression [28,32,33]. Overall, these data show that melatonin inhibits both cancer initiation and progression through several mechanisms, including estrogen pathway modulation, receptor-mediated and receptor-independent effects on different enzymatic processes, as well as antioxidant effects. It is well known that reactive oxygen species (ROS) participate in a variety of processes regulating cell growth, gene transcription, differentiation, and apoptosis [34]. In cancer cells, free radicals and ROS can act as tumor promoters, leading to cancer initiation or the growth enhancement of already transformed cells. Therefore, free radical scavengers and antioxidant molecules such as melatonin may display a significant role in preventing cancer and/or in hindering its progression [35,36].

Results obtained from research carried out on animals have received supporting data from studies performed on human. Besides some preliminary anecdotic reports [37,38] clinical trials carried out by Lissoni et al. [39] indicated appreciable benefits in treating cancer bearing patients with melatonin. In a pilot study, 14 women with metastatic breast cancer who had no clinical response to tamoxifen were given 20 mg of tamoxifen and 20 mg of melatonin in the evening. A partial response, defined as radiographic-confirmed reduction of lesions by greater than 50%, was observed in 4 (28.5%) out of 14 patients, with a median duration of 8 months. In two randomized clinical trials [40,41]—consisting of several cancer types, including breast tumors—melatonin had beneficial effects among patients with metastatic cancer. Panzer and Viljoen [42] have reviewed clinical studies with melatonin on patients with different types of cancer, provided evidence that melatonin therapy is beneficial, and showed that the indoleamine (a) increased survival in a few metastatic patients, (b) retarded cancer progression, (c) improved quality of life and performance status, and (d) decreased the incidence and severity of some side effects linked to conventional treatments (hypotension, thrombocytopenia, myelodysplastic syndrome, lymphocytopenia) [43–46]. However, these studies included several types of advanced cancer patients and only few cases of mammary tumors; thus, little information on the potential efficacy of melatonin treatment in breast cancer patients was provided. In addition, these findings require verification by independent and controlled replication studies, in order to overcome statistical bias and methodological deficiencies due to the limited number of patients under study [47].

18.3 MELATONIN EFFECTS ON BREAST CANCER: IN VITRO STUDIES

18.3.1 Inhibition of Breast Cancer Cell Growth

The melatonin's attributed anticancer effects have often derived from in vitro studies carried out on estrogen-responsive human breast cancer cell lines. The first in vitro experiments on MCF-7 cells demonstrated that melatonin, even at physiological concentrations, directly suppressed cancer cell growth [48,49]. Melatonin appears to exert an inhibitory effect by causing an accumulation of cells in the G0/G1 phase of the cell cycle [50] or, otherwise, by delaying the progression of MCF-7 cells from the G1 phase to the S phase of the cell cycle [51,52], allowing the cells to achieve greater differentiation. A similar pattern was observed for other estrogen-sensitive cancer cell lines (T47D and ZR75-1) [53–55]. Growth inhibition is accompanied by a significant decrease in DNA content and thymidine incorporation [56,57]. These effects seem to be related to both cancer cell characteristics and culture conditions.

18.3.2 Melatonin and Estrogen Receptors

Melatonin significantly inhibits cell growth only in breast cancer cells expressing estrogen receptors (ERα) [58,59]. Melatonin does not inhibit the proliferation of MDA-MB-231, MDA-MB-330, or BT-20 ERα-negative human breast tumor cells lines. However, the indoleamine has been demonstrated to inhibit growth proliferation on ERα-negative breast cancer and progesterone receptor-negative human breast tumor xenographs in nude rats [60]. Moreover, a significant oncostatic action has been observed in ER-negative, nonbreast tumors treated with melatonin [21]. These data suggest that some non-ER–mediated effects are likely to be elicited by the complex interplay between melatonin and living cells.

Furthermore, it has been shown that the effects of the indoleamine are mainly mediated by the interaction with a specific membrane-bound melatonin receptor. Several reports have demonstrated that melatonin can bind and activate the G protein–coupled membrane melatonin receptors 1 (MT1) and 2 (MT2) in a variety of tissues [62]. The oncostatic effects of melatonin on ER-positive breast cancer cells seem to be strictly dependent on the presence of the MT1, which has been found in both normal and cancerous tissues [63]. The MT1 receptor is differentially expressed in ERα-positive and ERα-negative breast cancer cells, with the higher MT1 levels found in the former cell lines [63]. The MT1 receptor couple with different Gαi proteins in multiple cell types, while also coupling with the Gq and G11 proteins in other cell types [62,64]. Selective MT1 antagonists (as luzindole) suppress melatonin-induced anticancer effects [52,65,66]. On the other hand, overexpression of MT1 receptor in MCF-7 cells significantly enhances the response of these cells to the growth inhibitory actions of melatonin, both in vitro and in vivo [67,68]. Similar results have been observed when treating MCF-7 cells with valproic acid, a MT1 receptor inducer [69]. Moreover, melatonin sensitivity of different MCF-7 strains is greatly dependent on MT1 expression [70]. MT2 receptor seems not to be involved in oncostatic effects triggered by melatonin, keeping in mind that MT2 activation has little influence in mediating the antiproliferative effects of melatonin on breast tumors [71]. Recent findings demonstrated that the MT1 receptor colocalizes with the Cav-1 antibody, indicating the MT1 receptor can also reside in the caveoli, a key membrane signaling platform [72].

MT1 and MT2 receptors are G-protein–coupled receptors, which are expressed in various parts of the central nervous system and in peripheral organs (blood vessels, mammary gland, gastrointestinal tract, liver, kidney and bladder, ovary, testis, prostate, skin, and the immune system). Melatonin receptors mediate a plethora of intracellular effects depending on the cellular milieu. These effects include changes in intracellular cyclic nucleotides (cAMP and cGMP) and calcium levels, activation of certain protein kinase C subtypes, intracellular localization of steroid hormone receptors, and regulation of G protein signaling proteins [73].

MT1 expression is regulated by both melatonin and estradiol, as first documented in experiments performed on cells of the pars tuberalis [74]. The steady-state level of MT1 mRNA is significantly enhanced in MCF-7 cells cultured in estradiol-depleted medium. In cancer cells cultured in the presence of fetal bovine serum (FBS), the MT1 receptor steady-state mRNA level is suppressed by the addition of estradiol (1 nM) or significantly diminished by the addition of melatonin, confirming the ability of melatonin to down-regulate the levels of its own receptor, at least at the steady-state mRNA levels [71,75]. Estradiol-induced down-regulation of MT1 receptor could explain some contradictory results, i.e., the lack of melatonin inhibition of estradiol-induced proliferation of breast cancer cells [76].

Although removal of estradiol from the culture media up-regulates MT1 levels, several reports were unable to demonstrate an enhanced growth inhibitory response to melatonin in MCF-7 cells growing in estradiol-deficient media, as the overall growth of those cells is generally slowed in the absence of estradiol [76]. These results imply that a number of other hormones, cytokines, or growth factor-related signaling pathways modulate MT1 expression, and the hormonal milieu of the tumor at the time of melatonin administration can dramatically impact the responsiveness of the tumor to the antiproliferative action of melatonin.

These actions are generally recognized as hormone-like effects. However, melatonin does not always act in this manner and several melatonin-induced effects are carried out without the intervention of a receptor. Melatonin should be rather considered as a tissue factor, behaving like a paracoid, an autocoid, an antioxidant, or a prooxidant factor depending on the physiological context [77]. The oncostatic effects triggered by melatonin are strictly context-dependent as well. Decreasing the fetal bovine serum concentration reduces the responsiveness of MCF-7 cells to melatonin, until cells are totally refractory in serum-free medium [78]; on the contrary, melatonin-induced inhibition is enhanced in both human [59] and animal cancer cells [57] cultured in charcoal-stripped serum supplemented with estradiol. Moreover, differences in MCF-7 cell strains and differences in their proliferation rate can account for the different sensitivity to the inhibitory effects induced by melatonin [79]. In addition, melatonin precursors, metabolites, or other pineal methoxyindoles do not exert any effect. The melatonin inhibitory activity is dependent on the pattern (continuous or pulsatile) of the exposure to the pineal indole in the culture media. The highest antiproliferative effects are obtained when the concentration of melatonin in culture media is changed every 12 h between 10^{-11} and 10^{-9} M, thus mimicking the physiological day/night oscillation of melatonin in the plasma of most mammals [80].

Culture conditions exert a relevant modulation on cell sensitivity to melatonin. In cells growing in anchorage-dependent monolayer culture with FBS, melatonin inhibits MCF-7 cells according to a bell-shaped curve, showing that the highest cytostatic effect is generally obtained around the physiological range (10^{-11} to 10^{-9} M), while higher or lower doses produce little or no inhibition [50]. Growth inhibition becomes evident after 48–72 hours and thereafter increases linearly up to 144 hours [52]. However, in an anchorage-independent culture system, the dose–response curve loses its characteristic form and becomes quite linear with increasing melatonin concentrations producing greater inhibition [81]. This result highlights that cellular attachment to a substratum, which is likely to modify both the cytoskeleton and cell shape, plays an important role in setting the level of sensitivity to melatonin.

18.3.3 Signaling Pathways Involved: Estrogen Pathways

Melatonin can influence estrogenic actions on mammary tissue in three different ways: [1] by down-regulating gonadal synthesis of steroids and, consequently, decreasing their circulating levels; thus, melatonin interferes with estrogen-related systemic effects; [2] by interacting with the ER, thus behaving as an antiestrogen; and [3] by down-regulating the activity of some enzymes, such as aromatase, involved in the synthesis of estrogens from androgens, i.e., behaving as a selective estrogen enzyme modulator.

18.3.4 Systemic Effects

Melatonin was formerly considered as a hormone controlling seasonal reproduction in wild animals [6,179]. In seasonally breeding mammalian species, melatonin controls reproductive function through the activation of receptor sites within the hypothalamic–pituitary axis, thus driving the levels of gonadal activity [84]. Namely, melatonin down-regulation of the ovarian estrogen secretion has been observed in a variety of mammals. It was initially [13] hypothesized that an impaired pineal secretion, which leads to reduced circulating melatonin levels, could result in unopposed estrogen secretion and thus to an increased susceptibility to breast cancer. In turn, normal or high serum melatonin levels, due to suppression of estrogen secretion or by direct inhibitory effects on breast tissue, might suppress induction of mammary cancer (Figure 18.1). Although, in humans, the role of melatonin on the reproductive system is not really understood, an inverse relationship between melatonin and ovarian activity [111] and a role of melatonin in the modulation of neuroendocrine–reproductive axis has been proposed [86,87]. Indeed, melatonin exerts some modulatory effects on steroidogenesis in human granulosa–luteal cells [88]; functional melatonin receptors have been also found in cells of antral follicles and corpora lutea of rat ovaries [89]. Together, these data suggest that melatonin could participate in the modulation of ovarian function by down-regulating the production of estrogens, thereby supporting the above-mentioned hypothesis of its role in breast cancer.

18.3.5 Melatonin–ER Interactions

Only ERα-positive breast tumor cell lines are growth-inhibited by physiological concentrations of melatonin, whereas ERα-negative cell lines are unaffected by the pineal hormone [58,90]. Various

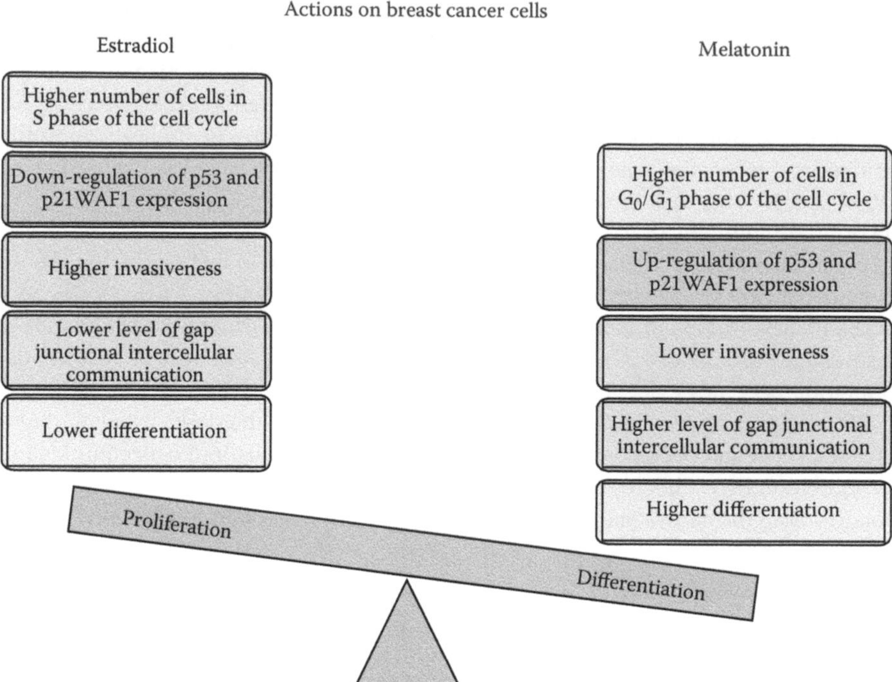

FIGURE 18.1 Interaction between melatonin and estrogens: action on breast cancer cells. Estradiol stimulates the cell proliferation while reducing differentiation processes. Melatonin promotes the differentiation and reduces breast cancer cells growth.

breast cancer cell lines have been reported to exhibit significant differences in their sensitivity to the antiproliferative effect of melatonin, which may be correlated with the degree of estrogen responsiveness [91] or the ERα/ERβ ratio [49,92]; indeed, MCF-7 sensitivity to melatonin is abolished by ERβ overexpression.

Since melatonin's inhibitory activity has been observed principally in estrogen-responsive breast cancer cells, it has been hypothesized that melatonin hinders cancer cell growth by antagonizing the intracellular estrogen response pathway. Melatonin blocks the mitogenic effects of estradiol as well as counteracts the estradiol-induced invasiveness of MCF-7 cells [93]. Furthermore, the indoleamine augments the sensitivity of MCF-7 cells to antiestrogens [94] and down-regulates the expression of proteins, growth factors, and proto-oncogenes regulated by estrogens [95]. Furthermore, the transfection of MT1 melatonin receptors into MCF-7 cells or MDA-MB-231 cells (Erα-negative) significantly enhances the growth-suppression effects of melatonin only in MCF-7 cells, that is, only in those also expressing the ER [67]. Indeed, melatonin significantly blunts estrogen-induced ERα transcriptional activity. The addition of pertussis toxin—a known uncoupler of $G_{\alpha i2}$ proteins—suppress the melatonin-induced inhibitory effects [96].

However, how melatonin interacts with the estrogen pathway remains an open question. Unlike antiestrogenic drugs, evidence indicates that melatonin does not bind to the ER or interfere with the binding of estradiol to its receptor [97]. Melatonin reduces the expression of ERα (both at the mRNA and protein level) and inhibits the binding of estradiol receptor complex to the estrogen response element (ERE) on DNA [29,98]. These effects are likely to depend on its binding to a high affinity membrane-bound receptor coupled to Gi proteins [63]. Via the activation of $G_{\alpha i2}$ protein, melatonin treatment decreases the basal phosphorylation level of the ERα. Thus, melatonin behaves as an antiestrogen, which does not bind to the ER, but to its own membrane receptors, and via binding to its specific receptors, melatonin interacts with the ER-signaling pathway. This effect is specific for ERα-mediated effects. One of the desirable properties of a selective estrogen modulator is its ability to specifically block the ERα but not ERβ. Indeed, it was demonstrated [34] that whereas melatonin is a specific inhibitor of estrogen-induced ERα-mediated transcriptional activation, the indoleamine does not inhibit ERβ-mediated transactivation.

18.3.6 Melatonin and Nuclear Receptors

The ligand-dependent nuclear transcription factors (NRs) play a multitude of essential roles in development, homeostasis, reproduction, and immune function [99]. NRs regulate transcription by several mechanisms and can both activate and inhibit gene expression [100]. The NRs include steroidal transcription factors such as the estrogen (ER), glucocorticoid (GR), thyroid hormone receptor (TR), liver X receptor (LXR), frasenoid X receptor (FXR), vitamin D receptor (VDR), retinoid acid receptor (RAR), retinoid X receptor (RXR), and peroxisome proliferators–activated receptors (PPARs) [101]. Through its role as a required heterodimeric partner, RXRs control the function of many other NRs, thus integrating a unique transcriptional network dependent on RXR responses [102,103]. RXR forms heterodimers with virtually all NRs including GR, ER, TR, PPAR, VDR, LXR, and FXR. NRs can activate transcription as monomers and/or dimers with the RXR. Once activated, NRs dissociate from corepressors and recruit coactivator proteins, which promote transcriptional activation [104,105]. Half of the NRs are so-called orphan receptors because the identity of their ligand is unknown. However, some of receptors belonging to RXRs are no longer "orphaned." Evidence of a genomic action of melatonin via nuclear RZR/ROR receptors was first hypothesized by Becker-Andre et al. in 1994 [106]. Subsequent studies have detected the nuclear melatonin receptor by using in situ hybridization neuronal tissue [107–109], including the pineal [110] and many other tissues as well [111,112].

Direct evidence of the epigenetic effect of melatonin has been provided by Sharma et al. [113]. In this study, melatonin significantly increased mRNA expression for various histone deacetylase (HDAC) isoforms and increased histone H3 acetylation in neural stem cell lines. As suggested by Korkmaz et al. [114], these effects are indicative of an epigenetic regulation exerted by melatonin at the NR/coregulator level rather than selective enzymatic inhibition or activation. We still do not know if melatonin effects are mediated via direct changes in phosphorylation of the nuclear receptor, regulation of coactivator or corepressor phosphorylation, or both. Regardless, these data clearly demonstrate the ability of melatonin, via signal transduction pathways, to affect gene expression in human breast cancer cells.

18.3.7 Melatonin as a Calmodulin and Calcium Modulator

Even if the molecular link between melatonin and estrogen pathways still has not been elucidated, it is likely that cyclic adenosine monophosphate (cAMP) could, at least in part, restore this function. Estrogens activate adenylate cyclase, thereafter increasing cAMP levels; in turn, cAMP synergizes with hormone receptors, enhancing ER-mediated transcription [115]. On the contrary, melatonin, after its binding to MT1, inhibits adenylate cyclase, reduces cAMP, and in turn protein kinase A (PKA) activity, leading to a diminished phosphorylation and activation of ERα and the coactivators CBP/P300, thus blocking the estrogenic effect [116,117].

Recently, it has been proposed that melatonin may hinder the estrogen pathway through the Ca^{2+}/calmodulin signaling pathway, either modifying the intracellular release of Ca^{2+} or by means of a direct interaction with calmodulin (CaM) [118]. Furthermore, melatonin causes subcellular CaM redistribution, stimulating its phosphorylation by protein kinase C (PKCα) [119]. It is known that CaM interacts with ER, stimulating the phosphorylation of the receptor and thus enhancing the binding of the estradiol–ER complex to the ERE [120]. On the other hand, anticalmodulin compounds inhibit breast cancer growth, probably by interfering with the CaM–ER interplay [121,122].

Since the structures of melatonin and calmodulin are phylogenetically well preserved, calmodulin–melatonin interaction probably represents a major mechanism for regulation and synchronization of cell physiology, and it is likely that melatonin interference with CaM function could contribute to modulate the estrogen receptor activation. Moreover, the melatonin-induced increase in both intracellular Ca^{2+} and membrane-bound CaM could enhance apoptosis and E-cadherin–mediated cell–cell adhesion [123]. Along these lines, Blask et al. [124] have reported that melatonin inhibits Ca^{2+}-stimulated MCF-7 cell growth via a glutathione-dependent mechanism. Indeed, once glutathione synthesis is inhibited through L-buthionine sulfoximine (LBSO) (an inhibitor of γ-glutamate cysteine ligase), the oncostatic action of 1 nM melatonin is subsequently blocked, indicating that glutathione is required for melatonin action [125]. In addition, glutathione depletion has been shown to cause a reduction in microtubule polymerization in cells that may relate to the oxidation of sulfhydryl groups [126]. In contrast, physiological concentrations of melatonin are known to stabilize microtubules by inhibiting Ca^{2+}/CaM depolymerization, which is itself a mitogenic signal transduction mechanism [17]. Thus, adequate levels of glutathione may be required to maintain sulfhydryl groups of microtubule-associated proteins in a reduced state in order for melatonin to suppress Ca^{2+}/CaM-mediated depolymerization of the cytoskeleton and thus cell proliferation. These effects are seemingly ER-independent, keeping in mind that they have been recorded also in ER-negative breast cancer cells, as well as in non–breast cancer cell lines devoid of the ER and, therefore, could provide a reliable explanation about how melatonin inhibits cell proliferation [25,128,129] (Figure 18.2).

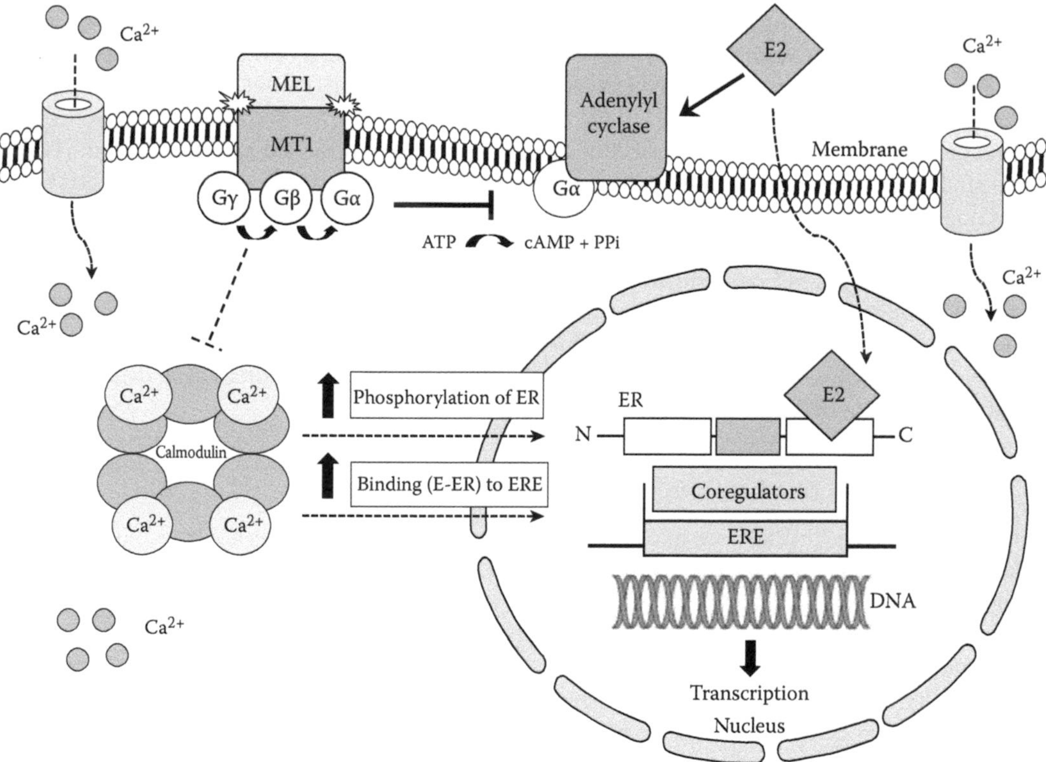

FIGURE 18.2 Calmodulin as a possible link between melatonin and estrogen signaling pathway. Melatonin interacts with the Ca^{2+}/calmodulin signaling pathway, either modifying the intracellular gathering of Ca^{2+} or by means of a direct interaction with calmodulin. Calmodulin interacts with ER, stimulating the phosphorylation of the receptor and enhancing the binding of the estradiol–ER complex to ERE (estrogens response elements). Estrogens activate adenylate cyclase, increasing c-AMP; on the contrary, melatonin, after binding to MT1, inhibits adenylate cyclase, thus reducing c-AMP.

Further studies are warranted in order to verify and better understand the physiological meaning of melatonin's modulation of CaM and intracellular calcium in breast cancer cells.

18.3.8 Aromatase Pathways

In MCF-7 breast cancer cells as well as in adipose tissue of tumor-bearing breasts, expression of the *CYP19* gene, which encodes aromatase P450, the enzyme responsible for estrogen biosynthesis, is regulated by two proximal promoters: I.3 and II [130], which are mainly modulated by intracellular cAMP [131]. Therefore, molecules or drugs that modulate cAMP levels could also influence aromatase expression in breast cancer cells. This is the case with prostaglandin E2 (PGE2), which increases intracellular cAMP levels and stimulates aromatase and estrogen biosynthesis [132].

Estrogens, in turn, increase cAMP, as previously mentioned. Thus, in breast cancer cells, but not in normal epithelial cells with different *CYP19* promoters, estrogens may induce through a paracrine loop the local biosynthesis of estrogens via the increase of cAMP and expression of aromatase. In contrast, melatonin, after its binding to MT1 membrane receptor linked to Gi proteins, decreases in a dose- and time-dependent manner the activity of adenylate cyclase and subsequently reduces cAMP synthesis thus leading to elevated cGMP levels and reduced aromatase concentration [133]. Indeed, it has been observed that melatonin, at both physiological (10^{-9} M) and pharmacological (10^{-4} M) concentrations, reduces the synthesis of estrogen in MCF-7 cells, through aromatase inhibition [134]. Furthermore, transfection of the MT1 melatonin receptor in MCF-7 cells significantly reduces aromatase activity and MT1-transfected cells show a level of aromatase activity that is 50% of control cancer cells when both are treated with melatonin [135]. Moreover, melatonin enhances the inhibitory effect of aminoglutethimide on aromatase activity in breast cancer cells through a significant reduction in aromatase mRNA expression [136]. Moreover, in MCF-7 cells, aromatase activity is stimulated by epidermal growth factor and transforming growth factor α [137], both of which are down-regulated by melatonin [138]; melatonin-dependent aromatase inhibition could be further achieved through inhibition of cyclooxygenase activity and reduced PGE2 synthesis [139].

As breast cancer occurs in regions of the mammary gland with the highest levels of aromatase expression, the inhibition of aromatase activity by melatonin may be an important mechanism in the ability of this indoleamine to control tumor growth. Further studies confirmed that melatonin efficiently inhibits local, tissue-based biosynthesis of estrogen. It is well recognized that mammary cancer tissue contains all the enzymatic machinery for the local biosynthesis of estrogens [140]. The presence of type 1 (17β-HSD1) isoform of 17β-hydroxysteroid dehydrogenases, which catalyse the conversion of the relatively weak estrone (E1), androstenedione, and 5-androstenedione into the more potent estradiol, has been documented in several human breast cancer cell lines, such as T47D and MCF-7 [140]. Estrogen production in normal mammary tissue is displaced toward the production of hormones with low activity (like estrone), whereas in breast adenocarcinomas, active estradiol formation predominates [141]. This effect is likely due to the different enzyme compositions of normal and cancerous tissues. The former possess a higher activity of both 17β-HSD type 2, which converts estradiol to estrone, and estrogen sulfotransferase, which inactivates both estrone and estradiol; on the other hand, opposite effects are mediate by aromatase and the type 2 isoform of 17β-hydroxysteroid dehydrogenase that are largely represented in cancer tissues. Melatonin reduces the synthesis of biologically active estrogens in MCF-7 cells through the simultaneous inhibition of sulfatases and 17β-HSD1 and the stimulation of estrogen sulfotransferase, the enzyme responsible for the formation of the biologically inactive estrogen sulfates; as a result, the production of estradiol from estrone in MCF-7 cells decreases twofolds to threefolds in the presence of 1 nM melatonin [142].

Moreover, it must be noted that the transcription factor nuclear factor kB (NFkB) is involved in *CYP19* activation by inducing several proinflammatory molecules (tumor necrosis factor-α [TNF-α], inducible nitric oxide synthase [iNOS], cyclooxygenase [COX-2], and PGE2) [143]. Overexpression of TNF-α, COX-2, and PGE2 has been demonstrated to induce increased aromatase expression in both human and mice breast cancer tissue [144,145]. It is noteworthy that melatonin inhibits every molecule in this pathway, mainly through its nuclear actions [146,147]. Moreover, melatonin inhibits p300 HAT activity, thus leading to a reduced COX-2 and iNOS synthase expression [148]. This effect is likely mediated by inhibition of p52 acetylation and binding of DNA. As expected, melatonin has been proven [149] to suppress NFkB binding to DNA through a reductionism in TNF-α, iNOS, COX-2, and PGE2 levels. Furthermore, melatonin interaction with PPARs and RXR hinders NFkB transcription, leading to cancer cell growth inhibition [150,151]. In turn, melatonin-induced activation of both PPARs and RXR receptor inhibits aromatase transcription via NFkB.

It has also been observed that melatonin inhibits the expression of other estrogen-regulated genes, like pS2 or cathepsine [152]. These findings are important, as pS2 is a differentiation factor in the gastrointestinal tract, as well as an inhibitor of adenocarcinoma cell proliferation [153,154].

18.3.9 Growth-Inhibitory Mechanisms

Melatonin significantly inhibits cancer proliferation in vitro. For melatonin to achieve these effects, it seems several mechanisms are involved, including effects on the expression of some proteins involved in the control of the G1-to-S transition, through the inhibition of cyclin D1 expression, and the increase in p53 release (Figure 18.3).

Cyclin D1 is a key protein of the G1-to-S transition and seems to mediate the steroid-dependent growth of both normal and malignant mammary epithelial cells [155]; moreover, down-regulation

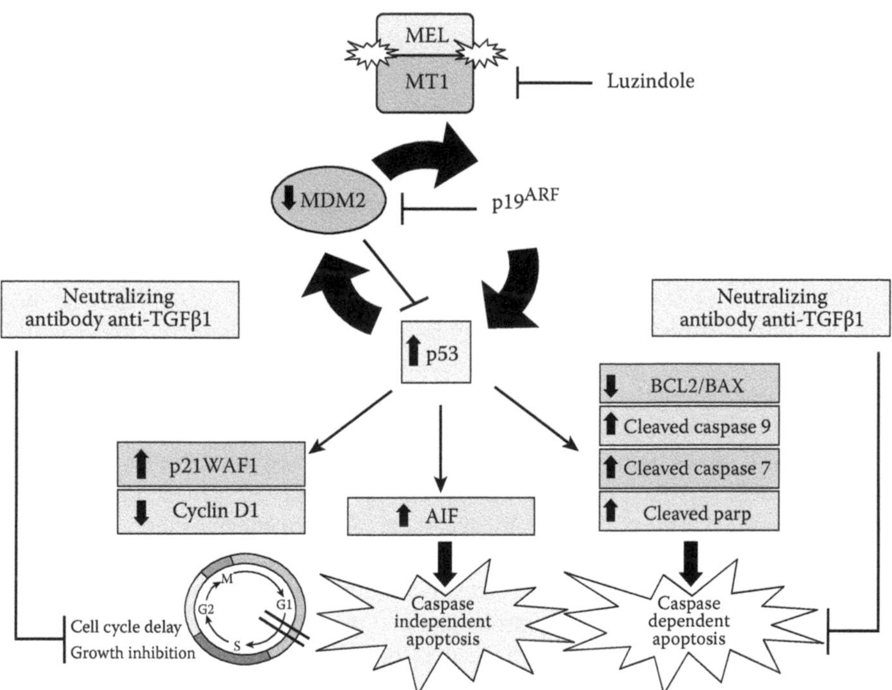

FIGURE 18.3 Apoptosis and growth inhibition induced by melatonin in MCF-7 cancer cells. Melatonin significantly inhibits cancer proliferation by increasing p53/MDM2 ratio. The *p53 gene* activates the expression of p21, which inhibits cyclin-dependent kinases, thus leading to a cell cycle arrest. In addition, melatonin induces apoptosis in MCF-7 cancer cells. Melatonin-induced early apoptosis is a caspase-independent process, involving the AIF. Melatonin-induced late apoptosis is a TGF-β1- and caspase-dependent process. During late apoptosis, activated caspases 9 and 7 and cleaved PARP increase significantly and concomitantly with a down-regulation of the Bcl/Bax ratio. By adding anti–TGF-β1-neutralizing antibodies, growth inhibition and late apoptosis triggered by melatonin are inhibited.

of cyclin D1 expression may drive the inhibitory effects displayed by antiestrogenic drugs [156]. Cyclin D1 interacts with several transcription factors as well as with nuclear receptors (including GR, ERα, and PPARs). NRs bind directly to cyclin D1 and their ligand-dependent transactivation is modulated by cyclin D1 [157]. It is noteworthy that cyclin D1 participates in the activation process of ERα transcription and cooperates in the down-regulation of both GR and PPARs [158]. Melatonin induces a significant transcriptional down-regulation of the *cyclin D1* gene through the inhibition of c-*jun* and ATF-2 proteins [159]. Both c-*jun* and ATF-2 proteins are known to transactivate the cAMP-responsive element present in the cyclin D1 promoter element [160].

The *p53 gene* is an important gene involved in both growth suppression and apoptosis pathways [159]. The *p53 gene* activates the expression of the *WAF1* gene (also known as p21), which inhibits cyclin-dependent kinases, thus leading to a failure of the phosphorylation of the retinoblastoma protein and the subsequent cell cycle arrest [161]. In breast cancer cells treated with physiological doses of melatonin, both p53 and p21 expression significantly increased. It is likely that up-regulation of p53 occurs downstream to enhance release of TGF-β1 induced by melatonin. Indeed, melatonin can up-regulate TGF-β1 mRNA expression in prostate [163] and breast cancer cells [164]. Moreover, the melatonin-inhibitory effect on breast cancer growth should be viewed as a TGF-β1–dependent process as it is completely prevented in several breast cancer cell lines by adding anti–TGF-β1 antibodies [52,57,165]. A significant rise in TGF-β1 levels in MCF-7 cells treated with melatonin is observed after 72 hours and an evident growth-inhibitory action can be documented only after this period. Adding anti–TGF-β1 antibodies, the growth inhibition induced by melatonin is completely suppressed. These data pointed out that melatonin-induced cell growth inhibition in MCF- 7 breast cancer cells is largely mediated through the involvement of the TGF-β1 pathway. Other mechanisms, however, may be supposed to be involved in melatonin-mediated inhibition of cancer cells.

The reduction in cAMP production caused by melatonin via MT1 and MT2 receptor interaction slows down the uptake of linoleic acid, an essential fatty acid, by specific fatty acid transporters [166]. Linoleic acid can be oxidized to 13-hydroxyoctadecadienoic acid by 15-lipoxygenase, serving as an energy source for tumor growth and tumor growth signaling molecules. Inhibition of linoleic acid uptake by melatonin is regarded as a mechanism of its antiproliferative effects.

Furthermore, melatonin hinders telomerase activity, induced by estrogens or cadmium, both in vitro and in vivo [167,168]. Melatonin-treated cells display a significant dose-dependent decrease in telomerase reverse transcriptase mRNA expression as well as the mRNA of telomerase-reverse, the RNA telomerase subunit. Similar results have been obtained with GP 52608—an agonist of melatonin nuclear receptors—while treatment with an agonist of melatonin membrane receptors was without effect, thus highlighting the relevance of epigenetic mechanisms triggered by melatonin [169]. Telomerase is a specialized ribonucleoprotein DNA polymerase that extends telomeres of eukaryotic chromosomes and its activity is under control of epigenetic regulation [170]. Telomerase is activated in most human cancers and its inhibition leads to cancer cell death. Therefore, it is tempting to speculate that such a mechanism could also be involved in melatonin-dependent cancer apoptosis [171].

18.3.10 Apoptosis Pathways

In contrast to the well-studied inhibition of apoptotic processes in normal cells [172], there is evidence that in cancer cells, melatonin may actually promote apoptosis. Melatonin induces apoptosis in colon cancer cells [173,174], hepatocarcinoma cells [175], neuroblastoma [176], Ehrlich ascites carcinoma cells [177], myeloid [178], lymphoma [179], and leukemia cells [180]. However, although inhibitory effects of melatonin on MCF-7 cells have been well documented, its apoptotic effects are still a matter of investigation. Cos et al. [181] did not find any apoptotic changes in MCF-7 cells treated with different concentrations of melatonin; meanwhile, some reports [182,183] documented a significant rise in MCF-7 cell apoptotic rate only when melatonin was administered together with retinoids. In the latter studies, melatonin enhances apoptosis by modulating the transcriptional activity of the retinoic acid receptors [184]. However, a recent study documented a significant increase in caspase 3 activity and DNA fragmentation in tumor tissues obtained from breast cancer-bearing rats treated with the pineal indole, therefore providing indirect proof of the apoptotic activity exerted by melatonin on breast cancer [185]. These preliminary results have been confirmed in vitro by treating MCF-7 cells with nanomolar concentration of melatonin [52]. Both flow cytometry and DNA fragmentation-based techniques documented an early (at 24 hours) and a late (at 96 hours) apoptosis in melatonin-treated MCF-7 cells. Early apoptosis is a caspase-independent process, and it is likely to be triggered by apoptosis inducing factor (AIF). A more complex pathway underlies late apoptosis, involving both TGF-β1 and terminal caspase effectors (caspases 7). Indeed, by adding anti–TGF-β1 antibodies, melatonin-induced late apoptosis is almost completely suppressed; however, early apoptosis remains unaffected. During late apoptosis, activated caspases 9 and 7 and cleaved PARP increased significantly and concomitantly with a down-regulation of the Bcl-2/Bax ratio. It is noteworthy that melatonin-triggered apoptosis involves both p53 and p73 release. In fact, melatonin-treated MCF-7 cells showed a significant increase in both p73 and p53, but only the p73 protein, the homologue of p53 protein, increased at 96 hours; at the same time, MDM2 levels were significantly reduced. These data seem to suggest that p53 is likely activated during early programmed cell death; however, only p73 is involved in caspase-dependent late apoptosis. It is worth noting that MDM2 is reduced as a consequence of melatonin treatment. MDM2 inhibits the transcriptional activity of p53 and promotes its degradation by the proteasome, thus representing the major physiological antagonist of p53 [186]. An autoregulatory negative feedback loop controls MDM2 expression, whereas p53 induces MDM2 expression and MDM2 represses p53 activity. Abrogation of MDM2 expression allows p53 to escape from the autoregulatory loop, becoming lethally active [187,188]. Therefore, melatonin, by inducing an early down-regulation of MDM2 expression concomitantly with p53 increase, causes a significant rise in the p53/MDM2 ratio (Figure 18.4). It is likely that the modified p53/MDM2 ratio could trigger the apoptotic cascade involving both caspase-dependent and caspase-independent pathways. In addition, we have recently found (unpublished results) that melatonin enhances the depolymerization of mitochondrial membrane, while inhibiting Akt-phosphorylation; these effects are probably involved in melatonin-dependent oncostatic effects and they participate in triggering the complex apoptotic cascade.

As highlighted by R.J. Reiter [172], "melatonin involvement in apoptotic processes is a new and relevant field of investigation. The results obtained to date appear promising, and if in fact melatonin uniformly induces apoptosis in cancer cells, the findings could have important clinical utility. Many tumors show resistance to drug treatment mainly due to their resistance to undergo apoptosis. Identifying agents which potentiate apoptosis in cancer cells is clearly of great interest." It may seem paradoxical that a substance could induce apoptosis in cancer cells, while preventing it in normal cells. However, melatonin shares this surprising behavior with other known antioxidant compounds, like epigallocatechins and procyanidins [189]. Therefore, it can be hypothesized that melatonin's ability to trigger apoptotic or antiapoptotic pathways is largely context-dependent; thus, an unknown environmental factor (e.g., electromagnetic fields) [190] and/or intracellular cues may drive melatonin's effects toward a specific pathway or in the opposite direction.

18.3.11 Malignant Behavior

Some preliminary observations suggest that melatonin can efficiently reduce the metastatic ability of MCF-7 cells. Mao et al. [191] have evaluated the potential anti-invasive actions of melatonin, employing three clones of MCF-7 cells with high metastatic potential including the MCF-7/6 clone derived by serial passages in nude mice, MCF-7 Her2.1 cells stably transformed with and overexpressing the Her2-neu/c-erbB2 construct, and MCF-7CXCR4 cells stably transformed with and overexpressing the CXCR4 cytokine G protein–coupled receptor. The invasive capacity of these clones was significantly reduced when they were treated with melatonin (10^{-8} or 10^{-9} M). Melatonin

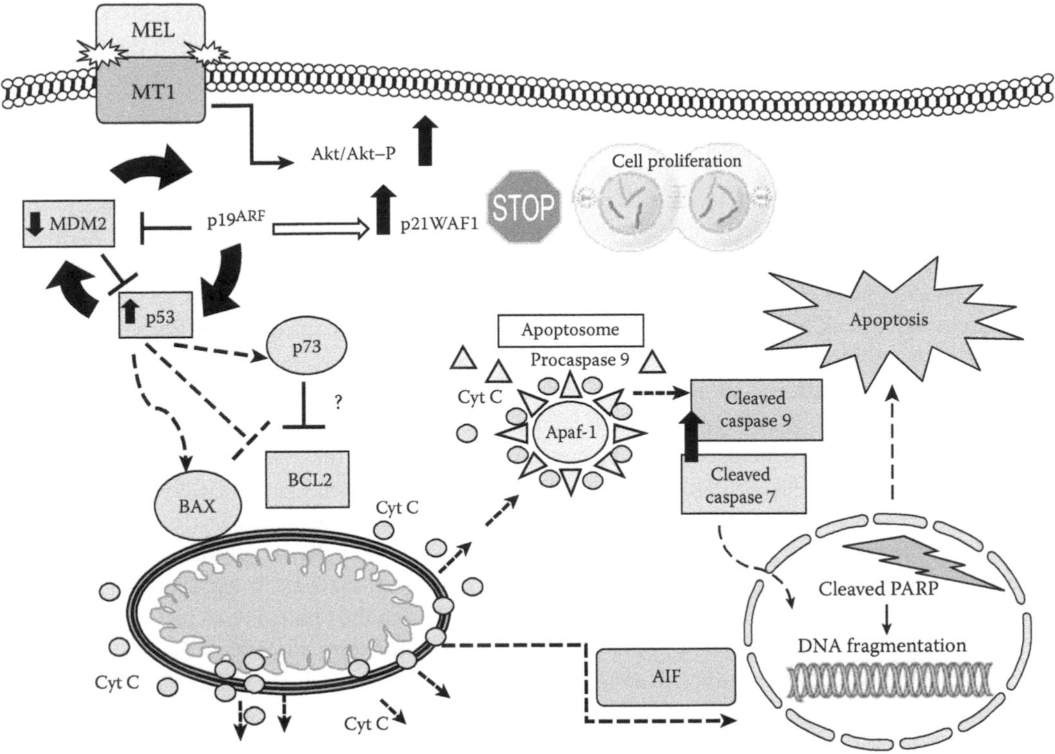

FIGURE 18.4 Apoptosis induced by melatonin in MCF-7 cancer cells. After binding to MT1 receptor, melatonin decreases MDM2 levels, thus allowing p53 to escape from the autoregulatory loop. The modified p53/MDM2 ratio triggers the apoptosis cascade involving both caspase-dependent and caspase-independent pathways. In addition, melatonin increases mitochondrial membrane depolarization, releasing cytochrome C and AIF. Melatonin is likely to inhibit Akt phosphorylation and subsequently the MAPK-related pathways.

treatment resulted in significant suppression (60% to 85% decrease) of cell invasion using a transwell assay system and matrigel-covered inserts.

In an in vitro study, Cos et al. [92] demonstrated that 1 nM melatonin reduced the invasiveness of cancer cells measured in Falcon invasion chambers and blocked estradiol-induced invasion; both subphysiological (0.1 pmol) and pharmacological concentrations (10 μM) of melatonin failed to inhibit cell invasion. It is likely that such effects could be attributed to an overall effect of melatonin on cell morphology, and they are mediated, at least in part, by a melatonin-induced rise in the expression of two cell surface adhesion proteins, E-cadherin and β1-integrin, as well as by an increased gap junctional intercellular communication between adjacent epithelial cells also induced by melatonin [192]. It has been hypothesized that if a cell were unable to perform gap junctional intercellular communication, normal growth control and cell differentiation would not be possible, thereby favoring the development of malignant neoplasia [193]. Because there is an inverse correlation between the ability of a cell to have gap junctional communication and its ability to metastasize [194], it is likely that melatonin could reduce metastatic behavior through inducing local gap junctional intercellular communication and reshaping the relationships between cancer cells and their microenvironment.

Estrogen treatment also induces a marked rearrangement of the cytoskeleton and adhesion structures and enhances the attachment of MCF-7 cells to laminin (a basement membrane component); likewise, melatonin completely abolished these effects of estradiol and shifted cancer cells to a lower invasive status [195]. These findings suggest that melatonin could exert an additional antitumor action by modulating the cross talk between cells and stromal components (stromal cells, laminin, collagen) and by increasing regulatory signals shared between adjacent cells through intercellular junctions.

18.3.12 Melatonin, Cytoskeleton, and Cell Morphology

From the initial studies carried out by Hill et al. [49], it was already observed that melatonin significantly modifies cell morphology and cytoskeleton architecture. The importance of these findings have been underestimated, and compelling evidence documenting the relevance of the melatonin's influence on the cytoskeleton has been only recently provided.

The cytoskeleton is an important cellular structure composed by an intricate fibrous network including microtubules, microfilaments, and intermediate filaments as well as associated proteins [196]. Dynamic and differential changes in cytoskeletal organization occur in different cellular processes according to the cell type and the specific function. Moreover, the cytoskeleton, together with integrins and other related adhesion proteins, orients much of the cell's metabolic and signal transduction machinery [197]. Indeed, cells are hardwired to respond immediately to mechanical stresses transmitted over cell surface receptors that physically couple the cytoskeleton to the extracellular matrix or to other cells [198]. The shape of cells and the structures they form is a consequence of physical forces generated in the cytoskeleton as well as in extracellular matrix. Shape, which reflects cytoskeleton organization [199], is linked to the repertoire of metabolic events that result from the right ordering in space of the enzymes catalyzing specific pathways. Physical forces (such as microgravity) induce dramatic changes in gene expression and alter cellular shape [200,201]. In particular, modifications in cell shape distortion can switch between distinct cell phenotypes, and this process can be viewed as a biological phase transition [202,203]. Moreover, tumor phenotype reversion is primarily associated to relevant shape modifications preceding molecular and metabolic "normalization" [204].

The cytoskeleton is a phylogenetically well-preserved structure allowing the cell to have a well-organized structure, a specific shape-associated phenotype, and an optimal function. By contrast, cancer is characterized by an abnormal cytoskeletal rearrangement with a poor organization and structure [205]. Therefore, the possibility that melatonin could preserve normal microfilament distribution, influencing cytoskeleton rearrangement and cell shape in cancerous tissues, requires further investigation [206].

Cancer cells show an abnormal microfilament organization, reduced stress fiber production, and loose focal contact adhesion. These changes enhance cell proliferation, cell migration [207], and foster resistance to anoikis [208]. Highly malignant metastatic cancer cells present poorly structured microfilaments and scarce anchorage to their substratum. These cells move by microfilaments and microtubules arranged in membrane ruffles, lamellipodia and filopodial formations at the leading edge, and a retraction of these cytoskeletal structures at the cell rear [209].

A bimodal effect of melatonin on microtubule organization was first described in 1994 in both in vitro polymerization assays and in an in situ preparation of cytoskeleton material [210]. Melatonin, in the presence of Ca^{2+}, augments tubulin polymerization, causing microtubule enlargement; conversely, melatonin without Ca^{2+} inhibits tubulin polymerization and causes microtubule disruption. Interestingly, in kidney epithelial cells (MDCK), melatonin's effects on cytoskeletal organization are not mediated by membrane MT receptors; in contrast, in breast cancer cells luzindole completely suppresses melatonin-induced effects on microfilaments. Furthermore, studies performed by Benitez-King et al. [211] have demonstrated how complex the interaction between melatonin and cytoskeleton is. In experimental conditions designed to measure cell anchorage, melatonin increases the number of focal adhesion contacts in MCF-7 cells, and microfilaments are arranged in thicker bundles of stress fibbers assembled with phosphovinculin to form focal adhesion contacts [212]. These results strongly suggest that melatonin inhibits cancer cell invasion and metastasis formation by changing microfilament phenotypes of migratory cells (ruffles and lamellipodia) to stress fibers that are microfilament phenotypes of attached cells. Melatonin-induced effects on stress fibers involve protein kinase C (PKC) [213] and the Rho-associated protein kinase (ROCK), downstream of the PKC pathway. In MDCK and MCF-7 cells treated with melatonin, addition of the PKC inhibitor abolished the increased number and thickening of stress fibers, as well as the augmented number of focal adhesion contacts elicited by the indoleamine in both cell lines [214]. It is noteworthy that calmodulin also participates in this process [215] and that melatonin modulates stress fiber formation by involving ROCK and Ca^{2+}/CaM balance: in MCF-7 cells, melatonin produces a redistribution of CaM and phosphorylated CaM, recruiting them to specific subcellular compartments, one of which is the cytoskeleton [216]. CaM is redistributed to the membrane cytoskeletal fraction where it becomes associated with myosin phosphorylation through the myosin light chain kinase [127].

18.4 CONCLUSION

Numerous studies have demonstrated the oncostatic properties of melatonin both in vivo using models of chemically induced rat mammary tumors as well as in vitro using MCF-7 human breast cancer cells. Melatonin exerts both inhibitory as well proapoptotic effects by interacting with several molecular pathways. Generally, melatonin's cytostatic effects are mediated by interactions of the indoleamine with both ERs and melatonin receptors. However, recently some receptor- and estrogen-independent signaling pathways activated by melatonin have been discovered. In particular, increasing attention should be directed to melatonin's effects on the cytoskeleton and cell shape, as well as understanding how melatonin could inhibit both Akt activation and MAPK-related pathways.

In light of its low toxicity, melatonin, either alone or in combination with chemoradiotherapy, should be considered as a potentially new anticancer treatment. There may be some difficulties in bringing a circadian rhythm-based melatonin chronotherapy to cancer clinics, but it is a challenge to use this indoleamine to derive its benefit in the practice of oncology.

18.5 SUMMARY POINTS

- Melatonin may reduce the incidence of experimentally induced breast tumors.
- Melatonin slows down estrogen-related effects at both systemic and cellular levels.
- Melatonin exerts both inhibitory as well as proapoptotic effects on breast cancer cells.
- Melatonin may affect cytoskeleton and cell shape.
- Melatonin could inhibit both Akt activation and MAPK-related pathways.

REFERENCES

1. Descartes, R. 1649. *Les passions de l'âme*, Amsterdam reprinted in AT, vol. XI *Passions of the Soul* Part One, Section 50, AT 369.
2. Lerner, A.B., Case, J.D., Takahashi, Y., et al. 1958. Isolation of melatonin, the pineal gland factor that lightens melanocytes. *J Am Chem Soc* 80:2587–2590.
3. Reiter, R.J., Tan, D.X., Manchester, L.C., et al. 2009. Melatonin and reproduction revisited. *Biol Reprod* 81(3):445–456.
4. Vijayalaxmi, T.C.R. Jr, Reiter, R.J., Herman, T.S. 2002. Melatonin: From basic research to cancer treatment clinics. *J Clin Oncol* 20(10):2575–2601.
5. Karasek, M., Reiter, R.J. 2002. Melatonin and aging. *Neuro Endocrinol Lett* 23(1):14–16.
6. Reiter, R.J. 2003. Melatonin: Clinical relevance *Best Pract Res Clin Endocrinol Metab* 17(2):273–285.
7. Reiter, R.J., Korkmaz, A. 2008. Clinical aspects of melatonin. *Saudi Med J* 29(11):1537–1547.
8. Manda, K., Reiter, R.J. 2010. Melatonin maintains adult hippocampal neurogenesis and cognitive functions after irradiation. *Prog Neurobiol J* 90(1):60–68.
9. Brzezinski, A. 1997. Melatonin in humans. *N Engl J Med* 336:186–195.

10. Georgiou, E. 1929. Uber die Natur und kie Pathogenese der Krebstumoren, Radiale Heilung des Krebses bei weiBen Mausen. *Zeitschr Kregsforsh* 38:562.
11. Lapin, V., Ebels, I. 1976. Effects of some low molecular weight sheep pineal fractions and melatonin on different tumours in rats and mice. *Oncology* 33:110–113.
12. Gupta, D., Attanasio, A., Reiter, R.J. 1988. Eds., The Pineal Gland and Cancer Brain Research Promotion, Tubingen.
13. Cohen, M., Lippman, M., Chabner, B. 1978. Role of pineal gland in aetiology and treatment of breast cancer. *Lancet* 2:814–816.
14. Srinivasan, V., et al. 2008. Therapeutic actions of melatonin in cancer: Possible mechanisms. *Integr Cancer Ther*. 7:189–203.
15. Srinivasan, V., Spence, D.W. Pandi-Perumal, S.R., et al. 2008. Melatonin, environmental light, and breast cancer. *Breast Cancer Res Treat* 108:339–350.
16. Reiter, R.J., Tan, D.X., Erren, T.C., Fuentes-Broto, L., Paredes, S.D. 2009. Light-mediated perturbations of circadian timing and cancer risk: A mechanistic analysis. *Integr Cancer Ther* 8:354–360.
17. Stevens, R.G. 1987. Electric power use and breast cancer: A hypothesis. *Am J Epidemiol* 125:556–561.
18. Bartsch, C., Bartsch, H. 2006. The anti-tumor activity of pineal melatonin and cancer enhancing life styles in industrialized societies. *Cancer Causes Control* 17:559–571.
19. Kerenyi, N.A., Pandula, E., Feuer, G. 1990. Why the incidence of cancer is increasing: The role of light pollution. *Med Hypotheses* 33:75–78.
20. Hansen, J. 2001. Increased breast cancer risk among women who work predominantly at night. *Epidemiology* 12:74–77.
21. Davis, S., Mirick, D.K., Stevens, R.G. 2001. Night shift work, light at night, and risk of breast cancer. *J Natl Cancer Inst* 93:1557–1562.
22. Bartsch, C., Bartsch, H., Jain, A.K., Laumas, K.R., Wetterberg, L. 1981. Urinary melatonin levels in human breast cancer patients. *J Neural Transm* 52:281–294.
23. Bartsch, C., Bartsch, H., Bellmann, O., Lippert, T.H. 1991. Depression of serum melatonin in patients with primary breast cancer is not due to an increased peripheral metabolism. *Cancer* 67:1681–1684.
24. Falkson, G., Falkson, H.C., Steyn, M.E., Rapoport, B.L., Meyer, B.J. 1990. Plasma melatonin in patients with breast cancer. *Oncology* 47:401–405.
25. Blask, D.E. 1984. The pineal: An oncostatic gland? In: *The Pineal Gland*. Ed. Reiter, R.J., 253–284. New York, Raven Press.
26. Saez, M.C., Barriga, C., Garcia, J.J., et al. 2005. Melatonin increases the survival time of animals with untreated mammary tumours: Neuroendocrine stabilization. *Mol Cell Biochem* 278:15–20.
27. Tamarkin, L., Cohen, M., Roselle, D., Reichert, C., Lippman, M., Chabner, B. 1981. Melatonin inhibition and pinealectomy enhancement of 7–12 dimethylbenz(*a*)anthracene-induced mammary tumors in the rat. *Cancer Res* 41:4432–4436.
28. Sanchez-Barcelo, E.J., Cos, S., Fernandez, R., Mediavilla, M.D. 2003. Melatonin and mammary cancer: A short review. *Endocr Relat Cancer* 10:153–159.
29. Kubatka, P., Bojková, B., Kalická, K., et al. 2001. Preventive effects of raloxifene and melatonin in *N*-methyl-*N*-nitrosourea–induced mammary carcinogenesis in female rats. *Neoplasma* 48(4):313–319.
30. Pawlikowski, M., Winczyk, K., Karasek, M. 2002. Oncostatic action of melatonin: Facts and question marks. *Neuro Endocrinol Lett* 23(1):24–29.
31. Cos, S., Mediavilla, D., Martínez-Campa, C., González, A., Alonso-González, C., Sánchez-Barceló, E.J. 2006. Exposure to light-at-night increases the growth of DMBA-induced mammary adenocarcinomas in rats. *Cancer Lett* 235:266–271.
32. Anisimov, V.N. 2003. The role of pineal gland in breast cancer development. *Crit Rev Oncol/Hematol* 46(3) 221–234.
33. Blask, D.E., Pelletier, D.B., Hill, S.M., et al. 1991. Pineal melatonin inhibition of tumor promotion in the *N*-nitroso-*N*-methylurea model of mammary carcinogenesis: Potential involvement of antiestrogenic mechanisms *in vivo*. *J Cancer Res Clin Oncol* 117:526–532.
34. Palmer, H.J., Paulson, K.E. 1997. Reactive Oxygen Species and Antioxidants in Signal Transduction and Gene Expression. *Nutr Rev* 55:353–361.
35. Cerutti, P.A. 1985. Prooxidant States and Tumor Promotion. *Science* 227:375–381.
36. Reiter, R.J., Tan, D.-X., Pilar, Terron, M., Czarnocki, Z. 2007. Melatonin and its metabolites: New findings regarding their production and their radical scavenging actions. *Acta Biochim Pol* 54:1–9.
37. Di Bella, L., Scalera, G., Rossi, M.T. 1979. Perspectives in pineal function. In: *The Pineal Gland of Vertebrates Including Man, Progress in Brain Research.* Eds. Kappers, J.A., and Pevet, P. 52:475–478. New York: Oxford Univ. Press.

38. Burns, J.K. 1973. Administration of melatonin to non-human primates and to women with breast carcinoma. *J Physiol* 229:38–39.
39. Lissoni, P., Barni, S., Meregalli, S., et al. 1995. Modulation of cancer endocrine therapy by melatonin: A phase II study of tamoxifen plus melatonin in metastatic breast cancer patients progressing under tamoxifen alone. *Br J Cancer* 71:854–856.
40. Lissoni, P., Barni, S., Tancini, G., et al. 1994. A randomised study with subcutaneous low-dose interleukin 2 alone vs interleukin 2 plus the pineal neurohormone melatonin in advanced solid neoplasms other than renal cancer and melanoma. *Br J Cancer* 69:196–199.
41. Lissoni, P., Barni, S., Cattaneo et al. 1991. Clinical results with the pineal hormone melatonin in advanced cancer resistant to standard antitumor therapies. *Oncology* 48:448–450.
42. Lissoni, P., Barni, S., Ardizzoia, A., et al. 1994. A randomized study with the pineal hormone melatonin versus supportive care alone in patients with brain metastases due to solid neoplasms. *Cancer* 73:699–701.
43. Lissoni, P., Barni, S., Crispino, S., Tancini, G., Fraschini, F. 1989. Endocrine and immune effects of melatonin therapy in metastatic cancer patients. *Eur J Cancer Clin Oncol* 25:789–795.
44. Lissoni, P., Barni, S., Tancini, G., et al. 1987. Clinical study of melatonin in untreatable advanced cancer patients. *Tumori* 73:475–480.
45. Lissoni, P., Barni, S., Ardizzoia, A., et al. 1992. Randomized study with the pineal hormone melatonin versus supportive care alone in advanced nonsmall cell lung cancer resistant to a first-line chemotherapy containing cisplatin. *Oncology* 49:336–339.
46. Mills, E., Wu, P., Seely, D., Guyatt, G. 2005. Melatonin in the treatment of cancer: A systematic review of randomized controlled trials and meta-analysis. *J Pineal Res* 39(4):360–366.
47. Bartsch, C., Bartsch, H., Karasek, M. 2002. Melatonin in clinical oncology. *Neuro Endocrinol Lett* 23(1):30–38.
48. Hill, S.M., Blask, D.E. 1985. Physiological concentrations of melatonin inhibit the proliferation of MCF-7 human breast cancer cells in vitro. *Endocr Soc* 1010:253.
49. Hill, S.M., Blask, D.E. 1988. Effects of the pineal hormone melatonin on the proliferation and morphological characteristics of human breast cancer cells (MCF-7) in culture. *Cancer Res* 48:6121–6126.
50. Cos, S., Blask, D.E., Lemus-Wilson, A., Hill, A.B. 1991. Effects of melatonin on the cell cycle kinetics and oestrogen rescue of MCF-7 human breast cancer cells in culture. *J Pineal Res* 10:36–42.
51. Cos, S., Recio, J., Sànchez-Barcelò, E.J. 1996. Modulation of the cell cycle time of MCF-7 human breast cancer cells by melatonin. *Life Sci.* 58:811–816.
52. Cucina, A., Proietti, S., D'Anselmi, F., Coluccia, P., Dinicola, S., Bizzarri, M.et al. 2009. Evidence for a biphasic apoptotic pathway induced by melatonin in MCF-7 breast cancer cells. *J Pineal Res* 46(2):172–180.
53. Molis, T., Muraoka, H.G., Castles, C., Blask, D.E., Hill, S.M. 1991. Growth regulatory effects of melatonin are linked to the oestrogen response pathway of human breast cancer cells. *Endocr Soc* 588:177.
54. L'Hermite-Baleriaux, M., L'Hermite, M., Pasteels, J.M., de Launoit, Y. 1990. Effect of melatonin on the proliferation of human mammary cancer cell lines. *Endocr Soc* 140:59.
55. Shellard, S.A., Whelan, R.D.H., Hill, B.T. 1989. Growth inhibitory and cytotoxic effects of melatonin and its metabolites on human tumour cell lines in vitro. *Br J Cancer* 60:288–290.
56. Cos, S., Fernandez, F., Sanchez-Barcelò. 1996. Melatonin inhibits DNA synthesis in MCF-7 human breast cancer cells in vitro. *Life Sci* 58:2447–2453.
57. Bizzarri, M., Cucina, A., Valente, M.G., et al. 2003. Melatonin and vitamin D3 increase TGF-beta1 release and induce growth inhibition in breast cancer cell cultures. *J Surg Res* 110(2):332–337.
58. Hill, S.M., Spriggs, L.L., Simon, M.A., Muraoka, H., Blask, D.E. 1992. The growth inhibitory action of melatonin on human breast cancer cells is linked to the estrogen response system. *Cancer Lett* 64:249–256.
59. Cos, S., Sanchez-Barcelo, E.J. 2000. Melatonin and mammary pathological growth. *Front Neuroendocrinol* 21:133–170.
60. Dauchy, R.T., Dauchy, E.M., Sauer, L.A., et al. 2004. Differential inhibition of fatty acid transport in tissue-isolated steroid receptor negative human breast cancer xenografts perfused in situ with isomers of conjugated linoleic acid. *Cancer Lett* 209:7–15.
61. Blask, D.E. 1993. Melatonin in oncology. In: *Melatonin. Biosynthesis, Physiological Effects, and Clinical Applications.* Eds. Yu, H.S., and Reiter, R.J. 447–475. Boca Raton, FL:CRC Press, Inc.
62. Brydon, L., Roka, F., Petit, L. 1999. Dual signaling of human Me11a melatonin receptors via G_{i2}, G_{i3} and $G_{q/11}$ proteins. *Mol Endocrinol* 13:2025–2038.
63. Ram, P.T., Dai, J., Yuan L et al. 2002. Involvement of the mt1 melatonin receptor in human breast cancer. *Cancer Lett* 179:141–150.

64. Roka, F., Brydon, L., Waldhoer, M. 1999. Tight association of the human Mel(1a)-melatonin receptor and G(i): Precoupling and constitutive activity. *Mol Pharmacol* 56:1014–1024.
65. Dubocovich, M.L., Masana, M.I., Iacob, S., et al. 1997. Melatonin receptor antagonists that differentiate between the human Mel1a and Mel1b recombinant subtypes are used to assess the pharmacological profile of the rabbit retina ML1 presynaptic heteroreceptor. *Naunyn Schmiedebergs Arch Pharmacol* 355:365–375.
66. Dubocovich, M.L. 1988. Luzindole (N-0774): A novel melatonin receptor antagonist. *J Pharmacol Exp Ther* Sept 246:902–910.
67. Yuan, L., Collins, A.R., Dai, J., Dubocovich, M.L., Hill, S.M. 2002. MT1 melatonin receptor overexpression enhances the growth suppressive effects of melatonin in human breast cancer cells. *Mol Cell Endocrinol* 192:147–156.
68. Collins, A., Yuan, L., Kiefer, T.L., Cheng, Q., Lai, L., Hill, S.M. 2003. Overexpression of the MT1 melatonin receptor in MCF-7 human breast cancer cells inhibits mammary tumour formation in nude mice. *Cancer Lett* 189:49–57.
69. Jawed, S., Kim, B., Ottenhof, T., Brown, G.M., Werstiuk, E.S., Niles, L.P. 2007. Human melatonin MT1 receptor induction by valproic acid and its effects in combination with melatonin on MCF-7 breast cancer cell proliferation. *Eur J Pharmacol* 560:17–22.
70. Bahia, H., Ashman, J.N., Cawkwell, L., et al. 2002. Karyotypic variation between independently cultured strains of the cell line MCF-7 identified by multicolour fluorescence in situ hybridization. *Int J Oncol* 20:489–494.
71. Lai, L., Yuan, L., Chen, Q., et al. 2008. The Gαi and Gαq proteins mediate the effects of melatonin on steroid/thyroid hormone receptor transcriptional activity and breast cancer cell proliferation. *J Pineal Res* 45:476–488.
72. Lai, L., Yuan, L., Cheng, Q., Dong, C., Mao, L., Hill, S.M. 2009. Alteration of the MT1 melatonin receptor gene and its expression in primary human breast tumors and breast cancer cell lines. *Breast Cancer Res Treat* 118:293–305.
73. Pandi-Perumal, S.R., Trakht, I., Srinivasan, V., et al. 2008. Physiological effects of melatonin: Role of melatonin receptors and signal transduction pathways. *Prog Neurobiol* 85:335–353.
74. Guerrero, H.Y., Gauer, F., Schuster, C., Pevet, P., Masson-Pevet, M. 2000. Melatonin regulates the mRNA expression of the MT1 melatonin receptor in the rat pars tuberalis. *Neuroendocrinology* 71:163–169.
75. Gerdin, M.J., Masana, M.I., Ren, D., Miller, R.J., Dubocovich, M.L. 2003. Short-term exposure to melatonin differentially affects the functional sensitivity and trafficking of the hMT1 and hMT2 melatonin receptors. *J Pharmacol Exp Ther* 304:931–939.
76. Baldwin, S.W., Travlos, G.S., Risinger, J.I., Barrett, J.C. 1998. Melatonin does not inhibit estradiol-stimulated proliferation in MCF-7 and BG-1 cells. *Carcinogenesis* 19:1895–1900.
77. Reiter, R.J., Tan, D.X., Manchester, L.C., Pliar Terron, M., Flores, L.J., Koppisepi, S. 2007. Medical implications of melatonin: Receptor-mediated and receptor-independent actions. *Adv Med Sci* 52:11–28.
78. Hill, S.M., Blask, D.E. 1986. Melatonin inhibition of MCF-7 breast cancer cell proliferation: Influence of serum factors prolactin and oestradiol. *Endocr Soc* 863:246.
79. Cos, S., Sanchez-Barcelo, E.J. 1995. Melatonin inhibition of MCF-7 human breast cancer cells: Influence of cell proliferation rate. *Cancer Lett* 93:207–212.
80. Cos, S., Sanchez-Barcelo, E.J. 1994. Differences between pulsatile or continuous exposure to melatonin on MCF-7 human breast cancer cell proliferation. *Cancer Lett* 85:105–109.
81. Cos, S., Blask, D.E. 1990. Effects of melatonin on the anchorage-independent growth of human breast cancer cells (MCF-7) in a clonogenic culture system. *Cancer Lett* 50:115–109.
82. Reiter, RJ. 1980. The pineal and its hormones in the control of reproduction in mammals. *Endocr Rev* 1:109–131.
83. Arendt, J. 1986. Role of the pineal gland and melatonin in seasonal reproductive function in mammals. *Oxf Rev Reprod Biol* 8:266–320.
84. Dubocovich, M.L., Rivera-Bermudez, M.A., Gerdin, M.J., et al. 2003. Molecular pharmacology, regulation and function of mammalian melatonin receptors. *Front Biosci* 8:1093–1108.
85. Kauppila, A., Kivela, A., Pakarinen, A., et al. 1987. Inverse seasonal relationship between melatonin and ovarian activity in humans in a region with a strong seasonal contrast in luminosity. *J Clin Endocrinol Metab* 65:823–828.
86. Aleandri, V., Spina, V., Morini, A. 1996. The pineal gland and reproduction. *Hum Reprod Update* 2:225–235.
87. Luboshitzky, R., Lavie, P. 1999. Melatonin and sex hormone interrelationships: A review. *J Pediatr Endocrinol Metab* 12:355–362.

88. Woo, M.M., Tai, C.J., Kang, S.K., et al. 2001. Direct action of melatonin in human granulose–luteal cells. *J Clin Endocrinol Metab* 86:4789–4797.
89. Soares, J.M., Masana, M.I., Ersahin, C., et al. 2003. Functional melatonin receptors in rat ovaries at various stages of the estrous cycle. *J Pharmacol Exp Ther* 306:694–702.
90. Sánchez-Barcelò, E.J., Cos, S., Mediavilla, D., Martınez-Campa, C., Gonzalez, A. and Alonso-Gonzalez, C. 2005. Melatonin–estrogen interactions in breast cancer. *J Pineal Res* 38:217–222.
91. Ram, P.T., Yuan, L., Dai, J., Kiefer, T., Klotz, D.M., Spriggs, L.L., Hill, S.M. 2000. Differential responsiveness of MCF-7 human breast cancer cell line stocks to the pineal hormone melatonin. *J Pineal Res* 28:210–218.
92. Del Rio, B., Garcia Pedrero, J.M., Martinez-Campa, C., Zuazua, P., Lazo, P.S., Ramos, S. 2004. Melatonin, an endogenous-specific inhibitor of estrogen receptor alpha via calmodulin. *J Biol Chem* 279:38294–38302.
93. Cos, S., Fernández, R., Güéuzmes, A., Sánchez-Barceló, E.J. 1998. Influence of melatonin on invasive and metastatic properties of MCF-7 human breast cancer cells. *Cancer Res* 58:4383–4390.
94. Wilson, S.T., Blask, D.E., Lemus-Wilson, A.M. 1992. Melatonin augments the sensitivity of MCF-7 human breast cancer cells to tamoxifen *in vitro*. *J Clin Endocrinol Metab* 75:669–670.
95. Mediavilla, M.D., Guezmez, A., Ramos, S., et al. 1997. Effects of melatonin on mammary gland lesions in transgenic mice overexpressing N-ras proto-oncogene. *J Pineal Res* 22:86–94.
96. Kiefer, T.L., Lai, L., Yuan, L., Dong, C., Burow, M.E., Hill, S.M. 2005. Differential regulation of estrogen receptor alpha, glucocorticoid, receptor and retinoic acid receptor alpha transcriptional activity by melatonin is mediated via different G proteins. *J Pineal Res* 38:231–239.
97. Garcìa-Rato, A., García-Pedrero, J.M., Martínez, M.A., Del Rio, B., Lazo, P.S., Ramos, S. 1999. Melatonin blocks the activation of estrogen receptor for DNA binding. *FASEB J* 13:857–868.
98. Lawson, N.O., Wee, B.E., Blask, D.E., Castles, C.G., Spriggs, L.L., Hill, S.M. 1992. Melatonin decreases estrogen receptor expression in the medial preoptic area of inbred (LSH/SsLak) golden hamsters. *Biol Reprod* 47:1082–1090.
99. Mangelsdorf, D.J., Thummel, C., Beato, M., et al. 1995. The nuclear receptor superfamily: The second decade. *Cell* 83:835–839.
100. Glass, C.K., Rosenfeld, M.G. 2000. The coregulator exchange in transcriptional functions of nuclear receptors. *Genes Dev* 14:121–141.
101. Benoit, G., Cooney, A., Giguere, V., et al. 2006. International Union of Pharmacology LXVI. Orphan nuclear receptors. *Pharmacol Rev* 58:798–836.
102. Mukherjee, R., Davies, P.J., Crombie, D.L., et al. 1997. Sensitization of diabetic and obese mice to insulin by retinoid X receptor agonists. *Nature* 386:407–410.
103. Mukherjee, R., Jow, L., Croston, G.E., Paterniti, J.R. 1997. Identification, characterization, and tissue distribution of human peroxisome proliferator–activated receptor (PPAR) isoforms PPARgamma2 versus PPARgamma1 and activation with retinoid X receptor agonists and antagonists. *J Biol Chem* 272:8071–8076.
104. McKenna, N.J., O'Malley, B.W. 2002. Minireview: Nuclear receptor coactivators—an update. *Endocrinology* 143:2461–2465.
105. McKenna, N.J., O'Malley, B.W. 2002. Combinatorial control of gene expression by nuclear receptors and coregulators. *Cell* 108:465–474.
106. Becker-Andre, M., Wiesenberg, I., Schaeren-Wiemers, N., et al. 1994. Pineal gland hormone melatonin binds and activates an orphan of the nuclear receptor superfamily. *J Biol Chem* 269:28531–28534.
107. Park, H.T., Baek, S.Y., Kim, B.S., Kim, J.B., Kim, J.J. 1996. Developmental expression of 'RZR beta, a putative nuclear-melatonin receptor' mRNA in the suprachiasmatic nucleus of the rat. *Neurosci Lett* 217:17–20.
108. Naji, L., Carrillo-Vico, A., Guerrero, J.M., Calvo, J.R. 2004. Expression of membrane and nuclear melatonin receptors in mouse peripheral organs. *Life Sci* 74:2227–2236.
109. Agez, L., Laurent, V., Pevet, P., Masson-Pevet, M., Gauer, F. 2007. Melatonin affects nuclear orphan receptors mRNA in the rat suprachiasmatic nuclei. *Neuroscience* 144:522–530.
110. Baler, R., Coon, S., Klein, D.C. 1996. Orphan nuclear receptor RZRbeta: Cyclic AMP regulates expression in the pineal gland. *Biochem Biophys Res Commun* 220:975–978.
111. Smirnov, A.N. 2001. Nuclear melatonin receptors. *Biochemistry* 66(1):19–26.
112. Bordji K, Grillasca JP, Gouze JN et al. (2000) Evidence for the presence of peroxisome proliferator–activated receptor (PPAR) alpha and gamma and retinoid Z receptor in cartilage. PPARgamma activation modulates the effects of interleukin-1beta on rat chondrocytes. *J Biol Chem* 275:12243–12250.

113. Sharma, R., Ottenhof, T., Rzeczkowska, P.A., Niles, L.P. 2008. Epigenetic targets for melatonin: Induction of histone H3 hyperacetylation and gene expression in C17.2 neural stem cells. *J Pineal Res* 45(3):277–284.
114. Korkmaz, A., Sanchez-Barcelo, E.J., Tan, D.X., Reiter, R.J. 2009. Role of melatonin in the epigenetic regulation of breast cancer. *Breast Cancer Res Treat* 115:13–27.
115. Aronika, S.M., Kraus, W.L., Katzenellenbogen, B.S. 1994. Estrogen action via the cAMP signalling pathway: Stimulation of adenylate cyclase and cAMP-regulated gene transcription. *Proc Nat Acad Sci USA* 91:8517–8521.
116. Ram, P.T., Kiefer, T., Silverman, M., Song, Y., Brown, G.M., Hill, S.M. 1998. Estrogen receptor transactivation in MCF-7 breast cancer cells by melatonin and growth factors. *Mol Cell Endocrinol* 141:53–64.119.
117. Kiefer, T., Ram, P.T., Yuan, L., Hill, S.M. 2002. Melatonin inhibits estrogen receptor transactivation and cAMP levels in breast cancer cells. *Breast Cancer Res Treatment* 71:37–45.
118. Benítez-King, G., Rios, A., Martinez, A., Anton-Tay, F. 1996. *In vitro* inhibition of Ca2+/calmodulin-dependent kinase II activity by melatonin. *Biochim Biophys Acta* 1290:191–196.
119. Soto-Vega, E., Ramirez-Rodriguez, G., Benitez-King, G. 2004. Melatonin stimulates calmodulin phosphorylation by protein kinase C. *J Pineal Res* 37:98–106.
120. Garcia-Pedrero, J.M., Martínez, M.A., Del Rio, B., et al. 2002. Calmodulin is a selective modulator of estrogen receptors. *Mol Endocrinol* 16:947–960.
121. Musgrove, E.A., Wakeling, A.E., Sutherland, R.L. 1989. Points of action of estrogen antagonist within the MCF-7 human breast cancer cell cycle. *Cancer Res* 49:2398–2404.
122. Dai J, Inscho EW, Yuan L & Hill SM. 2002. Modulation of intracellular calcium and calmodulin by melatonin in MCF-7 human breast cancer cells. *J Pineal Res* 32 112–119.
123. Li, Z., Kim, S.H., Higgins, J.M.G., Brenner, M.B., Sacks, D.B. 1999. IQGAP1 and calmodulin modulate E-cadherin function. *J Biol Chem* 274:37885–37892.
124. Blask, D.E. 1997. Systemic, cellular and molecular aspects of melatonin action on experimental breast carcinogenesis. In: *The Melatonin Hypothesis—Breast Cancer and Use of Electric Power*. Eds. Stevens, R.G., Wilson B.W., Anderson, L.E. 189–230. Columbus: Battelle Press.
125. Blask, D.E., Wilson, S.T., Zalatan, F. 1997. Physiological melatonin inhibition of human breast cancer cell growth in vitro: Evidence for a glutathione-mediated pathway. *Cancer Res* 57:1909–1914.
126. Leung, M.F., Chov, I.N. 1989. Relationship between L-chloro-2,4-diitrobenzene induced cytoskeletal perturbations and cellular glutathione. *Cell Biol Toxicol* 5:51–99.
127. Benítez-King, G., Anton-Tay, F. 1993. Calmodulin mediates melatonin cytoskeletal effects. *Experientia* 49:635–641.
128. Yang, Q.H., Xu, Y.N., Xu, R.K., Pang, S.F. 2007. Antiproliferative effects of melatonin on the growth of rat pituitary prolactin-secreting tumor cells in vitro. *J Pineal Res* 42:172–179.
129. Roth, J.A., Rabin, R., Agnello, K. 1997. Melatonin suppression of PC12 cell growth and death. *Brain Res* 768:63–70.
130. Zhou, D., Clarke, P., Wang, J., et al. 1996. Identification of a promoter that controls aromatase expression in human breast cancer and adipose stromal cells. *J Biol Chem* 271:15194–15202.
131. Michael, M.D., Michael, L.F., Simpson, E.R. 1997. A CRE-like sequence that binds CREB and contributes to cAMPdependent regulation of the proximal promoter of the human aromatase P450 (*CYP19*) gene. *Mol Cell Endocrinol* 134:147–156.
132. Zhao, Y., Agarwal, V.R., Mendelson, C.R., et al. 1996. Estrogen biosynthesis proximal to a breast tumor is stimulated by PGE2 via cyclic AMP, leading to activation of promoter II of the *CYP19* (aromatase) gene. *Endocrinology* 137:5739–5742.
133. Cardinali, D.P., Bonanni, Rey, R.A., Mediavilla, M.D., et al. 1992. Diurnal changes in cyclic nucleotide response to pineal indoles in murine mammary glands. *J Pineal Res* 13:111–116.
134. Cos, S., Martinez-Campa, C., Mediavilla, M.D., Sànchez-Barcelò, E.J. 2005. Melatonin modulates aromatase activity in MCF-7 human breast cancer cells. *J Pineal Res* 38:136–142.
135. González, A., Martínez-Campa, C., Mediavilla, M.D., et al. 2007. Effects of MT1 melatonin receptor overexpression on the aromatase-suppressive effect of melatonin in MCF-7 human breast cancer cells *Oncol Rep* 17:947–953.
136. Martinez-Campa, C., Gonzàlez, A., Mediavilla, M.D., Alonso-Gonzàlez, A., Sànchez-Barcelò, E.J., Cos, S. 2005. Melatonin enhances the inhibitory effect of aminoglutethimide on aromatase activity in MCF-7 human breast cancer cells. *Breast Cancer Res Treat* 94:249–254.
137. Ryde, C.M., Nicholls, J.E., Dowsett, M. 1992. Steroid and growth factor modulation of aromatase activity in MCF-7 and T47D breast carcinoma cell lines. *Cancer Res* 52:1411–1215.

138. Cos, S., Blask, D.E. 1994. Melatonin modulates growth factor activity in MCF-7 human breast cancer cells. *J Pineal Res* 17:25–32.
139. Martìnez-Campa, C., Gonzàlez, A., Mediavilla, M.D., et al. 2009. Melatonin inhibits aromatase promoter expression by regulating cyclooxygenases expression and activity in breast cancer cells. *Br J Cancer* 101:1613–1619.
140. Suzuki T, Miki Y, Nakamura Y et al. 2005. Sex steroid–producing enzymes in human breast cancer. *Endocr Relat Cancer* 12:701–720.
141. Suzuki, T., Miki, Y., Nakata, T., et al. 2003. Steroid sulfatase and estrogen sulfotransferase in normal human tissue and breast cancer. *J Steroid Biochem Mol Biol* 86:449–454.
142. Gonzalez, A., Cos, S., Martinez-Campa, C., Alonso-Gonzalez, C., Sanchez-Mateos, S., Mediavilla, M.D., Sanchez-Barcelo, E.J. 2008. Selective estrogen enzyme modulator actions of melatonin in human breast cancer cells. *J Pineal Res* 45:86–92.
143. Cai, Z., Kwintkiewicz, J., Young, M.E., Stocco, C. 2007. Prostaglandin E2 increases *cyp19* expression in rat granulosa cells: Implication of GATA-4. *Mol Cell Endocrinol* 263:181–189.
144. Irahara, N., Miyoshi, Y., Taguchi, T., Tamaki, Y., Noguchi, S. 2006. Quantitative analysis of aromatase mRNA expression derived from various promoters (I.4, I.3, PII and I.7) and its association with expression of TNF-alpha, IL-6 and COX-2 mRNAs in human breast cancer. *Int J Cancer* 118:1915–1921.
145. Subbaramaiah, K., Howe, L.R., Port, E.R., et al. 2006. HER-2/neu status is a determinant of mammary aromatase activity in vivo: Evidence for a cyclooxygenase-2–dependent mechanism. *Cancer Res* 66:5504–5511.
146. Mrnka, L., Hock, M., Rybova, M., Pacha, J. 2008. Melatonin inhibits prostaglandin E2 and sodium nitroprusside-induced ion secretion in rat distal colon. *Eur J Pharmacol* 581:164–170.
147. Dong, W.G., Mei, Q., Yu, J.P., Xu, J.M., Xiang, L., Xu, Y. 2003. Effects of melatonin on the expression of iNOS and COX-2 in rat models of colitis. *World J Gastroenterol* 9:1307–1311.
148. Deng, W.G., Tang, S.T., Tseng, H.P., Wu, K.K. 2006. Melatonin suppresses macrophage cyclooxygenase-2 and inducible nitric oxide synthase expression by inhibiting p52 acetylation and binding. *Blood* 108:518–5124.
149. Esposito, E., Iacono, A., Muia, C., et al. 2008. Signal transduction pathways involved in protective effects of melatonin in C6 glioma cells. *J Pineal Res* 44:78–87.
150. Crowe, D.L., Chandraratna, R.A. 2004. A retinoid X receptor (RXR)–selective retinoid reveals that RXR-alpha is potentially a therapeutic target in breast cancer cell lines, and that it potentiates antiproliferative and apoptotic responses to peroxisome proliferator–activated receptor ligands. *Breast Cancer Res* 6:R546–R555.
151. Fan, W., Yanase, T., Morinaga, H., et al. 2005. Activation of peroxisome proliferator–activated receptor-gamma and retinoid X receptor inhibits aromatase transcription via nuclear factor kappa B. *Endocrinology* 146:85–92.
152. Molis, T.M., Spriggs, L.L., Jupiter, Y., Hill, S.M. 1995. Melatonin modulation of estrogen-regulated proteins, growth factors, and proto-oncogenes in human breast cancer. *J Pineal Res* 18:93–103.
153. Henry, J.A., Piggott, N.H., Mallick, U.K., Nicholson, S., Farndon, J.R., Westley, B.R. 1990. PNR-2/pS2 immunohistochemical staining in breast cancer: Correlation with prognostic factors and endocrine response. *Br J Cancer* 4:615–622.
154. Calnaan, D.P.K., Westley, B.R., May, F.E.B., Floyd, D.N., Marchbank, T., Playford, R.J. 1999. The trefoil peptide TFF1 inhibits the growth of the human gastric adenocarcinoma cell line AGS. *J Pathol* 188:312–317.
155. Barnes, D.M., Gillett, C.E. 1998. Cyclin D1 in breast cancer. *Breast Cancer Res Treat* 52:1–15.
156. Cicatiello, L., Addeo, R., Sasso, A. 2004. Estrogens and progesterone promote persistent CCND1 gene activation during G1 by inducing transcriptional derepression via c-Jun/c-Fos/estrogen receptor (progesterone receptor) complex assembly to a distal regulatory element and recruitment of cyclin D1 to its own gene promoter. *Mol Cell Biol* 24:7260–7274.
157. Fu, M., Wang, C., Li, Z., Sakamaki, T., Pestell, R.G. 2004. Minireview: Cyclin D1: Normal and abnormal functions. *Endocrinology* 145:5439–5447.
158. Fu, M., Rao, M., Bouras, T., et al. 2005. Cyclin D1 inhibits peroxisome proliferator–activated receptor gamma-mediated adipogenesis through histone deacetylase recruitment. *J Biol Chem* 280:16934–16941.
159. Levine, A.J. 1997. p53, the Cellular Gatekeeper for Growth and Division. *Cell* 88:323–331.
160. Cini, G., Neri, B., Pacini, A., et al. 2005. Antiproliferative activity of melatonin by transcriptional inhibition of cyclin D1 expression: A molecular basis for melatonin-induced oncostatic effects. *J Pineal Res* 39:12–20.

161. Abbas, T., Dutta, A. 2009. p21 in cancer: Intricate networks and multiple activities. *Nature Reviews Cancer* 9:400–414.
162. Mediavilla, M.D., Cos, S., Sànchez-Barcelò, E.J. 1999. Melatonin increases p53 and p21WAF1 expression in MCF-7 human breast cancer cells in vitro. *Life Sci* 65:415–420.
163. Rimler, A., Matzkin, H., Zisapel, N. 1999. Cross talk between melatonin and TGF-1 in human benign prostate epithelial cells. *Prostate* 40:211.
164. Molis, T.M., Spriggs, L.L., Hill, S.M. 1994. Modulation of estrogen receptor mRNA expression by melatonin in MCF-7 human breast cancer cells. *Mol Endocrinol* 8:1683–1690.
165. Czeczuga-Semeniuk, E., Anchim, T., Dzieciol, J., et al. 2004. Can transforming growth factor–β1 and retinoids modify the acivity of estradiol and antiestrogens in MCF-7 breast cancer cells? *Acta Biochim Pol* 51:733–745.
166. Blask, D.E., Sauer, L.A., Dauchy, R.T. 2002. Melatonin as a chronobiotic/anticanceragent: Cellular, biochemical, and molecular mechanisms of action and their implications for circadian-based cancer therapy. *Curr Top Med Chem* 2:113–132.
167. Leon-Blanco, M.M., Guerrero, J.M., Reiter, J.R., Calvo, J.R., Pozo, D. 2003. Melatonin inhibits telomerase activity in the MCF-7 tumour cell line both in vitro and in vivo. *J Pineal Res* 35:204–211.
168. Martınez-Campa, C.M., Alonso-Gonzàlez, C., Mediavilla, M.D., Cos, S., Gonzalez, A., Sanchez-Barcelò, E.J. 2008. Melatonin down-regulates hTERT expression induced by either natural estrogens (17b-estradiol) or metalloestrogens (cadmium) in MCF-7 human breast cancer cells. *Cancer Lett* 268:272–277.
169. Leon-Blanco, M.M., Guerrero, J.M., Reiter, R.J., Pozo, D. 2004. RNA expression of human telomerase subunits TR and TERT is differentially affected by melatonin receptor agonists in the MCF-7 tumor cell line. *Cancer Lett* 216:73–80.
170. Blasco, M.A. 2007. The epigenetic regulation of mammalian telomeres. *Nat Rev Genet* 8:299–309.
171. Reiter, R.J. 2004. Mechanisms of cancer inhibition by melatonin. *J Pineal Res* 37:213–214.
172. Sainz, R.M., Mayo, J.C., Rodriguez, C., Tan, D.X., Lopez-Burillo, S., Reiter, R.J. 2003. Melatonin and cell death: Differential actions on apoptosis in normal and cancer cells. *Cell Mol Life Sci* 60:1407–1426.
173. Winczyk, K., Pawlikowski, M., Lawnicka, H., Kunert-Radek, J., Spadoni, G., Tarzia, G., et al. 2002. Effects of melatonin and melatonin receptors ligand *N*-[(4-methoxy-1*H*-indol-2yl) methyl] propanamide on murine Colon 38 cancer growth in vitro and in vivo. *Neuroendocrinol Lett* 1:50–54.
174. Karasek, M., Winczyk, K., Kunert-Radk, J., Wiesenberg, I., Pawlikowski, M. 1998. Antiproliferative effects of melatonin and CGP52608 on the murine colon 38 adenocarcinoma in vitro and in vivo. *Neuroendocrinol Lett* 19:71–78.
175. Martın-Renedo, J., Mauriz, J.L., Jorquera, F., Ruiz-Andres, O., Gonzàlez, P., Gonzàlez-Gallego, J. 2008. Melatonin induces cell cycle arrest and apoptosis in hepatocarcinoma HepG2 cell line. *J Pineal Res* 45:532–540.
176. Garcıà-Santos, G., Antolin, I., Herrera, F., et al. 2006. Melatonin induces apoptosis in human neuroblastoma cancer cells *J Pineal Res* 41:130–135.
177. El-Missiry, M.A., Abd El-Aziz, A.F. 2000. Influence of melatonin on proliferation and antioxidant system in Ehrlich ascites carcinoma cells. *Cancer Lett* 151:119–125.
178. Rubio, S., Estevez, F., Cabrera, J., Reiter, R.J., Loro, J., Quintana, J. 2007. Inhibition of proliferation and induction of apoptosis by melatonin in human myeloid HL-60 cells. *J Pineal Res* 42:131–138.
179. Trubiani, O., Recchioni, R., Moroni, F., Pizzicannella, J., Caputi, S., Di Primio, R. 2005. Melatonin provokes cell death in human B-lymphoma cells by mitochondrial-dependent apoptotic pathway activation. *J Pineal Res* 39:425–431.
180. Wolfler, A., Caluba, H.C., Abuja, P.M., Dohr, G., Schauenstein, K., Liebmann, P.M. 2001. Prooxidant activity of melatonin promotes fas-induced cell death in human leukemic Jurkat cells. *FEBS Lett* 502:127–131.
181. Cos, S., Mediavilla, M.D., Fernandez, R., et al. 2002. Does melatonin induce apoptosis in MCF-7 human breast cancer cells in vitro? *J Pineal Res* 32:90–96.
182. Eck-Enriquez, K.M., Yuan, L., Duffy, L., et al. 1998. A sequential treatment regimen with melatonin and all-*trans* retinoic acid induces apoptosis in MCF-7 tumour cells. *Br J Cancer* 77:2129–2137.
183. Czeczuga-Semeniuk, E., Wolczynski, S., Anchim, T., Dzieciol, J., Dabrowska, M., Pietruczuk, M. 2002. Effect of melatonin and all-*trans* retinoic acid on the proliferation and induction of the apoptotic pathway in the culture of human breast cancer cell line MCF-7. *Pol J Pathol* 53(2):59–65.
184. Eck-Enriquez, KM., Kiefer, T.L., Spriggs, L.L., Hill1, S.M. 2000. Pathways through which a regimen of melatonin and retinoic acid induces apoptosis in MCF-7 human breast cancer cells. *Breast Cancer Res Treatment* 61:229–239.

185. Abd El-Aziz, M.A., Hassan, H.A., Mohamed, M.H., et al. 2005. The biochemical and morphological alterations following administration of melatonin, retinoic acid and *Nigella sativa* in mammary carcinoma: An animal model. *Int J Exp Path* 86:383–396.
186. Momand, J., Wu, H.H., Dasgupta, G. 2000. MDM2—Master regulator of the p53 tumor suppressor protein. *Gene* 242:15–29.
187. De Rozieres, S., Maya, R., Oren, M., Lozano, G. 2000. The loss of MDM2 induces p53-mediated apoptosis. *Oncogene* 19:1691–1697.
188. Inoue, T., Geyer, R.K., Yu, Z.K., Maki, C.G. 2001. Downregulation of MDM2 stabilizes p53 by inhibiting p53 ubiquitination in response to specific alkylating agents. *FEBS Lett* 490:196–201.
189. Lopez-Burillo, S., Tan, D.X., Mayo, J.C., Sainz, R.M., Manchester, L.C., Reiter, R.J. 2003. Melatonin, xanthurenic acid, resveratrol, EGCG, vitamin C and a-lipoic acid differentially reduce oxidative DNA damage induced by Fenton reagents: A study of their individual and synergistic actions. *J Pineal Res* 34:269–277.
190. Harland, J.D., Liburdy, R.P. 1997. Environmental Magnetic Fields Inhibit the Antiproliferative Action of Tamoxifen and Melatonin in a Human Breast Cancer Cell Line. *Bioelectromagnetics* 18:555–562.
191. Mao, L., Yuan, L., Hill, S.M. Inhibition of cell proliferation and blockade of cell invasion by melatonin in human breast cancer cells mediated through multiple signaling pathways. Paper presented at the 97th Annual Meeting of the American Association for Cancer Research 2006 Washington, DC. Abstract 495.
192. Cos, S., Fernandez, R. 2000. Melatonin effects on intercellular junctional communication in MCF-7 human breast cancer cells. *J Pineal Res* 29:166–171.
193. Trosko, J.E., Chang, C.C., Madhukar, B.V., Klaunig, J.E. 1990. Chemical, oncogene and growth factor inhibition of gap junctional intercellular communication: An integrative hypothesis of carcinogenesis. *Pathobiology* 58:265–278.
194. Hamada, J., Takeichi, N., Kobayashi, H. 1987. Inverse correlation between the metastatic capacity of cell clones derived from a rat mammary carcinoma and their intercellular communication with normal fibroblasts. *Gann* 78:1175–1178.
195. Crespo, D., Fernàndez-Viadero, C., Verdura, R., Ovejero, V., Cos, S. 1994. Interaction between melatonin and estradiol on morphological and morphometric features of MCF-7 human breast cancer cells. *J Pineal Res* 16:215–222.
196. Roberts, K. 1974. Cytoplasmic microtubules and their functions. *Prog Biophys Mol Biol* 28:371–420.
197. Ingber, D.E. 2003. Tensegrity, II. How structural networks influence cellular information processing networks. *J Cell Sci* 116:1397–1408.
198. Wang, N., Tytell, J.D., Ingber, D.E. 2009. Mechanotransduction at a distance: Mechanically coupling the extracellular matrix with the nucleus. *Nat Rev Mol Cell Biol* 10(1):75–82.
199. Pourati, J., Maniotis, A., Speigel, D., et al. 1998. Is cytoskeletal tension a major determinant of cell deformability in adherent endothelial cells? *Am J Physiol* 274: C1283–C1289.
200. Hammond, T.G., Lewis, F.C., Goodwin, T.J., et al. 1999. Gene expression in space. *Nat Med* 5:359.
201. Stein, G.S., Van Wijnen, A.J., Stein, J.L., Lian, J.B., Pockwinse, S.H., McNeil, S. 1999. Implications for interrelationships between nuclear architecture and control of gene expression under microgravity conditions. *FASEB J.* 13: S157–S166.
202. Huang, S., Ingber, D.E. 2000. Shape-dependent control of cell growth, differentiation, and apoptosis: Switching between attractors in cell regulatory networks. *Exp Cell Res* 261:91–103.
203. Chen, C.S., Mrksich, M., Huang, S., Withesides, G.M., Ingber, D.E. 1997. Geometric control of cell life and death. *Science* 276:1425–1428.
204. D'Anselmi, F., Valerio, M.C., Cucina, A., et al. Metabolism and cell shape in cancer: A fractal analysis. *Int J Biochem Cell Biol* (in press).
205. Raz, A., Geiger, B. 1982. Altered organization of cell-substrate contacts and membrane-associated cytoskeleton in tumor cell variants exhibiting different metastatic capabilities. *Cancer Res* 42:5183–5190.
206. Benitez-King, G., Tunez, I., Bellon, A., et al. 2003. Melatonin prevents cytoskeletal alterations and oxidative stress induced by okadaic acid in N1E-115 cells. *Exp Neurol* 182:151–159.
207. Wang, L.H. 2004. Molecular signaling regulating anchorage independent growth of cancer cells. *Mt Sinai J Med* 71:361–367.
208. Bharadwaj, S., Thanawala, R., Bon, G., Falcioni, R., Prasad, G.L. 2005. Resensitization of breast cancer cells to anoikis by tropomyosin-1: Role of Rho kinase-dependent cytoskeleton and adhesion. *Oncogene* 24:8291–8303.
209. Raftopoulou, M., Hall, A. 2004. Cell migration: Rho GTPases lead the way. *Dev Biol* 265:23–32.

210. Huerto-Delgadillo, L., Anton-Tay, F., Benitez-King, G. 1994. Effects of melatonin on microtubule assembly depend on hormone concentration: Role of melatonin as a Calmodulin antagonist. *J Pineal Res* 17:55–62.
211. Benitez-King, G., Soto-Vega, E., Ramirez-Rodriguez, G. 2009. Melatonin modulates microfilament phenotypes in cancer cells: Implications for adhesion and inhibition of cancer cell migration. *Histol Histopathol* 24:789–799.
212. Ortiz-Lopez, L., Morales-Mulia, S., Ramirez-Rodriguez, G., Benítez-King, G. 2009. ROCK-regulated cytoskeletal dynamics participate in the inhibitory effect of melatonin on cancer cell migration. *J Pineal Res* 46:15–21.
213. Ramirez-Rodriguez, G., Meza, I., Hernandez, M.E., Castillo, A., Benítez-King, G. 2003. Melatonin induced cyclic modulation of vectorial water transport in kidney-derived MDCK cells. *Kidney Int* 63:1356–1364.
214. Ramirez-Rodriguez, G., Ortiz-Lopez, L., Benítez-King, G. 2007. Melatonin increases stress fibers and focal adhesions in MDCK cells: Participation of Rho-associated kinase and protein kinase C. *J Pineal Res* 42:180–190.
215. Yuan, J., Shi, G.X., Shao, Y., Dai, G., Wei, J.N., Chang, D.C., Li, C.J. 2008. Calmodulin bound to stress fibers but not microtubules involves regulation of cell morphology and motility. *Int J Biochem Cell Biol* 40:284–293.
216. Benítez-King, G. 2006. Melatonin as a cytoskeletal modulator: Implications for cell physiology and disease. *J Pineal Res* 40:1–9.

19 Melatonin in Mental Disorders: Treatment and Prevention

Maria D. Maldonado and Maria A. Pérez-San-Gregorio

CONTENTS

19.1 INTRODUCTION

Melatonin (*N*-acetyl-5-methoxytryptamine) is a molecule known for more than half a century as a mediator of biological and physiological rhythms in mammals. It was initially known to be produced exclusively in the pineal gland, but melatonin synthesis has been found in different sites of the organism, and the major sources of extrapineal melatonin are the central nervous system and immune system [1,2]. It is characterized by a wide spectrum of properties, including those involved in sleep and circadian rhythms [3], lipid metabolism [4], immune defense [5,6], tumor inhibition [7], drug detoxification [8], bone physiology [9], and free radical scavenger and antioxidant activities [10]. Some of these actions are receptor-mediated [4,7], while others are receptor-independent [11].

Mental disorders comprise a group of psychiatric illnesses (bipolar syndrome [BS], major depression, and schizophrenia) characterized by alterations in mood, cognition, and behaviors that cause substantial distress and interfere with daily functioning. These three mental disorders were chosen (a) because they are the only three for which there is clear evidence that neuroinflammation is involved, (b) because they are all marked by serious mood disturbances, and (c) they tend to be chronic and/or recurrent with changes in circadian rhythms and sleep loss as precipitating factors for relapses.

In normal subjects, the secretion of melatonin exhibits a circadian pattern synchronized with the day/night cycle. An alteration of this secretory pattern has been found in various psychiatric disorders (seasonal affective disorder, bipolar disorder, depression, bulimia, anorexia, schizophrenia, panic disorder, obsessive compulsive disorder), although it is still not known if such alterations have an etiological role or are secondary to the different disorders [12,13].

All living organisms maintain a complex dynamic equilibrium or homeostasis that is constantly challenged by internal or external adverse effects, termed *stressors* [14]. Epidemiological studies have confirmed that there is an increase in the incidence and prevalence of mental disorders linked, in most cases, with life habits (stressful life and bad diet) [15]; this is associated with an increased utilization of drugs and narcotics [16,17]. Their frequent use often disturbs the normal circadian rhythms of organs and systems. Additionally, the seasonality environmental changes cause alterations in all individuals but are more pronounced in patients with mental illnesses [12,18,19]. Melatonin plays an important role in influencing circadian rhythmicity and sleep [20], particularly seasonally at extreme latitudes where there are marked changes of day length and temperature [19,21]. Also, melatonin has proven immunomodulatory effects and acts on the immune system by regulating gene expression of several cytokines including tumor necrosis factor α (TNF-α), transforming growth factor β (TGF-β), and stem cell factor (SCF) by peritoneal macrophages as well as the levels of interleukin 1β (IL-1β), interferon γ (INF-γ), and SCF by splenocytes [20]. The effect of melatonin on the immune system is also supported by the existence of specific binding sites for melatonin in lymphocytes and monocytes, i.e., membrane (MT1 and MT2) and nuclear (RZR/ROR) receptors [2,22–24].

The immune and nervous systems use a common chemical language (neurotransmitters and cytokines) for intracommunication and intercommunication that provides a complex repertoire of mediators, receptors, and ligands between the two systems [16,25–27]. Work in this field has established that mental disorders disrupt the functional interaction between the nervous and immune systems [19]. This chapter of book provides a brief, albeit comprehensive, synthesis of information on the current understanding of mental disorders with objective depression, BS, and schizophrenia; this also summarizes some of the reasons for the use of melatonin on the mental health and on the immune and nervous systems of psychiatric patients. The review suggests the possible therapeutic use of melatonin as a cotreatment in mental disorders.

19.2 SLEEP LOSS IN PATIENTS WITH MENTAL DISORDERS: ROLE OF MELATONIN

In the *Diagnostic and Statistical Manual of Mental Disorders, Fourth Edition* (*DSM-IV*) [28], the appearance of disturbed sleep is one of the principal diagnostic criteria for major depressive disorder. Sleep is a necessary activity to maintain the internal homeostasis and for the overall health of organisms. Short sleep duration, poor sleep continuity, and poor sleep quality can disturb the psychological state and the susceptibility of an individual to illness or modify the course of the illness and its prognosis [25,29]. Psychiatric illnesses such as BS, major depression, and schizophrenia are associated with sleep disorders, and insomnia is one of the prodromal symptoms related with the decompensation and relapses of these illnesses [30]. In this way, many studies have established that insomnia is highly comorbid with psychiatric disorders and is a risk factor for the development of depression, anxiety, and suicide. Loss of sleep may be an index of the biological severity of the disorder, and people with insomnia are at high risk for adverse medical outcomes [31,32]. Patients who are clinically stable and medicated may continue to experience disturbed sleep, which may be enhanced or induced by the illness medication itself (antidepressant and antipsychotic drugs have adverse effects on the melatonergic system, thereby altering sleep) [33,34].

The regulation of the sleep/wakefulness rhythm is carried out by the hypothalamic suprachiasmatic nuclei (SCN) [35], and the fact that, on the one hand, the SCN expresses high levels of MT1 and MT2 melatonin receptors [36] and, on the other, the melatonin suppresses neuronal activity in the SCN [37] indicates why indoleamine is the key regulator of the sleep/wakefulness rhythm. The modifications in the rhythm and the amplitude of secretion of melatonin found in psychiatric illness could be responsible for the symptomatic disturbances of sleep and mood [12]. Studies in humans have shown that melatonin treatment (3–5 mg) not only improves the total sleep time but also decreases the depressive symptoms, documenting the close association between sleep and mood disorders [34,38–41]. These properties underline the use of melatonin and its analogous as a promising alternative for the treatment of depression.

19.3 DEPRESSION

During the past 25 years, numerous clinical trials have examined the therapeutic usefulness of melatonin in different fields of medicine including psychiatry and depression. Symptoms that are common to depression include altered mood (depressed mood, feelings of worthlessness, diminished ability to concentrate, recurrent thoughts of death or suicide), anxiety, sleep disturbance (insomnia, fatigue), loss of appetite, lack of motivation, loss of self-confidence, and decrease in self-esteem, as well as other symptoms as per the *DSM-IV* [28]. The link between clinical depression and immune function is well established [42]. A variety of indices used to score depression, e.g., the Beck Depression Inventory, document this relationship. There are three major theories that attempt to explain the biochemical and immune physiology of depression. These include (a) a deficiency of brain noradrenaline (NA) and serotonin (5-HT) plus an increased glutaminergic neurotransmission [43], (b) a disorder of the hypothalamic–pituitary–adrenal (HPA) axis [44], and (c) an abnormal secretion of some cytokines with the preponderance of an inflammatory state [45–47].

Prolonged chronic depression causes changes in the HPA axis and leads to an increase in the secretion of corticotrophin-releasing factor (CRF), adrenocorticotrophic hormone (ACTH), and cortisol release [48–50]. As mentioned above, epidemiological and biochemical studies have noted that insomnia and melatonin secretion are altered in patients as a prominent comorbidity of depression [51]. The deficiency of 5-HT and increased glutaminergic neurotransmission would be expected to cause elevated proinflammatory cytokines [44]; as a consequence, the chronic inflammatory state associated with depression would aggravate the depressive symptoms [49].

Depression and physiological and behavioral responses to infection have many common features [5,52]. Depression is a psychoneuroimmunological disorder in which an increased expression of adhesion molecules and the release of proinflammatory cytokines, which may have adverse consequences on immune defense and the neuroendocrine system, contribute to the symptoms of this condition (Figure 19.1). The rise in leukocyte adhesiveness/aggregation [50,53] and proinflammatory cytokine production in depressive patients [54,55] may account for a rapid recruitment of T cells from the blood compartment, causing a cell-mediated inflammation and a reduction of circulating T lymphocytes. As reported [56], patients with major depression exhibit accelerated apoptosis of leukocytes and blood oxidative stress levels resulting in fewer T-helper lymphocytes and neutrophils and a rise in reactive oxygen species (ROS) generation, infections, and proapoptotic proteins. This may explain the reduction in the number of lymphocytes in peripheral blood of these patients [57,58]. We propose that the immunodeficiency of depressive patients [53] is not an intrinsic

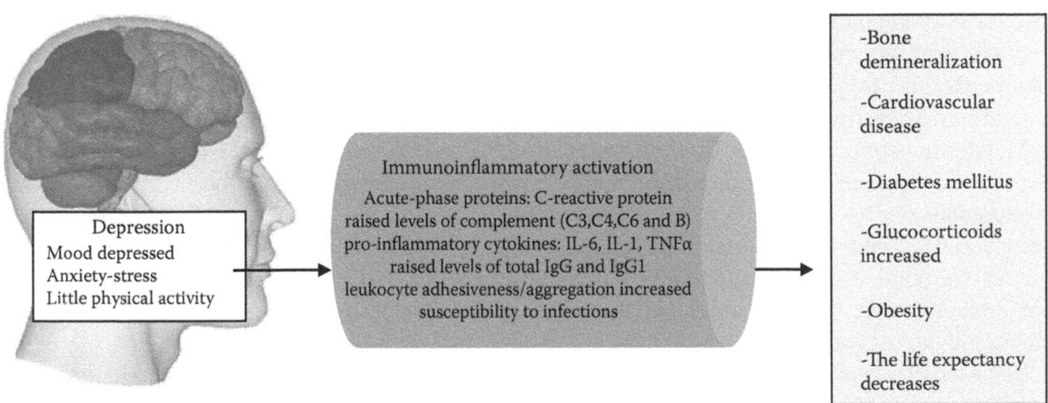

FIGURE 19.1 Major depression is associated with elevated systemic inflammation and may induce signs of metabolic syndrome. (From Maldonado, M.D. et al., *Recent Patents on CNS Drug Discovery*, 4, 61–69, 2009b. With permission.)

immunodeficiency but rather a consequence of the extensive T-cell activation–adhesion and oxidative stress. We suggest that the lymphocytes adhere to the walls of vessels and, therefore, they do not perform their normal defensive functions. This would explain why depressive patients possess a greater vulnerability to infections (flu, herpes viruses, pneumonia, etc.) [59]. Depression also enhances the risk for the development of certain inflammatory conditions, including cardiovascular disease (atherosclerosis and myocardial infarction) [60], metabolic syndrome (insulin resistance and obesity) [47], immune dysfunction (increased pro-inflammatory cytokines such as TNF-α, IL-1, IL-6; decreased anti-inflammatory cytokines such as IL-4 and IL-10; and susceptibility to infection) [50,53], and neuroendocrine disorders (elevated CRF, ACTH, and cortisol) [61].

The immunomodulatory properties of melatonin are well known; it acts on the immune system by regulating cytokine production of immunocompetent cells [62,63]. There are experimental and clinical data showing that melatonin reduces adhesion molecules and proinflammatory cytokines including IL-6, IL-8, and TNF-α and modifies serum inflammatory parameters. As a consequence, melatonin improves the clinical course of illnesses, which have an inflammatory etiology [64–66]. Melatonin and several of its metabolites neutralize free radicals and nonradical oxygen-based reactants [67]. The search for new antidepressive therapies should consider anti-inflammatory and antioxidant molecules, e.g., nonsteroidal anti-inflammatory drugs and melatonin, as a promising alternative for the treatment of depression [43,46,50,56].

19.3.1 Basis for Using Melatonin in Depression

Currently, the drugs used to treat depression include monoamine oxidase inhibitors (MAOI), tricyclic antidepressants (TCA), selective 5-HT reuptake inhibitors (SSRIs), and benzodiazepines. These drugs are used alone or in combination with psychological treatment (cognitive and interpersonal therapies) [68,69]. Although these treatments have obvious beneficial effects, they also inflict collateral damage. Thus, their benefits are counterbalanced by their negative effects on molecular physiology and cellular function to the extent that they eventually jeopardize the overall well-being of the organism. Because of this, the use of MAOIs declined when there were reports of hypertensive crises associated with ingestion of dietary tyramine (from red wine, chocolate, hard cheese, etc.) [70], while the TCAs, despite their poor record of safety, tolerability, and many adverse effects (sleep disturbances, anxiety, migraines, cognitive deficit, epilepsy, obesity, allergic reactions, photosensitivity, constipation, arrhythmias, etc.) were used as the major treatment. At present, a new generation of drugs of various classes has been developed with a variety of structures and mechanisms of action [44,71,72]; of these, the most widely prescribed are the SSRIs [69,73]. 5-HT transporters have recently been described in bones; this raises the possibility that medications that block 5-HT reuptake may influence bone metabolism [74]. In mice, 5-HT transporter gene disruption leads to osteopenia, and frequent SSRI use by older women increases the risk of hip fracture and loss of bone mineral density. This exceeds that caused by other antidepressants, e.g., TCA [75].

Melatonin is produced in the bone marrow [76,77]. This indoleamine is likely protective against oxidative damage in proliferating hematopoietic cells. Also, melatonin may be involved in bone development due to its influence on osteoblast differentiation [78,79]. Given these findings, the therapeutic treatment of depression using an SSRI in combination with melatonin may block the progressive bone loss resulting from the chronic use of SSRI. Melatonin also has anxiolytic, sedative, anticonvulsant [80], and antihypertensive properties [81]. This latter action may be helpful in alleviating depression in individuals who have to be treated with MAOIs.

Some psychotropic drugs used to treat psychiatric disorders have effects on the melatonergic system. Thus, the works of Hirsch-Rodriguez et al. [82] and Imbesi et al. [82,83] showed that the brain expresses MT1/MT2 receptors, which could determine the receptor-mediated biological effects of melatonin. Prolonged treatment with antidepressants, for example, desipramine, clomipramine, and fluoxetine, affects the distribution of melatonin receptor mRNAs in the brain, and also, the drugs increase the quantity of receptor mRNAs in the hippocampus (especially for the MT1 receptor).

The participation of melatonin receptors in these responses deserves investigation in randomized clinical trials to more clearly identify their role.

19.4 BIPOLAR SYNDROME

BS is defined by *DSM-IV* [28] as recurrent episodes of depression and mania. The patients exhibit depressive symptoms or elevated/irritable mood, grandiosity, decreased need for sleep, increased talking, racing thoughts, distractibility, overactivity, psychomotor agitation, and excessive involvement in risky activities. This chronic disease affects approximately 1%–2% of the world population and carries a substantial risk of suicide attempts that are often successful [84–86]. The illness has extreme episodes, but during the interepisodic (euthymic) periods, the patients may have a pharmacologically maintained normal life [87]. While the cause of this condition is unknown, some biochemical abnormalities include oversensitivity to acetylcholine, elevated acetylcholine receptor numbers, and supersensitivity to light [87].

In psychologically normal subjects, the blood melatonin rhythm exhibits a circadian pattern synchronized with the prevailing light/dark cycle. The neural pacemaker for this rhythm are SCN; they imposes 24-hour rhythm on both endocrine and autonomic function and determine the daily rhythmicity of organs and systems [88]. Bipolar patients reportedly have depressed melatonin levels [89] and melatonin secretion abnormalities (changes in the onset, duration, and offset of melatonin secretion) [13,90]. Whether these alterations have anything to do with this disorder or whether they are secondary to the neurotransmitter dysfunctions underlying BS is unknown. One report found plasma melatonin levels of BS patients are higher during a manic episode than in the depressive phase [91,92]. If this is verified, the amount of melatonin produced may reflect a state-dependent change in adrenergic function.

An association between BS and activation of the inflammatory response is supported by several findings [93,94], including elevated lymphocyte proliferation in response to mitogens [95], cytokines (T-helper type 1, Th1; T-helper type 2, Th2) [96] and cytokine receptors [97], complement, C-reactive protein, and immunoglobulins among others [94]. Each of these molecules transmits information from the immune system to the endocrine and nervous system and vice versa; in doing so, they activate brain functions in the hypothalamus and the hypothalamic–pituitary–adrenal axis, causing profound changes in the behavior [98]. Many of these responses are modulated by treatment with melatonin, which has receptors (MT1, MT2, and RZR/ROR) in the immune system and other organs where melatonin act as an intracrine, autocrine, or paracrine substance [2,24]. It is, therefore, not unreasonable to hypothesize that the deficits in baseline melatonin concentrations and the abnormalities in its secretion may contribute to the deficient immunological and inflammatory abnormalities.

19.4.1 Basis for Using Melatonin in BS

Numerous drugs including lithium, anticonvulsants (valproate, benzodiazepines), anticholinergic, antidepressant, and second-generation antipsychotic drugs are habitually used in the treatment of bipolar disorders [98]. These drugs have multiple beneficial effects including stabilization of neural activity, supporting neural plasticity, providing neuroprotection, and mood improvement [100,101]. Unfortunately, these drugs also negatively affect the neuroendocrine and immune systems, making their use less desirable [102,103].

Although its mechanism of action remains a mystery, lithium has been a highly effective treatment for BS. Lithium is the standard treatment for relapse prevention and it reduces the likelihood of suicide [85]. The negative consequences of lithium use includes dulled personality, reduced emotions, memory loss, tremors, and the possibility of the development of metabolic syndrome (obesity, diabetes, and increased blood pressure) [104,105]. Moreover, poor patient adherence to the treatment and dose uncertainty are reasons why it is often discontinued as a treatment. Melatonin

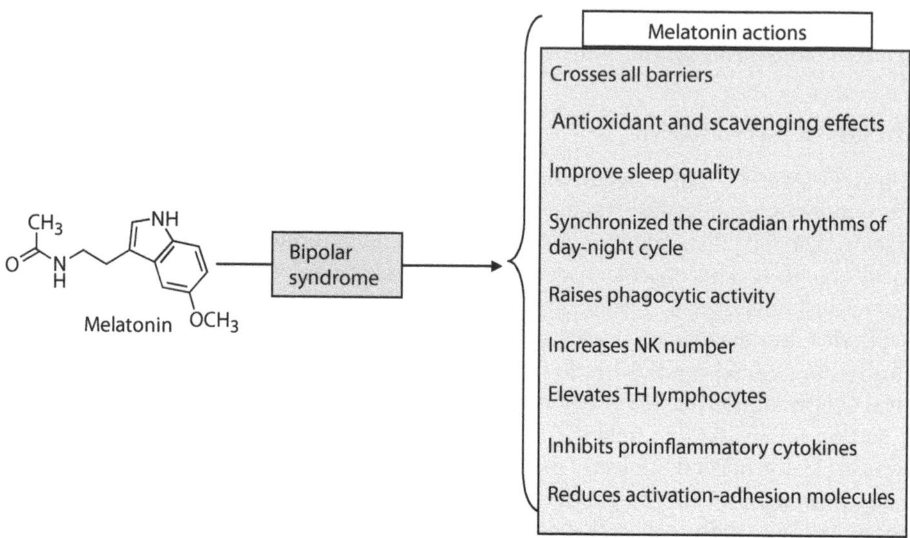

FIGURE 19.2 Properties of melatonin make it potentially useful in the treatment of BS. (From Maldonado, M.D. et al., *Recent Patents on CNS Drug Discovery*, 4, 61–69, 2009b. With permission.)

should be considered as a coalternative to/with lithium because of its anticonvulsant, anxiolytic, drug detoxification actions, and neuroprotective properties [8,79,106–111] (Figure 19.2).

Glucose utilization abnormalities, and eventually metabolic syndrome due to lithium use, are prevalent among patients with BS [112]. These patients are at increased risk for cardiovascular and cerebral infarction [105]. Melatonin may reduce the possibility of developing metabolic syndrome by reducing blood pressure [81,113] and enhancing cardiac and cerebral protection. The ability of the indoleamine to reduce hemodynamic load, as well as its antioxidant and radical scavenging effects, assists in limiting metabolic disturbances [10,114–116]. Daily administration of melatonin improves adaptation to a regular rest/activity cycle because of its chronotherapeutic effects. Its rapid onset of action and its effectiveness in improving the mood of bipolar depressed patients have been attributed to its ability to improve sleep quality [117,118]. This property of melatonin could be of importance to BS patients since they present before the manic episode with sleep loss and a frantic hyperactivity occurring before bipolar symptoms. The disturbances in circadian rhythms are major precipitating factors for BS, and they may respond to interventions that restore a normal sleep/wake cycle [13,118]. Whether the chronobiologic disturbances in BD patients are causal or only an epiphenomenon of the disease has not been established. A combination of melatonin with lithium or valproate is reportedly more efficacious than either lithium or valproate alone in the prevention of a manic relapse in patients with a partial or poor response to either monotherapy [119,122]. These observations suggest that melatonin is a viable option and an invaluable addition to the pharmacological armamentarium in the treatment of BD.

19.5 SCHIZOPHRENIA

Schizophrenia is a serious disorder with changes in neurophysiology that results in disruptions of an individual's normal perception of reality. Its frequency is estimated to be 1% of the world population [123]. Clinical characteristics include hallucinations, paranoia, delusions, speech/thought impairment, and poor sleep. The onset of these symptoms usually occurs during adolescence. Etiologically, the disorder is multifactorial and involves multiple genetic variants [124] and environmental influences [125]. Alterations in amino acid metabolism may be involved, specifically, in an impaired synthesis of 5-HT in the brain [126]. Additionally, serotonin 5-HT2A receptor up-regulation and glutamate receptor desensitization are characteristics of altered cortical processes of schizophrenia [123].

Immune system abnormalities (cellular and/or humoral) in schizophrenia and infective or autoimmune processes have been observed in patients with schizophrenia. High levels of circulating immune complexes are associated with the acute state (a relapse) of schizophrenia [127,128]. A number of the effects of antipsychotic medication on the immunological profile of schizophrenic patients are identified, and changes in cellular immune system are associated with treatment response. These changes are candidates for biological markers of the illness. An imbalance between Th1 and Th2 cytokines may occur. IL-6 and TNF-α production in schizophrenic patients was significantly higher than in normal controls, whereas IL-2, IL-4, and INF-γ production are significantly reduced in schizophrenic patients [129]. After 6 weeks of antipsychotic treatment, both IL-6 and TNF-α production dropped significantly while IL-4, INF-γ, and IL-2 production was unchanged by the treatment. An imbalance in inflammatory cytokines, with an increase in vivo of IL-1 receptor antagonist (IL-1RA), soluble IL-2 receptor (sIL-2R), and IL-6 and lower in vitro IL-2 levels, suggests the establishment of a chronic inflammatory syndrome in schizophrenia [130]. These alterations in cytokine levels may be involved with the immunopathogenesis of schizophrenia. They may explain the presence of activated astrocytes in the central nervous system. The possibility of successful prophylactic and therapeutic intervention at the immunological level against these proinflammatory cytokines using anti-inflammatory drugs, e.g., cyclooxygenase 2 inhibitors or ibuprofen, is suggested by these findings [43,131,132].

Melatonin has a documented role in neuroimmunomodulation. Specific melatonin receptors on lymphoid cells provide evidence for a direct effect of this indoleamine in the regulation of the immune system [22,24]. When neonates with sepsis, respiratory distress, or bronchopulmonary dysplasia were treated with melatonin, a significant reduction in proinflammatory cytokines including IL-6, IL-8, and TNF-α and modified serum inflammatory parameters occurred with an improvement in the clinical course [64,65]. Melatonin's ability to reduce inflammatory responses indicates protection at the endothelial level as well as a reduction in the infiltration of cerebral vascular wall by astrocyte-producing cytokines. These effects may be a result of a diminished NFκB activation [5,6,133]. The debilitating consequences of schizophrenia, and secondarily, the infective and autoimmune processes, are associated with the production and release of numerous proinflammatory biochemical mediators including the cytokines, IL-1, IL-6, IL-8, and TNF-α (Figure 19.3). The ability of melatonin to diminish proinflammatory cytokines and reduce the resulting tissue damage is substantial [62,63,134]. Melatonin readily passes through all biological membranes including the blood–brain barrier and it favorably alters the course of immunology disorders.

Patients with schizophrenia commonly have alterations with circadian rhythms and low melatonin levels [135]. Whether these changes are causal or secondarily related to the disease is unknown. In

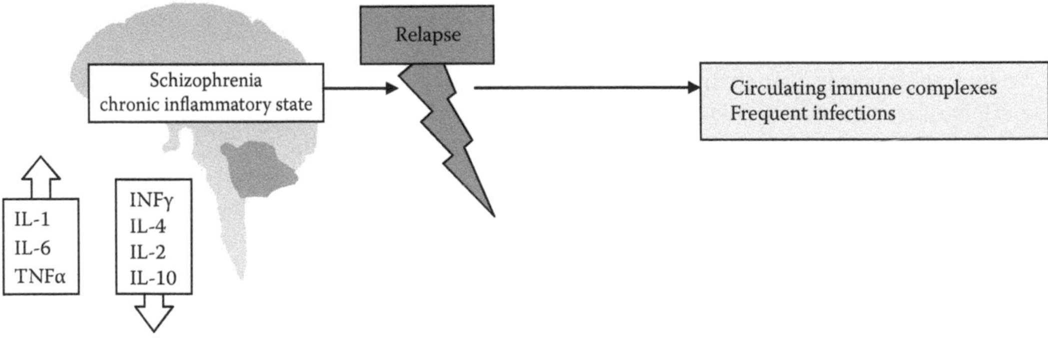

FIGURE 19.3 Summary of the immunological changes found in schizophrenia and consequences of repeated relapses of the illness. (From Maldonado, M.D. et al., *Recent Patents on CNS Drug Discovery*, 4, 61–69, 2009b. With permission.)

untreated schizophrenia, psychotic decompensation is associated with profound insomnia, one of the prodromal symptoms associated with a psychotic relapse. Antipsychotic medications (lithium or neuroleptics) are often an effective treatment for the insomnia, but the side effects include sedation, tardive dyskinesia, rabbit syndrome, or residual insomnia. Schizophrenia is associated with comorbid sleep disorders (increased in cancer risk, changes in cortisol levels, impaired immune responses, cognitive function, etc.), which may be a consequence of antipsychotic medications [33,136].

19.5.1 Basis for Using Melatonin in Schizophrenia

Patients with schizophrenia are treated with a variety of drugs to improve their condition and social life. Commonly used drugs include antipsychotics, classic neuroleptics (haloperidol) or atypical neuroleptics (e.g., risperidone, clozapine, olanzapine, ziprasidone), and lithium, as well as anti-inflammatory, antidepressant, and anticonvulsive drugs (e.g., phenobarbital, diazepam) [137,138]. While these treatments may have beneficial effects, they also inflict collateral damage, which causes the patients to discontinue their use; these noncompliant patients are at a higher risk for committing suicide or being institutionalized. To overcome this noncompliance, psychiatrists could consider alternative or complementary therapies including cotreatment with melatonin.

Sleep disorders in schizophrenia are typically aggressively treated since normalized sleep and its restorative processes may be important for a positive clinical outcome. Melatonin is an agent with the capacity of entraining circadian rhythms (chronobiotic effect) as well as having sleep-promoting effects and neuroprotective actions [13,109,111,133]. These properties have been documented in clinical trials with humans as well as in experimental animals [39,135,139]. Considering these effects, melatonin could be a viable strategy to reduce circadian disruption and improve the sleep of patients with schizophrenia. The side effects of even long term melatonin use are minimal [140].

The use of classic neuroleptic drugs is limited because of the eventual appearance of extrapyramidal symptoms, tardive dyskinesia, movement disorders, and a significant increase of peripheral blood mononuclear cell membrane lipid peroxidation [138]. Melatonin's protective effect against haloperidol was documented in patients. In a double-blind, placebo-controlled, crossover study, Shamir et al. [141] found that melatonin (10 mg daily), given for only 6 weeks to patients exhibiting tardive dyskinesia due to antipsychotic drug treatment, had markedly reduced movement disorders as assessed by the Abnormal Involuntary Movement Scale. The difference, relative to the placebo-treated controls, was highly statistically significant and no adverse side effects of melatonin therapy were noted. Besides tardive dyskinesia associated with haloperidol usage (13 patients), this study also showed that the abnormal involuntary movements induced by other antipsychotics (i.e., chlorpromazine, four patients; perphenazine, three patients; and zuclopenthixol, two patients), were also reduced when the patients were given melatonin. While the sample size was small and the treatments varied, the universal response of the patients lends support to the authors' suggestion that melatonin may be an effective treatment to attenuate tardive dyskinesia resulting from the use of antipsychotic medications by schizophrenic patients.

Weight gain, which may contribute to the development of metabolic syndrome, is an adverse side effect of treatment with atypical neuroleptics [137]. These treatments are sometimes discontinued due to dangerous effects including agranulocytosis and eosinophilia [142]. Melatonin has been related to the adipose tissue metabolism and obesity management, at least in animals [143]. Melatonin combined with these medicines may reduce the negative symptoms as much as possible, permitting the use of longer doses of the drugs [8].

19.6 CONCLUSIONS

Melatonin is a beneficial molecule that reduces neuronal deterioration and lowers the incidence and relapses of some mental disorders. It is involved in the control of numerous physiological functions including free radical scavenging, neuroimmunomodulation, elevated neurogenesis, circadian rhythms and sleep regulation, blood pressure reduction, and control of mood and behavior. Melatonin has several characteristics that make it clinically valuable: it does not cause hangover or withdrawal symptoms and is devoid of any addictive potential; it crosses all morphophysiological barriers; and it promotes sleep, which is highly important for the improvement of depressive disorders. Data are also accruing that the therapeutic effects of melatonin are in part due to their anti-inflammatory effects. While further research is required to determine the optimal recommended doses (3–12 mg of melatonin is currently commonly used to promote sleep), psychiatrists can recommend doses of melatonin based on previous and current efficacious studies and then adjust the doses based on the results obtained; most studies document the very low toxicity of melatonin over a wide range of doses [135,144–146]. The challenge for the future is to decide how and when it can best be employed, alone or in combination with other effective agents, to improve the outcome in psychiatric patients.

REFERENCES

1. Liu, Y.J., Zhuang, J., Zhu, H.Y., Shen, Y.X., Tan, Z.L., Zhou, J.N. 2007. Cultured rat cortical astrocytes synthesize melatonin: Absence of diurnal rhythm. *J Pineal Res* 43: 232–238.
2. Maldonado, M.D., Mora-Santos, M., Naji, L., Carrascosa-Salmoral, M.P., Naranjo, M.C., Calvo, J.R. 2010. Evidence of melatonin synthesis and release in mast cells. Possible modulator role on inflammation. *Pharmacol Res* 62: 282–287.
3. Agez, L., Laurent, V., Guerrero, H.Y., Pévet, P., Masson-Pévet, M., Gauer, F. 2009. Endogenous melatonin provides an effective circadian message to both the suprachiasmatic nuclei and the pars tuberalis of the rat. *J Pineal Res* 46: 95–105.
4. Maldonado, M.D., Siu, A.W., Sánchez-Hidalgo, M., Acuna-Castroviejo, D., Escames, G. 2006. Melatonin and lipid uptake by murine fibroblasts: Clinical implications. *Neuroendocrinol Lett* 27: 601–608.
5. Maldonado, M.D., Murillo-Cabezas, F., Terron, M.P., Flores, L.J., Tan, D.X., Manchester, L.C., Reiter, R.J. 2007. The potencial of melatonin in reducing morbidity–mortality after craniocerebral trauma. *J Pineal Res* 42: 1–11.
6. Maldonado, M.D., Murillo-Cabezas, F., Calvo, J.R., Lardone, P.J., Tan, D.X., Guerrero, J.M., Reiter RJ. 2007. Melatonin as pharmacologic support in burn patients: A proposed solution to thermal injury-related lymphocytopenia and oxidative damage. *Crit Care Med* 35: 1177–1185.
7. Garcia-Navarro, A., Gonzalez-Puga, C., Escames, G., López, L.C., López, A., López-Cantarero, M. et al. 2007. Cellular mechanisms involved in the melatonin inhibition of HT-29 human colon cancer cell proliferation in culture. *J Pineal Res* 43: 195–205.
8. Reiter, R.J., Tan, D.X., Sainz, R., Mayo, J.C., Lopez-Burillo, S. 2002. Melatonin reducing the toxicity and increasing the efficacy of drugs. *J Pharm Pharmacol* 54: 1299–1321.
9. Ostrowska, Z., Ziora, K., Kos-Kudła, B., Swietochowska, E., Oświecimska, J., Dyduch, A., Wołkowska-Pokrywa, K., Szapska, B. 2010. Melatonin, the RANKL/RANK/OPG system, and bone metabolism in girls with anorexia nervosa. *Endokrynol Pol* 61: 117–23.
10. Reiter, R.J, Tan, D.X., Maldonado, M.D. 2005. Melatonin as an antioxidant: Physiology versus pharmacology. *J Pineal Res* 39: 215–216.
11. Tomas-Zapico, C., Coto-Montes, A. 2005. A proposed mechanism to explain the stimulatory effect of melatonin on antioxidative enzymes. *J Pineal Res* 39: 99–104.
12. Pacchierotti, C., Iapichino, S., Bossini, L., Pieraccini, F., Castrogiovanni, P. 2001. Melatonin in psychiatric disorders: A review on the melatonin involvement in psychiatry. *Front Neuroendocrinol* 22: 18–32.
13. Srinivasan, V., Smits, G., Kayumov, L., Pandi-Perumal, S.R., Cardinali, D.P., Thorpy, M.J. 2006. Melatonin in circadian rhythm sleep disorders. *Neuroendocrine Correlates of Sleep–Wakefulness* 269–294. New York: Springer.
14. Chrousos, G.P. 2009. Stress and disorders of the stress system. *Nat Rev Endocrinol* 5: 374–381.
15. Lakhan, S.E., Vieira, K.F. 2008. Nutritional therapies for mental disorders. *Nutrition J* 7: 1–8.
16. Chakroun, N., Doron, J., Swendsen, J. 2004. Substance use, affective problems and personality traits: Test of two association models. *Encephale* 30: 564–569.
17. Haynes, J.C., Farrell, M., Singleton, N., Araya, R., Lewis, G., Wiles, N.J. 2007. Alcohol consumption as a risk factor for non-recovery from common mental disorder: Results from the longitudinal follow-up of the National Psychiatric Morbidity Survey. *Psychol Med* 1: 1–5.

18. Rosenthal, N.E., Sack, S.A., Gillin, J.C. 1984. Seasonal affective disorder. A description of the syndrome and preliminary finding with light therapy. *Arch Gen Psychiatr* 41: 72–80.
19. Morera, A.L., Abreu, P. 2006. Seasonality of psychopathology and circannual melatonin rhythm. *J Pineal Res* 41: 279–283.
20. Reiter, R.J. 2003. Melatonin: Clinical relevance. *Best Practice Res Clin Endocrinol Metab* 17: 273–285.
21. Witt-Enderby, P.A., Radio, N.M., John, S., Vicki, L.D. 2006. Therapeutic treatments potentially mediated by melatonin receptors: Potential clinical uses in the prevention of osteoporosis, cancer and as an adjuvant therapy. *J Pineal Res* 41: 297–305.
22. Garcia-Pergañeda, A., Pozo, D., Guerrero, J.M., Calvo, J.R. 1997. Signal transduction for melatonin in human lymphocytes. Involvement of a pertussis toxin-sensitive G protein. *J Immunol* 159: 3774–3781.
23. Garcia-Mauriños, S., Gonzalez-Haba, M.G., Calvo, J.R., Goberna, R., Guerrero, J.M. 1998. Involvement of molecular binding sites for melatonin in the regulation of, IL-2 and, IL-6 production by human blood mononuclear cells. *J Neuroimmunol* 92: 76–84.
24. Garcia-Mauriños, S., Pozo, D., Calvo, J.R., Guerrero, J.M. 2000. Correlation between nuclear melatonin receptor expression and enhanced cytokine production in human lymphocytic and monocytic cell lines. *J Pineal Res* 29: 129–137.
25. Leonard, B.E., Song, C. 1996. Stress and the immune system in the etiology of anxiety and depression. *Pharmacol Biochem Behav* 54: 299–303.
26. Maldonado, M.D., Perez-Sangregorio, M.A., Reiter R.J. 2009. The role of melatonin in the immuno-neuro-psychology of mental disorders. *Recent Pat CNS Drug Discov* 4: 61–69.
27. Maldonado, M.D., Reiter, R.J., Perez-Sangregorio, M.A. 2009. Melatonin as a potential therapeutic agent in psychiatric illness. *Hum Psychopharmacol Clin Exp* 24: 391–400.
28. American Psychiatric Association. 1994. *Diagnostic and Statistical Manual of Mental Disorders. 4th ed. (DSM-IV)*. American Psychiatric Press, Washington, DC.
29. Ancoli-Israel, S., Martin, J.L. 2006. Insomnia and daytime napping in older adults. *J Clin Sleep Med* 2: 333–342.
30. Perlis, M.L., Giles, D.E., Buysse, D.J., Tu, X., Kupfer, D.J 1997. Self-reporter sleep disturbance as a prodromal symptom in recurrent depression. *J Affect Disord* 42: 209–212.
31. Basta, M., Chrousos, G.P., Vela-Bueno, A., Vgontzas, A.N. 2007. Chronic insomnia and the stress system. *Sleep Med Clin* 2: 279–291.
32. Vgontzas, A.N., Liao, D., Bixler, E.O., Chrousos, G.P., Vela-Bueno, A. 2009. Insomnia with objective short sleep duration is associated with a high risk for hypertension. *Sleep* 32: 491–497.
33. Benson, K.L. 2006. Sleep in schizophrenia: Impairments, correlates, and treatment. *Psychiatr Clin North Am* 29: 1033–1045.
34. Srinivasan, V., Pandi-Perumal, S.R., Trakht, I., Spence, D.W., Hardeland, R., Poeggeler, B., Cardinali, D.P. 2009. Pathophysiology of depression: Role of sleep and the melatonergic system. *Psychiat Res* 165: 201–214.
35. Zee, P.C., Manthena, P. 2007. The brain's master circadian clock: Implications and opportunities for therapy of sleep disorders. *Sleep Medicine Reviews* 11: 59–70.
36. Ducovich, M.L., Markowska, M. 2005. Functional MT1 and MT2 melatonin receptors in mammals. *Endocrine* 27: 101–110.
37. Liu, C., Weaver, D.R., Jin, X., Shearman, L.P., Pieschl, R.L., Gribkoff, V.K., Reppert, S.M. 1997. Molecular dissection of two distinct actions of melatonin on the suprachiasmatic circadian clock. *Neuron* 9: 91–102.

ayumov, L., Brown, G., Jindal, R., Buttoo, K., Shapiro, C.M. 2001. A randomized double-blind, lacebo-controlled crossover study of the effect of exogenous melatonin on delayed sleep. *Psychosom Ied* 63: 40–48.

Vyatt, J.K., Dijk, D.J., Ritz-de Cecco, A., Ronda, J.M., Czeisler, C.A. 2006. Sleep-facilitating effect of xogenous melatonin in healthy young men and women is circadian-phase dependent. *Sleep* 29: 609–618.

arzón, C., Guerrero, J.M., Aramburu, O., Guzmán, T. 2009. Effect of melatonin administration on leep, behavioral disorders and hypnotic drug discontinuation in the elderly: A randomized, double-lind, placebo-controlled study. *Aging Clin Exp Res* 21: 38–42.

ahman, S.A., Kayumov, L., Shapiro, C.M. 2010. Antidepressant action of melatonin in the treatment of elayed sleep phase syndrome. *Sleep Med* 11: 131–136.

eonard, B.E., Song, C. 2002. Changes in the immune system in rodent models of depression. *Int J europsychopharmacol* 5: 345–356.

43. Muller, N., Schwarz, M.J. 2007. The immunological basis of glutamatergic disturbance in schizophrenia: Towards an integrated view. *J Neural Transm Suppl* 72: 269–280.
44. Frieling, H., Hillemacher, T., Demling, J.H., Kornhuber, J., Bleich, S. 2007. New options in the treatment of depression. *Fortschr Neurol Psychiatr* 75: 3–16.
45. Shelton, R.C., Claiborne, J., Sidoryk-Wegrzynowicz, M., Reddy, R., Aschner, M., Lewis, D.A., Mirnics, K. 2010. Altered expression of genes involved in inflammation and apoptosis in frontal cortex in major depression. *Mol Psychiatry*, doi:10.1038/mp.2010.52.
46. Muller, N., Schwarz, M.J. 2007. Inmunological aspects of depressive disoders. *Nervenarzt* 78: 1261–1273.
47. Mcintyre, R.S., Soczynska, J.K., Konarski, J.Z., Woldeyohannes, H.O., Law, C.W., Miranda, A. et al. 2007. Should depressive syndromes be reclassified as "metabolic syndrome type II"? *Ann Clin Psychiatry* 19: 257–264.
48. Leonard, B.E. 2006. HPA and immune axes in stress: Involvement of the serotonergic system. *Neuroimmunomodulation* 13: 268–276.
49. Leonard, B.E., Myint, A. 2006. Inflammation and depression: Is there a causal connection with dementia? *Neurotox Res* 10: 149–160.
50. Bruce, L.R. 2007. Worried sick: Antidepressants, stress and inflammation. *J Clin Psychiatry* 68: 10.
51. Srinivasan, V. Smits, M., Spence, W., Lowe, A.D., Kayumov, L., Pandi-Perumal S.R. 2006. Melatonin in mood disorders. *World J Biol Psychiatry* 7: 138–151.
52. Castanon, N., Leonard, B.E., Neveu, P.J., Yirmiya, R. 2002. Effects of antidepressants on cytokine production and actions. *Brain Behav Immun* 16: 569–574.
53. Leonard, B.E., Myint, A. 2009. The psychoneuroimmunology of depression. *Hum Psychopharmacol Clin Exp*, doi:10.1002/hup.1011.
54. Myint, A.M., Leonard, B.E., Steinbusch, H.W., Kim, Y.K. 2005. Th1, Th2, and Th3 cytokine alterations in major depression. *J Affect Disord* 88: 167–173.
55. Leonard, B.E. 2007. Psychopathology of depression. *Drugs Today* 43: 705–716.
56. Szuster-Ciesielska, A., Slotwinska, M., Stachura, A. Marmurowska-Michałowska, H., Dubas-Slemp, H., Bojarska-Junak, A., Kandefer-Szerszeń, M. 2008. Accelerated apoptosis of blood leucocytes and oxidative stress in blood of patients with major depression. *Prog Neuropsychopharmacol Biol Psychiatry* 32: 686–694.
57. Kronfol, Z., Nasrallah, H.A., Chapman, S., House, J.D. 1985. Depression, cortisol metabolism and lymphocytopenia. *J Affect Disord* 9: 169–173.
58. Darko, D.F., Rose, J., Gillin, J.C., Golshan, S., Baird SM. 1988. Neutrophilia and lymphopenia in major mood disorders. *Psychiatry Res* 25: 243–251.
59. Godbout, J.P., Glaser, R. 2006. Stress-induced immune dysregulation: Implications for wound healing, infectious disease and cancer. *J Neuroimmune Pharmacol* 1: 421–427.
60. Vaccarino, V., Johnson, B.D., Sheps, D.S., Reis, S.E., Kelsey, S.F., Bittner, V. et al. 2007. Depression, inflammation, and incident cardiovascular disease in women with suspected coronary ischemia: The National Heart, Lung and Blood Institute–sponsored WISE study. *J Am Coll Cardiol* 50: 2044–2050.
61. Holsboer, F., Ising, M. 2008. Central CRH system in depression and anxiety. Evidence from clinical studies with CRH1 receptor antagonists. *Eur J Pharmacol* 583: 350–357.
62. Carrillo-Vico. A., Lardone, P.J., Naji, L., Fernández-Santos, J.M., Martín-Lacave, I., Guerrero, J.M., Calvo, J.R. 2005. Beneficial pleiotropic actions of melatonin in an experimental model of septic shock in mice: Regulation of pro-/anti-inflammatory cytokine network, protection against oxidative damage and antiapoptotic effects. *J. Pineal Res* 39: 400–408.
63. Carrillo-Vico, A., Lardone, P.J., Fernández-Santos, J.M., Martín-Lacave, I., Calvo, J.R, Karasek, M., Guerrero, J.M. 2005. Human lymphocyte-synthesized melatonin is involved in the regulation of the interleukin 2/interleukin 2 receptor system. *J Clin Endocrinol Metab* 90: 992–1000.
64. Gitto, E., Reiter, R.J., Amodio, A., Romeo, C., Cuzzocrea, E., Sabatino, G. et al. 2004. Early indicators of chronic lung disease in preterm infants with respiratory distress syndrome and their inhibition by melatonin. *J Pineal Res* 36: 250–255.
65. Gitto, E., Reiter, R.J., Cordaro, S.P., La Rosa, M., Chiurazzi, P., Trimarchi, G. et al. 2004. Oxidative and inflammatory parameters in respiratory distress syndrome of preterm newborns: Beneficial effects of melatonin. *Am J Perinatol* 21: 209–216.
66. Gitto, E., Reiter, R.J., Sabatino, G., Buonocore, G., Romeo, C., Gitto, P. et al. 2005. Correlation among cytokines, bronchopulmonary dysplasia and modality of ventilation in preterm newborns: Improvement with melatonin treatment. *J Pineal Res* 39: 287–293.

67. Tan, D.X., Manchester, L.C., Terron, M.P. Flores, L.J., Reiter, R.J. 2007. One molecule, many derivatives: A never-ending interaction of melatonin with reactive oxygen and nitrogen species. *J Pineal Res* 42: 28–42.
68. Borda, M., Pérez-San-Gregorio, M.A., Blanco A. 2000. Conduct modification techniques manual in behavioral medicine. *Publications of the University of Seville* 1: 63–117.
69. Roger, M.P. 2007. New antidepressant or more of the same? Neuropsychiatric disease and treatment. *Editorial Foreword* 3–5.
70. Rapaport, M.H., 2007. Dietary restrictions and drug interactions with monoamine oxidase inhibitors: The state of the art. *J Clin Psychiatry* 68: 42–46.
71. Zupancic, M., Guilleminault, C. 2006. Agomelatine: A preliminary review of a new antidepressant. *CNS Drugs* 20: 981–992.
72. Pandi-Perumal, S.R., Trakht, I., Srinivasan, V., Spence, D.W., Poeggler, B., Harderland, R., Cardinali, D.P. 2009. The effect of melatonergic and non-melatonergic antidepressants on sleep: Weighing the alternatives. *World J Biol Psychiatry* 10: 342–354.
73. Battaglino, R., Vokes, M., Schulze, S., Sharma, A., Graves, D., Kohler, T. et al. 2007. Fluoxetine treatment increases trabecular bone formation in mice (fluoxetine affects bone mass). *J Cell Biochem* 10: 1387–1394.
74. Diem, S.J., Blackwell, T.L., Stone, K.L., Yaffe, K., Haney, E.M., Bliziotes, M.M., Ensrud, K.E. 2007. Use of antidepressnts and rates of hip bone loss in older women. *Arch Intern Med* 167: 1240–1245.
75. Haney, E.M., Chan, B.K., Diem, S.J., Ensrud, K.E., Cauley, J.A., Barrett-Connor, E. et al. 2007. Association of low bone mineral density with selective serotonin reuptake inhibitor use by older men. *Arch Intern Med* 167: 1231–1232.
76. Tan, D.X., Manchester, L.C., Reiter, R.J., Qi, W.B., Zhang, M., Weintraub, S.T., Cabrera, J., Sainz, R.M., Mayo, J.C. 1999. Identification of highly elevated levels of melatonin in bone marrow: Its origin and significance. *Biochim Biophys Acta* 1472: 206–214.
77. Cardinali, D.P., Ladizesky, M.G., Boggio, V., Cutrera, R.A., Mautalen, C. 2003. Melatonin effects on bone: Experimental facts and clinical perspective. *J Pineal Res* 34: 81–87.
78. Radio, N.M., Doctor, J.S., Witt-Enderby, P.A. 2006. Melatonin enhances alkaline phosphatase activity in differentiating human adult mesenchymal stem cells grow in osteogenic medium via MT2 melatonin receptors and the MEK/ERK (1/2) signalling cascade. *J Pineal Res* 40: 332–342.
79. Sánchez-Hidalgo, M., Lu, Z., Tan, D.X., Maldonado, M.D., Reiter, R.J., Gregerman, R.I. 2007. Melatonin inhibits fatty acid–induced triglyceride accumulation in ROS 17/2.8 cells: Implications for osteoblast differentiation and osteoporosis. *Am J Physiol Regul Integr Comp Physiol* 292: 2208–2215.
80. Lipartiti, M., Franceschini, D., Zanoni, R., Gusella, M., Giusti, P., Cagnoli, C.M. et al. 1996. Neuroprotective effects of melatonin. *Adv Exp Med Biol* 398: 315–321.
81. Simko, F., Paulis, L. 2007. Melatonin as a potential antihypertensive treatment. *J Pineal Res* 42: 319–322.
82. Hirsch-Rodriguez, E., Imbesi, M., Manev, R., Uz, T., Manev, H. 2006. The pattern of melatonin receptor expression in the brain may influence antidepressant treatment. *Med Hypotheses* 69: 120–124.
83. Imbesi, M., Uz, T., Yildiz, S. 2006. Drug and region-specific effects of protracted antidepressant and cocaine treatment on the content of melatonin MT1 and MT2 receptor mRNA in the mouse brain. *Int J Neuroprotect Neuroregen* 2: 185–189.
84. Judd, L.L., Akiskal, H.S. 2003. The prevalence and disability of bipolar spectrum disorders in the US population: Re-analysis of the ECA database taking into account subthreshold cases. *J Affect Disord* 73: 123–131.
85. Mcintyre, R.S., Muzina, D.J., Kemp, D.E., Blank, D., Woldeyohannes, H.O., Lofchy, J. et al. 2008. Bipolar disorder and suicide: Research synthesis and clinical translation. *Curr Psychiatry Rep* 10: 66–72.
86. Kovacsics, C.E., Gottesman, I.I., Gould TD. 2009. Lithium's antisuicidal efficacy: Elucidation of neurobiological targets using endophenotype strategies. *Annu Rev Pharmacol Toxicol* 49: 175–98.
87. Rihmer, Z., Gonda, X., Rhimer, A. 2006. Creativity and mental illness. *Psychiatr Hung* 21: 288–294.
88. Pandi-Perumal, S.R., Srinivasan, V., Maestroni, G.J., Cardinali, D.P., Poeggeler, B., Hardeland, R. 2006. Melatonin: nature's most versatile biological signal? *FEBS J* 273: 2813–2838.
89. Lam, R.W., Bercowitz, A.L., Berga, S.L., Clark, C.M., Kripke, D.F., Gillin, J.C. 1990. Melatonin suppression in bipolar and unipolar mood disorders. *Psychiatry Res* 33: 129–134.
90. Nurnberger, J.I., Adkins, S., Lahiri, D.K., Mayeda, A., Hu, K., Lewy, A. et al. 2000. Melatonin suppression by light in euthymic bipolar and unipolar. *Arch Gen Psychiatry* 57: 72–579.

91. Lewy, A.J., Wehr, T.A., Gold, P.W., Goodwin, F.K. 1979. Plasma melatonin in manic- depressive illness. In: E. Usdin, I.J. Kopin, J. Barchas, eds: *Catecholamines: Basic and Clinical Frontiers*. Vol 2, 1173–1175. New York: Pergamon Press.
92. Lewys, A.J., Wehr, T.A., Goodwin, F.K., Newsome, D.A., Rosenthal, N.E. 1981. Manic–depressive patients may be supersensitive to light. *Lancet* 1: 383–384.
93. Maes, M., Scharpe, S., Bosmans, E., Vandewoude, M., Suy, E., Uyttenbroeck, W. et al. 1992. Disturbances in acute phase plasma proteins during melancholia: Additional evidence for the presence of an inflammatory process during that illness. *Prog Psychopharmacol Biol Psychiatry* 16: 501–515.
94. Wadee, A.A., Kuschke, R.H., Wood, L.A., Berk, M., Ichim, L., Maes M. 2002. Serological observations in patients suffering from acute manic episodes. *Hum Psychopharmacol* 17: 175–179.
95. Tsai, S.Y., Lee, H.C., Chen, C.C., Huang, Y.L. 2007. Cognitive impairment in later life in patients with early-onset bipolar disorders. *Bipolar Disord* 9: 868–875.
96. Kim, Y.K., Myint, A.M., Lee, B.H., Han, C.S., Lee, S.W., Leonard, B.E., Steinbusch, H.W. 2004. T-helper types 1,2, and 3 cytokine interactions in symptomatic manic patients. *Psychiatry Res* 129: 267–272.
97. Maes, M., Bosmans, E., Calabrese, J., Smith, R., Meltzer, H.Y. 1995. Interleukin-2 and interleukin-6 in schizophrenia and mania: Effects of neuroleptics and mood stabilizers. *J Psychiatr Res* 29: 141–152.
98. Song, C., Horrobin, D.F., Leonard, B.E. 2006. The comparison of changes in behaviour, neurochemistry, endocrine, and immune functions after different routes, doses and durations of administrations of IL-1β in rats. *Pharmacopsychiatry* 39: 88–99.
99. van Winkel, R., De Hert, M., Van Eyck, D., Hanssens, L., Wampers, M., Scheen, A., Peuskens, J. 2008. Prevalence of diabetes and the metabolic syndrome in a sample of patients with bipolar disorder. *Bipolar Disord* 10: 342–348.
100. Zorrilla, Z.M. 2003. Mechanism of action of lithium: Intracellular signalling pathways. *Vertex* 14: 45–52.
101. Geddes, J.R., Burgess, S., Hawton, K., Jamison, K., Goodwin, G.M. 2004. Long-term lithium therapy for bipolar disorder: Systematic review and meta-analysis of randomized controlled trials. *Am J Psychiatry* 161: 217–222.
102. Surman, O.S. 1993. Possible immunological effects of psychotropic medication. *Psychosomatics* 34: 139–143.
103. Yolken, R.H., Torrey, E.F. 1995. Viruses, schizophrenia, and bipolar disorders. *Clin Microbiol Rev* 8: 131–145.
104. Teixeira, P.J., Rocha, F.L. 2007. The prevalence of metabolic syndrome among psychiatric inpatients in Brazil. *Rev Bras Psiquiatr* 29: 330–336.
105. van Winkel, R., De Hert, M., Wampers, M., Van Eyck, D., Hanssens, L., Scheen, A., Peuskens, J. 2008. Major changes in glucose metabolism, including new-onset diabetes, within 3 months after initiation of or switch to atypical antipsychotic medication in patients with schizophrenia and schizoaffective disorder. *J Clin Psychiatry* 69: 472–479.
106. Molina-Carballo, A., Muñoz-Hoyos A., Reiter, J.R., Sánchez-Forte, M., Moreno-Madrid, F., Rufo-Campos, M. et al. 1997. Utility of high doses of melatonin as adjunctive anticonvulsant therapy in a child with severe myoclonic epilepsy: Two years experience. *J Pineal Res* 23: 97–105.
107. Kabuto, H., Yokoi, I., Ogawa, N. 1998. Melatonin inhibits iron-induced epileptic discharges in rats by suppressing peroxidation. *Epilepsia* 39: 237–243.
108. Reiter, R.J., Tan, D.X., Terron, M.P., Flores, L.J., Czarnocki, Z. 2007. Melatonin and its metabolites: New findings regarding their production and their radical scavenging actions. *Acta Biochem Pol* 54: 1–9.
109. Reiter, R.J., Benitez-King G. 2009. Melatonin reduces neuronal loss and cytoskeletal deterioration: Implications for psychiatry. *Mental health* 32: 3–11.
110. Hung, M.W., Tipoe, G.L., Poon, A.M. 2008. Protective effect of melatonin against hippocampal injury of rats with intermittent hypoxia. *J Pineal Res* 44: 214–221.
111. Ramirez-Rodriguez, G., Klempin, F., Babu, H., Benitez-Kin, G., Kempermann G. 2009. Melatonin modulates cell survival of new neurons in the hippocampus of adult mice. *Neuropsychopharmacol* 34: 2180–2191.
112. Fagiolini, A., Frank, E., Scott, J.A., Turkin, S., Kupfer, D.J. 2005. Metabolic syndrome in bipolar disorder: Findings from the Bipolar Disorder Center for Pennsylvanians. *Bipolar Disord* 7: 424–430.
113. Simko, F., Paulis, L. 2008. Chronotherapy beyond blood pressure reduction? *J Pineal Res* 45: 227–228.
114. Moriya, T., Horie, N., Mitome, M., Shinohara, K. 2007. Melatonin influences the proliferative and differentiative activity of neural stem cells. *J Pineal Res* 42: 411–418.

115. Gutierrez-Cuesta, J., Sureda, F.X., Romeu, M., Canudas, A.M., Caballero, B., Coto-Montes, A. et al. 2007. Chronic administration of melatonin reduces cerebral injury biomarkers in SAMP8. *J Pineal Res* 42: 394–402.
116. Tengattini, S., Reiter, R.J., Tan, D.X., Terron, M.P., Rodella, L.F., Rezzani, R. 2008. Cardiovascular diseases: Protective effects of melatonin. *J Pineal Res* 44: 16–25.
117. Dowling, G.A., Burr, R.L., Van Someren, E.J., Hubbard, E.M., Luxenberg, J.S., Mastick, J., Cooper, B.A. 2008. Melatonin and bright-light treatment for rest activity disruption in institutionalized patients with Alzheimer's disease. *J Am Geriatr Soc* 56: 239–246.
118. Dallaspezia, S., Benedetti, F. 2009. Melatonin, circadian rhythms, and the clock genes in bipolar disorder. *Curr Psychiatry Rep* 11: 488–493.
119. Robertson, J., Peter, E. 1997. Case study: The use of melatonin in a boy with refractory bipolar disorder. *J Am Acad Child Adolesc Psychiatry* 36: 822–825.
120. Bersani, G., Garavini, A. 2000. Melatonin add-on in manic patients with treatment resistant insomnia. *Prog Neuropsychopharmacol Biol Psychiatry* 24: 185–191.
121. Gao, K., Calfbrese, J.R. 2005. Newer treatment studies for bipolar depression. *Bipolar Disord* 5: 13–23.
122. Nierenberg, A.A. 2009. Low-dose buspirone, melatonin and low-dose bupropion added to mood stabilizers for severe treatment-resistant bipolar depression. *Psychother Psychosom* 78: 391–393.
123. Gonzalez-Maeso, J., Ang, R.L., Yuen, T., Chan, P., Weisstaub, N.V., López-Giménez, J.F. et al. 2008. Identification of a serotonin/glutamate receptor complex implicated in psychosis. *Nature* 452: 38–39.
124. Walsh, T., McClellan, J., McCarthy, S.E., Addington, A.M., Pierce, S.B., Cooper, G.M., Nord, A.S. et al. 2008. Rare structural variants disrupt multiple genes in neurodevelopmental pathways in schizophrenia. *Science* 320: 539–543.
125. Shao, L., Vawter, M.P. 2008. Shared gene expression alterations in schizophrenia and bipolar disorder. *Biol Psychiatry* 64: 89–97.
126. van der Heijden, F.M., Fekkes, D., Tuinier, S., Sijben, A.E., Kahn, R.S., Verhoeven, W.M. 2005. Amino acids in schizophrenia: Evidence for coger tryptophan availability during treatment with atypical antipsychotics? *J Neural Transm* 112: 577–585.
127. Baskak, S.C., Ozsan, H., Baskak, B., Devrimci, O.H., Kinikli G. 2008. Peripheral blood T-lymphocyte and T-lymphocyte subset ratios before and after treatment in schizophrenia patients not taking antipsychotic medication. *Turk Psikiyatri Derg* 19: 5–12.
128. Koliaskina, G.I., Sekirina, T.P., Androsova, L.V., Kushner, S.G., Vasil'eva, E.F., Burbaeva, O.A., Morozova, M.A. 2007. The influence of atypical neuroleptics on the immune system of patient with schizophrenia. *Vestn Ross Med Nauk* 3: 14–19.
129. Na, K.S., Kim, Y.K. 2007. Monocytic, Th1 and Th2 cytokine alterations in the pathophysiology of schizophrenia. *Neuropsychobiology* 56: 55–63.
130. Potvin, S., Stip, E., Sepehry, A.A., Gendron, A., Bah, R., Kouassi, E. 2008. Inflammatory cytokine alterations in schizophrenia: A systematic quantitative review. *Biol Psychiatry* 63: 801–808.
131. Oken, R.J. 1995. Towards a unifiying hypothesis of neurodegenerative diseases and a concomitant rational strategy for their prophylaxis and therapy. *Med Hypotheses* 45: 341–342.
132. Oken, R.J. 2001. Obsessive–compulsive disorder: A neuronal membrane phospholipids hypothesis and concomitant therapeutic strategy. *Med Hypotheses* 56: 413–415.
133. Reiter, R.J., Tan, D.X., León, J. et al. 2005. When melatonin gets on your nerves: Its beneficial actions in experimental models of stroke. *Exp Biol Med* 230: 104–117.
134. Mattias, W., Zellweger, R., DeMaso., Ayala, A., Chaudry, I.H. 1996. Melatonin administration attenuates depressed immune functions after trauma–hemorrhage. *J Surg Res* 63: 256–262.
135. Suresh-Kumar, P.N., Andrade, C., Bhakta, S.G., Singh, N.M. 2007. Melatonin in schizophrenic outpatients with insomnia: A double-blind, placebo-controlled study. *J Clin Psychiatry* 68: 237–241.
136. Hocaoglu, C. 2009. Clozapine-induced rabbit syndrome: A case report. *Mental Illness* 1: 1–3.
137. Newcomer, J.W. 2005. Second-generation (atypical) antipsychotics and metabolic effects: A comprehensive literature review. *CNS Drugs* 1: 1–93.
138. Casademont, J., Garrabou, G., Miró, O., López, S., Pons, A., Bernardo, M., Cardellach, F. 2007. Neuroleptic treatment effect on mitochondrial electron transport chain: Peripheral blood mononuclear cells analysis in psychotic patients. *J Clin Psychopharmacol* 27: 284–288.
139. Paredes, S.D., Terrón, M.P., Valero, V., Barriga, C., Reiter, R.J., Rodríguez, A.B. 2007. Orally administered melatonin improves nocturnal rest in young and old ringdoves. *Basic Clin Pharmacol Toxicol* 100: 258–268.
140. Shamir, E., Rotenberg, V.S., Laudon, M., Zisapel, N., Elizur, A. 2000. First-night effects of melatonin treatment in patients with chronic schizophrenia. *J Clin Psychopharmacol* 20: 691–694.

141. Shamir, E., Barak, Y., Shalman, I., Laudon, M., Zisapel, N., Tarrasch, R. et al. 2001. Melatonin treatment in tardive dyskinesia: A double-blind, placebo-controlled, crossover study. *Arch Gen Psychiatr* 58: 1049–1052.
142. Zipris, P., Melamed, Y., Weizman, A., Bleich, A. 2007. Clozapine-induced eosinophilia and switch to quetiapine in a patient with chronic schizophrenia with suicidal tendencies. *Isr J Psychiatry Relat Sci* 44: 54–56.
143. Wolden-Hanson, T., Mitton, D.R., McCants, R.L., Yellon, S.M., Wilkinson, C.W., Matsumoto, A.M., Rasmussen, D.D. (2000). Daily melatonin administration to middle-aged male rats suppresses body weight, intraabdominal adiposity, and plasma leptin and insulin independent of food intake and total body fat. *Endocrinology* 141:487–497.
144. Cheung, R.T., Tipoe, G.L., Tam, S., Ma, E.S., Zou, L.Y., Chan, P.S. 2006. Preclinical evaluation of pharmacokinetics and safety of melatonin in propylene glycol for intravenous administration. *J Pineal Res* 41: 337–343.
145. Pignone, A.M., Rosso, D.A., Fiori, G., Matucci-Cerinic, M., Becucci, A., Tempestini, A. et al. 2006. Melatonin is a safe and effective treatment for chronic pulmonary and extrapulmonary sarcoidosis. *J Pineal Res* 41: 95–100.
146. Serfaty, M.A., Osborne, D., Buszewicz, M.J., Blizard, R., Raven, P.W. 2010. A randomized double-blind placebo-controlled trial of treatment as usual plus exogenous slow-release melatonin (6 mg) or placebo for sleep disturbance and depressed mood. *Int Clin Psychopharmacol* 25: 132–142.

20 Melatonin in Control of Gastric Secretion and Prevention of Gastric Mucosal Lesions

Peter C. Konturek, Iwona Brzozowska, Krzysztof Celinski, Stanislaw J. Konturek, and Tomasz Brzozowski

CONTENTS

20.1 INTRODUCTION

Melatonin, the principal secretory product of the pineal gland, is known to influence a variety of biological processes including circadian rhythms, neuroendocrine, cardiovascular or immune functions [1]. It is an indoleamine discovered by Lerner et al. in 1958 in the pineal gland [2], which was initially considered to be the primary source of this circulating hormone, but more recently, this indoleamine was found to be a ubiquitous molecule generated by neuroendocrine cells in various tissues, particularly in the gastrointestinal tract (GIT) [3], where it was found in many folds in amounts larger than those synthesized in the pineal gland. Experimental studies in animals demonstrated that melatonin acts in a paracrine fashion on GIT mucosa and, in part, it is released to portal circulation to be up-taken by the liver for metabolism and excretion with the bile to small bowel and then to go to enterohepatic circulation [4]. Melatonin is a derivative of an essential amino acid, L-tryptophan (L-Try), synthesized in a four-step pathway. First, L-Try is converted to 5-hydroxytryptophan by tryptophan 5-monooxygenase. The aromatic 1-amino acid decarboxylase then catalyzes the conversion of 5-hydroxytryptophan to serotonin (5-hydroxytryptamine). Arylalkylamine-*N*-acetyltrasferase (AANAT) acetylates serotonin to *N*-acetylserotonin, the immediate precursor of melatonin. The last step in this biosynthetic pathway is catalyzed by hydroxyindol-*O*-methyltransferase (HIOMT), which leads to the formation of melatonin [5]. All these melatonin biosynthetic pathway steps and involved enzymes have been identified in the rat gastric mucosa exposed to L-Try–rich diet, which accelerated the healing of gastric ulcerations [4].

Melatonin acts on target cells, at least in part, via specific receptors. To date, several mammalian melatonin receptors have been identified, including MT_1, MT_2, and MT_3 [6]. The first two receptors are G-protein–coupled membrane receptors, and their activation modulates a wide range of intracellular messengers, e.g., cAMP, cGMP, or an increase in cytosolic calcium ions [Ca^{2+}]. The MT_3 binding site has been identified as quinone reductase protein, and its physiological significance remains to be clarified [7]. Other actions of melatonin involve its direct scavenging of free radicals, but this effect occurs without contribution of specific receptors.

Human gastric mucosa is divided into three zones; cardiac, oxyntic, and pyloric. The hallmark of the oxyntic glands are the parietal cells secreting hydrochloric acid and that of pyloric glands are the G-cells releasing gastrin, which are responsible for the stimulation of the parietal cells through the direct activation of their CCK-2 receptors [8,9]. Gastrin acts mainly indirectly on acid secretion by excitation of enterochromaffin-like (ECL) cells and release of histamine, stimulating the parietal cells through the histamine H_2- receptors. A variety of neurocrine, endocrine, and paracrine signals regulate gastric acid secretion, including gastrin, histamine, acetylcholine, but most recently, the experimental studies provided evidence indicating that melatonin can also influence this secretion [9].

Gastric mucosa is exposed to various irritants of exogenous origin such as alcohol, hyperosmolar solutions, bacteria and their toxins present in the ingested foods, various drugs, especially non-steroidal anti-inflammatory drugs (NSAID), and of endogenous origin including bile salts refluxed from the duodenum into the stomach. Gastric mucosa exhibits the ability to self-defense, called gastroprotection, that is attributable to several lines of mucosal protection such as mucus bicarbonate secretion, mucosal hydrophobicity, gastric microcirculation, and release of gastroprotective substances, such as prostaglandins (PG), vasoactive neuropeptides, and nitric oxide (NO) originating from sensory nerves of the mucosa. Recent studies indicate that exogenous melatonin and that generated from tryptophan (L-Trp) in the enteroendocrine cells of the gastric mucosa also exerts highly gastroprotective action against lesions induced by ischemia–reperfusion, cold immobilization stress, ethanol, and NSAIDs [9]. This review is designed to describe the involvement of melatonin in the control of gastric acid secretion and in the mucosal protection.

20.2 MELATONIN IN THE CONTROL OF GASTRIC SECRETION

As mentioned in the introductory remarks, a variety of neurocrine, endocrine, and paracrine signals are involved in the regulation of gastric acid secretion, including gastrin, histamine, acetylcholine that are locally released in gastric mucosa, respectively, by pyloric G-cells, ECL cells, and the cholinergic neurons. Most of the initial studies related to the influence of melatonin on gastric secretion were performed in animals. Our group [10,11] was one of the first to report that melatonin applied intragastrically at doses of 2.5 to 10 mg/kg or L-Trp in doses 25–200 mg/kg inhibit gastric acid secretion and prevent acute gastric lesions induced by various irritants, but this prevention has been attributed mainly to the scavenging effect of this indoleamine on the reactive oxygen species (ROS) generation, stimulation of mucosal generation of PG, and increase in the gastric mucosal microcirculation. Kato et al. [12], who also specifically studied the influence of melatonin on gastric secretion, found that this indoleamine applied intracisternally in rats in doses ranging from 1 to 100 ng/rat caused a dose-dependent decrease of acid and pepsin secretion in conscious pylorus-ligated animals, while a higher (1 μg) dose administered intraperitoneally failed to affect this gastric secretion. The same group of investigators [13] reported later that larger doses of melatonin (1 or 10 mg/kg) given intraperitoneally caused gastric acid inhibition while preventing gastric lesions induced by stress or ischemia–reperfusion.

Brzozowska et al. [14], using rats with gastric fistulas and acetic acid–induced gastric ulcerations, confirmed that melatonin and L-Try accelerated ulcer healing and that this was accompanied not only by the inhibition of gastric acid secretion in fully awake chronic gastric fistula rats but also by the increase in plasma gastrin levels. This acceleration of ulcer healing by melatonin and L-Try was attributed to the rise in plasma gastrin, which could result from the fall in gastric acid secretion and contribute to the ulcer healing action of melatonin and L-Try. Thus, studies in animals revealed that melatonin and its precursor L-Try affect both gastric acid secretion and gastrin release. The question still remains whether these beneficial effects of melatonin and its precursor are of pharmacological character that can be documented in animals or whether they occur also in humans with the same therapeutic impact against gastric lesions. Recently, Kandiel et al. [15], who studied the possible therapeutic usefulness of orally given melatonin in patients with gastroesophageal disease, observed that such therapy increased significantly esophageal pH probably due to reduction of gastric acid secretion, suggesting that this indoleamine is capable of inhibiting gastric acid secretion also in humans and that this might contribute to the improvement of gastroesophageal disease symptoms. In another study on humans [16], it was found that orally administered melatonin or L-Try, which markedly reduced gastric mucosal lesions due to aspirin, caused a rise in serum levels of gastrin, which probably resulted from the inhibition of gastric acid secretion by this indoleamine, but the possible direct action of melatonin and L-Try on the pyloric G-cells cannot be excluded. The increase in fasting and postprandial plasma gastrin was also recently observed in healthy subjects and to greater extent in patients with liver cirrhosis who were orally given melatonin or L-Try, suggesting that both these substances may, indeed, directly stimulate gastrin release from the G-cells [17]. Thus, studies in both animals and humans seem to provide evidence that melatonin exerts significant inhibitory effect on gastric acid secretion and stimulatory influence on gastrin release, but the relationship between alterations in serum gastrin and gastric acid secretion caused by melatonin or L-Try, particularly in humans, requires further detailed examination.

20.3 GASTROPROTECTION BY EXOGENOUS AND ENDOGENOUS MELATONIN

The upper GIT, including the esophagus and the stomach, is involved not only in the transport and accumulation of ingested foods and their partial digestion but also exhibits self-defense from injury by a variety of irritants present in these foods, particularly bacteria and their toxins, drugs, and endogenous substances such as bile acids refluxed into the gastric lumen. This esophageal and gastric mucosal self-defense called *cytoprotection* or *mucosoprotection* has been attributed to the activation of several lines of mucosal protection including continuous mucus alkaline secretion, mucosal hydrophobicity, gastric microcirculation, generation of protective PG within the gastric mucosa, an increase in the mucosal sulfhydryls, and release of vasoactive neuropeptides from sensory afferent neurons. This phenomenon of "cytoprotection" was originally discovered by Robert et al. [18,19], who described the finding that PGs, the major products of arachidonate metabolism through cyclooxygenase (COX) pathway, are essential for the maintenance of mucosal integrity and protection. They provided convincing experimental evidence that exogenous PG applied topically on the gastric mucosa in minute, nonantisecretory doses almost completely prevented the appearance of gastric mucosal lesions induced by potent necrotizing substances such as ethanol, hyperosmolar solutions, strong acids (e.g., 0.6 N HCl), bases (e.g., 0.2 N NaOH), concentrated bile, or even the physical damage provoked by boiling water [18]. Major mechanisms implicated in this PG-induced "cytoprotection" in the stomach included the stimulation of gastric mucus and bicarbonate secretions, an increase in the gastric microcirculation, and the enhancement in the mucosal sulfhydryl compounds. Further studies revealed that an essential type of cytoprotection is "adaptive cytoprotection," the term that was also coined by Robert et al. [19] to describe the protective activity of endogenous PG generated within gastric mucosa by mild topical irritants such as 20% ethanol, 5 mM NaCl, or 5 mM taurocholate (TC) applied a few minutes prior to strong irritants, causing severe mucosal damage such as that induced by intragastric application of 100% ethanol, 25% NaCl, or 80 mM TC. The concept of cytoprotection pioneered by Robert's experimentations was further extended by the observation that mild irritants offer the cross-protective responses, e.g., 5% NaCl was effective in attenuation of damage induced not only by necrotizing concentration (25%) of NaCl but also by 100% ethanol or 80 mM TC, while 20% ethanol prevented the damage caused not only by 100% ethanol but also by 25% NaCl or 80 mM TC. Moreover, using the fine bioassay technique to measure a generation of prostacyclin (PGI_2) and PGE_2 in the gastric mucosa, it was demonstrated that the pretreatment of gastric mucosa with mild irritant resulted in an enhancement of the mucosal generation of PGI_2 and PGE_2, thus providing direct evidence for the role of endogenous PG in the mechanism of adaptive cytoprotection. Therefore, it was proposed that this protective mucosal mild irritation could be attributed to the local (paracrine) action of endogenous PG because mild irritants failed to exhibit the protective activity when applied systemically [20]. It is of interest that exogenous PGE_2 exhibited cytoprotective activity against the damage induced by ethanol and indomethacin to the isolated gastric mucosal cells or isolated gastric glands in vitro, indicating that this genuine "cytoprotective" activity of PG in in vitro conditions might contribute, at least in part, to the phenomenon of gastric protection observed in the stomach pretreated with PG in vivo [21–23]. These studies performed in vitro supported the notion that PG possessed the ability to directly attenuate the cell damage without the contribution of neural, vascular, or hormonal factors as well as gastric mucosal microcirculation responsible for the delivery of oxygen and nutrients to the damaged tissue. This PG-mediated cytoprotection in isolated cell systems has been for a long time a controversial issue because some experimental evidence suggested later on that PG protection does not exist in vitro and questioned also the notion that PG are primary mediators of adaptive cytoprotection. Instead of the primary mediatory role of PG in adaptive cytoprotection, other mechanisms were emphasized, including enhanced gastric blood flow and stimulation of viscous mucus secretion in the gastric mucosa due to the local irritating effect of the mild irritant [24,25].

Further studies revealed an important role in the mediation of cytoprotection of other compounds such as growth factors that were shown to share the gastroprotective properties of PG [26,27] because they were also capable of reducing mucosal damage induced by NSAID, such as aspirin, which causes gastric lesions in rats and cats under the conditions where biosynthesis of endogenous PG was completely inhibited by this NSAID.

The promise that potent pharmacological formulations containing PG may exert therapeutic efficacy in chronic peptic ulcer due to their gastroprotective activity observed in animals with acute mucosal injury had, however, not been fulfilled [28]. The healing of chronic gastric ulcerations is a complex process involving cell differentiation at the ulcer margin, the cell proliferation to cover the mucosal defect in gastric mucosa, and the formation of granulation tissue with new microvessels (angiogenesis). It become quickly evident that PGs, at nonantisecretory doses, are not efficient in the process of acceleration of experimental ulcer healing and are also ineffective in the prevention of ulcer recurrence and reflux esophagitis. Exogenous PGs such as misoprostol have been found to be effective in enhancing healing of chronic gastric or duodenal ulcer predominantly due to their gastric acid inhibitory action [29]. Second, by definition, PGs were originally believed to preserve all layers of the gastric mucosa injured by noxious and/or necrotizing substances. Later, it became apparent from detailed histological assessments of the gastric mucosa "protected" from the acute gastric injury by PG that these arachidonate metabolites failed to prevent morphologic disruption of surface epithelium and cell desquamation after ethanol administration [30]. Although PG prevented the macroscopic injury induced by ethanol, these arachidonate metabolites were incapable to prevent the destruction by this agent of superficial epithelial gastric mucosal cells but enhanced rapid restitution of the damaged mucosa by stimulation of mucosal cell migration from the intact foveolar and neck-gland area. The fact that the PG afforded protection to the deeper mucosal layers predominantly, including the regenerative zone of gastric glands, but failed to prevent injury to the superficial mucosal cells turned, however, into the question their "truly" cytoprotective properties [30]. This indicates that cytoprotective action of PG may involve preservation of gastric cells located in lower part of the gastric pits, but the surface epithelial cells are not protected despite of the presence of endogenous PG.

Besides PG, another important mediator, nitric oxide (NO), was later implicated as a mediator of adaptive cytoprotection [31,32]. The contribution of NO to adaptive cytoprotection was based on the finding that L-NNA reversed the effect of mild irritants with the extent similar to that observed with administration of indomethacin. Furthermore, concurrent treatment with L-arginine, a substrate for the NO synthase (NOS) activity, coadministration with L-NNA, or addition of exogenous PGE_2 analog to indomethacin counteracted the inhibitory effect of L-NNA and indomethacin on adaptive cytoprotection induced by 20% ethanol and diminished an increase in the gastric blood flow (GBF) induced by this mild irritant. Extensive experimental studies in the past decade revealed that NO released from the vascular endothelium, sensory afferent nerves, or gastric epithelium is essential not only for adaptive cytoprotection but also for the gastroprotection evoked by many physiological factors including growth factors such as gastrin, EGF, VEGF, bFGF, TGF-α, and PDGF, or gastrointestinal hormones, such as cholecystokinin (CCK), gastrin, leptin, and ghrelin [26,27,33–35]. EGF, when applied parenterally, markedly attenuated the gastric lesions evoked by ethanol and the protective activity of this peptide was inhibited by L-NNA, indomethacin, and DFMO, an inhibitor of ornithine decarboxylase (ODC)–polyamine pathways [35]. This study has indicated that growth factors may exert protective effect on the gastric mucosa injured by ethanol via mechanism involving mucosal NO and PG as well as enhanced mucosal polyamines and/or sulfhydryls biosynthesis.

Numerous recent studies showed that the GIT is the most abundant extrapineal source of circulating melatonin, with mucosal concentrations of this indoleamine exceeding its blood plasma levels by 100–400 times [3,4]. Oral application of L-Try, the melatonin precursor, causes a rapid elevation of circulating melatonin that is markedly higher than that obtained after systemic administration of this amino acid [10,11]. These results confirmed and extended previous findings that intragastric melatonin is a highly effective gastroprotector against stress-induced gastric lesions. Furthermore, the intragastric administration of L-Try, which results in a quick enzymatic conversion in the stomach of this amino acid into the melatonin, is highly effective in prevention of gastric stress–induced damage through an increase in gastric mucosal microcirculation possibly resulting from scavenging of free radicals, stimulation of antioxidative enzymes in the gastric mucosa, and reduction in lipid peroxidation [10]. This gastroprotective efficacy of melatonin against acute gastric lesions induced by stress are in keeping with other reports showing that this indoleamine or its precursor L-Try applied intragastrically attenuates the formation of acute gastric damage provoked by ethanol, aspirin, and hypoxia resulting from gastric ischemia followed by reperfusion. The mechanism of gastroprotection by melatonin or its precursor has been attributed to the scavenging of ROS and its ability to attenuate lipid membrane peroxidation, neutrophil-induced infiltration, and cytotoxicity caused by mucosal irritants. The beneficial effects of orally applied L-Try on gastric mucosa should be attributed to melatonin originating predominantly from the gastrointestinal tract mucosa because pinealectomy failed to affect the indole content in this mucosa [13].

20.4 MELATONIN AND NSAID-INDUCED GASTROPATHY

NSAIDs such as aspirin (acetyl salicylic acid) are known to provoke gastric mucosal damage and interfere with healing of acute or chronic gastric ulcerations. Despite these side effects, NSAID are among the most widely used medications in the world due to their high efficacy in reducing pain and inflammation and protection against stroke and myocardial infarction. Patients at risk for development of serious gastrointestinal side effects of NSAID are considered for prevention with PGE_2 or its stable analogs such as misoprostol and with gastric acid inhibitors such as proton pump inhibitors or COX-2 (coxibs)-selective inhibitor therapy [36]. Experimental studies in animals showed that the gastric mucosal lesions induced by NSAID are associated not only with their detrimental effect on PG biosynthesis but also with increased oxidative stress resulting from the neutrophil (PMN) activation (PMN) [37]. Administration of melatonin was reported to prevent and decrease acute gastric lesions induced by indomethacin [37], piroxicam [39], or aspirin [11]. Due to high free radical scavenging activity, melatonin and its precursor, L-Try, are natural candidates for the protection of the gastric mucosa against NSAIDs [38], but little is known whether NSAID-induced gastric mucosal lesions in humans can be prevented by the pretreatment with melatonin or its precursor, L-Try, and whether NSAID affect the biosynthesis of melatonin. According to our experience [16], aspirin administered in healthy volunteers for 11 days at a relatively large dose (2 g/day) induced marked increase in endoscopic mucosal lesions and gastric microbleeding observed mainly at day 3–7 upon the start of aspirin administration. Pretreatment with melatonin or L-Try (5 mg of melatonin or 0.5 g of L-Try twice daily 30 min before aspirin) remarkably reduced gastric lesions and gastric microbleeding. These protective effects were accompanied by the rise in plasma melatonin and almost complete suppression of gastric mucosal PG generation, suggesting that exogenous melatonin or its precursor, L-Try, exerts direct gastroprotective action that might be useful in prevention of acute gastric lesions provoked by oral application of aspirin. Further studies are needed to determine whether melatonin (or tryptophan) given for longer periods in humans could increase the gastric tolerance of aspirin in humans without or with peptic ulcer.

20.5 INVOLVEMENT OF MELATONIN TO THE MECHANISM OF ULCER HEALING

As documented above, melatonin and its precursor, L-Try, when applied exogenously, are highly effective in prevention of the formation of acute gastric lesions induced by ethanol, stress, aspirin, and ischemia–reperfusion [10–13]. Our recent studies [4,40], fully confirmed previous observations that both melatonin and its precursor, L-Try, administered intragastrically dose-dependently reduced the number of acute gastric lesions, attenuated lipid peroxidation, and enhanced activity of antioxidant enzymes in gastric mucosa in rats exposed to 3.5 hours of water immersion and restraint, representing typical oxidative stress–induced gastric disorder often leading to the micro-bleeding erosions in humans. These protective effects were accompanied by gradual increase in plasma melatonin levels, indicating that intragastric melatonin has local protective action on gastric mucosa acting via circulation following its absorption form the gut. L-Try, a highly hydrophobic substance, easily penetrates the GIT mucosal membrane to be quickly transformed into melatonin in the GIT mucosa, showing the same activity as exogenous melatonin itself applied topically to achieve similar plasma indole levels. Finally, liver causes marked metabolism and degradation of melatonin when passing from the gut lumen into the circulation [4,17].

The protective antistress effects and ulcer-healing efficacy of melatonin have been attributed not only to antioxidant action of this indole and restoration of microcirculation but also to the activation by this indole of mucosal COX–PG and NOS–NO systems, especially at the ulcer margin, as well as the activation of capsaicin-sensitive afferent nerves releasing gastroprotective and vasodilating neuropeptide calcitonin gene-related peptide (CGRP) [14]. This notion is supported by the evidence that inactivation of these nerves by a neurotoxic dose of capsaicin attenuated melatonin- and L-Try–induced protection and cotreatment with exogenous CGRP restored the beneficial action of melatonin and L-Try in gastroprotection against mucosal injury. Topically applied melatonin and L-Try administered intragastrically are known to enhance the release of gastrin that also might contribute to ulcer healing by stimulation of mucosal growth at the ulcer margin.

The mechanism of the gastroprotection afforded by melatonin and its precursor, L-Try, involves the stimulation of COX–PG system, the enhancement in GBF, and the scavenging of free radicals as described before [10,11,40,41]. If the GIT-originated melatonin is indeed involved in the local mucosal protection, it is expected that exogenous melatonin and its precursor, L-Try should also exert protection against the gastric mucosal lesions even in rats undergoing pinealectomy. Indeed, pinealectomy significantly reduced the basal plasma levels of melatonin and enhanced gastric ulcerogenicity of stress but failed to abolish the gastroprotective activity of exogenous melatonin and its precursor, L-Try [11,12]. Our finding that melatonin exerts the gastroprotective activity is in keeping with another study showing that central melatonin, through intracerebroventricular administration, afforded significant protection against stress-induced damage and reduced the severity of these lesions caused by a thyreotropin releasing hormone (TRH) analogue via interaction with its receptors localized in the central nervous system [43].

The healing of gastric ulcers is a time-dependent process and depends upon several components, including cell proliferation and differentiation at ulcer margin, formation of granulation tissue controlled by the expression of cytokines and growth factors, and the formation of new vessels (angiogenesis) at the ulcer bed. Gastroprotection has little in common with ulcer healing, even though ulcer healing may involve the common gastroprotective mediators that might contribute to both protective action and the process of ulcer healing by this indoleamine. In contrast to the gastroprotective mechanism of melatonin, its efficacy to influence ulcer healing mechanism has been little elucidated.

Bubenik et al. [43,44] were the first to observe the ulcer healing activity of melatonin in pigs, and then this effect was confirmed by our group in rats [14,45]. Bubenik et al. [43] demonstrated that 4-week administration of melatonin in the diet significantly reduced the incidence of spontaneous (chronic) gastric ulcers in young pigs. It is of interest that the pigs with such ulcers exhibited lower contents of melatonin in the gastric mucosa and in blood, suggesting that these spontaneous ulcers originate from the local deficiency of indoleamine. They also demonstrated that a coarsely ground diet, in contrast to finely ground diet, exerted stronger protective effects on the gastric mucosa by stimulating greater production of endogenous melatonin from the gastric mucosa [44].

Our group was particularly interested to examine whether melatonin that exerts a beneficial action against gastric injury due to the activation of the COX–PG system as well as the NOS–NO system [11,14] could also accelerate the healing of preexisting gastric ulcers induced by acetic acid. In previous reports from our laboratory, the suppression of COX by a nonselective COX inhibitor, i.e., indomethacin, attenuated the protective effects of melatonin against mucosal damage induced by stress and ischemia–reperfusion [10]. Based on these observations, the hypothesis has been put forward that PG and NO play a pivotal role in the acceleration of ulcer healing by melatonin [14,39]. The gastroprotective and ulcer healing effects of melatonin in the stomach are considered to be receptor-specific because not only melatonin-induced gastroprotection but also an acceleration of ulcer healing with an accompanying rise in the GBF in the ulcer area were abolished by luzindole, a specific antagonist of the membrane melatonin MT_2 receptors (MT_2R) [45,46].

The healing effects of melatonin involve hyperemia at the ulcer margin, and this circulatory effect may be attributed to melatonin per se or it may also be due to a potent vasodilators such as NO or PGE_2 originating from the vascular endothelium, gastric epithelium, or the capsaicin-sensitive nerve endings releasing the potent vasodilator CGRP [47,48]. The crucial role of NO in the action of melatonin is further supported by the observation that addition to L-NNA of L-arginine (but not D-arginine), the substrate for NOS, restored melatonin-induced ulcer healing, luminal release of NO, and mucosal hyperemia at the ulcer margin. Finally, both cNOS mRNA and iNOS mRNA were significantly up-regulated at the margin of the gastric ulcer in vehicle- and melatonin-treated gastric mucosa as compared with those in intact mucosa; however, only iNOS mRNA was significantly stimulated in melatonin-treated gastric mucosa, suggesting that overexpression of iNOS with subsequent excessive release of NO contributes to the acceleration of ulcer healing and the enhancement of the microcirculation at the ulcer edge [46].

These results remain in agreement with the existing evidence that the healing of preexisting ulcers involves an up-regulation of iNOS at the level of both mRNA and protein in the ulcer edge [49,50]. Furthermore, the importance of NO derived from the iNOS activity in a mechanism of ulcer healing was emphasized by the fact that selective suppression of iNOS expression and activity, accompanied by a reduction in NO generation, increased the number of inflammatory cells at the ulcer margin, resulting in a marked prolongation of ulcer healing [49]. These observations were contrary to the finding that the inhibition of NO biosynthesis via the suppression of iNOS by melatonin may contribute to the protective effect of this indole against lipopolysaccharide-induced endotoxemia in rats [51,52]. This possibly reflects different experimental conditions, suggesting that, under certain conditions such as endotoxemia, melatonin can exert a beneficial effect due to inhibition of iNOS expression and excessive release of NO, thus preventing the formation of the peroxynitrate anion, known to exhibit significant cell toxicity. An early rise in iNOS expression almost immediately after ulcer induction probably contributed to ulcerogenesis, which is the part of inflammatory response following ulcer induction. Since the treatment with melatonin and tryptophan actually significantly reduced iNOS expression as compared with that observed at the early phase (day 0) of healing, it is proposed that melatonin and its precursor have inhibitory action on the expression and probably activity of iNOS, thus eliminating its noxious influence on ulcer healing [45].

Based on these findings, it was reasonable to evaluate the alterations in the gene expression of factors possibly involved in the acceleration of ulcer healing by exogenous melatonin and L-Try, a major precursor of this indole. Melatonin- and L-Try–induced acceleration of ulcer healing involves an increase in the expression of specific melatonin receptors, and this is supported by the increase in gene expression of MT_2R and closely related enzymes, NAT and HIOMT, involved in biosynthesis of melatonin. The expression of both these enzymes was significantly increased mostly in the ulcer area and observed at the late (day 8) phase of ulcer healing, suggesting that locally generated melatonin in the ulcer bed could enhance the healing rate of this ulcer. Binding of labeled melatonin [45,53] reached the highest value in the ulcer base, and this binding was greatly inhibited by the administration of excessive amounts of exogenous melatonin and L-Try to the stomach with gastric ulcer. Interestingly, the administration of melatonin or tryptophan enhanced the gene expression of MT_2R, especially in the ulcer area, as compared to the nonulcerated mucosa [45]. The induction of chronic ulcer enhanced the gene expression of MT_2R, which is the prerequisite for the promotion of the binding of endogenous melatonin and helps the healing process by exhibiting antioxidative and anti-inflammatory actions. This was in keeping with previous results proving the beneficial influence of melatonin and L-Try on healing of chronic gastric ulcers in rats [14,39]. It is of interest that the ulcer induction by acetic acid coincided not only with a remarkable up-regulation of mRNA for MR_2R but also the up-regulation in the ulcer area of the major gastroprotective and antiulcer system, which is the COX–PG system. The overexpression of COX-2 mRNA was even further increased at day 8 of ulcer healing and the cotreatment with melatonin or L-Try further potentiated the enhancement of COX-2 expression in the ulcer area [45].

The involvement of cNOS/iNOS–NO system in ulcer healing and the possible role of melatonin in this process are not quite clear from this and other studies [50,54]. Although the nonspecific suppression of cNOS/iNOS–NO system by L-NNA an inhibitor of NO synthase delayed ulcer healing, there is no clear evidence whether melatonin and L-Try directly affect the expression and activity of iNOS or it could be due to inflammatory conditions associated with gastric ulcer induction. The partial explanation comes out from the evidence that the induction of an ulcer was accompanied by the overexpression of hypoxia inducible factor 1α (HIF-1α), which was detected almost immediately upon the application of ulcerogen, probably caused by severe tissue ischemia, resulting from the action of acetic acid on gastric mucosa [45]. This effect was followed by an overexpression of proinflammatory cytokines such as TNF-α and IL-1β and up-regulation of mRNA for iNOS, with excessive production of noxious NO possibly forming peroxynitrite likely contributing to early tissue damage and formation of ulceration [4,51]. As reported recently by Baatar et al. [55], vascular injury leading to ischemia is the major factor involved in the pathogenesis of chronic tissue injury and induction of ulceration, both in the esophagus and the stomach, where the acetic acid was applied. According to these authors, tissue ischemia and accompanying hypoxia trigger the angiogenesis and formation of network of new microvessels in the granulation tissue at the ulcer margin. These changes have been attributed to increased expression of HIF-1α that dramatically raises the expression of VEGF, activating the angiogenesis both under in vitro and in vivo conditions. Guo et al. [55] reported an early rise in the expression on iNOS, suggesting that this expression accompanied by excessive generation of NO was probably responsible for the enlargement of ulcer crater at the first days upon ulcer induction by acetic acid in rats. The expression of iNOS was observed to decline when the ulcer began to heal, indicating that NO generated by iNOS at a later phase of healing might contribute to ulcer healing by inducing apoptosis in inflammatory cells [49]. This is supported by the observation that HIF-1α overexpression during early mucosal damage is followed by angiogenesis in the granulation tissue as the major events contribute to the process of gastric tissue regeneration and ulcer healing. Indeed, after a relatively short period (3 hours) following the application of acetic acid, a marked rise in the expression of HIF-1α and VEGF were observed, and these changes were accompanied by a marked increase of expression of iNOS mRNA and overexpression of mRNA for proinflammatory cytokines, TNF-α and IL-1β, which could contribute to focal tissue damage caused by acetic acid application [45].

20.6 SUMMARY

- The upper part of the gastrointestinal tract, particularly the gastric mucosa, is an extremely rich source of melatonin released mainly after meals and exceeding about 400 times that produced by pineal gland.
- Exogenous melatonin or that derived from its precursor L-Try exhibits a potent gastroprotective activity against acute gastric lesions induced by a variety of damaging agents including ethanol, cold stress, aspirin, and ischemia–reperfusion in animals.
- Melatonin and L-Try applied orally to rats strongly increase plasma melatonin levels and inhibit gastric acid secretion, while increasing plasma gastrin concentrations.
- Both melatonin and its precursor, L-Try, administered orally in humans are also inhibitors of gastric acid secretion and stimulants of gastrin release.
- In humans, orally applied melatonin or tryptophan are highly effective in preventing the formation and enhancing the healing rate of the gastric lesions and gastric microbleeding induced by use of aspirin, suggesting that this indole or its precursor has potential in the treatment of gastric damage induced by aspirin-like drugs.

REFERENCES

1. Hardeland, R., Pandi-Perumal, R.S., and D.P. Cardinali. 2006. Melatonin. *Int J Biochem Cell Biol* 38(3):313–316.
2. Lerner, A.B., Case, J.D., and Y. Takahashi. 1958. Isolation of melatonin, a pineal factor that lightens melanocytes. *J Am Chem Soc*. 80:2057–2058.
3. Bubenik, G.A., 2002. Gastrointestinal melatonin: localization, function, and clinical relevance. *Dig Dis Sci* 47:2336–2348.
4. Konturek, S.J., Konturek, P.C., and I. Brzozowska. 2007. Localization and biological activities of melatonin in intact and diseased gastrointestinal tract (GIT). *J Physiol Pharmacol* 58(3):381–405.
5. Pandi-Perumal, S.R., Srinivasan, S., Maestroni, G.J.M., Cardinali, D.P., Poeggeler, B., and R. Hardeland. 2006. Melatonin: Nature's most versatile biological signal? *FEBS J* 273:2813–2838.
6. Audinot, V., Bonnaud, A., and Grandcolas, L. 2008. Molecular cloning and pharmacological characterization of rat melatonin MT1 and MT2 receptors. *Biochem Pharmacol* 75:2007–2019.
7. Carbajo-Pescador, S., Martin-Renedo, J., and A. Garcoa-Palomo. 2009. Changes in expression of melatonin receptors induced by melatonin treatment in hepatocarcinoma $HepG_2$ cells. *J Pineal Res* 47:330–338.
8. Schubert, M.L. 2009. Gastric exocrine and endocrine secretion. *Curr Opinion Gastroenterol* 25:529–578.
9. Konturek, S.J., Brzozowski, T., and Konturek, P.C. 2008. Brain-gut and appetite regulating hormones in the control of gastric secretion and mucosal protection. *J Physiol Pharmacol* 59(Suppl 2):7–31.
10. Konturek, P.C., Konturek, S.J., and T. Brzozowski. 1997. Gastroprotective activity of melatonin and its precursor, L-tryptophan, against stress-induced and ischemia-induced lesions is mediated by scavenge of oxygen radicals. *Scand J Gastroenterol* 52:433–438.
11. Brzozowski, T., Konturek, P.C., and S.J. Konturek. 1997. The role of melatonin and L-tryptophan in prevention of acute gastric lesions induced by stress, ethanol, ischemia and aspirin. *J Pineal Res* 23:79–89.
12. Kato, K., Murai, I., and S. Asai, S. 1998. Central nervous system action of melatonin on gastric acid and pepsin secretion in pylorus-ligated rats. *Neuroreport* 9:2447–2450.
13. Kato, K., Asai, S., and I. Murai. 2001. Melatonin's gastroprotective and anti-stress roles involve both central and peripheral effects. *J Gastroenterol* 36:91–95.
14. Brzozowska, I., Konturek, P.C., and T. Brzozowski. 2002. Role of prostaglandins, nitric oxide, sensory nerves and gastrin in acceleration of ulcer healing by melatonin and its precursor, L-tryptophan. *J Pineal Res* 32:149–162.
15. Kandil, T.S., Mousa, A.A., El-Gendy, A.A., and A. M. Abbas. 2010. The potential therapeutic effect of melatonin in gastro-esophageal reflux disease. *BMC Gastroenterol* 10:7–12.
16. Konturek, P.C., Celinski, K., and M. Slomka, M. 2008. Melatonin and its precursor L-tryptophan prevent acute gastric mucosal damage induced by aspirin in humans. *J Physiol Pharmacol* 59(Suppl 2):67–75.
17. Celinski, K., Konturek, P.C., and M. Slomka. 2009. Altered basal and postprandial plasma melatonin, gastrin, leptin and insulin in patients with liver cirrhosis and portal hypertension without and with oral administration of melatonin or tryptophan. *J Pineal Res* 46:408–414.

18. Robert, A., Nezamis, J.E., Lancaster, C., and A.J. Hanchar. 1979. Cytoprotection by prostaglandins in rats. Prevention of gastric necrosis produced by alcohol, HCl, NaOH, hypertonic NaCl and thermal injury. *Gastroenterology* 77:433–440.
19. Robert, A., Nezamis, I.E., Lancaster, C., Davies, I.P., Field, S.O., and A.J. Hanchar. 1983. Mild irritant prevent gastric necrosis through adaptive cytoprotection mediated by prostaglandins. *Am J Physiol* 245:113–116.
20. Brzozowski, T., Konturek, P.C., Konturek, S.J., Brzozowska, I., and T. Pawlik. 2005. Role of prostaglandins in gastroprotection and gastric adaptation. *J Physiol Pharmacol* 56(Suppl 5):33–55.
21. Tarnawski, A., Brzozowski, T., Sarfeh, J., Krause, W.J., Ulich, T.R., Gergely, H., and D. Hollander. 1998. Prostaglandin protection of human isolated gastric glands against indomethacin and ethanol injury. Evidence for direct cellular action of prostaglandin. *J Clin Invest* 81:1081–1089.
22. Tarnawski, A., Hollander, D., Stachura, J., Krause, W.J., and H. Gergely. 1985. Prostaglandin protection of the gastric mucosa against alcohol injury—a dynamic time related process. Role of the mucosal proliferative zone. *Gastroenterology* 88:334–352.
23. Terano, A., Mach, T., Stachura, J., Tarnawski, A., and K.J. Ivey. 1984. Effect of 16,16 dimethyl prostaglandin E_2 on aspirin induced damage to rat gastric epithelial cells in tissue culture. *Gut* 25:19–25.
24. Svanes, K., Gislason, H., and A. Guttu. Role of blood flow in adaptive protection of the cat gastric mucosa. *Gastroenterology* 100:1249–1258.
25. Smith, G.S., Myers, S.I., Bartula, L.L., and T.A. Miller. 1991. Adaptive cytoprotection against alcohol injury in the rat stomach is not due to increased prostanoid synthesis. *Prostaglandins* 41:207–223.
26. Konturek, S.J., Radecki, T., and T. Brzozowski. 1981 Gastric cytoprotection by epidermal growth factor. Role of endogenous prostaglandins and DNA synthesis. *Gastroenterology* 81:436–443.
27. Konturek, S.J., Brzozowski, T., Majka, J., Dembinski, A., Slomiany, A., and B.L. Slomiany. 1992. Transforming growth factor and epidermal growth factor in protection and healing of gastric mucosal injury. *Scand J Gastroenterol* 27:649–655.
28. Hawkey, C.J., and R.P. Walt. 1986. Prostaglandins for peptic ulcer: A promise unfulfilled. *Lancet* 85:1084–1087.
29. Hawkey, C.J. 1989. Prostaglandins; mucosal protection and peptic ulceration. *Methods Find Exp Clin Pharm* (Suppl 1) 11:45–51.
30. Hawkey, C.J., Kemp, R.T., Walt, R.P., Bhaskar, N.K., Davies, J., and B. Filipowicz. 1988. Evidence that adaptive cytoprotection in rats is not mediated by prostaglandins. *Gastroenterology* 94:948–954.
31. Whittle, B.J. 1995. Nitric oxide in physiology and pathology. *Histochem J* 27:727–737.
32. Whittle, B.J. 1997. Nitric oxide—a mediator of inflammation or mucosal defence. *Eur J Gastroenterol Hepatol* 9:1026–1032.
33. Konturek, S.J., Brzozowski, T., Bielanski, and A.V. Schally. 1995. Role of endogenous gastrin in gastroprotection. *Eur J Pharmacol* 278:203–212.
34. Mercer, D.W., Cross, J.M., Chang, L., and L.M. Lichtenberger. 1998. Bombesin prevents gastric injury in the rat: Role of gastrin. *Dig Dis Sci* 43:826–833.
35. Brzozowski, T., Drozdowicz, D., Majka, J., Polonczyk-Pytko, J., and S.J. Konturek. 1991. Role of polyamines in gastroprotection induced by epidermal growth factor. *J Physiol Pharmacol* 42:181–193.
36. Scheiman, J.M. 2008. Prevention of NSAID-induced ulcers. *Curr Treat Options Gastroenterol* 11:125–134.
37. Alarcon de la Lastra, C., Motilva, V., and M.J. Martin. 1999. Protective effect of melatonin on indomethacin-induced gastric injury in rats. *J Pineal Res* 26:101–107.
38. Bandyopadhyaya, D., Ghosh, G., Bandyopadhyaya, A., and R.J. Reiter. 2004. Melatonin protects against piroxicam-induced gastric ulceration. *J Pineal Res* 36:195–203.
39. Konturek, S.J., Konturek, P.C., and T. Brzozowski. 2006. Melatonin in gastroprotection against stress-induced acute gastric lesions and healing of chronic gastric ulcers. *J Physiol Pharmacol* 57(Suppl 5): 51–66.
40. Melchiorri, D., Sewerynek, E., and R.J. Reiter. 1997 Suppressive effect of melatonin administration on ethanol-induced gastroduodenal injury in rats in vivo. *Br J Pharmacol* 121:264–270.
41. Bandyopadhyay, D., Biswas, K., and U. Bandyopadhyay. 2000, Melatonin protects against stress-induced gastric lesions by scavenging the hydroxyl radical. *J Pineal R*es 29:143–151.
42. Kato, K., Murai, I., Asai, S., and S. Komuro. 1997. Central effect of melatonin against stress-induced gastric ulcers in rats. *Neuroreport* 8:2305–2309.
43. Bubenik, G.A., Ayles, H.L., and R.M. Frindship. 1998. Relationship between melatonin levels in plasma and gastrointestinal tissues and the incidence and severity of gastric ulcers in pigs. *J Pineal Res* 24:62–66.

44. Bubenik, G.A, Blask, D.E., and G.M. Brown. 1998. Prospects of the clinical utilization of melatonin. *Biol Signals Recept* 7:195–219.
45. Konturek, P.C., Konturek, S.J., and G. Burnat. 2008. Dynamic physiological and molecular changes in gastric ulcer healing achieved by melatonin and its precursor L-tryptophan in rats. *J Pineal Res* 45:180–190.
46. Dubocovich, M. 1988. Pharmacology and function of melatonin receptors. *FASEB J* 2:2765–2773.
47. Whittle, B.J.R., Lopez-Belmonte, J., and S. Moncada. 1999. Regulation of gastric mucosal integrity by endogenous nitric oxide, interactions with prostanoids and sensory neuropeptides in the rat. *Br J Pharmacol* 99:607–611.
48. Tramantama, M., Renzi, D., and A. Calabro. 1994. Influence of capsaicin-sensitive afferent fibers on acetic acid induced chronic gastric ulcers in rats. *Scand J Gastroenterol* 28:406–413.
49. Akiba, Y., Nakamura, M., and M. Mori. 1998. Inhibition of inducible nitric oxide synthase delays gastric ulcer healing in the rat. *J Clin Gastroenterol* 27: (Suppl 1):S64–S73.
50. Akimoto, M., Hashimoto, H., and M. Shigemoto. 2000. Changes of nitric oxide and growth factors during gastric ulcer healing. *J Cardiovasc Pharmacol* 36(Suppl 1):S282–S285.
51. Gilad, E., Wong, H.R., and B. Zingarelli. 1998. Melatonin expression of the inducible isoform of nitric oxide synthase in murine macrophages: Role of inhibition of NF-kappaB activation. *FASEB J* 12:685–693.
52. Crespo, E., Macias, M., and D. Pozo. 1999. Melatonin inhibits expression of the inducible NO synthase II in the liver and lung and prevents endotoxemia in lipopolysaccharide-induced multiple organ dysfunction syndrome in rats. *FASEB J* 13:1537–1546.
53. Poon, A.M., Chow, P.H., and A.S. Mak. 1997. Autoradiographic localization of 2[^{125}I]iodomelatonin binding sites in the gastrointestinal tract of mammals including humans and birds. *J Pineal Res* 23:5–14.
54. Guo, J.-S., Cho, C.-H., Wang, W.-P., Shen, X.-Z., Cheng, C.-L., and M.W. Koo. 2003. Expression and activities of three inducible enzymes in healing of gastric ulcers in rats. *World J Gastroenterol* 9:1767–1771.
55. Baatar, D., Jones, M.K., and K. Tsugawa. 2002. Esophageal ulceration triggers expression of hypoxia inducible factor-1 alpha and activates vascular epithelial growth factor gene: implication for angiogenesis and ulcer healing. *Am J Pathol* 161:1449–1457.

21 Melatonin for the Control of Reproduction in Small Ruminants

Luis Ángel Zarazaga, José Luis Guzmán, and Benoît Malpaux

CONTENTS

21.1 INTRODUCTION

Small ruminants from mid and high latitudes have a seasonal pattern of reproductive activity. These animals are sexually active during short days (autumn–winter), while during long days (spring), they enter a period of sexual rest—a mechanism of adaptation that allows birthing and lactation to occur at a time (normally spring) more favorable in terms of climatic conditions and food and water availability. Domestication has nearly abolished seasonal reproduction in cattle and pigs, but it is still seen in most breeds of sheep and goat originating from higher latitudes [1–4]. Melatonin has been shown as the hormone that controls such reproductive activity.

This reproductive model, however, determines seasonal variations in the market availability of small ruminant fresh products (meat, milk, and cheese), variations that lead to fluctuations in price. Reproductive seasonality can therefore be a problem for farmers. It can, however, be overcome by photoperiod manipulation. The control of daylength could be achieved by making use of lightproof buildings such as those employed at artificial insemination centers to maintain semen production. Specific treatments could adjust the breeding season to farmers' needs, e.g., making days longer by providing extra illumination during naturally short days and making days shorter during naturally long days by the administration of exogenous melatonin. Currently, however, light-only treatments enjoy greater producer support since they require no use of synthetic hormone treatments, something of particular concern to organic farmers.

This chapter describes the basic principles of and treatments used in photoperiod- and melatonin-based control of reproductive activity in small ruminants.

21.2 ROLE OF PHOTOPERIOD IN THE REGULATION OF SEASONAL REPRODUCTION

21.2.1 General Principles

The photoperiod is the main environmental factor responsible for the seasonality of reproduction in sheep and goats—both in males (Figure 21.1) [5] and females (Figure 21.2a and 21.2b) [6,7]. This assertion is based on two observations: the number of hours of light per day at different times of year varies strongly as one moves away from the equator and the higher the latitude, the stronger seasonality becomes. Further, unlike temperature, food availability, or social factors, photoperiod is reliably repeatable from one year to the next and is therefore the best indicator that the reproductive season has arrived.

Several models based on the modification of the natural light/dark cycle (with no changes in other environmental variables) have been proposed to demonstrate the regulation of the reproductive season by the photoperiod. In both sheep and goats, the reversal of the photoperiodic cycle causes the breeding season to shift phase by 6 months [8–12]. Using a light regimen that reproduces the annual variation of the photoperiod over 6 months induces two breeding seasons per year in sheep [13,14]. Similarly, reproductive activity can be controlled by alternating periods of 3 months of long days (16 hours light) with 3 months of short days (8 hours light). In ewes subjected to such a regimen, the onset of reproductive activity starts after 40–50 short days, while exposure to 20–30 long days inhibits reproductive activity [15]. Using a similar methodology, Chemineau et al. [16] compared the responses of ewes and goat does to changes in the photoperiod and indicated that the time between the shift from long to short days and the onset of reproductive activity was shorter in the former (52–53 days) than in the latter (74–85 days). These results suggest that ewes respond faster than female goats to photoperiod treatments. Recently, Celi et al. [12] showed that, in goats does living at Mediterranean latitudes, pituitary activity started after 46 days of short days, while pituitary rest started after 30 days of long days. In males, testicular growth begins after exposure to 30–40 short days, while the inhibition of reproductive activity occurs after 20–30 long days [17,18]. The alternation of 1 month of long days and 1 month of short days prevents seasonal changes in the activity of the male hypothalamopituitary axis [19].

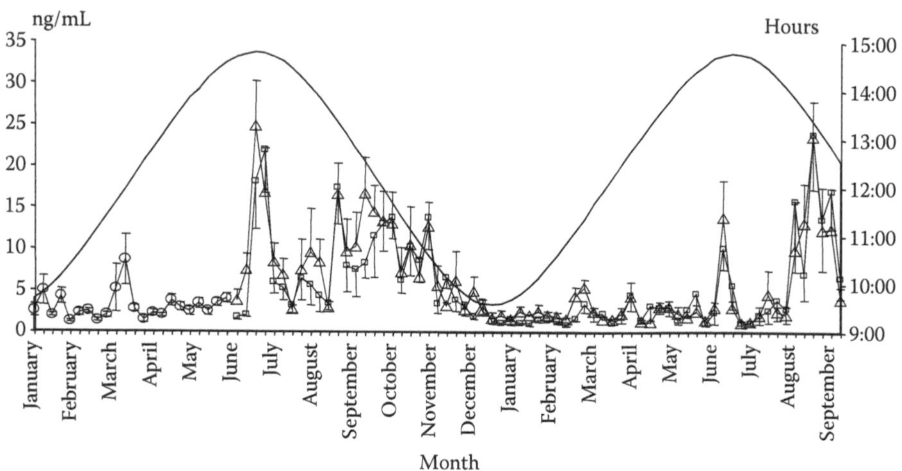

FIGURE 21.1 Mean (±SEM) plasma testosterone concentrations (ng/ml) in Spanish Payoya bucks fed 1.6 × maintenance (H) or 1.1 × their maintenance requirements. (From Zarazaga, L.A., et al., *Theriogenology* 2009;71:1316–1325. With permission.)

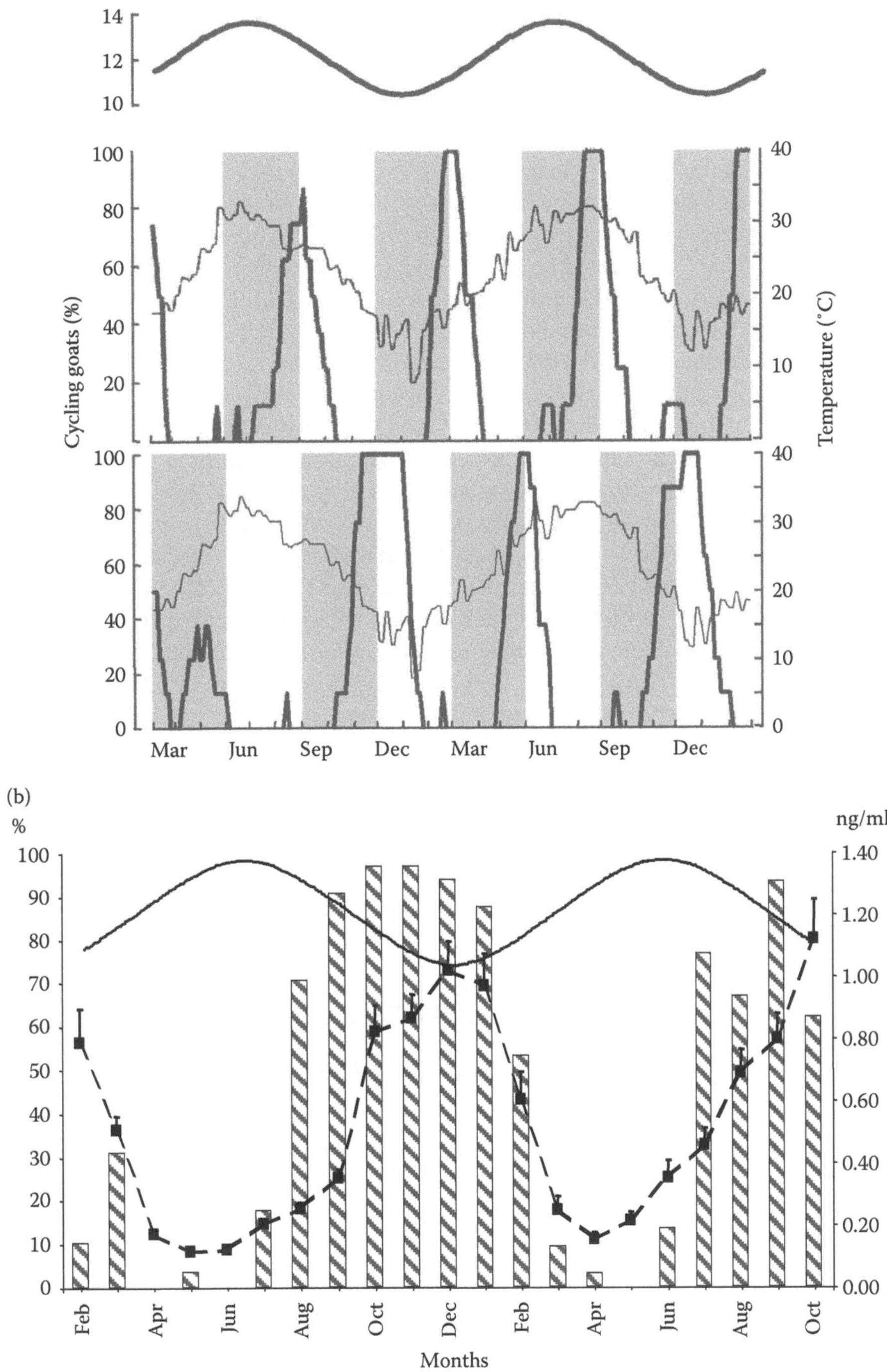

FIGURE 21.2 (a) Changes in percentage of cycling female goats in three groups subjected to alternating periods of 3 months of long days and 3 months of short days. (From Duarte, G., et al., *Anim. Reprod. Sci.* 2010;120:65–70. With permission.) (b) Monthly mean proportion of ovariectomized goats showing reproductive activity (estrous or ovulatory activity) and annual pattern of LH (ng/ml). (From Zarazaga, L.A., et al., *Anim. Reprod. Sci.* 2005;87:253–267. With permission.)

Together, the above data indicate that, in small ruminants, the onset of reproductive activity occurs after animals are exposed to short days, while reproductive rest occurs after the onset of long days.

21.2.2 Photorefractoriness: The Basis of the Control of Reproduction

Unfortunately, the regulation of the annual reproductive cycle is somewhat more complex than just "short days provide a stimulatory effect and long days provide an inhibitory effect." For example, reproductive activity ceases in ewes after exposure to 120–150 short days, with animals becoming refractory to this stimulus [20]. Similarly, after 6 months of exposure to long days, they become refractory to this photoperiod and resume reproductive activity [20]. In fact, it would appear that these mechanisms of photorefractoriness are actually those responsible for the seasonality of reproduction under natural conditions. In Suffolk ewes, it has been shown that the breeding season does not start because of the stimulation of decreasing daylength after the summer solstice. Rather, it would seem that these animals become refractory to the long days between the winter solstice and the summer solstice [21,22]. The same conclusion has been reached regarding the end of the breeding season, with animals becoming refractory to the stimulatory effects of short days and thus entering the anestrous season [23,24]. In other words, it is the loss of response to stimulatory daylength rather than any inhibition caused by increasing daylength that causes the cessation of breeding.

Particular segments of the annual photoperiodic cycle appear to be critical for the smooth running of reproduction [25]. Working with pinealectomized ewes, Wayne et al. [26] suggested the period of increasing days after the winter solstice to be responsible for the synchronization of the onset of the breeding season. Similarly, Jackson et al. [27] concluded this period to be responsible for breaking their refractoriness to short days, allowing animals to once again become sensitive to them and thus respond to the shortening days following the summer solstice. Sweeney et al. [28] indicate that, between the winter and summer solstices, "long days followed by short days" maintains the anestrous state and provides the cue for the initiation of reproductive activity. However, the shortening days between the summer solstice and the autumn equinox have been suggested as responsible for maintaining the reproductive season once initiated [26]. Sweeney et al. [28] concluded that, in ewes, the reproductive neuroendocrine axis is insensitive to "long days followed by short days" between the autumn equinox and the winter solstice, with sensitivity being regained just after the winter solstice.

21.3 TRANSDUCTION OF PHOTOPERIODIC INFORMATION

21.3.1 The Pineal Gland: The Organ That Secretes Melatonin

The pineal gland is also known as the epiphysis, from the Latin *epiphysis cerebri*, or as the "third eye," reflecting its sensitivity to the light. It is the main melatonin-secreting organ, although in vertebrates, including humans, it is also synthesized in the retina, skin, gastrointestinal tract, and ovary. Rhythmic production, however, occurs only in the pineal gland and retina [29,30]. In sheep brain, the pineal gland occupies a central location between the two cerebral hemispheres in front of the cerebellum at the posterodorsal area of the diencephalon [31]. Photoperiodic information is relayed to the pineal gland by a neural pathway involving several steps. After photoreception by the retina, impulses pass through the retinohypothalamic tract to the suprachiasmatic nuclei [32]. The role of this structure is to synchronize melatonin secretion to the light cycle. Lesions of the suprachiasmatic area of the hypothalamus have been shown to impair the rhythm of melatonin secretion in the ram [33]. The next step involves the passage of information from the suprachiasmatic nuclei to the superior cervical ganglia. These are involved in the synthetic activity of the pineal gland (their removal abolishes melatonin synthesis) [34–36]. The final step involves the movement of information from the superior cervical ganglia to the pineal gland itself. Pinealectomy renders animals unable to respond to changes in photoperiod [37].

21.3.2 Melatonin Synthesis and Secretion

Melatonin is an indoleamine, the initial precursor of which is the amino acid tryptophan. Tryptophan arrives at the pinealocytes from the blood and is converted into serotonin, which in turn is converted into *N*-acetyl-serotonin by the enzyme arylalkylamine *N*-acetyltransferase (AANAT). *N*-Acetyl-serotonin is subsequently methylated to form melatonin, a step that requires the enzyme hydroxy-indole-*O*-methyltransferase (HIOMT) [38]. Daily rhythms in melatonin production are controlled by AANAT activity rhythms, but the level of production may be limited by HIOMT activity. This idea developed when it was shown that elevated AANAT activity, when stimulated by adrenergic α and β receptor agonists, failed to promote melatonin production, whereas the increased activity of HIOMT positively correlated with pineal melatonin production [39].

After its synthesis, melatonin is delivered to the brain via the cerebrospinal fluid and to the peripheral tissues via the rich vasculature of the pineal gland, which flows into the vein of Galen or the cerebri magna vein. It then reaches the superior sagittal sinus. This sinus divides into two branches (the transverse sinuses), which are connected to the sigmoid sinuses and finally the internal jugular veins [40]. Recently, it has been shown that melatonin concentrations may vary considerably between the two jugular veins (the difference remaining stable throughout the night) in sheep and goats. The dominant side can be different among individuals. The origin of this difference does not appear to lie in the jugular veins themselves, but rather in the distribution of blood from the sagittal sinus to the jugular veins. This observation has practical implications since the accurate assessment of melatonin production by the pineal gland requires either melatonin concentrations be recorded in both jugular veins simultaneously or always in the same jugular vein [41,42].

21.3.3 The Light/Dark Cycle and Melatonin

Melatonin synthesis starts only after the onset of darkness. Melatonin secretion, however, depends on the photoperiod regime. Thus, in ewes under a long-day regime (16 hours light/8 hours darkness), melatonin secretion starts about 11 minutes after the onset of darkness. However, when the same animals are maintained under a short-day photoperiod (8 hours light/16 hours darkness), secretion starts 20 minutes after the lights are turned off [43]. This marked day/night rhythm is characterized by low or undetectable concentrations (around 4 pg/ml) during the day, increasing to 26–981 pg/ml at night in ewes [44] and 30–140 pg/ml in goats [41], and it persists even under constant darkness, indicating that melatonin synthesis has an endogenous rhythm under the control of the internal clock. Under continuous darkness, the period of melatonin secretion is almost 24 hours per day, although wide interanimal variability appears after several weeks [34,45–47]. When animals are maintained under constant light, the rhythm of melatonin release disappears and secretion occurs erratically [48]. The limits of entrainment of this rhythm have been studied experimentally using cycles of light/dark shorter or longer than 24 hours. The adjustment of melatonin release to nights of ahemeral light/dark cycles is remarkable when ewes have been kept under a long-day regimen; more disparity is seen, however, when they have been kept under a short-day regimen [49].

The exposure to extra light or the provision of a pulse of light during the night produces a decline in melatonin secretion in sheep and goats. However, depending on the exact time during the night when this pulse is given, normal melatonin release may (early or mid-night pulse) or may not (late pulse) manage to recover [45,50–54].

After its release, melatonin is metabolized in the liver and kidney with a mean half life of 17.8 minutes in the ewe [55].

21.4 CONTROL OF REPRODUCTION WITH MELATONIN

The aim of many studies on the use of artificial photoperiods and/or exogenous melatonin has been to overcome the seasonality of reproduction (for reviews, see refs. [4,57,58]). Such an objective is feasible through the use of lightproof buildings and using alternating periods of long and short days. However, keeping animals housed for many months during the year increases the cost of meat and milk production, a problem that limits the use of such techniques. The only situation in which animals are currently permanently housed in lightproof buildings is at artificial insemination centers, where valuable genetically improved males are reared for semen production. Exogenous melatonin, however, can mimic short days and therefore stimulate reproductive activity without the need for such special housing. Melatonin, discovered in 1958 by A. E. Lerner of Yale University, began to be used in reproductive control following its identification as the link between light and reproduction [58,59].

21.4.1 The Use of Exogenous Melatonin

The earliest works on the use of exogenous melatonin in the control of reproductive activity in sheep tried to determine the efficacy of different administration regimens. Daily administration is now known to be a prerequisite for stimulating reproductive activity; administration involving longer intervals reduces the efficacy of treatment [60]. Administration via food, intravaginal pessaries [61], injection [62], and even intraruminal soluble glass boluses [63] has been investigated, but the insertion of subcutaneous implants has been found to be the most efficient in sheep [64] and goats [16,65]. This method of administration has become widely used since it guarantees continuous liberation and requires only one intervention.

After a period of long days, ewes need about 40–60 short days for luteinizing hormone (LH) secretion to be stimulated [66]. For this reason, rams are introduced to ewes about 35 days after performing an implantation. However, in goats, there are important differences between breeds from the Mediterranean area and those from higher latitudes in terms of the time from implantation/number of short days required until the beginning of reproductive activity. In Mediterranean goats, LH and progesterone concentrations during the sexual rest period increase about 30 days after the insertion of the melatonin implant [65], but in Saanen dairy goats, Chemineau et al. [67] observed no ovulation before the introduction of males after 71 days of melatonin treatment. The introduction of males to females is now recommended to take place 45 days after implantation [68].

The efficiency of implantation treatment also depends on the moment when it is performed. Implants inserted around the time of the summer solstice have been widely used to advance the breeding season in adult ewes from high latitudes [69,70]. However, the breeding season starts earlier in Mediterranean breeds than in those from higher latitudes, even when both are subjected to the same photoperiod treatment [71]. Commercial melatonin implantation in Mediterranean ewes and goats is therefore usually performed around the time of the spring equinox [65,68,72]. In ewes, it has recently been demonstrated that melatonin implants inserted immediately after the winter solstice can advance reproductive activity in the absence of males and improve reproductive performance under field conditions [73].

Differences exist between sheep and goats in terms of the direct effect of melatonin on the stimulation of LH secretion. In ovariectomized and estradiol-treated goats, Zarazaga et al. [65] showed that melatonin implants inserted around the spring equinox were by themselves able to stimulate LH secretion during seasonal anestrus, without any contact with males being necessary. However, in ewes, Forcada et al. [74] observed that melatonin implantation at a similar date was unable to lead to the resumption of reproductive activity before the onset of the natural breeding season. This suggests that goats and sheep differ in their sensitivity to the photoperiod or melatonin implants.

Commercially, melatonin treatment is recommended in association with the male effect. Since the 1940s, it has been assumed that females must be kept from any contact with males for the male effect to occur. However, little experimental data are available on the minimum period of isolation or the minimum distance between males and females required, but normally, a separation of at least 3 weeks is recommended. Thereafter, the sudden reintroduction of males causes an increase in the frequency of gonadotropin-releasing hormone/LH pulses in anovulatory females and the strongly synchronous induction of ovulation.

Melatonin treatments that begin 30 and 45 days prior to the joining of the sexes in sheep and goats, respectively, have been shown the most efficient in many breeds in terms of increasing fertility and litter size and in advancing and compacting lambing patterns [75].

Gatica et al. [76] recently showed reproductive performance to be slightly greater when both sexes received melatonin compared with the treatment of females alone and much better than treating males alone. The exogenous dose, however, needs to be sufficient to maintain elevated plasma melatonin concentrations [74]. Commercial melatonin implants contain 18 mg of the hormone and release it for about 10 weeks, raising daytime concentrations to about 100 pg/ml in goats [77] and ewes [78].

Treatment with exogenous melatonin has been shown to increase fecundity, although the degree to which this occurs varies widely depending on the breed and the moment of treatment; the number of extra kids born per 100 treated females ranges from 15 to 40 [69,78–81]. This increase in prolificacy seems to be due to a direct effect of melatonin on the ovaries, increasing the ovulation rate by reducing the rate of atresia of preovulatory follicles [82].

Rodriguez-Osorio et al. [83] report melatonin (10 nM) to have a positive effect on porcine embryo cleavage rates and blastocyst total cell numbers. In addition, adding melatonin in a culture medium improved the rate of development of thawed ovine blastocysts, with higher hatching rates after 24 hours of culture [84]. Recently, it has been shown that in vivo melatonin treatment is beneficial for increasing ovarian follicle turnover and improving oocyte developmental competence and blastocyst kinetics [85]. Melatonin has also been successfully used to promote in vitro embryo development in mice [86], buffaloes [87], heifers [88], and sows [83,89]. Finally, Soares et al. [90] indicate that rat ovaries show an increase in the number of atretic follicles after pinealectomy.

21.4.2 Association between Light and Exogenous Melatonin

In high latitudes, melatonin implants need to be inserted closer to the summer solstice [68]. However, at Mediterranean latitudes, implanting at the spring equinox efficiently induces reproductive activity during seasonal anestrous in goats [65] and advances the onset of the breeding season in sheep [74]. The failure of melatonin to induce sexual activity in early spring at higher latitudes is thought to be due to the existence of a state of photorefractoriness to short days that impairs the animals' ability to respond to melatonin treatment. For this reason, treatment with long days is recommended before melatonin implantation when attempting to advance the breeding season in goats and sheep living at high latitudes. Under field conditions, the long-day part of the treatment is easy, as extra illumination can be provided either indoors or outdoors (Figure 21.3) [68]. The duration of the long-day treatment needs to be at least 2.5 months [91]. The effect on reproductive performance of this combination has been shown in sheep and goats. It appears that long days plus melatonin is more efficient than melatonin alone, which in turn is more effective than no treatment [92].

21.5 CONCLUDING REMARKS

The photoperiod is the main environmental factor that controls reproductive activity in small ruminants, melatonin being the hormone that transduces photoperiodic information.

To induce reproductive activity, a transition from long to short days is necessary; long days treatment is feasible under field conditions using an artificial photoperiod or using the natural photoperiod with a light pulse during the night. Short days can be simulated using exogenous melatonin implants.

Melatonin implants strongly induce reproductive activity during seasonal anestrus in sheep and goats, although in different ways. More studies are needed to determine the most efficient protocols for this treatment.

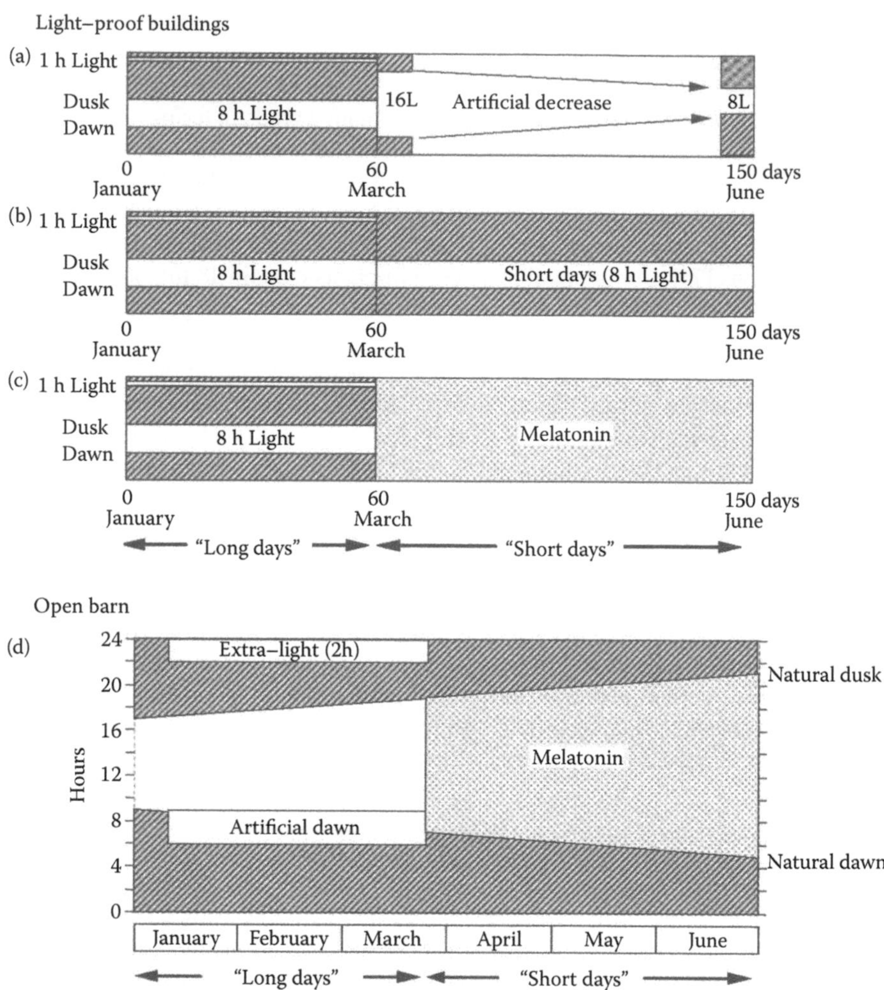

FIGURE 21.3 Photoperiod and melatonin treatments used to control the seasonality of reproduction in sheep and goats. (From Chemineau, P., et al., *INRA Prod. Anim.* 1996;9:45–60. With permission.)

REFERENCES

1. Shelton, M. 1978. Reproduction and breeding of goats. *Journal of Dairy Science* 61: 994–1010.
2. Ortavant, R., Pelletier, J., Ravault, J.P., Thimonier, J., Voland-Nail, P. 1985. Photoperiod: Main proximal and distal factor of the circannual cycle of reproduction in farm animals. In: Clarke, J.R. (Ed.), *Oxford Reviews of Reproductive Biology*. Oxford University Press, Oxford, pp. 305–345.
3. Chemineau, P., Daveau, A., Maurice, F., Delgadillo, J.A. 1992. Seasonality of estrus and ovulation is not modified by subjecting female alpine goats to a tropical photoperiod. *Small Ruminant Research* 8: 299–312.
4. Malpaux, B., Chemineau, P., Pelletier, J. 1992. Melatonin and reproduction in sheep and goats. In: Hing-Sing Yu and Reiter, R.J. (Ed.). *Melatonin Biosynthesis, Physiological Effects, and Clinical Applications*. CRC Press, Boca Raton, FL, pp. 253–289.
5. Zarazaga, L.A., Guzmán, J.L., Domínguez, C., Pérez, M.C., Prieto, R. 2009. Effects of season and feeding level on reproductive activity and semen quality in Payoya buck goats. *Theriogenology* 71: 1316–1325.
6. Duarte, G., Nava-Hernández, M.P, Malpaux, B., Delgadillo, J.A. 2010. Ovulatory activity of female goats adapted to the subtropics is responsive to photoperiod. *Animal Reproduction Science* 120: 65–70.
7. Zarazaga, L.A., Guzmán, J.L., Domínguez, C., Pérez, M.C., Prieto, R. 2005. Effect of plane of nutrition on seasonality of reproduction in Spanish Payoya goats. *Animal Reproduction Science* 87: 253–267.

8. Yeates, N.T.M. 1949. The breeding season of the sheep with particular reference to its modification by artificial light. *Journal of Agricultural Science, Cambridge*, 39: 1–43.
9. Thwaites, C.J. 1965. Photoperiodic control of breeding activity in the Southdown ewe with particular reference to the effects of an equatorial light regime. *Journal of Agricultural Science, Cambridge* 65: 57–64.
10. Thimonier, J., Mauléon, P. 1969. Variations saisonnières du comportement d'oestrus et des activités ovarienne et hypophysaire chez les ovins. *Annales de Biologie Animale, Biochimie, Biophysique* 9: 223–250.
11. Pelletier, J., Ortavant, R. 1970. Influence du photopériodisme sur les activités sexuelle, hypophysaire et hypothalamique du bélier Ile-de-France. *Colloque International CNRS* 172: 483–495.
12. Celi, I., Guzmán, J.L., Gatica, M.C., Malpaux, B., Zarazaga, L.A. 2010. Photoperiodic control of luteinizing hormone secretion is influenced by nutrition in Mediterranean goats. *10th International Conference on goats, International Goat Association, IGA,* Recife (Brasil) 19–23 September 2010.
13. Ortavant, R., Thibault, C. 1956. Influence de la durée d'éclairement sur les productions spermatiques du bélier. *Comptes Rendus des Séances de la Société de Biologie* 150: 358–362.
14. Mauléon, P., Rougeot, J. 1962. Régulation des saisons sexuelles chez des brebis de races différentes au moyen de divers rythmes lumineux. *Annales de Biologie Animale, Biochimie, Biophysique* 2: 209–222.
15. Karsch, F.J., Bittman, E.L., Foster, D.L., Goodman, R.L., Legan, S.J., Robinson, J.E. 1984. Neuroendocrine basis of seasonal reproduction. *Recent Progress in Hormone Research* 40: 185–232.
16. Chemineau, P., Pelletier, J., Guérin, Y. et al. 1988. Photoperiodic and melatonin treatments for the control of seasonal reproduction in sheep and goats. *Reproduction Nutrition Development* 28: 409–422.
17. D'Occhio, M.J., Schanbacher, B.D., Kinder, J.E. 1984. Profiles of luteinizing hormone, follicle-stimulating hormone, testosterone and prolactin in rams of diverse breeds: Effects of contrasting short (8L:16D) and long (16L:8D) photoperiods. *Biology of Reproduction* 30: 1039–1054.
18. Zarazaga, L.A., Gatica, M.C., Celi, I., Guzmán, J.L., Malpaux, B. 2010. Effect of artificial long days and/or melatonin treatment on the sexual activity of Mediterranean. *Small Ruminant Research*, in press. doi:10.1016/j.smallrumres.2010.05.008.
19. Delgadillo, J.A., Chemineau, P. 1992. Abolition of the seasonal release of Luteinizing Hormone and testosterone in Alpine male-goats (*Capra hircus*) by short photoperiodic cycles. *Journal of Reproduction and Fertility* 94: 45–55.
20. Thimonier, J. 1989. Contrôle photopériodique de l'activité ovulatoire chez la brebis. Existence de rythmes endogénes. Thèse Doctorale Université de Tours, 112 pp.
21. Robinson, J.E., Wayne, N.L., Karsch, F.J. 1985. Refractoriness to inhibitory daylength initiates the breeding season of the Suffolk ewe. *Biology of Reproduction* 32: 1024–1030.
22. Malpaux, B., Robinson, J.E., Wayne, N.L., Karsch, F.J. 1989. Regulation of the onset of the breeding season of the ewe: Importance of long days and of an endogenous reproductive rhythm. *Journal of Endocrinology* 122: 269–278.
23. Worthy, K., Haresign, W. 1983. Evidence that the onset of seasonal anoestrus in the ewe may be independent of increasing prolactin concentrations and daylenght. *Journal of Reproduction and Fertility* 69: 41–48.
24. Robinson, J.E., Karsch, F.J. 1984. Refractoriness to inductive day lengths terminates the breeding season of the Suffolk ewe. *Biology of Reproduction* 31: 656–663.
25. Robinson, J.E., Karsch, F.J. 1988. Timing the breeding season of the ewe: What is the role of daylength? *Reproduction Nutrition Development* 28: 365–374.
26. Wayne, N.L., Malpaux, B., Karsch, F.J. 1990. Photoperiodic requirements for timing onset and duration of the breeding season of the ewe: Synchronization of an endogenous rhythm of reproduction. *Journal of Comparative Physiology A: Sensory, Neural, and Behavioral Physiology* 166: 835–842.
27. Jackson, G.L., Gibson, M., Kuehl, D. 1988. Photoperiodic disruption of photorefractoriness in the ewe. *Biology of Reproduction* 38: 127–134.
28. Sweeney, T., Donovan, A., Roche, J.F., O'Callaghan, D. 1997. Variation in the ability of a long day followed by a short day photoperiod signal to initiate reproductive activity in ewes at different times of the year. *Journal of Reproduction and Fertility* 109: 121–127.
29. Cassone, V.M., Natesan, A.K. 1997. Time and time again: The phylogeny of melatonin as a transducer of biological time. *Journal of Biological Rhythms* 12: 532–534.
30. Itoh, M.T., Ishizuka, B., Kuribayashi, Y., Amemiya, A., Sumi, Y. 1999. Melatonin, its precursors, and synthesizing enzyme activities in the human ovary. *Molecular Human Reproduction* 5: 402–408.
31. Møller, M., Baeres, F.M.M. 2002. The anatomy and innervation of the mammalian pineal gland. *Cell and Tissue Research* 309: 139–150.

32. Legan, S.J., Winans, S.S. 1981. The photoneuroendocrine control of seasonal breeding in the ewe. *General and Comparative Endocrinology* 45: 317–328.
33. Tessonneaud, A., Locatelli, A., Caldani, M., Viguier-Martinez, M.C. 1995. Bilateral lesions of the suprachiasmatic nuclei alter the nocturnal melatonin secretion in sheep. *Journal of Neuroendocrinology* 7: 145–152.
34. Buttle, H.L., 1977. The effect o anterior cervical ganglionectomy on the seasonal variation in prolactin concentration in goats. *Neuroendocrinology* 23: 121–128.
35. Barrell, G.K., Lapwood, K.R. 1979. Effects of modifying olfactory and pineal gland function on the seasonality of semen production and plasma luteinizing hormone, testosterone and prolactin levels in rams. *Animal Reproduction Science* 1: 229–243.
36. Lincoln, G.A. 1979. Photoperiodic control of seasonal breeding in the ram: Participation of the cranial sympathetic nervous system. *Journal of Endocrinology* 82: 135–147.
37. Bittman, E.L., Karsch, F.J., Hopkins, J.W. 1983. Role of the pineal gland in ovine photoperiodism: Regulation of seasonal breeding and negative feedback effects of estradiol upon luteinizing hormone secretion. *Endocrinology* 113: 329–336.
38. Klein, D.C., Coon, S.L., Roseboom, P.H. et al. 1997. The melatonin rhythm-generating enzyme: Molecular regulation of serotonin *N*-acetyltransferase in the pineal gland. *Recent Progress in Hormone Research* 52: 307–358.
39. Ceinos, R.M., Chansard, M., Revel, F., Calgary, C., Míguez, J.M., Simonneaux, V. 2004. Analysis of adrenergic regulation of melatonin synthesis in Siberian hamster pineal emphasizes the role of HIOMT. *Neurosignals* 13: 308–317.
40. Duvernoy, H.M., Parratte, B., Tatu, L., Vuillier, F. 2000. The human pineal gland: Relationships with surrounding structures and blood supply. *Neurological Research* 22: 747–790.
41. Zarazaga, L.A., Celi, C., Guzmán, J.L., Malpaux, B. 2010. Melatonin concentrations in the two jugular veins, and relationship with the seasonal reproductive activity in goats. *Theriogenology* 74: 221–228.
42. Zarazaga, L.A., Todini, L., Chemineau, P., Marnet, P.-G., Locatelli, A., Malpaux, B. 2010. Nocturnal melatonin concentrations vary dramatically between the two jugular veins in most individual sheep maintained under mimicked or natural photoperiod. *Research in Veterinary Science* 88: 233–238.
43. Ravault, J.P., Chesneau, D. 1999. The onset of increased melatonin secretion after the onset of darkness in sheep depends on the photoperiod. *Journal of Pineal Research* 27: 1–8.
44. Coon S.L., Zarazaga L.A., Malpaux B. et al. 1999. Genetic variability in plasma melatonin in sheep is due to pineal weight, not to variations in enzyme activities. *American Journal of Physiology* 277: E792–E797.
45. Lincoln, G.A., Ebling, F.J.P., Almeida, O.F.X. 1985. Generation of melatonin rhythms. In: *Photoperiodims, Melatonin and the Pineal. Ciba Foundation Symposium*, 117, Pittman, London, 129.
46. Viguier-Martínez, M.-C., Ravault, J.-P. 1989. *Circadian rhythms in the Ile-de-France rams: Influence of the light.* Presented at 20ème congrès Groupe d'études des Rythmes Biologiques, Besançon, France, March 30 to 31, 1989.
47. Ravault, J.P., Arendt, J., Tobler, I., Chesneau, I., Moulin, O. 1989. Entrainment of melatonin rhythms in rams by symmetrical light–dark cycles of different period length. *Chronobiology International* 6: 329–339.
48. Ebling, F.J.P., Lincoln, G.A., Wollnik, F., Anderson, N. 1988. Effects of constant darkness and constant light on circadian organization and reproductive responses in the ram. *Journal of Biological Rhythms* 3: 365–384.
49. English, J., Arendt, J., Symons, A.M., Poulton, A.L., Tobler, I. 1988. Pineal and ovarian response to 22- and 24-h days in the ewe. *Biology of Reproduction* 39: 9–18.
50. Brinklow, B.R., Forbes, J.M., Rodway, R.G. 1984. Melatonin in the plasma of growing sheep subjected to short and skeleton long photoperiods. *Experientia* 40: 758–760.
51. Maeda, K., Mori, Y., Sawasaki, T., Kano, Y. 1984. Diurnal changes in peripheral melatonin concentration in goats and effects of light or dark interruption. *Japanese Journal of Veterinary Science* 46: 837–842.
52. Earl, C.R., D'Occhio, M.J., Kennaway, D.J., Seamark, R.F. 1985. Serum melatonin profiles and endocrine responses of ewes exposed to a pulse light late in the dark phase. *Endocrinology* 117: 226–230.
53. Ravault, J.P., Thimonier, J. 1988. Melatonin patterns in ewes maintained under skeleton or resonance photoperiodic regimens. *Reproduction Nutrition Development* 28: 473–486.
54. Earl, C.R., D'Occhio, M.J., Kennaway, D.J., Seamark, R.F. 1990. Mechanisms controlling the offset of melatonin secretion in the ewe. *Journal of Pineal Research* 8: 49–56.
55. Zarazaga, L.A., Malpaux, B., Guillaume, D., Bodin, L., Chemineau, P. 1998. Genetic variability in melatonin cocentrations in ewes originates in its synthesis, not in its catabolism. *American Journal of Physiology* 274: E1086–E1090.

56. Chemineau, P., Malpaux, B., Brillard, J.P., Fostier, A. 2007. Seasonality of reproduction and production in farm fishes, birds and mammals. *Animal* 1: 419–423.
57. Chemineau, P., Guillaume, D., Migaud, M., Thiéry, J.C., Pellicer-Rubio, M.T., Malpaux, B. 2008. Seasonality of reproduction in mammals: Intimate regulatory mechanisms and practical implications. *Reproduction in Domestic Animals* 43: 40–47.
58. Arendt, J., Symons, A.M., Laud, C.A., Pryde, S.J. 1983. Melatonin can induce early onset of the breeding season in ewes. *Journal of Endocrinology* 97: 395–400.
59. Bittman, E.L., Dempsey, R.J., Karsch, F.J. 1983. Pineal melatonin secretion drives the reproductive response to daylength in the ewe. *Endocrinology* 113: 2276–2283.
60. Ronayne, E., Jordan, B., Quirke, J.F., Roche, J.F. 1989. The effect of frequency of administration of melatonin on the time of onset of the breeding season in anoestrous ewes. *Animal Reproduction Science* 18: 13–24.
61. Nowak, R., Rodway, R.G. 1985. Effect of intravaginal implants of melatonin on the onset of ovarian activity in adult and prepubertal ewes. *Journal of Reproduction and Fertility* 74: 287–293.
62. Kumar, S., Purohit, G.N. 2009. Effect of a single subcutaneous injection of melatonin on estrous response and conception rate in goats. *Small Ruminant Research* 82: 152–155.
63. Poulton, A.L., Symons, A.M., Kelly, M.I., Arendt, J. 1987. Intraruminal soluble glass boluses containing melatonin can induce early onset of ovarian activity in ewes. *Journal of Reproduction and Fertility* 80: 235–239.
64. English, J., Poulton, A.L., Arendt, J., Symons, A.M. 1986. A comparison of the efficiency of melatonin treatments in advancing oestrus in ewes. *Journal of Reproduction and Fertility* 77: 321–327.
65. Zarazaga L.A., Gatica, M.C., Celi, I., Guzmán, J.L., Malpaux, B. 2009. Effect of melatonin implants on sexual activity in Mediterranean goat females without separation from males. *Theriogenology* 72: 910–918.
66. Bittman, E.L., Kaynard, A.H., Olster, D.H. 1985. Pineal melatonin mediates photoperiodic control of pulsatile luteinizing hormone secretion in the ewe. *Neuroendocrinology* 40: 409–418.
67. Chemineau, P., Normant, E., Ravault, J.P., Thimonier, J. 1986. Induction and persistence of pituitary and ovarian activity in the out-of-season lactating dairy goats after a treatment combining a skeleton photoperiod, melatonin and the male effect. *Journal of Reproduction and Fertility* 78: 497–504.
68. Chemineau, P., Malpaux, B., Pelletier, J. et al. 1996. Use of melatonin implants and photoperiodic treatments to control seasonal reproduction in sheep and goats. *INRA Productions Animales* 9: 45–60 (in French, with English abstract).
69. McMillan, W.H., Sealey, R.C. 1989. Do melatonin implants influence the breeding season in Coopworth ewes? *Proceedings of the New Zealand Society of Animal Production* 49: 43–46.
70. Haresign, W., Peters, A.R., Staples, L.D., 1990. The effect of melatonin implants on breeding activity and litter size in commercial sheep flocks in the UK. *Animal Production* 50: 111–121.
71. Martin, G.B., Tjondronegoro, S., Boukhliq, R. et al. 1999. Determinants of the annual pattern of reproduction in mature male Merino and Suffolk sheep: Modification of endogenous rhythms by photoperiod. *Reproduction, Fertility and Development* 11: 355–366.
72. Forcada, F., Abecia, J.A., Lozano, J.M., Ferrer, L.M., Lacasta, D. 1999. The effects on reproductive performance in the short and medium term of the combined use of exogenous melatonin and progestagen pessaries in ewes with a short seasonal anoestrous period. *Veterinary Research Communications* 23: 257–263.
73. Forcada, F., Abecia, J.A., Zúñiga, O., Lozano, J.M. 2002. Variation in the ability of melatonin implants inserted at two different times after the winter solstice to restore reproductive activity in reduced seasonality ewes. *Australian Journal of Agricultural Research* 53: 167–173.
74. Forcada, F., Zarazaga L., Abecia, J.A. 1995. Effect of exogenous melatonin and plane of nutrition after weaning on estrous activity, endocrine status and ovulation rate in Salz ewes lambing in the seasonal anestrus. *Theriogenology* 43: 1179–1193.
75. Chemineau, P., Vandaele, E., Brice, G., Jardon, C. 1991. Utilisation des implants de mélatonine pour l'amélioration des performances de reproduction chez la brebis. *Recueil de Médicine Vétérinaire* 167: 227–239.
76. Gatica, M.C., Guzmán, J.L., Celi, I., Malpaux, B., Zarazaga, L.A. 2010. Breed effect on the use of melatonin implants in Mediterranean goats. 10th International Conference on goats, International Goat Association, IGA, Recife (Brasil) 19–23 September 2010.
77. Delgadillo, J.A., Carrillo, E., Morán, J., Duarte, G., Chemineau, P., Malpaux, B. 2001. Induction of sexual activity of male creole goats in subtropical northern Mexico using long days and melatonin. *Journal of Animal Science* 79: 2245–2252.

78. Staples, L., McPhee, S., Reeve, J., Williams, A. H. 1991. Practical applications for controlled release melatonin implants in sheep. In: Foldes, A., Reiter, R. J. (Ed.). *Advances in Pineal Research.* 6th ed. John Libbey & Co., London, pp. 199–208.
79. Moore, R.W., Miller, C.M., Dow, B.W., Staples, L.D. 1988. Effects of melatonin on erarly breeding of F+ and ++ Boorola x Perendale and Romney ewes. *Proceedings of the New Zealand Society of Animal Production* 48: 109–111.
80. Maqueda, A., Portero, F., Deletang, F., Martino. 2001. Utilización de implantes de melatonina en corderas merinas durante el anoestro estacional. Comparación de su uso en la Sierra Norte de Sevilla en dos rebaños distintos. *XXVI Jornadas Científicas y V Internaciones de la Sociedad Española de Ovinotecnia y Caprinotecnia, (SEOC)*, pp. 1046–1051.
81. Puntas, J., Rodríguez, B., Azor, M^{a}D. et al. 2001. Melatonina en ovino segureño. *XXVI Jornadas Científicas y V Internaciones de la Sociedad Española de Ovinotecnia y Caprinotecnia, (SEOC)*, pp. 1085–1090.
82. Bister, J.L., Noël, B., Perrad, B., Mandiki, S.N.M., Mbayahaga, J., Paquay, R. 1999. Control of ovarian follicles activity in the ewe. *Domestic Animal Endocrinology* 17: 315–328.
83. Rodriguez-Osorio N, Kim IJ, Wang H, Kaya A, Memili E. 2007. Melatonin increases cleavage rate of porcine preimplantation embryos in vitro. *Journal of Pineal Research* 43: 283–288.
84. Abecia, J.A., Forcada, F., Zúñiga, O. 2002. The effect of melatonin on the secretion of progesterone in sheep and on the development of ovine embryos in vitro. *Veterinary Research Communications* 26: 151–158.
85. Berlinguer, F., Leoni, G.G., Succu, S. et al. 2009. Exogenous melatonin positively influences follicular dynamics, oocyte developmental competence and blastocyst output in a goat model. *Journal of Pineal Research* 46: 383–391.
86. Ishizuka, B., Kuribayashi, Y., Murai, K., Amemiya, A., Itoh, M.T. 2000. The effect of melatonin on in vitro fertilization and embryo development in mice. *Journal of Pineal Research* 28: 48–51.
87. Manjunatha, B.M., Devaraj, M., Gupta, P.S.P., Ravindra, J.P., Nandi, S. 2009. Effect of taurine and melatonin in the culture medium on buffalo in vitro embryo development. *Reproduction in Domestic Animals* 44: 12–16.
88. Papis, K., Poleszczuk, O., Wenta-Muchalska, E., Modlinski, J.A. 2007. Melatonin effect on bovine embryo development in vitro in relation to oxygen concentration. *Journal of Pineal Research* 43: 321–326.
89. Kang, J.-T., Koo, O.-J., Kwon, D.-K. et al. 2009. Effects of melatonin on in vitro maturation of porcine oocyte and expression of melatonin receptor RNA in cumulus and granulosa cells. *Journal of Pineal Research* 46: 22–28.
90. Soares JM Jr, Simões MJ, Oshima CT, Mora OA, De Lima GR, Baracat EC. 2003. Pinealectomy changes rat ovarian interstitial cell morphology and decreases progesterone receptor expression. *Gynecological Endocrinology* 17: 115–123.
91. Delgadillo, J.A., Flores, J.A., Véliz, F.G. et al. 2002. Induction of sexual activity in lactating anovulatory female goats using male goats treated only with artificially long days. *Journal of Animal Science* 80: 2780–2786.
92. Chemineau, P., Malpaux, B., Delgadillo, J.A. et al. 1992. Control of sheep and goat reproduction: Use of light and melatonin. *Animal Reproduction Science* 30: 157–184.

22 Melatonin in the Pancreatic Protection and Modulation of Pancreatic Exocrine Secretion

Jolanta Jaworek

CONTENTS

22.1 INTRODUCTION

Melatonin (5-methoxy-*N*-acetyltryptamine) has been discovered in the pineal gland by Aaron Lerner, a dermatologist from Yale University, more than 50 years ago [1]. This indoleamine is produced from the amino acid L-tryptophan in a reaction controlled by specific enzymes, two of them are arylalkylamino-*N*-acetyl-serotonin-transferase (AA-NAT) and hydroxyindolo-*O*-methyl-transferase (HIOMT) [2]. Secretion of this pineal product is directed by the suprachiasmatic nucleus in response to light/dark cycles, with a peak at night and reduction during the day [3]. Melatonin is best known as a regulator of seasonal and circadian rhythms, but the physiological role of this substance has been unclear for many years [4].

Melatonin remains the subject of many studies because of its unique anti-inflammatory and antioxidative properties [5,6]. It received considerable attention as scavenger of reactive oxygen and nitrogen species (ROS and RNS, respectively) protecting the cells from the injury caused by these free radicals [5–8]. In healthy organisms, low amounts of ROS are generated in the mitochondria and immediately neutralized by natural nonenzymatic scavengers (one of them is melatonin) or by the antioxidant enzymes such as superoxide dismutase (SOD), catalase (CAT), or glutathione peroxidase (GPx) [6–8]. Increased production of ROS and RNS during inflammatory reactions leads to the oxidants/antioxidants imbalance in the inflamed tissue [9]. Melatonin as a lipophilic substance easily penetrates inside the cells to preserve antioxidant enzyme activities, protect the mitochondria from oxidative damage, and stabilize lipid membranes from peroxidation [10]. It is worth to remember that beside its antioxidative properties, melatonin is also able to improve the immune defense of the organism. Currently recognized anti-inflammatory activities of melatonin include promotion of macrophages and B lymphocytes, modulation of nitric oxide, prostaglandins generation, and reduction of proinflammatory interleukin (IL), such as tumor necrosis factor α (TNF-α), IL-1β, IL-6, or IL-8 [11–15]. It was also reported that melatonin stimulates the production of vascular endothelial growth factor (VEGF), promotes angiogenesis, accelerates the wound healing, and decreases the scar formation [16,17]. Recent reports have shown that melatonin could influence the processes of apoptosis [18].

Melatonin binds to the specific G-protein-coupled receptors (MT): MT_1R, MT_2R, and MT_3R [19]. Intracellular orphan receptors for melatonin (ROR/RZR) have also been detected in the nucleus, cytoplasm, and mitochondria; however, the physiological significance of these receptors remains unclear [20]. In addition, melatonin, being highly lipophilic, could cross the cell membranes to influence the intracellular processes in the receptor-independent way [10].

22.2 PRESENCE OF MELATONIN IN THE GASTROINTESTINAL TRACT AND PANCREAS

Melatonin is produced in many tissues, and the gastrointestinal tract (GIT) appears as the main source of this substance [21]. As was calculated by Huether [22], the amount of this indoleamine in the gastrointestinal system exceeds 400 times the content of melatonin in the pineal gland. In the GIT, melatonin is synthesized in the enteroendocrine cells and released in response to food ingestion independent of the light/dark cycle [23,24]. Oral administration of the melatonin precursor L-tryptophan resulted in the increase of melatonin plasma level, and this observation has been stated also in the pinealectomized animals, indicating that synthesis of melatonin in the GIT is independent from the pineal gland [25,26].

Recently, melatonin has been localized in the pancreas by radioimmunoassay; however, melatonin immunolabeling in the pancreatic tissue was somewhat lower than that observed in the stomach and in the duodenum [27]. In our previous study, we have shown the presence of gene expression for AA-NAT, an enzyme involved in the synthesis of melatonin from L-tryptophan in the rat pancreas [28]. Subsequently, we have demonstrated the signal for HIOMT, another enzyme controlling the above reaction in the human pancreas, confirming the ability of the pancreatic gland to produce melatonin [29]. It is interesting that melatonin content in the pancreas undergoes rhythmic diurnal/nocturnal fluctuations, and in diabetic patients, the concentration of melatonin in the pancreas was significantly lower than in healthy individuals [30].

Melatonin membrane receptors MT_1 and MT_2 have been detected in the human pancreatic tissue in the islet of Langerhans, and it is very likely that melatonin takes part in the regulation of insulin release [31–33]. Melatonin receptors undergoes up-regulation in the diabetic patients, and recent data suggest that increased expression of MT_1B receptors may contribute to the pathogenesis of type 2 diabetes [34–36].

Despite the presence of melatonin in the pancreas and melatonin receptors in the pancreatic tissue, the role of this substance in the physiological regulation of pancreatic functions is still not complete.

22.3 PROTECTIVE EFFECTS OF MELATONIN IN ACUTE PANCREATITIS

Beneficial effect of melatonin has been demonstrated in many tissues [37–40]. Because of this antioxidative and anti-inflammatory activities, melatonin appears highly effective protector against the damage caused by oxidative stress and inflammation [41–43].

In the pancreas, protective effect of melatonin was first observed by Qi et al. about 10 years ago [44]. Our subsequent study in the rat supported and reinforced the above observations and revealed that pretreatment with the melatonin precursor L-tryptophan attenuated pancreatic tissue damage caused by acute inflammation and reduced lipid peroxidation in two models of acute pancreatitis: cerulein-induced and ischemia/reperfusion pancreatitis [28]. Protective effect of L-tryptophan was similar to melatonin. In addition, intraduodenal administration of this amino acid melatonin precursor produced significant and dose-dependent rise of plasma melatonin level (Figure 22.1). The above observations led to the conclusion that endogenous melatonin produced from L-tryptophan can protect the pancreas against acute inflammation [28]. The beneficial effect of melatonin or L-tryptophan on acute pancreatitis was manifested by dose-dependent reduction in lipase blood

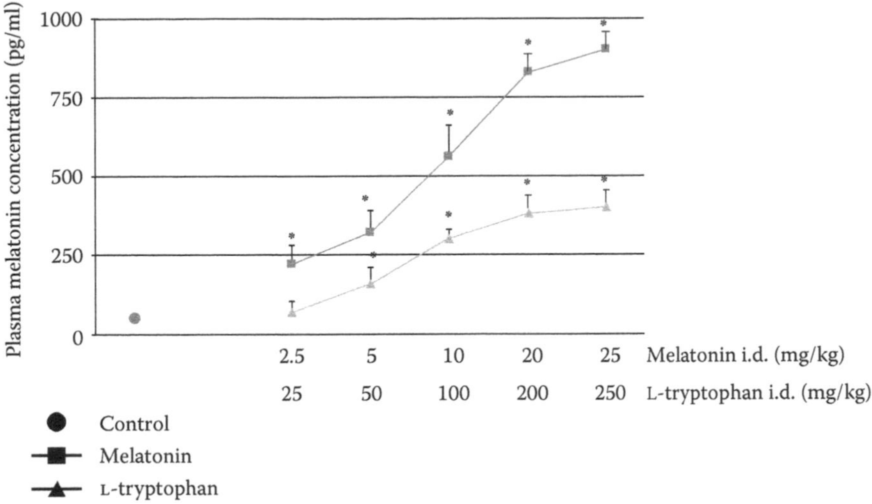

FIGURE 22.1 Effect of intraduodenal administration of various doses of melatonin or its precursor, L-tryptophan, on plasma concentration of melatonin. Means ± SEM from the separate experiments, each performed on six to eight rats. *Significant ($p < 0.01$) increase above the control value.

levels (Figure 22.2). Administration of melatonin or its amino acid precursor to the animals prior to the induction of acute pancreatitis resulted in the marked decrease of the lipid peroxidation product MDA + 4HNE in the pancreatic tissue. It was correlated with significant reduction of pro-inflammatory IL-1β and marked rise of anti-inflammatory IL-10 blood level observed in the animals with acute pancreatitis pretreated with melatonin or with L-tryptophan (Figures 22.3 and 22.4). Pretreatment with melatonin or with its precursor resulted in the significant and dose-dependent increase of antioxidant enzyme GPx activity in the pancreatic tissue taken from the rats with acute

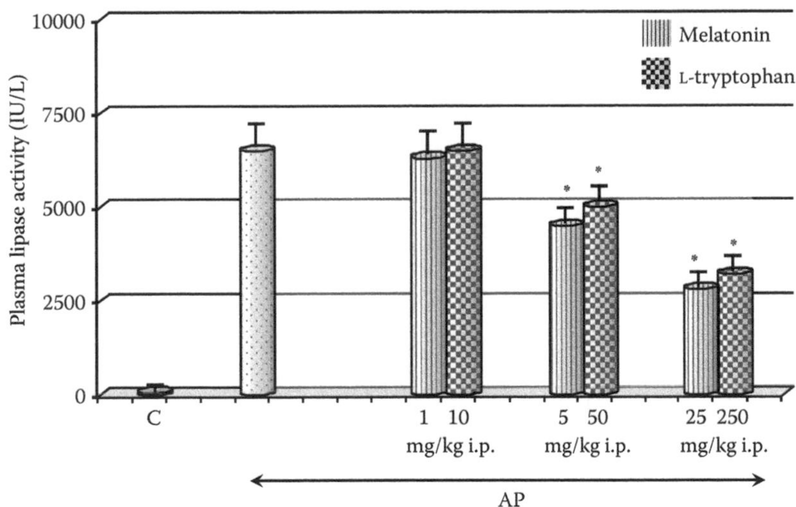

FIGURE 22.2 Effects of increasing doses of melatonin or L-tryptophan given intraperitoneally on plasma lipase activity in the rats with acute cerulein-induced pancreatitis (AP). Means ± SEM from the separate experiments, each performed on eight rats. *Significant decrease ($p < 0.01$) below the value detected in AP rats alone. C = intact control.

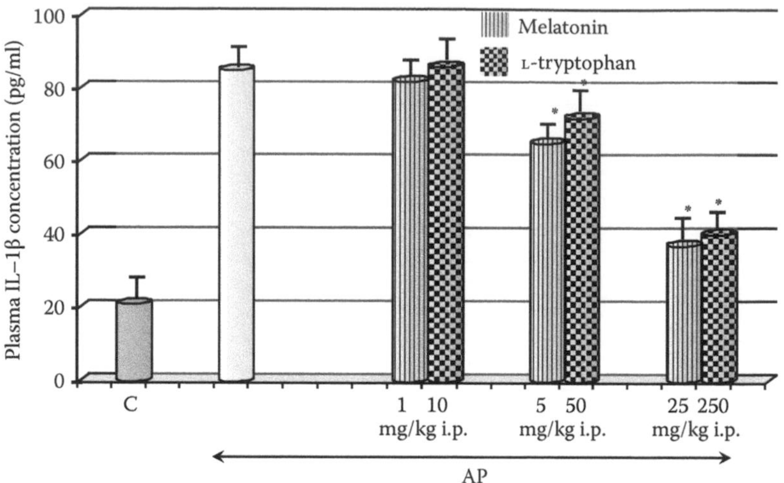

FIGURE 22.3 Effects of various concentrations of melatonin or L-tryptophan given intraperitoneally on plasma concentration of IL-1β in the rats with acute pancreatitis induced by cerulein overstimulation (AP). Means ± SEM from the separate experiments, each performed on 8–10 rats. Significant ($p < 0.01$) decrease below the value detected in AP rats alone. C = intact control.

pancreatitis (Figure 22.5). The protective effects of these substances were verified by the significant attenuation of histological manifestations of pancreatitis [28].

Subsequent studies, using different models of experimental pancreatitis, confirmed the notion that melatonin attenuates acute pancreatitis severity and the diminished harmful effects of acute inflammation. Melatonin is effective in pancreatic protection against the damage induced by L-arginine [45], ischemia/reperfusion, and cerulein overstimulation [18,28,44–47]. However, in pancreatitis induced by glycodeoxycholic acid, melatonin did not influence the serum amylase and failed

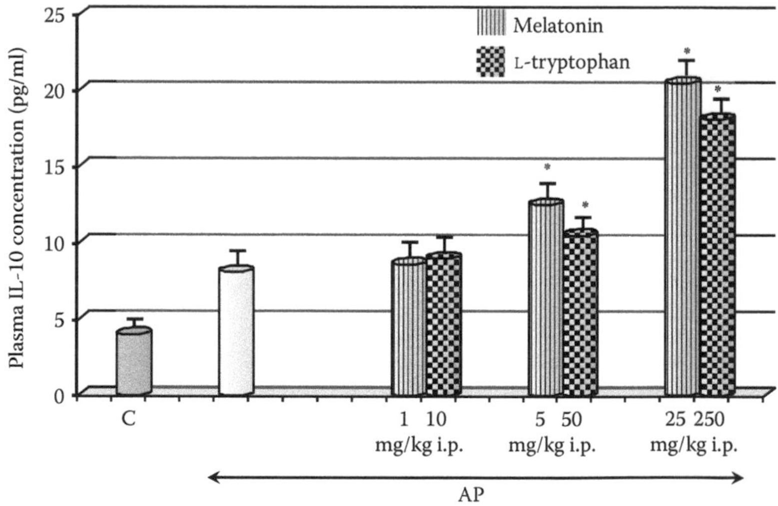

FIGURE 22.4 Plasma concentration of IL-10 in the rats with acute cerulein-induced pancreatitis (AP) alone or in the animals with acute pancreatitis pretreated with various concentrations of melatonin or L-tryptophan given intraperitoneally. Means ± SEM from the separate experiments, each performed on 8 to 10 rats. *Significant ($p < 0.01$) increase above the value detected in AP rats alone. C = intact control.

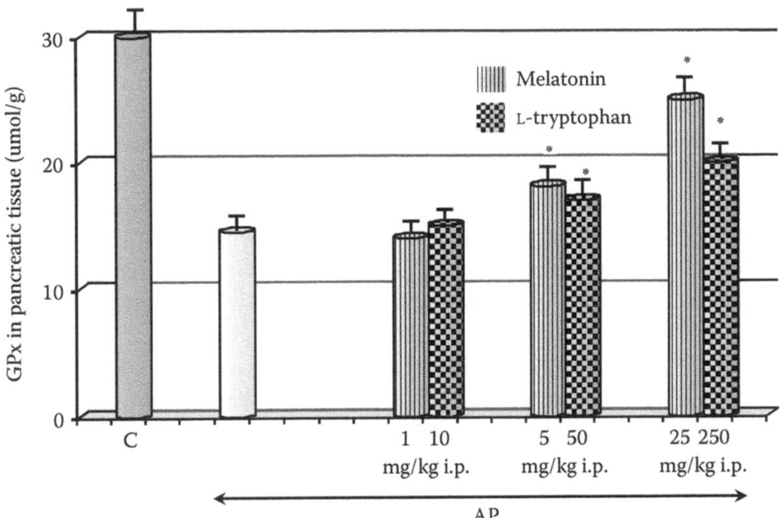

FIGURE 22.5 Pancreatic content of GPx in the rats subjected to cerulein-induced pancreatitis (AP) with or without pretreatment with melatonin or L-tryptophan given intraperitoneally. Means ± SEM from the separate experiments, each performed on 8 to 10 rats. *Significant increase above the value detected in AP rats alone. C = intact control.

to affect the mortality rate [48]. Melatonin has been reported to protect the pancreas against the damage caused by taurocholic acid [49] or by obstruction of pancreatic duct [50,51].

The beneficial effect of melatonin could be explained on several ways:

1. Melatonin acts as an antioxidant that can directly scavenge free radicals in many tissues including the pancreas [15,18,44,45,47,48,50,52].
2. Melatonin can improve the oxidative status of the pancreatic tissue indirectly through the activation of antioxidant enzymes such as SOD, CAT, GPx, GSH [13,18,45–47,50–52].
3. The pancreatoprotective effect of melatonin could be also attributed to the modulation of immune system because this indoleamine has been demonstrated to modulate lymphocyte proliferation [53], and recent report has shown that melatonin reduced mRNA expression of numerous proinflammatory cytokines such as IL-1 β, IL-6, IL-8, and TNF-α in the inflamed pancreas [13]. The influence of melatonin on the cytokine production was evidenced by the observation that melatonin and L-tryptophan, increased blood level of anti-inflammatory IL-10, and reduced proinflammatory IL-1β in animals with acute pancreatitis [11,49,54]. It was also shown that, in these animals, pretreatment with melatonin resulted in the decrease of proinflammatory TNF-α [28,49,55,56]. Protective effects of melatonin have also been related to the inhibition of neutrophil infiltration [28,49,52], improvement of pancreatic blood flow [28,52,56], decrease of myeloperoxidase level [13,48,50], reduction of prostaglandin generation [47], and limitation of apoptosis and necrosis in the inflamed pancreas [13].
4. In pancreatic acinar cell line AR42J incubated with melatonin, a significant increase of mRNA expression for heat shock protein (HSP60) was reported [57]. HSPs (chaperones), stimulated by high temperature, oxidative stress, or inflammation, are known to protect the cell compartment against damage [58]. It is likely that melatonin could directly affect the pancreatic acinar cells to protect them from the damage through the stimulation of HSP production. In pancreatic acinar cells, melatonin reduced the ultrastructural changes

caused by acute pancreatitis. Administration of this indoleamine prevented mitochondrial and nuclear damage, reduced the dilatation of endoplasmic reticulum and Golgi apparatus, and diminished formation of autophagosomes [45].

To date, little is known about the signaling pathway involved in the induction of defense mechanism directed by melatonin in acute pancreatitis. Recent study of Jung et al. demonstrated that melatonin increased expression of nuclear factor erythroid 2 (Nrf2)–related factor and reduced the nuclear binding of NFκB. Melatonin reduced the expression of iNOS, TNF-α, and others pro-inflammatory cytokines and increased antioxidant enzyme activities. It is proposed that activation of the Nrf2 pathway and inhibition of NFκB could be implicated in the curtailing of inflammation by melatonin [13].

It is noteworthy that pretreatment with melatonin, besides pancreatic protection, could reduce other organ damage induced by acute pancreatitis [5]. Under these conditions, administration of melatonin attenuated hepatic damage, which in turn might be beneficial for the prognosis of acute pancreatitis [59].

Recent report demonstrated that melatonin administration not only reduced the severity of acute pancreatitis but also promoted the spontaneous regeneration process of pancreatic tissue that was manifested by the improvement of nucleic acid content and rate of DNA synthesis in the melatonin-treated group of animals [54].

The beneficial effect of exogenous melatonin on acute pancreatitis has been confirmed in several studies. The question is: does endogenous melatonin produced in the organism take part in the physiological defense mechanisms of the pancreatic tissue?

Studies with luzindole, an antagonist of MT_2R, revealed that blockade of these receptors significantly aggravated pancreatic tissue damage in acute experimental pancreatitis. Pretreatment with luzindole produced significantly higher rises of amylase, lipase, and TNF-α blood levels in rats with acute pancreatic inflammation compared with those subjected to acute pancreatitis alone. This was accompanied by a huge accumulation of lipid peroxidation products in the pancreas, providing the

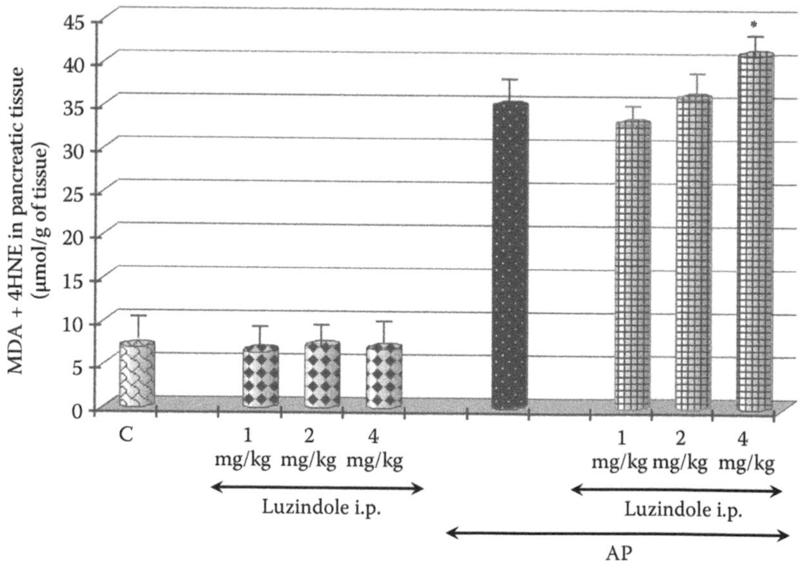

FIGURE 22.6 Pancreatic content of lipid peroxidation products MDA + 4HNE in the rats pretreated with luzindole, MT_2R antagonist, with or without cerulein-induced pancreatitis (AP). Means ± SEM from the separate experiments, each performed on six rats. Significant ($p < 0.05$) increase above the value detected in AP rats alone. C = intact control.

evidence of intense ROS generation [56] (Figure 22.6). Melatonin MT_2 receptors have been detected in the blood vessels, and activation of these receptors improved tissue blood flow [55,60]. It is very likely that beside its antioxidative properties, endogenous melatonin, through its MT_2 receptor, could ameliorate the pancreatic tissue from toxic inflammatory products such as cytokines and free radicals and thus could reinforce the pancreatic tissue resistance against acute damage.

The above observations suggest that endogenous melatonin could be the natural protector of the pancreatic tissue against the acute damage and could attenuate the intensity of the inflammatory processes in these gland. However, it is not clear if melatonin of pineal origin normally participates in the protection against acute pancreatitis. To answer this question, a study on rats with surgically removed pineal gland has been performed.

Pinealectomy significantly increased the severity of acute pancreatitis, aggravated histological manifestations of pancreatic inflammation, reduced antioxidant enzyme activity, and markedly augmented lipid peroxidation products in the pancreatic tissue of rats with acute pancreatitis as compared with sham-pinealectomized animals (Figure 22.7). In rats with removed pineal gland, melatonin blood level was undetectable. The above harmful effects of pinealectomy have been reversed by pretreatment with exogenous melatonin [61].

The hypothesis that pineal melatonin could be the natural protector of the pancreatic tissue against the acute damage is supported by previous data showing that circadian rhythm modulates the severity of acute pancreatitis. In experimental pancreatitis that was induced during the dark period, all morphological and biochemical parameters were less severe, compared with that observed during the day (Figure 22.8). Attenuation of pancreatitis observed at night was highly correlated with a high pancreatic SOD activity measured in the pancreas [52].

The above observations indicate that pineal melatonin contributes to pancreatic protection through the activation of the natural defense mechanism of pancreatic tissue as well as its direct and indirect antioxidant effects.

In conclusion, melatonin appears to be the natural pancreatic protector against the damage caused by acute inflammation. The beneficial effect of this indoleamine on acute pancreatitis involves several mechanisms such as (1) improvement of antioxidant defense of the pancreatic tissue (depending

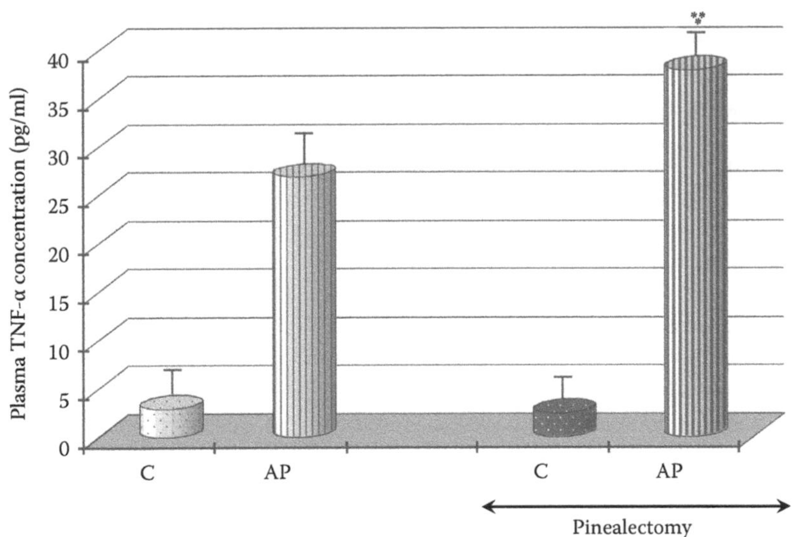

FIGURE 22.7 Effect of pinealectomy on TNF-α plasma concentration in the rats subjected to cerulein-induced pancreatitis (AP). Control = intact animals. Means ± SEM from the separate experiments, each performed on eight rats. *Significant ($p < 0.05$) increase above the values detected in the rat with intact pineal gland. C = intact control.

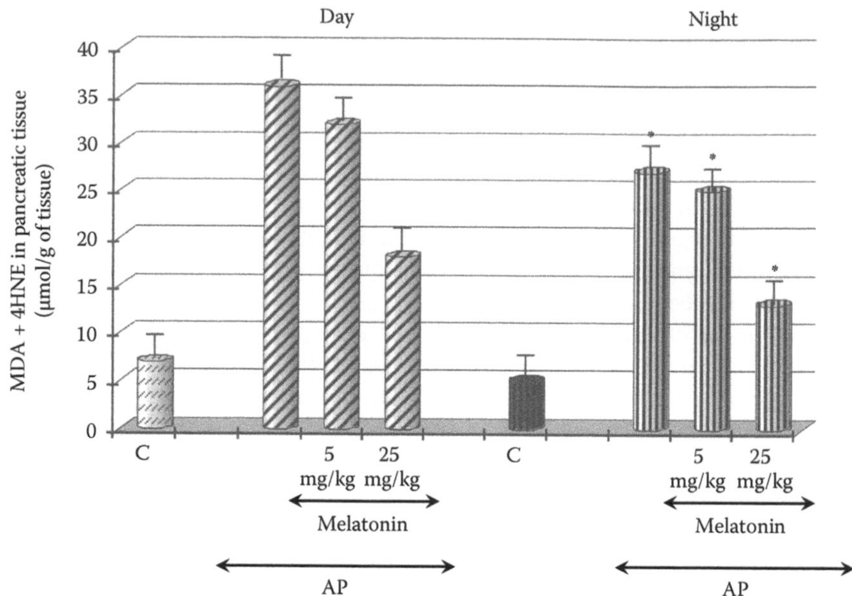

FIGURE 22.8 Pancreatic content of lipid peroxidation products MDA + 4HNE in the rats subjected to cerulein-induced pancreatitis (AP) pretreated with melatonin during the day or night. Means ± SEM from the separate experiments, each performed on six rats. *Significant ($p < 0.05$) decrease below the value detected in diurnal pancreatitis. C = intact control.

on the ability of melatonin to scavenge the ROS and increase the activity of antioxidant enzymes), (2) reduction of neutrophil infiltration and modulation of cytokine production, (3) limitation of apoptosis and necrosis in the inflamed pancreas, (4) increase of pancreatic blood flow, (5) stimulation of HSP production, and (6) activation of other yet unknown effects.

22.4 MELATONIN STIMULATES PANCREATIC ENZYME SECRETION

Administration of melatonin resulted in the spectacular increase in pancreatic enzyme secretion. In experimental studies, melatonin was given to the rats intraperitoneally or into the duodenal lumen. Both ways of application produced significant and dose-dependent increase in pancreatic amylase output [62–64]. It should be emphasized that intraluminally administered melatonin appears to be a more potent pancreatic secretagogue. A melatonin dose of 20 mg/kg administered into the duodenum augmented pancreatic amylase secretion to about 60% of maximal secretion obtained with 1 µg/kg of cholecystokinin (CCK) (Figure 22.9). The melatonin precursor L-tryptophan, when administered into the duodenal lumen or intraperitoneally, was shown to stimulate pancreatic secretory function, indicating that endogenous melatonin produced from this amino acid is able to activate pancreatic exocrine secretion [64].

Surprisingly, melatonin appears completely ineffective in the direct stimulation of pancreatic amylase release from isolated pancreatic acini. Also, L-tryptophan failed to affect pancreatic enzyme secretion in vitro [62]. This indicates that the mechanism of the stimulatory action of melatonin on exocrine pancreas is indirect and depends on the release of hormonal mediators or activation of neural pathway. To answer this question, the involvement of the sensory and vagal nerves and the implication of CCK or serotonin in the stimulatory effect of melatonin on the pancreatic enzyme secretion have been examined.

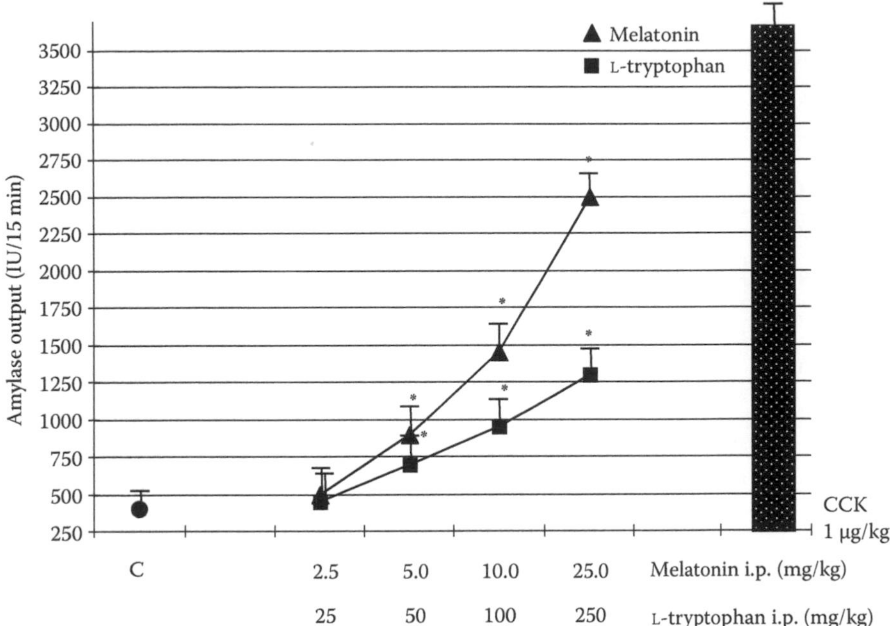

FIGURE 22.9 Effects of increasing concentrations of melatonin or L-tryptophan given into the duodenal lumen (i.d.) on pancreatic secretion of amylase in the rats. Means ± SEM from the separate experiments, each performed on six to eight rats. *Significant ($p < 0.05$) increase above the control value. C = unstimulated control.

Pancreatic exocrine function is regulated by complex neurohormonal mechanisms involving the central nervous system, vagal nerves, sympathetic nerves, and enteric nervous system operating in the gastrointestinal tract and the pancreas [65,66]. Food present in the duodenal lumen stimulates cholinergic vagovagal enteropancreatic reflexes [67]. Information from the gastrointestinal tract is delivered via afferent vagal fibers to the dorsal vagal complex (DVC) in the brainstem, and from the central nervous system, the efferent signals pass to the pancreas to stimulate pancreatic enzyme secretion [68]. Afferent nerves, which act as a part of these reflex pathway, are stimulated by CCK, serotonin, and perhaps other substances released by the digestive products into gut lumen [69,70].

Melatonin, which is present in the duodenal lumen, could be one of these substances that are responsible for the activation of enteropancreatic reflexes and stimulation of pancreatic exocrine function. Ingested food is the main source of melatonin, which is present in many plants [71]. Melatonin could also be accumulated from the circulation and released into the duodenum with the bile [72]. In addition, this indoleamine is synthesized in the intestinal mucosa in enteroendocrine cells from L-tryptophan and released in response to food ingestion [21–23].

The stimulatory effect of melatonin or L-tryptophan on pancreatic exocrine function was completely reversed by the deactivation of sensory nerves with capsaicin, bilateral vagotomy, or blockade of CCK1 receptors by tarazepide (Figure 22.10). In addition, administration of melatonin or L-tryptophan to the rats resulted in significant and dose-dependent rise in CCK plasma immunoreactivity, leading to the conclusion that melatonin, as well as L-tryptophan, exerts a stimulatory effect on the pancreatic enzyme secretion through the activation of vagal sensory nerves and stimulation of CCK release [62,64].

Subsequent study revealed that ketanserin, an antagonist of serotonin 5-HT_2 receptors, could also inhibit pancreatic amylase secretion afforded by melatonin (Figure 22.10). On the contrary, the stimulation of pancreatic exocrine function caused by L-tryptophan was much more resistant

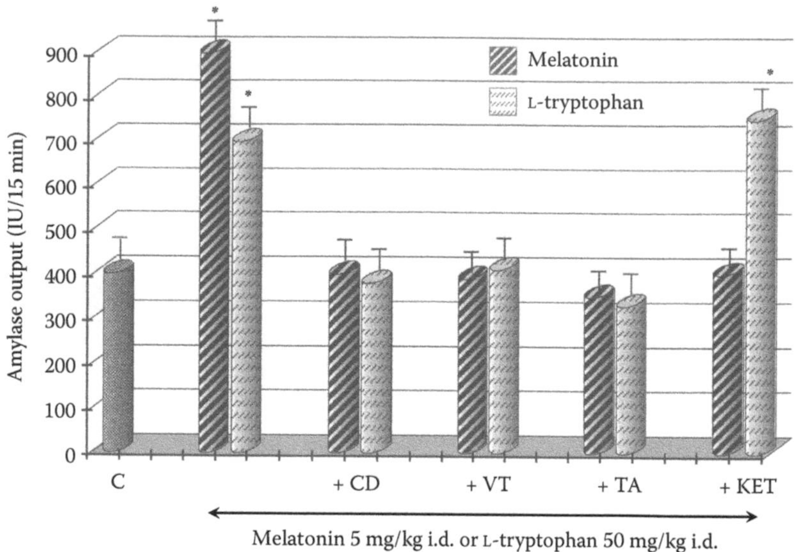

FIGURE 22.10 Pancreatic secretion of amylase in response to intraduodenal administration of melatonin or L-tryptophan in the rats with intact sensory and vagal nerves and in the animals subjected to deactivation of sensory nerves with capsaicin (CD) or to bilateral vagotomy (VT) in the rats pretreated with CCK1 receptor antagonist, tarazepide (TA), or with serotonin 5-HT_2 receptor antagonist, ketanserin (KET). Means ± SEM from the separate experiments, each performed on six rats. *Significant increases above the control value. C = unstimulated control.

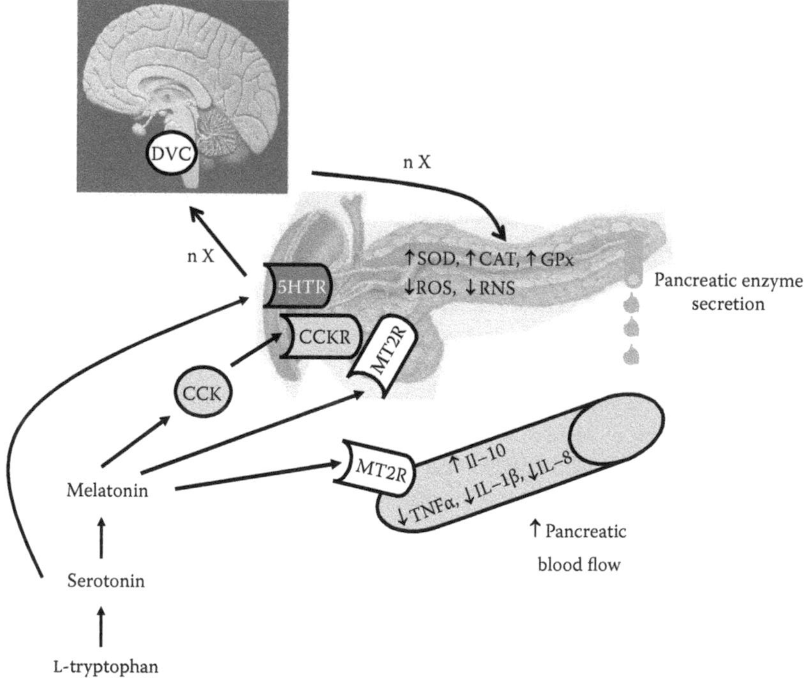

FIGURE 22.11 Proposed mechanisms of melatonin influence on the pancreas: beneficial action on acute pancreatitis and stimulation of pancreatic enzyme secretion. CCKR = CCK receptor; n X = vagal nerve; 5HTR = serotonin receptor; NO = nitric oxide.

to ketanserin than that caused by melatonin. This is because serotonin and its 5-HT_2 receptors are involved in the melatonin-induced pancreatic enzyme secretion, whereas L-tryptophan stimulates pancreatic exocrine function via different mechanisms, perhaps acting through a different receptor subtype that is not antagonized by ketanserin [73]. Further studies are needed to clarify the difference between the stimulatory effect of melatonin and that of L-tryptophan on the exocrine pancreas.

In conclusion, melatonin, which is present in relatively high concentrations in the gut, could provide an important stimulatory mechanism for the intestinal phase of pancreatic enzyme secretion. After food ingestion, melatonin content in the gut lumen increases, originating partially from the meal and from L-tryptophan, and this could create the potent signal initiating the secretion of pancreatic enzymes and activation of entire duodenal cluster unit.

22.5 SUMMARY

Melatonin produced in high amounts in the gastrointestinal system, as well as that secreted from the pineal gland, could be considered as the natural factor protecting the pancreas and other tissue from the damage caused by acute pancreatitis. The above pancreatoprotective influence of melatonin could be related to the antioxidant, immunomodulatory, and circulatory effects exerted by this substance on the pancreatic gland. In all probability, melatonin, which is present in high amounts in the gut lumen after food ingestion, could be implicated in the stimulation of pancreatic enzyme secretion though the activation of cholinergic enteropancreatic reflex involving the DVC in the brainstem (Figure 22.11).

REFERENCES

1. Lerner, AB, Case, JD, Lee, TH, Mori, W. 1958. Isolation of melatonin, the pineal factor, that lightens melanocytes. *J. Am. Chem. Sci.* 80:2587.
2. Stefluj, J, Horner, M, Ghosh, M et al. 2001. Gene expression of the key enzymes in melatonin synthesis in extrapineal tissues in the rat. *J. Pineal Res.* 30:243–247.
3. Perreau-Lentz, S, Kalsbeek, A, Garidou, ML. 2003. Suprachiasmatic control of melatonin synthesis in rats: inhibitory and stimulatory mechanism. *Eur. J. Neurosci.* 17:221–228.
4. Zawilska, JB, Skene, DJ, Arendt, J. 2009. Physiology and pharmacology of melatonin in relation to biological rhythms. *Pharmacol. Rep.* 61:383–410.
5. Huang, SH, Cao, XJ, Liu, W, Shi, XY, Wei, W. 2010. Inhibitory effect of melatonin on lung oxidative stress induced by respiratory syncytial virus infection in mice. *J. Pineal Res.* 48:109–116.
6. Hu, S, Yin, S, Jiang, X, Huang, D, Shen, G. 2009. Melatonin protects against alcoholic liver injury by attenuating oxidative stress, inflammatory response, and apoptosis. *Eur. J. Pharmacol.* 616:289–292.
7. Rodriquez, C, Mayo, JC, Sainz, RM et al. 2004. Regulation of antioxidative enzymes; a significant role for melatonin. *J. Pineal Res.* 36:1–9.
8. Domingues-Rodriguez, A, Abreu-Gonzales, P, Garcia-Gonzales, MJ, Samimi-Fard, S, Reiter, RJ, Kaski, JC. 2008. Association of ischemia-modified albumin and melatonin in patients with ST-elevated myocardial infarction. *Atherosclerosis.* 199:193–198.
9. Gałecka, E, Mrowicka, M, Malinowska, M, Gałecki, P. 2008. Wolne rodniki tlenu i azotu w fizjologii. *Pol. Merkur. Lek.* 143:446–448.
10. Reiter, RJ, Tan, DX, Manchester, LC, Pilar-Terron, M, Flores, LJ, Koppisepi, S. 2007. Medical implications of melatonin: receptor-mediated and receptor-independent actions. *Adv. Med. Sci.* 52:11–28.
11. Lahiri, S, Singh, P, Singh, S, Rashed, N, Palit, G, Pant, KK. 2009. Melatonin protects against experimental reflux esophagitis. *J. Pineal Res.* 46:207–213.
12. Petrosillo, G, Moro, N, Ruggiero, FM, Paradies, G. 2009. Melatonin inhibits cardiolipin peroxidation in mitochondria and prevents the mitochondrial permeability transition and cytochrome c release. *Free Radic. Biol. Med.* 47:969–974.
13. Jung, KH, Hong, SW, Zheng, HM et al. 2010. Melatonin ameliorates cerulein-induced pancreatitis by the modulation of nuclear erythroid 2-related factor 2 and nuclear factor-κB in rats. *J. Pineal Res.* 48(3):239–250.

14. Chen, HM, Hsu, JT, Chen, JC, Ng, CJ, Chiu, DF, Chen, MF. 2005. Delayed neutrophil apoptosis attenuated by melatonin in human acute pancreatitis. *Pancreas.* 31:560–364.
15. Gulben, K, Ozdemir, H, Berberoglu, U et al. 2010. Melatonin modulates the severity of taurocholate-induced acute pancreatitis. *Dig. Dis. Sci.* 55:941–946.
16. Pugazhenthi, K, Kapor, M, Clarkson, AM, Hall, I, Appleton, I. 2008. Melatonin accelerates the process of wound repair in full-thickness incisional wounds. *J. Pineal Res.* 44:387–396.
17. Soybir, G, Topuzlu, C, Odabas, O, Dolay, K, Bilir, A, Koksoy, F. 2003. The effects of melatonin on angiogenesis and wound healing. *Surg. Today.* 33:896–901.
18. Munoz-Casares, FC, Padillo, FJ, Briceno, J et al. 2006. Melatonin reduces apoptosis and necrosis induced by ischemia/reprfusion injury of the pancreas. *J. Pineal Res.* 40:195–203.
19. Jockers, R, Maurice, P, Boutin, JA, Delagrange, P. 2008. Melatonin receptors, hetero-dimerization, signal transduction and binding sites: what's new? *Br. J. Pharmacol.* 154:1182–1195.
20. Hardeland, R. 2009. Melatonin: signaling mechanisms of pleiotrophic agent. *Biofactors* 35:183–192.
21. Bubenik, GA. 2008. Thirty years since the discovery of gastrointestinal melatonin. *J. Physiol. Pharmacol.* 59, Suppl. 2:33–51.
22. Huether, G. 1994. The contribution of extrapineal sites of melatonin to circulating melatonin levels in higher vertebrates. *Experientia* 49:665–670.
23. Raikhlin, NT, Kvetnoy, IM, Tolkahev, VN. 1975. Melatonin may be synthetized in enterochromaffine cells. *Nature* 255:344–345.
24. Bubenik, GA, Pang, SF, Hacker, RR. 1996. Melatonin concentrations in serum and tissues of porcine gastrointestinal tract and their relationship to the intake and passage of food. *J. Pineal Res.* 21:251–256.
25. Huether, G, Poeggler, B, Reimer, A, George, A. 1992. Effects of tryptophan administration on circulating melatonin levels in chicks and rats: evidence for stimulation of melatonin synthesis and release in the gastrointestinal tract. *Life Sci.* 51:945–953.
26. Bubenik, GA, Brown, GM. 1997. Pinealectomy reduces melatonin levels in the serum but not in the gastrointestinal tract of the rat. *Biol Signal.* 6:40–44.
27. Stebelova, K, Anttila, K, Manttari, S, Saarela, SI, Zeman, M. 2010. Immunohistochemical definition of MT(2) receptors and melatonin in the gastrointestinal tissues of rat. *Acta Histochem.* 112:26–33.
28. Jaworek, J, Leja-Szpak, A., Bonior, J et al. 2003. Protective effect of melatonin and its precursor L-tryptophan on acute pancreatitis induced by caerulein overstimulation or ischemia/reperfusion. *J. Pineal Res.* 34:40–52.
29. Jaworek, J, Nawrot-Porąbka, K, Leja-Szpak, A et al. 2007. Melatonin as modulator of pancreatic enzyme secretion and pancreatoprotector. *J. Physiol. Pharmacol.* 58, Suppl. 6:65–80.
30. Stebelova, K, Herichova, I, Zeman, M. 2007. Diabetes induces changes in melatonin concentration in peripheral tissues of rat. *Neurol. Endocrinol. Lett.* 28:159–165.
31. Peschke, E, Stumpf, I, Bazwinsky, I, Litvak, L, Dralle, H, Muhlbauer, E. 2007. Melatonin and type 2 diabetes—A possible link? *J. Pineal Res.* 42:350–358.
32. Ramracheya, RD, Muller, DS, Squires, PE et al. 2008. Function and expression of melatonin receptors on human pancreatic islets. *J. Pineal Res.* 44:273–279.
33. Langenberg, C, Pascoe, L, Mari, A et al. 2009. Common genetic variation in the melatonin receptor 1B gene (MTNR1B) is associated with decreased early-phase insulin response. *Diabetologia.* 52:1537–1542.
34. Picinato, MC, Hirata, AC, Cipolla-Neto, J et al. 2008. Activation of insulin and IGF-1 signaling pathways by melatonin through MT1 receptor in isolated rat pancreatic islets. *J. Pineal Res.* 44:88–94.
35. Peschke, E, Stumpf, I, Bazwinsky, I, Litvak, L, Dralle, H, Muhlbauer, E. 2007. Melatonin and type 2 diabetes—A possible link? *J. Pineal Res.* 42:350–358.
36. Mulder, H, Nagorny, CL, Lyssenko, V, Groop, L. 2009. Melatonin receptors in pancreatic islets: good morning to a novel type 2 diabetes gene. *Diabetologia* 52:1240–1249.
37. Rezzani, R, Buffoli, B, Rodelia, R, Stacchiotti, A, Bianchi, R. 2005. Protective role of melatonin in cyclosporine A–induced oxidative stress in rat liver. *Int. J. Immunopharmacol.* 5:1397–1405.
38. Kurcer, Z, Oguz, E, Ozbilge, H et al. Melatonin protects from ischemia/reperfusion renal injury in rats: this effect is not mediated by proinflammatory cytokines. *J. Pineal Res.* 2007, 43;172–178.
39. Rodriguez, MI, Escames, G, Lopez, LC et al. 2007. Chronic melatonin treatment reduces the age-dependent inflammatory process in senescence-accelerated mice. *J. Pineal Res.* 42:1272–279.
40. Brzozowska, I, Konturek PCh, Brzozowski, T et al. 2002. Role of prostaglandins, nitric oxide, sensory nerves and gastrin in acceleration of ulcer healing by melatonin and its precursor. *J. Pineal Res.* 100:32:149–162.

41. Miller, SC, Pandi-Perumal, SR, Esquifino, AI, Cardinali, DP, Maestroni, GJ. 2006. The role of melatonin in immuno-enhancement: potential application in cancer. *Int. Exp. Pathol.* 87:81–87.
42. Carillo-Vico, A, Reiter, RJ et al. 2006. The modulatory role of melatonin on immune responsiveness. *Curr. Opin. Invest. Drugs*. 7:423–431.
43. Paredes, SD, Sanchez, S, Parvez, H, Rodriquez, AB, Barriga, C. 2007. Altered circadian rhythms of corticosterone, melatonin, and phagocytic activity in response to stress in rats. *Neurol. Endocrinol. Lett.* 11:489–495.
44. Qi, W, Tan, RX, Reiter, RJ. 1999. Melatonin reduces lipid peroxidation and tissue edema in caerulein-induced acute pancreatitis in the rats. *Dig. Dis. Sci.* 44:2257–2262.
45. Esrefoglu, M, Gul, M, Ates, B, Selimoglu, MA. 2006. Ultrastructural clues for the protective effect of melatonin against oxidative damage in cerulein-induced pancreatitis. *J. Pineal Res.* 40:92–97.
46. Szabolcs, A, Reiter, RJ, Letoha, T et al. 2006. Effect of melatonin on the severity of L-arginine–induced experimental pancreatitis in rats. *World J. Gastroenterol.* 12:251–258.
47. Chen, HM, Chen, JC, Ng, CJ, Chiu, DF, Chen, MF. 2006. Melatonin reduces pancreatic prostaglandins production and protects against caerulein-induced pancreatitis. *J. Pineal Res.*40:34–39.
48. Allahan, K, Kalyoncu, NI, Kural, BV, Ercin, C. 2004. Effect of melatonin on acute necrotizing pancreatitis in rats. *Z. Gastroenterol.* 42:967–972.
49. Gulben, K, Ozdemir, H, Berberoglu, U et al. 2010. Melatonin modulates the severity of taurocholate-induced acute pancreatitis in the rat. *Dig. Dis. Sci.* 55:941–946.
50. Barlas, A, Cevik, H, Arbak, S et al. 2004. Melatonin protects against pancreatobiliary inflammation and associated remote organ injury in rats: role of neutrophils. *J. Pineal Res.* 37:267–275.
51. Col, C, Dinler, K, Hasdemir, AO, Bugdayci, G. 2009. The effect of intraperitoneal injection of melatonin on serum amylase levels in acute pancreatitis. *JOP.* 10:306–309.
52. Jaworek, J, Konturek, SJ, Tomaszewska, R et al. 2004. The circadian rhythm of melatonin modulates the severity of caerulein-induced pancreatitis in the rat. *J. Pineal Res.* 37:161–170.
53. Zhou, W, Wang, P, Tao, L. 2009. Effect of melatonin on proliferation of neonatal cord blond mononuclear cells. *World J. Pediatr.* 5:300–303.
54. Sidhu, S, Pandhi, P, Malhortra, S, Vaiphei, K, Khanduya, KL. 2010. Melatonin treatment is beneficial in pancreatic repair process after experimental acute pancreatitis. *Eur. J. Pharmacol.* 628:282–289.
55. Baykal, A, Iskit, AB, Hamaloglou, E, Oguz, M, Hascelik, G, Sayek, Y. 2000. Melatonin modulates mesenteric blood flow and TNF-α cncentrations after lipopolysaccharide challenge. *Eur. J. Surg.* 166:722–727.
56. Jaworek, J, Konturek, SJ, Leja-Szpak, A. 2002. Role of endogenous melatonin and its MT2 receptor in the modulation of caerulein-induced pancreatitis in the rat. *J. Physiol. Pharmacol.* 53:791–804.
57. Bonior, J, Jaworek, J, Konturek, SJ, Pawlik, WW. 2005. Increase of heat shock protein gene expression by melatonin in AR42J cells. *J. Physiol. Pharmacol.* 56:471–481.
58. Joly, AL, Wettstein, G, Mignot, G, Ghiringhelli, F, Garrido, C. 2010. Dual role of heat shock proteins as regulators of apoptosis and innate immunity. *J. Innate Immun.* 2:238–247.
59. Esrefoglu, M, Gul, Turan, F. 2008. Comparative effects of several therapeutic agents on hepatic damage induced by acute experimental pancreatitis. *Dig. Dis. Sci* 53:1303–1310.
60. Anwar, MM, Meki, AR, Rahma, HH. 2000. Inhibitory effect of melatonin on vascular reactivity: possible role of vasoactive mediators. *Comp. Biochem. Physiol. Toxicol. Pharmacol.* 130:357–367.
61. Jaworek, J, Zwirska-Korczala, K, Szklarczyk, J et al. 2010. Pinealectomy aggravates acute pancreatitis in the rat. *Pharmacol. Rep* 62(5):864–873.
62. Jaworek, J, Nawrot, K, Konturek, SJ et al. 2004. Melatonin and its precursor; L-tryptophan: influence on pancreatic amylase secretion in vivo and in vitro. *J. Pineal Res.* 36:156–164.
63. Jaworek, J. 2006. Ghrelin and melatonin in the regulation of pancreatic exocrine secretion and maintaining of integrity. *J. Physiol. Pharmacol.* 57:83–96.
64. Leja-Szpak, A, Jaworek, J, Nawrot, K et al. 2004. Modulation of pancreatic enzyme secretion by melatonin and its precursor, L-tryptophan. Role of CCK and afferent nerves. *J. Physiol. Pharmacol.* 55:441–451.
65. Konturek, SJ, Zabielski, R, Konturek, JW, Czarnecki, J. 2003. Neuroendocrinology of the pancreas; role of brain–gut axis in pancreatic secretion. *Eur. J. Pharmacol.* 481:1–14.
66. Jaworek, J, Konturek, SJ, Szlachcic, A. 1997. The role of CGRP and afferent nerves in the modulation of pancreatic enzyme secretion in the rat. *Int. J. Pancreatol.* 22:137–146.
67. Niebergall-Roth, E, Siger, MV. 2006. Enteropancreatic reflexes mediating the pancreatic enzyme response to nutriens. *Auton. Neurosci.* 30:62–69.

68. Li, Y, Wu, X, Zhu, J, Yan, J, Owyang, C. 2003. Hypothalamic regulation of pancreatic secretion is mediated by central cholinergic pathways in the rat. *J. Physiol.* 52:571–587.
69. Li, Y, Owyang, C. 1997. High affinity CCK-A receptors on the vagus nerve mediate CCK-stimulated pancreatic secretion in the rat. *Am. J. Physiol.* 273:G679–G685.
70. Li, Y, Hao, Y, Zhu, J, Owyang, C. 2000. Serotonin released from intestinal enterochromaffin cells mediates luminal non-cholecystokinin–stimulated pancreatic secretion in rats. *Gastroenterology* 118:1197.
71. Caniato, R, Filipini, R, Piovan, A. 2003. Melatonin in plants. *Adv. Exp. Med. Biol.* 527:593–597.
72. Messner, M, Huether, G, Lorf, T et al. 2004. Presence of melatonin in the human hepatobiliary tract. *Life Sci.* 69:543–551.
73. Nawrot-Porąbka, K, Jaworek, J, Leja-Szpak, A et al. 2007. Involvement of vagal nerve in the pancreatostimulatory effects of luminal melatonin, or its precursor, L-tryptophan. Study in the rats. *J. Physiol. Pharmacol.* 58, Suppl. 6:81–95.

23 Life Environment and Sleep: Melatonin Production Affected by Light and Ambient Temperature in Humans

Masayuki Kondo and Tomoko Wakamura

CONTENTS

23.1 INTRODUCTION

23.1.1 Nighttime Melatonin Production Suppressed by Light

The melatonin rhythm is generated by an endogenous clock located in the suprachiasmatic nuclei (SCN) of the hypothalamus.

The melatonin secretion phase is entrained to the dark period, and it can be acutely suppressed by light exposure during the night. There are reports that melatonin inhibition occurs even under low light intensity.[1,2] In 1980, Lewy et al.[3] demonstrated that melatonin secretion in humans could be inhibited by artificial light of sufficient intensity and duration. A dose-dependent effect of the suppression was observed between 500 and 2500 lux given for 2 hours from 0200 to 0400 h. In addition, the bright light acutely affected the core body temperature (T_{core}) rhythm.[4] Even in adolescent participants (14–15 years), bright-light intensity (2000 lux) from fluorescent lamps (white-light type) in the evening (1930–2230 h) could suppress the saliva melatonin production in comparison with dim light (60 lux) from an incandescent lamp (yellow-light type) based on a field experiment.[5] Vandewalle et al.[6] reported that the change in electrophysiological activity, which was induced by light exposure in the daytime, was detected in the thalamus, and it was reported to be in direct relation to the enhancement of subjective alertness also stimulated by light exposure; however, the neural changes and their time courses induced by light exposure during the daytime are largely unknown.

23.1.2 Influence of Diurnal Bright/Dim Light Exposure on Melatonin Production

Due to the earth's rotation on its axis, the alternative stimulation of light and dark on the retina synchronizes the SCN to a matching 24-hour period; however, in modern life, the increased use of electric power for lighting during the night and a sun-free environment during the daytime inside buildings could lead to diminished amplitude of the light/dark cycle, which is the most important circadian zeitgeber for humans.

It is known that light intensity during the first half of the subjective night regulates the secretion of melatonin and delays the circadian phase; however, it has not been clarified whether light intensity in the daytime influences the melatonin secretion level. Midday (1100–1700 h) exposure to bright light (5000 lux) for three consecutive days changed the circadian organization of the plasma melatonin rhythm in humans.[7] Nighttime melatonin in urine after bright-light (5000 lux) exposure during the daytime (0630–1930 h) was excreted at a significantly higher concentration than after dim-light exposure (50 lux).[8] Although melatonin production was not measured, three consecutive daytime exposures to bright light from a fluorescent lamp (6000 lux, white-light type) increased the amplitude of the rectal temperature rhythm under a self-determined sleep/wake schedule, while 3-day exposure to dim light (200 lux) during the daytime could not increase the circadian rhythm amplitude in humans. In addition, the quality of nighttime sleep and daytime alertness was significantly higher after bright-light exposure than after dim-light exposure.[9] Takasu et al.[10] confirmed that repeated daytime bright exposure (5000 lux) increased the maximum value of plasma nocturnal melatonin and that the increased melatonin profile linked to a higher amplitude of T_{core} rhythm and decreased daytime sleepiness. These findings imply that enough exposure to bright light (including sunlight) during the daytime is important for the health, by maintaining the high amplitude of the circadian clock.

23.1.3 Lights with Various Wavelengths Affecting Melatonin Production

It should be pointed out that the two light sources used in the experiment performed by Lewy et al.[3] were different. The 500-lux light was from a fluorescent lamp called Vita-Lite, which had full-spectrum distribution, and the 2500-lux light was from an incandescent floodlight of 150 W. The article did not show the spectral distribution of the light source used in the experiment. As a matter of course, the composition of the light wavelengths from the incandescent lamp differed from the wavelength composition of the fluorescent lamp. This showed that consideration was not paid to the distribution of spectrum components three decades ago. In early experimental days, it was thought that only illumination (intensity) was important in this research field.

Light with a short wavelength was more effective in modifying the melatonin rhythm in chickens[11] and other species than that with a long wavelength; therefore, the wavelength of the artificial light used after sunset until sunrise is an important factor in melatonin rhythm. However, there are few studies on the effect of light wavelengths on the human melatonin rhythm. When an adult human was exposed to green and blue light for 5 hours during the night (2100–0200 h), melatonin production was suppressed in comparison with when exposed to red light.[12] The relatively high color temperature light from the fluorescent lamp (6500 K) administered during the night (2100–0200 h) also suppressed melatonin production more than the relatively low color temperature light from the warm-white fluorescent lamp (3000 K).[13] Blue light (460 nm, peak of sensitivity of melanopsin) was more powerful for resetting the circadian phase of melatonin in humans than green light (550 nm, peak sensitivity of visual system) in the same photon density conditions during the subjective night of the biological clock.[14] In another experiment under similar light conditions, again during the subjective night exposure to blue light (460 nm) was shown to extend the performance more than green light (550 nm) in a simple reaction time task.[15]

On the other hand, morning (0400–0900 h) exposure to light of 1000 lux consisting of different wavelengths had no significant effects on nighttime melatonin production; however, exposure to green light (545 nm, 1.683 W/Sr m^2) of 2500 lux in the morning suppressed melatonin production at night.[16] Although sunlight during the daytime includes all wavelengths, artificial light includes only specific wavelengths. It is necessary to study the role of the composition of various light wavelengths during the daytime in the regulation of the melatonin level at night in the near future.

23.2 INFLUENCE OF CYCLIC CHANGE OF LIGHT AND AMBIENT TEMPERATURE IN HUMANS

In recent years, it has been studied whether melatonin secretion is related to diurnal and seasonal cyclic changes in light and temperature conditions derived from the rotation/revolution rhythm of the earth. Humans have evolved the circadian clock system over millions of years, being always immersed in dusk and dawn and under cyclic alterations in environmental air temperatures in the evening and early morning. Here, we wish to highlight a new aspect of the inner fluctuation of the biological clock in the human body, which is linked to cyclic environmental fluctuations.

23.2.1 Influences of Twilight on Diurnal Variation of Circadian Rhythms in Humans

It was reported that the circadian phase of melatonin production could be advanced and therefore morning wakefulness improved more markedly by dawn simulation,[17,18] which was developed as a treatment for winter seasonal affective disorder patients.[19] In addition, it was reported that a gradual increase in light intensity for healthy participants in the morning caused natural arousal and the patients woke up in a better mood.[20,21]

A study[22] has been carried out concerning the influence of cyclic light changes in the evening and early morning on the circadian rhythm of T_{core}, urinary 6-hydroxymelatonin sulfate during sleep and the awakening sensation. Two kinds of light exposure were provided for each participant: (1) rectangular light change with an abrupt decrease from 3000 to 100 lux at 1800 h, abrupt increase from 0 to 3000 lux at 0700 h (rectangular condition) (Figure 23.1g). (2) Twilight-mimicking light change with a gradual decrease from 3000 to 100 lux starting at 1700 h (twilight period about 2 hours), with a gradual increase from 0 to 3000 lux starting at 0500 h (twilight period also about 2 hours) (twilight condition) (Figure 23.1e). The nadir time of T_{core} advanced significantly under the influence of twilight conditions. 6-Hydroxymelatonin sulfate production in urine collected at 0200 h was significantly higher under twilight conditions than under rectangular conditions (Figure 23.1e versus Figure 23.1g). Drowsiness in the morning was hardly felt under twilight conditions (Figure 23.1e). These results suggest that it is important to have twilight conditions in the evening and early morning to achieve a good sleep at night and fresh wakefulness in the morning.

23.2.2 Physiological Significance of Cyclic Changes in the Ambient Temperature around Dusk and Dawn for Circadian Rhythms in Humans

Haskell et al.[23] reported that the thermoregulation system was triggered by the ambient temperature (T_a) during REM sleep in humans. It is well known that the upper and lower extremities play an important role in heat-loss mechanisms[24] and in the rapid onset of sleep.[25] A gradual decrease in T_a from 27°C to 25.5°C over the 4 hours from midnight to 0400 h, when compared with opposite gradual changes of

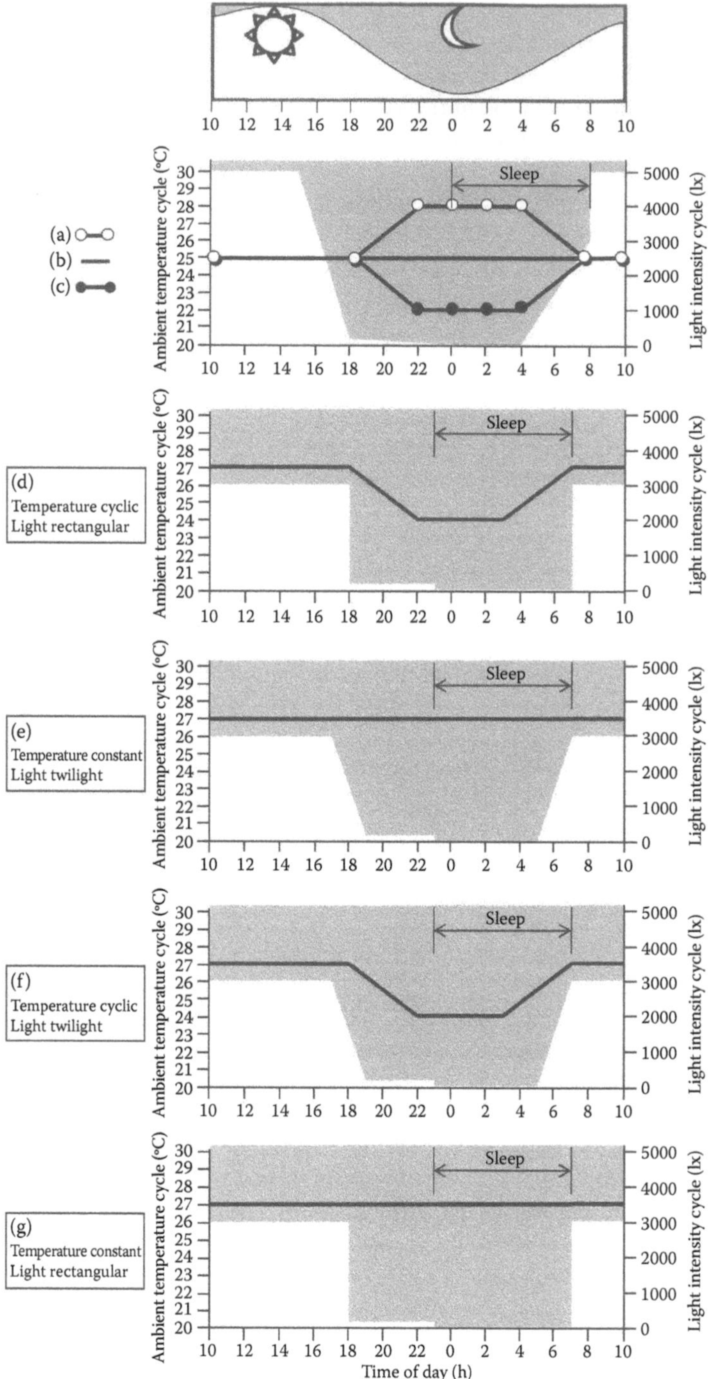

FIGURE 23.1 Experimental protocols. Ambient temperature (°C) is shown as a line. Light intensity (lux) is shown in the white area. Left vertical axis: ambient temperature (°C), right vertical axis: light intensity (lux). There were seven experimental conditions: (a) high ambient temperature (28°C) during the night, (b) constant ambient temperature (25°C) all day, (c) low ambient temperature (22°C) during the night, (d) cyclic ambient temperature and rectangular light change, (e) constant ambient temperature and twilight light change, (f) cyclic ambient temperature and twilight light change, and (g) constant ambient temperature and rectangular light change.

T_a in the room, induced a deeper fall of T_{core} and was accompanied by the subjective feeling of having had a better sleep in the morning.[26] Wakamura and Tokura[27] showed that T_{core} during the night's sleep was significantly lower when T_a decreased gradually from 25°C to 22°C between 1800 and 2200 h followed by a gradual increase from 22°C to 25°C between 0400 and 0800 h (Figure 23.1c), compared with either a constant T_a of 25°C over the 24 hours (Figure 23.1b) or a gradual increase of T_a from 25°C to 28°C between 1800 and 2200 h followed by a gradual decrease of T_a from 28°C to 25°C between 0400 and 0800 h (Figure 23.1a). In other words, a gradual decrease of T_a in the evening and a gradual increase in the morning, mimicking natural T_a changes under the lighting cycle with mimicking twilights, could promote the deepest fall of T_{core} during nocturnal sleep.

Furthermore, Kondo et al.[28] found that nocturnal 6-hydroxymelatonin sulfate levels in overnight urine were significantly higher under cyclic T_a conditions (Figure 23.1d) than constant T_a conditions (Figure 23.1g). This result was an important finding, i.e., the cyclic change of T_a could influence not only the circadian T_{core} rhythm but also melatonin secretion in humans.

23.2.3 Combined Influences of Gradual Changes in the Ambient Temperature and Light Intensity around Dusk and Dawn in Humans

In addition, it was studied whether the circadian rhythms of T_{core} and 6-hydromelatonin in humans would react to the combined conditions of gradual changes of T_a and light intensity in the evening and morning. Kondo et al.[29] reported that under gradual changes of T_a and light intensity around dusk and dawn (Figure 23.1f), T_{core} fell more quickly in the evening and rose faster toward the morning, and the level of urinary 6-hydroxymelatonin sulfate became higher during nocturnal sleep than constant T_a and rectangular light intensity (Figure 23.1g). Moreover, the feeling at waking was better under the influence of gradual changes of T_a and light intensity than constant T_a and rectangular light intensity.

As shown in Figure 23.2, the circadian phase of the nadir in T_{core} rhythm was significantly advanced by 71 min under the influence of cyclic changes of T_a than under constant T_a (Figure 23.1d versus Figure 23.1g),[28] and was advanced by 49 min under twilight changes of light than under rectangular changes of light (Figure 23.1e versus Figure 23.1g).[22] Under the influence of cyclic changes of T_a and twilight changes of light, the nadir phase in T_{core} rhythm was advanced by 56 min compared with under constant T_a and rectangular changes of light (Figure 23.1f versus Figure 23.1g).[29] Under the influence of cyclic changes of T_a and twilight changes of light, the nadir phase in T_{core} rhythm was advanced by 35 min compared with under constant T_a and twilight changes of light (Figure 23.1c versus Figure 23.1b).[27] Thus, the advance of nadir seemed to be suppressed under the influence of cyclic changes of T_a and light, compared with cyclic changes of only T_a, suggesting that twilight changes of light seem to have been powerful enough to turn back an advanced circadian phase. The physiological mechanisms of why twilight changes of light could turn back an advanced circadian phase remain to be studied. Liu et al.[30] found that T_a was a more effective entraining agent than light in *Neurospora*, and its ecological significance is plausible. Because the time of dawn is completely predictable and precise, we can set the nadir time of T_{core} to be not so early that it prevents too early waking and to avoid too short sleep hours.

23.3 Application of the Effects of Daytime Light and Ambient Temperature of Circadian Variation Based on the Natural Environment

23.3.1 Trend of Recent Studies

It became clear that the influence of daytime light exposure affects humans as described above, and there have been some clinical reports in which this evidence was applied. Mishima et al.[31] reported that morning bright light (0900–1100 h) prolonged the nocturnal sleep time and diminished nap times in older patients with dementia. Moreover, in hospitalized elderly patients with more frequent

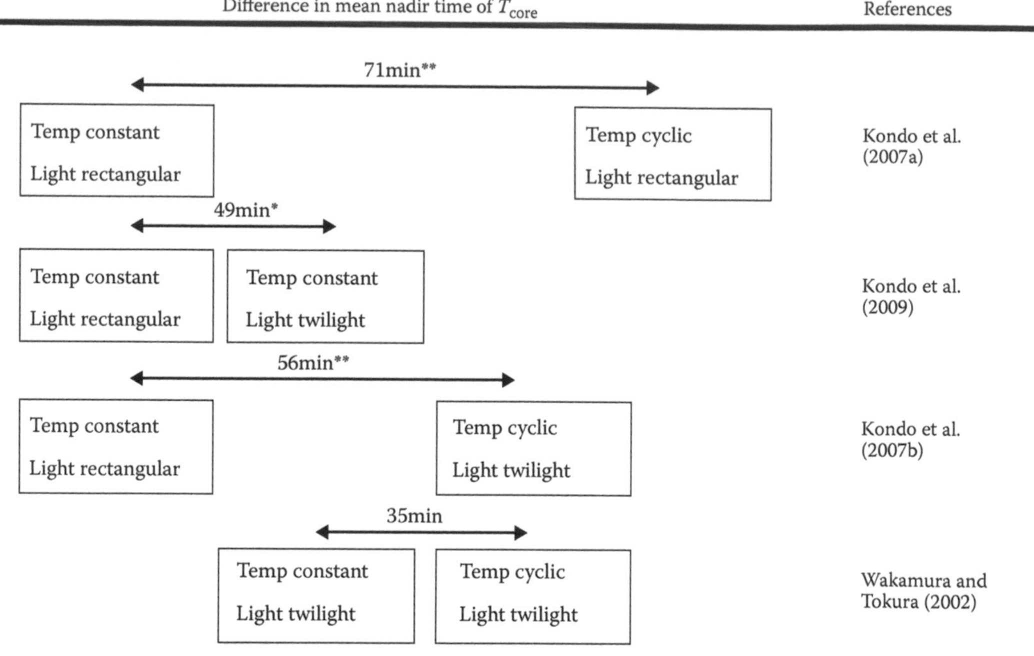

FIGURE 23.2 Summary of results: comparison of the difference in circadian nadir time between two conditions.

social contact than dementia patients, daytime light exposure improved their subsequent sleep structure and melatonin production during the night.[32] Recently, in an experiment in dementia patients using a randomized controlled trial, the effect of light exposure during the daytime (0900-1800 h) was reported as a treatment to improve their QOL.[33]

Further, healthy older participants had greater daytime light exposure than younger participants.[34] As a matter of course, the circadian phase of the older participants gradually advanced, and their awakening time was also more advanced; however, based on this result, we should be aware of the importance of the natural environment, including sunlight for our health. A study on the effects of exposure to daytime lighting to advance the circadian phase in shift workers[35] still could not describe its general importance of promoting physical and mental health in humans. In addition, although many studies on the thermal environment related to air-conditioning have been performed, few studies have focused on the reaction of melatonin to it.

23.3.2 Improving the Bedroom Environment to Improve the Quality of Sleep

A deeper fall and earlier phase advance of T_{core} and higher secretion of urinary melatonin sulfate during nocturnal sleep was demonstrated under twilight conditions than with the rectangular change of light. Furthermore, cyclic T_a showed similar influences to twilight light conditions, compared with constant T_a. Furthermore, T_{core} falls more quickly in the evening and rises more quickly in the early morning under the influence of the gradual reduction of T_a and light intensity in the evening, and the gradual rise of T_a and light intensity in the early morning, compared with constant T_a and light intensity. The nocturnal rise of melatonin was accelerated under such gradual environmental changes. These physiological changes could accelerate better sleep efficiency. Consequently, nocturnal sleep of higher quality with a better mood on awakening can be achieved.

With this in mind, when architects, interior designers, lighting designers, element designers, and others design indoor environments, it is important that they design for sleep promotion. Therefore, cyclic T_a and light intensity in the sleep space should not be kept constant during the night, but should fluctuate regularly during the evening and early morning.

A circadian control system of air-conditioning and light intensity should be incorporated as a completely automatic system, including a timer. If a timer could be incorporated into the system, a control system of T_a and light intensity (including various color temperatures) in the bedroom could be developed for the consumer.[36] This should not be restricted to the sleeping area but should also be applied in all rooms, including the living room, dining room, toilet, bathroom, and hallways.

Control of the sleep/wake cycle is influenced by the sleep duration/activity time according to individual wishes and social restrictions. It is impossible to return to following a natural life in our present situation. Therefore, our proposal for a dwelling environment on the basis of this experimental data could have profound effects on health maintenance and its promotion. These findings should be utilized in the design of dwelling environments promptly.

23.3.3 New Illuminating Device: Light-Emitting Diode

Recently, due to their low electric cost and lower impact on the environment, light-emitting diode (LED) lights have become popular. LED devices are so small that they can be used in small spaces; for example, a personal light-treatment device (attached to the glasses) is useful for light therapy equipped with low brightness blue LEDs.[37] It is also useful as illumination in housing. It is known from using LED electric bulbs that we can considerably reduce electric power usage, leading to a reduced amount of CO_2 emitted into the environment compared with an incandescent lamp. Moreover, there are mixed issue whether LEDs should be used for illumination in housing because LEDs are monochromatic; however, not enough research has been performed on the impact of LED lights on circadian rhythm, core body temperature, and melatonin secretion in humans, so further research is needed.

23.4 CONCLUSION

Humans are diurnally active animals and are usually exposed to light while engaged in cognitive tasks. The light/dark cycle is a good synchronizer of the circadian pacemaker of mammalians, including humans. Melatonin is a circulating hormone that is essential for regulating several biological functions, including the sleep/wake cycle.

The point that should be emphasized most in this chapter is that the natural environment at this latitude (Japan, 26–43°N), where the rotation of the globe in relation to the sun changes ambient temperature and light is critically important for the promotion of human health from a physical and mental point of view. We should pay attention to the daylight hours at each latitude, which is necessary to generalize the research results introduced in this chapter. It may be necessary to reconsider the circumstances of humans living in sunlight.

23.5 SUMMARY

- Twilight as a diurnal variation influences the circadian rhythms of melatonin production in humans.
- Cyclic changes in the ambient temperature around dusk and dawn influence the circadian rhythm in humans.
- Gradual changes in the ambient temperature, and light intensity around dusk, and dawn also influence circadian rhythm in humans.

- To improve the bedroom environment in order to improve the quality of sleep, the cyclic ambient temperature and light intensity in living spaces (including the bedroom) should be studied further, and the results of such studies could be considered and incorporated into the normal life of citizens.

ACKNOWLEDGMENTS

We particularly and sincerely thank Dr. Hiromi Tokura (Professor Emeritus at Nara Women's University, Japan), who is our special supervisor in the field of chronobiology and physiological anthropology. This chapter is dedicated to him in the hope that it will improve his health.

REFERENCES

1. Boivin, Diane B., Jeanne F. Duffy, Richard E. Kronauer, and Charles A. Czeisler. 1994. Sensitivity of the human circadian pacemaker to moderately bright light. *J Biol Rhythms*, 9(3–4): 315–331.
2. Boivin, Diane B., Jeanne F. Duffy, Richard E. Kronauer, and Charles A. Czeisler. 1996. Dose–response relationships for resetting of human circadian clock by light. *Nature*, 379(6565): 540–542.
3. Lewy, Alfred. J., Thomas A. Wehr, Frederick K. Goodwin, David. A. Newsome, and S. P. Markey. 1980. Light suppresses melatonin secretion in humans. *Science*, 210(4475): 1267–1269.
4. Badia, Philippe, Brent Myers, Maren Boecker, Janice Culpepper, and John R. Harsh. 1991. Bright light effects on body temperature, alertness, EEG and behavior. *Physiol Behav*, 50(3): 583–588.
5. Harada, Tetsuo. 2004. Effects of evening light conditions on salivary melatonin of Japanese junior high school students. *J Circ Rhythms*, 2: 1–5.
6. Vandewalle, Gilles, Steffen Gais, Manuel Schabus, Evelyne Balteau, Juilie C. Carrier, Annabelle Darsaud, Virginie Sterpenich, Genevieve Albouy, D.erk Jan Dijk, and Pierre Maquet. 2007. Wavelength-Dependent Modulation of Brain Responses to a Working Memory Task by Daytime Light Exposure. *Cereb Cortex*, 17: 2788–2795.
7. Hashimoto, Satoko, Masako Kohsaka, Kouji Nakamura, Hiroshi Honma, Sato Honma, and Ken-Ichi Honma. 1997. Midday exposure to bright light changes the circadian organization of plasma melatonin rhythm in humans. *Neurosci Lett*, 221(2–3): 89–92.
8. Park, Shin-Jung, and Hiromi Tokura. 1999. Bright light exposure during the daytime affects circadian rhythms of urinary melatonin and salivary immunoglobulin A. *Chronobiol Int*, 16: 359–371.
9. Wakamura, Tomoko, and Hiromi Tokura. 2000. The influence of bright light during the daytime upon circadian rhythm of core temperature and its implications for nocturnal sleep. *Nurs Health Sci*, 2: 41–49.
10. Takasu, N. Nana, Satoko Hashimoto, Yujiro Yamanaka, Yusuke Tanahashi, Ayano Yamazaki, Sato Honma, and Ken-Ichi Honma. 2006. Repeated exposures to daytime bright light increase nocturnal melatonin rise and maintain circadian phase in young subjects under fixed sleep schedule. *Am J Physiol Regul Integr Comp Physiol*, 291: R1799–1807.
11. Csernus, Valér, Paul Becher, and Béla Mess. 1999. Wavelength dependency of light-induced changes in rhythmic melatonin secretion from chicken pineal gland in vitro. *Neuro Endocrinol Lett*, 20(5): 299–304.
12. Morita, Takeshi, Yumiko Teramoto, and Hiromi Tokura. 1995. Inhibitory effect of light of different wavelengths on the fall of core temperature during the nighttime. *Jpn J Physiol*, 45: 667–671.
13. Morita, Takeshi, and Hiromi Tokura. 1996. Effects of lights of different color temperature on the nocturnal changes in core temperature and melatonin in humans. *Appl Human Sci*, 15: 243–246.
14. Lockley, Steven W, George C. Brainard, and Charles Czeisler. 2003. High sensitivity of the human circadian melatonin rhythm to resetting by short wavelength light. *J Clin Endocrinol Metab*, 88(9): 4502–4505.
15. Lockley, Steven W., Erin E. Evans, Frank AJ. Scheer, George C. Brainard, Charles A. Czeisler, and Daniel Aeschbach. 2006. Short-wavelength sensitivity for the direct effects of light on alertness, vigilance, and the waking electroencephalogram in humans. *Sleep*, 29: 161–168.
16. Morita, Takeshi, Hiromi Tokura, Tomoko Wakamura, Shin-Jung Park, and Yumiko Teramoto. 1997. Effects of the morning irradiation of light with different wavelengths on the behavior of core temperature and melatonin in humans. *Appl Human Sci*, 16: 103–105.
17. Norden, Michael J., and David H. Avery. 1993. A controlled study of dawn simulation in subsyndromal winter depression. *Acta Psychiatr Scand*, 88: 67–71.

18. Terman, Michael, David Schlager, Stephen Fairhurst, and Bill Perlman. 1989. Dawn and dusk simulation as a therapeutic intervention. *Biol Psychiatry*, 25: 966–970.
19. Terman, Michael, Jiuan Su Terman, Fredric M Quitkin, Patrick J. McGrath, Jonathan W Stewart, and Brian Rafferty, B. 1989. Light therapy for seasonal affective disorder. A review of efficacy. *Neuropsychopharmacology*, 2: 1–22.
20. Arakawa, Kazushige, Shuichiroh Shirakawa, Toshinori Kobayashi, Mitsugu Oguri, Yuichi Kamei, and Tumuta, Toyoaki. 1998. Effects of the gradually increasing dawn light stimuration on sleep feeling. *Psychiatry Clin Neurosci*, 52(2): 247–248.
21. Noguchi, Hiroki, Syuichiro Shirakawa, Yoko Komada, Emi Koyama, and Toshihiko Sakaguchi. 2001. Improved quality of awakening by simulating dawn lighting with an ordinary ceiling light. *J Illum Eng Inst Jpn*, 8: 315–321 [in Japanese, with English abstract].
22. Kondo, Masayuki, Hiromi Tokura, Tomoko Wakamura, Ki–ja Hyun, Satoshi Tamotsu, Takeshi Morita, and Tadashi Oishi. 2009. Influences of twilight on diurnal variation of core temperature, its nadir, and urinary 6-hydroxymelatonin sulfate during nocturnal sleep and morning drowsiness. *Coll Antropol*, 33: 193–199.
23. Haskell, Edwin H., Joseph W. Palca, Jim Michael Walker, Ralph J. Berger, and Horace Craig Heller. 1981. The effects of high and low ambient temperatures on human sleep stages. *Electroencephalogr Clin Neurophysiol*, 51: 494–501.
24. Aschoff, Jürgen. 1958. Hauttemperatur und hautdurchblutung im diesnst der temperaturregulation. [Skin temperature and blood circuration in the service of temperature regulation]. *Klin Wochenschr*, 36(5): 193–202.
25. Kräuchi, Kurt, Christain Cajochen, Ester Werth, and Anna Wirz-Justice. 1999. Warm feet promote the rapid onset of sleep. *Nature*, Sep 2;401(6748): 36–37.
26. Teramoto, Yumiko, Hiromi Tokura, Ikuko Ioki, Satsuki Suho, Ryo Inoshiri, and Masaaki Masuda. 1998. The effect of room temperature on rectal temperature during night sleep. *J Thermal Biol*, 23: 15–21.
27. Wakamura, Tomoko, and Hiromi Tokura. 2002. Circadian rhythm of rectal temperature in humans under different ambient temperature cycles. *J Thermal Biol*, 27(5): 439–447.
28. Kondo, Masayuki, Hiromi Tokura, Tomoko Wakamura, Ki-Ja Hyun, Satoshi Tamotsu, Takeshi Morita, and Tadashi Oishi. 2007. Combined influences of gradual changes in room temperature and light around dusk and dawn on circadian rhythms of core temperature, urinary 6-hydroxymelatonin sulfate and waking sensation just after rising. *Coll Anthropol*, 31: 587–593.
29. Kondo, Masayuki, Hiromi Tokura, Tomoko Wakamura, Ki-ja Hyun, Satoshi Tamotsu, Takeshi Morita, and Tadashi Oishi. 2007. Physiological significance of cyclic changes in room temperature around dusk and dawn for circadian rhythms of core and skin temperature, urinary 6-hydroxymelatonin sulfate, and waking sensation just after rising. *J Physiol Anthropol*, 26: 429–436.
30. Liu, Yi, Martha Merrow, Jennifer J. Loros, Jay C. Dunlap. 1998. How temperature changes reset a circadian oscillator. *Science*, 281(5378): 825–829.
31. Mishima, Kazuo, Masako Okawa, Yasuo Hishikawa, Satoshi Hozumi, Hiroshi Hori, and Kiyohisa Takahashi. 1994. Morning bright light therapy for sleep and behavior disorders in elderly patients with dementia. *Acta Psychiatr Scand*, 89: 1–7.
32. Wakamura, Tomoko, and Hiromi Tokura. 2001. Influence of bright light during daytime on sleep parameters in hospitalized elderly patients. *J Physiol Anthropol Appl Human Sci*, 20(6): 345–351.
33. Riemersma-van der Lek, Rixt F., Dick F. Swaab, Jos Twisk, Elly M. Hol, Witte J. G. Hoogendijk, and Eus J. W. Van Someren. 2008. Effect of bright light and melatonin on cognitive and noncognitive function in elderly residents of group care facilities: A randomized controlled trial. *JAMA*, 299(22): 2642–2655.
34. Scheuermaier, Karine, Alison M. Laffan, and Jeanne F. Duffy. 2010. Light exposure patterns in healthy older and young adults. *J Biol Rhythms*, 25: 113–122.
35. Dumont, Marie, Hélène Blais, Joanie Roy, and Jean Paquet. 2009. Controlled patterns of daytime light exposure improve circadian adjustment in simulated night work. *J Biol Rhythms*, 24: 427–437.
36. Sekisuihouse, Co. Ltd. 2005. Research development/pilot development of living space producing sleep. Available at http://www.sekisuihouse.co.jp/company/data/current/newsobj-1514-datafile.pdf (accessed August 23, 2010)
37. Figueiro, Mariana G., Andrew Bierman, John D. Bullough, and Mark S. Rea. 2009. A personal light-treatment device for improving sleep quality in the elderly: dynamics of nocturnal melatonin suppression at two exposure levels. *Chronobiol Int*, 26(4): 726–739.

24 Decreased Light Transmittance Because of Aging and Melatonin

Takeshi Morita

Aging causes qualitative and quantitative change in nocturnal sleep. Many studies, including those by Feinberg[1] and Bliwise,[2] reported decrease of slow-wave sleep (SWS) and sleep efficiency during sleep and increase of frequency of waking episodes in older persons. Light in the morning, daytime, and nighttime influences sleep-awakening rhythm,[3,4] and sleep deterioration, such as poor sleep, frequent awakenings, and difficulty to fall asleep after awakening at night, is often observed in older people with visual impairment.[5] The results of these studies suggest that the quantitative and qualitative change of light entering from an eye to the retina could be one of the reasons of sleep disorder with aging.

Light reaches the retina through the cornea, pupil, crystalline lens, and vitreous body. Beems and van Best[6] concluded that the change of light transmittance in the cornea is not significantly affected by age. One of the factors for the quantitative change is reduction of pupil diameter. Yang et al.[7] reported that the pupil diameter and age had negative correlation under photopic, mesopic, and dilated conditions.

Lens opacity caused by aging brings more quantitative and qualitative change than reduction of pupil diameter. Among visible lights, short-wavelength lights such as violet and blue rays have lower spectral transmittance than long-wavelength lights in the human optical route even for the healthy eyes of younger population, and the transmittance especially of the short-wavelength lights significantly decreases with aging.[8] Brainard et al.[9] concluded that the decreased level was remarkable in subjects with cataract, where the protein molecule in crystalline lens is denatured to sequence anomaly and polymer and they are accumulated and browning with age. Cataract is one of the major visual impairment symptoms that occurs in about 5% of subjects 50–65 years old, about 25% in subject 65–75 years old, and as high as 40%–60% in subjects 75–85 years old according to a study by Klein et al.[10]

Short-wavelength lights, whose transmittance decreases with age, is important for nonvisual information processing such as circadian rhythms (melatonin, body temperature, sleep/wake rhythms) as well as ocular vision and color perception.

Melanopsin-expressing retinal ganglion cells (mRGCs) are a recently discovered photoreceptor for nonvisual information processing.

Several groups of researchers studied the spectral sensitivity of melanopsin, a photopigment in mRGCs, with its peak at approximately 480 nm. Berson et al.,[11] Hatter et al.,[12] Dacey et al.,[13] Hankins et al.,[14] and Zaidi et al.[15] studied this theme in rats, mice, primates, and humans from a photopigment point of view. Brainard et al.[16] and Thapan et al.[17] reported that its peak was 460 nm based on their analysis on monochromatic light-induced melatonin suppression.

On the other hand, the spectral sensitivity of mRGCs in humans has not yet been studied thoroughly; however, previous researchers reported that its peak ranges from 450 to 500 nm, and this range agrees with the belief that the extent of transmittance of visible light that reaches the retina decreases with age. This explains the occurrence of various circadian rhythm disorders in older persons.

Turner and Mainster[18] calculated the circadian photoreception from the decrease of spectral transmittance caused by reduction of pupil diameter, age-related opacity of crystalline lens, and characteristics of spectral sensitivity of nonvisual photoreceptor mRGCs. In this study, a 25-year-old adult has a decreased circadian photoreception by 20%, a 65-year-old by 70%, a 75-year-old by 80%, and an over 85-year-old by 90% compared with a 10-year-old child.

However, sensitivity variations in photoreceptors should also be added to the study. Charman[19] had a similar discussion as Turner and Mainster[18] but also pointed out that these calculations did not take sensitivity variations of mRGCs into consideration. Morita et al.[20] suggested that cone sensitivity might have diurnal variations based on the study on the color discriminatory capability using a 100-hue test. In this context, mRGCs sensitivity may also have similar diurnal variations. The correlation of light sensitivity of mRGCs with aging was suggested by Curcio and Drucker[21] in their report that the density of RGC of older persons is reduced by one fourth compared with that of the young controls and by Semo et al.[22] who observed a 40% reduction in mRGCs in old mice compared with younger mice controls. Moreover, aging-related sensitivity variations may occur within the suprachiasmatic nucleus itself as an animal test suggests, causing sleep disorder.[23]

In cataract surgery, the aged opaque crystalline lens are removed by laser and replaced with intraocular lenses (IOLs). Surgery brings significant improvement in transmittance to the crystalline lens—it restores lens with opacification and remarkably deteriorated transmittance of short-wavelength lights to normal, increases information for visual system, and dramatically increases the amount of light to a nonvisual photoreceptor. While patients examined themselves qualitatively (i.e., whether they recovered rich colors, vitality, and satisfactory sleep), few studies analyze the reality quantitatively as evidence.

Hollwich's group delivered the first physiological report: they revealed that presurgical ACTH and cortisol secretion defects and impaired metabolism of water balance, blood sugar, and blood cell count were restored to a normal level by the surgery, pointing out the influence of decline in light transmittance caused by cataract.[24–26]

Asplund and Lindblad[27] examined sleep improvement at both 1 and 9 months after cataract surgery in 407 aged patients. One month after the surgery, 28.3% of the men and 37.5% of the women reported poor sleep, but after 9 months, the figures decreased to 15.8% and 31.3%, respectively, which is a comparable level with a poor sleep rate for subjects with healthy eyes (13.1% of the men and 28.8% of the women, respectively). However, some points still remain unclear, for example, subjects younger than 80 years showed improvement in sleepiness in the morning, but that development was not found in subjects 80 years and older.

Morita's group also discussed these issues comparing the influences on sleep by decreasing light transmittance caused by aging and change in sleep and melatonin behaviors before and after cataract surgery.

The elderly subjects were classified into three groups using color chips with regard to blue–yellow color discrimination of desaturated 15-hue test (Lanthony, France): normal (N), slight error (L), and marked error (H). Their physical activities, quantities of light received, and sleep quality in daily lives were examined.[28]

The level of transmittance of the short-wavelength light in the lens deteriorated by aging was measured by blue–yellow color discrimination, and the subjects were classified into normal (N; no decline in color discrimination, i.e., transmittance of short wavelength is retained), slight error (L; with some mistakes in color discrimination, i.e., transmittance is slightly declined), and marked error (H; with remarkable number of mistakes in color discrimination, i.e., transmittance is significantly declined). Decline level and physical activities, history of light received, and sleep quality in the daily lives were compared in these three groups. Group H showed higher actual wake rate (i.e., actual sleep rate is low) during sleep than group N. The report suggested the possibility that developed opacity of the lens caused declined transmittance of short-wavelength light, and they are unable to acquire light adequately in the daily lives, which is important for their circadian rhythms.

They also compared sleep and behavior of melatonin secretion before and after cataract surgery with the lifestyle of the subjects such as light received and physical activities in the daily lives.[29] No difference was found in the behavior of melatonin secretion before and after the surgery; however, there are some findings in sleep efficiency. There was no correlation between wake-up or retiring times and sleep efficiency before surgery, but negative correlation appeared after the surgery (i.e., earlier wake-up or retiring time brought better sleep efficiency and later caused worse efficiency). The authors discussed that the patients were able to acquire enough short-wavelength light in their daily lives through surgery, and it brought a different influence according to their lifestyles—an increase in short-wavelength light received in the daytime had a good influence on the biological rhythms of patients with early wake-up time and resulted in sleep improvement, whereas an increase in short-wavelength light received at nighttime brought bad influence on the biological rhythms of the patients with late retiring time and caused their sleep disorders. This result suggests that the time of day should be taken into account as well as the change in light transmittance based on its amount when considering the influence of short-wavelengths light on nonvisual information processing.

The choice of the IOL types is also controversial: UV-only–blocking IOL or blue-blocking IOL. UV-only–blocking IOL cuts the UV radiation but retains clear sight for visible light; blue-blocking IOL cuts both UV and blue radiations considering disturbance by short wavelengths light (blue light) on eye functions. Turner and Mainster[18] indicated the change of circadian photoreception caused by aging crystalline lens while comparing the circadian photoreception by both blue- and UV-only–blocking IOL. Blue-blocking IOL has less improvement for circadian photoreception, as it cuts the short wavelengths light; however, UV-only IOL is expected to bring significant improvement, as it transmits the short-wavelengths light.

Patel and Dacey[30] computed the influence of four light sources with six types of lens using three action spectra for circadian photoentrainment reported between 2001 and 2007. The result showed that UV-only–blocking IOL has approximately 40% higher effectiveness in circadian photoentrainment than blue-blocking IOL under natural light (5000K), cool white fluorescent lamp, and incandescent lamp (3000K).

Landers et al.[31] examined the influence of blue-blocking IOL on the circadian rhythms of patients 6 months after surgery and the photoreceptor damage of blue light (approximately 475 nm) using the Pittsburgh Sleep Quality Index questionnaire and compared the results with UV-only–blocking IOL. The study concluded that there was no need to consider the influence of circadian rhythms, as no statistically significant differences were observed between the two IOLs.

However, sleep efficiency differs depending on the chronotype (morning and evening types), even for the youth,[32] and daily life light history should be taken into consideration when studying the influence of IOLs.

REFERENCES

1. Feinberg, I. 1989. Effects of maturation and aging on slow wave sleep in man. In *Slow Wave Sleep. Physiological, Phathophysiolosical, and Functional Aspects.* ed. Wauquier, A, Dugovic, C, Radulovacki, M. 31–48. New York: Raven Press.
2. Bilwise, DL. 1994. Normal aging. In *Principle and Practice of Sleep Medicine.* ed. Kryger, MH, Roth, T, Dement, WC. 26–39. New York: Saunders.
3. Mishima, K, Okawa, M, Shimizu, T, Hishikawa, Y. 2001. Diminished melatonin secretion in the elderly caused by insufficient environmental illumination. *J Clin Endocrinol Metab.* 86:129–134.
4. Van Someren, EJ, Riemersma, RF, Swaab, DF. 2002. Functional plasticity of the circadian timing system in old age: Light exposure. *Prog Brain Res.* 138:205–231.
5. Asplund, R. 2000. Sleep, health and visual impairment in the elderly. *Arch Gerontol Geriatr.* 30:7–15.
6. Beems, EM, van Best, JA. 1990. Light transmission of the cornea in whole human eyes. *Exp Eye Res.* 50:393–395.

7. Yang, Y, Thompson, K, Burns, SA. 2002. Pupil location under mesopic, photopic, and pharmacologically dilated conditions. *Invest Ophthalmol Vis Sci.* 43:2508–2512.
8. Weale, RA. 1988. Age and the transmittance of the human crystalline lens. *J Physiol.* 395:577–587.
9. Brainard, GC, Rollag, MD, Hanifin, JP. 1997. Photic regulation of melatonin in humans: Ocular and neural signal transduction. *J Biol Rhythms.* 12:537–546.
10. Klein, B, Klein, R, Linton, K. 1992. Prevalence of age-related lens opacities in a population. *Ophthalmology.* 99:546–552.
11. Berson, DM, Dunn, FA, Takao, M. 2002. Phototransduction by retinal ganglion cells that set the circadian clock. *Science.* 295:1070–1073.
12. Hatter, S, Lucas, RJ, Mrosovsky, N, Thompson, S, Douglas, RH, Hankins, MW, Lem, J, Bie, M, Hofmann, F, Foster, RG, Yau, KW. 2003. Melanopsin and rod–cone photoreceptive systems account for all major accessory visual function in mice. *Nature.* 424:76–81.
13. Dacey, DM, Liao, HW, Peterson, BB, Robinson, FR, Smith, VC, Pokorny, J, Yau, KW, Gamlin PD. 2005. Melanopsin-expressing ganglion cells in primate retina signal color and irradiance and project to the LGN. *Nature.* 433:749–754.
14. Hankins, MW, Lucas, RJ. 2002. The primary visual pathway in humans is regulated according to long-term light exposure through the action of a nonclassical photopigment. *Curr Biol.* 12:191–198.
15. Zadi, FH, Hull, JT, Peirson, SN, Wulff, K, Aeschbach, D, Gooley, JJ, Brainard, GC, Gregory-Evans, K, Rizzo, JF III, Czeisler, CA, Foster, RG, Moseley, MJ, Lockley, SW. 2007. Short-wavelength light sensitivity of circadian, papillary, and visual awareness in humans lacking an outer retina. *Curr Biol.* 17:2122–2128.
16. Brainard, GC, Hanifin, JP, Greeson, JM, Byrne, B, Glickman, G, Gerner, E, Rollag, MD. 2001. Action spectrum for melatonin regulation in humans: Evidence for novel circadian photoreceptor. *J Neurosci.* 21:6405–6412.
17. Thapan, K, Arendt, J, Skene, DJ. 2001. An action spectrum for melatonin suppression: Evidence for a novel non-rod, non-cone photoreceptor system in humans. *J Physiol.* 535:261–267.
18. Turner, PL, Mainster, MA. 2008. Circadian photoreception: Ageing and the eye's important role in systemic health. *Br J Ophthalmol.* 92:1439–1444.
19. Charman, WN. 2003. Age, lens transmittance, and the possible effects of light on melatonin suppression. *Ophthal Physiol Opt.* 23:181–187.
20. Morita, T, Ohyama, M, Tokura, H. 1994. Diurnal variation of hue discriminatory capability under artificial constant illumination. *Experientia.* 50:641–643.
21. Curcio, CA, Drucker, DN. 1993. Retinal ganglion cells in Alzheimer's disease and aging. *Ann Neurol.* 33:248–257.
22. Semo, M, Lupi, D, Peirson, SN, Butler, JN, Foster, RG. 2003. Light-induced c-fos in melanopsin retinal ganglion cells of young and aged rodless/coneless (*rd/rd cl*) mice. *Eur J Neurosci.* 18:3007–3017.
23. Zhang, Y, Brainard, GC, Zee, PC, Pinto, LH, Takahashi, JS, Turek, FW. 1998. Effects of aging on lens transmittance and retinal input to the suprachiasmatic nucleus in golden hamsters. *Neurosci Lett.* 258:167–170.
24. Hollwich, F, Dieckhues, B. 1980. The effect of natural and artificial light via the eye on the hormonal and metabolic balance of animal and man. *Ophthalmologica.* 180:188–197.
25. Hollwich, F, Dieckhues, B. 1989. Effect of light on the eye on metabolism and hormones. *Klin Monbl Augenheilkd.* 195:284–290.
26. Hollwich, F, Hartmann, C. 1990. Influence of light through the eyes on metabolism and hormones. *Ophtalmologie.* 4:385–389.
27. Asplund, R, Lindblad, BE. 2004. Sleep and sleepiness 1 and 9 months after cataract surgery. *Arch Gerontol Geriatr.* 38:69–75.
28. Norimatsu, K, Sato, M, Morita, T. 2007. The effect of acquired colour deficiency in elderly people on some aspects of sleep. *Biol Rhythm Res.* 38:333–338.
29. Tanaka, M, Hosoe, K, Hamada, T, Morita, T. 2010. Changes in sleep state of the elderly before and after cataract surgery. *J Physiol Anthropol.* 29:219–224.
30. Patel, AS, Dacey, DM. 2009. Relative effectiveness of a blue light–filtering intraocular lens for photoentrainment of the circadian rhythm. *J Cataract Refract Surg.* 35:529–539.
31. Landers, JA, Tamblyn, D, Perriam, D. 2009. Effect of blue-light–blocking intraocular lens on the quality of sleep. *J Cataract Refract Surg.* 35:83–88.
32. Lehnkering, H, Siegmund, R. 2007. Influence of chronotype, season, and sex of subject on sleep behavior of young adults. *Chronobiol Int.* 24:875–888.

25 Melatonin and Treatment of Disorders Related to Jet Lag and Shift Work

Gregory M. Brown, Seithikurippu R. Pandi-Perumal, Ilya Trakht, D. Warren Spence, Daniel P. Cardinali, and Alexander Samel

CONTENTS

25.1 INTRODUCTION

In both jet lag disorder (JLD) and shift work disorder (SWD), there is an imposed or voluntary shift in the timing of the sleep/wake cycle resulting in a misalignment of the cycle and associated symptoms.

25.2 JET LAG DISORDER

Rapid travel across time zones has become an accepted component of our modern "24-hour society." Compared to previous decades, air travel is now a primary mode of transportation for both long-distance and intermediate distance journeys [1–4]. Extended air travel typically involves flights across multiple time zones and consequently results in JLD.

JLD defines the responses to an abrupt change in time zones following rapid travel across multiple time zones (in the form of transmeridian, transatlantic, transoceanic, or transequatorial travel); this response includes a constellation of bodily and psychological symptoms, which although transient are nevertheless unpleasant [5–7]. A second component of JLD is travel fatigue resulting from several causes including sleep loss, change in meal timing, low cabin pressure, and immobility among other factors [8]. Travel fatigue also occurs in extended travel that does not cross time zones (translatitudinal travel).

25.2.1 Symptoms of JLD

Almost all individuals who travel over multiple time zones are subject to transient physiological and psychological symptoms. Surveys of air travelers confirm that jet lag symptoms can persist for a few days, and for about half of those surveyed, the symptoms were regarded as severely bothersome. Normally, JLD symptoms remit after a few days following the flight. For some, however, the symptoms reportedly persisted for over a week, particularly when time zone differences were greater than 8 hours. Age, individual differences, number of time zones crossed, and direction of travel all contribute to the severity of the symptoms [9–11].

According to the *International Classification of Sleep Disorders* (ICSD) [12] and the *DSM-IV-TR* [13], JLD falls under the category of circadian rhythm sleep disorders (CRSD). The symptoms of JLD (also known as *time zone change syndrome*) include both physiological and psychological disturbances [7,14,15]. Women may experience delays in ovulation and menstrual dysregulation [16,17]. One study suggests that the chronic or repeated JLD exposure can lead to cognitive decline and temporal lobe atrophy in humans if there is a short recovery time between flights [18]. Model JLD is also associated with tumor progression in rodents [19] and elevated mortality rate in aged mice [20].

Both the severity and duration of JLD symptoms are affected by the total number of time zones crossed as well as by the direction of air travel (eastward or westward) [10,21]. Generally, there is a reduction in the symptoms as the number of time zones crossed decreases [22].

JLD symptoms may have important consequences if there are the mental and physical demands which occur immediately after the flight. For holiday travelers, such symptoms may only be a minor inconvenience. However, for business travelers, pilots, and others who are frequent fliers, the cognitive and physical impairments following JLD can be significant [23,24]. Among the consequences are the environmental costs of making poor decisions as well as the subjective distress that inevitably accompanies such experiences.

25.2.2 Determinants of JLD

JLD symptoms show considerable interindividual and intraindividual variability [5–8,25]. Age is one important factor. In simulated JLD, middle-aged male subjects (ages 37–52 years) had more symptoms than younger men (ages 18–25 years) [26]. Moreover, those older than 60 years are reported to have greater difficulty in adapting to JLD [9,11]. Another important variable is the individual's *chronotype*, a term relating the time of day when alertness is at its peak. Individuals who are "morning chronotypes" generally have less difficulty in phase-advancing their body rhythms (i.e., adjusting after a flight from west to east) than "evening chronotypes," and vice versa, if there were a phase delay [27]. Yet another study reported that those who had "rigid" sleep habits had more severe symptoms after transmeridian flight [21]. Among other factors that may play a role are unplanned exposure to light, fatigue from time spent in travel preparation, and the habitual activity and sleep schedule of the traveler.

Almost every physiological function has a circadian "phase map" consisting of an ordered sequence of peaks and valleys. While the period of the phase map for different physiological functions may be similar, the peaks and valleys of the maps frequently do not coincide [22]. Phase maps are also sensitive to environmental changes and can be transiently affected by temporal disruptions such as JLD or shift work. Under these circumstances, the recovery time for restoring the normal rhythm profile (period of re-entrainment) can differ significantly from one physiological function to another. Although during the period of re-entrainment individual circadian rhythms generally move in a direction that corresponds with that of the environmental time shift [22], in some cases, the circadian system moves in a direction that is opposite to that of the environmental change, giving rise to a phenomenon called "splitting." Phase map "partitioning" is more complex and involved a partial re-entrainment by some phase maps in a direction that is opposite to that of other phase maps [22]. Resynchronization typically requires several days (about 1 day per hour of phase-shift), and it is during this transition period that the symptoms of JLD are most pronounced.

The severity of phase desynchronization can be affected by the direction of jet travel. As noted above, eastward travelers (who are subjected to a phase-advance) usually require more time to adjust to altered sleep/wake schedules than westward jet travelers (subjected to phase delay). This difference in adjustment time is usually attributed to the internal body clock's greater ability to adapt to a longer rather than to a shorter delay.

25.2.3 Clinical Presentation

The myriad of physiological and psychological complaints associated with JLD (Table 25.1) can pose a temporary but significant disruption to the lives of the travelers who experience these complaints. Most of the symptoms involve sleep and biological rhythm desynchronization. The somatic complaints include, but are not limited to, anxiety and depressed mood, cardiovascular complaints, dizziness, gastrointestinal discomforts, glucose metabolism dysregulation, headaches, and menstrual irregularity in women [28,29].

25.2.3.1 Fatigue

Many studies have shown that fatigue is the most commonly reported consequence of JLD [4,6,15] (Figure 25.1). Bourgeois-Bougrine et al. [30] measured self-reported fatigue-related incidents among pilots from four airline industries following short- and long-haul flights. The authors found that the acute fatigue and sleep deprivation were mainly due to the pilots' work schedules, night flights, JLD, and successive early wake-ups. The authors concluded that these job-related factors were important contributors to accidents and incidents in the airline industry [30].

Studies of the performance of air crews using neuropsychological testing clearly indicate performance is reduced during long-haul flights and flights across many time zones [31–34]. For example, in a study of airline pilots on 5-day long-haul Madrid–Mexico–Madrid flights (seven time zones) and Madrid–Tokyo–Madrid flights (eight time zones), activity/rest and heart rate rhythms were linked to a "weak oscillator" while body temperature rhythms, which are closely related to the biological clock, showed a rigid response after the phase-shifts of the light/dark (LD) cycle [4]. Psychometric evaluation showed that all of the pilots showed signs of rhythm desynchronization.

TABLE 25.1
General Symptoms of Jet Lag

Anorexia or loss of appetite
Apathy
Bowel irregularities (constipation or frequent defecation)
Clumsiness
Daytime somnolence
Decreased vigilance and attention domains
Depression
Diminished mental abilities (i.e., cognitive performance, concentration, judgment, decision making, memory lapses)
Diminished physical performance
Disorientation
Fuzziness
Generalized fatigue and lethargy
Gastrointestinal symptoms (e.g., bloating, upset stomach)
General feeling of malaise
Headache
Impaired alertness
Impaired task performance (increased accidents and errors)
Inappropriate timing of defecation and urination
Irritability
Glucose metabolism dysregulation
Headaches
Mood disturbances
Muscular pain
Menstrual irregularity
Tiredness (traveler's fatigue)
Tumor progression is noted in chronic animal model
Trouble initiating and maintaining sleep
Sleeping difficulties (inappropriate sleep at local time)
Sleep loss
Slowed reflexes
Stress
Traveler's thrombosis (deep vein thrombosis)
Weakness

Note: Given the interindividual variability and susceptibility, the core symptoms vary and not necessarily each and every individual experiences or exhibits the entire spectrum of symptoms at a given point.

In both flight directions, pilots maintained the pattern of excretion of 6-sulfatoxymelatonin that prevailed in the time zone of their homes [35]. This evidence thus confirms that airline crew members, who constantly travel across multiple international time zones, experience significant disruptions to internal bodily rhythms.

25.2.3.2 Psychoimmunoneuroendocrine Correlates of JLD

McEwen coined the terms *allostasis* and *allostatic load* to describe the dynamic process by which the body maintains homeostasis [36,37]. The mediators of allostasis work as a nonlinear network meaning that too much or too little of each mediator can have harmful consequences by perturbing the entire network. The term *allostatic overload* is applied to the wear and tear produced by imbalances in the mediators of allostasis.

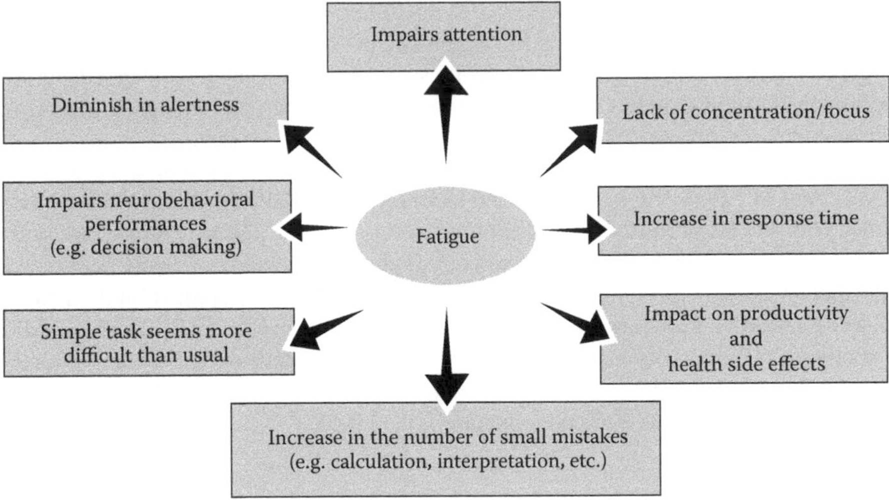

FIGURE 25.1 The several effects of fatigue.

Indeed, sleep deprivation produces an allostatic overload that can have deleterious consequences [37]. Restriction of sleep to 4 hours per night is associated with increases in blood pressure, decreases in parasympathetic tone, increases in evening cortisol and insulin levels, and increases in appetite, possibly through the elevation of ghrelin, a proappetitive hormone, and decreases in the levels of leptin, which has anorexic activity [38–41]. Proinflammatory cytokine levels are increased, along with decreases in performance on tests of psychomotor vigilance (after a modest sleep restriction to 6 hours per night), effects that are reversible by a nap [42,43].

Allostatic overload in animal models causes atrophy of neurons in the hippocampus and prefrontal cortex, brain regions involved in memory, selective attention, and executive function, and causes hypertrophy of neurons in the amygdala, a brain region involved in fear and anxiety, as well as aggression [44]. Thus, the ability to learn and remember and to make decisions may be compromised and may be accompanied by increased levels of anxiety and aggression. In this context, the results of Cho et al. [45] on chronic JLD exposure are very relevant. The investigators presented evidence showing that stress related neurochemical changes that were attributable to the experience of chronic JLD could actually affect the structure of the brain [18]. Further support for the hypothesis that JLD, in addition to promoting transient symptoms of fatigue, is also a significant physiological stressor, was provided by Iglesias et al. [16]. The investigators found that dysregulation of circadian timing systems could postpone ovulation and cause menstrual disturbances in 30%–35% of a female cabin crew.

25.2.4 The Circadian System and Melatonin

Humans, along with many other mammals, are a diurnal species with most body functions displaying a 24-hour rhythm that are chiefly controlled by the timing of exposure to light. In brief, this rhythm is controlled by a master clock located in the suprachiasmatic nucleus (SCN) of the hypothalamus, which coordinates the rhythms of other cells and tissues of the body [46,47]. This clock in turn is controlled primarily by the environmental LD cycle [48] (and see an earlier chapter in this volume by Verster et al.). Recent studies have shown that a unique circadian photoreception pathway exists, which employs light-sensitive retinal ganglion cells and which has direct neural connections to the SCN. This pathway uses a novel photopigment, melanopsin, that is maximally responsive to short-wavelength light (460–480 nm) [49–51]. The SCN acts on the pineal gland via a complex multisynaptic pathway projecting to the cervical sympathetic outflow to the pineal and causing the synthesis and release of melatonin. During light exposure of sufficient intensity, the SCN's output to the pineal gland is suppressed and melatonin synthesis ceases [46]. The action spectrum for melatonin suppression by light matches that of melanopsin [52] as does that of light's alerting effects [53,54]. Melatonin is the primary hormonal output of the circadian system.

Melatonin acts on the brain as well as peripheral sites via two Gi-protein–coupled membrane receptors MT1 and MT2 [55,56]. A third related receptor, called GPR50, shares 45% of the amino acid sequence with MT1 and MT2 but does not bind melatonin [57]. These receptors are both found in the SCN [58], although MT1 is located extensively in the brain outside of the SCN [59,60] as well as in the periphery, notably the retina [61]. In SCN slices, the MT1 receptor inhibits firing acutely while both MT1 and MT2 may contribute to phase-shifting in these slices [62]. MT1 and MT2 have also been shown to differentially regulate GABAA receptor function in SCN [63]. A fourth ^{125}I-2-iodomelatonin binding site has been identified in mammals [64] but is of considerably lower affinity. It has now been characterized as quinone reductase type 2 [65].

25.2.5 Prevention of JLD

An early study showed that bright light exposure resets the human circadian pacemaker, which controls daily variations in physiological, behavioral, and cognitive function, suggesting that it could be beneficial for alleviating the symptoms of JLD [66]. The effectiveness of light therapy is critically dependent on the timing and intensity of the exposure. Light treatment in the early morning can produce phase-advances before an eastbound flight [67]. Westward flights normally contain their own adjustment promoters given by traveler's subjective evening and early night exposure to the natural light in the new location, which will phase delay the circadian system.

It is now established that the effect of light on the circadian system can be measured by a phase response curve (PRC) in which the minimum in core body temperature is used as an estimate for the crossover point of the curve. Light pulses administered before this time point will delay the circadian clock while light pulses after the point will phase-advance the clock. Light exposure occurring close to the time of minimum core body temperature produces the greatest phase shift [68]. Phase delays of approximately 2.5–3 hours per day and phase-advances of 1.5–2 hours per day have been observed following carefully timed exposure to bright light [69,70]. As mentioned above, light is a pervasive and prominent zeitgeber that synchronizes the biological clock in mammals [71–73]. Inasmuch as bright light (2500 lux) almost completely suppresses melatonin production while dim light (500 lux or less) affects it only slightly, melatonin levels can be used as an alternative marker of the circadian phase position. In several studies, the onset of melatonin secretion in the evening under dim light (DLMO) has been used as a marker of the phase position of the circadian rhythm [74].

It is surprising that few definitive studies have been carried out using light pretreatment to prevent or reduce JLD symptoms. In 1995, Stewart et al. [75] exposed NASA pay load workers to 10,000 lux for 1 week prelaunch in a protocol designed to phase shift their body clocks to better suit their work schedule during launch. Treated subjects reported better sleep, performance, and physical and emotional well-being, thus supporting endorsement of the treatment for preadaptation of NASA workers. In 1996, Deacon and Arendt [76] established that light treatment could have a potent effect shifting the circadian system. Subjects were treated in semicontrolled conditions 9 hours westward by exposing them to circa 1000 lux broad-spectrum white light for 9 hours daily. They then delayed exposure 3 hours per day for 3 days and maintained the new schedule for 2 days at 9 hours west. The procedure produced a steady and consistent shift of core body temperature, melatonin rhythm (as 6-sulfatoxymelatonin), and sleep, and, with the exception of a small suppression of endogenous melatonin production during light treatment, there were no adverse effects. Burgess et al. [77] tested treatments that travelers could use to phase-advance their circadian rhythms prior to eastward flight. The aim was to determine if travelers could arrive with their circadian rhythms already partially re-entrained to local time. Participants phase-advanced their habitual sleep schedule by 1 hour per day for 3 days.

Exposure to light occurred during the first 3.5 hours after waking on each of the 3 days and under the following conditions: ordinary dim indoor light (<60 lux), intermittent bright light (>3000 lux, 0.5 hour on, 0.5 hour off, etc.), or continuous bright light (>3000 lux). The endogenous salivary DLMO was used as an indicator of phase changes. Mean DLMO phase-advances occurred in the dim, intermittent, and continuous light groups of 0.6, 1.5, and 2.1 hours, respectively. Side effects as assessed with actigraphy and subject logs were limited. The loss of sleep was minimal (on average, less than 1 hour) and occurred primarily on the first day of treatment when the sleep opportunity was shortened by 1 hour [77]. In a further study, Eastman et al. compared 1- and 2-hour sleep advances combined with 3 hours of intermittent bright light treatment (5000 lux 30 min on, 30 min off) and concluded that the 1-hour sleep schedule advance was as effective as a 2-hour advance schedule [78]. Paul et al. [79,80] used a light tower emitting monochromatic light of 500 nm to compare various timings of light treatment in hastening adaptive preflight circadian phase-advance and delay. This wavelength is close to the most effective range for activating melanopsin. The largest phase-advances resulted from light treatment that was initiated between 0600 and 0800 h, while greatest phase delays resulted from light treatment started between 0200 and 0300 h in entrained subjects with a regular sleep/wake cycle (2300 to 0700 h). A software program for calculating timing of light administration has been developed, but this program requires validation in actual studies [81].

Although there is good evidence that preflight light treatment could be beneficial, field studies of effects during actual flight have yet to be reported to our knowledge. The practicality of such extensive changes is questionable for the casual traveler, although preadaptive changes of 1 to 2 hours of sleep time and wake time (thus altering light exposure) could be useful for reducing jet lag symptoms. However, for major movements of personnel, such as troops or teams that can be preplanned and organized, strategic changes in schedule could be of considerable benefit.

An early study showed a significant effect of melatonin pretreatment on the circadian system before and after a 9-hour phase shift [82]. Similarly, but in the opposite direction to the effects of environmental light, it is now established that melatonin produces a PRC in the circadian system that is approximately 12 hours out of phase with the light PRC [83–85]. In contrast to light, melatonin will produce phase-advances in the circadian clock if it is administered during the early or late evening hours. Postponements of melatonin administration to the second part of the night or early morning will phase delay the clock. Optimal doses, type of melatonin (regular versus sustained release) and timings of melatonin treatment are still under investigation [86]. The common doses used in various studies have ranged from 0.5 to 5 mg regular melatonin by mouth. Although 5 mg is the most common dose used, this dosage can produce drowsiness [87–92]. Doses of 0.5 mg have been reported to be effective for producing phase shifting with less drowsiness [93]. It has been reported that larger doses produce greater phase shifts than lower doses [94,95]. However, it has also been reported that if a 3-mg dose is administered 4.8 hours prior to the DLMO and a 0.5-mg dose is administered about 2.4 hours before the DLMO, the phase-advance response is equivalent [96]. Thus, as suggested by the authors [96] and further elaborated by others [84,86], optimal timing of treatment may be different with different melatonin doses.

Revell and Eastman have shown that the addition of afternoon exogenous melatonin administration to morning light exposure will produce greater phase-advances than either treatment alone [85].

One problem in these studies is that they avoid many of the actual conditions of long-haul flights such as poor air quality, noise, light, cabin pressure, inappropriate meal times, uncomfortable seats, and restrained leg movements. These factors may be major contributors to JLD symptoms but continue to be poorly studied.

25.2.6 Improving the Symptoms of JLD

Once they are present, the proper management of JLD symptoms and its effects involves a two step process: (a) accelerating re-entrainment of circadian rhythms and (b) management of transient sleep loss. These objectives can be achieved by nonpharmacological and pharmacological means.

25.2.6.1 Nonpharmacological Management of JLD

One proposal has suggested that behavioral interventions such as meals and exercise can effectively aid the adjustment to a new time zone [97,98]. In a study of rats, the restriction of feeding schedules to a specific time was found to entrain body rhythms including that of corticosterone but not of melatonin [99]. In a study of humans, a single carbohydrate-rich meal provided in the morning instead of the evening produced a phase-advance of the temperature and heart rhythms [100]. Moreover, in a study in mice, differences in pathways for light- and food-entrainable rhythms have been shown [101]. However, no consensus has been reached regarding the exact manner with which to implement these behavioral changes [25,102].

Postflight-timed exposure to daylight has been reported to improve JLD symptoms in two subjects in an early study by Daan and Lewy [103]. In a clinical trial, the efficacy of light therapy for JLD using a head-mounted light visor was evaluated [104]. Twenty experimental subjects received either bright light (3000 lux) or dim red light [10 lux) for 3 hours on the first two evenings after a westward transcontinental flight. The subjects were assessed for salivary DLMO for 2 days preflight and for 2 days postflight. Although the study revealed that moderate circadian re-entrainment had occurred, there was no significant improvement in sleep characteristics, performance, or subjective assessment of JLD symptoms [104].

25.2.6.2 Pharmacological Management of JLD

The effects of many pharmacological compounds have been assessed to determine their efficacy for overcoming the problem of JLD. Most of these studies have focused on improving sleep in an effort to reduce the homeostatic sleep drive. The various compounds researched range from the use of sedative antihistamines [105]; short-acting benzodiazepines such as triazolam [106], temazepam [107,108], and brotizolam [109]; imidazopyridine hypnotics such as zopiclone [110,111], zolpidem [112], and zaleplon [108,113]; and the chronobiotic melatonin [46,114–116]. The ability of the hypnotics to reduce JLD symptoms, combined with the fact that they are typically used only on a short-term basis, justifies their use clinically, despite the fact that some can have pronounced side effects [15].

25.2.7 Sedative Antihistamines

Antihistamines (H_1-receptor antagonists) are the mainstay of symptomatic therapy for allergic disorders. A major drawback of these agents, however, is their tendency to increase diurnal somnolence. Drugs such as fexofenadine are second-generation antihistamines that do not readily enter the brain from the blood and hence cause fewer disruptive effects on cognitive and psychomotor function [117], whereas others such as hydroxyzine are very effective sleep inducers [118].

Although the risks associated with the consumption of sedating antihistamines have been extensively debated [119], such warnings are not always attended to by pilots, an inference supported by the finding that antihistamines are the leading agents found residually on autopsy in the systems of pilots who have crashed their aircraft [105]. Nevertheless, with the careful choice of agents in this class of drugs and with the proper dosage regimen, the central nervous system effects of antihistamines can be minimized or largely avoided while still preserving their therapeutic properties.

25.2.8 Short-Acting Benzodiazepines

Early studies showed that triazolam induced major shifts in the circadian clock of golden hamsters, as evidenced by changes in their locomotor activity [120]. While the ability of this drug to alter human circadian cycles has not been demonstrated, it has nevertheless been shown to benefit adaptation to a new LD cycle [106]. The ability of triazolam to improve sleep architecture over that of placebo allowed a faster adaptation to the new LD cycle, thus suggesting that triazolam has chronobiotic properties. However, the incidence of travelers' amnesia, cognitive impairment, and rebound insomnia associated with triazolam discourages its use for the treatment of JLD [121,122].

Temazepam has also been examined, with studies showing that it promotes improvements in subjective sleep quality without altering rates of physiological entrainment to the new environment [107]. The effects of temazepam were also studied in a group of athletes who had flown from the United Kingdom to Florida. The subjects were given either 10 mg of temazepam or a placebo immediately before local bedtime during their first three nights in Florida [123]. The results indicated that temazepam improved subjective sleep quality but did not improve performance beyond levels shown in controls.

It must be stressed that none of these drugs have been shown to prevent maladjustment to either shift work or transmeridian travel; whether they can alleviate the sleep loss symptoms or shorten the time required for readaptation is still an open question. Thus, benzodiazepine receptor antagonists cannot be recommended for prescription to patients with symptoms of maladjustment to shift work or JLD. The effects of these compounds in humans and the strong addictive risk limit their use as chronobiotics, at least in chronic conditions requiring long-term and repeating phase-shifting treatment.

25.2.9 Imidazopyridine Hypnotics

The efficacy of zolpidem, zopiclone, and zaleplon for reducing the symptoms of JLD has been evaluated [111,124–126]. Zolpidem, in doses of 10 mg, has been found to improve subjective sleep quality, particularly during the flight [126].

In a study in which zopiclone (7.5 mg) was assessed in subjects with a 5-hour westward phase delay, Daurat et al. [124] showed that subjects in the experimental group had better sleep quality than those in the placebo group; however, subjective JLD scores did not differ between the drug group and the placebo group. This study thus supports the conclusion that zopiclone accelerates the readjustment of the rest/activity rhythm by facilitating sleep rather than via a chronobiotic effect.

25.2.10 Melatonin

Agents that influence the circadian apparatus are referred to as *chronobiotics* [127]. The prototype of this class of agents is the hormone melatonin [46,114–116]. In humans, melatonin plays a major role in the coordination of circadian rhythmicity, most notably that of the sleep/wake cycle [128,129]. The timing or rhythm of melatonin secretion indicates the status of the body's internal clock, both in terms of its phase (i.e., internal clock time relative to external clock time) and amplitude. Similar to the effects of environmental light, melatonin's regulatory influence is also time-dependent, thus showing a phase–response curve [83]. As noted above, in contrast to light, melatonin will produce phase-advances in the circadian clock if it is administered during the early or late evening hours. Postponements of melatonin administration to the second part of the night or early morning will phase delay the clock.

These characteristics were the basis for early speculations that melatonin might be useful clinically for treating circadian-related sleep disorders, including JLD. With few exceptions [5], a compelling amount of evidence now indicates that melatonin can significantly reduce JLD symptoms in air travelers [3,77,78,86,90,92,96,130–136].

In the first placebo-controlled study of melatonin's use for JLD, Arendt et al. [87] found that a 5-mg dose of melatonin administered in the evening (1800 h) for 3 days prior to departure and for 4 days following arrival at the destination was effective for alleviating a number of JLD symptoms. Compared with controls, the passengers receiving melatonin showed a much faster adaptation of self-recorded sleep parameters and mood ratings, as well as objective measures such as endogenous melatonin and cortisol rhythms. A larger study of 52 passengers traveling from the United Kingdom to Sydney, Australia (more than eight time zones), produced similar findings. Half of the sample, which had been asked to ingest melatonin 2 days prior to the flight and for 4 days following their arrival, demonstrated superior improvement over controls on a self-rating of JLD scores [137]. In a cross-over placebo study involving 36 subjects, postflight administration of 5 mg of melatonin accelerated the adaptation of cortisol rhythm and improved subjective JLD scores [89]. Improvement of JLD scores with postflight melatonin treatment was also confirmed in another study of 52 aircrew members [90]. The combined regimen of slow-release caffeine plus melatonin has also been found to alleviate daytime sleepiness [135].

In one of the largest double-blind controlled studies ever undertaken of melatonin's use for JLD, 257 physicians traveling from Oslo, Norway, to New York were evaluated. All study group participants, including the placebo subjects, showed improvements in JLD scores on the first day after travel, followed by progressive improvement over the next 5 days. The investigators speculated that the physicians' knowledge that they had three out of four chances of receiving melatonin probably accounted for the large placebo effect [5].

A meta-analysis of 10 trials (Cochrane database) concluded that melatonin taken at bedtime in the place of destination (2200 h to midnight) was effective for reducing JLD symptoms of air travelers who had crossed five or more time zones. Intake of melatonin daily at the doses from 0.5 to 5.0 mg was also found to be effective. It was concluded that melatonin is "remarkably" effective for preventing or reducing JLD symptoms [138].

Melatonin's essential lack of adverse effects has now been recognized by the European Medicines Agency. The agency has approved a prolonged-release 2-mg melatonin preparation (Circadin™) as monotherapy for the treatment of primary insomnia characterized by poor quality of sleep in patients who are 55 years or older. This is the first official recognition of melatonin as a useful medication in sleep disorders. Circadin improves quality of sleep, morning alertness, sleep onset latency, and quality of life in middle-aged and older patients with insomnia [139–141].

Taken together, the data reviewed here indicate that oral administration of melatonin is one of the best available pharmacological treatments for JLD [46,142–146]. Its effectiveness is probably due to both its phase-shifting effect and its sleep-inducing effect [7]. Since the adjustment of the body clock appears to be the major mechanism for alleviating the symptoms of JLD, exogenous melatonin administration represents the primary mediator of this effect.

In Table 25.2, we summarize tentative recommendations for flights covering more than 8 time zones.

25.2.11 Potential Use of Melatonin Agonists in JLD

25.2.11.1 Ramelteon

Ramelteon (Rozerem™) is a new, highly, specific MT1/MT2 melatonin receptor agonist synthesized by Takeda Chemical Industries, Japan [147,148]. Its half-life is much longer (1–2 hours) than that of melatonin. Ramelteon acts on both MT1 and MT2 melatonergic receptors present in the SCNs and

TABLE 25.2
Estimated Time of Day for Exposure to Natural or Artificial Bright Light (>1000 lux, 30 min) to Blunt the Circadian System of an Air Traveler in Long (>8 h) Time Shifts

Number of Time Zones Crossed	East Bound	West Bound
8	0400–0700 h and 0900–1200 h	1200–1500 h and 1700–2000 h
9	0500–0800 h and 1000–1300 h	1100–1400 h and 1600–1900 h
10	0600–0900 h and 1100–1400 h	1000–1300 h and 1500–1800 h
11	0700–1000 h and 1200–1500 h	0900–1200 h and 1400–1700 h
12	0800–1100 h and 1300–1600 h	0800–1100 h and 1300–1600 h

Note: The data are speculative and based on empirical evidence from refs. [84] and [128]. This table is based on an assumed core body temperature minimum occurring at about 0200 h.

other brain areas. Ramelteon is considered a new type of hypnotic that lacks the adverse effects that are typically associated with benzodiazepines.

Seven randomized, double-blind placebo controlled trials of melatonin were compared with three clinical trials of ramelteon involving a large number of patients with insomnia in a recent review [149]. Ramelteon was found to be well tolerated, increases total sleep time, and reduces sleep latency. It also had a limited side effect profile and no clinically significant next-day performance effects [150]. Ramelteon has been shown to produce a circadian phase-advance with repeated administration in a laboratory setting [151].

A recent placebo-controlled study included 110 healthy adults with a history of jet lag sleep disturbances who were flown eastward across five time zones from Hawaii to the East Coast of the United States [152]. Ramelteon (1 to 8 mg) was administered 5 min before bedtime (local time) for four nights after arrival. Sleep parameters were measured using polysomnography on nights 2, 3, and 4 while next-day residual effects were assessed using psychomotor and memory function tests. Compared with placebo, there was a significant decrease in mean latency to persistent sleep on nights 2–4 with ramelteon 1 mg but not with the higher doses. The lack of significant effects of the higher doses could be due to the small size of the ramelteon groups ($n = 27$). No consistent significant differences were observed with ramelteon versus placebo on measures of next-day residual effects except on day 4 on which participants in all ramelteon groups performed significantly worse on the immediate memory recall test compared with placebo ($p \leq 0.05$). The incidence of adverse events was similar for ramelteon and placebo. In view of its phase-shifting effects, ramelteon could be proposed as a potential treatment to induce rapid resynchronization following time zone transition of travelers. However, further studies with larger samples of jet travelers, with different doses and various time zone phase shifts, will be necessary to assess the use of ramelteon in improving sleep quality and enhancing daytime performance.

25.2.11.2 LY 156735

LY 156735 (Eli Lilly, Indianapolis, IN) is a b-substituted analog of melatonin with both higher potency and higher bioavailability than the parent compound. In a simulated jet lag study, LY 156735 enhanced entrainment of all physiological rhythms to the postshift target time [153]. LY 156735 has still to be developed for this purpose.

25.2.11.3 Tasimelteon

In a randomized controlled trial of the melatonin MT1/MT2 agonist tasimelteon (VEC-162) for transient insomnia after sleep time shift, the drug reduced sleep latency and increased sleep efficiency compared with placebo as assessed by polysomnography [154]. Although the drug appears effective, optimal timing and dosage remains to be determined.

25.2.11.4 Agomelatine

Agomelatine (Valdoxan™, Servier, France) is a novel antidepressant drug that acts as both as melatonin MT1 and MT2 receptor agonist as well as a 5-HT_{2c} antagonist [155–157]. This dual mechanism of action is unique and is the basis for its simultaneous antidepressant efficacy and its capacity to mitigate sleep/wakefulness rhythm disorders. This has been confirmed clinically in depressed patients, with agomelatine demonstrating efficacy for ameliorating depressive symptoms [158] as well as for improving sleep quality [159–162]. It is interesting that agomelatine has been found effective in restoring the disrupted circadian rhythmicity in patients with seasonal affective disorder, thus acting on the main pathophysiological cause recognized for this disorder [163]. In a recent study, it was reported that agomelatine increased the amplitude of the circadian rest–activity cycle in patients with major depressive disorder [164]. As compared with sertraline, there was a greater improvement in sleep latency and efficiency and a greater improvement in depressive and anxiety symptoms. It has been shown that agomelatine can cause a phase shift in the sleep/wake cycle in healthy older men [165].

In considering the potential application of agomelatine for the treatment of JLD, it is important to bear in mind the underlying biological features that are common to JLD and depressive illness. More than 25 years ago, Wehr and Wirz-Justice [166] proposed the possible link between biological rhythm disorders and depression, postulating a phase-advance theory of depression. An internal phase angle disturbance between sleep and circadian rhythms has been hypothesized to underlie the pathophysiology of depression [167,168] (for a review, see Pandi et al. [169]). This is in accord with the suggestion that correction of the phase angle disturbances between sleep/wake cycle and circadian rhythms could ameliorate the symptoms of depressive illness [166].

Depressive symptoms have been reported in westbound travelers, giving support to the phase-advance theory of depression [170–172]. The transient desynchronization seen in jet travelers may play a role in triggering exacerbation of affective disorders symptoms or even de novo affective disorders [173]. The possible association between JLD and psychiatric morbidity was explored in 152 patients who were divided into groups based upon the number of time zones crossed [170]. The direction of flight was mainly eastbound. Possible links between JLD with major affective disorder or psychotic disorder were evaluated based upon the following criteria: (a) absence of major mental problems before flight or good remission of an existing disorder 1 year or more before flight; (b) appearance of major affective syndromes or psychotic syndromes during the first 7 days after landing [170]. Although the number of first major affective episodes or psychotic symptoms associated with JLD was found to be similar among groups, the number of relapses conjoint with JLD in the seven or more time zone group was significantly greater [170]. In two other studies, reported depression was found to be related to westbound flights and mania was found more frequently associated with eastbound flights [171,172]. Collectively, these studies further support the hypothesis of a possible link between JLD and major affective disorders. Dysregulation of melatonin secretion may constitute the common underlying mechanism in JLD and major affective disorders. With this background, the possible application of agomelatine in JLD emerges. As noted, agomelatine is a novel antidepressant drug that acts simultaneously as a melatonin MT1 and MT2 receptor agonist and as a 5-HT_{2c} antagonist [157]. A study performed in healthy older men indicated that agomelatine phase-shifts 24-hour rhythms of hormonal release and body temperature [165] and as noted above increases the amplitude of the circadian rest–activity rhythm in patients with major depression [164]. The chronobiotic activity of agomelatine has been shown in preclinical studies. Data in rodents indicate that agomelatine accelerates re-entrainment of wheel running activity after phase shifts [174]. Agomelatine resynchronizes experimentally disrupted circadian rhythms [175] and resets the electrical activity of neurons in the SCN [176].

Agomelatine is efficient in treating patients with major depressive disorder [159,160,162,177]. Most of these patients have some form of sleep difficulty including insomnia [178]. Most of the antidepressants that are in clinical use today negatively affect sleep initiation and maintenance. Clinical trials have shown that agomelatine induces earlier improvement of nocturnal sleep with preservation of daytime alertness (for references, see ref. [157]). Since agomelatine is effective in improving nocturnal sleep from the very beginning of treatment and has also been found effective in correcting the disturbed circadian rhythms, including the sleep/wake cycle [164,179], it has been suggested that the drug could useful for treating CRSDs and JLD [180]. Melatonin itself could also be useful for treating the dual symptom complexes of JLD and exacerbation of depressive symptoms in individuals with major depressive disorder. This hypothesis remains to be investigated.

25.2.12 Guidelines for Effective Management of JLD

To successfully overcome the effects of JLD, there is a need for an integrated JLD prevention and management program. The following guidelines are derived from evidence provided by scientific investigations, conventional experience, and anecdotal observations. For a more effective management of JLD, it is recommended that a combination of treatment regimens be undertaken.

- Adjustment to a new time zone can be encouraged by adopting the social timing of life in the new time zone as soon as possible. This includes scheduling changes in meals, sleep, and exercise.
- There are also indications that the symptoms of JLD can be effectively reduced by altering the home sleep/wake pattern for a few days in the direction of the anticipated destination schedule prior to departure. It has been estimated that approximately 1 day is required for adaptation to each hour of time change. Thus, a change in schedule that anticipates the schedule at the destination will be helpful even if it is for 1 to 2 hours. Conversely, for eastward travel, 3 to 5 mg melatonin 3 to 4 hours prior to bedtime, and for westward travel, 1 mg or less on waking will help.
- In field and simulation studies, suitably timed melatonin administration has been shown to accelerate phase shifts and significantly improve self-rated JLD symptoms in large numbers of time zone travelers. As noted above, melatonin should be given in the evening for eastbound travel or in the morning for westbound travel. A dose of 3 to 5 mg can be used 3 to 4 hours prior to travel and at bedtime at the destination, while 0.5 to 1 mg should be used on waking in the morning prior to travel. This lower dose will produce shift change without undue drowsiness. By administrating melatonin before, during, and after rapid time zone transition, JLD symptoms can be minimized without undesirable side effects. The recently introduced melatonergic agonists may also be helpful in this respect.
- Exposure to light has also been shown to accelerate phase shifts. In contrast to melatonin during the pretrip phase, exposure to bright light in the evening (and avoiding bright light in early morning) for westward travel and exposure to bright light in the early morning (and avoiding it in the evening) for eastward travel would be helpful. Moreover, after travel in an easterly direction, light exposure should take place early in the morning but late in the afternoon and evening after westbound travel.
- The combination of melatonin and light exposure one in the evening and the other in the morning is expected to have more effect than either treatment alone.
- Due to individual differences in circadian rhythms, a personalized administration schedule, rather than a standard therapeutic dosing, will offer the best results. Administration of melatonin at inappropriate times may create more problems than are alleviated.
- To increase the amount of sleep obtained, and thus to reduce the homeostatic sleep drive, rapidly eliminated hypnotics can be successfully used for the first few nights upon arriving at the new destination.

25.3 SHIFT WORK DISORDER

There is a wide range of work schedules that is referred to as shift work. These include occasional on-call overnight duty, rotating schedules, and steady, permanent night work. Due to the overlap of these categories, it is difficult to generalize about shift work [146]. About one in five workers in the United States do some form of shift work, with women being represented in this activity more often than men [181].

25.3.1 Symptoms of SWD

Drake et al. [182], in an epidemiologic survey, reported that over 10% of night workers and of rotating workers met minimal criteria for SWD, although most published studies fail to use these criteria [146]. An essential feature of this diagnosis is social, occupational, or other impairment due to the misalignment of body rhythms with the environment because of the shift work [12]. Persistent excessive sleepiness and insomnia in patients who work nights or rotating shifts should raise suspicion of SWD, although other causes should be ruled out [183]. Diagnostic criteria for SWD are given in ICSD-2 [12] or DSM-IV-TR [13]. As is the case for jet lag, there are major individual differences in susceptibility to shift work [184], and susceptibility can lead to accidents and comorbidity [185].

25.3.2 Diseases Associated with SWD

In 1999, Boggild and Knutsson [186] calculated that shift workers have a 43% higher risk of developing ischemic heart disease. Several studies have now confirmed that there is a relationship of cardiovascular disease with shift work [187–190]. Yadegarfar [191], reporting on deaths from ischemic heart disease, found that social class was a major confound in the population he studied. Moreover, Frost et al. [192], following a review of the literature, concluded that epidemiological evidence for a causal relation between shift work and ischemic heart disease is limited. However, in 2001, Karlsson et al. [193] reported an association between shift work and metabolic syndrome, a major risk factor for cardiovascular disease [194,195]. It has now been confirmed that the metabolic syndrome is prominent in shift workers [196–203]. Hypertension has been reported to be higher in male shift workers than in day workers [204]. Furthermore, alternating shift work has been reported to be a significant independent risk factor for high blood pressure [205], an effect that was more pronounced than that of age or body mass index. Alternating shift work was also an independent risk factor for increasing body weight [205] as well as for hypercholesterolemia [206,207]. It has been reported that nurses have a moderately increased incidence of ischemic stroke after an extended period of rotating shift work [208].

In 2007, the International Agency for Research on Cancer classified shift work as a probable human carcinogen (2A) [209–212]. This conclusion was based on considerable animal evidence and some limited human studies [213,214]. Animal studies suggest that altered lighting and changes in melatonin secretory patterns impact on breast tissue. Women who work on rotating night shifts are reported to have a moderately increased risk of breast cancer after extended periods of working night shifts as compared with controls [215,216] as do female cabin crew [217]. One study reported that female night shift workers have a significantly increased risk of developing endometrial cancer, particularly if they are obese [218]. Because melatonin has oncostatic effects including effects on estrogen and fat metabolism, it may play a role in both breast and endometrial cancer [219]. Light exposure at night may reduce melatonin levels. The role of melatonin in both these cancers remains to be defined.

Effects of shift work on mental health were examined longitudinally using GHQ data from the British Household Panel Survey using people aged 21–73 years who had been followed annually from 1995 to 2005 [220]. Women's mental health was more adversely affected by varying shift patterns, while night work had a greater negative impact on men's mental health. A recent case report of a patient diagnosed as having bipolar II disorder as well as being an extreme morning type showed that the patient maintained a stable mood on a stable work cycle but developed depressive symptoms when placed on a night shift schedule [221]. Her mood normalized when the night shift schedule was stopped.

25.3.3 Management of SWD

Management of SWD is similar to that of JLD because desynchrony with the environment is also the underlying cause. However, in SWD, the condition persists over time in a way that jet lag does not. For instance, in continuing night shift work, the individual still exists in an external social and day/night environment that is out of phase with the work schedule. Management is therefore based on the current understanding of circadian rhythm science.

25.3.3.1 Guidelines for Effective Management of SWD

- Organizational level changes may be very important [222]. These authors recommended three types of intervention: (1) switching from slow to fast rotation, (2) changing from backward to forward rotation, and (3) self-scheduling of shifts. There is evidence that a rapidly rotating schedule is less detrimental since it minimizes the time spent in a desynchronized state [223]. Clockwise rotation, rather than counterclockwise rotation, was reported to be preferred by workers probably because the body clock is somewhat longer than 24 hours [224]. Longer duty shifts allow more time off work [146]. It is possible that a flexible approach is best because of major individual differences in workers.

- Planned napping just before or on the job combined with caffeinated drinks has been reported to reduce sleepiness and improve alertness while working [146,225].
- Melatonin treatment prior to daytime sleep has been used with variable results [146]; nevertheless, there are a number of theoretical reasons to expect it and especially the newer agonists (Ramelteon, Circadin) that have longer half-lives to be useful both by causing sleepiness and by inducing phase shifting.
- Appropriately timed bright light treatment has been shown to be helpful in simulated shift work by assisting in phase shifts [146,225] and may also be combined with dark sun glasses that limit exposure during commutes [226]. Partial entrainment to a permanent night shift schedule has been shown to be beneficial in a simulation study and warrants further exploration in the work situation [227].
- The wakefulness-promoting agents armodafinil [228,229] and modafinil have been approved by the FDA for treatment of excessive sleepiness in patients with SWD and may be very useful for that problem [225].

25.4 OTHER CIRCADIAN RHYTHM SLEEP DISORDERS

It is beyond the scope of this chapter to discuss the other CRSDs. These disorders include delayed sleep phase disorder, advanced sleep phase disorder, non–24 hour sleep/wake pattern, and irregular sleep/wake pattern, as well as other unspecified phase patterns [12,13,230]. However, it should be noted that similar circadian rhythm principles should apply to their treatment.

25.5 CONCLUSION

Both JLD and SWD share a similar cause and management and, therefore, have major similarities. In both cases, three factors are important: (1) sleep scheduling, (2) resetting the body clock with light and/or chronobiotics such as melatonin, and (3) use of drugs to promote sleep and/or wakefulness as needed [146].

25.6 CONFLICT OF INTEREST DISCLOSURES

All views expressed in this article are those of the authors and do not necessarily represent the views of the organizations that they are associated with. The authors further declare that they have no proprietary, financial, professional, or any other personal interest of any nature or kind in any product or services and/or company that could be constructed or considered a potential conflict of interest that might have influenced the views expressed in this manuscript.

Mr. Pandi-Perumal is a stockholder and the president and CEO of Somnogen Inc., New York, USA. He has declared that he has no competing interests that might be perceived to influence the content of this article.

REFERENCES

1. Wright JE, Vogel JA, Sampson JB, Knapik JJ, Patton JF, and Daniels WL. 1983. Effects of travel across time zones (jet-lag) on exercise capacity and performance. *Aviat. Space Environ. Med.* 54 (2): 132–137.

2. Jehue R, Street D, and Huizenga R. 1993. Effect of time zone and game time changes on team performance: National Football League. *Med. Sci. Sports Exerc.* 25 (1): 127–131.
3. Takahashi T, Sasaki M, Itoh H, Yamadera W, Ozone M, Obuchi K, Hayashida K, Matsunaga N, and Sano H. 2002. Melatonin alleviates jet lag symptoms caused by an 11-hour eastward flight. *Psychiatry Clin. Neurosci.* 56 (3): 301–302.
4. Ariznavarreta C, Cardinali DP, Villanua MA, Granados B, Martin M, Chiesa JJ, Golombek DA, and Tresguerres JA. 2002. Circadian rhythms in airline pilots submitted to long-haul transmeridian flights. *Aviat. Space Environ. Med.* 73 (5): 445–455.
5. Spitzer RL, Terman M, Williams JB, Terman JS, Malt UF, Singer F, and Lewy AJ. 1999. Jet lag: Clinical features, validation of a new syndrome-specific scale, and lack of response to melatonin in a randomized, double-blind trial. *Am. J. Psychiatry* 156 (9): 1392–1396.
6. Akerstedt T. 2007. Altered sleep/wake patterns and mental performance. *Physiol Behav.* 90 (2–3): 209–218.
7. Waterhouse J, Reilly T, Atkinson G, and Edwards B. 2007. Jet lag: Trends and coping strategies. *Lancet* 369 (9567): 1117–1129.
8. Reilly T, Atkinson G, and Waterhouse J. 1997. Travel fatigue and jet-lag. *J. Sports Sci.* 15 (3): 365–369.
9. Klein KE, Wegmann HM, and Hunt BI. 1972. Desynchronization of body temperature and performance circadian rhythm as a result of outgoing and homegoing transmeridian flights. *Aerosp. Med.* 43 (2): 119–132.
10. Monk TH, Buysse DJ, Reynolds CF, III, and Kupfer DJ. 1995. Inducing jet lag in an older person: Directional asymmetry. *Exp. Gerontol.* 30 (2): 137–145.
11. Monk TH. 2005. Aging human circadian rhythms: Conventional wisdom may not always be right. *J. Biol. Rhythms* 20 (4): 366–374.
12. American Academy of Sleep Medicine. 2005. *The International Classification of Sleep Disorders: Diagnostic and Coding Manual (2nd ed.)*. Westchester, IL: American Academy of Sleep Medicine.
13. American Psychiatric Association. 2000. *Diagnostic and Statistical Manual of Mental Disorders. 4th Ed (DSM-IV-TR).* Washington, D.C.: American Psychiatric Press.
14. Petrie KJ, Powell D, and Broadbent E. 2004. Fatigue self-management strategies and reported fatigue in international pilots. *Ergonomics* 47 (5): 461–468.
15. Herxheimer A, and Waterhouse J. 2003. The prevention and treatment of jet lag. *BMJ* 326 (7384): 296–297.
16. Iglesias R, Terres A, and Chavarria A. 1980. Disorders of the menstrual cycle in airline stewardesses. *Aviat. Space Environ. Med.* 51 (5): 518–520.
17. Lauria L, Ballard TJ, Caldora M, Mazzanti C, and Verdecchia A. 2006. Reproductive disorders and pregnancy outcomes among female flight attendants. *Aviat. Space Environ. Med.* 77 (5): 533–539.
18. Cho K. 2001. Chronic 'jet lag' produces temporal lobe atrophy and spatial cognitive deficits. *Nat. Neurosci.* 4 (6): 567–568.
19. Filipski E, Delaunay F, King VM, Wu MW, Claustrat B, Grechez-Cassiau A, Guettier C, Hastings MH, and Francis L. 2004. Effects of chronic jet lag on tumor progression in mice. *Cancer Res.* 64 (21): 7879–7885.
20. Davidson AJ, Sellix MT, Daniel J, Yamazaki S, Menaker M, and Block GD. 2006. Chronic jet-lag increases mortality in aged mice. *Curr. Biol.* 16 (21): R914–R916.
21. Flower DJ, Irvine D, and Folkard S. 2003. Perception and predictability of travel fatigue after long-haul flights: A retrospective study. *Aviat. Space Environ. Med.* 74 (2): 173–179.
22. Aschoff J, and Wever R. 1981. The circadian system of man. In *Biological Rhythms*, 311–331. New York: Plenum Press.
23. Caldwell JA, Mallis MM, Caldwell JL, Paul MA, Miller JC, and Neri DF. 2009. Fatigue countermeasures in aviation. *Aviat. Space Environ. Med.* 80 (1): 29–59.
24. Reilly T, Waterhouse J, and Edwards B. 2005. Jet lag and air travel: Implications for performance. *Clin. Sports Med.* 24 (2): 367–80, xii.
25. Waterhouse J, Kao S, Edwards B, Atkinson G, and Reilly T. 2006. Factors associated with food intake in passengers on long-haul flights. *Chronobiol. Int.* 23 (5): 985–1007.
26. Moline ML, Pollak CP, Monk TH, Lester LS, Wagner DR, Zendell SM, Graeber RC, Salter CA, and Hirsch E. 1992. Age-related differences in recovery from simulated jet lag. *Sleep* 15 (1): 28–40.
27. Duffy JF, Dijk DJ, Hall EF, and Czeisler CA. 1999. Relationship of endogenous circadian melatonin and temperature rhythms to self-reported preference for morning or evening activity in young and older people. *J. Investig. Med.* 47 (3): 141–150.
28. Samel A, Wegmann HM, and Vejvoda M. 1995. Jet lag and sleepiness in aircrew. *J. Sleep Res.* 4 (S2): 30–36.

29. Boivin DB, and James FO. 2002. Phase-dependent effect of room light exposure in a 5-h advance of the sleep–wake cycle: Implications for jet lag. *J. Biol. Rhythms* 17 (3): 266–276.
30. Bourgeois-Bougrine S, Carbon P, Gounelle C, Mollard R, and Coblentz A. 2003. Perceived fatigue for short- and long-haul flights: A survey of 739 airline pilots. *Aviat. Space Environ. Med.* 74 (10): 1072–1077.
31. Wegmann HM, Gundel A, Naumann M, Samel A, Schwartz E, and Vejvoda M. 1986. Sleep, sleepiness, and circadian rhythmicity in aircrews operating on transatlantic routes. *Aviat. Space Environ. Med.* 57 (12 Pt 2): B53–B64.
32. Beh HC, and McLaughlin PJ. 1991. Mental performance of air crew following layovers on transzonal flights. *Ergonomics* 34 (2): 123–135.
33. Beh HC, and McLaughlin P. 1997. Effect of long flights on the cognitive performance of air crew. *Percept. Mot. Skills* 84 (1): 319–322.
34. Preston FS, Bateman SC, Short RV, and Wilkinson RT. 1973. Effects of flying and of time changes on menstrual cycle length and on performance in airline stewardesses. *Aerosp. Med.* 44 (4): 438–443.
35. Tresguerres JA, Ariznavarreta C, Granados B, Martin M, Villanua MA, Golombek DA, and Cardinali DP. 2001. Circadian urinary 6-sulphatoxymelatonin, cortisol excretion and locomotor activity in airline pilots during transmeridian flights. *J. Pineal Res.* 31 (1): 16–22.
36. McEwen BS. 1998. Stress, adaptation, and disease. Allostasis and allostatic load. *Annals NY Acad. Sci.* 840: 33–44.
37. McEwen BS. 2006. Sleep deprivation as a neurobiologic and physiologic stressor: Allostasis and allostatic load. *Metabolism* 55 (10 Suppl 2): S20–S23.
38. Leproult R, Copinschi G, Buxton O, and Van CE. 1997. Sleep loss results in an elevation of cortisol levels the next evening. *Sleep* 20 (10): 865–870.
39. Spiegel K, Leproult R, L'Hermite-Baleriaux M, Copinschi G, Penev PD, and Van CE. 2004. Leptin levels are dependent on sleep duration: Relationships with sympathovagal balance, carbohydrate regulation, cortisol, and thyrotropin. *J. Clin. Endocrinol. Metab* 89 (11): 5762–5771.
40. Spiegel K, Knutson K, Leproult R, Tasali E, and Van CE. 2005. Sleep loss: A novel risk factor for insulin resistance and Type 2 diabetes. *J. Appl. Physiol.* 99 (5): 2008–2019.
41. Van CE, Holmback U, Knutson K, Leproult R, Miller A, Nedeltcheva A, Pannain S, Penev P, Tasali E, and Spiegel K. 2007. Impact of sleep and sleep loss on neuroendocrine and metabolic function. *Horm. Res.* 67 Suppl 1: 2–9.
42. Vgontzas AN, Zoumakis E, Bixler EO, Lin HM, Follett H, Kales A, and Chrousos GP. 2004. Adverse effects of modest sleep restriction on sleepiness, performance, and inflammatory cytokines. *J. Clin. Endocrinol. Metab.* 89 (5): 2119–2126.
43. Vgontzas AN, Pejovic S, Zoumakis E, Lin HM, Bixler EO, Basta M, Fang J, Sarrigiannidis A, and Chrousos GP. 2007. Daytime napping after a night of sleep loss decreases sleepiness, improves performance, and causes beneficial changes in cortisol and interleukin-6 secretion. *Am. J. Physiol. Endocrinol. Metab.* 292 (1): E253–E261.
44. McEwen BS. 2005. Glucocorticoids, depression, and mood disorders: Structural remodeling in the brain. *Metabolism* 54 (5 Suppl 1): 20–23.
45. Cho K, Ennaceur A, Cole JC, and Suh CK. 2000. Chronic jet lag produces cognitive deficits. *J. Neurosci.* 20 (6): RC66.
46. Brown GM, Pandi-Perumal SR, Trakht I, and Cardinali DP. 2009. Melatonin and its relevance to jet lag. *Travel. Med. Infect. Dis.* 7 (2): 69–81.
47. Moore RY. 2007. Suprachiasmatic nucleus in sleep–wake regulation. *Sleep Med.* 8 Suppl 3: 27–33.
48. Lee HS, Nelms JL, Nguyen M, Silver R, and Lehman MN. 2003. The eye is necessary for a circadian rhythm in the suprachiasmatic nucleus. *Nat. Neurosci.* 6 (2): 111–112.
49. Hankins MW, Peirson SN, and Foster RG. 2008. Melanopsin: An exciting photopigment. *Trends Neurosci.* 31 (1): 27–36.
50. Panda S, Sato TK, Castrucci AM, Rollag MD, DeGrip WJ, Hogenesch JB, Provencio I, and Kay SA. 2002. Melanopsin (Opn4) requirement for normal light-induced circadian phase shifting. *Science* 298 (5601): 2213–2216.
51. Ruby NF, Brennan TJ, Xie X, Cao V, Franken P, Heller HC, and O'Hara BF. 2002. Role of melanopsin in circadian responses to light. *Science* 298 (5601): 2211–2213.
52. Thapan K, Arendt J, and Skene DJ. 2001. An action spectrum for melatonin suppression: Evidence for a novel non-rod, non-cone photoreceptor system in humans. *J. Physiol.* 535 (Pt 1): 261–267.
53. Revell VL, Arendt J, Fogg LF, and Skene DJ. 2006. Alerting effects of light are sensitive to very short wavelengths. *Neurosci. Lett.* 399 (1–2): 96–100.

54. Cajochen C, Munch M, Kobialka S, Krauchi K, Steiner R, Oelhafen P, Orgul S, and Wirz-Justice A. 2005. High sensitivity of human melatonin, alertness, thermoregulation, and heart rate to short wavelength light. *J. Clin. Endocrinol. Metab.* 90 (3): 1311–1316.
55. Reppert SM, Weaver DR, and Ebisawa T. 1994. Cloning and characterization of a mammalian melatonin receptor that mediates reproductive and circadian responses. *Neuron* 13 (5): 1177–1185.
56. Reppert SM, Godson C, Mahle CD, Weaver DR, Slaugenhaupt SA, and Gusella JF. 1995. Molecular characterization of a second melatonin receptor expressed in human retina and brain: The Mel1b melatonin receptor. *Proc. Natl. Acad. Sci. USA* 92 (19): 8734–8738.
57. Reppert SM, Weaver DR, Ebisawa T, Mahle CD, and Kolakowski LJ. 1996. Cloning of a melatonin-related receptor from human pituitary. *FEBS Lett.* 386 (2–3): 219–224.
58. Rivera-Bermudez MA, Masana MI, Brown GM, Earnest DJ, and Dubocovich ML. 2004. Immortalized cells from the rat suprachiasmatic nucleus express functional melatonin receptors. *Brain Res.* 1002 (1–2): 21–27.
59. Wu YH, Zhou JN, Balesar R, Unmehopa U, Bao A, Jockers R, Van HJ, and Swaab DF. 2006. Distribution of MT1 melatonin receptor immunoreactivity in the human hypothalamus and pituitary gland: Colocalization of MT1 with vasopressin, oxytocin, and corticotropin-releasing hormone. *J. Comp. Neurol.* 499 (6): 897–910.
60. Mazzucchelli C, Pannacci M, Nonno R, Lucini V, Fraschini F, and Stankov BM. 1996. The melatonin receptor in human brain: Cloning experiments and distribution studies. *Mol. Brain Res.* 39: 117–126.
61. Meyer P, Pache M, Loeffler KU, Brydon L, Jockers R, Flammer J, Wirz-Justice A, and Savaskan E. 2002. Melatonin MT-1-receptor immunoreactivity in the human eye. *Br. J. Ophthalmol.* 86 (9): 1053–1057.
62. Liu C, Weaver DR, Jin X, Shearman LP, Pieschi RL, Gribkoff VK, and Reppert SM. 1997. Molecular dissection of two distinct actions of melatonin on the suprachiasmatic circadian clock. *Neuron* 19: 91–102.
63. Wan Q, Man HY, Liu F, Braunton J, Niznik HB, Pang SF, Brown GM, and Wang YT. 1999. Differential modulation of GABAA receptor function by Mel1a and Mel1b receptors. *Nat. Neurosci.* 2 (5): 401–403.
64. Pickering DS, and Niles LP. 1990. Pharmacological characterization of melatonin binding sites in Syrian hamster hypothalamus. *Eur. J. Pharmacol.* 175 (1): 71–77.
65. Nosjean O, Ferro M, Coge F, Beauverger P, Henlin JM, Lefoulon F, Fauchere JL, Delagrange P, Canet E, and Boutin JA. 2000. Identification of the melatonin-binding site MT3 as the quinone reductase 2. *J. Biol. Chem.* 275 (40): 31311–31317.
66. Czeisler CA, Allan JS, Strogatz SH, Ronda JM, Sanchez R, Rios CD, Freitag WO, Richardson GS, and Kronauer RE. 1986. Bright light resets the human circadian pacemaker independent of the timing of the sleep–wake cycle. *Science* 233 (4764): 667–671.
67. Samel A, and Wegmann HM. 1997. Bright light: A countermeasure for jet lag? [Review] [40 refs]. *Chronobiol. Int.* 14 (2): 173–183.
68. Reid KJ, and Burgess HJ. 2005. Circadian rhythm sleep disorders. *Prim. Care* 32 (2): 449–473.
69. Eastman CI, and Martin SK. 1999. How to use light and dark to produce circadian adaptation to night shift work. *Ann. Med.* 31 (2): 87–98.
70. Shanahan TL, and Czeisler CA. 2000. Physiological effects of light on the human circadian pacemaker. *Semin. Perinatol.* 24 (4): 299–320.
71. Czeisler CA, Kronauer RE, Allan JS, Duffy JF, Jewett ME, Brown EN, and Ronda JM. 1989. Bright light induction of strong (type 0) resetting of the human circadian pacemaker. *Science* 244 (4910): 1328–1333.
72. Honma K, and Honma S. 1988. A human phase response curve for bright light pulses, 167–168.
73. Honma K, Honma S, and Wada T. 1987. Phase-dependent shift of free-running human circadian rhythms in response to a single bright light pulse. *Experientia* 43 (11–12): 1205–1207.
74. Smits MG, Spence DW, Pandi-Perumal SR, and Brown GM. 2010. Dim light melatonin onset in psychiatric disorders. In *Sleep and Mental Illness*, eds SR Pandi-Perumal and M Kramer, 130–138. Cambridge: Cambridge University Press.
75. Stewart KT, Hayes BC, and Eastman CI. 1995. Light treatment for NASA shiftworkers. *Chronobiol. Int.* 12 (2): 141–151.
76. Deacon S, and Arendt J. 1996. Adapting to phase shifts, I. An experimental model for jet lag and shift work. *Physiol. Behav.* 59 (4–5): 665–673.
77. Burgess HJ, Crowley SJ, Gazda CJ, Fogg LF, and Eastman CI. 2003. Preflight adjustment to eastward travel: 3 days of advancing sleep with and without morning bright light. *J. Biol. Rhythms* 18 (4): 318–328.

78. Eastman CI, Gazda CJ, Burgess HJ, Crowley SJ, and Fogg LF. 2005. Advancing circadian rhythms before eastward flight: A strategy to prevent or reduce jet lag. *Sleep* 28 (1): 33–44.
79. Paul MA, Miller JC, Gray G, Buick F, Blazeski S, and Arendt J. 2007. Circadian phase delay induced by phototherapeutic devices. *Aviat. Space Environ. Med.* 78 (7): 645–652.
80. Paul MA, Miller JC, Love RJ, Lieberman H, Blazeski S, and Arendt J. 2009. Timing light treatment for eastward and westward travel preparation. *Chronobiol. Int.* 26 (5): 867–890.
81. Houpt TA, Boulos Z, and Moore-Ede MC. 1996. MidnightSun: Software for determining light exposure and phase-shifting schedules during global travel. *Physiol Behav.* 59 (3): 561–568.
82. Samel A, Wegmann HM, Vejvoda M, Maass H, Gundel A, and Schutz M. 1991. Influence of melatonin treatment on human circadian rhythmicity before and after a simulated 9-hr time shift. *J. Biol. Rhythms* 6 (3): 235–248.
83. Lewy AJ, Bauer VK, Ahmed S, Thomas KH, Cutler NL, Singer CM, Moffit MT, and Sack RL. 1998. The human phase response curve (PRC) to melatonin is about 12 hours out of phase with the PRC to light. *Chronobiol. Int.* 15 (1): 71–83.
84. Burgess HJ, Revell VL, and Eastman CI. 2008. A three pulse phase response curve to three milligrams of melatonin in humans. *J. Physiol* 586 (2): 639–647.
85. Revell VL, and Eastman CI. 2005. How to trick mother nature into letting you fly around or stay up all night. *J. Biol. Rhythms* 20 (4): 353–365.
86. Paul MA, Miller JC, Gray GW, Love RJ, Lieberman HR, and Arendt J. 2010. Melatonin treatment for eastward and westward travel preparation. *Psychopharmacology* (*Berl.*) 208 (3): 377–386.
87. Arendt J, Aldhous M, and Marks V. 1986. Alleviation of jet lag by melatonin: Preliminary results of controlled double blind trial. *British Medical Journal—Clinical Research* 292 (6529): 1170.
88. Arendt J, and Aldhous M. 1988. Further evaluation of the treatment of jet-lag by melatonin: A double-blind crossover study. *Annual Review of Chronopharmacology* 5: 53–55.
89. Nickelsen T, Lang A, and Bergau L. 1991. The effect of 6-, 9-, and 11-hour time shifts on circadian rhythms: Adaption of sleep parameters and hormonal patterns following the intake of melatonin or placebo. In *Advances in Pineal Research*, eds J Arendt and P Pevet, 303–306. London: John Libbey & Co.
90. Petrie K, Dawson AG, Thompson L, and Brook R. 1993. A double-blind trial of melatonin as a treatment for jet lag in international cabin crew. *Biol. Psychiatry* 33 (7): 526–530.
91. Petrie K, Conaglen JV, Thompson L, and Chamberlain K. 1989. Effect of melatonin on jet lag after long haul flights. *British Medical Journal* 298 (6675): 705–707.
92. Edwards BJ, Atkinson G, Waterhouse J, Reilly T, Godfrey R, and Budgett R. 2000. Use of melatonin in recovery from jet-lag following an eastward flight across 10 time-zones. *Ergonomics* 43 (10): 1501–1513.
93. Suhner A, Schlagenhauf P, Johnson R, Tschopp A, and Steffen R. 1998. Comparative study to determine the optimal melatonin dosage form for the alleviation of jet lag. *Chronobiol. Int.* 15 (6): 655–666.
94. Deacon S, and Arendt J. 1995. Melatonin-induced temperature suppression and its acute phase-shifting effects correlate in a dose-dependent manner in humans. *Brain Research* 688 (1–2): 77–85.
95. Sharkey KM, and Eastman CI. 2002. Melatonin phase shifts human circadian rhythms in a placebo-controlled simulated night-work study. *Am. J. Physiol. Regul. Integr. Comp Physiol* 282 (2): R454–R463.
96. Revell VL, Burgess HJ, Gazda CJ, Smith MR, Fogg LF, and Eastman CI. 2006. Advancing human circadian rhythms with afternoon melatonin and morning intermittent bright light. *J. Clin. Endocrinol. Metab.* 91 (1): 54–59.
97. Reynolds NC, Jr., and Montgomery R. 2002. Using the Argonne diet in jet lag prevention: Deployment of troops across nine time zones. *Mil. Med.* 167 (6): 451–453.
98. Ford BJ. 1988. More on avoiding jet lag. *Nature* (*London*) 331 (6154): 309.
99. Holloway WRJ, Tsui HW, Grota LJ, and Brown GM. 1979. Melatonin and corticosterone regulation: Feeding time or the light:dark cycle? *Life Sci.* 25 (21): 1837–1842.
100. Krauchi K, Cajochen C, Werth E, and Wirz-Justice A. 2002. Alteration of internal circadian phase relationships after morning versus evening carbohydrate-rich meals in humans. *J. Biol. Rhythms* 17 (4): 364–376.
101. Fuller PM, Lu J, and Saper CB. 2008. Differential rescue of light- and food-entrainable circadian rhythms. *Science* 320 (5879): 1074–1077.
102. Atkinson G, Edwards B, Reilly T, and Waterhouse J. 2007. Exercise as a synchroniser of human circadian rhythms: An update and discussion of the methodological problems. *Eur. J. Appl. Physiol.* 99 (4): 331–341.

103. Daan S, and Lewy AJ. 1984. Scheduled exposure to daylight: A potential strategy to reduce "jet lag" following transmeridian flight. *Psychopharmacol. Bull.* 20 (3): 566–568.
104. Boulos Z, Macchi MM, Sturchler MP, Stewart KT, Brainard GC, Suhner A, Wallace G, and Steffen R. 2002. Light visor treatment for jet lag after westward travel across six time zones. *Aviat. Space Environ. Med.* 73 (10): 953–963.
105. Kay GG, and Quig ME. 2001. Impact of sedating antihistamines on safety and productivity. *Allergy Asthma Proc.* 22 (5): 281–283.
106. Buxton OM, Copinschi G, Van OA, Karrison TG, and Van CE. 2000. A benzodiazepine hypnotic facilitates adaptation of circadian rhythms and sleep–wake homeostasis to an eight hour delay shift simulating westward jet lag. *Sleep* 23 (7): 915–927.
107. Donaldson E, and Kennaway DJ. 1991. Effects of temazepam on sleep, performance, and rhythmic 6-sulphatoxymelatonin and cortisol excretion after transmeridian travel. *Aviat. Space Environ. Med.* 62 (7): 654–660.
108. Paul MA, Gray G, Kenny G, and Pigeau RA. 2003. Impact of melatonin, zaleplon, zopiclone, and temazepam on psychomotor performance. *Aviat. Space Environ. Med.* 74 (12): 1263–1270.
109. Nicholson AN, Pascoe PA, Roehrs T, Roth T, Spencer MB, Stone BM, and Zorick F. 1985. Sustained performance with short evening and morning sleeps. *Aviat. Space Environ. Med.* 56: 105–114.
110. Paul MA, Gray G, Sardana TM, and Pigeau RA. 2004. Melatonin and zopiclone as facilitators of early circadian sleep in operational air transport crews. *Aviat. Space Environ. Med.* 75 (5): 439–443.
111. Paul MA, Brown G, Buguet A, Gray G, Pigeau RA, Weinberg H, and Radomski M. 2001. Melatonin and zopiclone as pharmacologic aids to facilitate crew rest. *Aviat. Space Environ. Med.* 72 (11): 974–984.
112. Roth T, Roehrs T, and Vogel G. 1995. Zolpidem in the treatment of transient insomnia: A double-blind, randomized comparison with placebo. *Sleep* 18 (4): 246–251.
113. Paul MA, Gray G, MacLellan M, and Pigeau RA. 2004. Sleep-inducing pharmaceuticals: A comparison of melatonin, zaleplon, zopiclone, and temazepam. *Aviat. Space Environ. Med.* 75 (6): 512–519.
114. Arendt J, and Skene DJ. 2005. Melatonin as a chronobiotic. *Sleep Med. Rev.* 9 (1): 25–39.
115. Cardinali DP, Furio AM, Reyes MP, and Brusco LI. 2006. The use of chronobiotics in the resynchronization of the sleep–wake cycle. *Cancer Causes Control* 17 (4): 601–609.
116. Touitou Y, and Bogdan A. 2007. Promoting adjustment of the sleep–wake cycle by chronobiotics. *Physiol Behav.* 90 (2–3): 294–300.
117. Ridout F, Shamsi Z, Meadows R, Johnson S, and Hindmarch I. 2003. A single-center, randomized, double-blind, placebo-controlled, crossover investigation of the effects of fexofenadine hydrochloride 180 mg alone and with alcohol, with hydroxyzine hydrochloride 50 mg as a positive internal control, on aspects of cognitive and psychomotor function related to driving a car. *Clin. Ther.* 25 (5): 1518–1538.
118. Spahr L, Coeytaux A, Giostra E, Hadengue A, and Annoni JM. 2007. Histamine H1 blocker hydroxyzine improves sleep in patients with cirrhosis and minimal hepatic encephalopathy: A randomized controlled pilot trial. *Am. J. Gastroenterol.* 102 (4): 744–753.
119. Mohler SR, Nicholson A, Harvey P, Miura Y, and Meeves SG. 2002. The use of antihistamines in safety-critical jobs: A meeting report. *Curr. Med. Res. Opin.* 18 (6): 332–337.
120. Turek FW, and Van RO. 1988. Altering the mammalian circadian clock with the short-acting benzodiazepine, triazolam. *Trends Neurosci.* 11 (12): 535–541.
121. Morris HH, III, and Estes ML. 1987. Traveler's amnesia. Transient global amnesia secondary to triazolam. *JAMA* 258 (7): 945–946.
122. Mitler MM. 2000. Nonselective and selective benzodiazepine receptor agonists—Where are we today? *Sleep* 23 Suppl 1: S39–S47.
123. Reilly T, Atkinson G, and Budgett R. 2001. Effect of low-dose temazepam on physiological variables and performance tests following a westerly flight across five time zones. *Int. J. Sports Med.* 22 (3): 166–174.
124. Daurat A, Benoit O, and Buguet A. 2000. Effects of zopiclone on the rest/activity rhythm after a westward flight across five time zones. *Psychopharmacology (Berl.)* 149 (3): 241–245.
125. Suhner A, Schlagenhauf P, Hofer I, Johnson R, Tschopp A, and Steffen R. 2001. Effectiveness and tolerability of melatonin and zolpidem for the alleviation of jet lag. *Aviat. Space Environ. Med.* 72 (7): 638–646.
126. Jamieson AO, Zammit GK, Rosenberg RS, Davis JR, and Walsh JK. 2001. Zolpidem reduces the sleep disturbance of jet lag. *Sleep Med.* 2 (5): 423–430.
127. Dawson D, and Armstrong SM. 1996. Chronobiotics—Drugs that shift rhythms. [Review] [204 refs]. *Pharmacol. Ther.* 69 (1): 15–36.

128. Kennaway DJ, and Wright H. 2002. Melatonin and circadian rhythms. *Curr. Top. Med. Chem.* 2 (2): 199–209.
129. Claustrat B, Brun J, and Chazot G. 2005. The basic physiology and pathophysiology of melatonin. *Sleep Med. Rev.* 9 (1): 11–24.
130. Claustrat B, Brun J, David M, Sassolas G, and Chazot G. 1992. Melatonin and jet lag: Confirmatory result using a simplified protocol. *Biol. Psychiatry* 32 (8): 705–711.
131. Lino A, Silvy S, Condorelli L, and Rusconi AC. 1993. Melatonin and jet lag: Treatment schedule [letter; comment]. *Biol. Psychiatry* 34 (8): 587.
132. Czeisler CA. 1997. Commentary: Evidence for melatonin as a circadian phase-shifting agent. *J. Biol. Rhythms* 12 (6): 618–623.
133. Arendt J. 1999. Jet-lag and shift work: (2). Therapeutic use of melatonin. *J. R. Soc. Med.* 92 (8): 402–405.
134. Samel A. 1999. Melatonin and jet-lag. *Eur. J. Med. Res.* 4 (9): 385–388.
135. Beaumont M, Batejat D, Pierard C, Van BP, Denis JB, Coste O, Doireau P, Chauffard F, French J, and Lagarde D. 2004. Caffeine or melatonin effects on sleep and sleepiness after rapid eastward transmeridian travel. *J. Appl. Physiol.* 96 (1): 50–58.
136. Nicholson AN. 2006. Sleep and intercontinental flights. *Travel. Med. Infect. Dis.* 4 (6): 336–339.
137. Arendt J, Skene DJ, Middleton B, Lockley SW, and Deacon S. 1997. Efficacy of melatonin treatment in jet lag, shift work, and blindness. *J. Biol. Rhythms* 12 (6): 604–617.
138. Herxheimer A, and Petrie KJ. 2002. Melatonin for the prevention and treatment of jet lag. *Cochrane. Database Syst. Rev.* (2): CD001520.
139. Garfinkel D, Laudon M, Nof D, and Zisapel N. 1995. Improvement of sleep quality in elderly people by controlled-release melatonin. *Lancet* 346 (8974): 541–544.
140. Lemoine P, Nir T, Laudon M, and Zisapel N. 2007. Prolonged-release melatonin improves sleep quality and morning alertness in insomnia patients aged 55 years and older and has no withdrawal effects. *J. Sleep Res.* 16 (4): 372–380.
141. Wade AG, Ford I, Crawford G, McMahon AD, Nir T, Laudon M, and Zisapel N. 2007. Efficacy of prolonged release melatonin in insomnia patients aged 55–80 years: Quality of sleep and next-day alertness outcomes. *Curr. Med. Res. Opin.* 23 (10): 2597–2605.
142. Barion A, and Zee PC. 2007. A clinical approach to circadian rhythm sleep disorders. *Sleep Med.* 8 (6): 566–577.
143. Arendt J. 2009. Managing jet lag: Some of the problems and possible new solutions. *Sleep Med. Rev.* 13 (4): 249–256.
144. Sack RL. 2010. Clinical practice. Jet lag. *N. Engl. J. Med.* 362 (5): 440–447.
145. Sack RL. 2009. The pathophysiology of jet lag. *Travel. Med. Infect. Dis.* 7 (2): 102–110.
146. Sack RL, Auckley D, Auger RR, Carskadon MA, Wright KP, Jr., Vitiello MV, and Zhdanova IV. 2007. Circadian rhythm sleep disorders: Part I, basic principles, shift work and jet lag disorders. An American Academy of Sleep Medicine review. *Sleep* 30 (11): 1460–1483.
147. Kato K, Hirai K, Nishiyama K, Uchikawa O, Fukatsu K, Ohkawa S, Kawamata Y, Hinuma S, and Miyamoto M. 2005. Neurochemical properties of ramelteon (TAK-375), a selective MT1/MT2 receptor agonist. *Neuropharmacology* 48 (2): 301–310.
148. Miyamoto M. 2009. Pharmacology of ramelteon, a selective MT1/MT2 receptor agonist: A novel therapeutic drug for sleep disorders. *CNS Neurosci. Ther.* 15 (1): 32–51.
149. Bellon A. 2006. Searching for new options for treating insomnia: Are melatonin and ramelteon beneficial? *J. Psychiatr. Pract.* 12 (4): 229–243.
150. Sateia MJ, Kirby-Long P, and Taylor JL. 2008. Efficacy and clinical safety of ramelteon: An evidence-based review. *Sleep Med. Rev.* 12 (4): 319–332.
151. Richardson GS, Zee PC, Wang-Weigand S, Rodriguez L, and Peng X. 2008. Circadian phase-shifting effects of repeated ramelteon administration in healthy adults. *J. Clin. Sleep Med.* 4 (5): 456–461.
152. Zee PC, Wang-Weigand S, Wright KP, Jr., Peng X, and Roth T. 2010. Effects of ramelteon on insomnia symptoms induced by rapid, eastward travel. *Sleep Med.* 11 (6): 525–533.
153. Nickelsen T, Samel A, Vejvoda M, Wenzel J, Smith B, and Gerzer R. 2002. Chronobiotic effects of the melatonin agonist LY 156735 following a simulated 9h time shift: Results of a placebo-controlled trial. *Chronobiol. Int.* 19 (5): 915–936.
154. Rajaratnam SM, Polymeropoulos MH, Fisher DM, Roth T, Scott C, Birznieks G, and Klerman EB. 2009. Melatonin agonist tasimelteon (VEC-162) for transient insomnia after sleep-time shift: Two randomised controlled multicentre trials. *Lancet* 373 (9662): 482–491.

155. Millan MJ, Gobert A, Lejeune F, Dekeyne A, Newman-Tancredi A, Pasteau V, Rivet JM, and Cussac D. 2003. The novel melatonin agonist agomelatine (S20098) is an antagonist at 5-hydroxytryptamine2C receptors, blockade of which enhances the activity of frontocortical dopaminergic and adrenergic pathways. *J. Pharmacol. Exp. Ther.* 306 (3): 954–964.
156. Yous S, Andrieux J, Howell HE, Morgan PJ, Renard P, Pfeiffer B, Lseieur D, and Guardiola-Lemaitre B. 1992. Novel napthalenic ligands with high affinity for the melatonin receptor. *J. Med. Chem.* 35: 1484–1486.
157. Pandi-Perumal SR, Srinivasan V, Cardinali DP, and Monti MJ. 2006. Could agomelatine be the ideal antidepressant? *Expert. Rev. Neurother.* 6 (11): 1595–1608.
158. Olie JP, and Kasper S. 2007. Efficacy of agomelatine, a MT1/MT2 receptor agonist with 5-HT2C antagonistic properties, in major depressive disorder. *Int. J. Neuropsychopharmacol.* 10 (5): 661–673.
159. Loo H, Hale A, and D'haenen H. 2002. Determination of the dose of agomelatine, a melatoninergic agonist and selective 5-HT (2C) antagonist, in the treatment of major depressive disorder: A placebo-controlled dose range study. *Int. Clin. Psychopharmacol.* 17 (5): 239–247.
160. Kennedy SH, and Emsley R. 2006. Placebo-controlled trial of agomelatine in the treatment of major depressive disorder. *Eur. Neuropsychopharmacol.* 16 (2): 93–100.
161. Lemoine P, Guilleminault C, and Alvarez E. 2007. Improvement in subjective sleep in major depressive disorder with a novel antidepressant, agomelatine: Randomized, double-blind comparison with venlafaxine. *J. Clin. Psychiatry* 68 (11): 1723–1732.
162. Goodwin GM, Emsley R, Rembry S, and Rouillon F. 2009. Agomelatine prevents relapse in patients with major depressive disorder without evidence of a discontinuation syndrome: A 24-week randomized, double-blind, placebo-controlled trial. *J. Clin. Psychiatry* 70 (8): 1128–1137.
163. Pjrek E, Winkler D, Konstantinidis A, Willeit M, Praschak-Rieder N, and Kasper S. 2007. Agomelatine in the treatment of seasonal affective disorder. *Psychopharmacology (Berl.)* 190 (4): 575–579.
164. Kasper S, Hajak G, Wulff K, Hoogendijk WJ, Montejo AL, Smeraldi E, Rybakowski JK, Quera-Salva MA, Wirz-Justice AM, Picarel-Blanchot F, and Bayle FJ. 2010. Efficacy of the novel antidepressant agomelatine on the circadian rest–activity cycle and depressive and anxiety symptoms in patients with major depressive disorder: A randomized, double-blind comparison with sertraline. *J. Clin. Psychiatry* 71 (2): 109–120.
165. Leproult R, Van OA, L'Hermite-Baleriaux M, Van CE, and Copinschi G. 2005. Phase-shifts of 24-h rhythms of hormonal release and body temperature following early evening administration of the melatonin agonist agomelatine in healthy older men. *Clin. Endocrinol. (Oxf.)* 63 (3): 298–304.
166. Wehr TA, and Wirz-Justice A. 1982. Circadian rhythm mechanisms in affective illness and in antidepressant drug action. *Pharmacopsychiatria* 15 (1): 31–39.
167. Healy D, Minors DS, and Waterhouse JM. 1993. Shiftwork, helplessness and depression. *J. Affect. Disord.* 29 (1): 17–25.
168. Healy D, and Waterhouse JM. 1995. The circadian system and the therapeutics of the affective disorders. *Pharmacol. Ther.* 65 (2): 241–263.
169. Pandi-Perumal SR, Moscovitch A, Srinivasan V, Spence DW, Cardinali DP, and Brown GM. 2009. Bidirectional communication between sleep and circadian rhythms and its implications for depression: Lessons from agomelatine. *Prog. Neurobiol.* 88 (4): 264–271.
170. Katz G, Knobler HY, Laibel Z, Strauss Z, and Durst R. 2002. Time zone change and major psychiatric morbidity: The results of a 6-year study in Jerusalem. *Comp. Psychiatry* 43 (1): 37–40.
171. Jauhar P, and Weller MI. 1982. Psychiatric morbidity and time zone changes: A study of patients from Heathrow Airport. *Br. J. Psychiatry* 140: 231–235.
172. Young DM. 1995. Psychiatric morbidity in travelers to Honolulu, Hawaii. *Comp. Psychiatry* 36 (3): 224–228.
173. Katz G, Durst R, Zislin Y, Barel Y, and Knobler HY. 2001. Psychiatric aspects of jet lag: Review and hypothesis. *Med. Hypotheses* 56 (1): 20–23.
174. Tuma J, Strubbe JH, Mocaer E, and Koolhaas JM. 2001. S20098 affects the free-running rhythms of body temperature and activity and decreases light-induced phase delays of circadian rhythms of the rat. *Chronobiol. Int.* 18 (5): 781–799.
175. Armstrong SM, McNulty OM, Guardiola-Lemaitre B, and Redman JR. 1993. Successful use of S20098 and melatonin in an animal model of delayed sleep-phase syndrome (DSPS). *Pharmacol. Biochem. Behav.* 46 (1): 45–49.
176. Ying SW, Rusak B, Delagrange P, Mocaer E, Renard P, and Guardiola-Lemaitre B. 1996. Melatonin analogues as agonists and antagonists in the circadian system and other brain areas. *Eur. J. Pharmacol.* 296 (1): 33–42.

177. Kennedy SH, Rizvi S, Fulton K, and Rasmussen J. 2008. A double-blind comparison of sexual functioning, antidepressant efficacy, and tolerability between agomelatine and venlafaxine XR. *J. Clin. Psychopharmacol.* 28 (3): 329–333.
178. Kupfer DJ. 2006. Depression and associated sleep disturbances: Patient benefits with agomelatine. *Eur. Neuropsychopharmacol.* 16 (Suppl 5): S639–S643.
179. Rouillon F. 2006. Efficacy and tolerance profile of agomelatine and practical use in depressed patients. *Int. Clin. Psychopharmacol.* 21 Suppl 1: S31–S35.
180. Jindal RD, and Thase ME. 2004. Treatment of insomnia associated with clinical depression. *Sleep Med. Rev.* 8 (1): 19–30.
181. Presser HB. 1995. Job, family, and gender: Determinants of nonstandard work schedules among employed Americans in 1991. *Demography* 32 (4): 577–598.
182. Drake CL, Roehrs T, Richardson G, Walsh JK, and Roth T. 2004. Shift work sleep disorder: Prevalence and consequences beyond that of symptomatic day workers. *Sleep* 27 (8): 1453–1462.
183. Schwartz JR. 2010. Recognition of shift-work disorder in primary care. *J. Fam. Pract.* 59 (1 Suppl): S18–S23.
184. Van Dongen HP, and Belenky G. 2009. Individual differences in vulnerability to sleep loss in the work environment. *Ind. Health* 47 (5): 518–526.
185. Drake CL. 2010. The characterization and pathology of circadian rhythm sleep disorders. *J. Fam. Pract.* 59 (1 Suppl): S12–S17.
186. Boggild H, and Knutsson A. 1999. Shift work, risk factors and cardiovascular disease. *Scand. J. Work Environ. Health* 25 (2): 85–99.
187. Haupt CM, Alte D, Dorr M, Robinson DM, Felix SB, John U, and Volzke H. 2008. The relation of exposure to shift work with atherosclerosis and myocardial infarction in a general population. *Atherosclerosis* 201 (1): 205–211.
188. Puttonen S, Harma M, and Hublin C. 2010. Shift work and cardiovascular disease—Pathways from circadian stress to morbidity. *Scand. J. Work Environ. Health* 36 (2): 96–108.
189. Puttonen S, Kivimaki M, Elovainio M, Pulkki-Raback L, Hintsanen M, Vahtera J, Telama R, Juonala M, Viikari JS, Raitakari OT, and Keltikangas-Jarvinen L. 2009. Shift work in young adults and carotid artery intima-media thickness: The Cardiovascular Risk in Young Finns study. *Atherosclerosis* 205 (2): 608–613.
190. Knutsson A. 2008. Shift work and ischaemic heart disease. *Occup. Environ. Med.* 65 (3): 152.
191. Yadegarfar G, and McNamee R. 2008. Shift work, confounding and death from ischaemic heart disease. *Occup. Environ. Med.* 65 (3): 158–163.
192. Frost P, Kolstad HA, and Bonde JP. 2009. Shift work and the risk of ischemic heart disease—a systematic review of the epidemiologic evidence. *Scand. J. Work Environ. Health* 35 (3): 163–179.
193. Karlsson B, Knutsson A, and Lindahl B. 2001. Is there an association between shift work and having a metabolic syndrome? Results from a population based study of 27,485 people. *Occup. Environ. Med.* 58 (11): 747–752.
194. Grundy SM. 2007. Metabolic syndrome: A multiplex cardiovascular risk factor. *J. Clin. Endocrinol. Metab.* 92 (2): 399–404.
195. Decode Study Group. 2007. Does diagnosis of the metabolic syndrome detect further men at high risk of cardiovascular death beyond those identified by a conventional cardiovascular risk score? The DECODE Study. *Eur. J. Cardiovasc. Prev. Rehab.* 14 (2): 192–199.
196. Scheer FA, Hilton MF, Mantzoros CS, and Shea SA. 2009. Adverse metabolic and cardiovascular consequences of circadian misalignment. *Proc. Natl. Acad. Sci. USA* 106 (11): 4453–4458.
197. Garaulet M, and Madrid JA. 2009. Chronobiology, genetics and metabolic syndrome. *Curr. Opin. Lipidol.* 20 (2): 127–134.
198. Pietroiusti A, Neri A, Somma G, Coppeta L, Iavicoli I, Bergamaschi A, and Magrini A. 2010. Incidence of metabolic syndrome among night-shift healthcare workers. *Occup. Environ. Med.* 67 (1): 54–57.
199. Lin YC, Hsiao TJ, and Chen PC. 2009. Shift work aggravates metabolic syndrome development among early-middle-aged males with elevated ALT. *World J. Gastroenterol.* 15 (45): 5654–5661.
200. Karlsson B. 2009. Commentary: Metabolic syndrome as a result of shift work exposure? *Int. J. Epidemiol.* 38 (3): 854–855.
201. De BD, Van RM, Clays E, Kittel F, De BG, and Braeckman L. 2009. Rotating shift work and the metabolic syndrome: A prospective study. *Int. J. Epidemiol.* 38 (3): 848–854.
202. Copertaro A, Bracci M, Barbaresi M, and Santarelli L. 2008. Assessment of cardiovascular risk in shift healthcare workers. *Eur. J. Cardiovasc. Prev. Rehabil.* 15 (2): 224–229.
203. Biggi N, Consonni D, Galluzzo V, Sogliani M, and Costa G. 2008. Metabolic syndrome in permanent night workers. *Chronobiol. Int.* 25 (2): 443–454.

204. Nazri SM, Tengku MA, and Winn T. 2008. The association of shift work and hypertension among male factory workers in Kota Bharu, Kelantan, Malaysia. *Southeast Asian J. Trop. Med. Public Health* 39 (1): 176–183.
205. Suwazono Y, Dochi M, Sakata K, Okubo Y, Oishi M, Tanaka K, Kobayashi E, and Nogawa K. 2008. Shift work is a risk factor for increased blood pressure in Japanese men: A 14-year historical cohort study. *Hypertension* 52 (3): 581–586.
206. Dochi M, Suwazono Y, Sakata K, Okubo Y, Oishi M, Tanaka K, Kobayashi E, and Nogawa K. 2009. Shift work is a risk factor for increased total cholesterol level: A 14-year prospective cohort study in 6886 male workers. *Occup. Environ. Med.* 66 (9): 592–597.
207. Dochi M, Sakata K, Oishi M, Tanaka K, Kobayashi E, and Suwazono Y. 2008. Relationship between shift work and hypercholesterolemia in Japan. *Scand. J. Work Environ. Health* 34 (1): 33–39.
208. Brown DL, Feskanich D, Sanchez BN, Rexrode KM, Schernhammer ES, and Lisabeth LD. 2009. Rotating night shift work and the risk of ischemic stroke. *Am. J. Epidemiol.* 169 (11): 1370–1377.
209. Straif K, Baan R, Grosse Y, Secretan B, El Ghissassi F, Bouvard V, Altieri A, Benbrahim-Tallaa L, and Cogliano V. 2007. Carcinogenicity of shift-work, painting, and fire-fighting. *Lancet Oncol.* 8 (12): 1065–1066.
210. Erren TC, Morfeld P, Stork J, Knauth P, von Mulmann MJ, Breitstadt R, Muller U, Emmerich M, and Piekarski C. 2009. Shift work, chronodisruption and cancer? The IARC 2007 challenge for research and prevention and 10 theses from the Cologne Colloquium 2008. *Scand. J. Work Environ. Health* 35 (1): 74–79.
211. Stevens RG. 2009. Light-at-night, circadian disruption and breast cancer: Assessment of existing evidence. *Int. J. Epidemiol.* 38 (4): 963–970.
212. Fritschi L. 2009. Shift work and cancer. *BMJ* 339: B2653.
213. Kolstad HA. 2008. Nightshift work and risk of breast cancer and other cancers—A critical review of the epidemiologic evidence. *Scand. J. Work Environ. Health* 34 (1): 5–22.
214. Erren TC, Pape HG, Reiter RJ, and Piekarski C. 2008. Chronodisruption and cancer. *Naturwissenschaften* 95 (5): 367–382.
215. Schernhammer ES, Laden F, Speizer FE, Willett WC, Hunter DJ, Kawachi I, and Colditz GA. 2001. Rotating night shifts and risk of breast cancer in women participating in the nurses' health study. *J. Natl. Cancer Inst.* 93 (20): 1563–1568.
216. Schernhammer ES, Kroenke CH, Laden F, and Hankinson SE. 2006. Night work and risk of breast cancer. *Epidemiology* 17 (1): 108–111.
217. Megdal SP, Kroenke CH, Laden F, Pukkala E, and Schernhammer ES. 2005. Night work and breast cancer risk: A systematic review and meta-analysis. *Eur. J. Cancer* 41 (13): 2023–2032.
218. Viswanathan AN, Hankinson SE, and Schernhammer ES. 2007. Night shift work and the risk of endometrial cancer. *Cancer Res.* 67 (21): 10618–10622.
219. Viswanathan AN, and Schernhammer ES. 2009. Circulating melatonin and the risk of breast and endometrial cancer in women. *Cancer Lett.* 281 (1): 1–7.
220. Bara AC, and Arber S. 2009. Working shifts and mental health—Findings from the British Household Panel Survey (1995–2005). *Scand. J. Work Environ. Health* 35 (5): 361–367.
221. Meyrer R, Demling J, Kornhuber J, and Nowak M. 2009. Effects of night shifts in bipolar disorders and extreme morningness. *Bipolar Disord.* 11 (8): 897–899.
222. Bambra CL, Whitehead MM, Sowden AJ, Akers J, and Petticrew MP. 2008. Shifting schedules: The health effects of reorganizing shift work. *Am. J. Prev. Med.* 34 (5): 427–434.
223. Hakola T, and Harma M. 2001. Evaluation of a fast forward rotating shift schedule in the steel industry with a special focus on ageing and sleep. *J. Hum. Ergol. (Tokyo)* 30 (1–2): 315–319.
224. Czeisler CA, Moore-Ede MC, and Coleman RM. 1982. Rotating shift work schedules that disrupt sleep are improved by applying circadian principles. *Science* 217: 460–463.
225. Thorpy MJ. 2010. Managing the patient with shift-work disorder. *J. Fam. Pract.* 59 (1 Suppl): S24–S31.
226. Yoon IY, Jeong DU, Kwon KB, Kang SB, and Song BG. 2002. Bright light exposure at night and light attenuation in the morning improve adaptation of night shift workers. *Sleep* 25 (3): 351–356.
227. Smith MR, Fogg LF, and Eastman CI. 2009. A compromise circadian phase position for permanent night work improves mood, fatigue, and performance. *Sleep* 32 (11): 1481–1489.
228. Czeisler CA, Walsh JK, Wesnes KA, Arora S, and Roth T. 2009. Armodafinil for treatment of excessive sleepiness associated with shift work disorder: A randomized controlled study. *Mayo Clin. Proc.* 84 (11): 958–972.

229. Garnock-Jones KP, Dhillon S, and Scott LJ. 2009. Armodafinil. *CNS Drugs* 23 (9): 793–803.
230. Sack RL, Auckley D, Auger RR, Carskadon MA, Wright KP, Jr., Vitiello MV, and Zhdanova IV. 2007. Circadian rhythm sleep disorders: Part II, advanced sleep phase disorder, delayed sleep phase disorder, free-running disorder, and irregular sleep–wake rhythm. *Am. Acad. Sleep Med. Rev. Sleep* 30 (11): 1484–1501.

26 Melatonin and Its By-Products on Age-Related Macular Degeneration

Dan-Ning Hu, Joan E. Roberts, and Richard B. Rosen

CONTENTS

26.1 THE EYE AND THE AGE-RELATED MACULAR DEGENERATION

Age-related macular degeneration (AMD) is a progressive degenerative disease of the macular region in the retina. The macula is the central area of the retina, which enables us to see the fine details of our central vision. AMD is the leading cause of blindness in older persons in the Western countries. The prevalence of AMD in Americans 40 years or older is 1.5%, and it has been estimated that 1.75 million persons experience this disease. The prevalence increases dramatically with age and is 10% or more among persons older than 80 years.[1–9] Considering the significant medical, personal, social, and economic costs of AMD, the need for novel therapeutic and preventative strategies for AMD is pressing. Study of the relationship between AMD and melatonin may be helpful in addressing this problem.

Before the discussion of AMD, it is helpful to briefly review the anatomy and physiology of the eye. The wall of the human eye consists of three distinct concentric layers (Figure 26.1): the outer layer (the transparent cornea and the opaque white sclera), the middle layer (the uveal tract), and the inner layer (the retina). The uveal tract is composed of three parts: the iris anteriorly, an intermediate ciliary body, and the choroid posteriorly. The choroid is a highly vascularized connective tissue that supports and nourishes the retina. The retina consists of two layers: the retinal pigment epithelium (RPE) and the neural retina. The neural retina contains neurons (light sensitive receptors and neuronal networks that encode and transfer the visual information to the brain) and glial cells. The light-sensitive receptors are photoreceptors, which consist of cones (for day-light vision) and rods (for dim-light vision). The neuronal networks in the retina consist of bipolar cells, horizontal cells, amacrine cells, and retinal ganglion cells, and these cells form a network that transfers the visual information to the brain. The RPE is a single layer of pigment cells that have various functions that are essential for the support and viability of the overlaying photoreceptors (Figure 26.2).

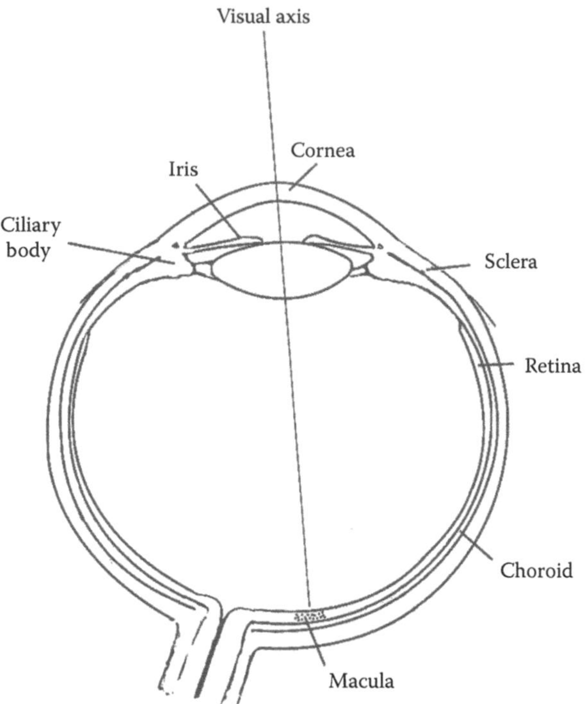

FIGURE 26.1 Anatomy of the eye. The wall of the human eye consists of three layers: the outer layer (the transparent cornea and the opaque white sclera), the middle layer (the uveal tract), and the inner layer (the retina). The uveal tract is composed of three parts: the iris anteriorly, an intermediate ciliary body, and the choroid posteriorly. The retina contains neurons that encode and transfer the visual information to the brain. The macula is the central area of the retina, which enables us to see the fine details of our central vision.

AMD is a disease mainly involving the RPE and photoreceptors in the central region of the retina (macula). Early stage of AMD is characterized by the appearance of drusen, yellow spots containing of cellular debris that accumulate between the retina and the choroid (Figure 26.3). Most people with these early changes still have good vision. The disease progresses when the drusen enlarge or as they are absorbed, leaving pigmentary disturbance in the RPE.

The advanced stages of AMD are described as being either dry or wet. The dry type progresses to geographic atrophy, which is characterized by pigmentary changes in the RPE and loss of overlaying photoreceptors, resulting in loss of central vision (Figure 26.4). No treatment is currently available for this type of AMD, with the exception of nutritional supplementation using antioxidants and zinc, which have been shown to help to slow the overall progression of the deterioration and preserve vision.[8–12]

The wet type of AMD (neovascular or exudative AMD) is characterized by the new vessels that develop from the choroidal vessels and progress to invade into the retina (Figure 26.5). This leads to retinal edema due to intravascular leakage, hemorrhage, and ultimately, scar formation in the macula, which causes permanent loss of central vision. Treatments for destruction of these new vessels have included laser photocoagulation, photodynamic therapy, and most recently intraocular injection of anti–vascular endothelial growth factor (VEGF) agents, which decrease the permeability of these new vessels and inhibit their growth. These agents have been most successful in reducing the swelling of the retina, inhibiting progression of the destruction of the macula, and in many cases, up to 40%, restoring visual function.

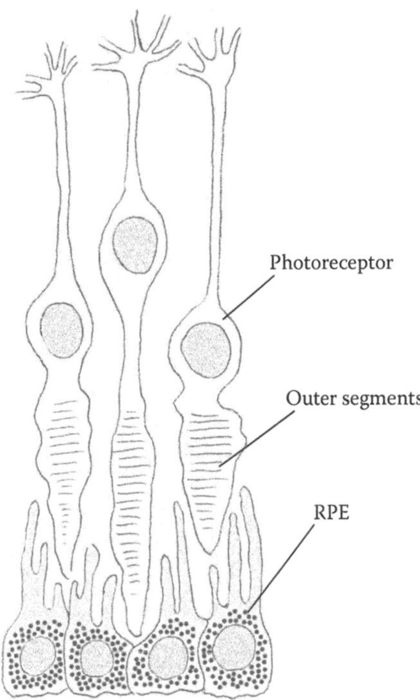

FIGURE 26.2 Photoreceptor and retinal pigment epithelium. Photoreceptors are the retinal cells that convert light energy into nerve impulses. RPE is a single layer of pigment cells that maintain the survival and function of photoreceptors. Photoreceptors and RPE are the most important cells involving the visual function and in the pathological processes of AMD.

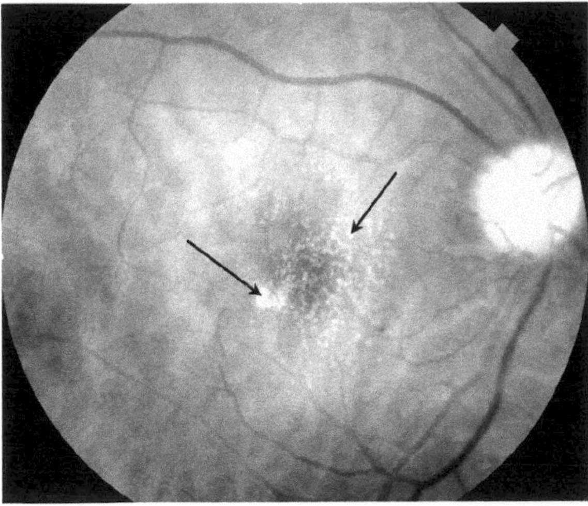

FIGURE 26.3 Early stage of AMD. Macula of a patient with early stage of AMD revealing drusen of various sizes (arrow).

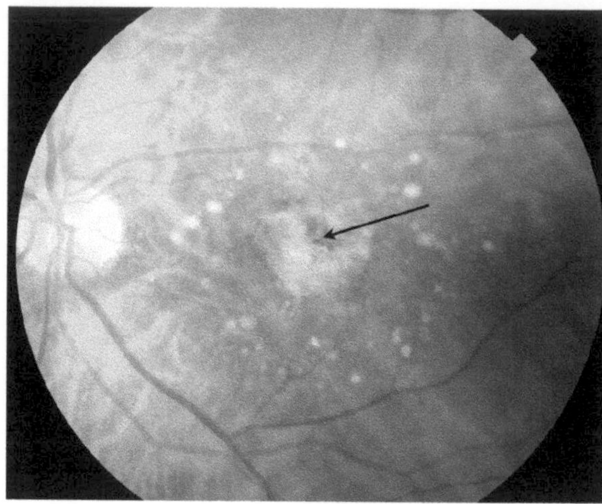

FIGURE 26.4 Advanced stages of dry type of AMD. Macula of a patient with advanced dry type of AMD showing large drusen and a central area of geographic atrophy (arrow).

26.2 PATHOGENESIS OF AMD

AMD is a multifactorial disease that is caused by both genetic and environmental factors. Individuals with a family history of AMD are at increased risk of developing the disease. Recently, association studies and experimental animal studies suggest that several genes are associated with the occurrence of AMD.[1–5] The strongest risk association are with polymorphisms of complement factor H (*CFH*, a proinflammatory gene related to immune and autoimmune reactions), *LOV387715/ARMS2* (a gene related to the function of mitochondria), and *HtrA1* (a stress-inducible member of a family of heat shock serine proteases).[1–5] On the other hand, certain polymorphisms of complement component 2 (*C2*) and *C3* gene (genes related to the immune response) may be protective for AMD.[1] Contributing environmental factors also increase the risk for AMD: these include advanced age, exposure to blue light (430 nm), cigarette smoking, high fat intake, obesity, and degree of

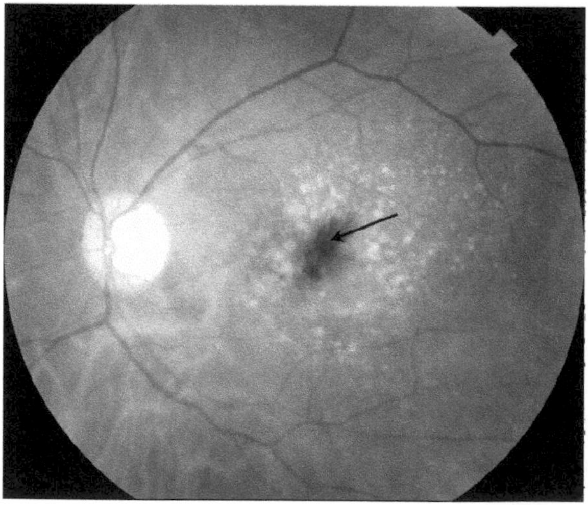

FIGURE 26.5 Advanced stages of wet type of AMD. Macula of a patient with advanced type of AMD showing large drusen and fresh hemorrhage (arrow) from choroidal neovascularization.

pigmentation (AMD is more frequent in whites as compared with blacks and Asians).[1,6] The age-associated increase in AMD risk may be mediated by gradual, cumulative damage to the retina from daily oxidative stress.[7–20]

In the past decades, there has been growing evidence that cumulative oxidative stress could play an important role in the development of AMD.[7–20] Oxidative stress has been implicated in many disease processes, especially age-related disorders. The retina is particularly vulnerable to oxidative stress due to its high consumption of oxygen, which can promote the formation of various reactive oxygen species (ROS).[8–10]

The photoreceptor (retinal cells that convert light energy into nerve impulses) and RPE (retinal pigment cells that maintain the survival and function of photoreceptors) are the most important cells involved in the visual function and pathogenesis of AMD. The photoreceptor/RPE complex contains several photosensitizers (e.g., lipofuscin), which can induce generation of singlet oxygen and other ROS after exposure to light. Membranes in the photoreceptor/RPE complex contain high levels of polyunsaturated fatty acids, which are readily oxidized to cause cellular damage.[8–10] Experimental animal and in vitro studies have demonstrated that various ROS can cause changes in the RPE and photoreceptors, resulting in increased production of various growth factors related to the angiogenesis process (e.g., VEGF[21]); altered extracellular matrix leads to sub-RPE deposits, which resemble drusen, and ultimately lead to damage and loss of function of the RPE and photoreceptors.[22–24] Increased lipid peroxidation products (malondialdehyde, or MDA) and change in various blood antioxidants and antioxidant enzymes have also been found in AMD patients.[9,14–18] Dietary intake and blood level of vitamin E, zinc, and natural carotenoid pigments located in the macula, lutein, and zeaxanthin are inversely correlated to the occurrence of AMD.[9,25–27] Several randomized controlled clinical trials found a beneficial effect with dietary supplementation of antioxidants on the occurrence or progression of AMD.[7,11–13]

Inflammation and aberrant complement activation also play a role in the pathogenesis of AMD.[2–5,28–39] Chronic inflammatory infiltrates have been demonstrated in the choroid and excised choroidal neovascular membranes from AMD.[28–30,35,36,40] Analysis of drusen composition in AMD patients and animal models have found various inflammatory proteins (e.g., acute phase proteins, cytokines), immunoglobulin, and components of the complement cascade.[5,10–12,18,19] *CFH*, a key inhibitor of the alternative pathway of complement activation, can bind and inactivate harmful complement components and prevent damage of intact host cells. In the past few years, *CFH* gene polymorphism, which causes loss of control of overactivated complement, has been reported to be an important risk factor for AMD.[1–5] Dysfunction of the complement system may result in local inflammation, autoimmune reactions, and tissue damage and may play an important role in the etiology of AMD.[2,29,30,33,37]

There are several possibilities linking ROS and inflammatory processes in AMD. ROS may cause damage of RPE cells and result in cell debris deposits between the RPE and Bruch's membrane, which may induce an inflammatory reaction.[28–30,40] Prolonged phagocytosis of oxidized photoreceptor outer segments may reduce the production of *CFH*, which could lead to impairment of regulation of overactivation of complement cascades.[38] Hollyfield et al.[39] demonstrated that AMD-like lesions in mice could be induced by immunization with an oxidant product in the retina, a mixture of docosahexaenoic acid, carboxyethylpyrrole, adducted with mouse serum albumin.

Furthermore, ROS have two different effects on the cells. Traditionally, they are thought to have cytotoxic effects and are implicated in causing cell death, but recent studies suggest that at subtoxic levels, they may influence signaling pathways and play a major role in various aspects of cell function.[41–44] Recently, we have studied the effects of low level H_2O_2 on the production of a proinflammatory cytokine, interleukin 6 (IL-6). Subtoxic levels of H_2O_2 (100 μM and less) increased the IL-6 mRNA levels and the release of IL-6 protein by the cultured human RPE cells in a dose- and time-dependent manner, which was accompanied with an increase in phosphorylated p38 MAPK. The p38 inhibitor completely abolished the H_2O_2-induced expression of IL-6 by the RPE cells (unpublished data). IL-6, which is known to modulate immune responses, inflammatory processes, and the occurrence of autoimmune diseases, has recently been documented to be increased in AMD. IL-6 may be the molecular linkage between increased oxidative stress and inflammatory/autoimmune reactions in AMD.

From these findings, it is clear that oxidative stress plays an important role in the occurrence of AMD and antioxidative substances may be protective against the progression of AMD.

26.3 MELATONIN AS AN ANTIOXIDANT AND FREE RADICAL SCAVENGER

Melatonin is a free radical scavenger and antioxidant that was first demonstrated by Ianas (1991). Since then, there have been hundreds of publications that demonstrate the free radical scavenging and antioxidant actions of melatonin in both in vitro and in vivo studies.[45–52] As with most tryptophan derivatives, melatonin interacts with hydroxyl radicals with a high rate constant ($1.2–7.5 \times 10^{10}$/M/s). Melatonin also quenches other ROS, such as singlet oxygen, peroxynitrite anion, and hypochlorous acid, but not superoxide.[45–52] Several melatonin oxidation products, i.e., N^1-acetyl-N^2-formyl-5-methoxykynuramine and N^1-acetyl-5-methoxykynuramine, are also potent free radical scavengers and antioxidants.[46,53] In addition to the direct effects, conjugates of melatonin to melatonin membrane receptors ($MT_{1/2}$ receptors) can induce the expression of various natural antioxidant enzymes or to increase their activity, e.g., superoxide dismutase, glutathione peroxidase, glutathione reductase.[46–47,52–54] Numerous in vitro and in vivo studies have documented the ability of both physiological and pharmacological concentrations of melatonin to protect various cells against oxidative stress.[55–64]

26.4 PRESENCE OF MELATONIN AND ITS RECEPTOR IN THE EYE

Melatonin can enter the retina and RPE from the circulation and can also be produced in the ocular tissues (e.g., retina, ciliary body). It has been reported that melatonin can be produced in the retina. Day retinal melatonin levels do not fall after pinealectomy, whereas day blood melatonin levels fall 60%. This suggests that the retina produces melatonin to maintain local melatonin levels despite the rhythm changes of systemic melatonin levels.[65] Tosni and Fukuhara[66] identified the production of melatonin in the photoreceptors. Melatonin is synthesized by the same pathway as that used in the pineal body. The melatonin levels in retina (rat) are 2 pg/gm.[67] Recently, Zmijewski et al.[68] detected the expression of key enzymes for melatonin synthesis, including hydroxylases, arylalkylamine *N*-acetyltransferase (AANAT), and hydroxyindole-*O*-methyltransferase (HIOMT) in cultured RPE, indicating that the RPE may be an additional source of melatonin in the eye.

The key enzymes for melatonin synthesis (AANAT and HIOMT) have been found in the human ciliary body,[65] strongly suggesting that melatonin is synthesized in the ciliary body. Furthermore, these enzymes also have been detected in the rabbit lens, indicating that melatonin may be also synthesized by the lens.[65] The aqueous humor, which fills the space located in the anterior segment of the eye, contains measurable amounts of melatonin. Chiquet (2006) reported that the morning melatonin levels in aqueous humor from healthy humans is 6.4 ± 9.3 pg/ml (mean ± SD),[69] which is similar to the 5.23 (daytime) and 22.1 pg/ml (nighttime) levels in the rabbits aqueous humor[70] but is lower than those reported by Rochrbach et al. (35 pg/ml in human aqueous humor)[71]; this discrepancy may be related to the different methods used for the measurement of melatonin.

The synthesis of melatonin in the eye is for local purposes and does not contribute significantly to plasma levels.[53,65,72–74] Melatonin receptors have been detected in various ocular cells. These reports include mainly Wiechman's study in the *Xenopus* and several other authors who have studied human tissues.[65,75–79] These findings have been summarized in Table 26.1.

In the retina and choroid, melatonin receptors are present in the RPE (MT_2), uveal melanocytes (MT_2), various retinal neurons, including photoreceptors (MT_1 and MT_2), horizontal cells (MT_1 and MT_2), retinal ganglion cells and amacrine cells (MT_1), and various vascular cells (MT_1).[65, 75–79] A subset of retinal ganglion cells express the photopigment melanopsin and are intrinsically photosensitive. These cells project to the suprachiasmatic nucleous of the hypothalamus and are implicated

TABLE 26.1
Melatonin Receptors in the Eye[65,75–79]

Melatonin Receptors Subtype	Species	Ocular Tissues and Cells
MT_1 (Mel_{1a})	*Xenopus*	Cornea (epithelium, keratocyte, endothelium); sclera (fibroblast, chondrocyte); retina (photoreceptors)
	Human	Cornea (epithelium, keratocyte, endothelium), retina (photoreceptor, horizontal cells, amacrine cells, ganglion cells), ocular vessels (retinal and choroidal vessels)
MT_2 (Mel_{1b})	*Xenopus*	Sclera (fibroblast), lens, retina (RPE, photoreceptor, horizontal cell)
	Human	Uvea (melanocyte), retina (RPE)
Mel_{1c}	*Xenopus*	Cornea (epithelium, keratocyte, endothelium), ciliary body (nonpigment epithelium [MT184], sclera [fibroblast, chondrocyte], retina [RPE, photoreceptors, amacrine cells])

in non-image–forming visual responses to environmental light, such as the papillary light reflex, seasonal adaptations in physiology, photic inhibition of nocturnal melatonin release, and modulation of sleep.[80]

Activation of melatonin receptors mainly leads to the down regulation of adenylate cyclase activity with subsequent decrease in activated protein kinase A and the induction of the expression of various natural antioxidant enzymes or an enhancement of their activity.[45–47,52–54,81–83] Activation of melatonin receptors also can activate or inhibit several other signaling pathways, including protein kinase C (PKC), phospholipase C, guanylate cyclase, etc., depending on the species, organs, and tissues.[45–47,51–54,65,81–83]

The effects of melatonin on the ocular physiology and pathology are a new area of research. Various reports have indicated that melatonin may stimulate the corneal wound healing, influence the production of aqueous humor and modulate intraocular pressure, protect the lens against UVB-induced cataract formation, modulate the growth of the eye and, thus, play a role in the occurrence of myopia, sensitize the retina for light sensation, and mediate ocular vessel constriction.[65,80,84]

The occurrence of AMD has been associated with the presence of increased ROS and is believed to contribute to the aging process. Melatonin can quench various ROS directly and indirectly by enhancing the expression of various natural antioxidant enzymes or increase their activity through the activation of melatonin receptors and, therefore, may protect ocular cells and tissues against ROS damage. Deficiency of melatonin in aging individuals may play a role in the pathogenesis of AMD, and therefore, it is worthwhile to study whether supplementation of melatonin may have a beneficial effect on the management of AMD.

26.5 CHANGES IN MELATONIN SECRETION IN AMD PATIENTS

The secretion of melatonin by the pineal body is circadian, with high levels at night and very low secretion during daylight. The measurement of melatonin secretion requires several collections of blood to measure plasma melatonin level at different times during the night. This procedure is inconvenient and requires hospitalization, which is seldom feasible.[85–88] Collection of the first morning urine and measurement of melatonin level in the urine makes the collecting procedure easier. However, less than 1% of melatonin appears unaltered in urine, and most of the melatonin undergoes conversion to metabolites prior to appearing in the urine.[86] Circulating melatonin undergoes hepatic metabolism to 6-hydroxymelatonin, which is immediately conjugated to yield 6-sulfatoxymelatonin (aMT6s). This product is then excreted in the urine and accounts for more than 70% of the melatonin secreted. Concentration of aMT6s in urine is two to three orders of magnitude higher than that of melatonin; therefore, it is very sensitive and no extraction is required.[85,86] There is also good correlation between nocturnal urinary aMT6s and plasma melatonin level during the night.[85–92] In order to compensate for the variation in the diluteness of urine, urinary creatinine should be measured, and aMT6s level is expressed as urine aMT6s/creatinine.[85,92] Estimation of nocturnal circulating melatonin levels by measuring nocturnal urine aMT6s/creatinine is a well-established, reliable, and most feasible procedure for clinical study, which has been used widely for the study of melatonin secretion and its relationship with various physiological and pathological situations.[85–89,93–96]

Recently, the levels of urine aMT6s/cre in AMD have been studied at the New York Eye and Ear Infirmary (NYEEI), and the results were compared with a group of age- and gender-matched controls.[74] The first urine of the morning was collected from 43 AMD patients and 12 controls without AMD. The level of aMT6s in specimens was measured by a commercial 6-sulfatoxymelatonin ELISA kit. The assay was performed by researchers that were masked to the clinical information.[74]

There was no statistically significant difference in age, gender, history of smoking, cancer, and coronary heart disease between AMD patients and the controls. The amount of aMT6s in nocturnal urine was 6.24 ± 3.45 ng aMT6/mg creatinine (mean ± SD) in AMD patients, which was 60% of the level in the age- and gender-matched controls (10.4 ± 4.51 ng/mg). The difference of aMT6 level in nocturnal urine between AMD patients and the controls was statistically significant ($p = 0.0128$). After adjustment for various factors (age, smoking, cancer, and coronary heart disease) that may influence the aMT6s level, the odds ratio of urinary aMT6s comparing AMD patients to controls was 0.65 (95% confidence interval = 0.48–0.88, $p = 0.0036$), indicating that urinary aMT6s level in AMD patients was lower than in controls even after multivariate adjustment.[74]

There are two possibilities in the causal relationship between the lower melatonin level and AMD. First, AMD interferes in the production of melatonin, and the pathologic process in the retina is the cause of the low circulating melatonin level in AMD. Second, deficiency of melatonin plays a role in the pathogenesis and is at least one of the risk factors for AMD.[74]

Melatonin is mainly produced in the pineal body, although there are other tissues where the production of melatonin has been detected, including ocular tissues.[65–67,72–74] However, the amount of melatonin produced in the eye is far less than that produced in the pineal body. It has been well documented that the blood melatonin level is derived exclusively from the pineal gland in mammals.[53–67,72–74] Therefore, it does not seem possible that the decrease of urinary aMT6s is due to the changes of melatonin production in the eye with AMD.[74]

Totally blind people may lose synchronization of circadian rhythms to the day/night cycle.[97] However, AMD almost never leads to total blindness. In the NYEEI series, none of the AMD patients had lost light perception. In four patients with vision of both eyes at hand movement to 20/400, their urinary aMT6s levels did not differ from patients with better vision, indicating that decrease of visual acuity due to AMD was not the cause of decrease of urinary aMT6s in AMD.[74]

Based on these facts, the role of oxidative stress in the pathogenesis of AMD, the antioxidative effects of melatonin, and the lower melatonin level in AMD may play a role in the pathogenesis of AMD rather than the pathologic process in the retina as the cause of the low circulating melatonin level in AMD. The mechanism of lower melatonin level in AMD, whether determined by genetic or environmental factors, is unknown and requires further investigation.

26.6 PROTECTIVE EFFECTS OF MELATONIN ON OCULAR CELLS AND TISSUES

Melatonin has been reported to protect the retina, the RPE, and the photoreceptors against oxidative processes.[98–103] The membranes of the outer part of the retinal photoreceptor are susceptible to lipid peroxidation because of their high content of polyunsaturated fatty acids. It has been suggested that lipid peroxidation participates in the oxidative damage leading to retinal photoreceptor degeneration.[8–10] Melatonin is a free radical scavenger and an antioxidant and has been reported to have a protective effect against lipid peroxidation.

Siu et al.[98] 1998 studied the efficacy of melatonin as an antioxidant against lipid peroxidation in rat retinal homogenates caused by iron (II) ions. The lipid peroxidation product MDA was used as a parameter for estimating the cell damage. Melatonin at concentrations from 0.5 to 4 mM shows a dose-dependent effect in the inhibition of MDA formation. The melatonin concentration required to inhibit lipid peroxidation by 50% (IC50) is 4.98 mM. These results indicate that melatonin can protect rat retinal homogenates against iron (II)-induced free radical damage. Vitamin E also decreases the formation of MDA, with an IC50 at 0.69 mM.

Marchiafava et al.[99] exposed single dark-adapted photoreceptors from the frog retina to saturating light to stimulate production of ROS. Melatonin at picomolar and low nanomolar concentrations (0.1–100 nM) effectively inhibited the light-induced oxidative processes, with a maximum effect at 1 nM. At this range of dosage, melatonin was 100 times more potent in inhibiting the light-induced oxidation than that of vitamin E. Both compounds exert pro-oxidant effects at 1 μM concentration or more, which is above the physiological levels of melatonin. This suggests that physiological levels of melatonin in a living cell may exert protective actions against a natural oxidant stimulus (light).

Guajardo et al.[101,102] studied the protective effect of melatonin on in vitro ascorbate–Fe^{2+}-dependent lipid peroxidation of rod outer segment membranes of bovine retina. Rod outer segment membranes were isolated from bovine retina. Ascorbate–Fe^{2+} was used to induce lipid peroxidation of polyunsaturated fatty acids located in rod outer segment membranes. Melatonin at concentrations from 0 to 10 mM showed a dose-dependent reduction of lipid peroxidation. Melatonin at 10 mM produced a reduction of 51% in the lipid peroxidation. The concentration of melatonin required to inhibit 50% of the lipid peroxidation (IC50) was 9.82 mM. Proteins, like lipids, can undergo chain oxidation and resulting in cell damage. Treatment of rod outer segment membranes with oxidative stress caused the formation of high molecular weight aggregates with partial or complete disappearance of many protein bands. Rhodopsin, the major integral protein of rod outer segment membranes, was reduced by 76% after the treatment with ascorbate–Fe^{2+}. Melatonin at 5 mM decreased the reduction of rhodopsin from 76% to 40%. These studies demonstrate that melatonin prevents both lipid peroxidation and protein oxidation.

Liang et al.[100] studied the protective effects of melatonin on human RPE cells subjected to hydrogen peroxide damage. Hydrogen peroxide at concentrations of 0.1–0.1 μM caused cell death of cultured human RPE cells. Pretreatment of melatonin at concentrations of 0.1–200 μM, 2–24 hours before the addition of hydrogen peroxide showed no significant protective effects. However, when melatonin was administered diurnally for three consecutive days, hydrogen peroxide–induced cell death and mitochondrial DNA damage was markedly reduced. Since melatonin was found to be effective only after prolonged administration, the stimulation of various antioxidant enzymes by melatonin was suggested as a possible mechanism for melatonin-induced reduction of oxidative stress.

Angiogenesis plays an important role in the occurrence of wet type of AMD. VEGF is the main growth factor that stimulated angiogenesis in the eye. Rosen and Hu[103] found that melatonin reduced the up-regulation of VEGF in human ocular melanocytes caused by PKC activation but did not suppress the normal secretion of VEGF by ocular melanocytes in vitro.

In an experimental animal study, Baydas et al.[104] reported that melatonin (10 mg/kg) prevented lipid oxidation (using MDA and 4-hydroxyalkenals as parameter) in diabetic rat retina. All of these studies indicate that melatonin may protect the retina, photoreceptors, and RPE against oxidative stress. The relative efficiency of antioxidative effects as compared with vitamin E varies widely among different experiments. This suggests that the antioxidative effects of melatonin may be cell-, species-, and stimulation-specific. Furthermore, whether the protective effect of melatonin on ocular cells is due to a direct antioxidant effect or to indirect receptor-mediated effect was not distinguished. Therefore, a comprehensive study of the protective effects of melatonin on various ocular cells against different oxidative stresses and the mechanisms that are involved in these processes is required.

26.7 MANAGEMENT OF AMD BY MELATONIN

There was only one clinical report dealing with the treatment of AMD by supplementation of melatonin. Yi et al.[105] reported on a clinical trial testing the effects of melatonin supplementation for the treatment of AMD. This was a case control study with a follow-up of 6–24 months. AMD patients (100 cases, including both dry and wet types) were treated with oral melatonin (3 mg/night at bedtime) for at least 3 months. Fifty-five patients were observed for six more months. At 6 months of treatment, the visual acuity remained stable. Changes of the fundus photos also remained stable or improved. Only eight eyes showed more retinal bleeding, six eyes showed more retinal exudates, and the majority had reduced pathologic changes. Therefore, they claimed that melatonin protected the retina and delayed progression of macular degeneration. While the results of this study are encouraging, this was a nonrandomized controlled study with only 6 months of follow-up and a follow-up rate of only 55%, which is relatively low. Therefore, a well-organized randomized clinical trial will be required for evaluating the therapeutic effects of melatonin on the treatment of AMD.

Additionally, it has been reported that melatonin treatment appears to have a detrimental effect on photoreceptor cell survival in response to bright light.[106,107] Wiechman et al.[106] hypothesized that the circadian rhythm of melatonin synthesis reflects a beneficial role during the dark period but is a potential hazard during exposure to light and suggested that it would be prudent for individuals to avoid chronic self-administration of melatonin in the presence of high levels of environmental illumination. While a dose-dependent detrimental effect of melatonin on the retina could not be established, most of the toxic effects of melatonin on the rat retina occurred at the dosages of 5000–50,000 µg/kg/day, which approximates a dosage of 300–3000 mg/day in a 60-kg weight human.[106,107] Therefore, the dosage of melatonin treatment should be lower than that; perhaps 1–3 mg/night is a safe dosage for the management of AMD. The time of day for melatonin application should also be considered in the organization of any clinical trial. Melatonin administration at night time appears optimal for efficacy and avoidance side effects and the potential hazard of melatonin taken in the presence of high illumination. Furthermore, melatonin as an endogenous sleep hormone will aid in overall sleep induction.

26.8 SUMMARY

1. The macula is the small central portion of the retina that is responsible for highest visual acuity. Macular degeneration is characterized by the breakdown of photoreceptors (which convert light energy into nerve impulses) and RPE (cells that maintain the survival and function of photoreceptors) in the macular area. AMD is the most common cause of legal blindness in the elderly population in the developed countries. The age-associated increase in AMD risk may be mediated by gradual, cumulative damage to the retina from daily oxidative stress, which causes chronic inflammation, angiogenesis, and damage of the photoreceptors and the RPE.
2. Melatonin is a free radical scavenger and antioxidant. Conjugates of melatonin to melatonin membrane receptors can induce the expression of various natural antioxidant enzymes or to increase their activities. Melatonin can enter the retina and RPE from the circulation and can also be produced in the ocular tissues (e.g., retina, ciliary body) and is present in the retina at relatively high levels. Melatonin membrane receptors have been found in the retina and RPE. Therefore, melatonin may have a protective effect on the retina and RPE against oxidative stress and thus prevent the occurrence of AMD.
3. Morning urinary 6-sulfatoxymelatonin levels (the major metabolite of melatonin representing the nighttime circulating melatonin levels) were significantly (40%) lower in AMD patients than in those age- and gender-matched controls. This suggests that deficiency of melatonin may play a role in the occurrence of AMD.

4. Melatonin has been reported to protect the RPE and photoreceptors against various oxidative processes in vitro and in experimental animal studies.
5. A clinical trial testing the effects of melatonin supplementation for the treatment of AMD showed that melatonin might protect the retina and delay progression of macular degeneration. Therefore, melatonin administrated orally at a dosage of 1–3 mg/night may have a role in the prevention and treatment of AMD. However, a well-organized randomized, double-blind, placebo-controlled clinical trial on the effect of melatonin in the management of AMD is still required for the final determination of the effectiveness of melatonin therapy in AMD.

REFERENCES

1. Ding X, Patel M, Chan CC. Molecular pathology of age-related macular degeneration. *Prog Retin Eye Res*. 2009; 28:1–18.
2. Bok D. Evidence for an inflammatory process in age-related macular degeneration gains new support. *Proc Natl Acad Sci USA*. 2005; 102:7053–4.
3. Klein RJ, Zeiss C, Chew EY et al. Complement factor H polymorphism in age-related macular degeneration. *Science*. 2005; 308:385–9.
4. Haines JL, Hauser MA, Schmidt S et al. Complement factor H variant increases the risk of age-related macular degeneration. *Science*. 2005; 308:419–21.
5. Thakkinstian A, Han P, McEvoy et al. Systematic review and meta-analysis of the association between complementary factor H Y402H polymorphisms and age-related macular degeneration. *Hum Mol Genet*. 2006;15:2784–90.
6. Roberts, J. E. Ocular Phototoxicity. *J Photochem Photobiol B*. 2001; 64:136–43.
7. Hogg R, Chakravarthy U. AMD and micronutrient antioxidants. *Curr Eye Res*. 2004; 29:387–401.
8. Winkler BS, Boulton ME, Gottsch JD, Sternberg P. Oxidative damage and age-related macular degeneration. *Mol Vis*. 1999; 5:32.
9. Beatty S, Koh H, Phil M, Henson D, Boulton M. The role of oxidative stress in the pathogenesis of age-related macular degeneration. *Surv Ophthalmol*. 2000; 45:115–34.
10. Ahmed SS, Lott MN, Marcus DM. The macular xanthophylls. *Surv Ophthalmol*. 2005; 50:183–93.
11. Age-Related Eye Disease Study Research Group. A randomized, placebo-controlled, clinical trial of high-dose supplementation with vitamins C and E and beta carotene for age-related cataract and vision loss: AREDS report no. 8. *Arch Ophthalmol*. 2001; 119:1417–36.
12. Richer S, Stiles W, Statkute L, Pulido J, Frankowski J, Rudy D, Pei K, Tsipursky M, Nyland J. Double-masked, placebo-controlled, randomized trial of lutein and antioxidant supplementation in the intervention of atrophic age-related macular degeneration: The Veterans LAST study (Lutein Antioxidant Supplementation Trial). *Optometry*. 2004; 75:216–30.
13. van Leeuwen R, Boekhoorn S, Vingerling JR, Witteman JC, Klaver CC, Hofman A, de Jong PT. Dietary intake of antioxidants and risk of age-related macular degeneration. *JAMA*. 2005; 294:3101–7.
14. Nowak M, Swietochowska E, Wielkoszyński T, Marek B, Karpe J, Górski J, Głogowska-Szelag J, Kos-Kudła B, Ostrowska Z. Changes in blood antioxidants and several lipid peroxidation products in women with age-related macular degeneration. *Eur J Ophthalmol*. 2003; 13:281–6.
15. Baskol G, Karakucuk S, Oner AO, Baskol M, Kocer D, Mirza E, Saraymen R, Ustdal M. Serum paraoxonase 1 activity and lipid peroxidation levels in patients with age-related macular degeneration. *Ophthalmologica*. 2006; 220:12–6.
16. Prashar S, Pandav SS, Gupta A, Nath R. Antioxidant enzymes in RBCs as a biological index of age related macular degeneration. *Acta Ophthalmol (Copenh)*. 1993; 71:214–8.
17. Cohen SM, Olin KL, Feuer WJ, Hjelmeland L, Keen CL, Morse LS. Low glutathione reductase and peroxidase activity in age-related macular degeneration. *Br J Ophthalmol*. 1994; 78:791–4.
18. Evereklioglu C, Er H, Doganay S, Cekmen M, Turkoz Y, Otlu B, Ozerol E. Nitric oxide and lipid peroxidation are increased and associated with decreased antioxidant enzyme activities in patients with age-related macular degeneration. *Doc Ophthalmol*. 2003; 106:129–36.
19. Frank RN, Amin RH, Puklin JE. Antioxidant enzymes in the macular retinal pigment epithelium of eyes with neovascular age-related macular degeneration. *Am J Ophthalmol*. 1999; 127:694–709.
20. Decanini A, Nordgaard CL, Feng X, Ferrington DA, Olsen TW. Changes in select redox proteins of the retinal pigment epithelium in age-related macular degeneration. *Am J Ophthalmol*. 2007; 143:607–15.

21. Kannan R, Zhang N, Sreekumar PG, Spee CK, Rodriguez A, Barron E, Hinton DR. Stimulation of apical and basolateral VEGF-A and VEGF-C secretion by oxidative stress in polarized retinal pigment epithelial cells. *Mol Vis.* 2006; 12:1649–59.
22. Marin-Castano ME, Csaky KG, Cousins SW. Nonlethal oxidant injury to human retinal pigment epithelium cells causes cell membrane blebbing but decreased MMP-2 activity. *Invest Ophthalmol Vis Sci.* 2005; 46:3331–40.
23. Curcio CA, Millican CL. Basal linear deposit and large drusen are specific for early age-related maculopathy. *Arch Ophthalmol.* 1999; 117:329–39.
24 Rakoczy PE, Zhang D, Robertson T, Barnett NL, Papadimitriou J, Constable IJ, Lai CM. Progressive age-related changes similar to age-related macular degeneration in a transgenic mouse model. *Am J Pathol.* 2002; 161:1515–24.
25. Beatty S, Murray IJ, Henson DB, Carden D, Koh H, Boulton ME. Macular pigment and risk for age-related macular degeneration in subjects from a Northern European population. *Invest Ophthalmol Vis Sci.* 2001; 42:439–46.
26. Moeller SM, Parekh N, Tinker L, Ritenbaugh C, Blodi B, Wallace RB, Mares JA. Associations between intermediate age-related macular degeneration and lutein and zeaxanthin in the Carotenoids in Age-related Eye Disease Study (CAREDS): An ancillary study of the Women's Health Initiative. *Arch Ophthalmol.* 2006; 124:1151–62.
27. Age-related eye disease study research group, SanGiovanni JP, Chew EY, Clemons TE, Ferris FL 3rd, Gensler G, Lindblad AS, Milton RC, Seddon JM, Sperduto RD. The relationship of dietary carotenoid and vitamin A,E and C intake with age-related macular degeneration in a case–control study: AREDS Report 22. *Arch Ophthalmol.* 2007; 125:1225–32.
28. Anderson DH, Mullins RF, Hageman GS, Johnson LV. A role for local inflammation in the formation of drusen in the aging eye. *Am J Ophthalmol.* 2002; 134:411–31.
29. Patel M, Chan CC. Immunopathological aspects of age-related macular degeneration. *Semin Immunopathol.* 2008; 30:97–110.
30. Kijlstra A, La Heij E, Hendrickse F. Immunological factors in the pathogenesis and treatment of age-related macular degeneration. *Ocul Immunol Inflamm.* 2005; 13:3–11.
31. Klein R, Knudtson MD, Klein BE et al. Inflammation, complement factor H, and age-related macular degeneration: The multi-ethnic study of atherosclerosis. *Ophthalmology.* 2008; 115:1742–9.
32. Seddon JM, George S, Rosner B, Rifai N. Progression of age-related macular degeneration: Prospective assessment of C-reactive protein, interleukin 6, and other cardiovascular biomarkers. *Arch Ophthalmol.* 2005; 123:774–82.
33. Moshfeghi MD, Blumenkranz MS. Role of genetic factors and inflammation in age-related macular degeneration. *Retina.* 2007; 27:269–75.
34. Donoso LA, Kim D, Frost A, Callahan A, Hageman G. The role of inflammation in the pathogenesis of age-related macular degeneration. *Surv Ophthalmol.* 2005; 51:137–52.
35. Hageman GS, Luthert PJ, Victor C, Johnson LV, Anderson DH, Mullins RF. An integrated hypothesis is that considers dursen as biomarkers of immune-mediated progresses at the RPE–Bruch's membrane interface in age-related macular degeneration. *Prog Retin Eye Res.* 2001; 20:705–2.
36. Lopez PF, Grossniklaus HE, Lambert HM et al. Pathologic features of surgically exised sub retinal neovascular membranes in age-related macular degeneration. *Am J Ophthalmol.* 1991; 112:647–56.
37. Meri S. Loss of self-control in the complement system and innate auto reactivity. *Ann NY Acad Sci.* 2007; 1109:93–105.
38. Chen M, Forrester JV, Xu H. Synthesis of complement factor H by retinal pigment epithelial cells is down-regulated by oxidized photoreceptor outer segments. *Exp Eye Res.* 2007; 84:635–45.
39. Hollyfield JG, Bonilha VL, Rayborn ME et al. Oxidative damage-induced inflammation initiates age-related macular degeneration. *Nat Med.* 2008; 14:194–8.
40. Zarbin MA. Current concepts in the pathogenesis of age-related macular degeneration. *Arch Ophthalmol.* 2004; 122:598–614.
41. McCubrey JA, Lahair MM, Franklin RA. Reactive oxygen species-induced activation of the MAP kinase signaling pathways. *Antioxid Redox Signal.* 2006; 8:1775–89.
42. Poli G, Leonarduzzi G, Biasi F, Chiarpotto F. Oxidative stress and cell signaling. *Curr Med Chem.* 2004; 11:1163–82.
43. Valko M, Leibfritz D, Moncol J, Cronin MT, Mazur M, Telser J. Free radicals and antioxidants in normal physiological functions and human disease. *Int J Biochem Cell Biol.* 2007; 39:44–84.
44. Martin KR, Barrett JC. Reactive oxygen species as double-edged swords in cellular processes: Low-dose cell signaling versus high-dose toxicity. *Hum Exp Toxicol.* 2002; 21:71–5.

45. Roberts, JE, Hu DN, Wishart, JR. Pulse radiolysis studies of melatonin and chloromelatonin. J. Photochem Photobiol B. 1998; 42:125–32.
46. Allegra M, Reiter RJ, Tan DX, Gentile C, Tesoriere L, Livrea MA. The chemistry of melatonin's interaction with reactive species. *J Pineal Res.* 2003; 34:1–10.
47. Reiter RJ, Tan DX, Mayo JC, Sainz RM, Leon J, Czarnocki Z. Melatonin as an antioxidant: biochemical mechanisms and pathophysiological implications in humans. *Acta Biochim Pol.* 2003; 50: 1129–46.
48. Reiter RJ, Tan DX, Manchester LC, Qi W. Biochemical reactivity of melatonin with reactive oxygen and nitrogen species: A review of the evidence. *Cell Biochem Biophys.* 2001; 34:237–56.
49. Roberts, JE, Hu, DN, Martinez L, Chignell CF. Photophysical studies on melatonin and its receptor agonists. *J Pineal Res.* 2000; 29:94–9.
50. Reiter RJ, Tan DX, Manchester LC, Lopez-Burillo S, Sainz RM, Mayo JC. Melatonin: Detoxification of oxygen and nitrogen-based toxic reactants. *Adv Exp Med Biol.* 2003; 527:539–48.
51. Reiter RJ, Tan DX, Terron MP, Flores LJ, Czarnocki Z. Melatonin and its metabolites: New findings regarding their production and their radical scavenging actions. *Acta Biochim Pol.* 2007; 54:1–9.
52. Rodriguez C, Mayo JC, Sainz RM, Antolín I, Herrera F, Martín V, Reiter RJ. Regulation of antioxidant enzymes: A significant role for melatonin. *J Pineal Res.* 2004; 36:1–9.
53. Pandi-Perumal SR, Srinivasan V, Maestroni GJ, Cardinali DP, Poeggeler B, Hardeland R. Melatonin: Nature's most versatile biological signal? *FEBS J.* 2006; 273:2813–38.
54. Tan DX, Manchester LC, Reiter RJ, Qi WB, Karbownik M, Calvo JR. Significance of melatonin in antioxidative defense system: Reactions and products. *Biol Signals Recept.* 2000; 9:137–59.
55. Radogna F, Paternoster L, Albertini MC, Cerella C, Accorsi A, Bucchini A, Spadoni G, Diamantini G, Tarzia G, De Nicola M, D'Alessio M, Ghibelli L. Melatonin antagonizes apoptosis via receptor interaction in U937 monocytic cells. *J Pineal Res.* 2007; 43:154–62.
56. Esposito E, Iacono A, Muià C, Crisafulli C, Mattace Raso G, Bramanti P, Meli R, Cuzzocrea S. Signal transduction pathways involved in protective effects of melatonin in C6 glioma cells. *J Pineal Res.* 2008; 44:78–87.
57. Molpeceres V, Mauriz JL, García-Mediavilla MV, González P, Barrio JP, González-Gallego J. Melatonin is able to reduce the apoptotic liver changes induced by aging via inhibition of the intrinsic pathway of apoptosis. *J Gerontol A Biol Sci Med Sci.* 2007; 62:687–95.
58. Koh PO. Melatonin attenuates the focal cerebral ischemic injury by inhibiting the dissociation of pBad from 14–3–3. *J Pineal Res.* 2008; 44:101–6.
59. Jou MJ, Peng TI, Reiter RJ, Jou SB, Wu HY, Wen ST. Visualization of the antioxidative effects of melatonin at the mitochondrial level during oxidative stress-induced apoptosis of rat brain astrocytes. *J Pineal Res.* 2004; 37:55–70.
60. Caballero B, Vega-Naredo I, Sierra V, Huidobro-Fernández C, Soria-Valles C, De Gonzalo-Calvo D, Tolivia D, Pallás M, Camins A, Rodríguez-Colunga MJ, Coto-Montes A. Melatonin alters cell death processes in response to age-related oxidative stress in the brain of senescence-accelerated mice. *J Pineal Res.* 2009; 46:106–14.
61. Das A, Belagodu A, Reiter RJ, Ray SK, Banik NL. Cytoprotective effects of melatonin on C6 astroglial cells exposed to glutamate excitotoxicity and oxidative stress. *J Pineal Res.* 2008; 45:117–24.
62. Chetsawang B, Chetsawang J, Govitrapong P. Protection against cell death and sustained tyrosine hydroxylase phosphorylation in hydrogen peroxide- and MPP-treated human neuroblastoma cells with melatonin. *J Pineal Res.* 2009; 46:36–42.
63. Montilla P, Cruz A, Padillo FJ, Túnez I, Gascon F, Muñoz MC, Gómez M, Pera C. Melatonin versus vitamin E as protective treatment against oxidative stress after extra-hepatic bile duct ligation in rats. *J Pineal Res.* 2001; 31:138–44.
64. Venkataraman P, Krishnamoorthy G, Vengatesh G, Srinivasan N, Aruldhas MM, Arunakaran J. Protective role of melatonin on PCB (Aroclor 1,254) induced oxidative stress and changes in acetylcholine esterase and membrane bound ATPases in cerebellum, cerebral cortex and hippocampus of adult rat brain. *Int J Dev Neurosci.* 2008; 26:585–91.
65. Alarma-Estrany P, Pintor J. Melatonin receptors in the eye: Location, second messengers and role in ocular physiology. 2007; 113:507–22.
66. Tosini G, Fukuhara C. Photic and circadian regulation of retinal melatonin in mammals. *J Neuroendocrinol.* 2003; 15:364–9.
67. Chanut E, Nguyen-Legros J, Versaux-Botteri C, Trouvin JH, Launay JM. Determination of melatonin in rat pineal, plasma and retina by high-performance liquid chromatography with electrochemical detection. *J Chromatogr B Biomed Sci Appl.* 1998; 709:11–8.

68. Zmijewski MA, Sweatman TW, Slominski AT. The melatonin-producing system is fully functional in retinal pigment epithelium (ARPE-19). *Mol Cell Endocrinol.* 2009; 307:211–6.
69. Chiquet C, Claustrat B, Thuret G, Brun J, Cooper HM, Denis P. Melatonin concentrations in aqueous humor of glaucoma patients. *Am J Ophthalmol.* 2006; 142:325–7.
70. Yu HS, Yee RW, Howes KA, Reiter RJ. Diurnal rhythms of immunoreactive melatonin in the aqueous humor and serum of male pigmented rabbits. *Neurosci Lett.* 1990; 116:309–14.
71. Rohrbach JM, Wollmann H, Heinze J, Gupta D, Thanos S. The role of melatonin in growth of malignant choroid melanoma. *Ophthalmologe.* 1993; 90:289–93.
72. Vanecek J. Cellular mechanisms of melatonin action. *Physiol Rev.* 1998; 78:687–721.
73. Chiquet C, Claustrat B, Thuret G, Brun J, Cooper HM, Denis P. Melatonin concentrations in aqueous humor of glaucoma patients. *Am J Ophthalmol.* 2006; 142:325–7.
74. Rosen R, Hu DN, Perez V, Tai K, Yu GP, Chen M, Tone Paul, McCormick SA, Walsh J. Urinary 6-sulfatoxymelatonin level in age-related macular degeneration patients. *Mol Vis.* 2009; 15:1673–9.
75. Wiechmann AF, Rada JA. Melatonin receptor expression in the cornea and sclera. *Exp Eye Res.* 2003; 77:219–25.
76. Wiechmann AF. Differential distribution of Mel(1a) and Mel(1c) melatonin receptors in *Xenopus laevis* retina. *Exp Eye Res.* 2003; 76:99–106.
77. Wiechmann AF, Udin SB, Summers Rada JA. Localization of Mel_{1b} melatonin receptor-like immunoreactivity in ocular tissues of *Xenopus laevis*. *Exp Eye Res.* 2004; 79:585–94.
78. Roberts JE, Wiechmann AF, Hu DN. Melatonin receptors in human uveal melanocytes and melanoma cells. *J Pineal Res.* 2000; 28:165–71.
79. Wiechmann AF, Wirsig-Wiechmann CR. Multiple cell targets for melatonin action in *Xenopus laevis* retina: Distribution of melatonin receptor immunoreactivity. *Vis Neurosci.* 2001; 18:695–702.
80. Lundmark PO, Pandi-Perumal SR, Srinivasan V, Cardinali DP. Role of melatonin in the eye and ocular dysfunctions. *Vis Neurosci.* 2006; 23:853–62.
81. Witt-Enderby PA, Bennett J, Jarzynka MJ, Firestine S, Melan MA. Melatonin receptors and their regulation: Biochemical and structural mechanisms. *Life Sci.* 2003; 72:2183–98.
82. Witt-Enderby PA, Radio NM, Doctor JS, Davis VL. Therapeutic treatments potentially mediated by melatonin receptors: Potential clinical uses in the prevention of osteoporosis, cancer and as an adjuvant therapy. *J Pineal Res.* 2006; 41:297–305.
83. Ekmekcioglu C. Melatonin receptors in humans: Biological role and clinical relevance. *Biomed Pharmacother.* 2006; 60:97–108.
84. Rada JA, Wiechmann AF. Melatonin receptors in chick ocular tissues: Implications for a role of melatonin in ocular growth regulation. *Invest Ophthalmol Vis Sci.* 2006; 47:25–33.
85. Graham C, Cook MR, Kavet R, Sastre A, Smith DK. Prediction of nocturnal plasma melatonin from morning urinary measures. *J Pineal Res.* 1998; 24:230–8.
86. Paakkonen T, Makinen TM, Leppaluoto J, Vakkuri O, Rintamaki H, Palinkas LA, Hassi J. Urinary melatonin: A noninvasive method to follow human pineal function as studied in three experimental conditions. *J Pineal Res.* 2006; 40:110–5.
87. Bojkowski CJ, Arendt J, Shih MC, Markey SP. Melatonin secretion in humans assessed by measuring its metabolite, 6-sulfatoxymelatonin. *Clin Chem.* 1987; 33:1343–8.
88. Benloucif S, Burgess HJ, Klerman EB, Lewy AJ, Middleton B, Murphy PJ, Parry BL, Revell VL. Measuring melatonin in humans. *J Clin Sleep Med.* 2008; 4:66–9.
89. Klante G, Brinschwitz T, Secci K, Wollnik F, Steinlechner S. Creatinine is an appropriate reference for urinary sulphatoxymelatonin of laboratory animals and humans. *J Pineal Res.* 1997; 23:191–7.
90. Nowak R, McMillen IC, Redman J, Short RV. The correlation between serum and salivary melatonin concentrations and urinary 6-hydroxymelatonin sulphate excretion rates: Two non-invasive techniques for monitoring human circadian rhythmicity. *Clin Endocrinol (Oxf).* 1987; 27:445–52.
91. Arendt J, Bojkowski C, Franey C, Wright J, Marks V. Immunoassay of 6-hydroxymelatonin sulfate in human plasma and urine: Abolition of the urinary 24-hour rhythm with atenolol. *J Clin Endocrinol Metab.* 1985; 60:1166–73.
92. Markey SP, Higa S, Shih M, Danforth DN, Tamarkin L. The correlation between human plasma melatonin levels and urinary 6-hydroxymelatonin excretion. *Clin Chim Acta.* 1985; 150:221–5.
93. Schernhammer ES, Kroenke CH, Dowsett M, Folkerd E, Hankinson SE. Urinary 6-sulfatoxymelatonin levels and their correlations with lifestyle factors and steroid hormone levels. *J Pineal Res.* 2006; 40:116–24.

94. Gogenur I, Middleton B, Kristiansen VB, Skene DJ, Rosenberg J. Disturbances in melatonin and core body temperature circadian rhythms after minimal invasive surgery. *Acta Anaesthesiol Scand.* 2007; 51:1099–106.
95. Nagata C, Nagao Y, Shibuya C, Kashiki Y, Shimizu H. Association of vegetable intake with urinary 6-sulfatoxymelatonin level. *Cancer Epidemiol Biomarkers Prev.* 2005; 14:1333–5.
96. Wood AW, Loughran SP, Stough C. Does evening exposure to mobile phone radiation affect subsequent melatonin production? *Int J Radiat Biol.* 2006; 82:69–76.
97. Sack RL, Lewy AJ, Blood ML, Keith LD, Nakagawa H. Circadian rhythm abnormalities in totally blind people: Incidence and clinical significance. *J Clin Endocrinol Metab.* 1992; 75:127–34.
98. Siu AW, Reiter RJ, To CH. The efficacy of vitamin E and melatonin as antioxidants against lipid peroxidation in rat retinal homogenates. *J Pineal Res.* 1998; 24:239–44.
99. Marchiafava PL, Longoni B. Melatonin as an antioxidant in retinal photoreceptors. *J Pineal Res.* 1999; 26:184–9.
100. Liang FQ, Green L, Wang C, Alssadi R, Godley BF. Melatonin protects human retinal pigment epithelial (RPE) cells against oxidative stress. *Exp Eye Res.* 2004; 78:1069–75.
101. Guajardo MH, Terrasa AM, Catalá A. Protective effect of indoleamines on in vitro ascorbate-Fe2+ dependent lipid peroxidation of rod outer segment membranes of bovine retina. *J Pineal Res.* 2003; 35:276–82.
102. Guajardo MH, Terrasa AM, Catalá A. Lipid–protein modifications during ascorbate–Fe2+ peroxidation peroxidation of photoreceptor membranes: Protective effect of melatonin. *J Pineal Res.* 2006; 41:201–10.
103. Rosen R, Hu DN. Melatonin suppresses the TPA induced up-regulation of VEGF by human uveal melanocytes in vitro. Present 2006 ARVO Meeting, May 4, 2006. Fort Lauderdale, FL.
104. Baydas G, Tuzcu M, Yasar A, Baydas B. Early changes in glial reactivity and lipid peroxidation in diabetic rat retina: Effects of melatonin. *Acta Diabetol.* 2004; 41:123–8.
105. Yi C, Pan X, Yan H, Guo M, Pierpaoli W. Effects of melatonin in age-related macular degeneration. *Ann N Y Acad Sci.* 2005; 1057:384–92.
106. Wiechmann AF, Chignell CF, Roberts JE. Influence of dietary melatonin on photoreceptor survival in the rat retina: An ocular toxicity study. *Exp Eye Res.* 2008; 86:241–50.
107. Wiechmann AF, O'Steen WK. Melatonin increases photoreceptor susceptibility to light-induced damage. *Invest Ophthalmol Vis Sci.* 1992; 33:1894–902.

27 Melatonin and Melanoma

Dan-Ning Hu, Joan E. Roberts, and Allan F. Wiechmann

CONTENTS

27.1 MELANOMAS (CLASSIFICATION, ETIOLOGY, PATHOGENESIS, CLINICAL MANIFESTATION, AND MANAGEMENT)

Melanoma is a malignant tumor that originates from melanocytes or their precursors.[1–4] Melanocytes are pigmented dendritic-like cells located in the skin, eye, mucous membrane, and other organs. During development, melanocyte precursors arise in the neural crest from where they migrate to various organs and tissues in the body. Melanocytes produce melanin. The color of the skin, hair, and iris is mainly determined by the quality and quantity of melanins produced by melanocytes.[5]

Melanomas can be divided into three main categories based on their anatomic locations: cutaneous, ocular, and mucosal melanomas. Cutaneous melanomas are the most common melanoma and account for 92%–94% of all melanomas.[6–8] Ocular melanomas are the second most common melanomas and account for approximately 5% of all melanomas. Ocular melanomas are further categorized by anatomical location as uveal melanoma and conjunctival melanoma. Uveal melanoma is much more frequent than conjunctival melanoma.[6–10] Mucosal melanomas occur in the mucosal lining of the nasal and oral cavities, anus, vagina, and urinary tract and account for less than 3% of all melanomas.[6–8,11]

The incidence of cutaneous melanoma has recently increased more rapidly than most adult onset malignant tumors in Whites. In the United States, the incidence of cutaneous melanoma is approximately 150 cases per million population per year.[2,6–8] Approximately 1 out of 85 Americans will develop melanoma in their lifetime. Cutaneous melanoma is the most dangerous form of skin cancer, with a mortality of 8000 people per year in the United States and accounting for most of the skin malignant tumor deaths.[2]

The incidence of uveal and mucosal melanoma has not increased during recent years. The prevalence of uveal melanoma is approximately 6–7 cases per million per year.[9,14]

Melanoma is most prevalent in Whites and is higher than that in the Blacks and Asians. Based on the White/Black incidence ratio, melanoma can be divided into two groups: high and low ratio groups. Cutaneous and uveal melanomas have a high White/Black incidence ratio (16:1), whereas mucosal and conjunctival melanomas have a low White/Black incidence ratio (2.5:1).[6,7,9–11]

Ultraviolet (UV) radiation is an important risk factor for the occurrence of cutaneous melanoma, but not for uveal and mucosal melanomas. This is due to the differences in the relative locations of the melanocytes in the various tissues in regard to their exposure to solar radiation. Solar UV radiation induces specific genetic mutations, which may increase the risk of melanoma.[15] Cutaneous and conjunctival melanocytes are directly exposed to solar UV radiation. The incidence of these melanomas increased during recent years, with an increased incidence of these melanomas in southern regions relative to those in northern regions in the United States and Europe.[8,13,14] Conversely, since uveal and mucosal melanocytes are not primarily exposed to solar radiation, the incidence of uveal and mucosal melanomas did not increase or even slightly decreased recently, and the incidence in southern regions is not greater or even lower than that in northern regions.[16–20]

Significant advancements have been recently made in our understanding of the molecular mechanisms in the etiology of various melanomas. Many mutations of genes have been found to be related with the development and progression of melanoma (Table 27.1).[3,14,16–23] Different types of melanomas differ not only on the epidemiologic and etiologic aspects but also on their molecular biological patterns (Table 27.1). Therefore, each melanoma subtype (cutaneous, uveal, mucosal, and conjunctival melanomas) must be considered as different and independent disease entities, with the possibility of each one having a unique oncogenetic pathway for tumor development. Independent studies are required for each type of melanoma to elucidate their pathogenesis and the subsequent development of effective therapies.[9–11]

Cutaneous melanoma can be divided into four main categories. Superficial spreading melanoma, which is mainly spread horizontally, is the most common type of cutaneous melanomas (accounting for 50%–75% of cutaneous melanomas) and is relevant to episodes of severe sunburn. Nodular melanoma is the second most common type (15%–35% of cutaneous melanomas) and is characterized by raised nodules or polypoid morphology. Lentigo maligna melanoma is rare (5%–15% of all cutaneous melanomas), generally flat in appearance, and occurs in aged people on sun-exposed regions. Acral lentiginous melanoma (5%–10% of cutaneous melanomas) occurs in the palms, soles, and nail bed and is not associated with solar radiation. There is no difference in the incidence of acral lentiginous melanoma between among racial/ethnic groups.[1,2]

The diagnosis of cutaneous melanoma depends on the clinical manifestations and pathological examination. Any cutaneous lesion suspected for melanoma should be biopsied for histological examination, which is the most reliable procedure for the diagnosis of melanoma.[1,2]

Uveal melanoma is the most common intraocular malignant tumor in the adults. Most uveal melanomas occur in the posterior part of the uvea (ciliary body and choroid), which is not exposed to solar radiation; only very few occur in the anterior part of the uvea (i.e., the iris, accounts for only

TABLE 27.1
Comparison of Epidemiology and Mutation of Oncogene between Various Melanomas[14,16–23]

	Cutaneous Melanoma		Ocular Melanoma		
	Non–Acral Lentiginous Melanoma	Acral Lentiginous Melanoma	Uveal Melanoma	Conjunctival Melanoma	Mucosal Melanoma
Exposure to sun radiation	Yes	No	No	Yes	No
Relationship between sun radiation and prevalence	Increase	No effect	No effect or slight decrease	Increase	No effect
Racial difference	++	No	++	+	No-+
BRAF mutation	50%–70%	10%–30%	0	20%–40%	0
NRAS mutation	15%–30%	10%	0		4%–24%
KIT mutation	2%	23%	0	8%	16%
GNAQ mutation	0	0	50%	0	0

3% of all uveal melanomas). Choroidal melanoma appears as an elevated pigment lesion that can be detected by ophthalmoscopic examination.

Surgical excision is the most important procedure for the treatment of various melanomas.[1,2] In cutaneous melanoma, radical (margin-free) excision is the treatment of choice for primary melanoma. If diagnosed early, most cutaneous melanomas can be effectively treated by surgical excision. However, metastatic cutaneous melanoma does occur. In single metastatic lesions (mainly in lungs, soft tissues, brain, and intestine), surgical excision is often performed, but the efficacy of surgery remains controversial. Systemic chemotherapy is the most widely used treatment for patients with metastatic melanoma. Dacarbazine (DTIC), the platinum analogs, and temozolomide (TMZ), which can spontaneously convert into its active metabolite DTIC, are the most frequently used drugs. However, metastatic melanoma is markedly resistant to chemotherapy and has a very poor prognosis, with a median survival rate of 6 months with a 5-year survival rate of less than 5%. None of the DTIC treatment, DTIC with temozolomide treatment or polychemotherapy, has been proven to prolong overall survival of disseminated melanoma tumor. To some extent, biotherapy (i.e., interferon α, or IFN-α) appears to improve patients' survival under certain clinical circumstances.[2]

The management of uveal melanoma depends on the tumor size, vision quality, and age of the patients. In small melanomas with useful vision in middle aged people, destruction of the tumor by transpupillary thermotherapy (using infrared diode laser to heat and destroy the tumor) may be an option. In medium-size tumors, plaque radiotherapy (using I^{125} in the United States and ^{106}Ru in Europe) or local surgical resection is the most frequent treatment option. For large-size tumors with poor vision, enucleation (excision of the whole eyeball) is usually suggested.[2,3,24,25]

Uveal melanoma has a poor prognosis as compared with the cutaneous melanoma. Uveal melanoma–related mortality is 31% after 5 years following diagnosis and approximately 50% after 25 years.[24] Systemic metastasis is common in uveal melanoma, and the liver is the most frequent organ for metastasis. Ten-year cumulative metastasis rate in uveal melanoma patients is 34%. Various procedures have been reported for the treatment of metastatic uveal melanoma, including chemotherapy, immunotherapy, local surgical excision, or intrahepatic chemoembolization, but the response rate is very poor. Most uveal melanoma patients with liver metastasis still die within 6 months, and the median survival time after diagnosis of metastasis is only 3.6 months.[2,3,24,25]

Because of the poor prognosis of metastatic melanoma, new therapies are urgently required.

27.2 MELATONIN AS AN ONCOSTATIC AGENT

Pinealectomy causes accelerated growth of transplanted tumors in experimental animals. The pineal gland is the most recognized organ that produces systemic melatonin. Therefore, it is postulated that deficiency of systemic melatonin following pinealectomy may be the cause of increased tumor growth. Administration of exogenous melatonin abolishes the accelerating effect of pinealectomy on the growth of tumors. This indicates that a deficiency of melatonin may lead to an increased growth of the tumors.[26–28] In humans, decreased melatonin levels have been correlated with increased cancer risk, including cancer of the breast, prostate, endometrium, lung, stomach, colon, and rectum.[29–32] Surgical removal of the tumor does not alter the levels of circulating melatonin, suggesting that lower levels of melatonin is not the result of tumor growth.[31] The increased incidence of breast and colorectal cancers seen in nurses engaged in night shift work suggests a possible link with the diminished secretion of melatonin associated with increased exposure to light at night.[32]

It has been reported that melatonin has oncostatic effects against a variety of tumor cells, including breast cancer, ovarian cancer, endometrial cancer, prostate cancer, and colon cancer cells.[29,32] Melatonin at physiological levels (10^{-11} to 10^{-9} M) inhibits the growth of a variety of cancer cells in vitro. The dose–response of tumor cells to inhibitory levels of melatonin displays either a bell-shaped or a linear pattern depending on the cell lines tested and the culture conditions. Many cell lines (human breast cancer, colon cancer, and neuroblastoma cells) exhibits a bell-shaped pattern, in which the cell growth is inhibited by melatonin at 10^{-12} M to 10^{-7} M, with a maximum inhibition at 10^{-10} to 10^{-9} M. These cell lines show no or little response to melatonin at subphysiological or pharmacological levels (10^{-6} M or more).[30] On the other hand, some cancer cells exhibit a linear response pattern, showing a dose-dependent decrease of cell numbers at different levels of melatonin.[30] At pharmacological levels, melatonin exhibits cytotoxic activity in several types of cancer cells. Furthermore, it has been reported that melatonin induces the differentiation of some cancer cells and lowers their invasive and metastatic status.[30]

Many different mechanisms have been suggested to involve the anticancer effects of melatonin. Various reactive oxygen species and free radicals can damage DNA and thus act as tumor promoters. Melatonin acts as a free radical scavenger (direct effects) and antioxidant (indirect effects by activation of melatonin receptors to stimulate the antioxidative enzyme systems) and may reduce DNA damage caused by oxidative stress thus decreasing the risk of development and progress of malignant tumors.[30,33,34]

Calmodulin is a calcium-binding protein that mediates many Ca^{2+}-dependent events and modulates cell growth via cell cycle progression and cytoskeletal integrity. The growth inhibition effects of melatonin on certain tumor cell lines may be due to increased degradation of calmodulin caused by melatonin binding to calmodulin. Melatonin also induces the movement of calmodulin from the cystol to the cytoskeletal membrane fraction. Therefore, the re-entry of quiescent cells from G0 into the cell cycle is blocked by melatonin and the growth stimulating effects of calmodulin are inhibited by melatonin.[30]

There are two different melatonin receptors present in mammalian cells, MT_1 and MT_2. Both of them belong to the superfamily of seven-pass transmembrane G-protein coupled receptors. Activation of these receptors by melatonin often results in inhibition of cyclic adenosine 3′,5′-monophosphate (cAMP) synthesis. Other signal transduction responses to melatonin activation of melatonin receptors include the regulation of cyclic guanosine monophosphate (cGMP) levels, protein kinase C (PKC), and mitogen-activated protein kinase inhibitor (MAPK) activity. These melatonin receptor-mediated signal transduction cascades may play a role in the anticancer effects of melatonin.[29,30] Circadian genes may also play a role in tumor suppression and tumor activation.[35]

Recently, it has been reported that linoleic acid is a specific tumor-growth signaling molecule. High linoleic acid levels increase the growth of several implanted tumors in experimental animals. Constant bright light irradiation 24 hours per day suppresses the production of melatonin and increases tumor linoleic acid uptake. The production of 13-hydroxyoctadecadienoic acid, a mitogenic metabolite of linoleic acid, is increased and the growth of the tumor is stimulated under such circumstances. Melatonin has a rapid inhibitory effect on tumor linoleic acid uptake and the growth of tumors. The inhibitory effects of melatonin on tumor cell growth can be blocked by melatonin receptor antagonists, indicating that this effect is receptor-dependent.[30]

There are two different types of breast cancer cells depending on the expression of estrogen receptor or not. Melatonin has no growth inhibiting effect on estrogen receptor–negative human breast cancer cells. In estrogen receptor–positive breast cancer cells, melatonin inhibits the mitogenic effects of estrogen and also down-regulates the expression of estrogen receptor. This indicates that the mechanism of anticancer effects of melatonin may be different in various tumor cell lines.[30]

Based on the oncostatic effects of melatonin detected from in vitro and in vivo studies, many clinical trials have been performed to test the clinical efficacy of melatonin in cancer patients in recent decades. In the majority of studies, melatonin was administrated to patients with advanced stage of malignant tumors in combination with other therapies, including chemotherapy, radiotherapy, and immunotherapy.[30,31,36,37] Only in a few instances was melatonin used alone. Many trials were nonrandomized studies, whereas a few trials were randomized. In nonrandomized trials, partial response was observed in a small percentage of patients receiving melatonin; the majority of tumor responses consisted of disease stabilization. Due to melatonin's ability to enhance the efficacy of some anticancer drugs, doses of these drugs could be adjusted to either reduce toxicities or enhance therapeutic effects. It has been reported that melatonin therapy reduces the toxicities associated with chemotherapy, including myelotoxicity, lymphocytopenia, thrombocytonia, nephrotoxicity, neuropathy, stomatitis, and cancer cachexia.[29–32]

Mills et al.[38] conducted a systemic review of randomized controlled trials and a meta-analysis on the effects of melatonin in the treatment of cancer. Ten randomized controlled clinical trials published between 1992 and 2003 that included 643 patients were analyzed. They found that melatonin reduced the risk of death at 1 year in cancer patients (relative risk: 0.66, 95% confidence interval: 0.59–0.73, $p < 0.0001$). This indicates that the risk of death at 1 year in cancer patients is decreased by 34% by the treatment of melatonin, which is statistically significant. The relative risks in the treatment of renal cancer, breast cancer, glioblastoma, and lung cancer are 0.43, 0.48, 0.61, and 0.67, respectively. Most of these clinical trials compared the results between conventional therapy and conventional therapy with melatonin; only a few trials compared the results between melatonin and no treatment. The most frequent dosage was 20 mg/day orally in the evening. This dosage is much higher than the 1.5–5.0 mg used for the treatment for insomnia and jet lag. However, no significant side effects were reported except the tendency to produce sedation or sleepiness in some patients.[38]

27.3 EFFECTS OF MELATONIN ON MELANOMA CELLS IN VITRO

Forty-three years ago, Das Gupta,[26] a pioneer in the study on the relationship of melatonin and melanoma, found that pinealectomy (surgical removal of the pineal organ) caused an increase in the growth and spread of transplanted melanoma in hamsters. The mammalian pineal organ is rich in biogenic amines, especially melatonin, serotonin, noradrenalin, and histamine. Administration of a small dose of exogenous melatonin to pinealectomized hamsters abolished the accelerating effect of pinealectomy on the growth of melanoma implants, indicating that the effect of pinealectomy on melanoma growth is due to a deficiency of melatonin.[27] Since then, numerous experiments have been performed in melanoma cells or immortal melanoma cell lines, from both human pathological specimens and experimental animals, to study the effects of melatonin on melanoma in vitro and in experimental animals.

There are mainly two different types of melanoma cell lines based on their origin, the cutaneous melanoma and uveal melanoma. Both types of melanoma cells have been studied in vitro for the investigation of effects and mechanisms of melatonin on melanoma cells.[39–48]

In cutaneous melanoma, Meyskens and Salmon[39] tested the effects of melatonin on cloning efficiency of melanoma cells obtained from 11 different patients and found that melatonin decreased cloning efficiency of melanoma cells in six cases, no effects in three cases, and stimulated colony formation in two cases. This indicates that melatonin may mainly have an inhibitory effect on the cloning efficiency of cutaneous melanoma cells and heterogeneous nature in human melanomas may determine the response of melanoma cells to melatonin.

Bartsch and Bartsch[40] reported that the effects of melatonin on melanoma cells showed a biphasic model with low concentrations of melatonin causing a 60% inhibition of human melanoma cells and a higher dose producing a moderate stimulation of cell growth. The biphasic effects of melatonin on melanoma cells were demonstrated by Slominske and Pruski.[41] They found that melatonin at low concentrations (10^{-10} to 10^{-8} M, which are within physiological concentration ranges) inhibited cell growth of two melanoma cells lines, S91 mouse melanoma cell line and AbC1 hamster melanoma cell line. Melatonin at higher concentrations (10^{-6} M or more) and very low concentrations (10^{-12} M) did not have effects on cell growth. Melatonin also affects melanogenesis. Melanin production as measured by tyrosinase activity is inhibited at high concentrations (10^{-6} M or more) but not by low concentrations (10^{-10} to 10^{-8} M). *N*-Acetylserotonin (precursor of melatonin) and 5-methoxytryptamine (metabolite of melatonin) do not have effects on cell growth and melanogenesis of melanoma cells.[41]

Yings et al.[42] studied the effects of melatonin on a human melanoma (M-6) cell line and also revealed that melatonin significantly inhibited the growth of melanoma cells in vitro. Cell viability in melatonin-treated cultures was similar to the controls and the growth inhibitory effect of melatonin could be reversed by its removal, indicating that cytotoxicity is not involved in producing the suppression of cell growth. However, the growth inhibitory effect of melatonin is dose-dependent at concentrations ranging from 10^{-9} to 10^{-4} M. Two melatonin analogous, 6-chloromelatonin and 2-iodomelatonin (melatonin receptor agonists), also inhibited the growth of melanoma cells in vitro.[42]

Cos et al.[38] examined the dose effect of melatonin (ranging from 10^{-13} to 10^{-5} M) on two metastatic cell sublines of mouse melanoma (B16BL6 and PG19). They found that melatonin at physiological concentrations (10^{-9} to 10^{-11} M) significantly inhibited cell growth on both cell lines, whereas supraphysiological (10^{-7} to 10^{-5} M) and subphysiological concentrations (10^{-13} M) lacked these effects.[43]

Souza et al.[44] studied the effects of melatonin and its precursors on two human melanoma cell lines. In the SK-Mel 28 cell line, melatonin inhibited cell growth in a dose-dependent manner at concentrations from 10^{-9} to 10^{-5} M. The precursors of melatonin, *N*-acetylserotonin and serotonin, also suppressed the cell growth with serotonin being the least potent. Two melatonin antagonists, luzindole (melatonin membrane receptor antagonist) and prazosin (MT_3 receptor antagonist), did not affect the growth inhibitory effects of melatonin. Cell growth of another human melanoma cell line (SK-Mel 23 cells) did not respond to melatonin and its precursors, indicating a heterogeneous response to melatonin in different cell lines.[44]

Recently, Cabrera et al.[45] also demonstrated that melatonin inhibited the cell growth and increased melanogenesis (estimated by measuring of tyrosinase activity) of a human melanoma cell line (SK-MEL-1). Antagonists of melatonin membrane receptors (luzindole and 4-P-PDOT) did not prevent the melatonin-induced cell growth arrest. In contrast, the melatonin-induced cell growth arrest could be abrogated by a p38 MAPK inhibitor (SB203580). Therefore, the authors suggested that a p38 MAPK signal pathway may play a role in cell growth inhibition by melatonin.[45]

In conclusion, most of these in vitro studies in cutaneous melanoma cells indicate that melatonin inhibits the growth of these cells; however, negative results were also obtained by certain studies on different melanoma cell lines or under different experiment circumstances. This indicates that the melatonin-induced cell growth arrest may be cell line-specific and the effects may also be influenced by different experimental circumstances. The dose effect of melatonin on cutaneous melanoma cell lines shows two different models. In several studies, melatonin inhibits cell growth of melanoma cells only at physiological concentrations, mostly from 10^{-11} to 10^{-9} M, whereas melatonin at lower (10^{-12} M and less) or higher concentrations (10^{-6} M or more) does not show significant inhibition of cell growth (the bell curve model).[40,41,43] Another model is the linear model, which shows that melatonin has a dose-dependent inhibitory effect (from 10^{-11} to 10^{-4} M) on the growth of several cutaneous melatonin cell lines, the higher the concentration, the greater inhibition of cell growth.[42,44] The mechanism of these two different models is not well understood. Several melatonin receptor agonists also inhibit the cell growth of cutaneous melanoma cells, but it has been reported that melatonin receptor antagonists do not prevent the melatonin-induced cell growth arrest. Conflicting results exist in the effects of melatonin precursors and metabolites on the growth of cutaneous melanoma cells. Studies on the expression of various melatonin receptors in different cutaneous melanoma cell lines revealed contradictory results. Further studies on the effects of melatonin, its precursors, metabolites, agonists, and antagonists on various cutaneous melanoma cell lines by using identical experimental methods and the detection of expression of various melatonin receptors in these cells are required for the clarification of these contradictory results.

Contrary to these studies, the effects of melatonin and its precursors, metabolites and analogs on uveal melanoma cells and the expression of different melatonin receptors on these cells have been studied systematically by us and revealed consistent results.[41–43] Melatonin inhibits the cell growth of several human uveal melanoma cell lines in a biphasic manner. Cell growth is suppressed by melatonin at physiological concentrations (10^{-10} to 10^{-8} M) with a mean inhibition rate of 50% after 5 days incubation at 10^{-9} M. Melatonin at lower (10^{-11} M and less) and higher (10^{-7} to 10^{-6} M) concentrations does not have significant effects on the growth of uveal melanoma cells. The precursors of melatonin (tryptophan and serotonin) and the abnormal metabolite of tryptophan (kynurenine)

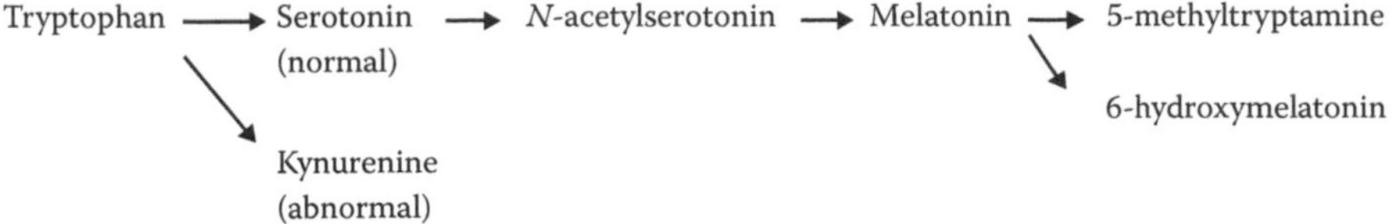

FIGURE 27.1 The pathway of synthesis and metabolism of melatonin.

do not inhibit the growth of uveal melanoma cells. The melatonin metabolite (6-hydroxymelatonin) inhibits the growth of melanoma cells to a lesser degree. [46–48]

The pathway of synthesis and metabolism of melatonin is illustrated in Figure 27.1.

Two melatonin membrane receptor agonists, 6-chlormelanoma (MT_1 and MT_2 receptors agonist) and S-20098 (MT_2 receptor agonist), inhibit the growth of uveal melanoma cells also in a biphasic manner. A putative melatonin nuclear receptor agonist (CGP-52608) does not inhibit the melanoma cell growth.[48] These results are consistent with the expression of various melatonin receptors in uveal melanoma cells. The expression of mRNA encoding the MT_2 receptor is detected in uveal melanoma cells, whereas MT_1 receptors mRNA could not be detected.[48] The growth inhibitory effects of various melatonin receptor agonists and the presence of MT_2 membrane receptors in uveal melanoma cells indicate that this effect is related to activation of the membrane MT_2 receptor and not related to the activation of MT_1 melatonin membrane receptors or the putative nuclear receptor.[48] The apparent decrease of effect of melatonin and its analogs at higher concentrations suggests that there may be a down-regulation of receptor levels. Cell viability is not affected by melatonin and its analogs, indicating that the effect is growth inhibition only. The signal pathways relevant to the growth inhibitory effects of melatonin require further investigation. It may be related to the activation of membrane receptors resulting in the modulation of cAMP, cGMP, PKC, and MAPK activity and intracellular redox status.

Tables 27.2 and 27.3 show the comparison of presence of various melatonin receptors and the effects of melatonin (including its precursor, metabolites, agonists, and antagonists) on the growth of melanoma cells between cutaneous and uveal melanoma cells in vitro.[39–48]

A few articles on the study of the effects of melatonin on experimental melanoma have been published.[27–29] Removal of the pineal organ resulted in an increase in the growth of transplanted melanoma in hamsters. Administration of melatonin to pinealectomized animals abolished this effect.[27,28] Administration of melatonin to intact animals revealed conflicting results. Early studies in transplanted melanoma in hamsters showed that administration of melatonin, even in a large dose (4 mg/day), did not influence the rate of tumor growth. There is considerable evidence that the mammalian pineal influences the functions of the brain, the endocrine glands, and the gonads. Therefore, some authors supposed that melatonin may not have a direct effect on tumor growth and that the changes produced by melatonin deficiency is perhaps due to a complex reaction involving the hypothalamus, brain stem, gonads, and various endocrine glands.[27,28]

TABLE 27.2
Presence of Melatonin Receptor and Effects of Melatonin in Various Melanoma Cells In Vitro[39–48]

	Cutaneous Melanoma	Uveal Melanoma
Tested cell lines	Human and experimental animals	Human
Effects	Inhibition of growth	Inhibition of growth
Mode of dose effects	Biphasic (10^{-11} to 10^{-9}M) or linear (10^{-9} to 10^{-5} M)	Biphasic (10^{-11} to 10^{-9}M)
Melatonin receptors	Conflicting	MT_2, no MT_1 or nuclear receptor

TABLE 27.3
Effects of Melatonin's Precursor, Metabolites, Agonists, and Antagonists on Growth of Melanoma Cells In Vitro[39–48]

		Cutaneous Melanoma	Uveal Melanoma
Precursor	Tryptophan		No effect
	Serotonin	Inhibition	No effect
	N-Acetylmelatonin	No effect or inhibition	
Metabolite	5-Methoxytryptamine	No effect	
	6-Hydroxymelatonin		Inhibition
Agonist	6-Choloromelatonin (MT_1,MT_2)		Inhibition
	2-Iodomelatonin (MT_1,MT_2)	Inhibition	
	S-20098 (MT_2)		Inhibition
	CGP-52608 (nuclear receptor)		No effect
Antagonist	Luzindole (MT_1,MT_2)	Prevent or no effect on melatonin's growth inhibition	
	4-P-PDOT (MT_2)	No effect on melatonin's growth inhibition	
	Prazosin (MT_3)	Prevent melatonin's growth inhibition	
Mechanism		Activation of membrane receptor (?)	Activation of MT_2 membrane receptor

One decade later, Narita and Kudo[49] studied the effects of melatonin on B16 mice melanoma cell lines transplanted to athymic mice. Animals were giving melatonin (5 μg/body weight/day) in their drinking water. The melatonin-treated mice had significantly smaller melanomas on day 40 as compared with control animals. The weights of the gonads and the adrenal glands of melatonin-treated mice were significantly reduced compared with control animals. Therefore, the authors supposed that the growth inhibitory effects of exogenous melatonin on transplanted melanoma in mice may involve a direct effect of melatonin on the melanoma cells and/or an indirect effect related to the role of melatonin in the regulation of both the pituitary–adrenal axis and the pituitary–gonadal axis.[49]

27.4 CLINICAL TRIALS OF MANAGEMENT OF MELATONIN ON METASTATIC MELANOMAS

Metastatic melanoma is poorly responsive to most conventional types of therapy. There is an obvious requirement for novel therapies that could be used in the treatment of metastatic melanoma. It has been reported that melatonin suppresses the growth of cutaneous and uveal melanoma cells in vitro.[29–34,39–48] Therefore, several oncology centers studied the potential role of melatonin as a therapeutic agent in metastatic melanoma.

Gonzalez et al.[50] studied the therapeutic effects of orally administered melatonin in patients with advanced melanoma. Forty patients received melatonin in doses from 5 to 700 mg/m²/day in four divided doses. Thirty patients had cutaneous melanoma and 10 had uveal melanoma. Twenty-nine patients were previously treated (8 with immunotherapy, 11 with chemotherapy, and 7 with radiotherapy) and 11 patients were previously untreated. The criteria used for the evaluation of therapeutic effects were (1) a complete response was defined as disappearance of all measurable disease, (2) a partial response was defined as a 50% decrease in the size of all measurable lesions, and (3) progressive disease was defined as a 25% increase of all measurable lesions. Patients who did not meet these criteria were classified as stable disease. After the observation for 10 weeks, 6 cases (15%, including one case suffering from uveal melanoma) had a partial response with a median response duration at 33+ weeks. Tumors metastasized to the brain, lymph nodes, and subcutaneous tissue responded in two cases. An additional six patients (15%, including one case suffering from uveal melanoma) had stable disease for a median of 20 weeks. Ten of 27 cases who were treated with 75 mg/m^2/day or more responded or remained stable compared with only 2 of 13 cases treated with lower doses.[50] The side effects encountered in this group were generally mild, consisting of fatigue (15 cases) or mild nausea (8 cases). No patients were removed from the study due to toxicity. The authors' conclusion is that melatonin can be administered safely to melanoma patients with a modest antitumor effect, and this study supports further investigation of the potential role of this agent.[50]

Lissoni et al.[51] performed a phase II clinical trials of melatonin plus a chemotherapy agent (tamoxifen) in 25 metastatic solid patients, including 4 melanoma patients. The working hypothesis for this combined therapy is that melatonin may enhance tamoxifen antitumor efficacy based on preliminary data. Both drugs were given orally each day (melatonin 20 mg/day in the evening and tamoxifen 20 mg per day at noon). Of the four melanoma patients treated, one patient had a partial response with a survival duration of 13 months; two patients had a stable disease with a duration of 13–16 months and one patient had a progressive disease and died after 4 months. No toxicity was found, and in particular, no melatonin-related toxicity was found. Most patients experienced a relief of depression symptoms (anxiety and asthenia). The authors concluded that melatonin combined with tamoxifen is a well-tolerated treatment, even in patients of poor clinical status, and this could be a potentially active therapy to induce stabilization of disease and objective tumor regression in at least a few cases in patients unable to receive more aggressive therapies. Melatonin may amplify tamoxifen efficacy, as suggested by the evidence of disease stabilization in patients previously progressing on tamoxifen alone. Alternatively, tamoxifen may amplify the oncostatic activity of melatonin, perhaps through a stimulation of transforming growth factor β release.[51]

Lissoni et al.[52] organized a randomized controlled trial to study the therapeutic effects of melatonin alone in melanoma patients with lymph node relapse. Thirty patients were randomized to receive no treatment or receive treatment of melatonin (20 mg/day orally in the evening). After a median follow-up of 31 months, the percent of disease-free survival was significantly higher in melatonin-treated patients than in controls. Melatonin reduced the risk of death at 1 year in this group of melanoma patients; the relative risk was 0.42 (melatonin reduced 58% risk of death) with 95% confidence intervals at 0.16–0.92. No melatonin-related toxicity was observed. The authors concluded that an adjuvant treatment with melatonin might be effective in preventing disease progression in node-relapsed melanoma patients.[52]

Lissoni et al.[53] organized a phase II study of combined treatment with melatonin, platinum (a chemotherapeutic agent), and interleukin 2 (IL-2, an immunotherapeutic agent) as a second-line therapy in metastatic melanoma patients progressing despite treatment with decarbazine plus IFN-α. During that time, the first-line therapy in metastatic melanoma patients was decarbazine plus IFN-α. However, many patients responded to this treatment poorly. Another choice was combined treatment of IL-2 with platinum; however, both drugs have to be used in high doses, with the consequence of considerable toxicity. The antitumor activity of IL-2 has been proven to be enhanced by the immunomodulating agent melatonin, which has also been shown to reduce its toxicity and increase the cytotoxicity of cancer chemotherapy. On this basis, a study was planned with low-dose IL-2 and platinum in association with melatonin. This study included 13 evaluable patients. Platinum was injected intravenously at 30 mg/m^2/day for 3 days every 21 days. IL-2 was administered subcutaneously at 3,000,000 IU/day from days 4–9 and from days 11–16 of the cycle. Finally, melatonin was given orally at 20 mg/day in the evening, every day without interruption. After this combined chemoneuroimmunotherapy, one patient obtained a complete response, while partial response was achieved in three other patients. Therefore, the objective tumor response rate was 4 (31%) out of 13. A stable disease occurred in five patients, whereas the remaining four patients had a progressive disease. The treatment was extremely well-tolerated in all patients, and in particular, no platinum-related neurotoxicity was observed. The authors concluded that low-dose platinum and IL-2 in association with melatonin, given as a second-line therapy, is an effective and well-tolerated treatment for metastatic melanoma, with a clinical efficacy at least comparable to that obtained with a first-line therapy of dacarbazine plus IFN-α.[53]

Based on the four clinical trials, a large dosage of melatonin administrated orally alone or combined with other anticancer drugs is effective in the treatment of metastatic melanoma. Melatonin could induce stabilization of disease and objective tumor regression in certain cases that failed to respond to the standard conventional treatments. In the combination of melatonin with other anticancer drugs, melatonin may enhance the anticancer effects of other drugs and reduce their toxicity. This dosage of melatonin used for the treatment of melanoma is much higher than the dosage (1–3 mg per day) used for the treatment of insomnia and jet lag. In three groups, 20 mg of melatonin was given orally at the evening, and no melatonin-related toxicity was observed.[51–53] In a group in which melatonin was administrated four times a day, slight side effects were encountered, including fatigue and slight nausea.[50] However, no patients were removed from the study due to toxicity.[50–53] A pharmacokinetic study found that orally administered melatonin was well absorbed, and a dosage of 50 mg every 4 hours (larger than that used in the treatment of melatonin in most treated groups) resulted in plasma melatonin levels 25–80 times higher than endogenous peak value and was well tolerated.[54]

In conclusion, the advantage of melatonin therapy is the low adverse events (especially administrated in the evening, 20 mg/day), low cost, and the substantial reduction in the risk of death.

There are several limitations in these studies. First of all, in these four studies published, only one study was a randomized controlled trial and none of these studies was a double-blind trial. The second limitation is that all four studies were performed by two groups of investigators only, one from the United States (one study) and one from Italy (three studies). Confirming the efficacy and safety of melatonin in melanoma treatment will require completion of double-blinded, independently conducted randomized controlled trials.

Furthermore, in experimental animal-transplanted melanoma models, removal of the pineal organ resulted in an increase in the growth of melanoma. Administration of melatonin to pinealectomized animals abolished this effect, indicating that a deficiency of melatonin can promote the growth of melanoma and administration of melatonin can reverse this process.[26–28] In humans, low serum melatonin levels or urinary excretion of melatonin metabolites have been found in several types of cancer patients as compared with age-matched controls.[29–32] Our knowledge on the melatonin levels in body fluid in melanoma patients is very limited. One study found that urinary 6-oxymelatonin (a melatonin metabolite) excretion in male cutaneous melanoma patients was lower than that of the control, whereas no difference in aqueous humor melatonin levels was found between ocular melanoma patients and the controls.[55,56] Therefore, it is required to study melatonin levels in the body fluids and urinary excretion of melatonin metabolite in melanoma patients and compare with age-matched controls. This study can clarify whether a deficiency of melatonin is present in melanoma patients. It will also be helpful in defining the role of melatonin in the occurrence of melanoma.

27.5 SUMMARY

1. Melanoma is a malignant tumor originating from melanocytes or their precursors. Melanoma can be divided into three main categories based on their anatomic locations: cutaneous (the most common type), ocular (the second common melanoma and the most common intraocular malignant tumor in the adults), and mucosal melanomas (the rarest). Cutaneous melanoma is the most dangerous form of skin cancer, with a mortality of 8000 people per year in the United States. Surgical excision is the most important procedure for the treatment of early-stage melanoma. However, metastatic melanoma is markedly resistant to chemotherapy or radiotherapy and has a very poor prognosis, with a median survival rate of less than 6 months. Therefore, new treatment procedures are urgently required.

2. Removal of the pineal organ results in increase in the growth of transplanted malignant tumors in hamsters. Administration of melatonin to pinealectomized animals abolishes this effect. Physiological doses of melatonin inhibit growth of cancer cells in vitro, whereas pharmacological dosages may cause apoptosis of cancer cells. Clinical trials using melatonin alone or combined with other anticancer drugs and immunotherapy have shown either a partial response or disease stabilization in a certain percentage of patients. Due to melatonin's ability to enhance the efficacy of some anticancer drugs, doses of these drugs could be adjusted to either reduce toxicities or enhance therapeutic effects. Meta-analysis on the randomized controlled clinical trials included 643 cancer patients found that melatonin reduced the risk of death at 1 year in cancer patients. No significant side effects were reported and this treatment is well accepted. The mechanisms of melatonin oncostatic effects may include receptor-mediated signal pathway cascades, intracellular redox status, reduced linoleic acid uptake or regulation of various hormone/growth factor receptors expression, modification of circadian tumor suppressor genes, etc.
3. In vitro studies indicate that melatonin inhibits the growth of melanoma cells, which may be biphasic (effectives at physiological dosages) or linear (dose-dependent at physiological and pharmacological dosages) in manner. In the study of ocular melanoma cells, melatonin membrane receptor agonists also suppressed the cell growth, whereas the studies in cutaneous melanoma cells revealed conflicting results. In experimental animal studies, administration of melatonin definitely reverses the increased growth of melanoma in pinealectomized animals and may or may not suppress melanoma growth in intact animals.
4. The results from four clinical trials for studying the effects of melatonin with or without other antitumor drugs in the treatment of metastatic melanoma patients showed the following: complete response (complete disappearance of tumor, only in combined therapy), partial response (50% decrease of tumor size), or stabilization of diseases occur in certain cases. Melatonin enhances the antitumor efficacy of other drugs so that a low dosage could be used to decrease the toxicity. In a random controlled study, melatonin alone significantly reduced the risk of death in 1 year by 58%. Melatonin treatment (orally 20 mg per day in the evening) is well accepted and no case was removed because of the melatonin-related toxicity.
5. Further studies on the effects of melatonin, its precursors, metabolites, agonists, and antagonists on various melanoma cell lines and the detection of expression of various melatonin receptors in these cells (in particular in cutaneous melanoma cells) are required. Studies on the effect of melatonin on experimental animal melanoma can verify the therapeutic effects of melatonin and reveal the oncostatic mechanisms. Studies on melatonin levels in the body fluids and urinary excretion of melatonin metabolite in melanoma patients are required for understanding the role of melatonin in the occurrence of melanoma. Further independently conducted double-blind randomized controlled trials on the effects of melatonin therapy (with or without other antitumor agents) in the treatment of melanoma can be helpful for the confirming and improvement of melatonin therapeutic efficacy.

REFERENCES

1. Balch CM, Houghton A, Sober A, Soong SJ. *Cutaneous Melanoma*. 4th ed. London: JB Lippincott Company; 2003.
2. Melanoma Molecular Project Map. 2010. Available at http://www.mmmp.org/MMMP/.
3. Jager MJ, Niederkorn JY, Ksander BR. *Uveal Melanoma*. London: Taylor & Francis; 2004.
4. Schatton T, Frank MH. Cancer stem cells and human malignant melanoma. *Pigment Cell Melanoma Res.* 2007; 21:39–55.
5. Wakamatsu K, Hu DN, McCormick SA, Ito S. Characterization of melanin in human iridal and choroidal melanocytes from eyes with various colored irides. *Pigment Cell Melanoma Res.* 2007; 21:97–105.

6. Neugut A, Kizelnik-Freilich S, Ackerman C. Black–white differences in risk for cutaneous, ocular, and visceral melanomas. *Am J Public Health.* 1994; 84:1828–1829.
7. McLaughlin CC, Wu XC, Jemal A, Martin HJ, Roche LM, Chen VW. Incidence of noncutaneous melanomas in the U.S. *Cancer* 2005; 103:1000–7.
8. Chang AE, Karnell LH, Menck HR. The National Cancer Base report on cutaneous and noncutaneous melanoma: A summary of 84,836 cases from the past decade. *Cancer.* 1998; 83:1664–1678.
9. Hu DN, Yu GP, McCormick SA, Schneider S, Finger PT. Population-based incidence of uveal melanoma in various races and ethnic groups. *Am J Ophthalmol.* 2005; 140:612–617.
10. Hu DN, Yu G, McCormick SA, Finger PT. Population-based incidence of conjunctival melanoma in various races and ethnic groups and comparison with other melanomas. *Am J Ophthalmol.* 2008; 145:418–423.
11. Hu DN, Yu GP, McCormick SA. Population-based incidence of vulvar and vaginal melanoma in various races and ethnic groups with comparisons to other site-specific melanomas. *Melanoma Res.* 2010; 20:153–158.
12. Scotto J, Fraumeni JF, Lee JAH. Melanomas of the eye and other noncutaneous sites: Epidemiologic aspects. *J Natl Cancer Inst.* 1976; 56:489–491.
13. Yu GP, Hu DN, McCormick S, Finger PT. Conjunctival melanoma: Is it increasing in the United States? *Am J Ophthalmol.* 2003; 135:800–806.
14. Jemal A, Devesa SS, Hartge P, Tucker MA. Cancer surveillance series. *J Natl Cancer Inst.* 2001; 93:678–683.
15. Abdel-Malek ZA, Kadekaro AL, Swope VB. Stepping up melanocytes to the challenge of UV exposure. *Pigment Cell Melanoma Res.* 2010; 23:171–186.
16. Yu GP, Hu DN, McCormick SA. Latitude and incidence of ocular melanoma. Photochem Photobiol. 2006; 82:1621–6.
17. Stang A, Streller B, Eisinger B, Jockel KH. Population-based incidence rates of malignant melanoma of the vulva in Germany. *Gynecol Oncol.* 2005; 96:216–221.
18. Bergman L, Seregard S, Nilsson Bo, Ringborg U, Lundell G, Ragnarsson-Olding B. Incidence of uveal melanoma in Sweden from 1960 to 1998. *Invest Ophthalmol Vis Sci.* 2002; 43:2579–2583.
19. Hu DN, McCormick SA, Yu GP. Latitude and incidence of veal melanoma. *Ophthalmology.* 2008; 115:757.
20. Hu DN, Simon JD, Sarna T. Role of ocular melanin in ophthalmic physiology and pathology. *Photochem Photobiol.* 2008; 84:639–644.
21. Gray-Schopfer V, Wellbrock C, Marais R. Melanoma biology and new targeted therapy. *Nature.* 2007; 445:851–857.
22. Beadling C, Jacobson-Dunlop E, Hodi FS, Le C, Warrick A, Patterson J, Town A, Harlow A, Cruz F, Azar S, Rubin BP, Muller S, West R, Heinrich MC, Corless CL. KIT gene mutations and copy number in melanoma subtypes. *Clin Cancer Res.* 2008; 14:6821–6828.
23. Van Raamsdonk CD, Bezrookove V, Green G, Bauer J, Gaugler L, O'Brien JM, Simpson EM, Barsh GS, Bastian BC. Frequent somatic mutations of GNAQ in uveal melanoma and blue naevi. *Nature.* 2009; 457:599–602.
24. Kujala E, Makitie T, Kivela T. Very long-term prognosis of patients with malignant uveal melanoma. *Invest Ophthalmol Vis Sci.* 2003; 44:4651–4659.
25. Augsburger JJ, Correa ZM, Shaikh AH. Effectiveness of treatments for metastatic uveal melanoma. *Am J Ophthalmol.* 2009; 148:119–127.
26. Das Gupta TK, Terz J. Influence of pineal gland on the growth and spread of melanoma in the hamster. *Cancer Res.* 1967; 27:1306–1311.
27. El-Domeiri AA, Das Gupta TK. Reversal by melatonin of the effect of pinealectomy on tumor growth. *Cancer Res.* 1973; 33:2830–2833.
28. El-Domeiri AA, Das Gupta TK. The influence of pineal ablation and administration of melatonin on growth and spread of hamster melanoma. *J Surg Oncol.* 1976; 8:197–205.
29. Witt-Enderby PA, Radio NM, Doctor JS, Davis VL. Therapeutic treatments potentially mediated by melatonin receptors: Potential clinical uses in the prevention of osteoporosis, cancer and as an adjuvant therapy. *J Pineal Res.* 2006; 41:297–305.
30. Blask DE, Sauer LA, Dauchy RT. Melatonin as a chronobiotic/anticancer agent: Cellular, biochemical, and molecular mechanisms of action and their implications for circadian-based cancer therapy. *Curr Topic Med Chem.* 2002; 2:113–132.

31. Bartsch C, Bartsch H. Melatonin in cancer patients and in tumor-bearing animals. *Adv Exp Med Biol.* 1999; 467:247–264.
32. Pandi-Perumal SR, Srinivasan V, Maestroni GJ, Cardinali DP, Poeggeler B, Hardeland R. Melatonin: Nature's most versatile biological signal? *FEBS J.* 2006; 273:2813–2838.
33. Reiter RJ. Preface. *Curr Topic Med Chem.* 2002; 2(2):1p.
34. Roberts JF, Hu DN, Wishart JF, Pulse radiolysis studies of melatonin and chloromelatonin. *J Photochem Photobiol B—Biol.* 1998; 42:125–132.
35. Gery S, Koeffler HP. The Role of Circadian Regulation in Cancer. *Cold Spring Harb Symp Quant Biol.* 2007; 72:459–464.
36. Conti A, Maestroni GJM. The clinical neuroimmunotherapeutic role of melatonin in oncology. *J Pineal Res.* 2001; 19:103–110.
37. Brivio F, Fumagalli F, Fumagalli G, Pescia S, Brivio R, Di Fede G, Rovelli F. Lissoni P. Synchronization of cortisol circadian rhythm by the pineal hormone melatonin in untreatable metastatic solid tumor patients and its possible prognostic significance on tumor progression. *In Vivo* 2010; 24:239–241.
38. Mills E, Wu P, Seely D, Guyatt G. Melatonin in the treatment of cancer: A systematic review of randomized controlled trials and meta-analysis. *J Pineal Res.* 2005; 39:360–366.
39. Meyskens FL, Salmon SE. Modulation of clonogenic human melanoma cells by follicle-stimulating hormone, melatonin, and nerve growth factor. *Br J Cancer.* 1981; 43:111.
40. Bartsch C, Bartsch H. The link between the pineal gland and cancer: An interaction involving chronobiological mechanisms. *Chronobiol Approach Social Med.* 1984; 105–126.
41. Slominski A, Pruski D. Melatonin inhibits proliferation and melanogenesis in rodent melanoma cells. *Exp Cell Res.* 1993; 206:189–194.
42. Ying SW, Niles LP, Crocker C. Human malignant melanoma cells express high-affinity receptors for melatonin: Antiproliferative effects of melatonin and 6-chloromelatonin. *Eur J Pharmacol.* 1993; 246:89–96.
43. Cos S, Garcia-Bolado A, Sanchez-Barcelo EJ. Direct antiproliferative effects of melatonin on two metastatic cell sublines of mouse melanoma (B16BL6 and PG19). *Melanoma Res.* 2001; 11:197–201.
44. Souza AV, Visconti MA, Castrucci AM. Melatonin biological activity and binding sites in human melanoma cells. *J Pineal Res.* 2003: 34:242–248.
45. Cabrera J, Negrin G, Estevez F, Loro J, Reiter RJ, Quintana J. Melatonin decreases cell proliferation and induces melanogenesis in human melanoma SK-MEL-1 cells. *J Pineal Res.* 2010; Epub.
46. Hu DN, Roberts JE. Melatonin inhibits growth of cultured human uveal melanoma cells. *Melanoma Res.* 1997; 7:27–31.
47. Hu DN, McCormick SA, Roberts JE. Effects of melatonin, its precursors and derivatives on the growth of cultured human uveal melanoma cells. *Melanoma Res.* 1998; 8:205–210.
48. Roberts JE, Wiechmann AF, Hu DN. Melatonin receptors in human uveal melanocytes and melanoma cells. *J Pineal Res.* 2000; 28:165–171.
49. Narita T, Kudo H. Effect of melatonin on B16 melanoma growth in athymic mice. *Cancer Res.* 1985; 45:4175–4177.
50. Gonzalez F, Sanchez A, Ferguson JA, Balmer C, Danieal C, Cohn A, Robinson WA. Melatonin therapy of advanced human malignant melanoma. *Melanoma Res.* 1991; 1:237–243.
51. Lissoni P, Paolorossi F, Tancini G, Ardizzoia A, Barni F, Maestroni GJ, Chilelli M. A phase II study of tamoxifen plus melatonin in metastatic solid tumour patients. *Br J Cancer.* 1996; 74:1466–1468.
52. Lissoni P, Brivio O, Brivio F, Barni S, Tancini G, Crippa D, Meregalli S. Adjuvant therapy with the pineal hormone melatonin in patients with lymph node relapse due to malignant melanoma. *J Pineal Res.* 1996; 21:239–242.
53. Lissoni P, Vaghi M, Ardizzoia A, Malugani F, Fumagalli E, Bordin V, Fumagalli L, Bordoni A, Mengo S, Gardani GS, Tancini G. A phase II study of chemoneuroimmunotherapy with platinum, subcutaneous low-dose interleukin-2 and the pineal neurohormone melatonin (P.I.M.) as a second-line therapy in metastatic melanoma patients progressing on dacarbazine plus interferon-alpha. *In Vivo.* 2002; 16:93–96.
54. Kane MA, Johnson A, Nash AE, Boose D, Mathai G, Balmer C, Yohn JJ, Robinson WA. Serum melatonin levels in melanoma patients after repeated oral administration. *Melanoma Res.* 1994; 4:59–65.
55. Grinevich YA, Labunetz IF. Melatonin, thymic serum factor, and cortisol levels in healthy subjects of different age and patients with skin melanoma. *J Pineal Res.* 1986; 3:263–275.
56. Rohrbach JM, Wollmann H, Heinze J, Gupta D, Thanos S. The role of melatonin in growth of malignant choroid melanoma. *Ophthalmology.* 1993; 90:289–293.

28 Melatonin and Inflammation—The Role of the Immune–Pineal Axis and the Sympathetic Tonus

Pedro A. Fernandes and Regina P. Markus

CONTENTS

28.1 INTRODUCTION

Coordination between the immune and neuroendocrine system is crucial for mammalian immune response. Besides the well known cross-talk among hormones and cytokine at the level of immune-competent cells, endocrine glands, and the central nervous system [1], the circadian temporization of the immune, endocrine, and nervous systems is relevant for a proper immune response. This interconnection is based on both positive and negative feedback loops, which regulate the timing of parallel and sequential events during immune responses. Lethargy, weakness, and decreased food intake show a circadian profile [2]. The effect of cytokines, such as tumor necrosis factor (TNF) and interleukin 1-β (IL1-β), responsible for the development of these effects, known as sickness behavior [3], show a rhythm profile [4–6].

The internal circadian timing is organized by the synchronization of an internal free oscillator, which delivers information to the whole organism via nervous and endocrine routes. The central oscillator is composed of thousands of oscillatory neurons capable of generating and transmitting coherent signals for synchronizing physiological and behavioral responses, and is located within the suprachiasmatic nuclei (SCN) of the hypothalamus. The heterogeneous neurons of the

SCN generate several stimulatory waves. Each neuronal output extends to a specific body structure, allowing targets to be stimulated in a time-controlled manner [7].

The central oscillator is synchronized by the light/dark alternation of the external environment. The ganglionar layer of the retina projects on the SCN, which transmits information to the paraventricular nuclei of the hypothalamus (PVN) and controls the secretion of hypophyseal and pineal hormones via a multisynaptic pathway. The nocturnal secretion of melatonin by the pineal gland and the direct neural outputs of the SCN are highly conserved mechanisms that control rest/activity cycles, food intake, reproduction, and also the immune system.

Cells and molecules linked to the immune system act in a collective and coordinated manner in response to foreign substances, organisms, or injuring physical agents. The immune response is a time-controlled process, and the early and late events are called innate immune response and adaptive immunity. Most infection agents induce inflammatory responses by activating innate immunity. The inflammatory process is characterized by the accumulation of fluid, plasma proteins, and white blood cells in response to physical injury, infection, or a local immune response. It can be divided into acute inflammation, which is an early and transient episode, and chronic inflammation, which occurs when the infection persists.

The inflammatory response is a sequential and coordinated process. The detection of structures that are shared by microbes but absent in mammals by professional phagocytes is followed by secretion of specific cytokines and chemokines that mediate the progress of the inflammatory response and promote tissue remodeling. Lipopolysaccharide (LPS), a component of the wall of gram-negative bacteria, triggers the synthesis of proinflammatory cytokines, such as TNF followed by interleukin 1beta (IL-1β) and IL-6 [8]. The interaction of cytokines with the endothelial cells adjacent to the site of infection induces the expression of adhesion molecules that promote the rolling and the stable attachment of neutrophils and monocytes to the endothelium layer [9]. These cells migrate to the tissue, in order to combat infection. The newly arrived cells also produce the abovementioned cytokines, amplifying the defense.

Macrophages also synthesize IL-12 and IL-18 [10], which trigger interferon-gamma (IFN-γ) production by natural killer (NK) cells and T lymphocytes [11]. IFN-γ, the macrophage-activating cytokine, induces the production of reactive oxygen intermediates and nitric oxide, which participate in killing phagocyted microbes. In addition, IFN-γ amplifies the production of IL-12 by macrophages directing the adaptive immune response toward Th1 response [12,13].

Although cytokines mainly act in an autocrine or paracrine manner, during early phases of the inflammatory response, their production may be high enough to allow circulatory detection and, therefore, act in a systemic endocrine manner. Systemic manifestations of infections are due to the macrophage-derived production of TNF, IL-1β, and IL-12 [9]. One of the most important actions of these cytokines is the activation of the hypothalamic–pituitary–adrenal axis (HPA). TNF and IL-1β directly activate HPA, inducing the increase of plasma glucocorticoids, potent anti-inflammatory hormones produced by the adrenal glands that are stimulated by the adrenal corticotropin hormone (ACTH) released by the pituitary [14,15]. Since those cytokines are produced in the earliest phase of the inflammatory process, the rise in circulatory glucocorticoids is also an early event. For example, in rats, the increase in blood corticosterone in rats treated with LPS occurs 30 minutes after administration [16]. Glucocorticoids also have an immunosuppressive effect mediated by several mechanisms, such as induction of apoptosis, inhibition of cytokine release, and inhibition of leukocyte migration [17].

Besides the temporal profile of the inflammatory response per se, the circadian timing of the organisms interferes in the development of the defense response. The bidirectional communication between the immune and neuroendocrine systems mounts different initial scenarios that may result in controversial responses of the inflammatory mediators [18–20]. Specifically, the bidirectional modulation between the immune system and the pineal gland, known as the immune–pineal axis [19], predicts a transient inhibition of the nocturnal melatonin surge, in order to equalize diurnal and nocturnal conditions regarding the hormonal signaling of darkness. In fact, this inhibition of melatonin production during the mounting of an inflammatory response was also predicted by mathematical modeling of the influence of the circadian rhythm on the acute inflammatory response [21].

The hormonal scenario, regarding the levels of melatonin and glucocorticoids at the beginning of the inflammatory response, also is implied in different responses according to the hour of the day. In such context, the crosstalk between adrenal and pineal hormones may be a key point for understanding the proper mounting and resolution of an inflammatory response.

This review outlines the information in the literature that supports the existence of the immune–pineal axis and raises the hypothesis of a new concept, which advocates that the relative strength of the activation of the hypothalamic–pituitary axis (HPA) and the sympathetic nervous system leads to the potentiation or inhibition of melatonin production.

28.2 THE IMMUNE–PINEAL AXIS

One of the earliest events of the inflammatory response, triggered by tissue injury or infection, is the migration of leukocytes to the affected region to neutralize and eliminate the offending stimulus. Leukocytes migrate through the endothelial layer via the postcapillary venules by several processes. Whereas the hemodynamic forces, imposed by the blood flow and by red blood cells, push leukocytes toward the endothelium, the expression of membrane molecules in both endothelial and leukocytes promotes physical adhesion between these cells. The process of migration is initiated by the rolling of the blood cells on the endothelial layer due to low-affinity adhesive molecules mediated by selectins. The expression of high-affinity adhesive molecules, known as integrins, allows the adherence necessary for triggering cell migration [22].

Previous studies have described changes in cell rolling, adhesion, and migration at different stages in the circadian rhythm and particularly with the nocturnal surge of melatonin. Migration is found to be facilitated during the daytime compared to nighttime [23,24]. Furthermore, pharmacologically applied melatonin stimulates an anti-inflammatory effect, attributed to the putative antioxidant and radical scavenger action of melatonin [25–29].

To determine the cellular target for melatonin's effect on leukocyte migration, we evaluated its influence on rolling and adherence of leukocytes to the endothelial layer [30,31]. Melatonin and the partial agonist of MT2 melatonin receptors, 4-phenyl-2-propionamidotetralin (4PPDOT), inhibit rolling, whereas melatonin, N-acetylserotonin, and the selective agonist for MT3 melatonin receptors, 5-methoxycarbonylamino-N-acetyl-tryptamine (5-MCA-NAT), inhibit the adherence of leukocytes (Figure 28.1). The affinity of melatonin for both receptors was in the pM to nM range, providing a potential mechanism for reducing cell migration during nighttime.

All the experiments described above were performed in rats, which are active at night. Therefore, it was not logical to propose that, when the animals are free in nature, their ability to mount an immune response is reduced by the nocturnal hormone. Therefore, we proposed a working hypothesis called the immune–pineal axis, summarized in Figure 28.2.

Under normal conditions, melatonin produced at night would impair the rolling and adherence of leukocytes to the endothelial layer, avoiding nondesired migration of leukocytes. In this context, melatonin can be considered one of the surveillance molecules that facilitate the maintenance of a proper concentration of cells in the blood by avoiding unnecessary migration to the tissue.

In the proinflammatory phase, we hypothesize that suppression of the nocturnal melatonin surge would occur during the inflammatory response. The pineal gland should be able to sense the so-called "danger-associated molecule patterns" (DAMPs) [32], which represent the pathogen-associated molecule pattern (PAMPs), such as gram-negative bacteria LPS and the endogenous molecules that bind to PAMPs receptors. These molecules would inhibit nocturnal melatonin production to allow a full mounting of the innate immune response, even at night.

Another factor that could contribute to the suppression of the nocturnal melatonin surge is the concomitant elevation of the sympathetic tonus and the release of adrenal cortical hormone, which

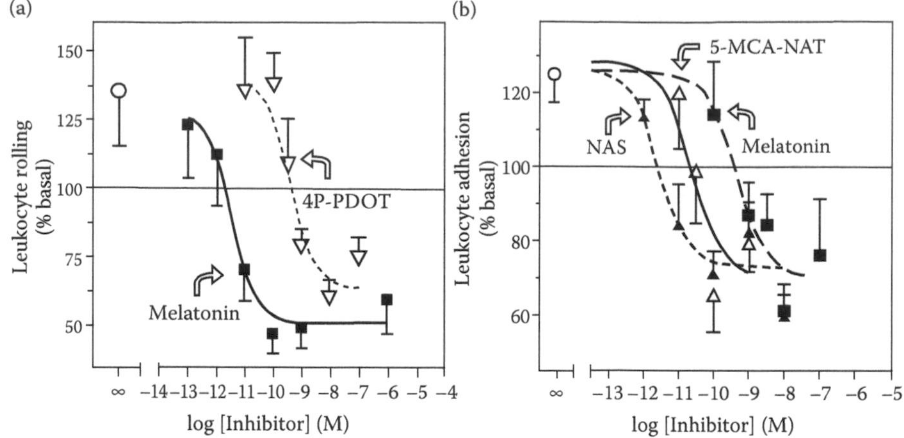

FIGURE 28.1 Melatonin inhibits leukocyte rolling and adhesion. Melatonin has inhibitory effects on both the rolling and adherence of leukocytes to the endothelial layer accessed by intravital microscopy of the microcirculation. (a) Melatonin and the analogous 4P-PDOT inhibit leukocyte rolling. Leukocyte rolling was determined 10 min after topical application of melatonin, 4P-PDOT, or vehicle (open circle). (b) Melatonin, its precursor N-acetylserotonin (NAS), and the MT3 agonist 5-MCA-NAT inhibited leukocyte adherence. Adherence was stimulated by 0.3 mM leukotriene B4. The treatments were performed topically 10 min after leukotriene B4 stimulation. Data are shown as mean ± SEM of 3–7 animals per point. The pD2 values for melatonin inhibition of rolling and adherence were 11.47 ± 0.37 and 9.33 ± 0.41, respectively (Reprinted from *Eur J Pharmacol*, 430, Lotufo, C.M., Lopes, C., Dubocovich, M.L., Farsky, S.H. and Markus, R.P., 351–357, 2001, with permission from Elsevier.)

block melatonin synthesis. In addition, activated cells, which migrate to the tissue, initiate the production of melatonin in a tonic manner. In this case, melatonin has a paracrine or even an autocrine role and is one of the mediators that contribute to the recovery phase of the inflammatory response.

Finally, during the resolution phase, the reduction of the sympathetic tonus would favor the potentiating effect of glucocorticoids, helping to restore the nocturnal melatonin surge.

Modeling the interaction between neuroendocrine–immune responses according to the timing organization of the organisms provided a new way to understand the development of defenses with the circadian rhythm. This approach showed that the pineal gland is not only driven by environmental lighting but is regulated by endogenous mediators of the immune system. Therefore, the pineal gland transduces the timing of a defense response.

28.2.1 Normal Conditions: Melatonin, the Hormone of Darkness

Melatonin is an indolamine synthesized by acetylation and methylation of serotonin by the action of the enzyme arylalkylamine-N-acetyltransferase (AA-NAT), which converts 5-HT into N-acetylserotonin (NAS) [33,34], and hydroxyindole-O-methyltransferase (HIOMT), which converts NAS into melatonin [33].

The SCN controls the daily melatonin synthesis. During the day, activation of GABA-ergic projections from the SCN to the PVN inhibits SCN activity [35]. At nighttime, glutamate stimulation of the PVN activates the intermediolateral column of the spinal cord, a preganglionar sympathetic fiber that innervates the superior cervical ganglia [36] and noradrenergic neurons that project on the pineal gland. In the rat pineal gland, two sympathetic neurotransmitters are released in response: noradrenaline and ATP [37].

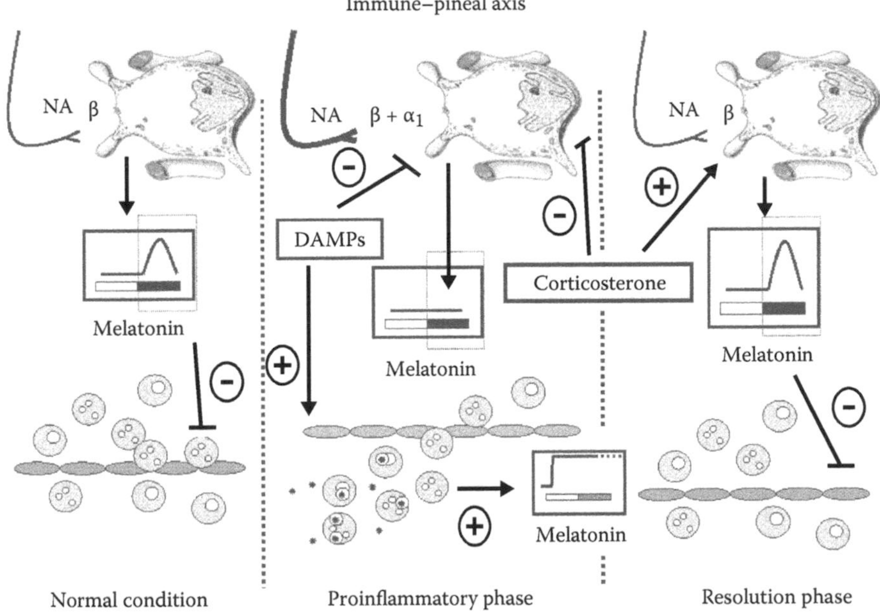

FIGURE 28.2 The immune–pineal axis—a working hypothesis. In normal conditions, the pineal rhythmic production of melatonin is triggered by β-adrenoceptors. Melatonin inhibits the migration of leukocytes through the endothelial layer. In the proinflammatory phase, DAMPs inhibit pineal nocturnal melatonin production and induce the synthesis of melatonin by activated immune-competent cells. This local tonic production of melatonin plays anti-inflammatory roles. The increase in sympathetic output during the proinflammatory phase leads to a concomitant activation of α- and β-adrenoceptors, creating a scenario where corticosterone inhibits pineal melatonin production, favoring leukocyte migration. In the resolution phase, the reduction in the sympathetic output results in the stimulation of β-, but not α-adrenoceptors. This scenario is compatible to a synergic interaction between corticosterone and noradrenaline, resulting in an increasing nocturnal melatonin synthesis.

Activation of β_1 adrenoceptors triggers melatonin synthesis by inducing the transcription and/or enhancing the activity of the enzyme AA-NAT. In nocturnal animals, the transcription factor phsophorylated cyclic AMP response element-binding protein (CREB-P), formed by the transduction pathway β-adrenoceptor → adenylylcyclase → cyclic AMP → protein kinase A, interacts with CRE sequences located in the promoter and the first intron of the *Aa-nat* gene, inducing its transcription [38, 39]. In diurnal animals, the protein is constitutively expressed [40]. In addition, the protein AA-NAT is degraded by the proteasome as soon as it is synthesized. The phosphorylation of AA-NAT by CREB-P stabilizes the protein due to its conjugation with the chaperone 14-3-3 [41,42].

Transpineal perfusion of propranolol, a β-adrenoceptor antagonist, inhibits nocturnal melatonin surge in rats [43], and treating humans with propranolol or atenolol reduces the nocturnal excretion of the melatonin metabolite, 6-sulfatoximelatonin [44].

Activation of α_1-adrenoceptors or $P2Y_1$ purinergic receptors triggers the release of calcium from the endoplasmic reticulum, leading to the potentiation of the activity of AA-NAT [45,46]. The effects of the activation of α_1 and $P2Y_1$ receptors are well understood in vitro [47] but poorly characterized in in vivo models.

HIOMT, the final enzyme in the melatonin biosynthetic pathway, is the rate-limiting factor of the pathway [48]. When AA-NAT is active, modulation of melatonin production can be achieved by regulation of HIOMT. Therefore, AA-NAT is responsible for the nocturnal melatonin surge, and the activity of both enzymes determines the amount of melatonin that signals darkness.

As described above, plasma melatonin under normal conditions reduces the rolling and adherence of leukocytes to the endothelial layer by approximately 50% [30]. This effect is similar to that observed with glucocorticoids [49]. Endogenous corticosterone increases neutrophilia [49] by accelerating neutrophil maturation in bone marrow [50] and enhancing neutrophil transference into the blood [51]. Corticosterone also blocks the rolling and adherence of neutrophils to the endothelial layer [49]. Conversely, melatonin impairs rolling and adhesion of neutrophils [30] by acting directly on the endothelial cells [31]. Therefore, both hormones are synergistically involved in proper surveillance and maintenance of stable steady state under normal conditions.

28.2.2 Proinflammatory Phase: Switch between Endocrine and Paracrine Melatonin Production

At the proinflammatory phase, when the defensive immune response begins, molecules that signal injury suppresses the nocturnal melatonin surge in the pineal gland. This is a transient process, as restoration of the melatonin rhythm is essential for maintaining normal circadian rhythm of the organism. The suppression of the nocturnal melatonin surge, besides allowing for migration of cells to the site of lesion, also isolates the organism from environmental cycling, providing the necessary interval of time for the defense response. Sickness behavior, which comprises fever, depression, restriction of food intake, and alteration in the sleep/wake cycle, occurs when the body is not receiving the proper information from the environmental photic cycle.

DAMPs and proinflammatory cytokines trigger the NFKB pathway, whereas glucocorticoids and anti-inflammatory cytokines inhibit the pathway. The NFKB pathway induces transcription of genes related to adhesion molecules; proinflammatory cytokines and receptors for mediators of inflammation, such as B1 bradykinin and prostaglandin receptors; and enzymes for synthesizing inflammatory mediators, such as cyclooxygenase-2 and inducible nitric oxide synthase [52]. More recently, this pathway was shown to be important in other physiological or constitutive responses. Besides the well-known role of NFKB in regards to the immune responses that require a stimulus-driven activation, in neuronal cells, the NFKB pathway is constitutively activated, playing an important role in neuroprotective and neurodegenerative conditions [53], neuronal sprouting, and the construction of new synapses [54]. In addition, cancer, atherosclerosis, diabetes, and Alzheimer's disease are all associated with dysregulation of NFKB [55].

The NFKB family, composed of five different coded proteins, RelA (also known as p65), RelB, c-Rel, NFKB1 (or p50), and NFKB2 (p52), has in common the REL homology domain (RHD), which is essential for dimerization, and a nuclear localization sequence (NLS), which guarantees the translocation of the dimer to the nucleus and its interaction with DNA [56,57]. Inhibitory proteins, known as NFKBI or IκB, cover the NLS, retaining the dimers in the cytoplasm [58]. The nomenclature of these proteins is under review, and here, we follow the nomenclature put forth by the "HUGO Gene Nomenclature Committee at the European Bioinformatics Institute" (http://www.genenames.org).

The NFKB subunits can be grouped according to their distribution and function. RelA and NFKB1 are ubiquitous proteins, whereas c-Rel, RelB, and NFKB2 are preferentially found in the hematopoietic tissue [59]. Regarding functionality, the subunits that have the transactivating domain (TAD) in the C-terminal (RelA, RelB, and c-Rel) are gene activators, whereas the others, NFKB1 (p50) and NFKB2 (p52), inhibit gene transcription. Homodimers formed by p50/p50 are repressors of gene transcription, whereas heterodimers, like p50/RelA, are activators [52].

28.2.2.1 Suppression of Melatonin Production by DAMPs

The pineal gland constitutively expresses NFKB in the nucleus, [60], which presents a daily variation with the nuclear accumulation peaking just before lights off and the lowest values maintained during the dark period [61]. In rat pineal glands, we observed a rapid decrease in the nuclear content of NFKB right at the light/dark transition [61]. The nuclear content was low during the night and slowly increased throughout the day, reaching a peak just before darkness.

The only NFKB dimer found in normal rat pineal glands, p50/p50, inhibits the transcription of the *Aanat* gene. Cultured glands incubated with inhibitors of NFKB activity increase N-acetylserotonin production [60]. It is interesting to note that "in silica" analysis showed that the 5′ upstream regulatory region of the rat *Aanat* gene contains four different putative NFKB responsive elements [19]. Thus, it was hypothesized that the nuclear translocation of p50/p50 leads to inhibition of noradrenaline-induced melatonin production.

Rat pinealocytes express CD-14, toll-like receptor-4 (TLR-4), and tumor necrosis factor receptor 1 (TNFR1), which are membrane receptors that recognize lipopolysaccharide (LPS) and TNF [62]. LPS triggers the nuclear translocation of the dimers p50/p50 and p50/RelA, resulting in the transcription of some and inhibition of other genes. Specifically, LPS induces the synthesis of TNF and inhibits melatonin production in vitro and in vivo [62,63]. In addition, TNF inhibits *Aanat* transcription [64]. Thus, during an inflammatory response, the activation of the NFKB pathway by DAMPs leads to the suppression of the nocturnal melatonin surge (Figure 28.2). Whether or not other DAMPs act on the pineal glands was not yet tested. However, it is important to mention that in some neurodegenerative disorders, such as Alzheimer's disease, the production of melatonin is suppressed in the early stages of the disease. A hallmark of Alzheimer's disease is the expression of β-amyloid protein, an endogenous DAMP that triggers the receptor TLR-4 [20].

Clinical data observed in patients that show higher levels of TNF with no nocturnal production of melatonin reinforce the hypothesis of a cross-talk between innate immune response and pineal gland activity. This is exemplified in women with mastitis or who delivered by cesarean section and present a suppression of the nocturnal melatonin surge accompanied by an increase in TNF level [65,66]. In addition, only mothers who had nonmeasurable values of TNF recovered nocturnal plasma melatonin levels [66].

Therefore, the pineal gland is instrumental in recognizing DAMPs, which trigger the pivotal pathway of the innate and acquired immune response and present pinealocytes, mediating the suppression of nocturnal melatonin production in the acute phase of an innate immune response.

28.2.2.2 Production of Melatonin by Immune-Competent Cells

Much research has considered melatonin as an anti-inflammatory agent, and here, we will mention some cases that are important for evaluating the immune–pineal axis [67,68]. In septic shock induced by LPS, melatonin reduces TNF, IL-12, and IFN-γ at the site of injection, and increased IL-10 both at the site of injection and in the plasma [69]. The ability of melatonin to reduce proinflammatory cytokines was also observed in septic shock induced by cecal ligation [70], diabetic rats facing a severe inflammation induced by LPS [71], and human preterm newborns with respiratory distress [72].

The effect of endogenous melatonin produced at the locus of injury in very high concentrations could mimic the response to an exogenous drug. In the context of the immune–pineal axis, the switch between central and local production of melatonin should have a temporal profile according to the passage between the pro- and anti-inflammatory phases of an innate immune response.

The production of melatonin by the immune system is well documented. Human lymphocytes [73], colostral mononuclear and polymorphonuclear cells [65], rat and human thymocytes [74], rat macrophages [75], and mast cells [76] have all been shown to produce high levels of melatonin.

Melatonin produced by immune-competent cells has either a paracrine or autocrine role and is important in the resolution phase of an immune response. Splenocytes from melatonin-treated mice exhibited increased mitogenic responses and produced higher levels of IFN-γ and IL-2 [77]. Exogenous melatonin increased the production of IL-2, IL-6, and INF-γ by human lymphocytes [78]; blocked lymphocyte melatonin production; and reduced IL-2 [69]. Therefore, at the cellular level, both endogenous and exogenous melatonin induced IL-2 production. More interesting was the observation that melatonin, TNF, and IL-2 in the colostrum and milk of women who had vaginal or cesarean delivery showed a clear day/night rhythm in IL-2 levels after vaginal delivery. In contrast,

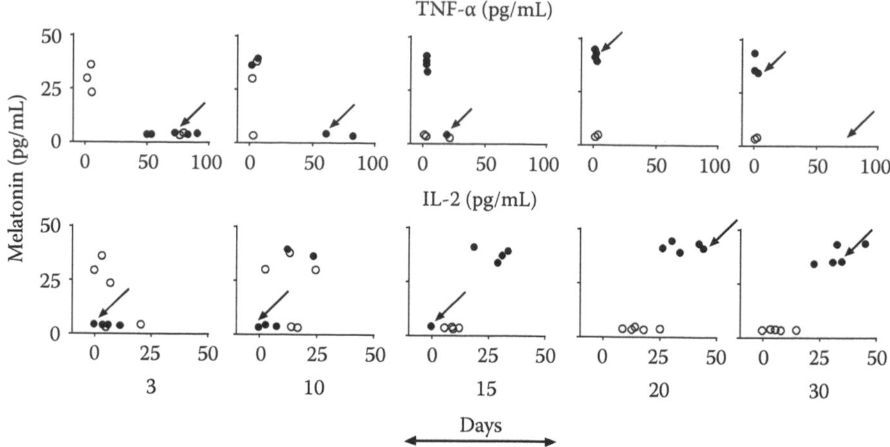

FIGURE 28.3 Daily variation of melatonin, TNF, and IL-2 in mothers who delivered by cesarean section. Correlation between melatonin and TNF (top panel) and melatonin and IL-2 (bottom panel) in the colostrum (3 days) and the milk (10, 15, 20, and 30 days) of mothers who delivered by cesarean section. Both day (open symbols) and night (closed symbols) are shown. While TNF is high, melatonin production is impaired, and the difference between daytime and nighttime IL-2 is decreased. When the level of TNF is below the detection limit of the method, indicating the recovery from the surgical section, the IL-2 rhythm is restored: low levels at daytime and high levels at nighttime. The black arrow points to a single mother who showed a delayed recovery, highlighting the importance of reducing TNF in the recovery of melatonin and IL-2 rhythms. (Pontes, G.N., Cardoso, E.C., Carneiro-Sampaio, M.M. and Markus, R.P. *J. Pineal Res.* 2007; 43: 365–371. Copyright Wiley-VCH Verlag GmbH and Co. KGaA. Reproduced with permission.)

the daily rhythm of IL-2 was interrupted immediately after cesarean delivery, accompanied by high levels of TNF and no nocturnal melatonin surge. After 10 to 15 days, when the melatonin rhythm was restored, and TNF level was below detectable levels, a significantly high nighttime value for IL-2 was finally observed [66] (Figure 28.3). The immune stimulating effect of melatonin, described by Maestroni and colleagues [79], could be exerted either by endocrine- or paracrine-produced melatonin. According to our model, the paracrine production, relevant in the absence of pineal command, is independent of the external light/dark cycle.

28.3 CORTICOSTERONE AS A MODULATOR OF THE IMMUNE–PINEAL AXIS

28.3.1 The Dual Effect of Corticosterone on Pineal Melatonin Production

Corticosterone has a dual effect on the pineal gland, either activating or inhibiting sympathetic-induced melatonin synthesis. In the context of the immune–pineal axis, it is important to take into account the magnitude of sympathetic stimulation because the activation of β- or β+α- adrenoceptors could result in different responses.

There is an anatomical relationship between the pineal and adrenal glands, as sympathetic innervation for both arises from the PVN. In the case of the pineal gland, nocturnal activation of the PVN stimulates sympathetic activation and the production of melatonin. In the case of the adrenal gland, both neural and hormonal stimulation lead to the release of cortical hormones. The neural stimulation of the adrenal gland is mediated by an increase in sympathetic output driven by neurons originating in the PVN, whereas hormonal stimulation is related to the activation of the HPA axis that is also triggered by the PVN [80,81]. The existence of a crosstalk between the adrenal

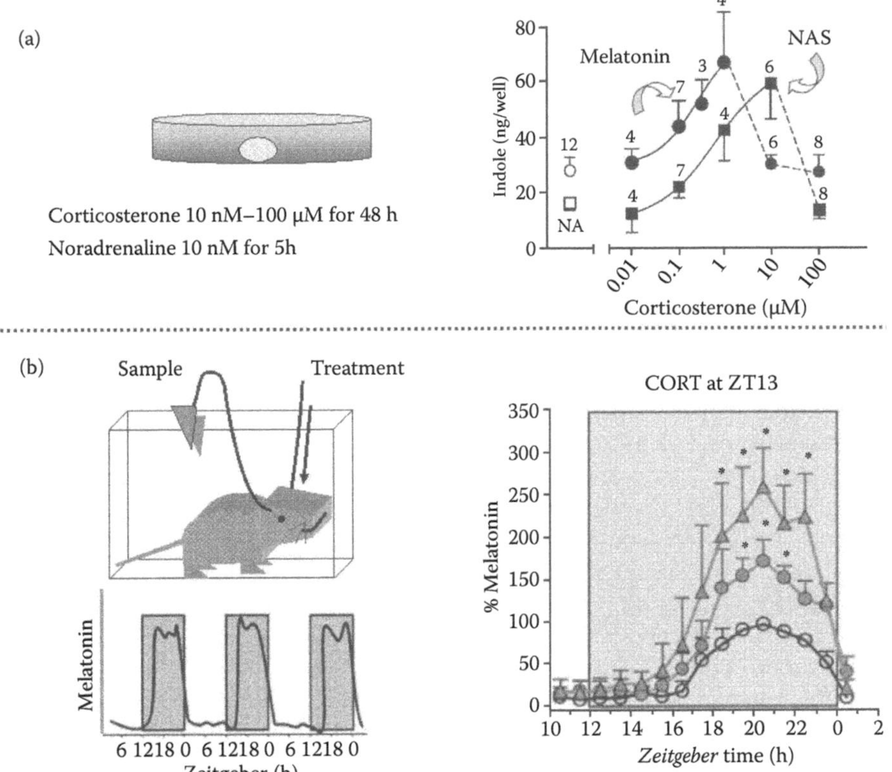

FIGURE 28.4 Corticosterone potentiates pineal melatonin production. (a) Two-day cultivated pineal glands were exposed to corticosterone (0.01–100 μM) for 48 h and then stimulated by noradrenaline (NA, 10 nM) for 5 h. These glands presented a bell-shaped increase in the production of N-acetylserotonin (squares) and melatonin (circles). The points represent the mean ± SEM of the indicated number of experiments. (b) Rhythmic pineal melatonin production can be followed by intrapineal microdialysis. Infusion of corticosterone beginning at ZT13 (6 mg/mL; flux: 3 μL/min; gray lines represent corticosterone infusion, gray circles represent the time points of the second day of experiment, and gray triangles represent the time points of the third day of experiment) on the second day and lasting until the end of the experiment increased nocturnal pineal production. The data were normalized to the peak of melatonin found during the control day (black lines represent infusion of Ringer's solution, and open circles the time points of the first day of the experiment) for each animal. Data are expressed as the mean ± SEM, $n = 3$–6 animals; *$P < 0.05$ compared to control day time point. The gray boxes represent the dark phase of the day. (Ferreira, Z.S., Fernandes, P.A.C.M., Duma, D., Assreuy, J., Avellar, M.C.W., and Markus, R.P. *J. Pineal. Res.* 2005; 38: 182–188. Copyright Wiley-VCH Verlag GmbH & Co. KGaA. Reproduced with permission. Fernandes, P.A., Bothorel, B., Clesse, D., Monteiro, A.W., Calgari, C., Raison, S., Simonneaux, V., and Markus, R.P. *J. Neuroendocrinol.* 2009; 21: 90–97. Copyright Wiley-VCH Verlag GmbH & Co. KGaA. Reproduced with permission.)

and pineal glands was difficult to establish because glucocorticoids either enhances [60,64,82] or reduces [83–85] nocturnal melatonin output, depending on the experimental protocol.

The synthesis of N-acetylserotonin and melatonin induced by noradrenaline is modified in a bell-shaped manner by corticosterone (Figure 28.4a). Low concentrations (10 nM–10 μM) potentiate, whereas higher concentrations (100 μM) did not change the noradrenaline-induced response [60]. The potentiating effect of corticosterone observed in cultured glands was confirmed by transpineal perfusion of corticosterone in rats, as corticosterone increased nocturnal melatonin output without changing daytime values [86] (Figure 28.4b). Administration of corticosterone at ZT2 or ZT13 led to similar effects, strongly indicating that corticosterone is able to modulate, but not trigger, melatonin production. This ability of corticosterone to increase the nocturnal melatonin surge was confirmed in a model of mildly stressed rats where plasma corticosterone levels reached 350 ng/mL [82], which is similar to that introduced by transpineal perfusion [86]. In these experiments, restraining the rats was not sufficient to activate the sympathetic nervous system, since no sudoresis or development of gastric ulcers was detected, but was enough to increase plasma corticosterone level and pineal melatonin output. Therefore, in either cultured pineals or in vivo glands stimulated by applied or endogenous corticosterone, the adrenal hormone in concentrations compatible with those found in mildly stressed animals increases nocturnal melatonin surge.

In contrast, some other authors have shown that incubation of cultured pineal glands with corticosterone and sympathomimetic drugs inhibit melatonin synthesis [84]. Although the method for cultivating the glands [87] was similar to that used by Ferreira and collaborators [60], the concentrations of corticosterone and noradrenaline used by Yuwiler [84] were higher. Experiments ex vivo confirmed that high concentrations of corticosterone inhibited melatonin production, whereas moderate concentrations had no effect [85]. In addition, adrenalectomy abolished the reduction of the nocturnal melatonin surge induced by stress [83].

Comparing these controversial results strongly suggests that the level of circulating corticosterone is critical for modulating pineal gland activity. Indeed, high concentrations of glucocorticoids inhibit cortisol or corticosterone negative feedback on the hypothalamus and hypophysis, due to desensitization of glucocorticoid receptors [88]. Taking together data from different labs, we hypothesized that, under moderate stress, the hormonal information of nighttime is reinforced, whereas under a great deal of stress, the organism loses the hormonal difference between day and night. Therefore, nocturnal melatonin surge is reduced or even abolished.

The difference between low and high concentrations of glucocorticoids was due to the sensitivity of transcription and the modulation of the activity of the enzymes aryl-alkyl-N-acetyltransferase (AA-NAT) and hydroxindole-O-methyltransferase (HIOMT). Corticosterone (1 μM) enhanced the transcription and the activity of AA-NAT but not the transcription and activity of HIOMT [64,86]. Higher levels of corticosterone (10 μM) had no effect on AA-NAT activity but enhanced HIOMT activity. In contrast, a 10-fold higher concentration reduced AA-NAT activity [84]. Therefore, the mechanism underlying the controversial effects of corticosterone on melatonin synthesis is probably the ability of this hormone to potentiate or inhibit the activity of this key enzyme in melatonin synthesis.

28.3.2 The Role of the Sympathetic Tonus

The pineal gland has a dense noradrenergic innervation [89], and the 100-fold increase in the release of noradrenaline at night [90] by the sympathetic nerve fibers triggers pineal melatonin synthesis [91]. In pinealocytes, the expression of β_1-adrenoceptors (600 fmol/mg protein) [92] is higher than that of α_1-adrenoceptors (180 fmol/mg protein) (92). The density of β_1-, but not α_1-adrenoceptors [94], varies during the day, with acrophase at the light/dark transition [95].

The activation of β_1-adrenoceptor is known to initiate melatonin synthesis, and activation of α_1-adrenoceptors in cultured glands works synergistically with β_1-adrenoceptors, amplifying the signal 10-fold [96]. However, the relative role played by the activation of β_1- and α_1-adrenoceptors in physiological and pathophysiological conditions is unclear. Some in vivo studies suggested a small synergistic effect of only 15% [97], whereas ex vivo studies indicated that α_1-adrenoceptors did not participate in sympathetic-induced melatonin synthesis [98]. More controversy was created by developmental studies, as experiments with young rats with aging between 2 to 4 weeks pointed to an antagonistic interaction between the stimulation of α_1- and β_1-adrenoceptors [99].

During an inflammatory process, there is activation of the HPA and sympathetic–adrenal–medullar axes, which are two major pathways that can alter immune function by the action of their neuroendocrine products, such as glucocorticoids and catecholamine [100]. The peptides corticotrophin-releasing hormone (CRH) and ACTH liberated by HPA axis activation are able to transiently increase noradrenaline production by the superior cervical ganglion [101,102], resulting in an enhancement of the sympathetic output on the pineal gland. Since β_1-adrenoceptors have a higher affinity for noradrenaline than $\alpha 1$-adrenoceptors [103], increasing the release of noradrenaline by the sympathetic terminals could stimulate both β_1- and α_1-adrenoceptors. Considering that, under inflammatory conditions, the level of circulating corticosterone also increases, we hypothesized that when both adrenergic receptors are stimulated, corticosterone inhibits melatonin synthesis. In contrast, when only β_1-receptors are activated, corticosterone potentiates melatonin production. In this case, as happens in other organs, α and β stimulation will prepare the organism for physiological or pathophysiological antagonistic responses.

In conclusion, the level of sympathetic tonus on the pineal gland could determine the effect of corticosterone on the synthesis of melatonin. Normal tonus or low-stress conditions activate only β_1-adrenoceptors, a scenario where corticosterone potentiates nocturnal melatonin output. In contrast, a high-stress situation results in the activation of both α_1- and β_1-adrenoceptors, a condition that will suppress the nocturnal melatonin surge and, according to the immune–pineal axis hypothesis, would facilitate the migration of cells through the endothelial layer, even when migration is not appropriate. As the inflammatory response progresses from the pro inflammatory to the resolution phase, the sympathetic tonus decreases, and the modulation of circulating adrenal cortical hormones will change from inhibiting to potentiating pineal melatonin production.

28.3.3 Chronic Inflammation

The light/dark rhythm of melatonin during chronic inflammatory disorders does not show a general pattern; in other words, it depends on the experimental model or the diseases. While in some models, a complete suppression of nocturnal melatonin surge is observed, in others, daily melatonin rhythm is maintained.

An important example for suppression of nocturnal melatonin production either in animal models [104] or humans [105] is Alzheimer's disease, which is considered a chronic inflammation of the central nervous system. It is interesting to note that the key marker for Alzheimer's disease is the β-amyloid protein, which is known to interact with TLR-4 receptors [20]. These are the receptors that trigger the NFKB pathway leading to inhibition of melatonin synthesis.

Chronic inflammation induced by injection of Bacillus Calmette–Guerin (BCG) in the paws of mice did not affect the normal daily rhythm of melatonin. Here, circulating corticosterone was essential for maintaining melatonin rhythm, as chemical or surgical adrenalectomy abolished the nocturnal melatonin surge [106,107]. In addition, the size of the paw varied throughout the day, being smaller at night. Adrenalectomy or pinealectomy abolished the daily rhythm of paw edema, which was recovered in both cases by injecting melatonin at night [107]. Similarly, melatonin rhythm is maintained in rheumatoid arthritis [108], a disorder that expresses high levels of TNF and glucocorticoid.

Thus, the understanding of the role of the immune–pineal axis during chronic inflammatory disorders is still an open field, as the cross-talk between inflammatory mediators and melatonin is analyzed in an integrated manner.

28.4 CONCLUSION

The immune–pineal axis predicts a progressive change in pineal gland activity during the course of an acute inflammatory response, taking into account the ability of this gland to interact with

DAMPs, cytokines, and hormones related to inflammation. This hypothesis predicts that a persistent stimulation of the NFKB pathway results in a blockage of nocturnal melatonin synthesis, whereas a tonic increase in circulating cortical adrenal hormones may restore the melatonin rhythm, even in the presence of an inflammatory response. This model accommodates different changes in pineal activity over the course of an inflammatory response and the anti-inflammatory properties of locally produced melatonin.

REFERENCES

1. Besedovsky, H.O. and del Rey, A. 2002. Introduction: immune–neuroendocrine network. *Front Hormon Res.* 29: 1–14.
2. Coogan, A.N. and Wyse, C.A. 2008. Neuroimmunology of the circadian clock. *Brain Res.* 1232: 104–112.
3. Dantzer, R. 2009. Cytokine, sickness behavior, and depression. *Immunol Allergy Clin North Am.* 29: 247–264.
4. Taishi, P., Bredow, S., Guha-Thakurta, N., Obál, F. Jr. and Krueger, J.M. 1997. Diurnal variations of interleukin-1 beta mRNA and beta-actin mRNA in rat brain. *J Neuroimmunol.* 75: 69–74.
5. Cearley, C., Churchill, L. and Krueger, J.M. 2003. Time of day differences in IL1beta and TNFalpha mRNA levels in specific regions of the rat brain. *Neurosci Lett.* 352: 61–63.
6. Sadki, A., Bentivoglio, M., Kristensson, K. and Nygard, M. 2007. Suppressors, receptors and effects of cytokines on the aging mouse biological clock. *Neurobiol Aging.* 28: 296–305.
7. Kalsbeek, A., Perreau-Lenz, S. and Buijs, R.M. 2006. A network of (autonomic) clock outputs. *Chronobiol Int.* 23: 521–535.
8. Kakizaki, Y., Watanobe, H., Kohsaka, A. and Suda, T. 1999. Temporal profiles of interleukin-1beta, interleukin-6, and tumor necrosis factor-alpha in the plasma and hypothalamic paraventricular nucleus after intravenous or intraperitoneal administration of lipopolysaccharide in the rat: estimation by push–pull perfusion. *Endocr J.* 46: 487–496.
9. Abbas, A.K. and Lichtman, A.H. (eds.). 2005. *Cellular and Molecular Immunology*, Updated Edition. Philadelphia: Elsevier Saunders.
10. Salazar-Mather, T.P., Hamilton, T.A. and Biron, C.A. 2000. A chemokine-to-cytokine-to-chemokine cascade critical in antiviral defense. *J Clin Invest.* 105: 985–993.
11. Boehm, U., Klamp, T., Groot, M. and Howard, J.C. 1997. Cellular responses to interferon-gamma. *Annu Rev Immunol.* 15: 749–795.
12. Yoshida, A., Koide, Y., Uchijima, M. and Yoshida, T.O. 1994. IFN-gamma induces IL-12 mRNA expression by a murine macrophage cell line, J774. *Biochem Biophys Res Commun.* 198: 857–861.
13. Murphy, T.L., Cleveland, M.G., Kulesza, P., Magram, J. and Murphy, K.M. 1995. Regulation of interleukin 12 p40 expression through a NF-kappa B half-site. *Mol Cell Biol.* 15: 5258–5267.
14. Chrousos, G.P. 1995. The hypothalamic–pituitary–adrenal axis and immune-mediated inflammation. *N Engl J Med.* 332: 1351–1362.
15. McCann, S.M., Lyson, K., Karanth, S., Gimeno, M., Belova, N., Kamat, A. and Rettori, V. 1995. Mechanism of action of cytokines to induce the pattern of pituitary hormone secretion in infection. *Ann N Y Acad Sci.* 771: 386–395.
16. Nadeau, S. and Rivest, S. 2002. Endotoxemia prevents the cerebral inflammatory wave induced by intraparenchymal lipopolysaccharide injection: role of glucocorticoids and CD14. *J Immunol.* 169: 3370–3381.
17. Baschant, U. and Tuckermann, J. 2010. The role of the glucocorticoid receptor in inflammation and immunity. *J Steroid Biochem Mol Biol.* 120: 69–75.
18. Skwarlo-Sonta, K., Majewski. P., Markowska, M., Oblap, R. and Olszanska, B. 2003. Bidirectional communication between the pineal gland and the immune system. *Can J Physiol Pharmacol.* 81: 342–349.
19. Markus, R.P., Ferreira, Z.S., Fernandes, P.A. and Cecon, E. 2007. The immune–pineal axis: a shuttle between endocrine and paracrine melatonin sources. *Neuroimmunomodulation.* 14: 126–33.
20. Markus, R.P., Silva, C.L., Franco, D.G., Barbosa, E.M. Jr. and Ferreira, Z.S. 2010. Is modulation of nicotinic acetylcholine receptors by melatonin relevant for therapy with cholinergic drugs? *Pharmacol Ther.* 126: 251–62.

21. Scheff, J.D., Calvano, S.E., Lowry, S.F. and Androulakis, I.P. 2010. Modeling the influence of circadian rhythms on the acute inflammatory response. *J Theor Biol.* 264: 1068–1076.
22. Granger, D.N. and Kubes P. 1994. The microcirculation and inflammation: modulation of leukocyte–endothelial cell adhesion. *J Leukoc Biol.* 55: 662–675.
23. Bureau, J.P., Labrecque, G., Coupe, M. and Garrelly, L. 1986. Influence of BCG administration time on the in-vivo migration of leukocytes. *Chronobiol Int.* 3: 23–28.
24. Garrelly, L., Bureau, J.P. and Labreque, G. 1991. Temporal study of carrageenan-induced PMN migration in mice. *Agents Actions.* 33: 225–228.
25. Bertuglia, S., Marchiafava, P.L. and Colantuoni, A. 1996. Melatonin prevents ischemia reperfusion injury in hamster cheek pouch microcirculation. *Cardiovasc Res.* 31: 947–952.
26. Maestroni, G.J. 1996. Melatonin as a therapeutic agent in experimental endotoxic shock. *J Pineal Res.* 20: 84–89.
27. Cuzzocrea, S., Zingarelli, B., Gilad, E., Hake, P., Salzman, A.L. and Szabo, C. 1997. Protective effect of melatonin in carrageenan-induced models of local inflammation: relationship to its inhibitory effect on nitric oxide production and peroxynitrite scavenging activity. *J Pineal Res.* 23: 106–116.
28. Cuzzocrea, S., Zingarelli, B., Costantino, G. and Caputi, A.P. 1998. Protective effect of melatonin in a non-septic shock model induced by zymosan in the rat. *J Pineal Res.* 25: 24–33.
29. Costantino, G., Cuzzocrea, S., Mazzon, E. and Caputi, A.P. 1998. Protective effects of melatonin in zymosan-activated plasma-induced paw inflammation. *Eur J Pharmacol.* 363: 57–63.
30. Lotufo, C.M., Lopes, C., Dubocovich, M.L., Farsky, S.H. and Markus, R.P. 2001. Melatonin and N-acetylserotonin inhibit leukocyte rolling and adhesion to rat microcirculation. *Eur J Pharmacol.* 430: 351–357.
31. Lotufo, C.M., Yamashita, C.E., Farsky, S.H. and Markus, R.P. 2006. Melatonin effect on endothelial cells reduces vascular permeability increase induced by leukotriene B4. *Eur J Pharmacol.* 534: 258–263.
32. Zhang, Q., Raoof, M., Chen, Y., Sumi, Y., Sursal, T., Junger, W., Brohi, K., Itagaki, K. and Hauser, C.J. 2010. Circulating mitochondrial DAMPs cause inflammatory responses to injury. *Nature.* 464: 104–107.
33. Axerold, J. and Weissbach, H. 1960. Enzymatic O-methylation of N-acetylserotonin to melatonin. *Science.* 131: 1312.
34. Voisin, P., Namboodiri, M.A.A. and Klein, D.C. 1984. Arylamine N-acetyltransferase and aryl-alkylamine N-acetyltransferase in the mammalian pineal gland. *J Biol Chem.* 259: 10913–10918.
35. Kalsbeek, A., Garidou, M.L., Palm, I.F., van Der Vliet, J., Simonneaux, V., Pévet, P. and Buijs, R.M. 2000. Melatonin sees the light: blocking GABA-ergic transmission in the paraventricular nucleus induces daytime secretion of melatonin. *Eur J Neurosci.* 12: 3146–3154.
36. Teclemariam-Mesbah, R., Ter Horst, G.J., Postema, F., Wortel, J. and Buijs, R.M. 1999. Anatomical demonstration of the suprachiasmatic nucleus–pineal pathway. *J Comp Neurol.* 406: 171–182.
37. Mortani-Barbosa, E.J.M., Ferreira, Z.S. and Merkus, R.P. 2000. Purinergic and noradrenergic cotransmission in the rat pineal gland. *Eur J Pharmacol.* 401: 59–62.
38. Burke, Z., Wells, T., Carter, D., Klein, D.C. and Baler, R. 1999. Genetic targeting: the serotonin N-acetyltransferase promoter imparts circadian expression selectively in the pineal gland and retina of transgenic rats. *J Neurochem.* 73: 1343–1349.
39. Chen, W. and Baler, R. 2000. The rat arylalkylamine N-acetyltransferase E-box: differential use in a master vs. a slave oscillator. *Mol Brain Res.* 81: 43–50.
40. Schomerus, C., Korf, H.W., Laedtke, E., Weller, J.L. and Klein, D.C. 2000. Selective adrenergic/cyclic AMP-dependent switch-off of proteasomal proteolysis alone switches on neural signal transduction: an example from the pineal gland. *J Neurochem.* 75: 2123–2132.
41. Gastel, J.A., Roseboom, P.H., Rinaldi, P.A., Weller, J.L., and Klein, D.C. 1998. Melatonin production: proteosomal proteolysis in serotonin N-acetyltransferase regulation. *Science (Wash DC).* 279: 1358–1360.
42. Ganguly, S., Coon, S.L. and Klein, D.C. 2002. Control of melatonin synthesis in the Mammalian pineal gland: the critical role of serotonin acetylation. *Cell Tissue Res.* 309: 127–137.
43. Sun, X., Deng, J., Liu, T. and Borjigin, J. 2002. Circadian 5-HT production regulated by adrenergic signaling. *Proc Natl Acad Sci U S A.* 99: 4686–4691.
44. Stoschitzky, K., Sakotnik, A., Lercher, P., Zweiker, R., Maier, R., Liebmann, P. and Lindner, W. 1999. Influence of beta-blockers on melatonin release. *Eur J Clin Pharmacol.* 55: 11–115.
45. Klein, D.C. 1985. Photoneural regulation of the mammalian pineal gland. In: Everet, D. and Clark, D. (eds.), *Photoperiodism, Melatonin and the Pineal. Ciba Foundation Symposium 117.* Pittman Press: London, 38–56.

46. Ferreira, Z.S., Garcia, C.R., Spray, D.C. and Markus, R.P. 2003. P2Y(1) receptor activation enhances the rate of rat pinealocyte-induced extracellular acidification via a calcium-dependent mechanism. *Pharmacology*. 69: 33–37.
47. Ferreira, Z.S. and Markus, R.P. 2001. Characterisation of P2Y(1)-like receptor in cultured rat pineal glands. *Eur J Pharmacol*. 415: 151–156.
48. Liu, T. and Borjigin, J. 2005. N-acetyltransferase is not the rate-limiting enzyme of melatonin synthesis at night. *J Pineal Res*. 39: 91–96.
49. Farsky, S.P., Sannomiya, P. and Garcia-Leme, J. 1995. Secreted glucocorticoids regulate
50. Cavalcanti, D.M., Lotufo, C.M., Borelli, P., Ferreira, Z.S., Markus, R.P. and Farsky, S.H. 2007. Endogenous glucocorticoids control neutrophil mobilization from bone marrow to blood and tissues in non-inflammatory conditions. *Br J Pharmacol*. 152: 1291–1300.
51. Cavalcanti, D.M., Lotufo, C.M., Borelli, P., Tavassi, A.M., Pereire, A.L., Markus, R.P. and Farsky, S.H. 2006. Adrenal deficiency alters mechanisms of neutrophil mobilization. *Mol Cell Endocrinol*. 249: 32–39.
52. Hayden, M.S. and Ghosh, S. 2008. Shared principles in NF-kappaB signaling. *Cell*. 132: 344–362.
53. Kaltschmidt, B. and Kaltschmidt, C. 2000. Constitutive NF-kappa B activity is modulated via neuron–astroglia interaction. *Exp Brain Res*. 130: 100–104.
54. Kaltschmidt, B., Widera, D. and Kaltschmidt, C. 2005. Signaling via NF-kappaB in the nervous system. *Biochim Biophys Acta*. 1745: 287–299.
55. Sethi, G. and Tergaonkar, V. 2009. Potential pharmacological control of the NF-kappaB pathway. *Trends Pharmacol Sci*. 30: 313–321.
56. Ghosh, S. and Hayden, M.S. 2008. New regulators of NF-kappaB in inflammation. *Nat Rev Immunol*. 11: 837–848.
57. Verma, I.M., Stevenson, J.K., Schwarz, E.M., Van Antwerp, D. and Miyamoto, S. 1995. Rel/NF-kappaB/I kappa B family: intimate tales of association and dissociation. *Genes Dev*. 9: 2723–2735.
58. Vallabhapurapu, S. and Karin, M. 2009. Regulation and function of NF-kappaB transcription factors in the immune system. *Annu Rev Immunol*. 27: 693–733.
59. Liou, H.C. and Hsia, C.Y. 2003. Distinctions between c-Rel and other NF-kappaB proteins in immunity and disease. *Bioessays*. 25: 767–780.
60. Ferreira, Z.S., Fernandes, P.A.C.M., Duma, D., Assreuy, J., Avellar, M.C.W. and Markus, R.P. 2005. Corticosterone modulates noradrenaline-induced melatonin synthesis through inhibition of nuclear factor kappaB. *J Pineal Res*. 38: 182–188.
61. Cecon, E., Fernandes, P.A., Pinato, L., Ferreira, Z.S. and Markus, R.P. 2010. Daily variation of constitutively activated nuclear factor kappa B (NFKB) in rat pineal gland. *Chronobiol Int*. 27: 52–67.
62. da Silveira Cruz-Machado, S.S., Carvalho-Sousa, C.E., Tamura, E.K., Pinato, L., Cecon, E., Fernandes, P.A., Avellar, M.C.W., Ferreira, Z.S. and Markus, R.P. 2010. TLR4 and CD14 receptors expressed in rat pineal gland triggers NFKB pathway. *J Pineal Res*. 49: 183–192.
63. Tamura, E.K., Fernandes, P.A., Marçola, M., da Silveira Cruz-Machado, S. and Markus, R.P. 2010. Long-lasting priming of endothelial cells by plasma melatonin levels. *PLoS One*. 5:e13958.
64. Fernandes, P.A., Cecon, E., Markus, R.P. and Ferreira, Z.S. 2006. Effect of TNF-alpha on the melatonin synthetic pathway in the rat pineal gland: basis for a 'feedback' of the immune response on circadian timing. *J Pineal Res*. 41: 344–350.
65. Pontes, G.N., Cardoso, E.C., Carneiro-Sampaio, M.M. and Markus, R.P. 2006. Injury switches melatonin production source from endocrine (pineal) to paracrine (phagocytes)—melatonin in human colostrum and colostrum phagocytes. *J Pineal Res*. 41: 136–141.
66. Pontes, G.N., Cardoso, E.C., Carneiro-Sampaio, M.M. and Markus, R.P. 2007. Pineal melatonin and the innate immune response: the TNF-alpha increase after cesarean section suppress nocturnal melatonin production. *J Pineal Res*. 43: 365–371.
67. Srinivasan, V., Spence, D.W., Trakht, I., Pandi-Perumal, S.R., Cardinali, D.P. and Maestroni, G.J. 2008. Immunomodulation by melatonin: its significance for seasonally occurring diseases. *Neuroimmunomodulation*. 15: 93–101.
68. Srinivasan, V., Pandi-Perumal, S.R., Spence, D.W., Kato, H. and Cardinali, D.P. 2010. Melatonin in septic shock: some recent concepts. *J Crit Care*. 25: 656.e6.
69. Carrillo-Vico, A., Lardone, P. J., Naji, L., Fernandez-Santos, J. M., Martin-Lacave, I., Guerrero, J.M. and Calvo, J.R. 2005. Beneficial pleiotropic actions of melatonin in an experimental model of septic shock in mice: regulation of pro-/anti-inflammatory cytokine network, protection against oxidative damage and anti-apoptotic effects. *J Pineal Res*. 39: 400–408.

70. Wu, J.Y., Tsou, M.Y., Chen, T.H., Chen, S.J., Tsao, C.M. and Wu, C.C. 2008. Therapeutic effects of melatonin on peritonitis-induced septic shock with multiple organ dysfunction syndrome in rats. *J Pineal Res.* 45: 106–116.
71. Zhong, L.Y., Yang, Z.H., Li, X.R., Wang, H. and Li, L. 2009. Protective effects of melatonin against the damages of neuroendocrine–immune induced by lipopolysaccharide in diabetic rats. *Exp Clin Endocrinol Diabetes.* 117: 463–469.
72. Gitto, E., Pellegrino, S., Gitto, P., Barberi, I. and Reiter, R.J. 2009. Oxidative stress of the newborn in the pre- and postnatal period and the clinical utility of melatonin. *J Pineal Res.* 46: 128–139.
73. Carrillo-Vico, A., Calvo, J.R., Abreu, P., Lardone, P.J., García-Mauriño, S., Reiter, R.J, and Guerrero, J.M. 2004. Evidence of melatonin synthesis by human lymphocytes and its physiological significance: possible role as intracrine, autocrine, and/or paracrine substance. *FASEB J.* 18: 537–539.
74. Naranjo, M.C., Guerrero, J.M., Rubio, A., Lardone, P.J., Carrillo-Vico, A., Carrascosa-Salmoral, M.P., Jiménez-Jorge, S., Arellano, M.V., Leal-Noval, S.R., Leal, M., Lissen, E. and Molinero, P. 2007. Melatonin biosynthesis in the thymus of humans and rats. *Cell Mol Life Sci.* 64: 781–790.
75. Martins, E. Jr., Ferreira, A.C., Skorupa, A.L., Afeche, S.C., Cipolla-Neto, J. and Costa Rosa, L.F. 2004. Tryptophan consumption and indoleamines production by peritoneal cavity macrophages. *J Leukoc Biol.* 75: 1116–1121.
76. Maldonado, M.D., Mora-Santos, M., Naji, L., Carrascosa-Salmoral, M.P., Naranjo, M.C. and Calvo, J.R. 2009. Evidence of melatonin synthesis and release by mast cells. Possible modulatory role on inflammation. *Pharmacol Res.* 62: 282–287.
77. Pioli, C., Caroleo, M.C., Nistico, G. and Doria, G. 1993. Melatonin increases antigen presentation and amplifies specific and non specific signals for T-cell proliferation. *Int J Immunopharmacol.* 15: 463–468.
78. Garcia-Mauriño, S., Gonzalez-Haba, M.G., Calvo, J.R., Rafii-el-Idrissi, M., Sanchez-Margalet, V., Goberna, R. and Guerrero, J.M. 1997. Melatonin enhances IL-2, IL-6, and IFN-gamma production by human circulating CD4+ cells: a possible nuclear receptor-mediated mechanism involving T helper type 1 lymphocytes and monocytes. *J Immunol.* 159: 574–581.
79. Miller, S.C., Pandi-Perumal, S.R., Esquifino, A.I., Cardinali, D.P. and Maestroni, G.J. 2006. The role of melatonin in immuno-enhancement: potential application in cancer. *Int J Exp Pathol.* 87: 81–87.
80. Buijs, R.M., Wortel, J., Van Heerikhnuize, J.J., Feenstra, M.G., Ter Horst, G.J., Romijn, H.J. and Kalsbeek, A. 1999. Anatomical and functional demonstration of a multisynaptic suprachiasmatic nucleus adrenal (cortex) pathway. *Eur J Neurosci.* 11: 1535–1544.
81. Ulrich-Lai, Y.M., Arnhold, M.M. and Engeland, W.C. 2006. Adrenal splanchnic innervation contributes to the diurnal rhythm of plasma corticosterone in rats by modulating adrenal sensitivity to ACTH. *Am J Physiol Regul Integr Comp Physiol,.* 290: 1128–1135.
82. Couto-Moraes, R., Palermo-Neto, J. and Markus, R.P. 2009. The immune–pineal axis: stress as a modulator of pineal gland function. *Ann N Y Acad Sci.* 1153: 193–202.
83. Troiani, M.E., Reiter, R.J., Vaughan, M.K., Gonzalez-Brito, A. and Herbert, D.C. 1988. The depression in rat pineal melatonin production after saline injection at night may be elicited by corticosterone. *Brain Res.* 450: 18–24.
84. Yuwiler, A. 1989. Effects of steroids on serotonin-N-acetyltransferase activity of pineals in organ culture. *J Neurochem.* 52: 46–53.
85. Zhao, Z.Y. and Touitou, Y. 1993. Kinetic changes of melatonin release in rat pineal perifusion at different circadian stages. Effect of corticosteroids. *Acta Endocrinol Copenh.* 129: 81–88.
86. Fernandes, P.A., Bothorel, B., Clesse, D., Monteiro, A.W., Calgari, C., Raison, S., Simonneaux, V. and Markus, R.P. 2009. Local corticosterone infusion enhances nocturnal pineal melatonin production in vivo. *J Neuroendocrinol.* 21: 90–97.
87. Parffitt, A., Weller, J.L. and Klein, D.C. 1976. Beta-adrenergic blockers decrease adrenergically stimulated n-acetyltransferase activity in pineal glands in organ culture. *Neuropharmacology.* 15: 353–358.
88. Marques, A.H., Silverman, M.N. and Sternberg, E.M. 2009. Glucocorticoid dysregulations and their clinical correlates. From receptors to therapeutics. *Ann N Y Acad Sci.* 1179: 1–18.
89. Kappers, J.A. 1960. The development, topographical relations and innervation of the epiphysis cerebri in the albino rat. *Zeitschrift fur Zellforschung.* 52: 163–215.
90. Drijfhout, W.J., Grol, C.J. and Westerink, B.H.C. 1996. Parasympathetic inhibition of pineal indole metabolism by prejunctional modulation of noradrenaline release. *Eur J Pharmacol.* 20: 24–32.
91. Moore, R.Y. and Klein, D.C. 1974. Visual pathways and the central neural control of a circadian rhythm in pineal serotonin N-acetyltransferase activity. *Brain Res.* 71: 17–33.

92. Zatz, M., Kebabian, J.W., Romero, J.A., Lefkowitz, R.J. and Axelrod, J. 1976. Pineal beta adrenergic receptor: correlation of binding of 3H-l-alprenolol with stimulation of adenylate cyclase. *J Pharmacol Exp Ther.* 196: 714–22.
93. Sugden, D. and Klein, D.C. 1984. Rat pineal alpha 1-adrenoceptors: identification and characterization using [^{125}I]iodo-2-[beta-(4-hydroxyphenyl)-ethylaminomethyltetralone. *Endocrinology.* 114: 435–440.
94. Sugden, D. and Klein, D.C. 1985. Development of the rat pineal alpha 1-adrenoceptor. *Brain Res.* 325: 345–348.
95. Roomero, J.A. and Axelod, J. (1974). Pineal beta-adrenergic receptor: diurnal variation in sensitivity. *Science.* 184: 1091–1092.
96. Vanecek, J., Sugden, D., Weller, J. and Klein, D.C. 1985. Atypical synergistic α1 and β-adrenergic regulation of adenosine 3′,5′-monophosphate and guanosine 3′,5′-monophosphate in rat pinealocytes. *Endocrinology.* 116: 2167–2173.
97. Nilsson, K.J. and Reiter, R. J. 1989. In vivo stimulation of Syrian hamster pineal melatonin levels by isoproterenol plus phenylephrine is not accompanied by a commensurate large increase in N-acetyltransferase activity. *Neuroendocrinol Lett.* 11: 63–68.
98. Tobin, V.A. McCance, I., Coleman, H.A. and Parkington, H.C. 2002. How important is stimulation of alpha-adrenoceptors for melatonin production in rat pineal glands? *J Pineal Res.* 32: 219–224.
99. Wagner, G., Brandstätter, R. and Hermann, A. 2000. Adrenergic and cholinergic regulation of in vitro melatonin release during ontogeny in the pineal gland of Long Evans rats. *Neuroendocrinology.* 72: 154–161.
100. Padgett, D.A. and Glaser, R. 2003. How stress influences the immune response. *Trends Immunol.* 24: 444–448.
101. Sabban, E.L., Nankova, B.B., Serova, L.I., Kvetnansky, R. and Liu, X. 2004. Molecular regulation of gene expression of catecholamine biosynthetic enzymes by stress: sympathetic ganglia versus adrenal medulla. *Ann N Y Acad Sci.* 1018: 370–377.
102. Serova, L.I., Gueorguiev, V., Cheng, S.Y. and Sabban, E.L. 2008. Adrenocorticotropic hormone elevates gene expression for catecholamine biosynthesis in rat superior cervical ganglia and locus coeruleus by an adrenal independent mechanism. *Neuroscience.* 153: 1380–1389.
103. Molinoff, P.B. 1984. Alpha- and beta-adrenergic receptor subtypes properties, distribution and regulation. 28: 1–15.
104. Olcese, J.M., Cao, C., Mori, T., Mamcarz, M.B., Maxwell, A., Runfeldt, M.J., Wang, L., Zhang, C., Lin, X., Zhang, G. and Arendash, G.W. 2009. Protection against cognitive deficits and markers of neurodegeneration by long-term oral administration of melatonin in a transgenic model of Alzheimer disease. *J Pineal Res.* 47: 82–96.
105. Cardinali, D.P., Brusco, L.I., Liberczuk, C. and Furio, A.M. 2002. The use of melatonin in Alzheimer's disease. *Neuro Endocrinol Lett.* 23: 20–23.
106. Lopes, C., deLyra, J.L., Markus, R.P. and Mariano, M. 1997. Circadian rhythm in experimental granulomatous inflammation is modulated by melatonin. *J Pineal Res.* 23: 72–78.
107. Lopes, C., Mariano, M. and Markus, R.P. 1998. Interaction between the adrenal and the pineal gland in chronic experimental inflammation induced by BCG in mice. *Inflamm Res.* 50: 6–11.
108. Cutolo, M., Otsa, K., Aakre, O. and Sulli, A. 2005. Nocturnal hormones and clinical rhythms in rheumatoid arthritis. *Ann N Y Acad Sci.* 1051: 372–381.

29 Neuroendocrinological Effects of Antidepressants: Is There a Role for Melatonin?

Marco Antonioli, Joanna Rybka, and Livia A. Carvalho

CONTENTS

29.1 INTRODUCTION

Major depressive disorder (MDD) is a highly prevalent disorder, with lifetime prevalence reported at 16.2% in a U.S. epidemiological survey.[1] It has great socioeconomic importance as it is the psychiatric disorder that most frequently causes psychosocial disability. Indeed, according to the World Health Organization, it will be the second leading cause of disability worldwide in terms of burden of disease. Although there is a range of medications offered to subjects with MDD that have demonstrated the efficacy of several classes of antidepressants, it is still unknown exactly how antidepressants exert their therapeutic benefit. Currently available pharmacotherapy is associated with a delayed onset of several weeks and causes side effects, and still, only around 30%–45% of MDD subjects typically attain remission. The majority of subjects are at risk for chronic depression and other morbidity factors, including suicide, substance abuse, and other serious medical conditions. These unmet needs highlight the importance of investigating novel treatment options for depression.

In mammals, the temporal organization presents a daily adjustment to the environmental light/dark cycle. Environmental light detected by the retina adjusts the central clock in the suprachiasmatic nuclei, which innervates the pineal gland through a polysynaptic pathway. During the night, the pineal gland produces and releases the nocturnal hormone melatonin, which circulates throughout the whole body and adjusts its functions according to the existence and duration of darkness.[2]

The activity of the pineal gland is modulated by the immune–endocrine system. During an activation of the inflammatory response system (IRS), proinflammatory cytokines, such as tumor necrosis factor (TNF)-α, inhibit while anti-inflammatory mediators, such as glucocorticoids, enhance the synthesis of melatonin, interfering in the daily adjustment of the light/dark cycle. Mood disorder patients have neuroendocrine abnormalities including reduced levels of the pineal hormone melatonin and circadian rhythm dysregulations. They also show an activation of the IRS in the presence of glucocorticoid resistance. Therefore, the activated IRS in these patients may be involved in the biological mechanism by which depressed patients show a disconnection of the organism from environmental cycling. In this review, we will discuss the main mechanisms that support the hypothesis that melatoninergic disturbances are part of the pathophysiology of depression, and that antidepressants may exert their therapeutic benefit in part by correcting immune–endocrine disturbances.

29.1.1 Pineal Axis in Depression

Melatonin, a physiological index for noradrenergic function, has been investigated in the pathophysiology of major depression.[3] Since melatonin production occurs from serotonin after stimulation of beta-adrenoreceptors, it has been hypothesized that a disturbance in melatonin secretion could be present in the acute phase of depressive illness and be related to its pathophysiology.[4] Several authors have investigated the interplay between major depression and melatonin, but the literature remains controversial. Many earlier studies showed lower concentration of melatonin in depressed patients compared with healthy volunteers.[5–7]

Melatonin disturbances in depressed patients seem to be more prevalent in the severely ill. Melatoninergic disturbances in depression may be related to treatment severity as no differences were found in mildly ill patients when compared with a carefully screened group of healthy volunteers.[6–8] Indeed, most of work conducted so far investigated moderately to severely ill depressive patients. Crasson et al. showed decreased nighttime plasma melatonin levels in severely ill inpatients with major depression.[9] When compared with healthy volunteers, these patients also had a phase shift in melatonin production in the morning compared to nighttime levels.

Accordingly, Paparrigopoulos found the lowest levels of melatonin after atenolol in the most severely ill depressive patients.[10] These results suggest that the reduced levels of melatonin in depression may be due to decreased sensitivity of β-adrenergic receptors. Reduced levels of melatonin, together with other neuroendocrine markers like cortisol levels, were predictors of depression severity in postmenopausal women.[11] Melatonin levels in depressed patients may also depend on the subtype of depression. Brown et al. were one of the first to report blunted melatonin levels in a small group of melancholic depressed patients when compared with nonmelancholic subtypes.[12] This finding was later confirmed by Fountoulakis et al. who also found lower levels of aMT6s, the main urinary melatonin metabolite, in melancholic depressive patients when compared with other depression subtypes.[13] On the other hand, melatonin levels were found to be increased in bipolar depression or in the presence of psychotic features. Apart from the disturbance in the levels of melatonin, circadian rhythm alterations have also been reported. Tuunainen et al.[12] found an association between current major depression and delayed offset and later nocturnal peak of aMT6s excretion in a large group of postmenopausal women.[11] Parry et al. also showed a delayed offset of melatonin in postmenopausal women.[14] It should be noted, however, that the different detection methods between the various studies do not allow direct comparison, and other results have also been reported.[15,17–20] Finally, the variability of results in previous studies may also be explained at least in part by the influence of factors such as age, body mass index,[15] latitude,[16] and season.[17]

To date, only one study has investigated the effect of melatonin receptor knockout in depressive-like behavior, and results support the findings in humans. Mice which are knockout for melatonin receptor type I (MT1) show increased depressive-like behavior as shown by severely impaired prepulse inhibition in the acoustic startle response as well as increased immobility time in the forced swim test.[18] Apart from the pineal gland, MT1 is also widespread in the hypothalamus[19]; MT1 colocalization with corticotropin-releasing hormone (CRH) neurones in the hypothalamus possibly allows for neuroendocrine modulation and regulation of the circadian rhythms.[19]

Why exactly melatoninergic disturbances occur in mood disorder is not well known, but familial vulnerability may play a role. In this regard, a shift on the production of melatonin is associated with a positive family history for depression in postmenopausal women.[11] More recently, Gałecki et al. showed that depression is associated with at-risk polymorphisms of the *ATMS* gene that configures lower levels of the acetylserotonin methyltransferase (ASMT), the reported rate-limiting melatonin synthesis enzyme, in the presence of concomitant reduction of ASMT gene expression levels.[20] Taking together these results suggests that neuroendocrine disturbances in depressive patients involve melatoninergic dysregulation.

29.1.2 HPA Axis in Depression

In addition to the melatoninergic disturbances in major depression, clinical studies have also demonstrated an impairment of the hypothalamus–pituitary–adrenal (HPA) axis in patients with major depression [glucocorticoid receptor (GR) resistance] and its resolution by antidepressant treatment. Indeed, one of the most consistent findings in psychiatry is the activation of the HPA axis. CRH produced by the hypothalamus stimulates the release of adrenocorticotropic hormone (ACTH) from the pituitary gland, which, in turn, stimulates the release of cortisol from the adrenal gland. Cortisol will then interact with its own receptors GR and mineralocorticoid receptors (MRs) to exert its biological functions, which include immunosuppressive properties. Cortisol inhibits its own production via glucocorticoid-mediated negative feedback. In depressed patients, the hyperactivity of the HPA axis is characterized by high cortisol levels in the plasma, urine, and cerebrospinal fluid,[21] impairment in the negative feedback,[22,23] and hyperplasia of the adrenal and pituitary glands.[24] Consistent with these findings, increased volume of the pituitary in patients with affective and nonaffective psychosis was shown by our group using brain magnetic resonance imaging.[25,26] Other HPA axis abnormalities have been found in victims of suicide—many of whom were presumably depressed—including a down-regulation of CRH receptors in the frontal cortex[27] and increased weight of adrenal glands.[28] The disturbance of the HPA axis has been reliably verified directly or indirectly by a multitude of studies. Directly, the hyperactivity has been seen by hypercortisolemia in the plasma, urine, and cerebrospinal fluid. Indirectly, it has been seen after tests designed to measure the HPA axis activity and the integrity of the GR-mediated negative feedback mechanism. Why exactly depressed patients have an impairment of the HPA axis negative feedback is not well known, but a dysfunction of the GR and MR may play a role. Indeed, reduced GR function has also been demonstrated in vitro, in peripheral tissues of depressed patients, as shown by reduced sensitivity to the effects of glucocorticoids on immune and metabolic functions.[29]

29.1.3 Immune–Pineal–HPA Axis

The classical control of pineal melatonin production by the environmental light/dark cycle is modified during the development of an inflammatory response as mediators of inflammation found in the plasma interfere with pineal melatonin synthesis.[30] The rat pineal gland expresses GR, which mediates the potentiation of noradrenaline-induced melatonin production in pineal glands in vitro[31] and in vivo.[32] Corticosterone, the hormone in animals that is equivalent to cortisol in humans, enhances NA-induced melatonin production at lower concentrations. Corticosterone acts through the GRs and the nuclear factor kappa B (NF-κB) pathway[31] and enhances the transcription of the *aa-nat* gene, the rate-limiting enzyme in the production of melatonin.[33] Circulating corticosterone could play a role in modulating the nocturnal melatonin surge. Chronic inflammation in animals increases the release of corticosterone and is of utmost importance for maintaining the nocturnal melatonin surge. Indeed, chronic inflammation itself presents a diurnal variation that is abolished by conditions that prevent melatonin surge like constant light or pinealectomy and is restored by exogenous administration of melatonin.[34] Adrenalectomy (surgical or pharmacological) also abolishes the diurnal rhythm of the inflammatory lesion, and this effect is also restored by exogenous administration of melatonin.[35] Finally and in support to the idea of the immune–pineal–HPA axis is the fact that nocturnal rise in 6-sulfatoximelatonin excretion was abolished by adrenalectomy.[35] Therefore, the nocturnal rise of melatonin in the presence of a chronic inflammatory response requires not only sympathetic neural input but also the presence of glucocorticoids. The nocturnal production of melatonin is also modulated by cytokines that interfere with the NF-κB pathway.[30] TNF-α inhibits the NA-induced transcription of the *aa-nat* gene and the production of NAS. In addition, in women with acute inflammation (mastitis), suppression of the nocturnal melatonin surge is significantly correlated with an increase in circulating TNF-α. At the beginning of inflammation when TNF-α values are high, the nocturnal surge of melatonin is suppressed, and as soon as TNF-α levels return to values that are below detection, the nocturnal melatonin surge is restored. In summary, both proinflammatory and anti-inflammatory mediators modulate the nocturnal melatonin surge, with proinflammatory mediators reducing or even suppressing melatonin production and anti-inflammatory mediators increasing pineal activity, at least within a certain concentration range. All these findings suggest that neuroendocrine impairments may work together in the development of the whole constellation of neurobiological alterations found in depression.

Depressed patients show an activation of the IRS in the presence of glucocorticoid resistance as shown by increased levels of cortisol. As presented above, depressed patients also present disturbances in both melatonin levels and rhythm. Why exactly depressed patients have circadian rhythm disturbances is not known, but glucocorticoid resistance may play a role. Few studies, so far, have investigated the hypothesis that the increased cortisol levels impair melatonin production in depression. Beck-Friis et al. analyzed glucocorticoid-mediated negative feedback of the HPA axis via the dexamethasone suppression test and melatonin surge in depressed patients.[6] Accordingly, they found only those patients whose presented glucocorticoid resistance also presented melatoninergic disturbances, which suggests that there is a dysregulation in the neuroendocrine cross-talk in these patients.

29.1.4 Melatonin, Inflammatory System, and Depression

In the past ten years, an increasing amount of evidence suggests that activation of the inflammatory system is involved in the pathogenesis of depression. First, depressed patients have high levels of proinflammatory cytokines including TNF-α, IL-1-β, and interleukin-6 (IL-6). The increased level of IL-6 has been most frequently observed.[36–40] Furthermore, major depression is also strongly associated with the increased level of acute phase proteins including CRP.[41,42] Second, clinical administration of cytokines or agents which increase production of proinflammatory cytokines can induce depressive symptoms in patients with no previous mental health issues[43–45] and inflammation-induced depression can also be treated with antidepressants.[46] Finally, activation of the immune system and administration of proinflammatory cytokines to laboratory animals induce a behavior that is similar to depression in humans.[47] The activation of the inflammatory system is one possible mechanism that could bring about neuroendocrine abnormalities in depression.

A number of studies have demonstrated that treatment with proinflammatory cytokines induces glucocorticoid resistance, an effect that can be reversed by antidepressants. For example, cytokines induce decrease in GR function as evidenced by decreased sensitivity to the effects of glucocorticoids on functional endpoints and decreased GR affinity for its ligand. Cytokines can activate the HPA axis, causing an elevation of systemic glucocorticoid levels, and inhibit GR function at multiple levels, including GR translocation and induction of GR isoforms with reduced capacity to bind ligand.[44,48] IL-6 has been reported to induce a prolonged increase in plasma concentrations of ACTH and cortisol in healthy men.[49] IL-1 directly blocks GR translocation and function in vitro,[44] an effect that is virtually opposite to that of antidepressants in the same experimental system.[50] The in vitro studies are supported by studies in humans showing that, on peripheral cells and tissues of patients with inflammatory diseases such as asthma, ulcerative colitis, acquired immunodeficiency syndrome, and rheumatoid arthritis, especially those showing resistance to the therapeutic effects of glucocorticoids, reductions in GR function and affinity that are similar to those induced by cytokines are also demonstrated.

As previously discussed, neuro-immune–endocrine interactions also involve the pineal gland, which, in turn, influences the development and function of the immune system. Moreover, membrane-bound melatonin receptors are found in lymphoid glands and immune cells.[51,52] In addition to mediating immune reactions and GR function, cytokines have been shown to alter sleep architecture significantly[49] supporting the hypothesis that circadian rhythm dysregulation in depressed patients involves the immune–pineal–HPA axis. Inflammatory agents can also regulate melatonin synthesis. As previously discussed, TNF leads to inhibition of AA-NAT transcription and the production of N-acetylserotonin and melatonin in cultured glands. Negative modulation of norepinephrine-induced melatonin production by TNF-α is a transient phenomenon in the sequence of the inflammatory response, and the self-regulatory response in the pineal gland would allow the restoration of the nocturnal melatonin surge.[30] This regulatory mechanism is disrupted when very high systemic TNF-α levels are present, resulting in abnormalities in the secretion of circadian melatonin, mainly related to an absence of the diurnal rhythm. Therefore, melatonin cycle impairments reported in depression[11,53–55] may occur at the onset of an inflammatory response; if the melatonin circadian rhythm cannot be restored shortly thereafter, it is possible that the high systemic TNF-α levels are present. AA-NAT is considered to play a key role in the regulation of melatonin biosynthesis, as changes in its activity are paralleled by alterations in melatonin levels.[56] The interaction of endogenous norepinephrine with β-adrenoceptors to increase AA-NAT activity and melatonin release has been suggested.[57] β-adrenoceptor stimulation has been shown to increase gene expression and protein production of TNF-α as well as IL-1β and IL-6[58]; however, data suggesting that an enhanced adrenergic tonus leads to immunosuppression primarily via alpha 2-receptor-mediated mechanisms are also available.[59] Consequently, chronic β-receptor blockade reduces plasma levels of IL-6.[60] Also, stress-induced activation of NF-κB in peripheral blood mononuclear cells appears to be dependent on norepinephrine and can be brought down by α1-adrenoceptor blockade.[61] It has been reported that mice kept under constant light or receiving injections of β-adrenergic blockers (propranolol) to inhibit melatonin synthesis exhibited an inability to mount a primary antibody response to sheep red blood cells, a decreased cellularity in thymus and spleen, and a depressed autologous mixed lymphocyte reaction, and all of those were reversed by melatonin administration when given in the late afternoon.[62] β-adrenoceptor blockers, which depress melatonin secretion, exert immunosuppressive effects only when given in the evening[10] when the immunoenhancing effect of melatonin is highest. Exogenous melatonin reverses beta-blocker-induced immunosuppression and enhances immune parameters (Figure 29.1).

Melatonin promotes inflammation; however, there are times when melatonin counteracts it. These effects, in fact, can be dependent on melatonin interaction with NF-κB. The hormone has been reported to inhibit NF-κB in various animal models.[63,64] As a matter of fact, melatonin is also able to activate NF-κB, thus regulating the expression of adhesion molecules on circulating leukocytes.[65,66] NF-κB, a determinant factor of inflammatory responses, is constitutively expressed in the pineal gland and the latter possesses receptors to trigger the NF-κB pathway.[30] Activation of NF-κB exaggerates inflammatory response including the release of the proinflammatory cytokines TNF-α, IL-1, and IL-6, whereas inhibition of pineal NF-κB leads to an enhancement of melatonin production.[30] In turn, melatonin inhibits the translocation of NF-κB to the nucleus[64] and inflammation mediated by NF-κB. It has been suggested that NF-κB inhibition can be achieved through activation of transcription factor Nrf2 which protects cells and tissues from oxidative stress by activating protective antioxidant and detoxifying enzymes. Reports that Nrf2 disruptions are associated with increased NF-κB further support this hypothesis.[67,68] The above mechanism further expands and integrates the complex role of melatonin in having both inflammatory and anti-inflammatory properties.

In addition to cytokines, glucocorticoids also transmit signals through a common NF-κB pathway to induce and turn off inflammatory responses[69] which can suggest even more profound effect

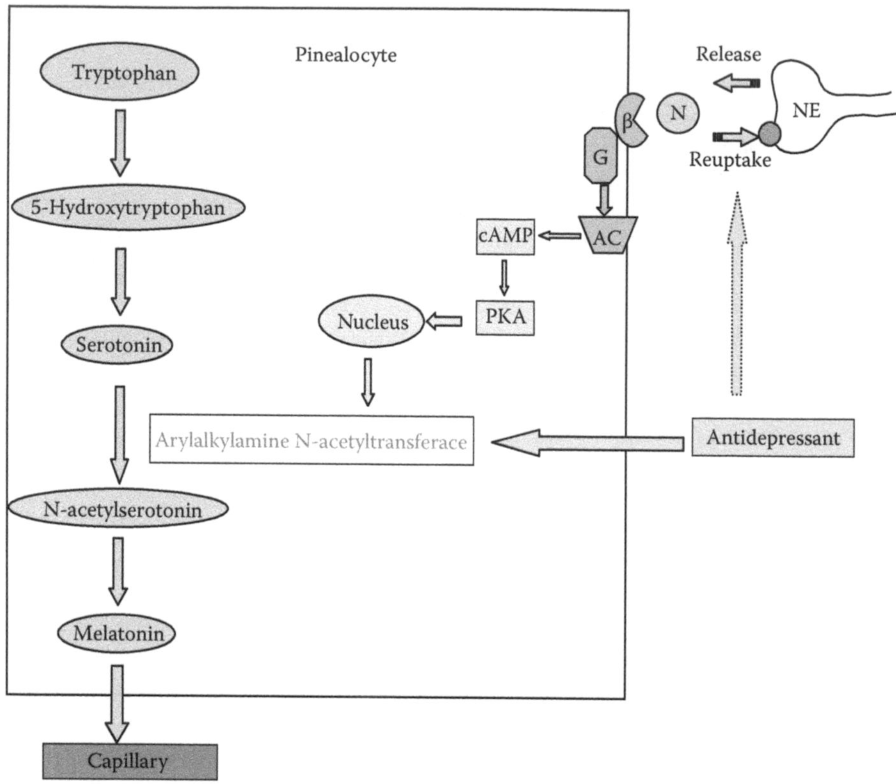

FIGURE 29.1 Possible mechanism of antidepressants in regulating melatoninergic function. Antidepressants have shown to increase melatonin levels directly by increasing arylalkylamine N-acetyltransferase,[134] and indirectly by inhibiting the reuptake of noradrenaline and thus increasing PKA.

of melatonin on inflammatory response. Melatonin has been shown to abolish several effects of exogenous corticoids inducing immunosuppression[62] and is believed to work as an anti-adrenocortical or antistress factor.[70] The melatonin/corticoid relationship is significant because high absolute levels of corticoids and disorganization of the normal rhythm of corticoid release are also involved in the pathogenesis of depression. In line with these findings, melatonin acts against the negative effects of stress on immune homeostasis.

Such characteristics as sleep duration can also entail variations in inflammatory markers. There are remarks on the elevated levels of IL-6 and CRP in women who are short sleepers.[71] Furthermore, abnormal IL-6 production is apparent across the melatonin circadian cycle in patients with major depression[38] which can suggest the immunoregulatory effect of the pineal gland and melatonin. Indeed, melatonin plays an important role in modulating humoral and cellular immune responses.[72] Leukocytes possess melatonin-specific receptors including both MT1/MT2 and high-affinity nuclear receptor RZR, and this provides the molecular basis for the sensitivity of leukocytes to melatonin. Moreover, leukocytes possess the enzymatic machinery necessary to synthesize melatonin.[73] Effects exerted by melatonin on immune parameters depend on many factors, including sex, age, immune system maturation, way of immune system activation, and stressful conditions.[74] Moreover, the differential proinflammatory and anti-inflammatory roles of melatonin might promote, regulate, and counteract inflammation simultaneously.[73]

Another main pathway by which cytokines can induce neuroendocrine abnormalities in depression involves tryptophan metabolism. Tryptophan leads either to the synthesis of serotonin and

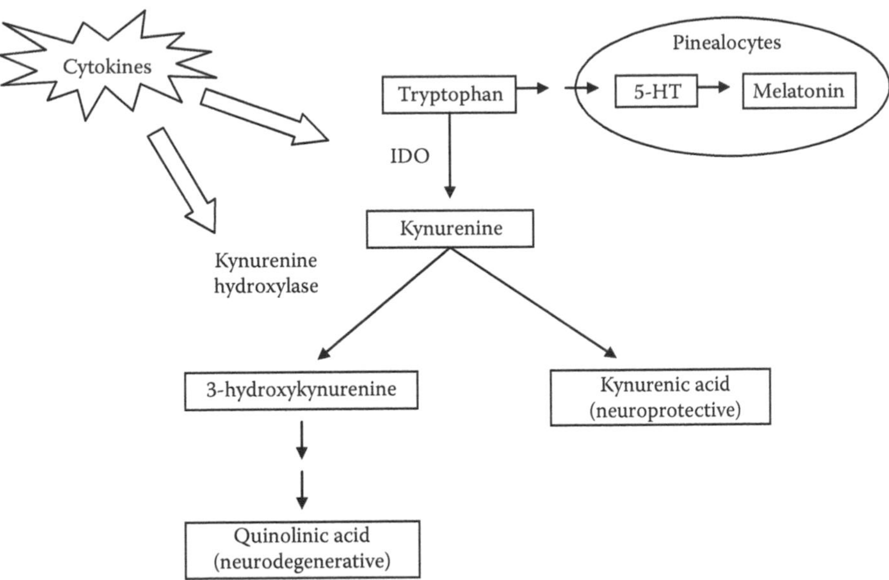

FIGURE 29.2 The effect of cytokines on the kynurenine pathway may be involved in the reduced levels of melatonin found in depressed patients.

melatonin or to the kynurenine pathway. Tryptophan via indoleamine 2,3-dioxygenase (IDO) is converted into kynurenine, which, in turn, can take two different pathways: One leads to a neuroprotective metabolite kynurenic acid and the other through kynurene-3-monooxigenase (KMO) to neurotoxic metabolites (3-hydroxykynurenine and then quinolinic acid).[75] Proinflammatory cytokines are able to shift tryptophan metabolism toward a neurotoxic pathway: They enhance KMO, which degrades kynurenine into 3-hydroxykynurenine and thus diverts the kynurenine pathway more into the neurotoxic path.[76–78] The cytokine hypothesis suggests that external or psychosocial stressors and internal stressors such as organic inflammatory conditions may trigger depression via inflammatory processes.[79] The importance of IDO as a critical molecular mediator in the development of inflammation-induced depressive-like behavior has been recently reinforced by studies conducted by O'Connor and colleagues. They showed that peripheral administration of lipopolysaccharide (LPS) in mice activates IDO to induce a depressive-like behavioral syndrome and to increase the brain serotonin turnover. On the contrary, blockade of IDO activation either indirectly with an anti-inflammatory drug that attenuates LPS-induced expression of proinflammatory cytokines or directly with an IDO antagonist prevents the development of depressive-like behavior. Interestingly, both the anti-inflammatory drug and the IDO antagonist are able to normalize the kynurenine/tryptophan ratio. Moreover, administration of kynurenine to naive mice dose-dependently induces depressive-like behavior.[80]

All these findings, taken together, contribute to the idea that depression is the symptomatic manifestation of a multifactorial disease, which involves, in addition to the well-known psychological and social factors, underlying abnormalities in the complex constellation of neuroendocrine pathways and possibly the intercommunications among all these systems (Figure 29.2).

29.2 ANTIDEPRESSANT ACTION

How do antidepressants exert their therapeutic action? Although the exact etiopathogenesis of depression is not clear, to date, pharmacotherapy has targeted and modulated various sites of actions believed to be impaired in this major disease: monoamine levels, serotonin transporters, receptor abnormalities, neuropeptide systems, glutamatergic neurotransmission, HPA axis, and circadian rhythm misalignment.[81] In this chapter, we will focus the attention on the possible effects of antidepressants on the main neuroendocrine abnormalities found in depression, in particular, melatonin, cortisol, and immune system impairments.

29.2.1 Antidepressants on Melatonin

Many studies investigating the effects of antidepressants on melatonin synthesis, circulating levels, and metabolism have been done so far; almost all subtypes of antidepressants were tested, tricyclic antidepressants, tetracyclic, MAO inhibitors, serotonin–norepinephrine reuptake inhibitors (SNRIs), and selective serotonin reuptake inhibitors (SSRIs). We will elicit the major findings with regards to these effects starting with studies conducted on animals, then in depressed patients, and finally on healthy subjects. A summary of the findings on the effect of antidepressants on melatonin in depressed patients and in healthy subjects are shown in Tables 29.1 and 29.2, respectively. In 1977, Parfitt et al. showed that isolated pineal glands incubated with tryptophan and TCA desipramine showed increased levels of melatonin concentration and increased activity of N-acetyltransferase compared with controls.[82] Franklin et al. investigated the effects of the SNRI venlafaxine acute treatment on the levels of melatonin in rat pineal glands and found increased levels of melatonin after acute treatment.[83] These levels were then attenuated in subchronic treatment, possibly for adaptive desensitization of pinealocyte β-adrenoceptors. These findings are confirmed also by Cowen et al.[84] but they also showed that the night phase of melatonin is kept normal after 10 days of desipramine, which means that reduction of the sensibility of the adrenoceptors may be a part of the pineal adaptive process that keeps the pineal function normal after modification of the overall pineal synaptic function. Recently, one study conducted involving mice has showed a positive effect of the SSRI fluoxetine on the gene expression of AA-NAT hippocampus and striatum;[85] this suggests a possible way of modulating melatonin synthesis with antidepressants. In another study, fluvoxamine, another SSRI, showed an inhibitory effect on cytochrome peroxidase CYP450, implicated in melatonin catabolism,[86,87] but this was not confirmed by other antidepressants. Also, the SSRI paroxetine, given to supratherapeutic concentration, had an effect on CYT although without the magnitude of fluvoxamine. It is possible that one of the effects of antidepressants on melatonin is via inhibition of the melatonin catabolism (Figure 29.1). These previous studies of antidepressants on melatonin suggest a direct and indirect involvement; some putative mechanisms are shown here (Figure 29.2).

Also, some antidepressants seem to inhibit tryptophan catabolism, leading to a rise in its circulating levels: One study showed that paroxetine, in addition to inhibiting brain 5-HT turnover, enhanced 5-HT synthesis by increasing brain tryptophan concentration secondarily to inhibition of liver tryptophan pyrrolase (main tryptophan degrading enzyme) activity.[88] This mechanism may indirectly give to the pineal gland more substrate for the melatonin synthesis (Figure 29.2). Antidepressants may increase melatonin synthesis by shifting tryptophan metabolism towards the synthesis of serotonin and consequently melatonin. Studies conducted on depressed patients seem to confirm the idea that antidepressants modulate melatonin. Thompson et al. conducted a study on six depressed patients and six healthy volunteers and measured differences on melatonin levels after three weeks of treatment with desipramine: They found that melatonin was significantly increased after treatment compared to the control group.[89] Golden et al. measured the mean levels of aMT6s in 24-hour urinary samples in a court of 27 depressed patients, at baseline and after treatment, following three to six weeks of treatment with MAO inhibitors, tranylcypromine or clorgiline, or desipramine. They showed that all the three antidepressants significantly increased urinary aMT6s levels.[90] Eight depressed patients were treated for three weeks with desipramine and again showed increased urinary aMT6s after the first week.[91] Kennedy et al. conducted a study on 15 depressed females after one and six weeks, and they also found that antidepressants increased urinary aMT6s levels after one week[3]; interestingly, they showed normalization after six weeks. This normalization after the long-term treatment can be explained by a sort of adaptive mechanism by the pineal

TABLE 29.1
The Effect of Antidepressants on Melatonin in Depressed Patients

Name		Antidepressant	Treatment	Plasma Melatonin	Urinary aMT6s
Thompson	1985	Desipramine	3 weeks	↑	
Golden	1988	Tranylcypromine	3 to 6 weeks		↑
		Clorgiline			↑
		Desipramine			↑
Bearn	1989	Desipramine	1 day		=
			1 week		↑
			2 weeks		↑
			3 weeks		↑
Kennedy	1992	Desipramine	1 week		↑
			6 weeks		=
Palazidou	1992	Desipramine	After 1 day	↑	
			Six weeks	↑	
Brown	1996	Desipramine	5 weeks		↑
Jolanta Rabe-Jabłońska	2001	Clomipramine	8 weeks	↓	
Miller	2001	Fluvoxamine	6 weeks		↑ In responders
					↓ In nonresponders
		Imipramine	6 weeks		↑ In responders
					↓ In nonresponders
Schmidt	2006	Mirtrazapine	Long term (28 days)	↑	
Carvalho	2008	Fluoxetine	8 weeks		=
		Duloxetine			↑
					↑
					↑

TABLE 29.2
The Effect of Antidepressants on Melatonin in Healthy Subjects

Name		Antidepressant	Treatment	Plasma Melatonin	Urinary aMT6s
Cowen	1985	Desipramine	Acute	↑	
			3 weeks	=	
Demisch	1986	Fluvoxamine	Acute (Once)	↑	
Demish	1987	Tranylcypromine	Baseline–3 weeks	= - =	
		Pirlindole	"	= - =	
		Maprotiline	"	= - =	
		Fluvoxamine	"	↑ - ↑	
Franey	1986	Desipramine	Acute	↑	↑
Palazidou	1989	Mirtazapine	Acute	↑	
Palazidou	1992	(+)Oxaprotiline	3 weeks	↑	
		(-)Oxaprotiline	3 weeks	=	
D.J. Skene	1994	Fluvoxamine	Acute	↑	↓
		Desipramine	Acute	=	↑
Markus	2010	Clomipramine	Acute		↑
			3 weeks		=

gland β1-adrenoceptors to the constant high levels of noradrenaline in the synaptic cleft. Palazidou et al. also tested desipramine in eight patients with endogenous depression and found an increase in plasma melatonin after one day and after six weeks of treatment.[92] In contrast, a study measured plasma melatonin before and after eight weeks of TCA clomipramine treatment in 20 depressed patients compared with 14 healthy subjects; surprisingly, the study showed that depressed patients had a higher level of both diurnal and nocturnal melatonin compared with control. Additionally, previous studies showed that clomipramine treatment significantly increased diurnal melatonin while controversially decreased nocturnal secretion, but this latter finding was not significant.[93] Miller et al. showed melatonin response after treatment of 24 outpatients meeting Diagnosis and Statistical Manual for Mental Health III (DSM-III-R) criteria for major depression with either SSRI fluvoxamine or TCA imipramine for six weeks and measured urinary aMT6s; the results divided responders who showed an increase in the metabolite and nonresponders who showed instead a decrease; this suggests that pineal reactivity may be a potential biomarker of the patient response to the treatment.[94] Schmid et al. analyzed 10 depressed patients' melatonin secretion after 28 days of treatment with mirtazapine and saw a significant increase in plasma melatonin.[95] Carvalho et al. showed an increase in melatonin production after treatment with fluoxetine and SNRI duloxetine in drug-free depressed patients compared with placebo; both groups had the same improvement in emotional states, suggesting a pharmacological effect of antidepressants on melatonin, but possibly not directly related to their therapeutic action. Similar results were found observing melatonin modulation by antidepressants in healthy subjects.[96] Cowen et al. showed the effect of desipramine on 10 healthy volunteers for three weeks: They measured an initial increase in plasma melatonin (first week) and a progressive decrease for the other days of treatment until it reached again the normal levels.[97] They also measured a rebound after the treatment was withdrawn, which was explained as follows: Desipramine causes an adaptive inhibition of the presynaptic junction firing rate that leads to a desensitization of the presynaptic a2 adrenoceptors, implicated in the control of the negative feedback on the presynaptic portion; when desipramine is withdrawn, there is an increased firing rate of the prejunctional synapses, which, in the presence of reduced negative feedback, leads to an increased NA outflow and, thus, in plasma melatonin secretion. Another study showed an increase in plasma melatonin after one single administration of fluvoxamine in six healthy subjects measured one and two days after administration.[98] One year after, the same authors showed the effect of MAO inhibitors tranylcypromine and pirlindole, the TeAC maprotiline, the fluvoxamine, and the serotonin S2-receptor antagonist mianserin administered each to groups of four to seven healthy subjects for three weeks. They showed a significant increase in plasma melatonin only with fluvoxamine.[99] Moreover, Franey et al. analyzed the desipramine effect on eight male volunteers administered at 16:00 hours and showed an increase in plasma melatonin at 21:00, 22:00, 23:00, and 24:00 hours after administration and an increase in nocturnal aMT6s at 23:00 and 24:00 hours; no significant effect on the total aMT6s in one day was shown, so it is likely that these effects of desipramine were due to the increase in synaptic noradrenaline availability in consequence of the inhibition of noradrenaline (NE) reuptake into pineal synaptic junctions. In this study, the increase in plasma melatonin was not significant at late hours; this can be due to the fact that the maximum functional pineal gland capacity of synthesizing melatonin was reached, or due to pineal β-adrenoceptors' adaptive desensitization to high levels of noradrenaline.[100] Another study in favor of this is that by Palazidou et al. who gave a selective inhibitor of noradrenaline reuptake in either (+) oxaprotiline, the active form, or (–) oxaprotiline, the inactive form, to 10 male volunteers for three weeks; their study showed an increase in night plasma melatonin in the group who received the active form, measured at baseline, first, seventh, and at the end of the three weeks.[101] This was in accordance to what they found some years before after giving mirtazapine to 10 healthy volunteers: again, melatonin increased.[102] Some other interesting findings come from Skene et al. in their study on fluvoxamine and desipramine administration to eight healthy volunteers. They found an acute increase in plasma melatonin with both drugs, markedly with fluvoxamine; these drugs also increased the duration of the whole melatonin secretion: desipramine by advancing the onset and fluvoxamine by delaying the offset. Fluvoxamine also delayed the acrophase, whereas with desipramine, it came earlier. Moreover, their study showed an increase in aMT6s after desipramine, whereas it showed a decrease in the metabolite by fluvoxamine in night samples.[103] These findings are in accord with the idea that desipramine, a noradrenaline reuptake inhibitor, increases melatonin synthesis, and suggest that fluvoxamine interferes mostly with melatonin catabolism. Markus et al. showed an acute increase in the melatonin metabolite after clomipramine administration in 32 healthy subjects. However, the same subjects showed a normalization of the pineal activity after long-term administration. The increase in melatonin seemed also associated with an improvement of the emotional state.[104] This long list of findings supports the idea that antidepressants can modulate the production of melatonin: Possible mechanism seems to be the increased stimulation of pineal β-adrenoceptors from the increased concentration of noradrenaline in the synaptic cleft; this effect though seems regulated by an adaptive desensitization of the receptors; another mechanism of action can be the increased stimulation of SNC by the serotonergic projection from the raphe nucleus, which modulates the response of the suprachiasmatic nucleus to the light signals from the retinohypothalamic tract; a third mechanism can involve the regulation of melatonin catabolism. Moreover, there are suggestions of interactions between antidepressant and expression of enzymes involved in melatonin synthesis. Melatonin can also be modulated by a possible increase in circulating serotonin: Some antidepressants like fluoxetine and MAO inhibitors increase plasma serotonin.[105,106]

Few studies have been performed looking at the SSRI effect on melatonin. Apart from the study by Carvalho et al.[96] elicited before, Childs et al.[107] studied the effect of fluoxetine on 10 patients with seasonal affective disorder and found an increase in melatonin levels. Contrary to this result, Nathan et al.[108] tested paroxetine on eight healthy controls and measured no differences in melatonin levels before and after treatment. Recently, Tan et al.[109] have shown no particular effect of fluoxetine on melatonin levels in 13 depressed patients compared with control, but interestingly, they have found a positive correlation between the amplitude of melatonin secretion and the improvement of the recovery of depression.

29.2.2 Antidepressant and GR Function

Glucocorticoids exert their physiological action through GR, and since the HPA axis impairment is implicated in the development of depression, we believe that antidepressants may have an effect on these receptors. There are several studies that demonstrate that antidepressants up-regulate GR: Peiffer et al. showed an increase in hippocampal and hypothalamic GR mRNA levels in rats after administration of desipramine or imipramine[110]; also, Pariante et al. showed that antidepressant treatment for four weeks increased GR expression, promoted GR nuclear translocation, and enhanced GR function.[50,111] The same effect has been shown also by Okugawa et al. who studied the antidepressant effects on tricyclic and SSRI antidepressants on animal neuronal cells.[112] Also, Carvalho et al. showed an up-regulation in the peripheral red blood cells of the GR function.[113] We saw that glucocorticoids interact with the pineal gland stimulating the production of melatonin through GR binding and consequent inhibition of NF-κB. It is possible that abnormalities in the GR function can partially explain the melatonin impairments found in depressed patients, and the restoration of the GR function can be related to their therapeutic effect. Antidepressants have shown to also have an effect on the circulating levels of corticosteroids as reported by many recent studies. Fluoxetine effectively decreased cortisol levels in alcohol-treated rats.[114] Binder et al. measured cortisol levels, as an indication of HPA activity, in 194 patients with major depression and found an association between remission and restoration of the HPA axis hyperactivity; moreover, they found that the integrity of the HPA axis negative feedback, assessed with the dexamethasone suppression test, predicted the responsiveness to antidepressants in male patients.[115] Another study showed that five weeks of administration of mirtazapine in 23 patients with major depression decreased levels of cortisol and dehydroepiandrosterone (DHEA), an androgen secreted by the adrenal gland; in addition, the increase in DHEA was correlated with the score in the Hamilton questionnaire.[116] In another study,[117] 70 depressed patients received either venlafaxine or mirtazapine for four weeks, and responders had a decline in the levels of DHEA-sulfate, which can be used to assess the HPA axis function.[118]

In 2009, Juruena et al. compared 45 inpatients with major depression who are treatment-resistant to at least two antidepressants, after 20 weeks of treatments, with 46 controls and found that patients with severe depression had hyperactivity of the HPA axis but had normal negative feedback functionality, whereas treatment-resistant patients had an abnormal negative feedback response assessed by prednisolone activation of glucocorticoid and MR.[119] In spite of this, two studies[120,121] measuring the effects of venlafaxine or sertraline on cortisol and showing no effect or even an increased level; however, these studies analyzed are limited by the small size of their cohorts, whereas previous studies refer to a much bigger sample size and are thus more reliable. In this review, we saw how glucocorticoids can interact with the pineal gland stimulating the production of melatonin through GR binding and consequent inhibition of NF-κB. It is thus possible that abnormalities in the GR function can partially explain the melatonin impairments found in depressed patients and the capacity.

Finally, a new antidepressant drug called Agomelatine has recently entered in the market, and it gives promising results: It has both a 5-HT 2c receptor antagonist and melatonergic properties, combining the effect of the melatonergic and serotonergic systems and having antidepressant activity.[122,123] It also has the capacity of re-entraining disrupted circadian rhythms, as shown in studies on rats,[124,125] on healthy subjects,[126,127] and on depressed patients[128–130]; also, it has been shown to have a good safety pattern of a side effect,[131] in particular, a side effect related to sexual impairment found in other antidepressants[132]; finally, it has shown a few discontinuation symptoms after withdrawal compared to SSRI paroxetine.[133]

29.3 CONCLUSIONS

Throughout this review, we have analyzed the neuroendocrinological point of view. Melatonin, circadian rhythms, HPA axis, and proinflammatory cytokines seem to be impaired in depressed patients. Compared to the normal population, melatonin seems to have lower nocturnal levels, phase shifts, or amplitude variations of its circadian rhythms, and impaired β-adrenoceptors have been found; these abnormalities have been positively correlated to the severity of depression. A recent study has also tried to find some genetic bases of these alterations, and interesting results have associated depression with the presence of particular polymorphism in genes of enzymes for melatonin synthesis. Depressed patients have shown impaired circadian rhythms like sleep/wake cycles, core body temperature, and cortisol and melatonin diurnal variation; interestingly, the severity of depression has been correlated with alteration in the amplitude of these circadian rhythms and with phase angles between the onset of melatonin and the nadir of the core body temperature.

Furthermore, HPA axis abnormalities are revealed in depression: in particular, altered GR function, impaired negative feedback, and HPA hyperactivity resulting in chronic high levels of cortisol, which is known to negatively affect the central nervous system. Finally, depressed patients show high levels of proinflammatory cytokines, which chronically can induce depressive-like behavior, and low levels of anti-inflammatory cytokines. This hyperactivity of the immune system can interact with tryptophan metabolism, leading to an increased production of neurodegenerative compounds. All these main neuroendocrine alterations seem to be linked together: Melatonin, as well as its known properties of modulating circadian rhythms, has shown to modulate the immune system activity, showing proinflammatory and anti-inflammatory actions, and to interfere with the HPA axis and cortisol secretion; corticosteroids, apart from their established immunosuppressive action, seem to have an up-regulatory action upon melatonin synthesis; cytokines have proven to down-regulate GR, and inflammation has shown to down-regulate the synthesis of melatonin. Antidepressants, apart from their well-established modulation of the synaptic monoamine levels, seem to have positive effects on the neuroendocrine alteration found in depressed patients. In the majority of studies, they have shown to increase nocturnal melatonin levels mainly because of their noradrenergic action and stimulation, and, in some part, also for a serotonergic action. It seems also that the capacity of antidepressants to normalize the HPA activity is a key component of their therapeutic action: Decreasing cortisol levels and restoration of the negative feedback by up-regulating the GR function seem to be the peculiar effects to responders of the treatment, whereas a lack of these effects is found among nonresponders. Finally, antidepressants have shown an anti-inflammatory effect, decreasing proinflammatory and increasing anti-inflammatory cytokines. Interesting results have recently come up from the discovery of the antidepressant activity of Agomelatine, a molecule with both melatonergic and serotonergic activities, and its capacity in restoring circadian rhythms which we will now summarize. Melatonin, cortisol, and proinflammatory cytokine levels have shown to be impaired in depressive patients: low nocturnal melatonin levels, high cortisol levels, and high proinflammatory cytokines. In conclusion, we can say that, one possible therapeutic action that seems restored after treatment with antidepressants may lie in the antidepressants' capacity of positively affecting neurobiological impairments: stimulating pineal synthesis of melatonin, which has shown beneficial effects on depression, modulating the hyperactivity of the immune system, and, in responders, restoring the HPA axis function, possibly modulating the GR function. Further research in this field will help in understanding the reasons underlying the responsiveness to treatments and in developing more effective treatments. How can this be possible? Is this a part of the therapeutic effect of the antidepressant treatments? We saw that tryptophan metabolism plays a central role in connecting these three systems. Tryptophan can take different metabolic pathways. Through one, it produces serotonin and melatonin, and is controlled, among other factors, by the activity of the Aa-Nat enzyme. Another, controlled by the IDO enzyme, produces kynurenine that can be transformed into either neuroprotective or neurotoxic metabolites. Proinflammatory cytokines can induce a shift of the tryptophan metabolism toward the production of neurotoxic compounds. Moreover, inflammation has proved to inhibit melatonin production through NF-κB and TNF-α. Overall, depressed patients show high levels of these cytokines. Therefore, we can think that these patients have high levels of neurotoxic metabolites and low levels of melatonin. The monoamine theory of depression states that a low level of neurotransmitters, such as serotonin and noradrenaline, is an evidence of the disease; we know that most antidepressants increase the synaptic levels of these neurotransmitters. Since melatonin is under the circadian noradrenergic control of the hypothalamus, we can speculate that depressed patients possibly show low levels of melatonin because of a decrease in NE neurotransmission, and melatonin increases after treatment because of an increased availability of NE. Glucocorticoids should play an inhibitory role on the immune systems, but in depressed patients, this function is impaired. We showed that a possible explanation of this lies on the decreased function of their receptors (GR). GR has also been found on pineal glands, and we know that cortisol can stimulate melatonin synthesis, so the GR impairment theory could also explain the coexistence of high cortisol and low melatonin levels found in depressed patients. Melatonin has shown a wide range of activities: controls sleep, is neuroprotective, is antioxidant, and, in some cases, inhibits proinflammatory cytokines. What do antidepressants have to do with all of this? Studies showed that they can restore GR function, can inhibit cytokine levels, and directly stimulate melatonin metabolism. Therefore, restoring the GR function can play a role in solving HPA axis impairment, glucocorticoid resistance can be counteracted, and corticosteroids can exert their immunosuppressive action. This is in fact shown in depressed patients who, after treatment, have low levels of inflammatory cytokines. Having said this, we can consider that perhaps there is more circulating tryptophan which can go into the pinealocytes and take the serotonin–melatonin pathway. Antidepressants have shown also both a direct positive effect on melatonin enzyme Aa-nat, stimulating its synthesis, and an indirect (fluvoxamine) effect on melatonin catabolism by inhibiting liver enzymes. Antidepressants, moreover, exert their main action by inhibiting reuptake of either serotonin or noradrenaline, and in some cases both. Therefore, it is clear that they can increase either pineal noradrenergic stimulation, serotonin availability, or both. These ideas can explain the findings by many studies about antidepressant action on depressed patients which showed an increase in either nocturnal melatonin or urinary aMT6s after treatment. Studies on healthy volunteers confirm this hypothesis. The pineal gland seems also to have a sort of adaptive mechanism in regulating pinealocyte adrenoceptor sensitivity in a way that hyperstimulation by noradrenaline can, in the long term, desensitize the receptors. Studies on isolated rat pineal glands focus mainly on this, stating that antidepressants act mainly in desensitizing beta adrenoceptors, but the treatment administrations in rats are not exactly comparable with human studies: The length of the administration is much shorter, and isolated pineal glands from rats may not take into consideration all the neurobiological mechanisms underlying depression in humans. In conclusion, this review confirms the existence of an interrelationship between immune–pineal–HPA axis and suggests that this system is involved in depression. This hypothesis opens a new avenue to the fact that melatonin may be a sensor and a player in depression.

ACKNOWLEDGMENTS

Some of the work presented here has been funded by the NARSAD – Brain and Behaviour Research Foundation, formerly, National Alliance for Research on Schizophrenia and Depression and the Commission of European Communities 7th Framework Programme Collaborative Project Grant Agreement no. 22963 (Mood Inflame). Marco Antonioli was funded by ERASMUS Placement Grant within the LLP/ERASMUS Placement Programme. Livia A. Carvalho is funded by the NARSAD Young Investigator Award 2009, the European College of Psychopharmacology (ECNP) Young Investigator Award 2010, and the British Council Partnership in Science with Platform Beta Techniek. The authors have no relevant financial interest to disclose.

REFERENCES

1. Kessler RC. Epidemiology of women and depression. J Affect Disord 2003; 74:5–13.
2. Maronde E, Stehle JH. The mammalian pineal gland: known facts, unknown facets. Trends Endocrinol Metab 2007 May;18(4):142–9.
3. Kennedy SH, Brown GM. Effect of chronic antidepressant treatment with adinazolam and desipramine on melatonin output. Psychiatry Res 1992; 43:177–85.
4. Demisch L. Clinical pharmacology of melatonin regulation. In: Yu H-SRRJ, editor. Melatonin, Biosynthesis, Physiological Effects and Clinical Applications. Boca Raton, Florida: CRC Press; 1993. pp. 513–40.
5. Beck-Friis J, Kjellman BF, Aperia B, Unden F, von Rosen D, Ljunggren JG, et al. Serum melatonin in relation to clinical variables in patients with major depressive disorder and a hypothesis of a low melatonin syndrome. Acta Psychiatr Scand 1985; 71:319–30.
6. Beck-Friis J, Ljunggren JG, Thoren M, von RD, Kjellman BF, Wetterberg L. Melatonin, cortisol and ACTH in patients with major depressive disorder and healthy humans with special reference to the outcome of the dexamethasone suppression test. Psychoneuroendocrinology 1985; 10:173–86.
7. Claustrat B, Chazot G, Brun J, Jordan D, Sassolas G. A chronobiological study of melatonin and cortisol secretion in depressed subjects: plasma melatonin, a biochemical marker in major depression. Biol Psychiatry 1984; 19:1215–28.
8. Carvalho LA, Gorenstein C, Moreno RA, Markus RP. Melatonin levels in drug-free patients with major depression from the southern hemisphere. Psychoneuroendocrinology 2006; 31:761–8.
9. Crasson M, Kjiri S, Colin A, Kjiri K, L'Hermite-Baleriaux M, Ansseau M, et al. Serum melatonin and urinary 6-sulfatoxymelatonin in major depression. Psychoneuroendocrinology 2004 Jan;29(1):1–12.
10. Paparrigopoulos T. Melatonin response to atenolol administration in depression: indication of beta-adrenoceptor dysfunction in a subtype of depression. Acta Psychiatr Scand 2002 Dec;106(6):440–5.
11. Tuunainen A, Kripke DF, Elliott JA, Assmus JD, Rex KM, Klauber MR, et al. Depression and endogenous melatonin in postmenopausal women. J Affect Disord 2002; 69:149–58.
12. Brown R, Kocsis JH, Caroff S, Amsterdam J, Winokur A, Stokes PE, et al. Differences in nocturnal melatonin secretion between melancholic depressed patients and control subjects. Am J Psychiatry 1985; 142:811–6.
13. Fountoulakis KN, Karamouzis M, Iacovides A, Nimatoudis J, Diakogiannis J, Kaprinis G, et al. Morning and evening plasma melatonin and dexamethasone suppression test in patients with nonseasonal major depressive disorder from northern Greece (latitude 40–41.5 degrees). Neuropsychobiology 2001; 44:113–7.

14. Parry BL, Meliska CJ, Sorenson DL, López AM, Martínez LF, Nowakowski S, et al. Increased melatonin and delayed offset in menopausal depression: role of years past menopause, follicle-stimulating hormone, sleep end time, and body mass index. J Clin Endocrinol Metab 2008; 93:54–60. Epub 2007 Nov 27.
15. Ostrowska Z, Zwirska-Korczala K, Buntner B, Pardela M, Drozdz M. Association of body mass and body fat distribution with serum melatonin levels in obese women either non-operated or after jejunoileostomy. Endocr Regul 1996 Mar;30(1):33–40.
16. Wetterberg L, Bratlid T, von Knorring L, Eberhard G, Yuwiler A. A multinational study of the relationships between nighttime urinary melatonin production, age, gender, body size, and latitude. Eur Arch Psychiatry Clin Neurosci 1999;249(5):256–62.
17. Arendt J, Wirz-Justice A, Bradtke J. Annual rhythm of serum melatonin in man. Neurosci Lett 77 A.D.;7:327–30.
18. Weil ZM, Hotchkiss AK, Gatien ML, Pieke-Dahl S, Nelson RJ. Melatonin receptor (MT1) knockout mice display depression-like behaviors and deficits in sensorimotor gating. Brain Res Bull 2006 Feb 15;68(6):425–9.
19. Wu YH, Zhou JN, Balesar R, Unmehopa U, Bao A, Jockers R, et al. Distribution of MT1 melatonin receptor immunoreactivity in the human hypothalamus and pituitary gland: colocalization of MT1 with vasopressin, oxytocin, and corticotropin-releasing hormone. J Comp Neurol 2006 Dec 20;499(6):897–910.
20. Gałecki P, Szemraj J, Bartosz G, Bieńkiewicz M, Gałecka E, Florkowski A, et al. Single-nucleotide polymorphisms and mRNA expression for melatonin synthesis rate-limiting enzyme in recurrent depressive disorder. J Pineal Res 2010; 48:311–7.
21. Gold PW, Goodwin FK, Chrousos GP. Clinical and biochemical manifestations of depression. Relation to the neurobiology of stress (1). N Engl J Med 1988; 319:348–53.
22. Nemeroff CB. The corticotropin-releasing factor (CRF) hypothesis of depression: new findings and new directions. Mol Psychiatry 1996; 1:336–42.
23. Carroll BJ, Feinberg M, Greden JF, Tarika J, Albala AA, Haskett RF, et al. A specific laboratory test for the diagnosis of melancholia. Standardization, validation, and clinical utility. Archives of General Psychiatry 1981; 38:15–22.
24. Axelson DA, Doraiswamy PM, Boyko OB, Rodrigo EP, McDonald WM, Ritchie JC, et al. In vivo assessment of pituitary volume with magnetic resonance imaging and systematic stereology: relationship to dexamethasone suppression test results in patients. Psychiatry Res 1992; 44:63–70.
25. Pariante CM, Vassilopoulou K, Velakoulis D, Phillips L, Soulsby B, Wood SJ, et al. Pituitary volume in psychosis. Br J Psychiatry 2004; 185:5–10.
26. Pariante CM, Dazzan P, Danese A, Morgan KD, Brudaglio F, Morgan C, et al. Increased pituitary volume in antipsychotic-free and antipsychotic-treated patients of the AEsop first-onset psychosis study. Neuropsychopharmacology 2005; 30:1923–31.
27. Merali Z, Du L, Hrdina P, Palkovits M, Faludi G, Poulter MO, et al. Dysregulation in the suicide brain: mRNA expression of corticotropin-releasing hormone receptors and GABA(A) receptor subunits in frontal cortical brain region. J Neurosci 2004; 24:1478–85.
28. Dumser T, Barocka A, Schubert E. Weight of adrenal glands may be increased in persons who commit suicide. Am J Forensic Med Pathol 1998; 19:72–6.
29. Carvalho LA, Juruena MF, Papadopoulos A, Poon L, Cleare A, Pariante CM. Clomipramine and Glucocorticoid receptor Function. Neuropsychopharmacology 2009;34(9):2194–5.
30. da SC-M, Carvalho-Sousa CE, Tamura EK, Pinato L, Cecon E, Fernandes PA, et al. TLR4 and CD14 receptors expressed in rat pineal gland trigger NFKB pathway. J Pineal Res 2010 Sep;49(2):183–92.
31. Ferreira ZS, Fernandes PA, Duma D, Assreuy J, Avellar MC, Markus RP. Corticosterone modulates noradrenaline-induced melatonin synthesis through inhibition of nuclear factor kappa B. J Pineal Res 2005; 38:182–8.
32. Fernandes PA, Bothorel B, Clesse D, Monteiro AW, Calgari C, Raison S, et al. Local corticosterone infusion enhances nocturnal pineal melatonin production in vivo. J Neuroendocrinol 2009; 21:90–7.
33. Iuvone PM, Tosini G, Pozdeyev N, Haque R, Klein DC, Chaurasia SS. Circadian clocks, clock networks, arylalkylamine N-acetyltransferase, and melatonin in the retina. Prog Retin Eye Res 2005 Jul;24(4):433–56.
34. Lopes C, deLyra JL, Markus RP, Mariano M. Circadian rhythm in experimental granulomatous inflammation is modulated by melatonin. J Pineal Res 1997; 23:72–8.
35. Lopes C, Mariano M, Markus RP. Interaction between the adrenal and the pineal gland in chronic experimental inflammation induced by BCG in mice. Inflamm Res 2001; 50:6–11.

36. Brietzke E, Stertz L, Fernandes BS, Kauer-Sant'Anna M, Mascarenhas M, Escosteguy VA, et al. Comparison of cytokine levels in depressed, manic and euthymic patients with bipolar disorder. J Affect Disord 2009 Aug;116(3):214–7.
37. Jehn CF, Kuhnhardt D, Bartholomae A, Pfeiffer S, Schmid P, Possinger K, et al. Association of IL-6, Hypothalamus-Pituitary-Adrenal Axis Function, and Depression in Patients With Cancer. Integr Cancer Ther 2010 Aug 11.
38. Alesci S, Martinez PE, Kelkar S, Ilias I, Ronsaville DS, Listwak SJ, et al. Major depression is associated with significant diurnal elevations in plasma interleukin-6 levels, a shift of its circadian rhythm, and loss of physiological complexity in its secretion: clinical implications. J Clin Endocrinol Metab 2005 May;90(5):2522–30.
39. Bouhuys AL, Flentge F, Oldehinkel AJ, van dB. Potential psychosocial mechanisms linking depression to immune function in elderly subjects. Psychiatry Res 2004 Jul 15;127(3):237–45.
40. Tiemeier H, Hofman A, van Tuijl HR, Kiliaan AJ, Meijer J, Breteler MM. Inflammatory proteins and depression in the elderly. Epidemiology 2003 Jan;14(1):103–7.
41. Ford DE, Erlinger TP. Depression and C-reactive protein in US adults: data from the Third National Health and Nutrition Examination Survey. Arch Intern Med 2004 May 10;164(9):1010–4.
42. Danner M, Kasl SV, Abramson JL, Vaccarino V. Association between depression and elevated C-reactive protein. Psychosom Med 2003 May;65(3):347–56.
43. Capuron L, Miller AH. Cytokines and psychopathology: lessons from interferon-alpha. Biol Psychiatry 2004 Dec 1; 56(11):819–24.
44. Pariante CM, Pearce BD, Pisell TL, Sanchez CI, Po C, Su C, et al. The proinflammatory cytokine, interleukin-1alpha, reduces glucocorticoid receptor translocation and function. Endocrinology 1999 Sep;140(9):4359–66.
45. Orru MG, Baita A, Sitzia R, Costa A, Muntoni E, Landau S, et al. [Interferon-alpha-induced psychiatric side effects in patients with chronic viral hepatitis: a prospective, observational, controlled study]. Epidemiol Psichiatr Soc 2005 Jul;14(3):145–53.
46. Musselman DL, Lawson DH, Gumnick JF, Manatunga AK, Penna S, Goodkin RS, et al. Paroxetine for the prevention of depression induced by high-dose interferon alfa. N Engl J Med 2001 Mar 29;344(13):961–6.
47. Huang Y, Henry CJ, Dantzer R, Johnson RW, Godbout JP. Exaggerated sickness behavior and brain proinflammatory cytokine expression in aged mice in response to intracerebroventricular lipopolysaccharide. Neurobiol Aging 2008 Nov;29(11):1744–53.
48. Maddock C, Pariante CM. How does stress affect you? An overview of stress, immunity, depression and disease. Epidemiol Psichiatr Soc 2001 Jul;10(3):153–62.
49. Spath-Schwalbe E, Hansen K, Schmidt F, Schrezenmeier H, Marshall L, Burger K, et al. Acute effects of recombinant human interleukin-6 on endocrine and central nervous sleep functions in healthy men. J Clin Endocrinol Metab 1998; 83:1573–9.
50. Pariante CM, Pearce BD, Pisell TL, Owens MJ, Miller AH. Steroid-independent translocation of the glucocorticoid receptor by the antidepressant desipramine. Mol Pharmacol 1997; 52:571–81.
51. Pierpaoli W. Neuroimmunomodulation of aging. A program in the pineal gland. Ann N Y Acad Sci 1998 May 1;840:491–7.
52. Skwarlo-Sonta K, Majewski P, Markowska M, Oblap R, Olszanska B. Bidirectional communication between the pineal gland and the immune system. Can J Physiol Pharmacol 2003 Apr;81(4):342–9.
53. Branchey L, Weinberg U, Branchey M, Linkowski P, Mendlewicz J. Simultaneous study of 24-hour patterns of melatonin and cortisol secretion in depressed patients. Neuropsychobiology 1982;8(5): 225–32.
54. Buckley TM, Schatzberg AF. A pilot study of the phase angle between cortisol and melatonin in major depression - a potential biomarker? J Psychiatr Res 2010 Jan;44(2):69–74.
55. Hasler BP, Buysse DJ, Kupfer DJ, Germain A. Phase relationships between core body temperature, melatonin, and sleep are associated with depression severity: further evidence for circadian misalignment in non-seasonal depression. Psychiatry Res 2010 Jun 30;178(1):205–7.
56. Blomeke B, Golka K, Griefahn B, Roemer HC. Arylalkylamine N-acetyltransferase (AANAT) genotype as a personal trait in melatonin synthesis. J Toxicol Environ Health A 2008;71(13-14):874–6.
57. Cardinali DP, Vacas MI, Keller Sarmiento MI, Etchegoyen GS, Pereyra EN, Chuluyan HE. Neuroendocrine integrative mechanisms in mammalian pineal gland: effects of steroid and adenohypophysial hormones on melatonin synthesis in vitro. J Steroid Biochem 1987;27(1-3):565–71.
58. Murray DR, Prabhu SD, Chandrasekar B. Chronic beta-adrenergic stimulation induces myocardial proinflammatory cytokine expression. Circulation 2000 May 23;101(20):2338–41.

59. Schauenstein K, Felsner P, Rinner I, Liebmann PM, Stevenson JR, Westermann J, et al. In vivo immunomodulation by peripheral adrenergic and cholinergic agonists/antagonists in rat and mouse models. Ann N Y Acad Sci 2000;917:618–27.
60. Mayer U, Wagenaar E, Dorobek B, Beijnen JH, Borst P, Schinkel AH. Full blockade of intestinal P-glycoprotein and extensive inhibition of blood-brain barrier P-glycoprotein by oral treatment of mice with PSC833. J Clin Invest 1997 Nov 15;100(10):2430–6.
61. Bierhaus A, Wolf J, Andrassy M, Rohleder N, Humpert PM, Petrov D, et al. A mechanism converting psychosocial stress into mononuclear cell activation. Proc Natl Acad Sci U S A 2003 Feb 18;100(4):1920–5.
62. Maestroni GJ, Conti A, Pierpaoli W. Role of the pineal gland in immunity. Circadian synthesis and release of melatonin modulates the antibody response and antagonizes the immunosuppressive effect of corticosterone. J Neuroimmunol 1986 Nov;13(1):19–30.
63. Chuang JI, Mohan N, Meltz ML, Reiter RJ. Effect of melatonin on NF-kappa-B DNA-binding activity in the rat spleen. Cell Biol Int 1996 Oct;20(10):687–92.
64. Mohan N, Sadeghi K, Reiter RJ, Meltz ML. The neurohormone melatonin inhibits cytokine, mitogen and ionizing radiation induced NF-kappa B. Biochem Mol Biol Int 1995 Dec;37(6):1063–70.
65. Cristofanon S, Uguccioni F, Cerella C, Radogna F, Dicato M, Ghibelli L, et al. Intracellular prooxidant activity of melatonin induces a survival pathway involving NF-kappaB activation. Ann N Y Acad Sci 2009 Aug;1171:472–8.
66. Cecon E, Fernandes PA, Pinato L, Ferreira ZS, Markus RP. Daily variation of constitutively activated nuclear factor kappa B (NFKB) in rat pineal gland. Chronobiol Int 2010 Jan;27(1):52–67.
67. Jin W, Wang H, Yan W, Xu L, Wang X, Zhao X, et al. Disruption of Nrf2 enhances upregulation of nuclear factor-kappaB activity, proinflammatory cytokines, and intercellular adhesion molecule-1 in the brain after traumatic brain injury. Mediators Inflamm 2008;2008:725174.
68. Thimmulappa RK, Lee H, Rangasamy T, Reddy SP, Yamamoto M, Kensler TW, et al. Nrf2 is a critical regulator of the innate immune response and survival during experimental sepsis. J Clin Invest 2006 Apr;116(4):984–95.
69. Smoak KA, Cidlowski JA. Mechanisms of glucocorticoid receptor signaling during inflammation. Mech Ageing Dev 2004 Oct;125(10-11):697–706.
70. Konakchieva R, Mitev Y, Almeida OF, Patchev VK. Chronic melatonin treatment counteracts glucocorticoid-induced dysregulation of the hypothalamic–pituitary–adrenal axis in the rat. Neuroendocrinology 1998; 67:171–80.
71. Miller MA, Kandala NB, Kivimaki M, Kumari M, Brunner EJ, Lowe GD, et al. Gender differences in the cross-sectional relationships between sleep duration and markers of inflammation: Whitehall II study. Sleep 2009 Jul 1;32(7):857–64.
72. Carrillo-Vico A, Guerrero JM, Lardone PJ, Reiter RJ. A review of the multiple actions of melatonin on the immune system. Endocrine 2005 Jul;27(2):189–200.
73. Radogna F, Diederich M, Ghibelli L. Melatonin: A pleiotropic molecule regulating inflammation. Biochem Pharmacol 2010 Aug 7.
74. Skwarlo-Sonta K. Melatonin in immunity: comparative aspects. Neuro Endocrinol Lett 2002 Apr;23 Suppl 1:61–6.
75. Zunszain PA, Anacker C, Cattaneo A, Carvalho LA, Pariante CM. Glucocorticoids, cytokines and brain abnormalities in depression. Prog Neuropsychopharmacol Biol Psychiatry 2010 Apr 18.
76. Wichers MC, Maes M. The role of indoleamine 2,3-dioxygenase (IDO) in the pathophysiology of interferon-alpha-induced depression. J Psychiatry Neurosci 2004; 29:11–7.
77. Wichers MC, Koek GH, Robaeys G, Verkerk R, Scharpe S, Maes M. IDO and interferon-alpha-induced depressive symptoms: a shift in hypothesis from tryptophan depletion to neurotoxicity. Mol Psychiatry 2005; 10:538–44.
78. Muller N, Schwarz MJ. The immune-mediated alteration of serotonin and glutamate: towards an integrated view of depression. Mol Psychiatry 2007; 12:988–1000.
79. Maes M, Yirmyia R, Noraberg J, Brene S, Hibbeln J, Perini G, et al. The inflammatory & neurodegenerative (I&ND) hypothesis of depression: leads for future research and new drug developments in depression. Metab Brain Dis 2009; 24:27–53.
80. O'Connor JC, Lawson MA, Andre C, Moreau M, Lestage J, Castanon N, et al. Lipopolysaccharide-induced depressive-like behavior is mediated by indoleamine 2,3-dioxygenase activation in mice. Mol Psychiatry 2009; 14:511–22.
81. Racagni G, Popoli M. The pharmacological properties of antidepressants. Int Clin Psychopharmacol 2010; 25:117–31.

82. Parfitt A, Klein DC. Increase caused by desmethylimipramine in the production of [3H]melatonin by isolated pineal glands. Biochem Pharmacol 1977; 26:904–5.
83. Franklin M, Clement EM, Campling G, Cowen PJ. Effect of venlafaxine on pineal melatonin and noradrenaline in the male rat. J Psychopharmacol 1998; 12:371–4.
84. Cowen PJ, Fraser S, Grahame-Smith DG, Green AR, Stanford C. The effect of chronic antidepressant administration on beta-adrenoceptor function of the rat pineal. Br J Pharmacol 1983; 78:89–96.
85. Uz T, Ahmed R, Akhisaroglu M, Kurtuncu M, Imbesi M, Dirim AA, et al. Effect of fluoxetine and cocaine on the expression of clock genes in the mouse hippocampus and striatum. Neuroscience 2005; 134:1309–16.
86. Pastrakuljic A, Tang BK, Roberts EA, Kalow W. Distinction of CYP1A1 and CYP1A2 activity by selective inhibition using fluvoxamine and isosafrole. Biochem Pharmacol 1997; 53:531–8.
87. Hartter S, Wang X, Weigmann H, Friedberg T, Arand M, Oesch F, et al. Differential effects of fluvoxamine and other antidepressants on the biotransformation of melatonin. J Clin Psychopharmacol 2001; 21:167–74.
88. Badawy AA, Morgan CJ. Effects of acute paroxetine administration on tryptophan metabolism and disposition in the rat. Br J Pharmacol 1991; 102:429–33.
89. Thompson C, Mezey G, Corn T, Franey C, English J, Arendt J, et al. The effect of desipramine upon melatonin and cortisol secretion in depressed and normal subjects. Br J Psychiatry 1985; 147:389–93.
90. Golden RN, Markey SP, Risby ED, Rudorfer MV, Cowdry RW, Potter WZ. Antidepressants reduce whole-body norepinephrine turnover while enhancing 6-hydroxymelatonin output. Arch Gen Psychiatry 1988; 45:150–4.
91. Bearn J, Franey C, Arendt J, Checkley SA. A study of the effects of desipramine treatment alone and in combination with L-triiodothyronine on 6-sulphatoxymelatonin excretion in depressed patients. Br J Psychiatry 1989; 155:341–7.
92. Palazidou E, Papadopoulos A, Ratcliff H, Dawling S, Checkley SA. Noradrenaline uptake inhibition increases melatonin secretion, a measure of noradrenergic neurotransmission, in depressed patients. Psychol Med 1992; 22:309–15.
93. Rabe-Jablonska J, Szymanska A. Diurnal profile of melatonin secretion in the acute phase of major depression and in remission. Med Sci Monit 2001 Sep;7(5):946–52.
94. Miller HL, Ekstrom RD, Mason GA, Lydiard RB, Golden RN. Noradrenergic function and clinical outcome in antidepressant pharmacotherapy. Neuropsychopharmacology 2001; 24:617–23.
95. Schmid DA, Wichniak A, Uhr M, Ising M, Brunner H, Held K, et al. Changes of sleep architecture, spectral composition of sleep EEG, the nocturnal secretion of cortisol, ACTH, GH, prolactin, melatonin, ghrelin, and leptin, and the DEX-CRH test in depressed patients during treatment with mirtazapine. Neuropsychopharmacology 2006; 31:832–44.
96. Carvalho LA, Gorenstein C, Moreno R, Pariante C, Markus RP. Effect of antidepressants on melatonin metabolite in depressed patients. J Psychopharmacol 2009; 23:315–21.
97. Cowen PJ, Green AR, Grahame-Smith DG, Braddock LE. Plasma melatonin during desmethylimipramine treatment: evidence for changes in noradrenergic transmission. Br J Clin Pharmacol 1985; 19:799–805.
98. Demisch K, Demisch L, Bochnik HJ, Nickelsen T, Althoff PH, Schoffling K, et al. Melatonin and cortisol increase after fluvoxamine. Br J Clin Pharmacol 1986; 22:620–2.
99. Demisch K, Demisch L, Nickelsen T, Rieth R. The influence of acute and subchronic administration of various antidepressants on early morning melatonin plasma levels in healthy subjects: increases following fluvoxamine. J Neural Transm 1987; 68:257–70.
100. Franey C, Aldhous M, Burton S, Checkley S, Arendt J. Acute treatment with desipramine stimulates melatonin and 6-sulphatoxy melatonin production in man. Br J Clin Pharmacol 1986; 22:73–9.
101. Palazidou E, Skene D, Arendt J, Everitt B, Checkley SA. The acute and chronic effects of (+) and (-) oxaprotiline upon melatonin secretion in normal subjects. Psychol Med 1992; 22:61–7.
102. Palazidou E, Papadopoulos A, Sitsen A, Stahl S, Checkley S. An alpha 2 adrenoceptor antagonist, Org 3770, enhances nocturnal melatonin secretion in man. Psychopharmacology (Berl) 1989; 97:115–7.
103. Skene DJ, Bojkowski CJ, Arendt J. Comparison of the effects of acute fluvoxamine and desipramine administration on melatonin and cortisol production in humans. Br J Clin Pharmacol 1994; 37:181–6.
104. Markus RP, Franco DG, Carvalho LA, Gentil V, Gorenstein C. Acute increase in urinary 6-sulfatoximelatonin after clomipramine, as a predictive measure for emotional improvement. J Psychopharmacol 2010; 24:855–60.
105. Celada P, Perez J, Alvarez E, Artigas F. Monoamine oxidase inhibitors phenelzine and brofaromine increase plasma serotonin and decrease 5-hydroxyindoleacetic acid in patients with major depression: relationship to clinical improvement. J Clin Psychopharmacol 1992; 12:309–15.

106. Zolkowska D, Rothman RB, Baumann MH. Amphetamine analogs increase plasma serotonin: implications for cardiac and pulmonary disease. J Pharmacol Exp Ther 2006; 318:604–10.
107. Childs PA, Rodin I, Martin NJ, Allen NH, Plaskett L, Smythe PJ, et al. Effect of fluoxetine on melatonin in patients with seasonal affective disorder and matched controls. Br J Psychiatry 1995; 166:196–8.
108. Nathan PJ, Norman TR, Burrows GD. Nocturnal plasma melatonin concentrations in healthy volunteers: effect of single doses of d-fenfluramine, paroxetine, and ipsapirone. J Pineal Res 1996; 21:55–8.
109. Tan ZL, Bao AM, Zhao GQ, Liu YJ, Zhou JN. Effect of fluoxetine on circadian rhythm of melatonin in patients with major depressive disorder. Neuro Endocrinol Lett 2007; 28:28–32.
110. Peiffer A, Veilleux S, Barden N. Antidepressant and other centrally acting drugs regulate glucocorticoid receptor messenger RNA levels in rat brain. Psychoneuroendocrinology 1991; 16:505–15.
111. Pariante CM, Makoff A, Lovestone S, Feroli S, Heyden A, Miller AH, et al. Antidepressants enhance glucocorticoid receptor function in vitro by modulating the membrane steroid transporters. Br J Pharmacol 2001; 134:1335–43.
112. Okugawa G, Omori K, Suzukawa J, Fujiseki Y, Kinoshita T, Inagaki C. Long-term treatment with antidepressants increases glucocorticoid receptor binding and gene expression in cultured rat hippocampal neurones. J Neuroendocrinol 1999; 11:887–95.
113. Carvalho LA, Garner BA, Dew T, Fazakerley H, Pariante CM. Antidepressants, but not antipsychotics, modulate GR function in human whole blood: an insight into molecular mechanisms. Eur Neuropsychopharmacol 2010; 20:379–87.
114. Hu J, Xia Y, Wu Z, Liu L, Tang C. Fluoxetine might alleviate brain damage and hypercortisolemia related to chronic alcohol in rats. J Stud Alcohol Drugs 2010; 71:290–4.
115. Binder EB, Kunzel HE, Nickel T, Kern N, Pfennig A, Majer M, et al. HPA-axis regulation at in-patient admission is associated with antidepressant therapy outcome in male but not in female depressed patients. Psychoneuroendocrinology 2009; 34:99–109.
116. Schule C, Baghai TC, Eser D, Schwarz M, Bondy B, Rupprecht R. Effects of mirtazapine on dehydroepiandrosterone-sulfate and cortisol plasma concentrations in depressed patients. J Psychiatr Res 2009; 43:538–45.
117. Paslakis G, Luppa P, Gilles M, Kopf D, Hamann-Weber B, Lederbogen F, et al. Venlafaxine and mirtazapine treatment lowers serum concentrations of dehydroepiandrosterone-sulfate in depressed patients remitting during the course of treatment. J Psychiatr Res 2010; 44:556–60.
118. Fischli S, Jenni S, Allemann S, Zwahlen M, Diem P, Christ ER, et al. Dehydroepiandrosterone sulfate in the assessment of the hypothalamic–pituitary–adrenal axis. J Clin Endocrinol Metab 2008; 93:539–42.
119. Juruena MF, Pariante CM, Papadopoulos AS, Poon L, Lightman S, Cleare AJ. Prednisolone suppression test in depression: prospective study of the role of HPA axis dysfunction in treatment resistance. Br J Psychiatry 2009; 194:342–9.
120. Hallam KT, Begg DP, Olver JS, Norman TR. An investigation of the effect of immediate and extended release venlafaxine on nocturnal melatonin and cortisol release in healthy adult volunteers. Hum Psychopharmacol 2008; 23:129–37.
121. Ahrens T, Frankhauser P, Lederbogen F, Deuschle M. Effect of single-dose sertraline on the hypothalamus–pituitary–adrenal system, autonomic nervous system, and platelet function. J Clin Psychopharmacol 2007; 27:602–6.
122. Millan MJ, Gobert A, Lejeune F, Dekeyne A, Newman-Tancredi A, Pasteau V, et al. The novel melatonin agonist agomelatine (S20098) is an antagonist at 5-hydroxytryptamine2C receptors, blockade of which enhances the activity of frontocortical dopaminergic and adrenergic pathways. J Pharmacol Exp Ther 2003; 306:954–64.
123. de BC, Guardiola-Lemaitre B, Mocaer E, Renard P, Munoz C, Millan MJ. Agomelatine, the first melatonergic antidepressant: discovery, characterization and development. Nat Rev Drug Discov 2010; 9:628–42.
124. Martinet L, Guardiola-Lemaitre B, Mocaer E. Entrainment of circadian rhythms by S-20098, a melatonin agonist, is dose and plasma concentration dependent. Pharmacol Biochem Behav 1996; 54:713–8.
125. Van RO, Weibel L, Olivares E, Maccari S, Mocaer E, Turek FW. Melatonin or a melatonin agonist corrects age-related changes in circadian response to environmental stimulus. Am J Physiol Regul Integr Comp Physiol 2001; 280:R1582–R1591.
126. Cajochen C, Krauchi K, Mori D, Graw P, Wirz-Justice A. Melatonin and S-20098 increase REM sleep and wake-up propensity without modifying NREM sleep homeostasis. Am J Physiol 1997; 272:R1189–R1196.

127. Krauchi K, Cajochen C, Mori D, Graw P, Wirz-Justice A. Early evening melatonin and S-20098 advance circadian phase and nocturnal regulation of core body temperature. Am J Physiol 1997; 272:R1178–R1188.
128. Llorca PM. The antidepressant agomelatine improves the quality of life of depressed patients: implications for remission. J Psychopharmacol 2010; 24:21–6.
129. Quera-Salva MA, Lemoine P, Guilleminault C. Impact of the novel antidepressant agomelatine on disturbed sleep-wake cycles in depressed patients. Hum Psychopharmacol 2010; 25:222–9.
130. Kasper S, Hajak G, Wulff K, Hoogendijk WJ, Montejo AL, Smeraldi E, et al. Efficacy of the novel antidepressant agomelatine on the circadian rest-activity cycle and depressive and anxiety symptoms in patients with major depressive disorder: a randomized, double-blind comparison with sertraline. J Clin Psychiatry 2010; 71:109–20.
131. Olie JP, Kasper S. Efficacy of agomelatine, a MT1/MT2 receptor agonist with 5-HT2C antagonistic properties, in major depressive disorder. Int J Neuropsychopharmacol 2007; 10:661–73.
132. Serretti A, Chiesa A. Treatment-emergent sexual dysfunction related to antidepressants: a meta-analysis. J Clin Psychopharmacol 2009; 29:259–66.
133. Montgomery SA, Kennedy SH, Burrows GD, Lejoyeux M, Hindmarch I. Absence of discontinuation symptoms with agomelatine and occurrence of discontinuation symptoms with paroxetine: a randomized, double-blind, placebo-controlled discontinuation study. Int Clin Psychopharmacol 2004; 19:271–80.
134. Uz T, Manev H. Chronic fluoxetine administration increases the serotonin N-acetyltransferase messenger RNA content in rat hippocampus. Biological Psychiatry 1999; 45:175–9.

30 Role of Melatonin in Collagen Synthesis

John E. Tidwell and Ming Pei

CONTENTS

30.1 INTRODUCTION

The human musculoskeletal system comprises different tissues including muscles, bones, tendons, ligaments, intervertebral discs, and cartilage. While other organ systems consist mostly of cellular material, the musculoskeletal system consists mostly of extracellular material and has physical properties that rely heavily on the properties of collagen, the major component of extracellular matrix (ECM). Within the musculoskeletal system, ECM production occurs at the cellular level primarily by chondrocytes, fibroblasts, osteocytes, and myocytes. Collagen is a protein that provides local tissue with support and strength with variability of structure in different tissues.[1,2] Additionally, collagen synthesis has a strong impact on wound healing throughout the body with musculoskeletal implications for skin wound healing, cartilage intervertebral disc repair, and fracture repair.

Melatonin, N-acetyl-5-methoxytryptamine, is a derivative of the essential amino acid tryptophan and is produced primarily in the pineal gland in mammals. Known as a regulator of circadian rhythm, it also has physiologic roles in blood pressure regulation, oncogenesis, seasonal reproduction, immune function, and retinal physiology. Because melatonin synthesis is under the control of the sympathetic nervous system, it is not considered a classic endocrine hormone, but rather, a neuroendocrine hormone with action extending far beyond the pineal gland.[3] Melatonin research has dramatically increased over the past decade with regard to physiologic and pathologic human conditions. Its role within the musculoskeletal system has only been partially elucidated to date with some favorable evidence for a positive impact on human health.

Melatonin's role as an antioxidant and free radical scavenger (receptor independent function) is well established, and its receptor-mediated activity at the cellular membrane and nuclear level has shown increased support for cellular healing and collagen synthesis.[4–7] Although produced primarily in the pineal gland, extrapineal melatonin synthesis has been documented in the intestine, skin, platelets, retinas, lymphocytes, and bone marrow.[8] While systemic melatonin levels are relatively unaffected by extrapineal synthesis, local cellular concentrations and a more autacoid or paracoid function more likely explain its extrapineal effects, especially with regard to tissue healing.[9] Not only is its synthesis widespread, but its receptors have been discovered in various tissue types, including the musculoskeletal tissues.[3]

The mechanism of action for melatonin is not completely understood regarding collagen synthesis, but current studies point to melatonin's upstream effects on a variety of growth factors and cytokines, primarily transforming growth factor beta (TGF-β), through regulation of cellular proliferation and differentiation. A link was first established between TGF-β1 and melatonin in benign prostate epithelial cells.[10] TGF-β1 is a growth factor known to stimulate chondrocyte ECM synthesis and inhibit catabolic cytokines like interleukin-1.[11,12] It is also known that collagen is a protein that is susceptible to oxidative damage by reactive oxygen species such as ·OH and O_2· resulting in fragmentation of collagen strands,[13] creating a simpler explanation for melatonin's effects on collagen synthesis via free radical scavenging.

30.2 MELATONIN-MEDIATED COLLAGEN SYNTHESIS IN CARTILAGE HEALING

Articular cartilage is composed of chondrocytes (1% by volume) and the ECM (99% by volume) it produces, which mostly consists of collagens, proteoglycans, and other noncollagenous proteins. Found in the tissue surrounding joints, cartilage provides cushion for loading and joint motion while the chondrocytes are repopulating the necessary matrix macromolecules and providing joint lubrication. As these functions slow or fail with aging, osteoarthritis develops. Collagen is a significant macromolecule for cartilage, contributing 60% of its dry weight and providing the tissue's structure and tensile strength.[1,2] Collagen synthesis from chondrocytes remains poorly understood, but cytokines are believed to play a primary role in cellular stimulation and regulation.[14] Anabolic effects are largely due to insulin-like growth factor I and TGF-β1.[11,15,16]

Melatonin is just beginning to be studied as an up-regulator of ECM synthesis by chondrocytes. Our recent study described melatonin's effects on an in vitro pellet culture system of porcine articular chondrocytes. ECM expressions of cartilage collagen type II along with other ECM proteins at the mRNA and protein levels were positively affected by melatonin administration in a non-dose-dependent manner with peak effect between 1- and 10-ng/mL concentrations. TGF-β1 is the leading cytokine candidate and was investigated for its potential as a signaling pathway for melatonin, given that internal TGF-β1 increased protein levels after 10 days of melatonin treatment, primarily affecting expression at a concentration of 1 ng/mL.[16] It is already known that high amounts of TGF-β1 are stored in healthy cartilage and that human osteoarthritic cartilage expresses less TGF-β1 than does normal healthy cartilage.[17] However, previous in vivo studies in murine knee joints concluded intra-articular TGF-β1 at higher doses can produce osteoarthritic changes in the knee, making this a problematic candidate for the direct treatment of osteoarthritis in humans.[18] Melatonin does have a role in the regulation of TGF-β1, but no conclusive data are available to determine if melatonin's effects are antioxidative or receptor mediated in nature. The latter is more likely if further correlation with cytokine TGF-β1 could be proven. However, this study, combined with the abundance of literature on antioxidative properties, makes a combination of the two most likely. In vivo experimentation in a rabbit knee osteoarthritis model concerning intra-articular melatonin's ability to decrease cartilage damage and stimulate cartilage healing is currently being performed in our laboratory. Preliminary morphological data are promising for melatonin's ability to protect degenerating cartilage regardless of mechanism of action.

Intervertebral discs (IVD) are another relatively newly studied tissue with regard to melatonin. IVDs are also cartilaginous structures with low cellular density and high ECM density that, in vertebrate animals, separate the spine's vertebral bodies from each other by balancing flexibility and stability. They allow for motion between vertebrae and absorb energy under compression. Like cartilage, the annulus fibrosus (outer ring) is composed primarily of collagen, while proteoglycans predominantly make up the nucleus pulposus (inner substance). These are the extracellular structural components accounting for its mechanical properties.[1]

Recent studies link exogenous melatonin administration with a slower degeneration process in IVD studies in a surgical rat model. Histomorphometric analysis concluded that melatonin partially prevented the bone trabecular width and longitudinal thickness decreases seen in the surgically created degeneration group. Histopathologically, the annulus fibrosus showed more regular structure and alignment than the nontreated discs, although no quantitative information regarding collagen was provided. Moreover, TGF-β1 was again identified as a potential mediator for melatonin's mechanism of action given its increased expression shown by immunohistochemistry.[19] Earlier, this same group found an increase in higher-density tissue of the endplates in degenerated IVDs in a melatonin-treated group using the same rat model.[20] These results suggest that melatonin may be involved in chondrocyte differentiation and cartilage regeneration.

IVD degeneration plays a role in the pathogenesis of idiopathic scoliosis, as studied over the last decade,[21] although there still exists evidence supporting the contrary.[22] One group discovered that type II collagen was increased in scoliotic IVD compared to normal discs.[23] Additionally, research in chickens showed a trend toward increased hydroxyproline (a fairly specific component of collagen) without statistical significance eight weeks after surgical pinealectomy.[24] These chickens all developed scoliosis and showed IVD degeneration both macro- and microscopically as well as on magnetic resonance imaging (MRI).

30.3 MELATONIN-MEDIATED COLLAGEN SYNTHESIS IN BONE HEALING

Bone, like cartilage, is provided structure mostly through its ECM; however, a few key structural differences exist. The matrix is produced by osteocytes rather than chondrocytes and is 60–70% inorganic material, primarily calcium and phosphate. Organic bone ECM is primarily collagen type I, providing most of its tensile strength rather than collagen type II. Bone has excellent blood supply compared to cartilage and contains a relatively higher proportion of cellular material than cartilage. These two facts combined explain why bone heals better than does cartilage when damaged. The bone marrow, the site of synthesis of red and white blood cells, platelets, and stem cells, is also stored within the long bones of the body. Bone contains a wider variety of cells than does cartilage. Osteoblasts are the bone-forming cells, while osteoclasts break down bone. The balance between these two constitutes bone homeostasis.[1,2]

The first studies of melatonin that sparked interest in melatonin's effects on bone were in vitro and revealed a dose-dependent increase in collagen synthesis and cellular proliferation as shown by increased procollagen type 1 c-peptide production, while cellular differentiation remained unaffected.[25] Other early studies showed in vitro potential for melatonin to promote osteoblast differentiation and bone formation.[26] Using luzindole, a melatonin receptor antagonist, they provided a plausible explanation for the mechanism of action through melatonin transmembrane receptors. These investigations spawned much work on melatonin as a regulator of bone metabolism both in vivo and in vitro. Because melatonin steadily decreases in humans as we age, which is even more dramatic in females at menopause,[27] researchers have studied melatonin and its role in preventing osteoporosis and increasing bone mass alone and in combination with estrogen therapy.[28,29]

Naturally, melatonin became of orthopedic interest for fracture healing and bone fusion. Interestingly, one group found that long-term studies on pinealectomized rats maintained high levels of melatonin within the bone marrow.[30] Additionally, it was shown that bone marrow cells have the necessary enzymes to create melatonin from serotonin.[31] Together, these studies suggest that melatonin can function as an autacoid with local paracrine function in addition to the effects on bone metabolism that may be realized from systemic pineal melatonin.[29] Other studies showed that melatonin's effects on bone metabolism were related to decreased osteoclast activity secondary to down-regulated RANKL expression from osteoblasts,[32] providing yet another potential mechanism.

Further in vitro research on human osteoblasts from mandibles concluded that melatonin promotes osteoblastic differentiation in a dose-dependent manner. Melatonin receptor expression was confirmed in these human osteoblasts, and significantly more receptors were found within the younger patients' bone samples. Furthermore, other markers of up-regulation of osteoblasts, including type I collagen, were shown to be significantly increased. In vitro, the effects of melatonin were blocked with the administration of luzindole and other inhibitors of this receptor-mediated pathway.[33] This strengthens the position that melatonin's mechanism of action is based on its receptor-mediated cascade. The same investigators also studied in vivo effects on bone in mice, concluding systemic daily melatonin administration stimulated bone growth by measuring volume of nonhealing bone growth over a 21-day period.[33] The dental community investigated similar local application of melatonin to stimulate osteointegration within dental implants with favorable results.[34] Our laboratory has begun research into the effects of local and systemic melatonin administration on fracture healing in an osteoporotic and nonosteoporotic fracture rat model given these previous findings and the lack of in vivo studies to date. Further studies will be required to elucidate the mechanism of action of melatonin in bone.

30.4 MELATONIN-MEDIATED COLLAGEN SYNTHESIS IN WOUND HEALING

Melatonin's effects on wound healing and collagen synthesis have been studied over the past two decades in vitro as well as in different animal models.[35] These studies began as increased fibrosis was noted after beta-blocker administration, which notably blocks melatonin synthesis, showed increased collagen tissue content.[36] Another group found increased fibrosis within pinealectomized animals' retroperitoneal space.[37] Wound healing relies on the attraction of inflammatory cytokines and immune cells which promote healing and angiogenesis in addition to sufficient collagen production. Collagen is the predominant feature of the skin's ECM that determines its tensile strength and structure. There are currently conflicting reports with regard to collagen production in wound healing models. In general, no specific mechanism of action of melatonin has been delineated but many have been proposed with some correlations.

Intradermal injections of melatonin (120 ug/100 g daily) with an incisional wound rat model was shown to stimulate angiogenesis as well as improve qualitative histological collagen alignment and density, with the scar more closely resembling normal skin. This research proposed that the increased vascular endothelial growth factor (VEGF), cyclooxygenase-2, arginase, and hemoxygenase (HO) activity levels locally with decreased inducible nitric oxide synthase (iNOS) during the inflammatory phase are responsible. Although quantitative collagen studies were not performed, increased arginase, which generates proline for use in collagen synthesis, provides a potential mediator for melatonin's effects.[38]

Similar reports of increased collagen production were found in rat wound healing models given daily melatonin intramuscular injections at 23:00 h. Increased quantitative hydroxyproline and collagen levels, angiogenesis, and immune response cells with melatonin administration were found within the healing incisions. A specific mechanism of action again was not studied except to show through microscopy that fibroblasts were denser and that endothelial cell proliferation was increased without causality. The authors also believe that immunomodulation may play a role in improved results because increased macrophage and lymphocyte infiltration on electron microscopy were found in the acute phase of healing.[39]

Quantitative studies have shown increased collagen production in healing rat myofibroblasts within the site of myocardial infarction after subcutaneous administration of melatonin (3–300 ug/100 g). Both surgical and pharmacologic pinealectomy decreased collagen accumulation, while melatonin administration significantly reversed those effects. Results were dose dependent with positive effects seen at 30 and 60 ug/100 g. The author proposed that melatonin influences collagen through direct cellular mechanisms as shown by the in vitro portions of this experiment, where isolated rat myofibroblasts from these scars showed no increased proliferation of cells but specifically an increase in collagen production.[40]

The same group previously studied other wound healing models in the skin with opposite quantitative collagen results, suggesting that melatonin's effects are target organ dependent. Contrary to others' findings,[38,39] they reported in older studies that, in normal skin and wound healing rat models, pinealectomy actually increased collagen content in the skin, while melatonin reversed those increases.[41,42] Alternative studies in wound healing in rat intestinal anastamosis and skin healing models found a decrease in collagen synthesis and epithelial proliferation with melatonin given at 30 ug/100 g subcutaneously daily at 17:00 h. Hydroxyproline levels in both skin and intestine were lowered by melatonin compared to control and pinealectomized rats.[43] The dosing, route of administration, and timing of administration may provide a source of explanation for these differences. In fact, one study found conflicting quantitative collagen counts in wound healing with morning and evening administration of melatonin systemically.[44]

30.5 CONCLUSIONS

A link has been established across the tissue types discussed for melatonin to play a role in repair and collagen synthesis. No specific mechanism of action has been defined, although the most studied and promising link between collagen synthesis, tissue healing, and melatonin has been the growth factor TGF-β1 as a cell stimulator. Presumably, this mechanism would prove similar between different tissue types. Given its role as an antioxidant and free radical scavenger, it is also likely that, during the repair process, melatonin acts to keep cellular damage to a minimum, allowing for improved healing. Other considerations are melatonin's immunologic role as a stimulator of immune cell function and synthesis.[45] This has not been studied specifically with regard to repair as a potential mechanism for collagen synthesis. More cell types containing transmembrane and nuclear receptors specific for melatonin are being discovered, which will add to literature support for collagen synthesis as a function of receptor-mediated activity.

The role of melatonin for clinical use has yet to be determined, but its role in wound healing of skin, bone, and cartilage is beginning to be studied in depth and in in-vivo animal models. Given its natural history as one of the earliest biologic signaling transducers found in all major taxa of organisms,[46] there are likely to be more clinical uses outside of sleep medicine and within the tissue repair world.

For future studies, there are a few study design details that should be monitored closely. Timing of administration of melatonin may prove to be important in the clinical use of melatonin. Previous studies in a sponge granuloma revealed melatonin's effects on wound healing, and collagen synthesis was dependent on morning or evening administration.[44] Additionally, across the literature, there is a variety of administration techniques from intraperitoneal, intramuscular, subcutaneous, oral, and other local applications, as well as extremely variable dosing. When studying tissue healing and repair outside of the pineal gland and brain, local applications of melatonin would seem to offer the most benefit; however, systemic applications should still be considered. The dose-dependent activity of melatonin is also questioned,[16] presenting further challenges in the development of receptor-mediated and antioxidant mechanisms of action. Additional in-vivo model consideration should be given for studies to determine whether or not melatonin is serving to prevent damage or actually stimulating repair of tissues, and this may be tissue dependent as well as mechanism-of-action dependent.

REFERENCES

1. Einhorn, Thomas et al. *Orthopaedic Basic Science: Foundations of Clinical Practice*. Illinois: AAOS, 2007.
2. Gelse, Kolja et al. "Collagens—structure, function, and biosynthesis." *Advanced Drug Delivery Reviews* 55 (2003): 1531–1546.
3. Reiter, Russell J et al. "Medical implications of melatonin: receptor-mediated and receptor-independent actions." *Advances in Medical Sciences* 52 (2007): 11–28.
4. Altun, Armagan and Betul Ugur–Altun. "Melatonin: therapeutic and clinical utilization." *The International Journal of Clinical Practice* 61, no. 5 (2007): 835–845.
5. Pandi-Perumal, Seithikurippu Ratnas et al. "Melatonin: nature's most versatile biological signal?" *FEBS Journal* 273 (2006): 2813–2838.
6. Reiter, Russell J et al. "Reducing oxidative/nitrosative stress: a newly-discovered genre for melatonin." *Critical Reviews in Biochemistry and Molecular Biology* 44, no. 4 (2009): 175–200.

7. Tan, Dun–Xian et al. "One molecule, many derivatives: a never-ending interaction of melatonin with reactive oxygen and nitrogen species?" *Journal of Pineal Research* 42 (2007): 28–42.
8. Claustrat, Bruno et al. "The basic physiology and pathophysiology of melatonin." *Sleep Medicine Reviews* 9 (2005): 11–24.
9. Reiter, Russell J. "Pineal melatonin—cell biology of its synthesis and of its physiological interactions." *Endocrine Reviews* 12, no. 2 (1991): 151–180.
10. Rimler, Avi et al. "Cross talk between melatonin and TGFβ1 in human benign prostate epithelial cells." *The Prostate* 40 (1999): 211–217.
11. Redini, Françoise et al. "Transforming growth factor beta exerts opposite effects from interleukin-1 beta on cultured rabbit articular chondrocytes through reduction of interleukin-1 receptor expression." *Arthritis & Rheumatism* 36 (1993): 44–50.
12. Van Beuningen, Henk et al. "Transforming growth factor-beta 1 stimulates articular chondrocyte proteoglycan synthesis and induces osteophyte formation in the murine knee joint." *Laboratory Investigations* 71 (1994): 279–290.
13. Henroitin, Yves et al. "Biochemical biomarkers of oxidative collagen damage." *Advances in Clinical Chemistry* 49 (2009): 31–55.
14. Guerne, Pierre–André et al. "Growth factor responsiveness of human articular chondrocytes: distinct profiles in primary chondrocytes, subcultured chondrocytes, and fibroblasts." *Journal of Cellular Physiology* 158 (1994): 476–484.
15. Allen, Janice et al. "Rapid onset synovial inflammation and hyperplasia induced by transforming growth factor beta." *Journal of Experimental Medicine* 171 (1990): 231–247.
16. Pei, Ming et al. "Melatonin enhances cartilage matrix synthesis by porcine articular chondrocytes." *Journal of Pineal Research* 46 (2009): 181–187.
17. Pedrozo, Hugo et al. "Growth plate chondrocytes store latent transforming growth factor (TGF)-beta 1 in their matrix through latent TGF-beta 1 binding protein-1." *Journal of Cell Physiology* 177 (1998): 343–354.
18. Van Beuningen, Henk et al. "Osteoarthritis-like changes in the murine knee joint resulting from intra-articular transforming growth factor-beta injections." *Osteoarthritis Cartilage* 8 (2000): 25–33.
19. Turgut, Mehmet et al. "The effect of exogenous melatonin administration on trabecular width, ligament thickness and TGF-β_1 expression in degenerated intervertebral disc tissue in the rat." *Journal of Clinical Neuroscience* 13 (2006): 357–363.
20. Turgut, Mehmet et al. "Changes in vascularity of cartilage endplate of degenerated intervertebral discs in response to melatonin administration in rats." *Neurosurgery Review* 26 (2003): 133–138.
21. Kouwenhoven, Jan–Willem and Rene M Castelein. "The pathogenesis of adolescent idiopathic scoliosis." *Spine* 33 (2008): 2898–2908.
22. Cheung, Kenneth et al. "The effect of pinealectomy on scoliosis development in young nonhuman primates." *Spine* 30 (2005): 2009–2013.
23. Antoniou, John et al. "Elevated synthetic activity in the convex side of scoliotic intervertebral discs and endplates compared with normal tissues." *Spine* 26 (2001): E1980–E206.
24. Turgut, Mehmet et al. "Surgical pinealectomy accelerates intervertebral disc degeneration process in chicken." *European Spine Journal* 15 (2006): 605–612.
25. Nakade, Osamu et al. "Melatonin stimulates proliferation and type 1 collagen synthesis in human bone cells in vitro." *Journal of Pineal Research* 27 (1999): 106–110.
26. Roth, Jerome et al. "Melatonin promotes osteoblast differentiation and bone formation." *Journal of Biologic Chemistry* 274 (1999): 22041–22047.
27. Sack, Robert et al. "Human melatonin production decreases with age." *Journal of Pineal Research* 3 (1986): 379–388.
28. Cardinali, Daniel P et al. "Melatonin effects on bone: experimental facts and clinical perspectives." *Journal of Pineal Research* 34 (2003): 81–87.
29. Suzuki, Nobuo et al. "Novel bromomelatonin derivatives as potentially effective drugs to treat bone diseases." *Journal of Pineal Research* 45 (2008): 229–234.
30. Conti, Ario et al. "Evidence for melatonin synthesis in mouse and human bone marrow cells." *Journal of Pineal Research* 28 (2000): 193–202.
31. Tan, Dun–Xian et al. "Identification of highly elevated levels of melatonin in bone marrow: its origin and significance." *Biochimica et Biophysica Acta* 1472 (1999): 206–214.
32. Koyama, Hiroki et al. "Melatonin at pharmacologic doses increases bone mass by suppressing resoprtion through down-regulation of the RANKL-mediated osteoclast formation and activation." *Journal of Bone and Mineral Research* 17, no. 7 (2002): 1219–1229.

33. Satomura, Kazuhito et al. "Melatonin at pharmacologic doses enhances human osteoblastic differentiation in vitro and promotes mouse cortical bone formation in vivo." *Journal of Pineal Research* 42 (2007): 231–239.
34. Cutando, Antonio et al. "Melatonin stimulates osteointegration of dental implants." *Journal of Pineal Research* 45 (2008): 174–179.
35. Slominski, Andrzej et al. "Melatonin in the skin: synthesis, metabolism and functions." *TRENDS in Endocrinology and Metabolism* 19 (2007): 17–24.
36. Elkind, Arthur et al. "Silent retroperitoneal fibrosis with methysergide therapy." *Journal of the American Medical Association* 205 (1968): 1041–1044.
37. Cunnane, Stephen et al. "The pineal and regulation of fibrosis—pinealectomy as a model of primary biliary dirrhosis: roles of melatonin and prostaglandins in fibrosis and regulation of T lymphocytes." *Medical Hypothesis* 5 (1979): 403–414.
38. Pugazhenthi, Kamali et al. "Melatonin accelerates the process of wound repair in full-thickness incisional wounds." *Journal of Pineal Research* 44 (2008): 387–396.
39. Soybir, Gursel et al. "The effects of melatonin on angiogenesis and wound healing." *Surgery Today* 33 (2003): 896–901.
40. Drobnik, Jacek et al. "Regulatory influence of melatonin on collagen accumulation in the infracted heart scar." *Journal of Pineal Research* 45 (2008): 285–290.
41. Drobnik, Jacek and Ryszard Dabrowski. "Melatonin suppresses the pinealectomy-induced elevation of collagen content in a wound." *Cytobios* 85 (1996): 51–58.
42. Drobnik, Jacek and Ryszard Dabrowski. "Pinealectomy-induced elevation of collagen content in the intact skin is suppresses by melatonin application." *Cytobios* 100 (1999): 49–55.
43. Bulbuller, Nurullah et al. "Effect of melatonin on wound healing in normal and pinealectomized rats." *Journal of Surgical Research* 123 (2005): 3–7.
44. Drobnik, Jacek and Ryszard Dabrowski. "The opposite effect of morning or afternoon application of melatonin on collagen accumulation in the sponge-induced granuloma." *Neuroendocrinology Letters* 21 (2000): 209–212.
45. Carillo–Vico, Antonio et al. "A review of the multiple actions of melatonin on the immune system." *Endocrine* 27 (2005): 189–200.
46. Hardeland, Ruediger and Birgit Fuhrberg. "Ubiquitous melatonin: presence and effects in unicells, plants, and animals." *Trends in Comparative Biochemistry and Physiology* 2 (1996): 25–45.

31 Melatonin and DNA Protection

Luis Sarabia, Carlos Ponce, María José Munuce, and Héctor Rodríguez

CONTENTS

31.1 INTRODUCTION

Melatonin—the principal hormone of the vertebrate pineal gland—is a promising molecule that rightly deserves to be the focus of future research efforts. Produced by the pineal gland and secreted in a well-described temporal variation, melatonin is released into the cerebrospinal fluid and the plasmatic circulation, and performs various biological actions upon reaching melatonin receptor–rich target tissues, thus driving up a wide range of rhythmic physiology. In recent years, melatonin has been attracting some attention because of its antioxidant properties: it is a highly lipophilic substance that easily penetrates organic membranes and therefore is able to protect important intracellular structures including mitochondria and DNA from oxidative damage directly at the sites where such damage occurs.

In addition, melatonin contributes in the regulation of multiple pathophysiological processes, such as oxidation, tissue inflammation, cancer, and apoptosis, and it has been proposed that it may act through the indirect regulation of gene expression. Thus, considering melatonin as an immune modulator agent with multiple anti-inflammatory and antioxidant effects would seemingly favor its clinical application in some of these conditions. Further studies should also try to establish the beneficial combination of antioxidants, as well as their doses, and the timing of administration. When such problems will be resolved, hopeful results about antioxidant therapy in critical illnesses will be more univocal and promising.

There are three different melatonin receptors: Mel_{1a} or MT_1, Mel_{1b} or MT_2, and Mel_{1c}. In addition to the membrane-bound melatonin receptors, it has been demonstrated that melatonin binds to receptors from the retinoid-related orphan nuclear hormone receptor family (RZRα/ROR and RZRβ/ROR) [1].

Numerous factors or physiological stimuli are capable of influencing the number and functional status of the MT1 and MT2 receptors, such as melatonin, the photoperiod, the circadian clock, or the phenomena of receptor dimerization [2].

31.2 MELATONIN AND GENE EXPRESSION UP-REGULATION

Intriguingly, melatonin up-regulates gene expression and the activity of several antioxidative enzymes such as Cu/Zn superoxide dismutase (CuZn SOD), Mn superoxide dismutase (Mn SOD), catalase, and glutathione peroxidase (GPx). Thus, melatonin not only acts as a potent antioxidant itself, but is also capable of activating an entire endogenous enzymatic protective system against oxidative stress [3]. This includes gene expression, protein synthesis, and enzymatic activity for arylalkylamine *N*-acetyltransferase (AANAT) and hydroxyindole-*O*-methyltransferase (HIOMT), as well as for tryptophan hydroxylase with its isoforms TPH1 and TPH2 [3].

In parallel, the combination of elevated nitric oxide (NO) plus excess O_2 with the formation of high levels of peroxynitrite ($ONOO^-$) could contribute to the pathophysiology of many molecular diseases. The activation of the DNA repair enzyme poly(ADP ribose)polymerase-1 (PARP-1), a member of PARP enzyme family, mediates $ONOO^-$-induced necrosis. From a physiological viewpoint, PARP-1 activity and poly(ADP-ribosyl)ation reactions are implicated in DNA repair, genomic stability maintenance, gene-transcription regulation, and DNA replication. An important function of PARP-1 is to allow DNA repair and cell recovery under conditions associated with a low level of DNA damage [4]. It has been reported that a single melatonin molecule is able to scavenge up to 10 ROS/RNS (reactive oxygen and nitrogen species), and melatonin scavenging capacity extends to its secondary, tertiary, and quaternary metabolites. Using the Comet assay, it has been shown in vitro that melatonin exhibited a protective effect on rat brain cells exposed to ionizing radiation [5], mice testis cells treated with genotoxic agents [6], and rat lymphocytes exposed to magnetic fields (50 Hz) [7]. Moreover, DNA damage was diminished in patients diagnosed with Graves' disease, in whom lymphocytes were exposed in vitro to melatonin (100 mM, 4 h) [8]. Melatonin shows antiproliferative activity in a number of cells including tumor cells, serves as a trap for free radicals, and might act in many other yet unstudied ways. In experiments with transfection of RORE (retinoic acid receptor–related orphan receptor response element) containing reporter constructions, melatonin and its analogs that interact predominantly with nuclear receptors of the ROR/RZR subfamily significantly increased the transactivating effects of these receptors [9,10]. Therefore, secretion, movement, and action of melatonin are highly sensitive to the processes of body homeostasis. This feature allows melatonin to become a highly effective guardian of an individual's health, with functions ranging from participating in DNA protection to the processes of inflammation and cancer, in addition to classical regulatory actions.

31.2.1 Experience from Our Laboratory

Organophosphates have demonstrated alkylating and clastogenic properties; thus, they are capable of inducing changes in the genetic material, and they are potentially mutagenic and/or carcinogenic [11]. The effects of pesticides on male fertility began to generate interest after the publication of the report of Whorton et al. [12], who associated exposure to the nematocide dibromochloropropane (DCBP) with male infertility and DNA toxicity on human beings. Several steps of spermatogenesis—from the early phase of spermatogonial proliferation, through the formation of spermatocytes, their conversion into spermatids and subsequent differentiation—constitute potentially susceptible targets for the deleterious action of environmental toxicants or DNA-damaging agents (such as drugs or radiation). These agents can produce cellular or genomic damage in the germinal epithelium generating carcinomas and/or inheritable defects [13]. Moreover, epididymal spermatozoa showed an increment in the rate of teratozoospermia and chromatin quality alterations, with an increase of apoptosis in the germ cell line [14,15]. When human and mice seminiferous tubules cultured in vitro were exposed to parathion (OP) and its metabolite, paraoxon, spermatogonial proliferation was inhibited [16]. These effects are partially due to the overproduction of free oxygen radicals [17], which causes multiple ruptures in DNA molecule and deoxyribose degradation—both are likely consequences of the formation of the hydroxyl radical (OH). Serious damage on DNA initiates the beginning of mutagenic and carcinogenic processes [18]. In fact, diazinon-induced oxidative stress and ROS generation have been shown in a murine model after acute toxicity [19–21]. The well-demonstrated antioxidant properties of melatonin make it an efficient molecule for cell protection from oxidative damage. For instance, 2 mM melatonin reduced by 70% the damage induced by ionizing radiations on DNA in comparison to dimethylsulfoxide (DMSO, another well-known radioprotective agent), of which a concentration of 1 M is required to produce a similar protection level [22].

Diazinon (*O,O*-diethyl[*O*-2-isopropyl-6-methylpyrimidine-4-yl]-phosphorothioate) [23] is a synthetic chemical substance with a broad-spectrum of insecticide activity [24]. Although the protective mechanism of melatonin has not been completely clarified in most cases—according to the exhaustive review of Reiter [25]—our interest has been to investigate whether melatonin can prevent the cytotoxic and/or genotoxic effects of the organophosphorous pesticide diazinon on both mouse somatic (evaluated by the micronucleus test on bone marrow cells) and sperm cells under conditions of acute toxicity.

31.3 PROTECTIVE EFFECT OF MELATONIN ON DNA FRAGMENTATION IN CELLS EXPOSED TO A GENOTOXIC AGENT

A total of 72 adult CF-1 mice that were 12 weeks of age were maintained in our laboratory's animal housing facilities under controlled lighting conditions (12 h light:12 h darkness) and temperature maintained between 18 and 20°C. Animals were provided with pelleted food and water ad libitum. All animal studies were conducted in accordance with the principles and procedures outlined by the bioethics committee of the University of Chile Medical School. Mice were housed in 12 cages of 6 individuals each. All mice were injected with 200 µl of solution in a single injection. Mice from the control group were injected intraperitoneally (ip) with vehicle (3% ethanol in 0.9% NaCl). The experimental groups were ip injected with diazinon (dz) properly diluted in vehicle to reach 1/3 of the lethal dose 50 [1/3 LD_{50}, or 2/3 LD_{50}, or with melatonin (mlt) alone, mlt + dz 1/3 LD_{50} or mlt + dz 2/3 LD_{50}]. All groups were sacrificed on days 1 and 32 postinjection (pi). The groups injected with melatonin plus diazinon received melatonin 30 min before diazinon application. The dose of melatonin was 10 mg/kg of body weight (b.w.); for diazinon, the LD_{50} was previously determined in 65 mg/kg b.w. via intraperitoneal injection.

The mice testes were extracted, freed from the tunica, and cut with a scalpel blade until pieces that were approximately 1 mm^3 or less were obtained. The macerated tissue was placed in an Eppendorf tube containing 1.5 ml of a trypsin solution (8 mg/ml trypsin in 0.1% PBS/BSA) for enzymatic digestion. After mechanical disgregation with a Pasteur pipette, a 5-min centrifugation step at 1800 × *g* was carried out. The pellet was resuspended in an Eppendorf tube containing 3 mg hyaluronidase and 0.9 mg colagenase for a second digestion for 30 min at 34°C in a thermoregulated bath using an agitation rate of 90 cycles/min. The pellet was resuspended to a final concentration of 2×10^6 cells/ml.

31.4 MELATONIN AND DNA PROTECTION

One of the mechanisms by which a toxic substance can alter the male reproductive function is by altering the DNA or its associated proteins in the testis [26]. According to the findings reported in our study, the hydrogen bonds of the DNA double chain are the most sensitive structures to chromatin-damaging agents [27]. In our results, germinal cells exhibited chromosomal fragmentation only at day 1 after treatment (Figure 31.1) [28]. In addition, diazinon provoked a nonlethal, cytotoxic damage on germ cells that could induce mutations in the genetic material of spermatocytes and permanent genetic changes in sperm, as observed on subsequent days.

Briefly, for comet assay, spermatogenic cells obtained from treated animals were treated according to Haines et al. [29]; cells were visualized at 400× using an epifluorescence microscope (Carl Zeiss, Germany) with an excitement filter of 510–560 nm and a filter barrier of 590 nm. Positive comet cells had the appearance of a comet, with a brightly fluorescent head and a tail to one side formed by DNA, which contained broken strands that were drawn away during electrophoresis. Samples were run in duplicate, and 50 cells were randomly analyzed per slide for a total of 100 cells

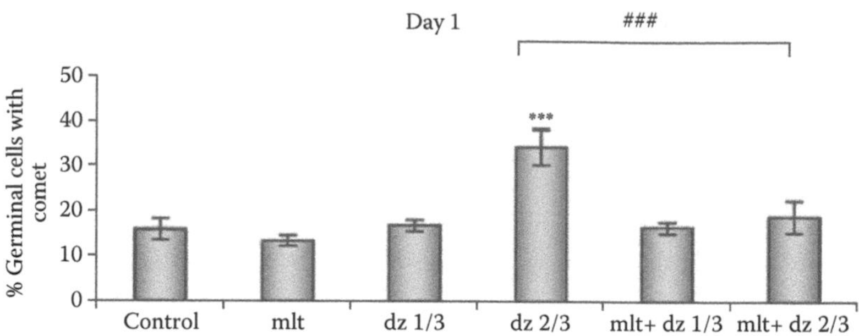

FIGURE 31.1 Fragmentation of DNA in cells of germinal epithelium (% germ cells with comet) of testis at day 1 pi determined in samples with more than 68% of primary spermatocytes (germ cells). (Reprinted from *Ecotoxicol. Environ. Saf.*, 72, Sarabia, L., Maurer, I., Bustos Obregón, L., 663–668, Copyright (2009), with permission from Elsevier.)

per sample to determine the percentage of nuclei with fragmented DNA in the control and treated groups.

It has been demonstrated elsewhere that organophosphates are able to alter the homeostatic balance between cell proliferation and apoptosis [6,30]. On the other hand, some studies have revealed that organophosphates have alkylating and clastogenic properties [11]. Our results demonstrated the potential of diazinon to induce fragmentation of DNA in cells of the testicular spermatogenic tissue in vivo and the ability of melatonin to prevent it (Figures 31.1 and 31.2), in agreement with the findings reported by Tan et al. [31]. In their study, the most interesting result was that the protection provided by melatonin against other genotoxicants such as safrole was obtained with a very low dose of melatonin. The appearance of nuclei with broken DNA into small fragments in the control group can be explained by the fact that the spermatogenic cells have a high proliferation rate and, therefore, mechanisms of population regulation and homeostasis preservation—such as apoptosis—will normally occur [15,30]. In our studies, we found that diazinon produced a significant decrease in the percentage of spermatozoa with compacted chromatin (compacted chromatin test with sodium thioglycolate [15]) in the group treated with an elevated dose of the pesticide, but it was prevented with a pretreatment using melatonin (Figures 31.3 and 31.4). Briefly, spermatozoa from cauda epididymis were obtained by mechanical disgregation of the tissue in PBS, then filtered and washed twice with PBS, and the thioglycolate assay was performed. This test analyzes the state of the sperm chromatin condensation by exposing the cell to a strongly reducing substance such as sodium thioglycolate (0.4 M, pH 9.0). For this test, 0.9 ml reducing reagent was mixed with 0.1 ml

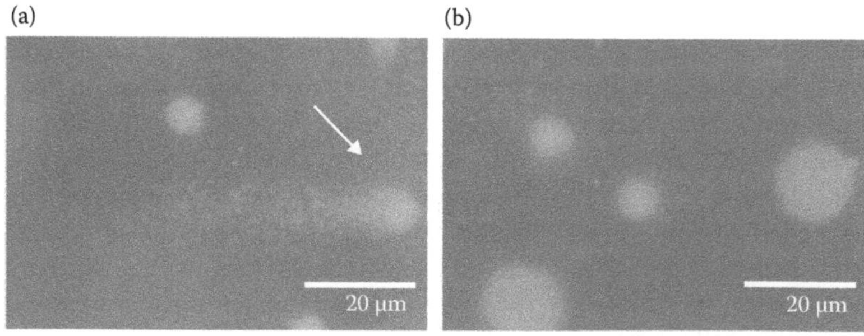

FIGURE 31.2 Comet assay. (a) Primary spermatocyte, diazinon 2/3 LD_{50} at day 1 pi. Arrow indicates a nucleus with fragmented DNA. (b) Normal nuclei of four primary spermatocytes with intact DNA protected by melatonin. (Reprinted from *Ecotoxicol. Environ. Saf.*, 72, Sarabia, L., Maurer, I., Bustos Obregón, L., 663–668, Copyright (2009), with permission from Elsevier.)

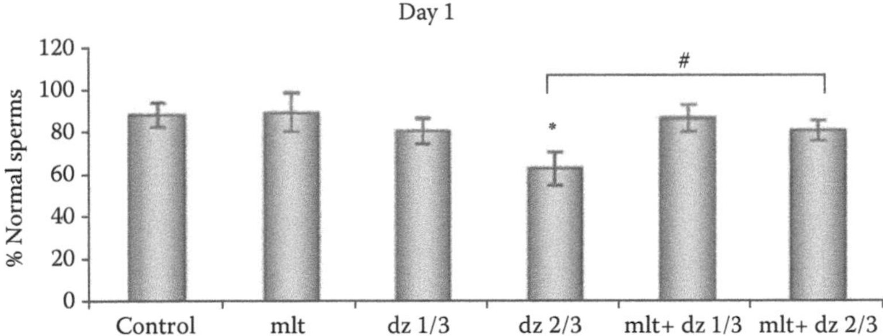

FIGURE 31.3 State of chromatin compaction at day 1 pi in sperm treated with sodium thioglycolate. (Reprinted from *Ecotoxicol. Environ. Saf.*, 72, Sarabia, L., Maurer, I., Bustos Obregón, L., 663–668, Copyright (2009), with permission from Elsevier.)

of a sperm suspension at room temperature for 10 min. A smear was made and stained with aniline blue 5% during 5 min, dried, and mounted for microscope observation with high magnification. Two patterns were observed: (1) condensed sperm chromatin, with a head of habitual size; and (2) decondensed sperm chromatin, when the head swelling reaches 50% or more than the normal head volume. Spermatozoa were observed at 100× and the size of the sperm heads was measured with a 1 mm^2 reticulated ocular. Two hundred spermatozoa were evaluated per animal, according to Fornés and Bustos-Obregón [32].

Diazinon, in a dose of 1/3 of its LD_{50}, produced openings in the double strand of spermatic DNA as determined with the acridine orange test (Figure 31.5; based on the method described by Tejada et al. [33]), but no alteration in the binding of protamines to DNA (as determined by the sodium thioglycolate test; Figures 31.3 and 31.4). At day 1 pi, we observed damage in sperm present in the epididymis and in testicular spermatocytes; however, on day 32 pi, the maturation of spermatocytes into epididymal spermatozoa may explain the recovery on all tested parameters we found. Spermatozoa were obtained by mechanical disgregation of cauda epididymis in PBS; they were filtered to remove debris, washed twice with PBS, boiled at 90°C for 6 min, and immediately fixed in Carnoy solution overnight. Thick smears were made and the slides were immediately read

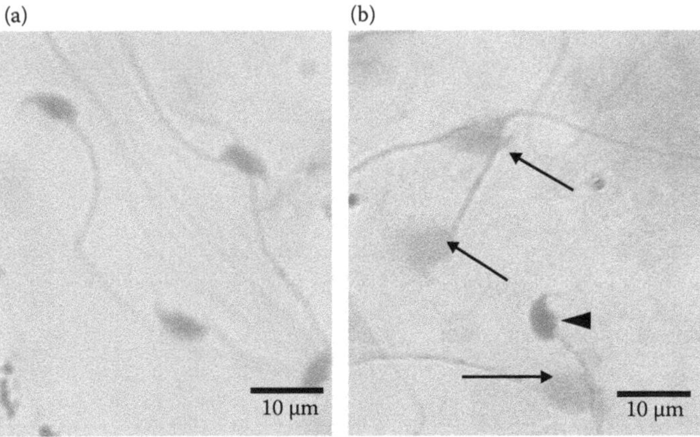

FIGURE 31.4 (a) Sperm with normal condensed chromatin. Control at day 1 pi. (b) Arrows show spermatozoa with decondensed chromatin and one sperm with condensed chromatin (arrowhead). (Reprinted from *Ecotoxicol. Environ. Saf.*, 72, Sarabia, L., Maurer, I., Bustos Obregón, L., 663–668, Copyright (2009), with permission from Elsevier.)

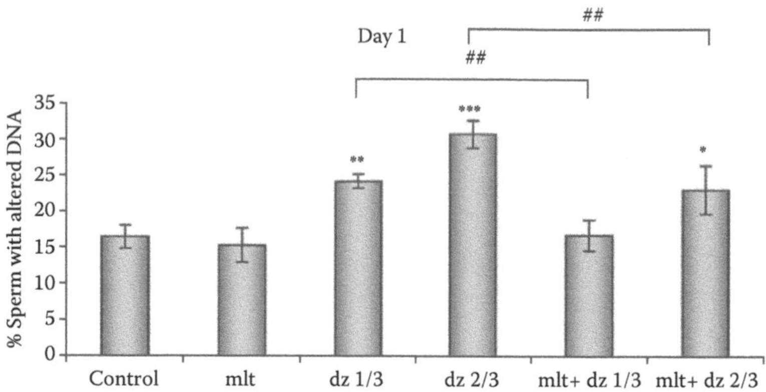

FIGURE 31.5 Effect of diazinon and melatonin on stability of sperm DNA. (Reprinted from *Ecotoxicol. Environ. Saf.*, 72, Sarabia, L., Maurer, I., Bustos Obregón, L., 663–668, Copyright (2009), with permission from Elsevier.)

on a fluorescence Zeiss M 01 microscope in epifluorescence configuration. The procedure was previously described by Tejada et al. [33].

The micronucleus test has been widely used to detect the effects of genotoxicity of environmental mutagens, and it has been proposed as a "screening method" to determine the clastogenic potential or aneuploidy produced by toxic substances [28]. In our study, we found that diazinon increases the quantity of polychromatic erythrocytes with micronuclei; at the same time, we observed that in animals pretreated with melatonin before diazinon administration, there was no increase in micronuclei rates (Figure 31.6). These results are congruent with a previous report in which melatonin prevented the increment of micronuclei in polychromatic erythrocytes in peripheral blood as a consequence of the use of the OP paraquat, both 24 and 48 h after injection [34]. Therefore, diazinon also produces DNA alterations in somatic cells. Tan et al. [35] demonstrated highly elevated levels of melatonin in the bone marrow of mice; this fact is interesting for a possible major level of protection against toxic agents in this tissue. In mammals, during their passage through the epididymis, sperm acquires a mature motility pattern and fertilizing ability (Hamilton, 1972). These and other sperm changes are influenced by absorptive and secretory functions of the epididymal epithelium

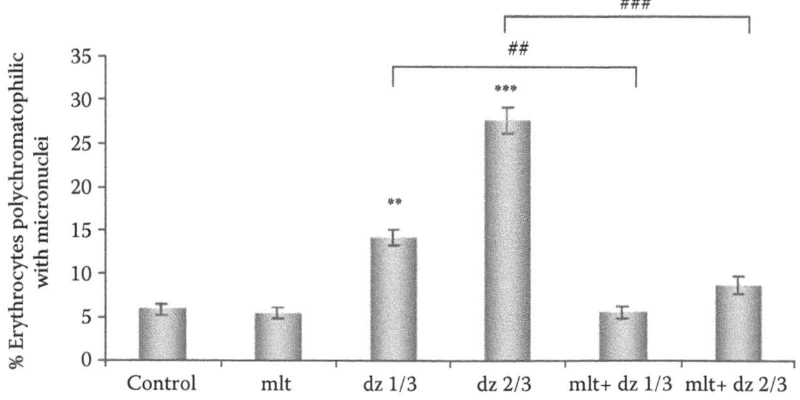

FIGURE 31.6 Percentage of polychromatophilic erythrocytes with micronuclei determined in bone marrow smears on day 1 pi. (Reprinted from *Ecotoxicol. Environ. Saf.*, 72, Sarabia, L., Maurer, I., Bustos Obregón, L., 663–668, Copyright (2009), with permission from Elsevier.)

that permits the passage of substances of different chemical structures, such as glycerylphosphorylcholine, carnitine, steroids, and sialic acid [36]. The possibility that diazinon may cross the epididymal epithelium based on its lipophilic properties reaching sperm stored could explain the effects on chromatin compaction, DNA stability observed on day 1. Moreover, there are reports about the local production of melatonin and its metabolites in testicular tissues [37]. In conclusion, melatonin may prevent the damage on DNA and the adverse effects of toxicants on germ cells by conserving the quality and integrity of chromatin.

The pineal gland is not an exclusive site of melatonin production. The enterochromaffin cells of the gastrointestinal tract produce 400 times as much melatonin as the pineal gland with a protective role against ulcerations of the gastric mucosa because of its antioxidant properties. In gastric infection, melatonin significantly reduces the oxidative DNA damage of the gastric mucosa. The antioxidant effects of melatonin, with the subsequent protective effects on gatrointestinal tract (GIT) mucosa, makes melatonin an excellent treatment choice when associated with drugs that cause mucosa damage. Melatonin should be also taken into consideration for the treatment of GIT motility problems. The results of the clinical trials are least conclusive concerning GIT diseases in which the inflammatory or even autoimmune component is important. In addition, the role of melatonin as an oncostatic drug has been widely documented in in vivo and in vitro experimental investigations, covering a large number of different neoplasias including breast, prostate or colorectal cancer, glioblastoma, leukemia, etc. Melatonin's oncostatic properties depend on: (1) its antiproliferative effects; (2) its ability to increase p53; (3) its capacity to induce cell differentiation; (4) its antimetastatic effects; (5) its ability to modulate gene expression; (6) its interaction with estrogen receptors, down-regulating their expression, binding to DNA, and transactivation; (7) its modulation of the immune response; (8) its capacity to decrease telomerase activity; (9) its function as a free radical scavenger; and (10) its anti-aromatase actions [38].

31.5 CONCLUSION

In conclusion, our results and other authors' data show that melatonin prevents DNA damage and the adverse effects on cells induced by genotoxicants in vivo and in vitro, thus conserving the quality of chromatin and protecting the germinal epithelium from the clastogenic action of toxic agents. More studies are necessary to determine the precise molecular mechanism for melatonin protective action, which—as we hypothesize—might be based on its powerful antioxidant properties.

REFERENCES

1. Steinhilber D, Brungs M, Werz O, Wiesenberg I, Danielsson C, Kahlen JP, Nayeri S et al. (1995). The nuclear receptor for melatonin represses 5-lipoxygenase gene expression in human B lymphocytes. *J. Biol. Chem.*, 270, 7037–7040.
2. Schuster C. (2007) Sites and mechanisms of action of melatonin in mammals: the MT1 and MT2 receptors. *J. Soc. Biol.*, 1, 85–96.
3. Fischer T, Slominski A, Zmijewski M, Reiter R, Paus R. (2008). Melatonin as a major skin protectant: from free radical scavenging to DNA damage repair. *Exp. Dermatol.*, 17, 713–730.
4. Korkmaz A, Reiter R, Topal T, Manchester L, Oter S, Tan. (2009) Melatonin: an established antioxidant worthy of use in clinical trials. *Mol. Med.*, 15(1–2), 43–50.
5. Undeger B, Zorlu G, Oge K, Bacaran N. (2004) Protective effects of melatonin on the ionizing radiation induced DNA damage in the rat brain. *Exp. Toxicol. Pathol.* 55, 379–384.
6. Sarabia L, Maurer I, Bustos Obregón L. (2009) Melatonin prevents damage elicited by the organophosphorous pesticida diazinon on mouse sperm DNA. *Ecotoxicol. Environ. Saf.*, 72, 663– 668.
7. Jajte J, Zmyslony M, Palus J, Dziubaltowska E, Rajkowska E. (2001) Protective effect of melatonin against in vitro iron ions and 7 mT 50 Hz magnetic field-induced DNA damage in rat lymphocytes. *Mutat. Res.*, 483, 57–64.
8. Tang X, Liu X, Sun W, Zhao J, Zheng R. (2005). Oxidative stress in Graves' disease patients and antioxidant protection against lymphocytes DNA damage in vitro. *Pharmazie*, 60, 696–700.

9. Schrader M, Danielsson C, Wiesenberg I, Carlberg C. (1996) Identification of natural monomeric response elements of the nuclear receptor RZR/ROR. They also bind COUP-TF homodimers. *J. Biol. Chem.*, 27, 19732–19736.
10. Missbach M, Jagher B, Sigg I, Nayeri S, Carlberg C, Wiesenberg I. (1996) Thiazolidine diones, specific ligands of the nuclear receptor retinoid Z receptor/retinoid acid receptor-related orphan receptor alpha with potent antiarthritic activity. *J. Biol. Chem.*, 271, 13515–13522.
11. Wild D. (1995) Mutagenicity studies on organophosphorous insecticides. *Mutat. Res.*, 16, 359–363.
12. Whorton D, Krauss R, Marshall S, Milby T. (1977) Infertility in male pesticide workers. *Lancet*, 2, 1259–1261.
13. Bjørge C, Brunborg G, Wiger R, Holme J, Scholz T, Dybing E, Soderlund E. (1996) A comparative study of chemically-induced DNA damage in isolated human and rat testicular cells. *Reprod. Toxicol.*, 10, 509–519.
14. Sobarzo C, Bustos-Obregón E. (2000) Efecto agudo del Parathion sobre el epitelio seminıferos de ratones inmaduros. *Rev. Chil. Anat.*, 18 (1), 61–68.
15. Bustos-Obregón E, Díaz O, Sobarzo C. (2001) Parathion induces mouse germ cells apoptosis. *Ital. J. Anat. Embryol.*, 106, 199–204.
16. Rodríguez H, Bustos-Obregón E. (1998) An in vitro model to evaluate the effect of an organophosphoric agropesticide on cell proliferation in mouse seminiferous tubules. *Andrología*, 32, 1–5.
17. Melchiorri D, Reiter R, Attia A, Hara M, Burgos A, Nistico G. (1995) Potent protective effect of melatonin on in vivo paraquat-induced oxidative damage in rats. *Life Sci.*, 56, 83–85.
18. Meneghini R, Martins E. (1993) Hydrogen peroxide and DNA damage. In: Halliwell B, Aruoma OI (Eds.), *DNA and Free Radicals*. Harwood, London, pp. 83–86.
19. Teimouri F, Amirkabirian N, Esmaily H, Mohammadirad A, Aliahmadi A, Abdollahi M. (2006) Alteration of hepatic cells glucose metabolism as a noncholinergic detoxication mechanism in counteracting diazinon-induced oxidative stress. *Hum. Exp. Toxicol.*, 25, 697–703.
20. Giordano G, Afsharinejad Z, Guizzetti M, Vitalote A, Kavanagh T, Costa L. (2007) Organophosphorus insecticides chlorpyrifos and diazinon and oxidative stress in neuronal cells in a genetic model of glutathione deficiency. *Toxicol. Appl. Pharmacol.*, 219, 181–189.
21. Sutcu R, Altuntas I, Buyukvanli B, Akturka O, Ozturka O, Koylu H, Delibas N. (2007) The effects of diazinon on lipid peroxidation and antioxidant enzymes in rat erythrocytes: role of vitamins E and C. *Toxicol. Ind. Health.*, 23, 13–17.
22. Reiter R, Melchiorri D, Sewerynek E, Poeggeler B, Barlow-Walden L, Chuang J et al. (1995) A review of the evidence supporting melatonin's role as an antioxidant. *J. Pineal Res.*, 18, 1–11.
23. Agency for Toxic Substances and Disease Registry (ATSDR) (1997). Available from: http://www.atsdr.cdc.gov/es/es_index.html (accessed June 8, 2010).
24. World Health Organization (WHO). (1998) PNUMA. International Program on Chemical Safety, Diazinon. Geneva Editions.
25. Reiter R. (2002). Melatonin: lowering the high price of free radicals. *News Physiol. Sci.*, 15, 246–250.
26. Wyrobek A, Bruce W. (1975) Chemical induction of sperm abnormalities in mice. *Proc. Natl. Acad. Sci. U. S. A.*, 72, 4425–4429.
27. Bustos-Obregón E, Valenzuela M, Rojas M. (1998) Agropesticides and testicular damage. In: Martínez-García F, Regadera J (Eds.), *Male Reproduction. A Multidisciplinary Overview*. School of Medicine, Autonoma University, Madrid, Spain (Churchill Communications, Spain).
28. Ellahueñe M, Pérez L, Orellana M, Muñoz C, Lafuente N. (1994) Genotoxic evaluation of eugenol using the bone marrow micronucleus assay. *Mutat. Res.*, 105, 413–416.
29. Haines G, Hendry J, Daniel C, Morris I. (2002) Germ cell and dose-dependent DNA damage measured by the comet assay in murine spermatozoa after testicular X-irradiation. *Biol. Reprod.*, 67, 854–861.
30. Billing H, Chum S, Eisenhauer K, Hsueh A. (1996). Gonad cell apoptosis: hormone-regulated cell demise. *Hum. Reprod. Update*, 2, 103–117.
31. Tan D, Poeggeler B, Reiter R, Chen L, Chen S, Manchester L, Barlow-Walden L. 1993. The pineal hormone melatonin inhibits DNA-adduct formation induced by the chemical carcinogen safrole in vivo. *Cancer Lett.*, 70, 65–71.
32. Fornés M, Bustos-Obregón E. (1994) Study of nuclear decondensation of the rat spermatozoa by reducing agents during epididymal transit. *Andrologia*, 26, 87–92.
33. Tejada R, Mitchell J, Norman A, Marik J, Friedman S. (1984) A test for the practical evaluation of male fertility by acridine orange (AO) fluorescence. *Fertil. Steril.*, 42, 87–91.
34. Ortiz G, Reiter R, Zuñiga G, Melchiorri D, Sewerynek E, Pablos M, Oh C, García J, Bitzer-Quintero O. (2000) Genotoxicity of paraquat: micronuclei induced in bone marrow and peripheral blood are inhibited by melatonin. *Mutat. Res.*, 464, 239–245.

35. Tan D, Manchester L, Reiter R, Qi W, Zhang M, Weintraub ST et al. (1999). Identification of highly elevated of melatonin in bone marrow: its origin and significance. *Biochim. Biophys. Acta*, 1472, 206–214.
36. Hamilton D. (1972) The mammalian epididimys. In: Balin, H., Glassner, S. (Eds.), *Reproductive Biology*. Excerpta Medica, Amsterdam, pp. 268–337.
37. Tijmes M, Pedraza R, Valladares L. (1996) Melatonin in the rat testis: evidence for local synthesis. *Steroids*, 61, 65–68.
38. Sánchez-Barceló E, Mediavilla M, Tan D, Reiter R. (2010) Clinical uses of melatonin: evaluation of human trials. *Curr. Med. Chem.*, 7, 2070–2095.

32 Melatonin Modulation of Vascular Structure and Function

Mustafa Yildiz

CONTENTS

Melatonin (5-methoxy-*N*-acetyltryptamine) is a neurohormone synthesized in the pineal gland, which is located on the midline, attached to the posterior end of the roof of the third ventricle in the brain, mainly during the night, and it affects a number of heart functions such as cardiac rhythms, arterial blood pressure, and heart rate [1,2]. Light has an inhibitory effect on pineal melatonin secretion [1]. Melatonin release is synchronized with daylight cycle by a multisynaptic pathway. Sympathetic nerve stimulation from the intermediolateral nucleus occurs after interpolation in the superior cervical ganglion is finally directed to the epiphysis to induce melatonin synthesis [3]. The activity of rate-limiting enzymes in the epiphysis is regulated by norepinephrine binding to pineal β_1 and α_1 adrenoceptors [4,5]. The local renin–angiotensin system may also effect melatonin secretion [6]. Nonspecific mechanisms of melatonin action can also reside in direct interaction with calmodulin, a small, acidic protein approximately 148 amino acids long (16,706 Da), inhibition of calcium (Ca^{2+}) channels, or calcium pump stimulation observed in cardiomyocytes [7–9]. The interference of melatonin synthesis and action with other neurohumoral systems plays a crucial role in the regulation of cardiovascular functions by melatonin. The physiological actions of melatonin depend on membrane receptors in melatonin-responsive cells and tissues [10]. Melatonin mainly has two membrane receptors called MT1 and MT2, which are G protein–coupled receptors, and has intracellular signaling proteins such as quinon reductase 2, calmodulin, calreticulin, and tubulin. The third receptor type, MT3, which has a lower affinity, is probably not coupled with G protein [11]. In the cardiovascular system, whereas the MT1 receptor was found in chicken and human coronary arteries as well as in rat heart [12,13], the MT2 receptor was identified in the human heart, coronary arteries, and the aorta [14]. When melatonin receptors are activated, some interactions start in the cell including alterations in the levels of cyclic nucleotides (cAMP, cGMP) and calcium, activation of protein kinase C subtypes, intracellular localization of steroid hormone receptors, and regulation of G protein signaling proteins.

32.1 MECHANISMS OF MELATONIN'S EFFECT ON BLOOD PRESSURE

Arterial blood pressure is the force that drives blood to flow through the arteries, capillaries, and finally veins back to the heart. Blood pressure is determined by the cardiac output and the resistance of the blood vessels to blood flow. Cardiac output is the volume of blood pumped by the heart per minute (ml blood/min). It is a function of heart rate and stroke volume:

$$\text{Cardiac output (ml/min)} = \text{Heart rate (beats/min)} \times \text{Stroke volume (ml/beat)}$$

The resistance is mainly produced in the arterioles and is known as the systemic or peripheral vascular resistance. The interactions between blood flow, pressure, and peripheral vascular resistance are shown in the equation:

$$\text{Blood pressure} = \text{Cardiac output} \times \text{Peripheral vascular resistance}$$

Melatonin can affect blood pressure in different ways. The effects of melatonin on blood pressure may be explained by central regulatory mechanisms. Improved baroreflex responses, decreased sympathetic output or norepinephrine levels, and association of decreased heart rate or cardiac output with decreased blood pressure after melatonin administration support the idea of the central action of melatonin [15–17]. Intravenous administration of melatonin (30–60 mg/kg) decreases brain serotonin release in both the corpus striatum and the hypothalamus and results in sympathetic inhibition or parasympathetic stimulation, which leads to hypotension and bradycardia in rats [18]. Holmes and Sugden [19] investigated the effect of melatonin administration on hypertension produced by electrolytic lesion of the pineal gland in the rat. Administration of melatonin prevented the emergence of pinealectomy-induced hypertension and significantly decreased blood pressure. Kawashima et al. [20] studied the effects of melatonin on blood pressure and heart rate of 23-week-old male primary hypertensive rats. Melatonin infusion using an osmotic minipump produced a significant reduction in blood pressure and a slight but significant decrease in heart rate. These cardiovascular effects of melatonin developed gradually. Plasma renin concentration tended to decrease after melatonin treatment [20].

Although the mechanisms involved in the central effect of melatonin are still unknown, some pathways can be suggested [2]. First, the suprachiasmatic nuclei, paraventricular nucleus, and intermediolateral nucleus are responsible for the excitation of sympathetic neurons in the superior cervical ganglion that regulates pineal melatonin synthesis [3]. It can be hypothesized that the modulation of suprachiasmatic nuclei activity by melatonin alters sympathetic tone and thus represents a protective mechanism against excessive sympathetic activation [21]. Second, gamma-aminobutyric acid (GABA)-ergic signalization is involved in the inhibition of paraventricular nucleus by suprachiasmatic nuclei and in the inhibition of rostral ventrolateral medulla by caudal ventrolateral medulla [22,23]. Melatonin was reported to enhance GABA-ergic signalization that may contribute to the inhibition of these nuclei and subsequent decrease in sympathetic tone [24]. Third, in nitric oxide formation, melatonin may improve nitric oxide production, which was shown to potentiate GABA-ergic inhibitory effects in rostral ventrolateral medulla and paraventricular nucleus [23,25].

32.2 EFFECT OF MELATONIN ON VASCULAR STRUCTURE

Melatonin, the principal hormone of the pineal gland, influences the catecholamine levels in perivascular nerves [26], influences pulmonary arteries and veins via endothelium-dependent factors [27], induces relaxation of the rat aorta [28], directly affects Ca^{2+}-dependent cardiac sarcolemma adenosinetriphosphatase [9], and modifies catecholamine metabolism in the heart [29]. Receptors for melatonin have been detected in the walls of cerebral and caudal arteries of rats [30,31], and melatonin both decreases blood flow to the animal brain [32] and enhances the constriction of rat caudal artery induced by norepinephrine [31].

In large arteries, the structure of the arterial wall determines the pulsatile hemodynamics of pressure and flow. Mechanical wall stiffness, wall thickness, and elastin and collagen content vary along the arterial tree, further contributing to regional differences in pressure and blood flow.

Pulse wave velocity is a technique in which large artery elasticity is assessed from analysis of the peripheral arterial waveform [33]. It is calculated from measurements of pulse transit time and the distance traveled by the pulse between two recording sites. Pulse wave velocity, which is an indicator of arterial stiffness, plays an important clinical role in identifying patients under high cardiovascular risk [33–35]. Pulse wave velocity is higher in hardened vessels and lower in vessels with high distensibility. Arterial stiffness can be affected by structural and functional changes [36]. Structural changes involve the composition of the arterial wall, hypertrophy of smooth muscle cells, and decrease in contents of the extracellular matrix. Arteries become wider and less elastic with advancing age as a consequence of age-related reduction in arterial elastin and increase in collagen content. Several studies have shown that arterial stiffness depends on variation in blood pressure level (stiffness becomes higher at high blood pressure and lower at low blood pressure), through mechanical changes in arterial wall stretching and resulting changes in contribution of elastin and collagen fibers to the elastic modulus [33,35]. Administration of melatonin significantly reduced the internal carotid artery pulsatility index, which is believed to reflect the downstream vasomotor state and resistance, and arterial stiffness by using carotid–femoral (aortic) pulse wave velocity measurements [17,37]. Also, endogenous melatonin may contribute to the nocturnal decrease in blood pressure and aortic pulse wave velocity via inhibition of the sympathetic system [38]. Sympathetic neural control affects small resistance arteries and the mechanical properties of large arteries; activation of the sympathetic nervous system has been shown to reduce distensibility of small- and medium-size arteries in animals [39,40]. Boutouyrie et al. [41] found that increases in sympathetic stimulation are associated with a reduction of radial artery distensibility in humans. The sympathetic nervous system exerts a marked tonic restraint on arterial distensibility, and this restraint involves large arteries with a predominant elastic structure and arteries with a predominant muscle structure. The decrease in aortic distensibility may increase the impedance to left ventricular ejection fraction and may thus reduce the effective coronary blood flow and myocardial oxygen supply, as well as further aggravate myocardial ischemia.

Melatonin can improve vascular morphology. It may provide an antiatherogenic effect via improved nitric oxide production and by protecting low-density lipoproteins from oxidative modification [28]. Oxidation of low-density lipoprotein plays a central role in the development and progression of atherosclerosis [42]. Oxidized low-density lipoprotein is taken into macrophages through scavenger receptors without going through down-regulation and causes formation of foam cells. Oxidation products of low-density lipoproteins are cytotoxic, and these cytotoxic products are especially dangerous for endothelial cells. Oxidized low-density lipoprotein may induce vasoconstriction through inhibition of nitric oxide production and stimulation of endothelin [43]. In hypertriglyceridemic rats, melatonin prevented intimal infiltration by foam cells induced by cholesterol in association with modified plasmatic fatty acid composition [44]. The prevention of early atheromatous changes and endothelial damage with direct impact on arterial function may help several organs, especially the brain, to cope with ischemia–reperfusion injury or other pathological conditions [2]. Régrigny et al. [45] showed that a deficit in melatonin induced by pinealectomy decreased the cross-sectional area, attenuated compliance, and increased stiffness of rat cerebral arterioles, whereas low-dose melatonin treatment prevented the development of these alterations. Elevated plasma homocysteine levels promote atherosclerosis in blood vessels because of the generation of reactive oxygen radicals and reduction in nitric oxide bioavailability. The relation between homocysteine level and melatonin has been researched. Melatonin administration with a methionine-rich diet decreased homocysteine concentrations and oxidative stress, and in one study [46] increased nitric oxide production was observed.

32.3 SUMMARY

Melatonin, a neurohormone produced in the pineal gland mainly during the night by stimulation of β_1 and α_1 adrenergic receptors, affects a variety of heart functions such as cardiac rhythms, arterial blood pressure, and heart rate. However, the mechanisms of melatonin effect on heart functions are still not completely understood. The activation of melatonin receptors on vascular endothelial and vascular smooth muscle cells and the antioxidant effects of melatonin could be responsible for this hormonal effect on vascular tone. The aim of this review is to argue for the melatonin modulation of vascular structure and function.

REFERENCES

1. Scheer, F.A., van Doornen, L.J., Buijs, R.M. 1999. Light and diurnal cycle affect human heart rate: possible role for the circadian pacemaker. *J Biol Rhythms* 14:202–212.
2. Paulis, L., Simko, F. 2007. Blood pressure modulation and cardiovascular protection by melatonin: potential mechanisms behind. *Physiol Res* 56:671–684.
3. Moore, R.Y. 1996. Neural control of the pineal gland. *Behav Brain Res* 73:125–130.
4. Klein, D.C., Sugden, D., Weller, J.L. 1983. Postsynaptic alpha-adrenergic receptors potentiate the beta-adrenergic stimulation of pineal serotonin *N*-acetyltransferase. *Proc Natl Acad Sci U S A* 80:599–603.
5. Ribelayga, C., Pevet, P., Simonneaux, V. 1997. Adrenergic and peptidergic regulations of hydroxyindole-*O*-methyltransferase activity in rat pineal gland. *Brain Res* 777:247–501.
6. Baltatu, O., Afeche, S.C., Dos Santos, S.H.J. et al. 2002. Locally synthesized angiotensin modulates pineal melatonin generation. *J Neurochem* 80:328–334.
7. Turjanski, A.G., Estrin, DA., Rosenstein, R.E., et al. 2004. NMR and molecular dynamics studies of the interaction of melatonin with calmodulin. *Protein Sci* 13:2925–2938.
8. Satake, N., Shibata, S., Takagi, T. 1986. The inhibitory action of melatonin on the contractile response to 5-hydroxytryptamine in various isolated vascular smooth muscles. *Gen Pharmacol* 17:553–558.
9. Chen, L.D., Tan, D.X., Reiter, R.J. et al. 1993. In vivo and in vitro effects of the pineal gland and melatonin on [Ca^{2+} + Mg^{2+}]-dependent ATPase in cardiac sarcolemma. *J Pineal Res* 14:178–183.
10. Dubocovich, M.L. 1995. Melatonin receptors: are there multiple subtypes? *Trends Pharmacol Sci* 16:50–56.
11. Mor, M., Plazzi, P.V., Spadoni, G., Tarzia, G. 1999. Melatonin. *Curr Med Chem* 6:501–518.
12. Ekmekcioglu, C., Haslmayer, P., Philipp, C. et al. 2001. Expression of the MT1 melatonin receptor subtype in human coronary arteries. *J Recept Signal Transduct Res* 21:85–91.
13. Abete, P., Bianco, S., Calabrese, C. et al. 1997. Effects of melatonin in isolated rat papillary muscle. *FEBS Lett* 412:79–85.
14. Ekmekcioglu, C., Thalhammer, T., Humpeler, S. et al. 2003. The melatonin receptor subtype MT2 is present in the human cardiovascular system. *J Pineal Res* 35:40–44.
15. Girouard, H., Denault, C., Chulak, C., de Champlain, J. 2004. Treatment by *N*-acetylcysteine and melatonin increases cardiac baroreflex and improves antioxidant reserve. *Am J Hypertens* 17:947–954.
16. K.-Laflamme, A., Wu, L., Foucart, S., de Champlain, J. 1998. Impaired basal sympathetic tone and alpha1-adrenergic responsiveness in association with the hypotensive effect of melatonin in spontaneously hypertensive rats. *Am J Hypertens* 11:219–229.
17. Arangino, S., Cagnacci, A., Angiolucci, M. et al. 1999. Effects of melatonin on vascular reactivity, catecholamine levels, and blood pressure in healthy men. *Am J Cardiol* 83:1417–149.
18. Chuang, J.I., Chen, S.S., Lin, M.T. 1993. Melatonin decreases brain serotonin release, arterial pressure and heart rate in rats. *Pharmacology* 47:91–97.
19. Holmes, S.W., Sugden, D. 1976. Proceedings: the effect of melatonin on pinealectomy-induced hypertension in the rat. *Br J Pharmacol* 56:360P–361P.
20. Kawashima, K., Miwa, Y., Fujimoto, K., Oohata, H., Nishino, H., Koike, H. 1987. Antihypertensive action of melatonin in the spontaneously hypertensive rat. *Clin Exp Hypertens A* 9:1121–1131.
21. Reppert, S.M., Weaver, D.R., Rivkees, S.A., Stopa, E.G. 1988. Putative melatonin receptors in a human biological clock. *Science* 242:78–81.
22. Kalsbeek, A., Garidou, M.L., Palm, I.F. et al. 2000. Melatonin sees the light: blocking GABA-ergic transmission in the paraventricular nucleus induces daytime secretion of melatonin. *Eur J Neurosci* 12:3146–154.
23. Patel, K.P., Li, Y.F., Hirooka, Y. 2001. Role of nitric oxide in central sympathetic outflow. *Exp Biol Med (Maywood)* 226:814–824.
24. Wang, F., Li, J., Wu, C., Yang, J., Xu, F., Zhao, Q. 2003. The GABA(A) receptor mediates the hypnotic activity of melatonin in rats. *Pharmacol Biochem Behav* 74:573–578.

25. Rossi, N.F., Black, S.M., Telemaque-Potts, S., Chen, H. 2004. Neuronal nitric oxide synthase activity in the paraventricular nucleus buffers central endothelin-1- induced pressor response and vasopressin secretion. *J Cardiovasc Pharmacol* 44 (Suppl 1):S283–S288.
26. Weekley, L.B. 1993. Effects of melatonin on pulmonary and coronary vessels are exerted through perivascular nerves. *Clin Auton Res* 3:45–47.
27. Weekley, L.B. 1993. Effects of melatonin on isolated pulmonary artery and vein: role of vascular endothelium. *Pulm Pharmacol* 6:149–154.
28. Weekley, L.B. 1991. Melatonin-induced relaxation of rat aorta: interaction with adrenergic agonists. *J Pineal Res* 11:28–34.
29. Viswanathan, M., Hissa, R., George, JC. 1986. Suppression of sympathetic nervous system by short photoperiod and melatonin in the Syrian hamster. *Life Sci* 38:73–79.
30. Capsoni, S.M., Viswanathan, M., De Oliveira, A.M., Saavedra, J.M. 1994. Characterization of melatonin receptors and signal transduction system in rat arteries forming the circle of Willis. *Endocrinology* 135:373–378.
31. Viswanathan, M.J., Laitinen, T., Saavedra, J.M. 1990. Expression of melatonin receptors in arteries involved in thermoregulation. *Proc Natl Acad Sci U S A* 87:6200–6203.
32. Capsoni, S., Stankov, B.M., Fraschini, F. 1995. Reduction of regional cerebral blood flow by melatonin in young rats. *Neuroreport* 6:1346–1348.
33. Asmar, R., Benetos, A., Topouchian, J. et al. 1995. Assessment of arterial distensibility by automatic pulse wave velocity measurement. Validation and clinical application studies. *Hypertension* 26:485–490.
34. Yildiz, M., Simsek, G., Uzun, H., Uysal, S., Sahin, S., Balci, H. 2010. Assessment of low-density lipoprotein oxidation, paraoxonase activity, and arterial distensibility in epileptic children who were treated with anti-epileptic drugs. *Cardiol Young* 2:1–8.
35. Yildiz, M. 2010. Arterial distensibility in chronic inflammatory rheumatic disorders. *Open Cardiovasc Med J* 4:83–88.
36. Guerin, A.P., Blacher, J., Pannier, B., Marchais, SJ., Safar, M.E., London, G.M. 2001. Impact of aortic stiffness attenuation on survival of patients in end-stage renal failure. *Circulation* 103:987–992.
37. Yildiz, M., Sahin, B., Sahin, A. 2006. Acute effects of oral melatonin administration on arterial distensibility, as determined by carotid–femoral pulse wave velocity, in healthy young men. *Exp Clin Cardiol* 11:311–313.
38. Yildiz, M., Akdemir, O. 2009. Assessment of the effects of physiological release of melatonin on arterial distensibility and blood pressure. *Cardiol Young* 19:198–203.
39. Cox, R.H. 1976. Effects of norepinephrine on mechanics of arteries in vitro. *Am J Physiol* 231:420–425.
40. Cox, RH., Bagshaw, R.J. 1980. Effects of pulsations on carotid sinus control of regional arterial hemodynamics. *Am J Physiol* 238:H182–H190.
41. Boutouyrie, P., Lacolley, P., Girerd, X., Beck, L., Safar, M., Laurent, S. 1994. Sympathetic activation decreases medium sized arterial compliance in humans. *Am J Physiol* 267:H1368–H1377.
42. Wakatsuki, A., Okatani, Y., Ikenoue, N., Shinohara, K., Watanabe, K., Fukaya, T. 2001. Melatonin protects against oxidized low-density lipoprotein-induced inhibition of nitric oxide production in human umbilical artery. *J Pineal Res* 31:281–288.
43. Davignon, J., Ganz, P. 2004. Role of endothelial dysfunction in atherosclerosis. *Circulation* 109 (23 Suppl 1):III27–32.
44. Pita, M.L., Hoyos, M., Martin-Lacave, I., Osuna, C., Fernández-Santos, J.M., Guerrero, J.M. 2002. Long-term melatonin administration increases polyunsaturated fatty acid percentage in plasma lipids of hypercholesterolemic rats. *J Pineal Res* 32:179–186.
45. Régrigny, O., Delagrange, P., Scalbert, E., Atkinson, J., Chillon, J.M. 2001. Melatonin increases pial artery tone and decreases the lower limit of cerebral blood flow autoregulation. *Fundam Clin Pharmacol* 15:233–238.
46. Murawska-Cialowicz, E., Januszewska, L., Zuwala-Jagiello, J. et al. 2008. Melatonin decreases homocysteine level in blood of rats. *J Physiol Pharmacol* 59:717–729.

33 Melatonin and Sleep Disturbances in Patients with End-Stage Renal Disease

Birgit C. P. Koch, Marije Russcher, and J. Elsbeth Nagtegaal

CONTENTS

33.1 INTRODUCTION

Sleep disturbances are much more prevalent in the dialysis population than in the general population [1]. Several studies on the impact and importance of sleep problems on quality of life in patients on dialysis revealed that sleep disturbances have a major effect on the vitality and general health of these patients [2]. Sleep disturbances in patients on dialysis might be caused by both the pathology of the renal disease and the dialysis treatment itself [3]. Although sleep disorders found in this population can be complex—for example, sleep apnea, restless legs syndrome, and periodic limb movement disorder can cause sleep problems for patients—this chapter will focus on disturbances in the circadian sleep–wake rhythm. Focusing on these disturbances is a novel field of interest in this patient population, but such disturbances can have a prominent role in the development of sleep disorders, and therefore in impairment of quality of life, in patients with end-stage renal disease (ESRD).

An overview of circadian sleep–wake rhythm, the scope of the problem regarding sleep disturbances in this population, the role of melatonin, possible external and internal influences on sleep–wake rhythmicity in patients with ESRD, and possible approaches for strengthening the synchronization of the circadian sleep–wake rhythm will be explored in the following sections.

33.2 DEFINITIONS OF RENAL DISEASE

Chronic kidney disease (CKD) is defined according to the presence of kidney damage and level of kidney function. Five stages of CKD are specified, although cut-off levels between stages are arbitrary [4]. Stage 1 CKD is mildly diminished renal function, with few overt symptoms, whereas stage 5 CKD is a severe illness and requires some form of renal replacement therapy (dialysis or renal transplant). CKD might be a progressive loss of renal function over a period of months or years through five stages, but a patient can also be first diagnosed with stage 5 CKD or progression of CKD can (fortunately) be halted before a more severe stage is reached. With each stage the glomerular filtration rate deteriorates, which is determined by the creatinine level in blood and the amount of proteins in urine (proteinuria). When CKD proceeds to stages 4–5, metabolic acidosis, abnormal levels of potassium, calcium, and phosphate, and anemia can occur. Long-term complications are cardiovascular disease (which is the primary cause of death in this population) and bone disease (e.g., osteodystrophy) [4].

In stage 5 of CKD, dialysis is indicated. Dialysis can be performed via hemodialysis and peritoneal dialysis (PD). In hemodialysis, the patient's blood is pumped through the blood compartment of a dialyzer, exposing it to a semipermeable membrane. The cleaned blood is then returned to the body. Ultrafiltration occurs by the hydrostatic pressure across the dialyzer membrane. This is usually done by applying a negative pressure to the dialysate compartment of the dialyzer. This pressure gradient causes water and dissolved solutes to move from blood to dialysate, and allows removal of several liters of excess fluid during a typical 3- to 5-h dialysis treatment. Hemodialysis treatments are typically given in a dialysis center three times per week (conventional daytime hemodialysis). However, recently different dialysis regimens have been introduced: nocturnal dialysis (slow dialysis 8 h a night for 4–6 days a week at home or in-center on different days) and short daily dialysis (5–6 times a week, for 2 h).

In PD, a sterile solution containing minerals and glucose is run through a tube into the peritoneal cavity, the abdominal body cavity around the intestine, where the peritoneal membrane acts as a semipermeable membrane. The dialysate is left there for a period of time to absorb waste products. Subsequently, it is drained out through the tube and discarded. This cycle or "exchange" can be repeated manually 4–5 times during the day, which is called continuous daytime peritoneal dialysis (CAPD), or can be performed overnight with an automated system (APD). Ultrafiltration occurs via osmosis; the dialysis solution used contains a high concentration of glucose, and the resulting osmotic pressure causes fluid to move from the blood into the dialysate. As a result, more fluid is drained than was instilled. PD is less efficient than conventional daytime hemodialysis, but because it is carried out each day and for a longer period, the net effect in terms of removal of waste products and of salt and water are often similar to hemodialysis [4].

33.3 SLEEP DISTURBANCES IN RENAL DISEASE

Studies have suggested that between 30% and 80% of individuals with ESRD report subjective sleep-related problems [5–8]. Information on circadian rhythm sleep disorders, such as delayed sleep phase syndrome (DSPS), is not available for patients with ESRD.

Patients on daytime hemodialysis and patients with CKD both have reduced total sleep time and reduced sleep efficiency in comparison with healthy subjects [9]. Patients on hemodialysis have less rapid eye movement (REM) sleep, a higher brief arousal index, a higher respiratory disturbance index, less total sleep time, increased wake time after sleep onset, lower sleep efficiency, a higher periodic limb movement index, and longer sleep onset latencies in comparison with patients with CKD [9]. These findings suggest that sleep problems experienced by patients with CKD and those experienced by individuals on hemodialysis might have different etiologies. Functional and psychological factors might have a greater role in patients with CKD, and intrinsic sleep disruption (e.g., arousal, apnea, and limb movements) secondary to the effects of intermittent daytime hemodialysis may play a more important role in individuals on hemodialysis [9]. Furthermore, low serum albumin and psychological stress have been associated with insomnia in individuals with CKD [10]. In our study on 120 daytime hemodialysis patients, we found that subjective sleep efficiency was significantly impaired in comparison with the control group. In addition, the classical hypnotics were not successfully used. We found relationships between decreased sleep efficiency and increased phosphate and urea. Furthermore, hemoglobin levels between 10 and 12 g/dl were associated with better sleep efficiency [11]. Population-specific sleep-promoting interventions might be needed.

Little data comparing the prevalence of sleep disorders in patients on daytime hemodialysis and on PD exist. In one study, hemodialysis patients reported more sleep disturbances than PD patients [12]. However, other studies have found that the type of dialysis and dialysis adequacy did not affect the prevalence of sleep disorders [13]. One study showed that patients on APD were more likely to experience sleep problems than patients on CAPD [14]. Another study showed that changing from CAPD to APD resulted in an alleviation of sleep apnea, possibly owing to the more vigorous clearance of fluid with APD [15]. Studies in which objective techniques of sleep measurement were used, such as actigraphy or polysomnography, have rarely been performed in PD patients. Using actigraphy, we found that patients on daytime hemodialysis experienced the worst sleep, in comparison with patients on nocturnal hemodialysis and automated PD [16].

To increase our knowledge about sleep disturbances in ESRD patients, more studies are needed. It may be hypothesized that the different dialysis techniques (the short but intense urea reduction in conventional daytime hemodialysis in comparison to the slow but constant urea reduction in PD patients) may have an important role in the difference in the prevalence of sleep problems in these populations. The influence of urea on melatonin and sleep–wake rhythm will be discussed later in this chapter.

33.4 FACTORS THAT MAY CAUSE SLEEP DISTURBANCES IN PATIENTS WITH RENAL DISEASE

In patients with renal disease, the circadian sleep–wake rhythm can be disrupted by both internal factors (e.g., biochemical parameters and melatonin) and external factors (e.g., dialysis and medications), as presented in Figure 33.1.

33.4.1 Effects of Dialysis

Daytime hemodialysis can increase daytime sleep propensity, which can lead to delayed sleep onset and decreased nighttime sleep. Several possible causes for these sleep disturbances exist. First, mononuclear cells produce interleukin (IL)-1, IL-6, and tumor necrosis factor (TNF) as a result of complement activation, interaction with the dialyzer, and/or exposure to bacteria wall fragments

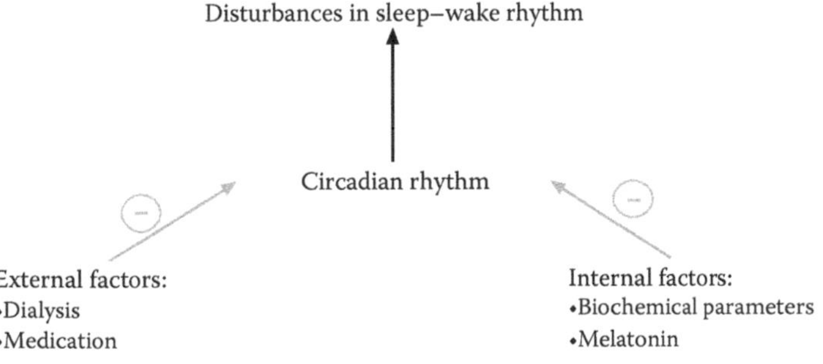

FIGURE 33.1 Overview of possible mechanisms of desynchronization of sleep–wake rhythm, leading to sleep disturbances in ESRD.

(muramyl peptides) [17–19]. IL-1 is involved in both fever production and sleep induction [17]. Fever and chills commonly occur during or after dialysis in the presence of endotoxin-contaminated dialysate. However, a slight increase in body temperature has also been observed in patients undergoing hemodialysis with uncontaminated dialysate [19]. It is suggested that IL-1, IL-6, or TNF produced by peripheral blood mononuclear cells in the bloodstream are recognized as a pyrogenic signal by specific centers within the central nervous system (CNS). Such signals induce the synthesis of prostaglandins that represent the central mediators of the coordinated response, which leads to a rise in core body temperature [3, 17–19].

Body temperature can also rise as a result of heat load from the dialysis bath. Because of the known association between body cooling and sleep onset [20, 21], hemodialysis-associated elevations in body temperature might activate cooling mechanisms that enhance daytime sleep propensity, particularly during the post-hemodialysis period. Chronic, episodic elevations in body temperature in association with hemodialysis might therefore alter the sleep propensity rhythm [22].

In addition, dialysis can induce imbalances in brain and serum osmolarity, resulting in shifts of water from the blood to the brain. This condition, known as disequilibrium syndrome, is associated with a paradoxical acidosis in the cerebrospinal fluid that results from the slow movement of bicarbonate across the blood–brain barrier. Disequilibrium syndrome causes cerebral edema, which can lead to depression of the CNS. This depression causes a decrease in alertness and arousal [23, 24]. Therefore, the depression of the CNS in dialysis patients can lead to daytime sleepiness and can therefore result in an impaired sleep–wake rhythm [25].

Moreover, the hemodialysis procedure is a significant physical and psychological stressor. The stress response triggered by emotional arousal can lead to reactions such as anxiety, depression, and increased daytime sleepiness [26, 27].

Finally, hemodialysis may also affect the sleep–wake cycle by altering exposure to *zeitgebers* (time cues) that help set or entrain the circadian system. The time of day the treatment is given can affect an individual's wake-up time, time for physical activity, meal times, light exposure, social activities [3], and even survival [28].

33.4.2 Effects of Medication

Several drugs commonly prescribed for patients on dialysis can have negative adverse effects on sleep such as insomnia and sedation [29]. This subsection focuses exclusively on medications with potentially sleep-disturbing effects, which are prescribed more often to ESRD patients than to individuals of the same age and gender in the general population [30]. Among the antihypertensive drugs, β adrenergic–receptor antagonists (β blockers) have been associated with tiredness, insomnia, nightmares and vivid dreams, depression, mental confusion, and psychomotor impairment [29, 31]. The severity of adverse effects is affected by the age of the patient and the administered dose: older patients are more sensitive to medication because of the altered absorption and metabolism of drugs in older age [32]. In general, sleep disturbances seem to be more common with the use of lipophilic β blockers (e.g., metoprolol) than with hydrophilic β blockers (e.g., atenolol). However, even atenolol, the most hydrophilic β blocker available, has been shown to increase total wake time at night [31]. β Blockers have also been associated with decline in nocturnal melatonin production [33].

Benzodiazepines can be used for their sleep-inducing effects. These drugs increase total sleep time, reduce sleep latency, and suppress REM and slow-wave sleep [34]. Benzodiazepines also decrease nocturnal melatonin production [35]. Benzodiazepines have been shown to have minimal efficacy in the general older population with sleep problems [36].

33.4.3 Rhythm of Endogenous Melatonin in ESRD Patients

Studies in patients with chronic renal failure, patients on daytime hemodialysis, and animal models of chronic renal failure have shown that the nocturnal surge in melatonin above dim light melatonin

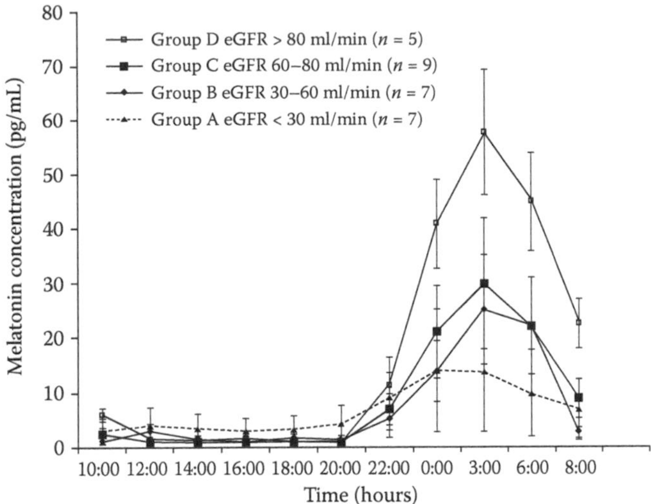

FIGURE 33.2 Melatonin concentration during 24 h in four groups of patients with different glomerular filtration rates. Group D represents best (and normal) renal function; group A presents worst renal function (pre-dialysis). The more renal function deteriorates, the more melatonin concentration decreases. Vertical axis: melatonin concentration in serum (in pg/ml), horizontal axis: time in hours (CREAM study, Koch et al., Impairment of endogenous melatonin rhythm is related to the degree of Chronic Kidney Diseases (CREAM study), *Nephrol. Dial. Transplant.*, 2, 513–519, 2010.)

onset (DLMO) is absent in chronic renal failure [37–41]. Our group found a relationship between decreasing renal function and decreased concentrations of melatonin in serum [42], as shown in Figure 33.2.

The melatonin rhythm was more likely to be abolished in patients on hemodialysis than in patients with chronic renal insufficiency, not on hemodialysis, suggesting an influence of hemodialysis on the rhythm [39]. Lower melatonin levels were associated with more severe sleep disturbances in hemodialysis patients [43]. Reports on melatonin levels during the daytime in patients with renal disease are conflicting as both increased and decreased melatonin levels have been reported in daytime hemodialysis patients [38–41].

A number of mechanisms can explain the disturbance of the circadian melatonin rhythm in patients with renal disease. As mentioned above, daytime dialysis can result in daytime sleepiness and nocturnal insomnia [1, 3]. The resulting disturbed sleep–wake rhythm can lead to the absence of the trigger that starts melatonin production at night [3]. The decline in melatonin levels in patients with renal insufficiency has been reported to be the result of an impairment in β adrenoreceptor–mediated responsiveness [39–44]. The adrenergic system plays an important role in the synthesis of NAT [45–46], a key enzyme in melatonin biosynthesis. Nocturnal levels of NAT activity are decreased in rats rendered uremic by partial nephrectomy [47]. In addition, sleep apnea is common in patients with ESRD [48]. During daytime, melatonin levels have been reported to be much higher in the general apnea patient population without ESRD than in healthy controls, but the nocturnal melatonin surge was absent in patients with apnea [49].

Although knowledge on the dialyzability of substances is important in ESRD, information on the dialysis properties of melatonin and its metabolites is scarce and contradictory. In one study [41], the concentration of serum melatonin and its main urinary metabolite, 6-sulfatoxymelatonin (6-SM), was measured 2 min after the onset of daytime hemodialysis (pre-dialysis), 90 minutes thereafter (mid-dialysis), and shortly before the end of the 3-h dialysis treatment (post-dialysis). The pre-dialysis melatonin concentration was not significantly different from that in the control group of normal volunteers. Serum melatonin concentration fell in the hemodialysis group approximately 25% during dialysis, whereas 6-SM remained virtually unchanged, probably because of the considerable binding of melatonin to albumin and the acute-phase protein α_1-acid glycoprotein [50]. The small change in melatonin concentration between pre-dialysis and post-dialysis was considered an attenuated variation of serum melatonin and metabolite in the morning hours [41]. Lüdemann et al. [51], however, found increased daytime melatonin levels and a significant dialyzability for melatonin (50%) and its metabolite, 6-SM (50%).

33.4.4 Effects of Biochemical Parameters

Blood urea nitrogen level is significantly higher in patients on conventional hemodialysis with pathological daytime sleepiness than in "alert" patients [48, 52]. In addition, sleep onset latency is negatively correlated with blood urea nitrogen level [52]. These findings indicate that excessive daytime sleepiness in patients with ESRD might be related to uremia [48, 52]. Furthermore, in plasma from uremic patients, the number of β_1 and β_2 adrenoreceptors is significantly decreased, as compared with normal values [53]. Such impairment in adrenergic function is associated with the decline in melatonin levels in patients with renal insufficiency [40].

The results of earlier studies in patients on hemodialysis investigating other possible associations between biochemical parameters and sleep disturbances show conflicting results. One study showed serum phosphate levels to correlate inversely with sleep disturbances [54], but another study showed that only urea showed a significant relationship with sleep disturbances [5]. Other researchers found no correlations at all between biochemical markers and sleep disturbances [6]. In one study investigating sleep disturbances among 694 patients on hemodialysis, plasma creatinine and urea levels were surprisingly higher in the control group (without insomnia) than in the insomnia group [7]. This finding was probably a result of an increased protein intake and a greater percentage of male individuals in the control group [7]. A study of 883 patients on maintenance dialysis found that advanced age, excessive alcohol intake, cigarette smoking, polyneuropathy, and a dialysis shift in the morning were independent risk factors for sleep disturbances [8]. Unfortunately, laboratory data were not reported in that study [8]. Erythropoietin deficiency seems to play a role in dysregulation of melatonin metabolism in chronic renal failure [37]. However, the precise role of erythropoietin in melatonin metabolism in renal failure, the existence of its circadian rhythm [55–58], and its relationship with melatonin need further investigation.

33.5 RESYNCHRONIZING THE SLEEP–WAKE RHYTHM

Various approaches have the potential to resynchronize a disrupted circadian sleep–wake rhythm, including nocturnal dialysis, lowering of dialysate temperature, administration of exogenous melatonin, administration of exogenous erythropoietin, bright light, and intradialytic exercise (Figure 33.3). Studies of these approaches in patients with ESRD, although limited, have been successful in strengthening the circadian sleep–wake rhythm in this population.

33.5.1 Nocturnal Hemodialysis

Several studies have investigated the effect of changing from conventional hemodialysis to nocturnal home hemodialysis. The prevalence of sleep apnea declined in patients switching from conventional hemodialysis to nocturnal home hemodialysis, but improvements in sleep efficiency, periodic limb movement disorder, and sleep fragmentation were not observed [59, 60]. Another study showed that conversion to nocturnal home hemodialysis resulted in a decrease in daytime sleepiness and an improvement in sleep onset latency, partly owing to improved control of uremia [52]. With respect to strengthening the sleep–wake rhythm, nocturnal hemodialysis has several advantages. Although anxiety, restricted positions, and alarms might have adverse effects on sleep

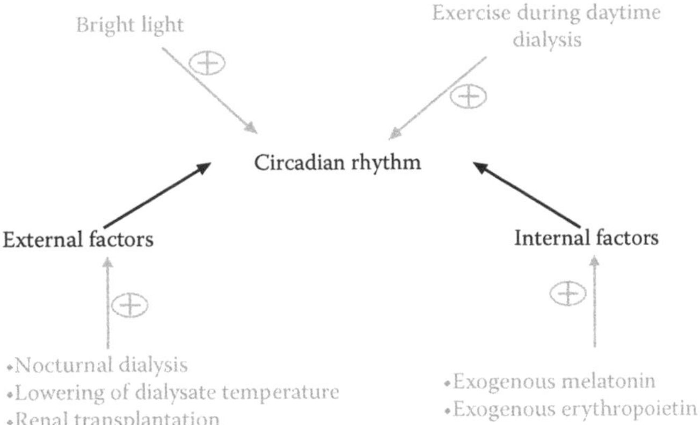

FIGURE 33.3 Various approaches for resynchronizing of circadian sleep–wake rhythm, outlined in gray text boxes and gray arrows.

during nocturnal dialysis, the sleep-promoting effects of dialysis described earlier coincide with the appropriate and conventional time of day. Therefore, a switch to nocturnal dialysis could restore the normal temporal relationship between the sleep period and the other circadian rhythms, and would likely result in an improved quality of both sleep and daytime functioning. The increased dialysis time of nocturnal hemodialysis leads to improved clearance of toxins, which might further enhance the improvements in sleep and daytime functioning. In addition, it is hypothesized that if the normal synchronization between sleep–wake behavior and the circadian system is restored, the endogenous melatonin concentration will exhibit its normal nocturnal surge. To the best of our knowledge, two studies investigating the melatonin rhythm in nocturnal dialysis have been published, and found no difference between melatonin rhythm on dialysis nights and nondialysis nights [43]. Furthermore, we have found increased slow-wave sleep, melatonin rhythm, and improved subjectively scored sleep after switching from daytime to nocturnal dialysis (after a period of 6 months of nocturnal dialysis) [61].

33.5.2 Effects of Exogenous Melatonin on Circadian Sleep–Wake Rhythm

One potential solution to circadian desynchronization problems is a chronobiotic, a drug that phase shifts circadian rhythms in the desired direction and acts as a *zeitgeber* to maintain this stable phase. Exogenous melatonin could presumably fulfill this role [35]. In studies on individuals without renal disease in whom normal melatonin rhythm was disturbed, administration of exogenous melatonin resulted in the recovery of the melatonin rhythm and an improved sleep rhythm [62, 63]. Subjective sleep quality improved and patients felt more refreshed after a night of sleep [62, 63]. Research on the effect of exogenous melatonin supplementation in patients on dialysis is limited. Exogenous melatonin has also been shown to have a beneficial effect on symptoms of insomnia in medically ill patients recently admitted to the hospital with diseases such as cardiovascular disease, diabetes, pulmonary disease, and liver disease [64]. Again, the study included no patients with renal disease and only subjective measurements of sleep evaluation were used.

In individuals with an inappropriately timed endogenous melatonin rhythm, exogenous melatonin can produce a phase advance or a phase delay in the melatonin rhythm, thereby resynchronizing the rhythm [65]. In individuals with an abolished melatonin rhythm and an absence of the nocturnal melatonin surge, however, exogenous melatonin might play another role. Exogenous melatonin bypasses a key enzyme in melatonin synthesis (NAT), which might result in a temporal recovery of enzymatic activity [63]. Therefore, after a period of exogenous melatonin administration, the endogenous enzymatic activity of NAT could be resensitized, enabling the synthesis and release of endogenous melatonin to be triggered at night [63]. We started the study on the Effects of Melatonin on Sleep Problems of Dialysis Patients (EMSCAP) in daytime hemodialysis patients to correct endogenous melatonin rhythm via exogenous melatonin. In this short-term (6 weeks) placebo-controlled crossover setting, exogenous melatonin (3 mg) improved sleep (objectively and subjectively measured) and the endogenous nocturnal melatonin rise was recovered [66].

33.5.3 Lowering Dialysate Temperature and Improved Sleep–Wake Rhythm

Patients on hemodialysis, who are typically hypothermic [67], often obtain a net heat load during a dialysis treatment session. This net heat load activates the cooling process in the body, which is associated with the onset of sleep propensity [23]. Subsequent daytime napping therefore increases, which may result in a disturbed sleep–wake rhythm [22, 26]. One study showed that decreasing dialysate temperature improved nocturnal sleep, by decreasing sympathetic activation and maintaining the normally elevated nocturnal skin temperature until later into the morning [68]. The time of sleep onset was earlier with cool dialysate (35°C) than with warm dialysate (37°C), and trends were seen in longer total sleep and shorter latencies to REM sleep. The heat load was significantly lower with cool dialysate than with warm dialysate during and after dialysis [68].

33.5.4 Correction of Erythropoietin by Exogenous Erythropoietin

A study conducted on rats with chronic renal failure showed that administration of erythropoietin resulted in the normalization of the defective melatonin rhythm [37]. Amelioration of melatonin metabolism with erythropoietin administration in rats with chronic renal failure appears to be consistent with the demonstrated effects of this therapy on various other neuroendocrinological disorders of uremia [69]. Erythropoietin therapy has been shown to restore thyroid-stimulating hormone response to thyroid-releasing hormone, improve follicle-stimulating hormone response to gonadotropin-releasing hormone, and normalize the basal levels of growth hormone and prolactin in patients with ESRD [69].

The available data do not allow any conclusion on the mechanism(s) with which erythropoietin replacement therapy improves the dysregulation of melatonin metabolism in chronic renal failure. Further studies are required to determine if the effect of erythropoietin therapy is mediated by correction of anemia or if it represents a direct action of the hormone on melatonin production [37].

Exogenous melatonin has been shown to prevent oxidative stress induced by iron and erythropoietin administration in patients on chronic hemodialysis [70].

A study of patients on hemodialysis showed that normalization of hematocrit level with recombinant human erythropoietin therapy resulted in improvements in periodic limb movement disorder, improvements in sleep quality, and less daytime sleepiness, probably owing to an increased sense of well-being and improved cognitive functioning [71].

Furthermore, a study investigating anemia correction in patients with congestive heart failure and anemia found that improvements in hemoglobin level (after treatment with erythropoietin and intravenous iron) significantly correlated with improvements in minimal oxygen saturation seen during sleep and with decreases in daytime sleepiness [72]. Anemia correction with erythropoietin treatment was also associated with a reduction in sleep-related breathing disorders in this patient population.

33.5.5 Exercise during HD Treatment

As daytime napping during hemodialysis treatment has been associated with disrupted nighttime sleep [48], exercise during hemodialysis treatment might have a beneficial effect on the sleep–wake rhythm. Indeed, improvements in physical functioning and health-related quality of life were seen after the initiation of exercise training in patients on hemodialysis [73]. In addition, transcutaneous electrical muscle stimulation and passive cycling movements have been shown to have beneficial effects on blood pressure and urea and phosphate removal during hemodialysis [74].

Symptoms of restless legs syndrome have also been shown to be attenuated when hemodialysis patients participate in intradialytic aerobic exercise training [75]. No studies investigating the association between exercise and the sleep–wake rhythm in patients with ESRD have yet been published, but studies in other groups have shown that physical exercise is associated with improved sleep, as measured by actigraphy [76].

33.5.6 Use of Bright Light

The circadian system is highly sensitive to environmental light and may not function optimally in the absence of its synchronizing effect. Use of bright light (±10,000 lux) has been shown to ameliorate sleep disturbances in the elderly population [77]. With advancing age, the circadian clock may initiate sleep-promoting mechanisms at an earlier time of day (phase advance) and the amplitude of the circadian variation in sleep propensity is lower. Bright light can influence circadian factors, and timed exposure to bright light can be used to alleviate insomnia in older individuals [78, 79]. Not all research initiatives on bright light in older individuals with insomnia, however, have shown positive results [80].

Bright light has not been studied yet in patients with ESRD. Since we expect that light as an important synchronizer can resynchronize the disturbed circadian thythm in ESRD patients, we have recently initiated the Study on Hemodialysis: Illumination Effects (SHINE). In this study, we compare melatonin rhythm, sleep, and mood in hemodialysis patients in a short-term crossover design with and without bright light (10,000 lux) during 2 h of dialysis, with light-to-eye distance measured at 60 cm.

33.5.7 Transplantation

Although kidney transplantation provides the best outcome for patients with ESRD in comparison to dialysis in terms of morbidity and mortality and quality of life, sleep disturbances continue to be observed [81]. In recent years, research has mainly focused on sleep-disordered breathing, obstructive sleep apnea syndrome, and restless legs syndrome before and after kidney transplantation. Results are conflicting. It was shown that improvements were seen compared to the period when the patient was still on dialysis. On the other hand, in some studies, the above-mentioned sleep disturbances were still found to be more prevalent in kidney transplant recipients than in the general population, possibly putting them at a higher risk for cardiovascular disease [82–86].

No reliable information is known about melatonin levels and circadian phase disturbances in kidney transplant recipients. It would be of interest to know whether the increase in kidney function after kidney transplantation coincides with an increase in melatonin production at night, a vice versa effect reported by the Circadian Rhythm of Erythropoietin and Melatonin (CREAM) in renal disease [42], in which a decrease in melatonin production was seen with decreasing kidney function. It is therefore not known whether a correlation exists between melatonin levels and sleep problems after kidney transplantation and if exogenous melatonin would alleviate the sleep problems of kidney transplant recipients.

33.6 DIRECTIONS FOR FUTURE RESEARCH/CONCLUSIONS

In summary, external and internal factors can impair the sleep–wake rhythms of patients with ESRD. These factors can lead to disruption of the circadian sleep–wake rhythm and sleep disturbances in this patient population. Various approaches for resynchronization of the biological clock in patients are promising, but further research is warranted, and a greater awareness of the problem is needed to improve the quality of life of patients with ESRD. Future research should be carried out to obtain more insight in circadian rhythm and renal disease and to seek out the most successful approach in resynchronizing rhythm. These studies should be subdivided in four categories of patients: hemodialysis patients, transplantation patients, patients with other forms of renal replacement therapy, and patients with CKD.

In the future, hemodialysis patients are projected to benefit from the results of an upcoming long-term placebo-controlled study on the effects of exogenous melatonin in daytime hemodialysis patients—the MELatOnin anD qualitY of life (MELODY study). This study might confirm the beneficial role of exogenous melatonin on sleep and quality of life. As described in the discussion, melatonin has a role in oxidative stress and circadian blood pressure profile. Therefore, cardiovascular outcomes will also be researched in this study. In relation to this topic, more research on endogenous melatonin, oxidative stress, the immune system, and blood pressure in hemodialysis patients is warranted.

In exogenous melatonin studies, endogenous melatonin levels are measured after a single day of stopping study medication. It would add to our knowledge on melatonin rhythm if day-to-day kinetic research is performed to evaluate the effect of melatonin, even after cessation of melatonin treatment for a longer period. If melatonin rhythm remains improved after medication is stopped, the circadian rhythm may be resynchronized, and the patient does not need to take the medication chronically.

Our research group is preparing a study in transplantation patients, called the Circadian Rhythm In Kidney Transplantation (CRIKT) study. In this study, we will investigate the circadian rhythm before and after transplantation. Since we already know that renal function significantly improves after transplantation, we expect that this may result in an improvement of circadian rhythm. In addition, the role of the donor might be important, as the donor may induce other diurnal rhythms in the acceptor of the graft after transplantation, compared to before transplantation.

We have learned from the CREAM study that renal dysfunction affects the levels of melatonin in patients with CKD. A wide range of research possibilities regarding the influence of renal function on other circadian rhythms is worth pursuing.

Even fewer studies have been performed on sleep and circadian rhythm in PD. This type of dialysis is quite different from hemodialysis, and research on this therapy can establish the impact of dialysis technique on circadian sleep–wake rhythm.

REFERENCES

1. Parker, K. 2003. Sleep disturbances in dialysis patients. *Sleep Med. Rev.* 7: 131–143.
2. Molzahn, A.E., Northcott, H.C., and Dossetor, J.B. 1997. Quality of life of individuals with end stage renal disease: perceptions of patients, nurses, and physicians. *ANNA J.* 24: 325–333.
3. Parker, K.P., Bliwise, D.L., and Rye, D.B. 2000. Hemodialysis disrupts basic sleep regulatory mechanisms: building hypotheses. *Nurs. Res.* 49: 327–332.
4. Leunissen, K.M.L., Kooiman, J.P., and Krediet, R.T. 2000. Hemodialysis and peritoneal dialysis. In *Clinical Nephrology*, edited by De Jong, P.E., Koomans, H.A., and Weening, J.J., 395–423. Maarssen: Elsevier Healthcare [Dutch].
5. Walker, S., Fine, A., and Kryger, M.H. 1995. Sleep complaints are common in a dialysis unit. *Am. J. Kidney Dis.* 26: 751–756.
6. Mucsi, I. et al. 2004. Sleep disorders and illness intrusiveness in patients on chronic dialysis. *Nephrol. Dial. Transplant.* 19: 1815–1822.
7. Sabbatini, M.A. et al. 2002. Insomnia in maintenance hemodialysis patients. *Nephrol. Dial. Transplant.* 17: 852–856.
8. Merlino, G. et al. 2006. Sleep disorders in patients with end-stage renal disease undergoing dialysis therapy. *Nephrol. Dial. Transplant.* 21: 184–190.
9. Parker, K.P. et al. 2005. Polysomnographic measures of nocturnal sleep in patients on chronic, intermittent daytime hemodialysis vs those with chronic kidney disease. *Nephrol. Dial. Transplant.* 20: 1422–1428.

10. Mendelssohn, D. et al. 2004. Sleep disorders and quality of life in chronic kidney disease patients in the predialysis stage. *J. Am. Soc. Nephrol.* 15:132A.
11. Koch, B.C. et al. 2008. Subjective sleep efficiency of haemodialysis patients. *Clin. Nephrol.* 70: 411–418.
12. Barrett, B.J. et al. 1990. Clinical and psychological correlates of somatic symptoms in patients on dialysis. *Nephron* 55: 10–15.
13. Holley, J.L., Nespor, S., and Rault, R. 1992. A comparison of reported sleep disorders in patients on chronic hemodialysis and continuous peritoneal dialysis. *Am. J. Kidney Dis.* 19: 156–161.
14. Bro, S. et al. 1999. A prospective, randomized multicenter study comparing APD and CAPD treatment. *Perit. Dial. Int.* 19: 526–533.
15. Tang, S.C. et al. 2006. Alleviation of sleep apnea in patients with chronic renal failure by nocturnal cycler-assisted peritoneal dialysis compared with conventional continuous ambulatory peritoneal dialysis. *J. Am. Soc. Nephrol.* 17: 2607–2616.
16. Koch, B.C. et al. 2010. Different melatonin rhythms and sleep–wake rhythms in patients on peritoneal dialysis, daytime hemodialysis and nocturnal hemodialysis. *Sleep Med.* 11: 242–246.
17. Dinarello, C.A. 1992. Interleukin-1 and tumor necrosis factor and their naturally occurring antagonists during hemodialysis. *Kidney Int.* 38 (Suppl): S68–S77.
18. Herbelin, A. et al. 1990. Influence of uremia and hemodialysis on circulating interleukin-1 and tumor necrosis factor alpha. *Kidney Int.* 37: 116–125.
19. Zaoui, P., and Hakim, R.M. 1994. The effects of the dialysis membrane on cytokine release. *J. Am. Soc. Nephrol.* 4: 1711–1718.
20. Lack, L.C., and Lushington, K. 1996. The rhythm of human sleep propensity and core body temperature. *J. Sleep Res.* 5: 1–11.
21. Lack, L.C. et al. 2008. The relationship between insomnia and body temperatures. *Sleep Med. Rev.* 12: 307–317.
22. Campbell, S.S., Dawson, D., and Zulley, J. 1993. When the human circadian system is caught napping: evidence for endogenous rhythms close to 24 hours. *Sleep* 16: 638–640.
23. Blagg, C.R. 1989. Acute complications associated with hemodialysis. In *Replacement of Renal Function by Dialysis: A Textbook of Dialysis*, edited by Maher, J.F., 750–771. Boston, MA: Kluwer Academic.
24. Plum, F., and Posner, J.B. 1985. Multifocal, diffuse, and metabolic brain diseases causing stupor or coma. In *The Diagnosis of Stupor and Coma,* edited by Plum, F., and Posner, J.B, 177–303. Philadelphia, PA: F.A. Davis.
25. DiFresco, V. et al. 2000. Dialysis disequilibrium syndrome: an unusual cause of respiratory failure in the medical intensive care unit. *Intensive Care Med.* 26: 628–630.
26. Claghorn, J.L. et al. 1981. Daytime sleepiness in depression. *J. Clin. Psychiatry* 42: 342–343.
27. Stapleton, S. 1992. Etiologies and indicators of powerlessness in persons with end-stage renal disease. In *Coping with Chronic Illness: Overcoming Powerlessness*, edited by Miller, J.F., 163–178. Philadelphia, PA: F.A. Davis.
28. Bliwise, D.L. et al. 2001. Survival by time of day of hemodialysis in an elderly cohort. *JAMA* 286: 2690–2694.
29. McAinsh, J. and Cruickshank, J.M. 1990. Beta-blockers and central nervous system side effects. *Pharmacol. Ther.* 46: 163–197.
30. Koch, B.C.P. et al. 2008. Prescription of hypnotics and potentially sleep-disturbing medication in hemodialysis patients. *Pharm. Weekblad.* [*Dutch*] 25: 132–134.
31. Van Den Heuvel, C.J., Reid, K.J., and Dawson, D. 1997. Effect of atenolol on nocturnal sleep and temperature in young men: reversal by pharmacological doses of melatonin. *Physiol. Behav.* 61: 795–802.
32. The Merck Manual Online, via http://www.merck.com/mmpe/index.html (accessed on 18 April 2009).
33. Brismar, K. et al. 1988. Melatonin secretion related to side effects of beta-blockers from the Central Nervous System. *Acta Med. Scand.* 223: 525–530.
34. Qureshi, A., and Lee-Chiong Jr., T. 2004. Medications and their effects on sleep. *Med. Clin. North Am.* 88: 751–66.
35. Nagtegaal, J.E., Kerkhof, G.A., and Smits, M.G. 2002. Chronobiological, clinical and cpharmacological aspects of melatonin in human circadian rhythm dysfunction. In *Treatise on Pineal Gland and Melatonin*, edited by Haldar, C. et al., 461–89. Enfield: Science Publishers.
36. Glass, J. et al. 2005. Sedative hypnotics in older people with insomnia: meta-analysis of risks and benefits. *BMJ* 331: 1169–1176.
37. Vaziri, N.D. 1996. Dysregulation of melatonin metabolism in chronic renal insufficiency: role of erythropoietin-deficiency anemia. *Kidney Int.* 50: 653–656.

38. Viljoen, M. et al. 1992. Melatonin in chronic renal failure. *Nephron* 60: 138–143.
39. Karasek, M. et al. 2005. Decreased melatonin nocturnal concentrations in hemodialyzed patients. *Neuro Endocrinol. Lett.* 26: 653–656.
40. Karasek, M. et al. 2002. Circadian serum melatonin profiles in patients suffering from chronic renal failure. *Neuro Endocrinol. Lett.* 23 (Suppl 1): 97–102.
41. Vaziri, N.D. et al. 1993. Serum melatonin and 6-sulfatoxymelatonin in end-stage renal disease: effect of hemodialysis. *Artif. Organs* 17: 764–769.
42. Koch B.C. et al. 2010. Impairment of endogenous melatonin rhythm is related to the degree of Chronic Kidney Disease (CREAM study). *Nephrol. Dial. Transplant.* 2: 513–519.
43. Geron, R. et al. 2006. Polymorphonuclear leucocyte priming in long intermittent nocturnal hemodialysis patients—is melatonin a player? *Nephrol. Dial. Transplant.* 21: 3196–3201.
44. Souchet, T. et al. 1986. Impaired regulation of beta 2-adrenergic receptor density in mononuclear cells during chronic renal failure. *Biochem. Pharmacol.* 35: 2513–2519.
45. Claustrat, B. Brun, J., and Chazot, G. 2005. The basic physiology and pathophysiology of melatonin. *Sleep Med. Rev.* 9: 11–24.
46. Scheer, F.A., and Czeisler, C.A. 2005. Melatonin, sleep, and circadian rhythms. *Sleep Med. Rev.* 9: 5–9.
47. Holmes, E.W. et al. 1989. Testicular dysfunction in experimental chronic renal insufficiency: a deficiency of nocturnal pineal *N*-acetyltransferase activity. *Br. J. Exp. Pathol.* 70: 349–356.
48. Hanly, P. 2004. Sleep apnea and daytime sleepiness in end-stage renal disease. *Semin. Dial.* 17: 109–114.
49. Ulfberg, J., Micic, S., and Strøm, J. 1998. Afternoon serum-melatonin in sleep disordered breathing. *J. Intern. Med.* 244: 163–168.
50. Morin, D. et al. 1997. Melatonin high-affinity binding to alpha-1-acid glycoprotein in human serum. *Pharmacology* 54: 271–275.
51. Lüdemann, P., Zwernemann, S., and Lerchl, A. 2001. Clearance of melatonin and 6-sulfatoxymelatonin by hemodialysis in patients with end-stage renal disease. *J. Pineal Res.* 31: 222–227.
52. Hanly, P. et al. 2003. Daytime sleepiness in patients with CRF: impact of nocturnal hemodialysis. *Am. J. Kidney Dis.* 41: 403–410.
53. Ferchland, A. et al. 1998. Effects of uremic plasma on alpha- and beta-adrenoceptor subtypes. *Nephron* 80: 46–50.
54. Unruh, M.L. et al. 2003. Sleep quality and clinical correlates in patients on maintenance dialysis. *Clin. Nephrol.* 59: 280–288.
55. Wide, L. Bengtsson, C., and Birgegård, G. 1989. Circadian rhythm of erythropoietin in human serum. *Br. J. Haematol.* 72: 85–90.
56. Koopman, M.G. et al. 1989. Circadian rhythm of glomerular filtration rate in normal individuals. *Clin. Sci. (Lond.)* 77: 105–111.
57. Roberts, D., and Smith, D.J. 1996. Erythropoietin does not demonstrate circadian rhythm in healthy men. *J. Appl. Physiol.* 80: 847–851.
58. Buemi, M. et al. 1992. The circadian rhythm of erythropoietin in subjects with pre-terminal uremia. *Clin. Nephrol.* 37: 159–160.
59. Hanly, P. Chan, C., and Pierratos, A. 2003. The impact of nocturnal hemodialysis on sleep apnea in ESRD patients. *Nephrol. News Iss.* 17: 19–21.
60. Hanly, P.J., and Pierratos, A. 2001. Improvement of sleep apnea in patients with chronic renal failure who undergo nocturnal hemodialysis. *N. Engl. J. Med.* 344: 102–107.
61. Koch, B.C. et al. 2009. Effects of nocturnal hemodialysis on melatonin rhythm and sleep-wake behavior: an uncontrolled trial. *Am. J. Kidney Dis.* 53: 658–664.
62. Kunz, D., and Bes, F. 2001. Exogenous melatonin in periodic limb movement disorder: an open clinical trial and a hypothesis. *Sleep.* 24: 183–187.
63. Nagtegaal, J.E. et al. 1998. Delayed sleep phase syndrome: A placebo-controlled cross-over study on the effects of melatonin administered five hours before the individual dim light melatonin onset. *J. Sleep Res.* 7: 135–143.
64. Andrade, C. et al. 2001. Melatonin in medically ill patients with insomnia: a double-blind, placebo-controlled study. *J. Clin. Psychiatry* 62: 41–45.
65. Arendt, J., and Skene, D.J. 2005. Melatonin as a chronobiotic. *Sleep Med. Rev.* 9: 25–39.
66. Koch, B.C. et al. 2009. The effects of melatonin on sleep–wake rhythm of daytime haemodialysis patients: a randomized, placebo-controlled, cross-over study (EMSCAP study). *Br. J. Clin. Pharmacol.* 67: 68–75.

67. Pérgola, P.E., Habiba, N.M., and Johnson, J.M. 2004. Body temperature regulation during hemodialysis in long-term patients: is it time to change dialysate temperature prescription? *Am. J. Kidney Dis.* 44: 155–165.
68. Parker, K.P. et al. 2007. Lowering dialysate temperature improves sleep and alters nocturnal skin temperature in patients on chronic hemodialysis. *J. Sleep Res.* 16: 42–50.
69. Ramirez, G. et al. 1992. Hypothalamo-hypophyseal, thyroid and gonadal function before and after erythropoietin therapy in dialysis patients. *J. Clin. Endocrinol. Metab.* 74: 517–524.
70. Herrera, J. et al. 2001. Melatonin prevents oxidative stress resulting from iron and erythropoietin administration. *Am. J. Kidney Dis.* 37: 750–757.
71. Benz, R.L. et al. 1999. A preliminary study of the effects of correction of anemia with recombinant human erythropoietin therapy on sleep, sleep disorders, and daytime sleepiness in hemodialysis patients (The SLEEPO study). *Am. J. Kidney Dis.* 34: 1089–1095.
72. Zilberman, M. et al. 2007. Improvement of anemia with erythropoietin and intravenous iron reduces sleep-related breathing disorders and improves daytime sleepiness in anemic patients with congestive heart failure. *Am. Heart J.* 154: 870–876.
73. Painter, P. et al. 2000. Physical functioning and health-related quality-of-life changes with exercise training in hemodialysis patients. *Am. J. Kidney Dis.* 35: 482–492.
74. Farese, S. et al. 2008. Effect of transcutaneous electrical muscle stimulation and passive cycling movements on blood pressure and removal of urea and phosphate during hemodialysis. *Am. J. Kidney Dis.* 52: 745–752.
75. Sakkas, G.K. et al. 2008. Intradialytic aerobic exercise training ameliorates symptoms of restless legs syndrome and improves functional capacity in patients on hemodialysis: a pilot study. *ASAIO J.* 54: 185–190.
76. Mauvieux, B. et al. 2003. A study comparing circadian rhythm and sleep quality of athletes and sedentary subjects engaged in night work. *Can. J. Appl. Physiol.* (*French*) 28: 831–887.
77. Van Someren, E.J., Riemersma, R.F., and Swaab, D.F. 2002. Functional plasticity of the circadian timing system in old age: light exposure. *Prog. Brain Res.* 138: 205–231.
78. Campbell, S.S., Dawson, D., and Anderson, M.W. 1993. Alleviation of sleep maintenance insomnia with timed exposure to bright light. *J. Am. Geriatr. Soc.* 41: 829–836.
79. Lack, L. et al. 2005. The treatment of early-morning awakening insomnia with 2 evenings of bright light. *Sleep* 28: 616–623.
80. Friedman, L. et al. 2009. Scheduled bright light for treatment of insomnia in older adults. *J. Am. Geriatr. Soc.* 57: 441–452.
81. Sabbatini, M. et al. 2008. Renal transplantation and sleep: a new life is not enough. *J. Nephrol.* 21 (Suppl 13): S97–S101.
82. O Rodrigues, C.J. et al. 2010. Sleep-disordered breathing changes after kidney transplantation: a polysomnographic study. *Nephrol. Dial. Transplant.* 25: 2011–2015.
83. Molnar, M.Z. et al. 2010. Sleep apnea is associated with cardiovascular risk factors among kidney transplant patients. *Clin. J. Am. Soc. Nephrol.* 5: 125–132.
84. Mallamaci, F. et al. 2009. Sleep disordered breathing in renal transplant patients. *Am. J. Transplant.* 9: 1373–1381.
85. Beecroft, J.M. et al. 2008. Improvement of periodic limb movements following kidney transplantation. *Nephron. Clin. Pract.*, 109: c133–c139.
86. Molnar, M.Z. et al. 2007. Restless legs syndrome, insomnia, and quality of life after renal transplantation. *J. Psychosom. Res.* 63: 591–597.

34 Melatonin and Traumatic Stress

Petr Bob

CONTENTS

34.1 INTRODUCTION

Melatonin is a small lipid- and water-soluble indoleamine (*N*-acetyl-5-methoxytryptamine) that can easily diffuse through cell membranes, and functions as an important signal molecule in unicellular organisms, plants, fungi, and also in animals and humans [1–5]. The primary site of its biosynthesis in humans is the pineal gland, but its production also occurs in the retina, gastrointestinal tract, skin, bone marrow cells, and lymphocytes [6–14]. Melatonin synthesis is closely related with sleep regulation (with nocturnal maximum) and other cyclic metabolic activities linked to biological clocks regulation, which enables order and temporal relationships in normal interactions of various bodily processes. Additionally, there is growing evidence that circulating hormones and other metabolic signals may modulate circadian oscillations via clock gene expression in some brain regions and peripheral structures, which in turn enable integration of circadian, hormonal, and metabolic information [15–18]. For example, melatonin modulates the rhythm of the clock gene *Per1* in the pituitary gland, striatum, and adrenal cortex [19–22]. These inner clocks are also necessary for collecting information and creating temporal order of mental experience. Typical changes in temporal order of mental experience may occur during stress that presents a moment of cognitive conflict associated with spatiotemporal disorganization and lack of order in mental experience including its temporal–episodic component. These disruptions of temporal integration likely play an important role in mental disorders and may cause dissociation of mental experience.

34.2 SPATIOTEMPORAL INTEGRATION AND COGNITIVE FUNCTIONS

More than three centuries ago, Rene Descartes intuitively postulated that information from various sensory sources is fused and thought that ". . . although the soul is joined to the whole body there is a certain part where it exercises its functions more than all the others." He also proposed that time is a basic mechanism of the universe and used the "clock" metaphor as an explanation for the basic mechanism of the brain and other physiologic functions [23, 24]. Descartes intuitively postulated that this information is fused and governed by clock mechanisms and described the mind as an extracorporeal entity expressed through the pineal gland [23, 24]. In his work, Descartes intuitively anticipated some issues related to the so-called "binding problem" of consciousness that has played an important role in recent cognitive neuroscience. This problem means that there must be a neural correlate of consciousness that, as a part of the nervous system, transforms neural activity to reportable subjective experience. Most likely, this neural correlate of consciousness enables us to compare and bind activity patterns only if they arrive simultaneously at the neural correlate of a conscious experience [25]. In addition, consciousness seems to be dependent on the temporal organization of neural activity, and there is clinical evidence that certain parts of the brain are more essential for consciousness than others. From this point of view, consciousness combines the present multimodal sensory information processed in distributed brain structures with the past processed information and creates spatiotemporal memory. Information from each modality is continuously distributed into distinct features, and locally processed in different relatively specialized brain regions and globally integrated by interactions among these regions. What seems to be most important is that information is not only locally processed but is represented by integration through levels of synchronization of functionally distinct cognitive modules connecting various neuronal populations that enable coherence among multiple brain regions that facilitate large-scale integration, or "binding" [26–29].

34.3 MELATONIN, SUPRACHIASMATIC NEURONS, AND NEUROCOGNITIVE BINDING

Recent data suggest that neurons of suprachiasmatic nuclei (SCN) play an important role in temporal integration and binding, and there is accumulating evidence that rhythmicity in the SCN is the product of a highly organized network of heterogeneous cells [30–32]. This unique and specialized network organization of SCN oscillators presents an integrative framework for individual neural oscillators with the temporal patterns of rhythmicity that are organized into a coherent activity and facilitate temporal synchronization that produces differentially timed waves specifically targeting the pineal gland and other structures, and controls neuroendocrine rhythms [30–32]. Melatonin also plays a unique role in this process as one of the endocrine output signals involved in circadian information processing, which—as an endogenous synchronizer—is able to stabilize and reinforce circadian rhythms and their mutual relationships. This highly organized integrative process occurs at various levels of the circadian network and through gene expression in some brain regions and peripheral structures influences integration of circadian, hormonal, and metabolic information and creation of temporal order of bodily and mental experiences [18, 33, 34]. The process of creating this specific temporal order is reflected in processes related to association of all processed information necessary for memory consolidation that must preserve all the information in the temporal causal order and synchrony or sequentiality of the internal cognitive maps.

In this context, there is evidence that melatonin plays a significant role in memory formation, long-term potentiation (LTP), and synaptic plasticity in the hippocampus and other brain regions [35–40]. A mechanism probably underlying the effects of melatonin on synaptic plasticity is a modulation of the intrinsic excitability, which influences both excitatory and inhibitory neurotransmitter systems [38, 41, 42]. In this context, various electrophysiological studies have reported that melatonin may regulate the electrical activities of hippocampal neurons [39, 43–50] and alter synaptic transmission between hippocampal neurons [51–53]. These findings provide evidence that melatonin may regulate learning and memory through its influence on synaptic connections and synaptic strength within the hippocampus and also the strength of excitatory synaptic transmission regulating LTP. In addition, melatonin may also influence rhythms in gene expression and second-messenger systems [21, 39, 48].

34.4 MELATONIN, CONSOLIDATION OF SPATIOTEMPORAL MEMORY, AND STRESS

Historical and recent findings indicate that repeated stress, and especially traumatic stressful experiences, may disturb mental integrity and lead to dissociation of memory and mental experience.

The concept of dissociation was developed by Pierre Janet, who found that dissociative reaction is most often a consequence of abuse or traumatic experiences that lead to a loss of inhibitory control over certain mental contents and may produce split fragments of the mind because of the intensely negative effects of stressful events [54–57]. This clinical experience of psychological fragmentation of memory contents is in agreement with experimental evidence of neural dissociability of memory processes [58–61]. The evidence supports the view that memory systems concerned with encoding emotion and context are dissociable at psychological, physiological, and anatomical levels [62]. In addition, there is evidence that stress disrupts normal activity and memory consolidation in the hippocampus and the prefrontal cortex, which may cause that memories consolidated under high levels of stress are stored without a contextual or spatiotemporal frame [63–65]. Together, these findings indicate that neurophysiological processes related to consolidation of stressful emotional experiences produce memories that are frequently fragmentary, and temporally and spatially disorganized [66]. For example, disturbed temporal memory related to stress conditions is evident from studies focusing on episodic and autobiographical memories in individuals who were exposed to a traumatic event and after the event or later experienced temporal disorganization, but not absence of emotions or dissociative amnesia [67]. Other studies also provide evidence demonstrating that exposure to a significant psychological stressor preserves or even enhances memory for emotional aspects of an event, and simultaneously disrupts memory for nonemotional aspects of the same event [65]. Together, these results provide evidence that stress may have differential effects on brain systems responsible for encoding and retrieving memories in the amygdala and the hippocampal formation, and cause typical forms of spatiotemporal disorganization, fragmentation, and incompleteness [65, 68].

34.5 MELATONIN AND STRESS

Recent experimental and clinical findings indicate that stressful events are related to melatonin alterations in animals and in humans, which suggest an association between stress, melatonin production, and neurodevelopment [69–75]. For example, there is evidence from animal models that repeated maternal separation and deprivation cause low blood melatonin levels, and there is also evidence that blood melatonin levels and spatial memory performance in both male and female adolescent rats are significantly negatively correlated [69]. Moreover, further studies have found that immobilization stress induces pinealocyte degeneration [75–78] and leads to a significant increase in pineal melatonin levels [79–81]. In addition, there is also evidence from animal models that psychosocial stress may induce a robust increase in the melatonin metabolite, 6-sulfatoxymelatonin, in subordinate animals [82, 83]. These findings are also in agreement with data indicating that melatonin receptors are also present in regions that participate in stress response, such as the hippocampus and the adrenal gland [50, 91], and vice versa that the pineal gland expresses a high density of the glucocorticoid receptor [88–90]. These data suggest that the pineal gland may be a target site for glucocorticoid damage during stress, as has been similarly observed in other regions, such as the hippocampus, which are highly sensitive to stress and prolonged glucocorticoid secretion during chronic stress, and this may induce deleterious effects [81]. The pineal gland may be affected by prolonged glucocorticoid secretion during chronic stress, which leads to deleterious effects by inhibition of glucose transport, and a faster decline in ATP concentrations and metabolism in pinealocytes, as has been proposed for hippocampal stress damage [81, 92]. Stress may impair the sympathetic innervation of the pineal gland and the rhythmic secretion of melatonin, which may influence the modulation of neurotransmitter release (especially serotonin and dopamine [70]) and may specifically influence the hippocampus (which has high levels of melatonin receptors) and regulate the limbic–HPA and sympatheticadrenergic–noradrenergic systems [50, 81].

Collectively, these findings suggest that melatonin probably has a specific role in mechanisms of consciousness, memory, emotional processes, and stress [93–95], which is consistent with studies indicating that melatonin induces alterations in psychopathology mainly in patients with depression, schizophrenia, anxiety disorders, eating disorders, and other mental disorders [87, 96]. Among the typical symptoms related to stress are sleep disturbances (e.g., insomnia) and reduced nocturnal peak of pineal melatonin secretion, which is often observed in depressed patients [84–87], in agreement with many studies reporting decreased melatonin levels in patients with depressive disorder although melatonin increase has also been documented [87, 97–100]. Typical melatonin alterations have also been found in patients with schizophrenia, which suggests that diminished melatonin secretion and subnormal plasma melatonin levels may be associated with the pathophysiology of some schizophrenic patients [87, 101–105]. In addition, characteristic alterations in rhythm of melatonin secretion have also been found in other mental diseases [87, 106–110], indicating its involvement in the pathophysiology of some psychiatric disorders.

34.6 CONCLUSION

According to recent evidence, melatonin represents an important aspect of the biological clock and, on many levels of living organisms, represents an embodied time that is a major factor of bodily and mental functioning that significantly influences encoding and contextual binding in memory processes and cognition. In this context, traumatic stress presents an event associated with spatiotemporal disorganization and lack of order in mental experience that has been identified as a significant factor in the pathogenesis of mental disorders [111–114]. In addition, it has been well documented that stress exposure in childhood may determine developmental abnormalities in the amygdala, hippocampus, cerebellum, anterior cingulate cortex, corpus callosum, and other brain structures that play a critical role in mediating the response to stress [111, 112, 115, 116]. Although at this time the relationship between stress and melatonin is only partially understood, it is likely that melatonin disturbances may reflect specific changes in temporal binding and encoding episodic memory related to traumatic stress and dissociation, and vice versa positive influences of melatonin on brain functions, memory, and cognition [117–120] seem to be particularly a promising topic for further research, which could be helpful in the treatment of several mental disorders.

ACKNOWLEDGMENTS

This work was supported by research grants MSM0021620849, MSM0021622404, and support of research project of Centre for Neuropsychiatric Research of Traumatic Stress 1M06039 by Czech Ministry of Education.

REFERENCES

1. Yu, H.S., Reiter, R.J. 1993. *Melatonin: Biosynthesis, Physiological Effects, and Clinical Applications*. CRC Press, Boca Raton, FL.
2. Reiter, R., Tan, D.X., Manchester, L.C. et al. 2007. Melatonin in edible plants (Phytomelatonin): identification, concentrations, bioavailability and proposed functions. *World Rev Nutr Diet* 97:211–230.
3. Afreen, F., Zobayed, S.M.A., Kozai, T. 2006. Melatonin in *Glycyrrhiza uralensis*: response of plant roots to spectral quality of light and UV-B radiation. *J Pineal Res* 41:108–115.
4. Fideleff, H.L., Boquete, H., Fideleff, G. et al. 2006. Gender-related differences in urinary 6-sulfatoxymelatonin levels in obese pubertal individuals. *J Pineal Res* 40:214–218.
5. Lerner, A.B., Case, J.D., Takahashi, Y. et al. 1958. Isolation of melatonin, the pineal gland factor that lightens melanocytes. *J Am Chem Soc* 80:2587.
6. Cardinali, D.P., Rosner, J.M. 1971. Metabolism of serotonin by the rat retina "in vitro." *J Neurochem* 18:769–1770.
7. Tosini, G., Menaker, M. 1998. The clock in the mouse retina: melatonin synthesis and photoreceptor degeneration. *Brain Res* 789:221–228.
8. Liu C., Fukuhara C., Wessel, J.H. III et al. 2004. Localization of Aa-nat mRNA in the rat retina by fluorescence in situ hybridization and laser capture microdissection. *Cell Tissue Res* 315:197–201.

9. Conti A., Conconi S., Hertens, E. et al. 2000. Evidence for melatonin synthesis in mouse and human bone marrow cells. *J Pineal Res* 28:193–202.
10. Champier J., Claustrat B., Besancon, R. et al. 1997. Evidence for tryptophan hydroxylase and hydroxy-indol-*O*-methyl-transferase mRNAs in human blood platelets. *Life Sci* 60:2191–2197.
11. Bubenik, G.A. 2002. Gastrointestinal melatonin: localization, function, and clinical relevance. *Dig Dis Sci* 47:2336–2348.
12. Slominski, A., Wortsman, J., Tobin, D.J. 2005. The cutaneous serotoninergic/melatoninergic system: securing a place under the sun. *FASEB J* 19:176–194.
13. Slominski, A., Fischer, T.W., Zmijewski, M.A. et al. 2005. On the role of melatonin in skin physiology and pathology. *Endocrine* 27:137–148.
14. Carrillo-Vico, A., Calvo, J.R., Abreu, P. et al. 2004. Evidence of melatonin synthesis by human lymphocytes and its physiological significance: possible role as intracrine, autocrine, and/or paracrine substance. *FASEB J* 18:537–539.
15. Cardinali, D.P., Furio, A.M., Reyes, M.P. et al. 2006. The use of chronobiotics in the resynchronization of the sleep–wake cycle. *Cancer Causes Control* 17:601–609.
16. Morin, L.P. 2007. SCN organization reconsidered. *J Biol Rhythms* 22:3–13.
17. Kalsbeek, A., Perreau-Lenz, S., Buijs, R.M. 2006. A network of (autonomic) clock outputs. *Chronobiol Int* 23:521–535.
18. Rutter, J., Reick, M., McKnight, S.L. 2002. Metabolism and the control of circadian rhythms. *Annu Rev Biochem* 71:307–331.
19. Messager, S., Garabette, M.L., Hastings, M.H. et al. 2001. Tissue specific abolition of Per1 expression in the pars tuberalis by pinealectomy in the Syrian hamster. *Neuroreport* 12:579–582.
20. Uz, T., Akhisaroglu, M., Ahmed, R. et al. 2003. The pineal gland is critical for circadian Period1 expression in the striatum and for circadian cocaine sensitization in mice. *Neuropsychopharmacology* 28:2117–2123.
21. Von Gall, C., Garabette, M.L., Kell, C.A. et al. 2002. Rhythmic gene expression in pituitary depends on heterologous sensitization by the neurohormone melatonin. *Nat Neurosci* 5:234–238.
22. Perrin, J.S., Segall, L.A., Harbour, V.L. et al. 2006. The expression of the clock protein PER2 in the limbic forebrain is modulated by the estrous cycle. *Proc Natl Acad Sci U S A* 103:5591–5596.
23. Barrera-Mera, B., Barrera-Calva, E. 1998. The Cartesian clock metaphor for pineal gland operation pervades the origin of modern chronobiology. *Neurosci Biobehav Rev* 23:1–4.
24. Smith, C.U. 1998. Descartes' pineal neuropsychology. *Brain Cogn* 36:57–72.
25. Van de Grind, W. 2002. Physical, neural, and mental timing. *Conscious Cogn* 11:241–264.
26. John, E.R. 2002. The neurophysics of consciousness. *Brain Res Rev* 39:1–28.
27. Singer, W. 2001. Consciousness and the binding problem. *Ann N Y Acad Sci* 929:123–146.
28. Crick, F., Koch, C. 2003. A framework for consciousness. *Nat Neurosci* 6:119–126.
29. Zeman, A. 2001. Consciousness. *Brain* 124 (Pt 7):1263–1289.
30. Kalsbeek, A., Palm, I.F., La Fleur, S.E. et al. 2006. SCN outputs and the hypothalamic balance of life. *J Biol Rhythms* 21:458–469.
31. Indic, P., Schwartz, W.J., Herzog, E.D. et al. 2007. Modeling the behavior of coupled cellular circadian oscillators in the suprachiasmatic nucleus. *J Biol Rhythms* 22:211–219.
32. Hamada, T., Antle, M.C., Silver, R. 2004. Temporal and spatial expression patterns of canonical clock genes and clock-controlled genes in the suprachiasmatic nucleus. *Eur J Neurosci* 19:1741–1748.
33. Pevet, P., Agez, L., Bothorel, B. et al. 2006. Melatonin in the multioscillatory mammalian circadian world. *Chronobiol Int* 23:39–51.
34. Saper, C.B., Lu, J., Chou, T.C. et al. 2005. The hypothalamic integrator for circadian rhythms. *Trends Neurosci* 28:152–157.
35. Baydas, G., Ozveren, F., Akdemir, I. et al. 2005. Learning and memory deficits in rats induced by chronic thinner exposure are reversed by melatonin. *J Pineal Res* 39:50–56.
36. Larson, J., Jessen, R.E., Zu, T. et al. 2006. Impaired hippocampal long-term potentiation in melatonin MT2 receptor-deficient mice. *Neurosci Lett* 393:23–26.
37. Chaudhury, D., Wang, L.M., Colwell, C.S. 2005. Circadian regulation of hippocampal long-term potentiation. *J Biol Rhythms* 20:225–236.
38. Ozcan, M., Yilmaz, B., Carpenter, D.O. 2006. Effects of melatonin on synaptic transmission and long-term potentiation in two areas of mouse hippocampus. *Brain Res* 1111:90–94.
39. Wang, L.M., Suthana, N.A., Chaudhury, D. et al. 2005. Melatonin inhibits hippocampal long-term potentiation. *Eur J Neurosci* 22:2231–2237.

40. Gorfine, T., Zisapel, N. 2007. Melatonin and the human hippocampus, a time dependent interplay. *J Pineal Res* 43:80–86.
41. Saenz, D.A., Goldin, A.P., Minces, L. et al. 2004. Effect of melatonin on the retinal glutamate/glutamine cycle in the golden hamster retina. *FASEB J* 18:1912–1913.
42. Skaper, S.D., Ancona, B., Facci, L. et al. 1998. Melatonin prevents the delayed death of hippocampal neurons induced by enhanced excitatory neurotransmission and the nitridergic pathway. *FASEB J* 12:725–731.
43. Shibata, S., Cassone, V.M., Moore, R.Y. 1989. Effects of melatonin on neuronal activity in the rat suprachiasmatic nucleus in vitro. *Neurosci Lett* 97:140–144.
44. Stehle, J., Vanecek, J., Vollrath, L. 1989. Effects of melatonin on spontaneous electrical activity of neurons in rat suprachiasmatic nuclei: an in vitro iontophoretic study. *J Neural Transm* 78:173–177.
45. Mason, R., Rusak, B. 1990. Neurophysiological responses to melatonin in the SCN of short-day sensitive and refractory hamsters. *Brain Res* 533:15–19.
46. Jiang, Z.G., Nelson, C.S., Allen, C.N. 1995. Melatonin activates an outward current and inhibits Ih in rat suprachiasmatic nucleus neurons. *Brain Res* 687:125–132.
47. Van den Top, M., Buijs, R.M., Ruijter, J.M. et al. 2001. Melatonin generates an outward potassium current in rat suprachiasmatic nucleus neurones in vitro independent of their circadian rhythm. *Neuroscience* 107:99–108.
48. Gerdin, M.J., Masana, M.I., Rivera-Bermudez, M.A. et al. 2004. Melatonin desensitizes endogenous MT2 melatonin receptors in the rat suprachiasmatic nucleus: relevance for defining the periods of sensitivity of the mammalian circadian clock to melatonin. *FASEB J* 18:1646–1656.
49. Zeise, M.L., Semm, P. 1985. Melatonin lowers excitability of guinea pig hippocampal neurons in vitro. *J Comp Physiol* 57:23–29.
50. Musshoff, U., Riewenherm, D., Berger, E. et al. 2002. Melatonin receptors in rat hippocampus: molecular and functional investigations. *Hippocampus* 12:165–173.
51. Wan, Q., Man, H.Y., Liu, F. et al. 1999. Differential modulation of GABAA receptor function by Mel1a and Mel1b receptors. *Nat Neurosci* 2:401–403.
52. Hogan, M.V., El-Sherif, Y., Wieraszko, A. 2001. The modulation of neuronal activity by melatonin: in vitro studies on mouse hippocampal slices. *J Pineal Res* 30:87–96.
53. El-Sherif, Y., Tesoriero, J., Hogan, M.V. et al. 2003. Melatonin regulates neuronal plasticity in the hippocampus. *J Neurosci Res* 72:454–460.
54. Bob, P. 2003. Dissociation and neuroscience: history and new perspectives. *Int J Neurosci* 113: 903–914.
55. Bob, P. 2008. Pain, dissociation and subliminal self-representations. *Conscious Cogn* 17:355–69.
56. Spiegel, D. 1997. Trauma, dissociation, and memory. *Ann N Y Acad Sci* 821:225–237.
57. Kihlstrom, J.F. 2005. Dissociative disorders. *Annu Rev Clin Psychol* 1:227–253.
58. Phillips, R.G., LeDoux, J.E. 1992. Differential contribution of amygdala and hippocampus to cued and contextual fear conditioning. *Behav Neurosci* 106:274–285.
59. LeDoux, J.E. 1992. Brain mechanisms of emotion and emotional learning. Curr *Opin Neurobiol* 2:191–198.
60. LeDoux, J.E. 1993. Emotional memory systems in the brain. *Behav Brain Res* 58:69–79.
61. LeDoux, J.E. 1994. Emotion, memory and the brain. *Sci Am* 70:50–57.
62. Bechara, A., Tranel, D., Damasio, H. et al. 1995. Double dissociation of conditioning and declarative knowledge relative to the amygdala and hippocampus in humans. *Science* 269:1115–1118.
63. Diamond, D.M., Rose, G.M. 1994. Stress impairs LTP and hippocampal-dependent memory. *Ann N Y Acad Sci* 746:411–414.
64. Ruel, J.M., De Kloet, E.R. 1985. Two receptor systems for corticosterone in rat brain: microdistribution and differential occupation. *Endocrinology* 117:2505–2512.
65. Payne, J.D., Jackson, E.D., Ryan, L. et al. 2006. The impact of stress on neutral and emotional aspects of episodic memory. *Memory* 14:1–16.
66. Nadel, L., Jacobs, W.J. 1998. Traumatic memory is special. *Curr Dir Psychol Sci* 7:154–157.
67. Kenardy, J., Smith, A., Spence, S.H. et al. 2007. Dissociation in children's trauma narratives: an exploratory investigation. *J Anxiety Disord* 21:456–466.
68. Brewin, C.R. 2007. Autobiographical memory for trauma: update on four controversies. *Memory* 15:227–248.
69. Uysal, N., Ozdemir, D., Dayi, A. et al. 2005. Effects of maternal deprivation on melatonin production and cognition in adolescent male and female rats. *Neuro Endocrinol Lett* 26:555–560.

70. Simonneaux, V., Ribelayga, C. 2003. Generation of the melatonin endocrine message in mammals: a review of the complex regulation of melatonin synthesis by norepinephrine peptides, and other pineal transmitters. *Pharmacol Rev* 55:325–395.
71. Sumaya, I.C., Masana, M.I., Dubocovich, M.L. 2005. The antidepressant-like effect of the melatonin receptor ligand luzindole in mice during forced swimming requires expression of MT2 but not MT1 melatonin receptors. *J Pineal Res* 39:170–177.
72. Lepage, O., Larson, E.T., Mayer, I. et al. 2005. Tryptophan affects both gastrointestinal melatonin production and interrenal activity in stressed and nonstressed rainbow trout. *J Pineal Res* 38:264–271.
73. Paredes, S.D., Sanchez, S., Parvez, H. et al. 2007. Altered circadian rhythms of corticosterone, melatonin, and phagocytic activity Min response to stress in rats. *Neuro Endocrinol Lett* 28:101–112.
74. Krskova, L., Vrabcova, M., Zeman, M. 2007. Effect of melatonin on exploration and anxiety in normotensive and hypertensive rats with high activity of renin–angiotensin system. *Neuro Endocrinol Lett* 28:295–301.
75. Bob, P., Fedor-Freybergh, P. 2008. Melatonin, consciousness, and traumatic stress. *J Pineal Res* 44:341–7.
76. Martinez, F., Hernandez, T., Sanchez, P. et al. 1992. Synaptic ribbon modifications in the pineal gland of the albino rat following 24 hours of immobilization. *Acta Anat* 145:430–433.
77. Milin, J. 1998. Stress-reactive response of the gerbil pineal gland: concretion genesis. *Gen Comp Endocrinol* 110:237–251.
78. Milin, J., Demajo, M., Todorovic, V. 1996. Rat pinealocyte reactive response to a long-term stress inducement. *Neuroscience* 73:845–854.
79. Lynch, H.J., Deng, M.H. 1986. Pineal responses to stress. *J Neural Transm Suppl* 21:461–473.
80. Vollrath, L., Welker, H.A. 1988. Day-to-day variation in pineal serotonin *N*-acetyltransferase activity in stressed and nonstressed male Sprague–Dawley rats. *Life Sci* 42:2223–2229.
81. Dagnino-Subiabre, A., Orellana, J.A., Carmona-Fontaine, C. et al. 2006. Chronic stress decreases the expression of sympathetic markers in the pineal gland and increases plasma melatonin concentration in rats. *J Neurochem* 97:1279–1287.
82. Fuchs, E., Schumacher, M. 1990. Psychosocial stress affects pineal function in the tree shrew (*Tupaia belangeri*). *Physiol Behav* 47:713–717.
83. Larson, E.T., Winberg, S., Mayer, I. et al. 2004. Social stress affects circulating melatonin levels in rainbow trout. *Gen Comp Endocrinol* 136:322–327.
84. Jindal, R.D., Thase, M.E. Treatment of insomnia associated with clinical depression. *Sleep Med Rev* 2004. 8:19–30.
85. Brown, R., Kocsis, J.H., Caroff, S. et al. Differences in nocturnal melatonin secretion between melancholic depressed patients and control subjects. *Am J Psychiatry* 1985. 142:811–816.
86. Frazer, A., Brown, R., Kocsis, J. et al. 1986. Patterns of melatonin rhythms in depression. *J Neural Transm (Suppl)* 21:269–290.
87. Pacchierotti, C., Iapichino, S., Bossini, L. et al. 2001. Melatonin in psychiatric disorders: a review on the melatonin involvement in psychiatry. *Front Neuroendocrinol* 22:18–32.
88. Warembourg, M. 1975. Radioautographic study of the rat brain and pituitary after injection of 3H dexamethasone. *Cell Tissue Res* 161:183–191.
89. Sarrieau, A., Dussaillant, M., Moguilewsky, M. 1988. Autoradiographic localization of glucocorticosteroid binding sites in rat brain after in vivo injection of [3H]RU 28362. *Neurosci Lett* 92:14–20.
90. Meyer, U., Kruhoffer, M., Flugge, G. et al. 1998. Cloning of glucocorticoid receptor and mineralocorticoid receptor cDNA and gene expression in the central nervous system of the tree shrew (*Tupaia belangeri*). *Brain Res Mol Brain Res* 55:243–253.
91. Torres-Farfan, C., Richter, H.G., Rojas-Garcia, P. et al. 2003. mt1 Melatonin receptor in the primate adrenal gland: inhibition of adrenocorticotropin-stimulated cortisol production by melatonin. *J Clin Endocrinol Metab* 88:450–458.
92. Sapolsky, R.M. 2000. The possibility of neurotoxicity in the hippocampus in major depression: a primer on neuron death. *Biol Psychiatry* 48:755–765.
93. Laudon, M., Hyde, J.F., Ben-Jonathan, N. 1989. Ontogeny of prolactin releasing and inhibiting activities in the posterior pituitary of male rats. *Neuroendocrinology* 50:644–649.
94. Boatright, J.H., Rubim, N.M., Iuvone, P.M. 1994. Regulation of endogenous dopamine release in amphibian retina by melatonin: the role of GABA. *Vis Neurosci* 11:1013–1018.
95. Hemby, S.E., Trojanowski, J.Q., Ginsberg, S.D. 2003. Neuron-specific age-related decreases in dopamine receptor subtype mRNAs. *J Comp Neurol* 456:176–183.

96. Webb, S.M., Pulg-Domingo, M. 1995. Role of melatonin in health and disease. *Clin Endocrinol* 42:221–234.
97. Kennedy, S.H., Kutcher, S.P., Ralevski, E. et al. 1996. Nocturnal melatonin and 24-h 6-sulphatoxymelatonin levels in various phases of bipolar affective disorder. *Psychiatr Res* 63:219–222.
98. Lieberman, H. 1984. The effects of melatonin on human mood and performance. *Brain Res* 323:201–207.
99. Little, K.Y., Ranc, J., Gilmore, J. et al. 1997. Lack of pineal betaadrenergic receptor alterations in suicide victims with major depression. *Psychoneuroendocrinology* 22:53–62.
100. Rubin, R.T., Heist, E.K., McGeoy, S.S. et al. 1992. Neuroendocrine aspects of primary endogenous depression: XI. Serum melatonin measures in patients and matched control subjects. *Arch Gen Psychiatr* 49:558–567.
101. Monteleone, P., Natale, M., La Rocca, A. et al. 1997. Decreased nocturnal secretion of melatonin in drug-free schizophrenics: no change after subchronic treatment with antipsychotics. *Neuropsychobiology* 36:159–163.
102. Sandyk, R., Kay, S.R. 1990. Pineal melatonin in schizophrenia: a review and hypothesis. *Schizophr Bull* 16:653–662.
103. Rao, M.L., Gross, G., Strebel, B. et al. 1994. Circadian rhythm of tryptophan, serotonin, melatonin, and pituitary hormones in schizophrenia. *Biol Psychiatry* 35:151–163.
104. Sandyk, R. 1992. The pineal gland and the mode of onset of schizophrenia. *Int J Neurosci* 67:9–17.
105. Monteleone, P., Natale, M., Fuschino, A. et al. 1997. Disruption of melatonin circadian rhythm in schizophrenia and obsessive compulsive disorder. *Biol Psychiatry* 42(Suppl 1):226–227.
106. Bandelow, B., Sengos, G., Wedeking, D. et al. 1997. Urinary excretion of cortisol, norepinephrine, testosterone, and melatonin in panic disorder. *Pharmacopsychiatry* 30:113–117.
107. Arendt, J., Bhanji, S., Francy, C. et al. 1992. Plasma melatonin levels in anorexia nervosa. *Br J Psychiatry* 161:361–364.
108. Kennedy, S.H. 1994. Melatonin disturbances in anorexia nervosa and bulimia nervosa. *Int J Eating Disord* 16:257–265.
109. Monteleone, P., Catapano, F., Del Buono, G. et al. 1994. Circadian rhythms of melatonin, cortisol and prolactin in patients with obsessive–compulsive disorder. *Acta Psychiatr Scand* 89:411–415.
110. Morera, A.L., Abreu, P. 2006. Seasonality of psychopathology and circannual melatonin rhythm. *J Pineal Res* 41:279–283.
111. Teicher, M., Andersen, S.L., Polcari, A. et al. 2003. The neurobiological consequences of early stress and childhood maltreatment. *Neurosci Biobehav Rev* 27:3–44.
112. Putnam, F. 1997. *Dissociation in Children and Adolescents. A Developmental Perspective*. Guilford Press, London.
113. Bob, P., Susta, M., Gregusova, A., Jasova, D. 2009. Dissociation, cognitive conflict and nonlinear patterns of heart rate dynamics in patients with unipolar depression. *Prog Neuropsychopharmacol Biol Psychiatry* 33:141–145.
114. Bob, P., Susta, M., Glaslova, K., Boutros, N.N. 2010. Dissociative symptoms and interregional EEG cross-correlations in paranoid schizophrenia. *Psychiatry Res* 177:37–40.
115. Teicher, M., Tomoda, A., Andersen, S.L. 2006. Neurobiological consequences of early stress and childhood maltreatment: are results from human and animal studies comparable? *Ann N Y Acad Sci* 1071:313–323.
116. Bremner, J.D. 2006. The relationship between cognitive and brainchanges in posttraumatic stress disorder. *Ann N Y Acad Sci* 1071:80–86.
117. Benitez-King, G. 2006. Melatonin as a cytoskeletal modulator: implications for cell physiology and disease. *J Pineal Res* 40:1–9.
118. Wu, Y.H, Swaab, D.F. 2005. The human pineal gland and melatonin in aging and Alzheimer's disease. *J Pineal Res* 38:145–152.
119. Lee, E.J, Lee, M.Y., Chen, H.Y. et al. 2005. Melatonin attenuates gray and white matter damage in a mouse model of transient focal cerebral ischemia. *J Pineal Res* 38:42–52.
120. Maldonado, M.D., Murillo-Cabezas, F., Terron, M.P. et al. 2007. The potential of melatonin in reducing morbidity–mortality after craniocerebral trauma. *J Pineal Res* 42:1–11.

35 Measurement of Melatonin in Other Body Fluids

Soyhan Bağcı

CONTENTS

35.1 INTRODUCTION

Melatonin (MT) is a lipophilic amino acid derivative and is not stored but directly released from the pineal gland by diffusion. About 60%–85% of the circulating MT is bound to albumin [1,2]. MT displays high lipid and water solubility and gains access to various fluids, tissues, and cellular compartments. It is therefore detected in saliva [3], urine [4], cerebrospinal fluid (CSF) [5], semen [6], amniotic fluid [7], and milk [8]. Just like the serum/plasma hormone profile, levels of MT likewise display a circadian rhythm in other body fluids. Besides measurements of MT levels in plasma or serum, measurements have also been carried out in all kinds of other body fluids both to monitor the circadian rhythm of MT and to understand the multiple molecular functions of MT, for example, in the ventricular system of the brain. Because the concentrations of proteins and other constituents can vary several folds in body fluids according to the presence of any kind of disease, the sampling time, or methods, the matrix effects of these constituents can be expected to influence the measurement of MT.

In this aspect, the purpose of this chapter is to review the literature on the analytical investigations of other body fluids besides serum and plasma. Topics to be covered include the analysis of the different body fluids for the measurement of MT levels. Furthermore, the review will discuss some of the advantages, disadvantages, and problems of the widely available measurement procedures in body fluids.

35.2 MEASUREMENT OF MT AND ITS METABOLITES IN URINE

Circulating MT has a very short half life and is predominantly metabolized by hydroxylation at the C-6 position to 6-hydroxymelatonin in the liver. This hydroxylated product can be conjugated with either sulfate, 6-sulfatoxymelatonin (aMT6s), or glucuronide [9]. These conjugates are then excreted into urine [10]. Less than 1% of endogenous MT is also excreted unchanged into urine [9,11].

35.2.1 Measurement of MT in Urine

Like serum MT, urinary MT excretion rates show a clear circadian rhythm, with low daytime and high nocturnal values [12–14]. A good correlation of urinary MT excretion and circulating MT concentration in blood was found in several studies [12,15–18]. Whereas aMT6s in urine has been widely used as a measurement of pineal MT secretion [19–26], only a few studies have measured urine MT concentration, since the total amount of MT excreted into urine was found to be about 360 times lower than that of aMT6s [11,12,16–18]. In cases with suspected or known metabolic or liver disease, urinary MT may be considered as a measurement of choice because of its independence of hepatic degradation pathways [27].

After oral application, absorbed MT is collected by the hepatic venous system and 30%–60% is immediately metabolized to 6-hydroxymelatonin in the liver during the first pass [28]. Thus, a certain portion of absorbed MT never appears in the systemic circulation or in body tissues, but is directly excreted as aMT6s into urine [18]. It has been demonstrated that aMT6s excretion increases after an oral MT administration; however, this has not been correlated with serum MT levels [18]. Because of the broad bioavailability and a strong first-pass hepatic metabolism of oral MT, which may result in serum MT concentrations differing up to 25-folds among subjects after the application of identical dose, urinary MT measurement, but not aMT6s, is a useful tool for drug monitoring after the oral MT application [18,28–30].

It has been demonstrated that urinary MT excretion was significantly elevated in the first nighttime urine sample (from 10 PM to 2 AM) and remained elevated until 9 AM [12]. Total urinary MT and aMT6s excretion correlated significantly with the area under the curve (AUC) of MT rhythm (0.67 versus 0.42 and 0.44 versus 0.39, at nighttime and at daytime, respectively) [12]. A good correlation between the plasma MT level at midnight and MT in the first morning urine (the correlation coefficient varied from 0.74 to 0.89) suggested that only morning urinary MT levels may be sufficient to establish the nocturnal pineal MT production [11,15].

A mean MT concentration of 64.4 pg/ml (range: 7.0–185.0 pg/ml) was reported in the morning urine [16]. In another study, similar results were found in the morning urine of older women (urinary MT ranged from 7.6 to 92.8 pg/ml; mean of 54.7 pg/ml) [17].

Because, so far, measurements of urinary MT have not been preferred over measurements of aMT6s in urine, only a few methods have been described to measure urinary MT, such as the 2-^{125}I-MT radioimmunoassay (RIA) method described previously by Vakkuri et al. [31] and a commercially available RIA kit, which uses the Kennaway G-280 anti-MT antibody [12,18]. An extensive validation of the assay of the urinary MT is especially required because of the unpredictable matrix effects of proteins and other constituents in the urine [15].

35.2.2 Measurement of aMT6s in Urine

MT's major urinary metabolite, aMT6s, is excreted in high amounts in the urine. It is a very stable metabolite which is not altered by storage for up to 15 years at –20°C [32] or for five days at room temperature [33]. Alternatively to the measurement of MT in blood, the measurement of aMT6s in urine appears to provide a robust, simple, and reliable assessment of the MT secretion and allows longitudinal noninvasive studies in humans [34]. Furthermore, other than single plasma or pineal MT measurements, which only reflect momentary pineal MT levels, the measurements of urinary aMT6s excretion provide an estimation of the integrated pineal MT production. There are several lines of evidence that total nocturnal MT production is well correlated with levels of urinary aMT6s excretion in 12- to 24-hour urine collections [12,20,33,35].

A clear circadian rhythm of the urinary aMT6s excretion has been previously described [12]. However, there is always a phase delay between the increase of MT in serum and the peak of aMT6s in urine, depending on the catabolic capacity of the respective species [4,35,36]. After the production of the endogenous MT by the pineal gland, the hormone is collected by the venous capillary system, emptying into the Galen vein and further into the venous portion of the systemic circulation [37]. A part of the circulated MT in the arterial part of the systemic circulation is metabolized to either aMT6s or a less abundant metabolite 6-hydroxymelatonin glucuronide in the liver, which are both water-soluble and excreted by the kidneys. The pattern of aMT6s in the urine reflects the pineal MT rhythm qualitatively as well as quantitatively [4,35,36]. Unlike endogenous MT, 30%–60% of exogenous (oral or intravenous) MT is metabolized to 6-hydroxymelatonin in the liver during the first pass, and this portion of MT never enters the general circulation [28]. Therefore, it is important to know that increased aMT6s excretion after oral MT application did not reflect the serum MT levels [18]. Therefore, the measurement of aMT6s in the urine is widely used as an index of the endogenous MT, but not exogenous MT.

The analysis of the relationship between blood MT levels and urinary aMT6s excretion indicated a high and consistent association between the concentrations of MT in blood and urinary aMT6s excretion in several studies [19,35]. The correlations between aMT6s and either AUC or peak plasma MT values ranged from $r = 0.62$ to $r = 0.84$ [16,19,20,33,38]. This correlation has also been confirmed in older subjects [17].

The collection of urine samples for research as well as for practice can be achieved in several ways such as a 24-hour urine sample, single isolated urine sample, or serial episodic samples collected over a specific time period. It is important to remember that the glomerular filtration rate and the volume of the urine production are different in each individual and over time. The patterns of aMT6s excretion are clearly affected by water consumption and renal function [39]. The osmolality and creatinine content are used as markers for the concentration of urine. Low creatinine and specific gravity levels may indicate diluted urine. If urine samples are not collected over a 24-hour period and the total urinary output is unknown, renal clearance can be estimated by measuring one of these parameters. Because osmolality strongly depends on actual osmoregulatory processes and is influenced by various physiological factors, e.g., salt intake, blood pressure, and hormones [39], the urine creatinine concentration is generally used as a more reliable parameter for detecting diluted urine samples. It was demonstrated that the morning urinary aMT6s values did not correlate with plasma MT levels unless corrected for creatinine [16]. Creatinine-corrected aMT6s values would be of interest in the study of MT. If the total volume of the voiding is unknown, aMT6s concentrations should be typically corrected using creatinine (amount of substance per milliliter divided by milligram creatinine per milliliter) and expressed as amount per milligram of creatinine [39]. It should be noted, however, that the urinary creatinine concentration itself can be influenced to some degree by physical activity [40], circadian changes [41], age [42–44], gender [42], race [42], body size and lean-body mass [42,45], and protein intake [46]. Therefore, a careful consideration of the effects of these factors on creatinine concentrations is required in the individual studies of the urinary aMT6s that are corrected for the urinary creatinine concentration. If the exact urine volume is known, there is no need to use urinary creatinine as a substitute for urine volume and aMT6s concentrations are corrected for volume and calculated per hour of the urine sampling (ng/hr) [38,47].

Initially, assays of aMT6s in urine were based on the gas chromatography–mass spectrometry (GC–MS) method [48,49]. These were later replaced by more specific and sensitive RIA, which used ^{125}I-labeled aMT6s, sheep anti-aMT6s antiserum, and the separation of bound and free fractions with charcoal [19,50]. It was demonstrated that there is a good correlation ($r = 0.93$, $p < 0.001$) between direct RIA and the GC–MS method for aMT6s [33]. As GC–MS measures the total (free and conjugated) aMT6s level, the values obtained by the GC–MS method were found 1.5-folds higher than those that were obtained by the specific aMT6s RIA method [33]. Finally, an enzyme immunoassay, which is a competitive immunoassay using a capture second antibody technique, was developed for the measurement of aMT6s in urine [51]. Assay performance has been extensively validated by the manufacturer and the results correlate well with the RIA ($r = 0.987$) [51]. The main advantages of enzyme immunoassay are avoidance of radioactivity, its stability after 15 months at −20°C, and a short processing time. However, compared with RIA, its lower detection limit is high (varied from 0.8 to 1.0 ng/ml for aMT6s by enzyme-linked immunosorbent assay (ELISA) using commercial KITs from different companies and, on average, about 0.25 ng/ml for RIA from Stockgrand).

GC–MS analysis of total urinary excretion of conjugated 6-hydroxymelatonin was found to be 12.9 ± 0.6 µg/day in young males (aged 4–16 years), 15.9 ± 0.8 µg/day in young females (aged 3–16 years), and 11.4 ± 0.75 µg/day in adults (>16 years) [52]. In another study, urinary aMT6s measured by a direct RIA in normal volunteers aged 2–80 years was reported to be 8 ± 4 µg/day (mean ±

TABLE 35.1
Urinary aMT6s Excretion in Healthy Adults for Different Age Groups

	Age Group (years)	aMT6s Mean (SD)	aMT6s Range
Nighttime period	20–35	2841 (1119)	1017–6074
2300–0700 hr aMT6s (ng/hr)	36–50	2136 (947)	598–3612
	51–65	1499 (468)	861–2421
	>65	1010 (580)	327–2396
	Total	2004 (1117)	327–6074
Morning period	20–35	1681 (666)	608–2987
0700–1100 hr aMT6s (ng/hr)	36–50	1363 (1060)	154–4172
	51–65	749 (530)	178–2282
	>65	611 (407)	2–1343
	Total	1175 (830)	2–4172
Daytime period	20–35	526 (252)	182–1130
1100–1800 hr aMT6s (ng/hr)	36–50	491 (278)	202–1140
	51–65	384 (179)	139–725
	>65	454 (219)	173–997
	Total	473 (239)	139–1140
Evening period	20–35	579 (354)	138–1706
1800–2300 hr aMT6s (ng/hr)	36–50	577 (556)	176–2425
	51–65	490 (432)	101–1578
	>65	371 (209)	209–887
	Total	525 (404)	101–2425
24-hr aMT6s (µg)	20–35	36.8 (12.3)	13.5–58.1
	36–50	29.6 (13.2)	9.9–52.9
	51–65	20.4 (5.5)	12.3–32.8
	>65	15.8 (6.8)	7.5–32.7
	Total	27.2 (13.3)	7.5–58.1
Night/day ratio	20–35	6.0 (2.1)	2.4–10.5
	36–50	4.8 (2.3)	0.7–9.8
	51–65	4.9 (3.2)	1.5–11.6
	>65	2.8 (1.6)	0.8–5.4
	Total	4.8 (2.6)	0.7–11.6

Source: Mahlberg, R., et al., *Psychoneuroendocrinology*, 31, 634–41, 2006.
Note: Abbreviation: hr, hour(s); ng, nanogram.

SD) in children aged 2–20 years [34]. There was an age-related decline in the total 24-hour aMT6s excretion with significantly lower values (4 ± 2 μg/day) in elderly subjects aged 60–80 years, as it was expected [34]. A recent study has provided normative data on the daily profile of urinary aMT6s in healthy subjects between the ages of 20 and 84 (Table 35.1) [53]. They concluded that the total amount of 24-hour aMT6s (range 7.5–58 μg) as well as the amount of aMT6s excreted during nighttime (range 327–6.074 ng/h) varied as much as 20-folds between individuals. Thus, variation in the 24-hour MT excretion can be explained by nighttime MT excretion to the extent of 94% [53].

The highest excretion rate of aMT6s was pointed out during the interval from 10 PM to 8 AM, with the first voided morning specimen containing 75%–90% of the daily total secretion in all age groups [52]. The afternoon samples from 3 PM to 10 PM contained only a small percentage (<5% of the total daily excretion in all age groups). It was demonstrated that both morning urinary MT and aMT6s account for approximately 70% of the total plasma MT measured during the night before [16]. The studies have demonstrated the efficacy of using a single morning voided urine sample to assess total and peak nocturnal MT values in healthy young men [16] and in older women [17]. This aspect seems to be important in newborn infants because of the limitations of the collection procedure for 24-hour urine samples. Although collection bags with the use of drainage tubes allow for sampling over a 24-hour period in newborn infants, this procedure is unpractical in preterm infants because of the inadequate adherence to skin and the potential stripping of epithelium and discomfort with bag removal. Alternatively, urine samples can be extracted from the diaper. However, diaper pad collection procedures may alter aMT6s values because of either the chemical reaction of aMT6s with the pad material or the influence of other substances in the urine [26]. Thus, although morning urinary aMT6s measurements do not provide information about the timing of the peak value, these measurements are still a reasonable indicator of nocturnal plasma MT and allow measurements in all age groups.

35.3 MEASUREMENT OF MT IN SALIVA

The use of saliva as a diagnostic fluid may offer a noninvasive, stress-free, and ethical alternative to repeated measurements in serum, suitable for even the most premature infants [3,35,54–57]. Both in adults and in newborn infants, highly significant, reproducible correlation between plasma and salivary MT concentrations has been reported previously [3,54,56,58–60]. The ratio of salivary to total blood (plasma or serum) MT in 24-hour patterns has been reported to vary from 0.21 to 0.91 in some studies [35,54–56,58]. The ratio of salivary MT to serum MT in newborns was found to be 0.78 (ranged from 0.58 to 1.03), which is in good agreement with values measured among adults [60]. It is possible that the individual differences in the saliva flow rate may account for some of the variation of the salivary/serum MT ratio in the newborn infants because of the high variability of their water balance during the first days of life [57].

Although the measurement of MT concentration in saliva is a widely accepted and convenient procedure to assess the circadian rhythm of MT, both in research and clinical settings [54,56,60,61], many physiological aspects such as the effect of the saliva flow rate or the mechanisms of the excretion of MT into the saliva have not been clearly studied. Therefore, it is important to establish the optimum procedure for saliva collection to obtain reproducible results and to know the limitations and the options of salivary MT diagnostics.

35.3.1 THE VARIABILITY OF SALIVA PRODUCTION AND EFFECT OF SALIVA PROPERTIES ON SALIVARY MT CONCENTRATION

Saliva is stored in secretion granules in the acini of the salivary glands. The volume and the composition of the saliva can vary during daytime and among individuals. Salivation can either be stimulated or reduced by several factors. Strong acidic stimulus, high-frequency chewing, and high bite force result in increased saliva output. Parasympathetic stimulation results in increased watery (less viscous) saliva, whereas sympathetic stimulation results in mucoid (more viscous) saliva secretions [62]. The other factor affecting saliva composition is the flow index, which varies in accordance with different factors such as water balance, body position, light stimulation, heart rhythm, medication, mechanic intraoral and extraoral stimulation, and gland size [63]. Unstimulated whole saliva showed significant circadian rhythms in the flow rate [64]. The average unstimulated whole salivary flow rate is 0.3–0.4 ml/min during waking hours, and the lowest flow rate, less than 0.1 ml/min, occurs during nighttime [63–65]. An unstimulated rate of 0.1 ml/min or less indicates hyposalivation in adults [65,66]. Furthermore, it has been demonstrated that the saliva flow rate of newborn infants was found to be 15 times lower compared to adolescents [67].

The influence of the saliva flow rate on MT concentrations in saliva is controversial in the literature. Although no significant effect of flow rate on salivary MT concentrations has been described [54], it has recently been reported that an increase in flow rate as a result of stimulation by citric acid for saliva collection resulted in a decrease in the salivary MT concentration [56]. Our results also demonstrated [57] that there was a significant difference in the salivary/serum MT ratio according to salivation degree. Infants with hyposalivation had higher salivary/serum MT ratios than infants with ideal saliva samples. Infants with hypersalivation had lower salivary/serum MT ratios than infants with ideal samples.

On the other hand, about 60%–85% of MT in serum is reversibly bound to plasma albumin with a low binding affinity [1,2]. Albumin-bound MT is not secreted into saliva and only minimal amounts of albumin and consequently albumin-bound MT appear in saliva. There is a highly significant correlation ($r = 0.84$, $p < 0.05$) between the unbound fraction of MT in plasma and the salivary MT levels, and this suggests that the salivary fraction of MT probably represents only the free plasma MT fraction [2]. However, the salivary MT concentration has been reported to be higher than 40% of the blood MT concentration in some studies [55,57,59,68]. It may be explained with the low and somewhat variable affinity and poor specificity of MT binding to albumin and variations in serum albumin concentrations in some subjects [69]. It is also unclear whether the affinity of MT to albumin is different in term and particularly preterm newborns and infants compared with adults. Furthermore, the effects of other factors such as drugs, other hormones, and hyperbilirubinemia on the affinity of MT to albumin have not been studied so far. However, it is well established that newborn infants (and particularly preterm infants) have lower albumin concentrations than adults, which may result in a higher proportion of unbound MT and, consequently, in part explain why the salivary/serum ratio found in newborn infants was higher than that reported in adults [2].

35.3.2 Effect of Saliva Collection Methods on MT Concentration

Saliva can be considered as gland-specific saliva or whole saliva. Total or whole saliva refers to the complex mixture of fluids from both the major and minor salivary glands. As several nonsalivary constituents including secretions of upper airways, gastrointestinal reflux, mucous of the nasal cavity and pharynx, food remainders, desquamated epithelial and blood cells, as well as traces of medications or chemical products may also exist in saliva, collection of saliva must ensure sample integrity [63,70,71].

The most commonly used method of saliva collection involves the use of cotton-based materials such as a sterile cotton dental roll, cotton-type Salivette device [72], or filter paper [61] to absorb saliva. As these devices either cannot be used in newborn infants or are impractical for routine use, alternatively, the feasibility of sampling saliva in newborn infants with cotton buds, available with wooden or plastic sticks, has been demonstrated [57]. Because the use of cotton buds with wooden sticks resulted in falsely low cortisol concentrations when the saliva was left uncentrifuged at room temperature for 24 hours or more [73], cotton buds with plastic sticks should be preferred for saliva sampling for MT studies. The mean recovery of MT from cotton-type Salivette is about 80% and salivary MT was perfectly stable for at least 3 days even when kept at room temperature (28°C) and for months when kept frozen (at –20°C or lower) [74]. Furthermore, storage of cotton buds uncentrifuged for 24 hours at 4°C or for 2 months at −40°C does not affect the recovery of MT from cotton buds, making it unnecessary to centrifuge the salivary samples within a short period of time after sampling [57].

Although some laboratories are collecting saliva by spitting into tubes, the recoveries of MT from spiked saliva samples may be low, most probably due to the hydrophobicity of MT [74]. This led to a high and irreversible binding of the MT, particularly to the cotton-type swabs. Therefore, it is ideal to place the cotton-based materials between the cheek and the gum for saliva sampling.

35.3.3 Analytical Methods for Measurement of MT in Saliva

For the determination of MT in saliva, several techniques have been described, including RIA [3], ELISA, use of an iodinated tracer and solid-phase second antibody [75], high-performance liquid chromatography tandem mass spectrometry (HPLC–MS) [76], column-switching semi-microcolumn liquid chromatography–mass spectrometry (LC–MS) [77], and recently, automated solid-phase extraction, HPLC, and fluorescence detection [78].

For the determination of MT in saliva, immunoassay methods such as RIA and ELISA are most commonly used. The saliva ELISA MT assay requires saliva samples to be pretreated, but saliva samples to be assayed by RIA do not require pretreatment. These methods are highly sensitive, even though the analysis takes a long time (16–24 hours), owing to the need for stages of incubation. The disadvantages of these methods are the possible cross-reactions with structurally similar substances or interference with the analysis by some nutrients present in saliva.

As an alternative to RIA, the HPLC–MS method showed a high sensitivity and specificity for MT and more reliable results compared with the RIA [76]. The analytical results demonstrated that the assay produced more reliable determinations of MT in saliva compared with a commercial RIA method [76].

The first chromatographic method, called the column-switching semi-microcolumn LC–MS method, enables direct determination of endogenous MT in human saliva. The method is highly selective and improves the sample throughput by minimum sample pretreatment and a relatively short run-time [77].

Recently, an automated solid-phase extraction followed by HPLC separation and fluorescence detection using the native fluorescence of MT has been developed and validated [78]. However, this method uses 2000 µl saliva, which is a larger volume than that used in other saliva methods with LC–MS [77] or LC–MS/MS [76], which uses 400–1000 µl, or compared with an HPLC method [79] with reinforced fluorescence of MT, which uses only 20 µl. It can be difficult to sample the required volume of 2000 µl in elderly subjects, who have reduced saliva excretion, and in newborn infants.

35.4 MT IN THE CSF

It is widely accepted that MT is present in the ventricular system and a significant amount of MT crosses the blood–brain barrier. Serial measurement of MT levels in humans demonstrated a clear diurnal MT rhythm in the CSF [80].

Nevertheless, questions about the main source of MT in the CSF remain unanswered. First studies on animals and humans showed that CSF MT is lower than the corresponding plasma MT levels, suggesting that MT reaches the CSF via the peripheral circulation [81–85]. Interestingly, although the diurnal CSF levels of MT in a study were about one fourth of the corresponding plasma levels, nocturnal CSF levels of MT were similar to the nocturnal plasma levels [83]. These reports usually are based on cisternal or lumbar CSF samples [80,81,83,86,87]. Although another study [84] demonstrated that MT levels were higher in serum compared with both those in lumbar and ventricular CSFs, CSF samples were also collected from patients undergoing neurosurgical operations at daytime due to occlusive hydrocephalus, or communicating hydrocephalus, or normal CSF flow.

Later, it has been shown that CSF MT levels are more concentrated than those in the blood [37,88]. According to these results, the first hypothesis was refined to suggest that the high MT content in the lateral ventricular CSF may be due to the simple diffusion of MT from the choroid plexus of the lateral ventricle after retrograde transport from the Galen vein, which drains into the sagittal sinus before entering the jugular vein [37].

Nevertheless, a recent study has shown that third ventricular levels of MT are 7-folds higher than those in the lateral ventricle and 20-folds higher than those in the jugular vein [89]. As a matter of fact, the major part of the CSF is produced in the brain by the choroid plexuses of the lateral ventricles. The fluid flows through the foramen of Monro from the lateral ventricles into the third ventricle and passes through the cerebral aqueduct of Sylvius to the fourth ventricle. It then enters from the fourth ventricle into the subarachnoid space through the foramina of Magendie and Luschka flowing downward around the spinal cord. However, the flow of the CSF may not be unidirectional in the ventricles. It was observed that the ventricular system (an observation during surgery) has a very strong pulsatility [89]. During each pulse, it is probable that at least some third ventricular CSF enters the lateral ventricle. In this respect, it has been shown that lateral ventricle MT concentrations started to rise after an increase was noted in the third ventricle [89]. This observation could explain the lower MT level in the lateral ventricle compared with that in the third ventricle. Also, it might explain why the MT concentration is still higher in the lateral ventricle than that in the plasma [89].

Most recently, it has been demonstrated that the levels of MT in the pineal recess, the evagination of the third ventricle into the pineal stalk, were even higher than in the ventral part of the third ventricle [90] and the endocrine cells in the superior part of the sheep pineal recess were in direct contact with the CSF [91].

Finally, these findings suggested that the majority of MT detectable in the CSF is secreted directly from the pineal gland to the ventricular lumen of the pineal recess [89–91]. Furthermore, it was observed in humans that MT levels were higher in the third ventricle than in the lateral one, which shows that MT may enter the CSF through the pineal recess, even during daytime [92].

As for ethical and practical reasons, it is difficult to obtain information on the levels or the circadian rhythm of MT in the CSF in humans, the majority of the studies are based on CSF samples in animals [37,83,88,93]. In the literature, CSF MT concentrations in humans and animals were reported very differently depending on both the site of sampling (simple point lumbar puncture [80–84,94–96], lateral ventricle [37,84,88,93,97], third ventricle [89,90,92,97], or pineal recess [90]) and the time of sampling (at the daytime [84,94,97] or at the night [81,90,96]). Furthermore, other factors such as main diseases of patients or sensitivity of the test may also affect the measurement of MT concentration in the CSF [84,95,97–99].

To measure the MT concentration in the CSF, RIA with extraction or direct RIA is a favorable and sensitive method (0.4 pg/ml) [5,81,89]. In addition to RIA, GC–MS [37,97] and, recently, HPLC (with a detection limit of 0.5 pg/ml) [96] were also used to measure the MT concentration in the CSF.

35.5 MT IN HUMAN MILK

As in other body fluids, MT also exhibits a circadian rhythm in the colostrum and human milk, with high levels during the night and undetectable levels during the day [8,100]. The presence of the rhythm in milk suggests that postnatal transfer of MT via the milk to the neonate may play a role in the entrainment of the newborn to the prevailing photic environment of the mother [101]. However, the evidence for milk as a source of MT to the infants is lacking.

The basic methods for measurement of MT in human milk include assay by either RIA or ELISA using the same protocol such as salivary MT determination, and commercial kits are available for both methods.

35.6 SUMMARY

- MT is a lipophilic molecule and gains access to various fluids, tissues, and cellular compartments so that it is detected in the saliva, urine, CSF, semen, amniotic fluid, and milk.
- Besides pineal production, an active synthesis of MT has been demonstrated in other peripheral tissues, such as the gastrointestinal tract, airway epithelium, liver, pancreas, kidney, adrenals, thymus, thyroid, and placenta.
- As an alternative to plasma or serum, measurements of MT in other body fluids are widely used in MT studies.
- Measurement of MT in saliva and MT/aMT6s in urine is a noninvasive, stress-free, and ethical alternative to repeated measurements in serum and allows the long-term studies of the circadian MT rhythm.
- The measurement of MT using other body fluids such as CSF, milk, intestinal fluid, or amniotic fluid may provide an understanding of the local physiological role of MT.

ACKNOWLEDGMENT

The author would like to thank Peter Bartmann, Heiko Reuter, and Halil Saglam for their contributions.

REFERENCES

1. Cardinali, D.P., H.J. Lynch, and R.J. Wurtman, Binding of melatonin to human and rat plasma proteins. *Endocrinology*, 1972. **91**(5): pp. 1213–8.
2. Kennaway, D.J. and A. Voultsios, Circadian rhythm of free melatonin in human plasma. *J Clin Endocrinol Metab*, 1998. **83**(3): pp. 1013–5.
3. Miles, A., et al., Salivary melatonin estimation in clinical research. *Clin Chem*, 1985. **31**(12): pp. 2041–2.
4. Fellenberg, A.J., G. Phillipou, and R.F. Seamark, Measurement of urinary production rates of melatonin as an index of human pineal function. *Endocr Res Commun*, 1980. **7**(3): pp. 167–75.
5. Smith, I., et al., Absolute identification of melatonin in human plasma and cerebrospinal fluid. *Nature*, 1976. **260**(5553): pp. 716–8.
6. van Vuuren, R.J., D.J. du Plessis, and J.J. Theron, Melatonin in human semen. *S Afr Med J*, 1988. **73**(6): pp. 375–6.
7. Mitchell, M.D., et al., Melatonin in amniotic fluid during human parturition. *Br J Obstet Gynaecol*, 1978. **85**(9): pp. 684–6.
8. Illnerova, H., M. Buresova, and J. Presl, Melatonin rhythm in human milk. *J Clin Endocrinol Metab*, 1993. **77**(3): pp. 838–41.
9. Kopin, I.J., et al., The fate of melatonin in animals. *J Biol Chem*, 1961. **236**: pp. 3072–5.
10. Young, I.M., et al., Melatonin is metabolized to N-acetyl serotonin and 6-hydroxymelatonin in man. *J Clin Endocrinol Metab*, 1985. **60**(1): pp. 114–9.
11. Wetterberg, L., et al., A simplified radioimmunoassay for melatonin and its application to biological fluids. Preliminary observations on the half-life of plasma melatonin in man. *Clin Chim Acta*, 1978. **86**(2): pp. 169–77.
12. Paakkonen, T., et al., Urinary melatonin: a noninvasive method to follow human pineal function as studied in three experimental conditions. *J Pineal Res*, 2006. **40**(2): pp. 110–5.
13. Lynch, H.J., et al., Daily rhythm in human urinary melatonin. *Science*, 1975. **187**(4172): pp. 169–71.
14. Akerstedt, T., et al., Melatonin excretion, body temperature and subjective arousal during 64 hours of sleep deprivation. *Psychoneuroendocrinology*, 1979. **4**(3): pp. 219–25.
15. Lang, U., et al., Radioimmunological determination of urinary melatonin in humans: correlation with plasma levels and typical 24-hour rhythmicity. *J Clin Endocrinol Metab*, 1981. **53**(3): pp. 645–50.
16. Graham, C., et al., Prediction of nocturnal plasma melatonin from morning urinary measures. *J Pineal Res*, 1998. **24**(4): pp. 230–8.
17. Cook, M.R., et al., Morning urinary assessment of nocturnal melatonin secretion in older women. *J Pineal Res*, 2000. **28**(1): pp. 41–7.

18. Kovacs, J., et al., Measurement of urinary melatonin: a useful tool for monitoring serum melatonin after its oral administration. *J Clin Endocrinol Metab*, 2000. **85**(2): pp. 666–70.
19. Arendt, J., et al., Immunoassay of 6-hydroxymelatonin sulfate in human plasma and urine: abolition of the urinary 24-hour rhythm with atenolol. *J Clin Endocrinol Metab*, 1985. **60**(6): pp. 1166–73.
20. Markey, S.P., et al., The correlation between human plasma melatonin levels and urinary 6-hydroxy-melatonin excretion. *Clin Chim Acta*, 1985. **150**(3): pp. 221–5.
21. Bojkowski, C.J. and J. Arendt, Annual changes in 6-sulphatoxymelatonin excretion in man. *Acta Endocrinol (Copenh)*, 1988. **117**(4): pp. 470–6.
22. Matthews, C.D., M.V. Guerin, and X. Wang, Human plasma melatonin and urinary 6-sulphatoxy melatonin: studies in natural annual photoperiod and in extended darkness. *Clin Endocrinol (Oxf)*, 1991. **35**(1): pp. 21–7.
23. Lushington, K., et al., Urinary 6-sulfatoxymelatonin cycle-to-cycle variability. *Chronobiol Int*, 1996. **13**(6): pp. 411–21.
24. Kennaway, D.J., et al., Urinary 6-sulfatoxymelatonin excretion and aging: new results and a critical review of the literature. *J Pineal Res*, 1999. **27**(4): pp. 210–20.
25. Schernhammer, E.S., et al., Urinary 6-sulfatoxymelatonin levels and their correlations with lifestyle factors and steroid hormone levels. *J Pineal Res*, 2006. **40**(2): pp. 116–24.
26. Thomas, K.A., 6-sulfatoxymelatonin collected from infant diapers: feasibility and implications for urinary biochemical markers. *Biol Res Nurs*, 2010. **11**(3): pp. 288–92.
27. Iguchi, H., K.I. Kato, and H. Ibayashi, Melatonin serum levels and metabolic clearance rate in patients with liver cirrhosis. *J Clin Endocrinol Metab*, 1982. **54**(5): pp. 1025–7.
28. Lane, E.A. and H.B. Moss, Pharmacokinetics of melatonin in man: first pass hepatic metabolism. *J Clin Endocrinol Metab*, 1985. **61**(6): pp. 1214–6.
29. Aldhous, M., et al., Plasma concentrations of melatonin in man following oral absorption of different preparations. *Br J Clin Pharmacol*, 1985. **19**(4): pp. 517–21.
30. Waldhauser, F., et al., Bioavailability of oral melatonin in humans. *Neuroendocrinology*, 1984. **39**(4): pp. 307–13.
31. Vakkuri, O., J. Leppaluoto, and O. Vuolteenaho, Development and validation of a melatonin radioimmunoassay using radioiodinated melatonin as tracer. *Acta Endocrinol (Copenh)*, 1984. **106**(2): pp. 152–7.
32. Griefahn, B., et al., Long-term stability of 6-hydroxymelatonin sulfate in 24-h urine samples stored at -20 degrees C. *Endocrine*, 2001. **15**(2): pp. 199–202.
33. Bojkowski, C.J., et al., Melatonin secretion in humans assessed by measuring its metabolite, 6-sulfatoxymelatonin. *Clin Chem*, 1987. **33**(8): pp. 1343–8.
34. Bojkowski, C.J. and J. Arendt, Factors influencing urinary 6-sulphatoxymelatonin, a major melatonin metabolite, in normal human subjects. *Clin Endocrinol (Oxf)*, 1990. **33**(4): pp. 435–44.
35. Nowak, R., et al., The correlation between serum and salivary melatonin concentrations and urinary 6-hydroxymelatonin sulphate excretion rates: two non-invasive techniques for monitoring human circadian rhythmicity. *Clin Endocrinol (Oxf)*, 1987. **27**(4): pp. 445–52.
36. Stieglitz, A., et al., Urinary 6-sulphatoxymelatonin excretion reflects pineal melatonin secretion in the Djungarian hamster (Phodopus sungorus). *J Pineal Res*, 1995. **18**(2): pp. 69–76.
37. Shaw, P.F., D.J. Kennaway, and R.F. Seamark, Evidence of high concentrations of melatonin in lateral ventricular cerebrospinal fluid of sheep. *J Pineal Res*, 1989. **6**(3): pp. 201–8.
38. Crasson, M., et al., Serum melatonin and urinary 6-sulfatoxymelatonin in major depression. *Psychoneuroendocrinology*, 2004. **29**(1): pp. 1–12.
39. Klante, G., et al., Creatinine is an appropriate reference for urinary sulphatoxymelatonin of laboratory animals and humans. *J Pineal Res*, 1997. **23**(4): pp. 191–7.
40. Calles-Escandon, J., et al., Influence of exercise on urea, creatinine, and 3-methylhistidine excretion in normal human subjects. *Am J Physiol*, 1984. **246**(4 Pt 1): pp. E334–8.
41. Singh, R., et al., Circadian periodicity of urinary volume, creatinine and 5-hydroxyindole acetic acid excretion in healthy Indians. *Life Sci*, 2000. **66**(3): pp. 209–14.
42. Barr, D.B., et al., Urinary creatinine concentrations in the U.S. population: implications for urinary biologic monitoring measurements. *Environ Health Perspect*, 2005. **113**(2): pp. 192–200.
43. Moriguchi, J., et al., Decreases in urine specific gravity and urinary creatinine in elderly women. *Int Arch Occup Environ Health*, 2005. **78**(6): pp. 438–45.
44. Hellerstein, S., J.L. Hunter, and B.A. Warady, Creatinine excretion rates for evaluation of kidney function in children. *Pediatr Nephrol*, 1988. **2**(4): pp. 419–24.
45. Mori, Y., et al., Urinary creatinine excretion and protein/creatinine ratios vary by body size and gender in children. *Pediatr Nephrol*, 2006. **21**(5): pp. 683–7.

46. Neubert, A. and T. Remer, The impact of dietary protein intake on urinary creatinine excretion in a healthy pediatric population. *J Pediatr*, 1998. **133**(5): pp. 655–9.
47. Hendrick, J.C., et al., [Urinary excretion of 6-sulphatoxymelatonin in normal subjects: statistical approach to the influence of age and sex]. *Ann Endocrinol (Paris)*, 2002. **63**(1): pp. 3–7.
48. Fellenberg, A.J., G. Phillipou, and R.F. Seamark, Specific quantitation of urinary 6-hydroxymelatonin sulphate by gas chromatography mass spectrometry. *Biomed Mass Spectrom*, 1980. **7**(2): pp. 84–7.
49. Tetsuo, M., et al., Quantitative analysis of 6-hydroxymelatonin in human urine by gas chromatography--negative chemical ionization mass spectrometry. *Anal Biochem*, 1981. **110**(1): pp. 208–15.
50. Harthe, C., et al., Direct radioimmunoassay of 6-sulfatoxymelatonin in plasma with use of an iodinated tracer. *Clin Chem*, 1991. **37**(4): pp. 536–9.
51. Peniston-Bird, J.F., et al., An enzyme immunoassay for 6-sulphatoxy-melatonin in human urine. *J Pineal Res*, 1996. **20**(2): pp. 51–6.
52. Tetsuo, M., M. Poth, and S.P. Markey, Melatonin metabolite excretion during childhood and puberty. *J Clin Endocrinol Metab*, 1982. **55**(2): pp. 311–3.
53. Mahlberg, R., et al., Normative data on the daily profile of urinary 6-sulfatoxymelatonin in healthy subjects between the ages of 20 and 84. *Psychoneuroendocrinology*, 2006. **31**(5): pp. 634–41.
54. Miles, A., D.R. Philbrick, and J.E. Grey, Salivary melatonin estimation in assessment of pineal-gland function. *Clin Chem*, 1989. **35**(3): pp. 514–5.
55. Laakso, M.L., et al., Correlation between salivary and serum melatonin: dependence on serum melatonin levels. *J Pineal Res*, 1990. **9**(1): pp. 39–50.
56. Voultsios, A., D.J. Kennaway, and D. Dawson, Salivary melatonin as a circadian phase marker: validation and comparison to plasma melatonin. *J Biol Rhythms*, 1997. **12**(5): pp. 457–66.
57. Bagci, S., et al., Saliva as a valid alternative in monitoring melatonin concentrations in newborn infants. *Early Hum Dev*, 2009. **85**(9): pp. 595–8.
58. Miles, A., et al., Diagnostic and clinical implications of plasma and salivary melatonin assay. *Clin Chem*, 1987. **33**(7): pp. 1295–7.
59. Vakkuri, O., Diurnal rhythm of melatonin in human saliva. *Acta Physiol Scand*, 1985. **124**(3): pp. 409–12.
60. Bagci, S., et al., Utility of salivary melatonin measurements in the assessment of the pineal physiology in newborn infants. *Clin Biochem*, 2010. **43**(10–11): pp. 868–72.
61. Nelson, F.A., L.A. Farr, and M. Ebadi, Salivary melatonin response to acute pain stimuli. *J Pineal Res*, 2001. **30**(4): pp. 206–12.
62. Navazesh, M., C. Christensen, and V. Brightman, Clinical criteria for the diagnosis of salivary gland hypofunction. *J Dent Res*, 1992. **71**(7): pp. 1363–9.
63. Humphrey, S.P. and R.T. Williamson, A review of saliva: normal composition, flow, and function. *J Prosthet Dent*, 2001. **85**(2): pp. 162–9.
64. Dawes, C., Circadian rhythms in human salivary flow rate and composition. *J Physiol*, 1972. **220**(3): pp. 529–45.
65. Dawes, C., Salivary flow patterns and the health of hard and soft oral tissues. *J Am Dent Assoc*, 2008. **139 Suppl**: pp. 18S–24S.
66. Navazesh, M., How can oral health care providers determine if patients have dry mouth? *J Am Dent Assoc*, 2003. **134**(5): pp. 613–20; quiz 633.
67. Seidel, B.M., et al., Secretory IgA, free secretory component and IgD in saliva of newborn infants. *Early Hum Dev*, 2001. **62**(2): pp. 159–64.
68. McIntyre, I.M., et al., Melatonin rhythm in human plasma and saliva. *J Pineal Res*, 1987. **4**(2): pp. 177–83.
69. Morin, D., et al., Melatonin high-affinity binding to alpha-1-acid glycoprotein in human serum. *Pharmacology*, 1997. **54**(5): pp. 271–5.
70. Edgar, W.M., Saliva: its secretion, composition and functions. *Br Dent J*, 1992. **172**(8): pp. 305–12.
71. Tabak, L.A., A revolution in biomedical assessment: the development of salivary diagnostics. *J Dent Educ*, 2001. **65**(12): pp. 1335–9.
72. Walker, R.F., et al., Experience with the Sarstedt Salivette in salivary steroid determinations. *Ann Clin Biochem*, 1990. **27(Pt 5)**: pp. 503–5.
73. Morelius, E., N. Nelson, and E. Theodorsson, Saliva collection using cotton buds with wooden sticks: a note of caution. *Scand J Clin Lab Invest*, 2006. **66**(1): pp. 15–8.
74. Weber, J.M., et al., Melatonin in saliva: sampling procedure and stability. *Poster presented at the 11th Annual Meeting of the Society for Light Treatment and Biological Rhythms (SLTBR)*, Old Town Alexandria, VA, USA, May 16–18, 1999.

75. English, J., et al., Rapid direct measurement of melatonin in saliva using an iodinated tracer and solid phase second antibody. *Ann Clin Biochem*, 1993. **30(Pt 4)**: pp. 415–6.
76. Eriksson, K., A. Ostin, and J.O. Levin, Quantification of melatonin in human saliva by liquid chromatography-tandem mass spectrometry using stable isotope dilution. *J Chromatogr B Analyt Technol Biomed Life Sci*, 2003. **794**(1): pp. 115–23.
77. Motoyama, A., T. Kanda, and R. Namba, Direct determination of endogenous melatonin in human saliva by column-switching semi-microcolumn liquid chromatography/mass spectrometry with on-line analyte enrichment. *Rapid Commun Mass Spectrom*, 2004. **18**(12): pp. 1250–8.
78. Romsing, S., F. Bokman, and Y. Bergqvist, Determination of melatonin in saliva using automated solid-phase extraction, high-performance liquid chromatography and fluorescence detection. *Scand J Clin Lab Invest*, 2006. **66**(3): pp. 181–90.
79. Hamase, K., et al., A sensitive internal standard method for the determination of melatonin in mammals using precolumn oxidation reversed-phase high-performance liquid chromatography. *J Chromatogr B Analyt Technol Biomed Life Sci*, 2004. **811**(2): pp. 237–41.
80. Bruce, J., et al., Sequential cerebrospinal fluid and plasma sampling in humans: 24-hour melatonin measurements in normal subjects and after peripheral sympathectomy. *J Clin Endocrinol Metab*, 1991. **72**(4): pp. 819–23.
81. Arendt, J., et al., Radioimmunoassay of melatonin: human serum and cerebrospinal fluid. *Horm Res*, 1977. **8**(2): pp. 65–75.
82. Vaughan, G.M., et al., Melatonin concentration in human blood and cerebrospinal fluid: relationship to stress. *J Clin Endocrinol Metab*, 1978. **47**(1): pp. 220–3.
83. Reppert, S.M., et al., A diurnal melatonin rhythm in primate cerebrospinal fluid. *Endocrinology*, 1979. **104**(2): pp. 295–301.
84. Tan, C.H. and J.C. Khoo, Melatonin concentrations in human serum, ventricular and lumbar cerebrospinal fluids as an index of the secretory pathway of the pineal gland. *Horm Res*, 1981. **14**(4): pp. 224–33.
85. Young, S.N., et al., Effect of oral melatonin administration on melatonin, 5-hydroxyindoleacetic acid, indoleacetic acid, and cyclic nucleotides in human cerebrospinal fluid. *Neuroendocrinology*, 1984. **39**(1): pp. 87–92.
86. Rollag, M.D., R.J. Morgan, and G.D. Niswender, Route of melatonin secretion in sheep. *Endocrinology*, 1978. **102**(1): pp. 1–8.
87. Perlow, M.J., et al., Daily rhythms in cortisol and melatonin in primate cerebrospinal fluid. Effects of constant light and dark. *Neuroendocrinology*, 1981. **32**(4): pp. 193–6.
88. Kanematsu, N., et al., Presence of a distinct 24-hour melatonin rhythm in the ventricular cerebrospinal fluid of the goat. *J Pineal Res*, 1989. **7**(2): pp. 143–52.
89. Skinner, D.C. and B. Malpaux, High melatonin concentrations in third ventricular cerebrospinal fluid are not due to Galen vein blood recirculating through the choroid plexus. *Endocrinology*, 1999. **140**(10): pp. 4399–405.
90. Tricoire, H., et al., Melatonin enters the cerebrospinal fluid through the pineal recess. *Endocrinology*, 2002. **143**(1): pp. 84–90.
91. Tricoire, H., B. Malpaux, and M. Moller, Cellular lining of the sheep pineal recess studied by light-, transmission-, and scanning electron microscopy: morphologic indications for a direct secretion of melatonin from the pineal gland to the cerebrospinal fluid. *J Comp Neurol*, 2003. **456**(1): pp. 39–47.
92. Longatti, P., et al., Ventricular cerebrospinal fluid melatonin concentrations investigated with an endoscopic technique. *J Pineal Res*, 2007. **42**(2): pp. 113–8.
93. Hedlund, L., et al., Melatonin: daily cycle in plasma and cerebrospinal fluid of calves. *Science*, 1977. **195**(4279): pp. 686–7.
94. Rousseau, A., et al., Serum and cerebrospinal fluid concentrations of melatonin: a pilot study in healthy male volunteers. *J Neural Transm*, 1999. **106**(9–10): pp. 883–8.
95. Smith, J.A., et al., Melatonin in serum and cerebrospinal fluid. *Lancet*, 1976. **2**(7982): p. 425.
96. Rizzo, V., et al., Determination of free and total (free plus protein-bound) melatonin in plasma and cerebrospinal fluid by high-performance liquid chromatography with fluorescence detection. *J Chromatogr B Analyt Technol Biomed Life Sci*, 2002. **774**(1): pp. 17–24.
97. Leston, J., et al., Melatonin is released in the third ventricle in humans. A study in movement disorders. *Neurosci Lett*, 2010. **469**(3): pp. 294–7.
98. Liu, R.Y., et al., Decreased melatonin levels in postmortem cerebrospinal fluid in relation to aging, Alzheimer's disease, and apolipoprotein E-epsilon4/4 genotype. *J Clin Endocrinol Metab*, 1999. **84**(1): pp. 323–7.

99. Zhou, J.N., et al., Early neuropathological Alzheimer's changes in aged individuals are accompanied by decreased cerebrospinal fluid melatonin levels. *J Pineal Res*, 2003. **35**(2): pp. 125–30.
100. Pontes, G.N., et al., Injury switches melatonin production source from endocrine (pineal) to paracrine (phagocytes) - melatonin in human colostrum and colostrum phagocytes. *J Pineal Res*, 2006. **41**(2): pp. 136–41.
101. Kennaway, D.J., Melatonin and development: physiology and pharmacology. *Semin Perinatol*, 2000. **24**(4): pp. 258–66.

36 Cell Studies with Melatonin Exposed to UV Light and Ionizing Radiation

Ilona Iżykowska, Marek Cegielski, and Piotr Dzięgiel

CONTENTS

36.1 INTRODUCTION

36.1.1 Influence of UV and Ionizing Radiation on Skin and Other Organs

UV radiation (UVR) with a wavelength in the range of 280 to 320 nm (UVB) and 320 to 400 nm (UVA) negatively influences the skin [1]. UVB affects keratinocytes and melanocytes of the epidermis; UVA affects the basal layer of keratinocytes and fibroblasts of the dermis [2–4]. Both types of UVR influence the cell DNA. UVB is absorbed by DNA and induces formation of cyclobutane pyrimidine dimers and pyrimidine [6–4] pyrimidone photoproducts. UVA generates large amounts of free radicals in cells, which, in effect, leads to oxidation of DNA bases and formation of 8-oxodeoxyguanosine [5]. Mutations in genes regulating proliferation, cell growth cycle, or apoptosis can lead to tumor transformation of skin cells [6,7]. Keratinocytes are more resistant to UVR compared to fibroblasts, since they have a more efficient genome repair system [8]. Damaged keratinocytes are eliminated through apoptosis (sunburn cells) or give rise to nonmelanoma cancer cells: basal cancer cells and squamous cancer cells [9,10]. To a lesser extent, abnormal melanocytes undergo apoptosis, accumulate mutations, and transform into melanoma cells [11]. UVA-induced oxidative stress leads to cell membrane lipid peroxidation, as well as reduction of endogenous antioxidant enzyme activity: superoxide dismutase (SOD), catalase (CAT), peroxidise (GSH-Px), and glutathione reductase (GSH-R) [12]. UVB activates apoptotic proteins and proinflammatory cytokines in the epidermis, destroys extracellular matrix proteins in the dermis, and is responsible for its photoaging [13–15].

In cells, ionizing radiation leads to formation of free radicals, which damage DNA, lipids, and proteins of cell membrane [16,17]. This type of radiation increases apoptotic gene expression in keratinocytes and fibroblasts, while reducing DNA repair gene expression [18,19]. Studies on animals demonstrate that ionizing radiation causes damage in liver, lung, brain, and bone cells [20–22].

36.1.2 Melatonin Functions

Melatonin is a commonly occurring compound in many organisms: bacteria, algae, plants, invertebrates, and vertebrates. In vertebrates, melatonin serves as a neurohormone of the pineal gland, which regulates the circadian rhythms. Extrapineal sites of melatonin synthesis include the brain, retina, gastrointestinal tract, skin, peripheral blood lymphocytes, and bone marrow. Specific structure enables melatonin to scavenge free radicals and diffuse through biological membranes. Thanks to this ability, melatonin can regulate the oxidoreductive status of the cell as well as influence the intracellular processes by affecting calmoduline and nuclear receptors RORα/RZR. Additionally, melatonin influences the cell by its membrane receptors MT1 and MT2 [23].

One of the most important functions of melatonin is its antioxidant and antiproliferating capacity. Melatonin detoxifies reactive oxygen species (hydroxyl radical—$^{\bullet}OH$, singlet oxygen—$^1O_2$, peroxy radicals—$ROO^{\bullet}$, hydrogen peroxide—H_2O_2) as well as reactive nitrogen species (nitric oxide—$NO^{\bullet}$, peroxynitrite—$ONOO^-$). Melatonin metabolites formed as a result of neutralization of reactive oxygen and nitrogen species also possess the radical-scavenging ability. They are the following: 6-hydroxymelatonin, cyclic 3-hydroxymelatonin, N1-acetyl-N2-formyl-5-methoxykynuramine (AFMK), and N-acetyl-5-methoxykynuramine (AMK). Because of them, melatonin deactivates free radicals through a cascade [24]. Melatonin can indirectly affect the oxidative status of the cell as a result of an increase in gene expression of antioxidant enzymes: SOD, CAT, GSH-Px, and GSH-R. Regulation of antioxidant enzymes involves MT1 and RORα receptors [25]. Melatonin regulates mitochondrial functions and prevents cell apoptosis as a result of deactivation of reactive oxygen and nitrogen species, an increase in activity of enzymes of the electron transport chain, and stabilization of mitochondrial membrane potential [26].

Melatonin has an oncostatic effect on malignant cells. Administration of melatonin together with anthracyclines, for example, intensifies their cytotoxic action on malignant cells, while protecting normal cells from oxidative stress [27–29]. Antiproliferative activity of melatonin was best recognized in studies on human breast adenocarcinoma cells (MCF7), in which melatonin decreased cell cycle gene expression and increased the expression of proapoptotic genes [30]. Studies on transgenic mice with *HER-2/neu* proto-oncogene overexpression showed that exogenous melatonin decreased the frequency of occurrence and magnitude of adenocarcinomas, prevented metastases to lymph nodes and lungs, and decreased expression of *HER-2/neu* [31].

36.2 IN VITRO STUDIES

36.2.1 The Influence of Melatonin on Normal and Malignant Cells Treated with UVR

Melatonin is synthesized in different layers of human skin: keratinocytes of the spinous and granular layer, as well as melanocytes of the epidermis, hair follicles, mast cells, and endothelium of blood vessels of the dermis. Also, expression of MT1 and MT2 melatonin receptors takes place in various skin cells [32]. *In vitro* studies on keratinocyte, fibroblast, melanocyte, and melanoma cell lines demonstrated expression of enzymes of the melatonin synthesis pathway as well as *MT1*, *MT2*, and *RORα/RZR* receptors expression [33–36]. Melatonin concentration in keratinocytes surpasses its concentration in blood serum. High melatonin concentration serves elimination of UVR-induced free radicals. Under UVR influence, the transformation of melatonin to 2-hydroxymelatonin and AFMK takes place in the skin. Both metabolites possess the capability to interact with free radicals. Therefore, melatonin and its metabolic products form an antioxidant system protecting the skin from UVR [37]. At the same time, UVR can disturb the function of the skin melatoninergic system. UVB in various doses (5, 20, 50, 100 mJ/cm^2) changes the expression of genes encoding for enzymes participating in melatonin synthesis as well as *MT1*, *MT2*, and *RORα*/RZR melatonin receptor gene expression [33,34].

In vitro studies showed protective action of melatonin on normal cells exposed to UVR. Melatonin inhibited formation of reactive oxygen species in cells of the cornea and leukocytes exposed to UVB radiation [38,39]. Using liposomes as a model of the cell membrane, it has been revealed that melatonin deactivated free radicals, increased membrane fluidity, and prevented lipid peroxidation [40]. In cells exposed to UVC radiation, melatonin scavenged •OH and prevented damages to DNA [41].

The time of melatonin administration is significant. In in vivo and in vitro studies, melatonin applied to the skin of patients or added to cell culture medium 15 to 30 minutes before UV irradiation prevented erythema formation and decreased the number of cells undergoing apoptosis. The addition of melatonin immediately after the exposition did not protect the skin from erythema or merely delayed cell apoptosis [42,43]. A 30-minute preincubation with 10^{-3} M melatonin increased the survival rate of keratinocytes exposed to 30 and 60 mJ/cm^2 UVB and 15 J/cm^2 UVA by 11%, 19%, and 15% respectively. Additionally, melatonin at concentration of 10^{-6} M increased survival rate of cells irradiated with 30 mJ/cm^2 by 11% [44]. Similarly, in another study, melatonin added at 10^{-3} or 10^{-4} M 30 minutes before irradiation of HaCaT keratinocytes with 50 mJ/cm^2 UVR significantly increased cell survival rate assessed in DNA synthesis tests and ability of colony formation as well as decreased the number of cells undergoing apoptosis [45]. In irradiated keratinocytes, melatonin restored the proper potential in the mitochondrial membrane; inhibited the activation of the endogenous pathway of apoptosis; and decreased the expression of genes involved in the apoptotic process, tumor-related genes, and cell cycle regulatory genes; while at the same time stimulated antioxidant enzyme gene expression [46,47]. In a similar model of in vitro cell irradiation, melatonin inhibited the apoptosis of U937 human leukemia cells exposed to UVB and led to stabilization of mitochondrial membrane potential, prevention of the cytochrome c release into cytoplasm, and inhibition of apoptosis activation [42]. Moreover, it has been demonstrated that melatonin regulated apoptosis of the above-mentioned cells also through activation of ERK and MAPK kinases, as well as deactivation of kinases p38 MAPK and JNK activated by oxidative stress [48].

In UVB-irradiated fibroblasts, melatonin decreased the expression of genes involved in carcinogenesis [49]. After irradiating the fibroblasts with a 140-mJ/cm^2 dose of UVB, only 56% of all cells survived. Melatonin added to the medium at a concentration of 10^{-7} or 10^{-9} M, one hour before and 24 hours after irradiation, inhibited membrane lipid peroxidation and decreased the number of cells arrested in the G1 phase of cell cycle and undergoing apoptosis. The number of undamaged fibroblasts increased to 92.5% [50]. Another study showed, however, that 30-minute incubation with melatonin at the concentration of 10^{-3} or 10^{-4} M only slightly increased survival of fibroblasts irradiated with 30 mJ/cm^2 and 60 mJ/cm^2 doses of UVB or a 15 J/cm^2 dose of UVA [44].

The protective effect of melatonin on irradiated cells may depend on its membrane receptors, MT1 and MT2. It has been agreed that melatonin protects the U937 line cells exposed to UVB from apoptosis by its receptors, MT1 or MT2 [51]. Melatonin, through the MT1 or MT2 receptor, as well as bcl-2 protein, inhibited activation of bax protein and related processes, e.g., release of cytochrome c into the cytoplasm and activation of caspase 3 and 9 [52].

Unpublished data presenting the influence of melatonin on keratinocytes and fibroblasts exposed to UVB doses of 30 and 60 mJ/cm^2 and a UVA dose of 15 J/cm^2 proved that melatonin, depending on its concentration at 10^{-3}, 10^{-6}, or 10^{-9} M, changed the expression of the *MT1* receptor gene. For some melatonin concentrations, increased or unchanged expression of *MT1* was related to increased survival rate of keratinocytes: cells incubated with 10^{-3} M melatonin and irradiated with 30 mJ/cm^2, 60 mJ/cm^2, or 15 J/cm^2 as well as cells incubated with 10^{-6} M melatonin and irradiated with 30 mJ/cm^2 (Figures 36.1 and 36.2). Melatonin, to a lesser extent, influenced the survival rate and expression of *MT1* in fibroblasts. Doses of 60 mJ/cm^2 and 15 J/cm^2 led to a total decline in *MT1* gene expression. *MT1* gene expression was maintained after addition of melatonin at 10^{-6} M. We observed an increase in *MT1* expression for a smaller dose of UVB, also together with melatonin at 10^{-9} M (Figures 36.3 and 36.4) [53]. Further research investigating the role of the MT1 receptor or other melatonin receptors in protection of irradiated cells is necessary.

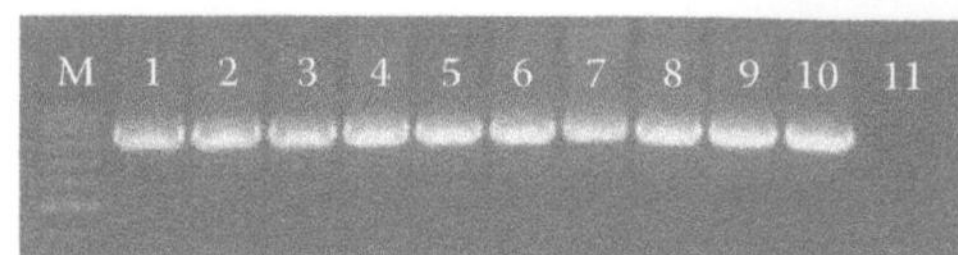

FIGURE 36.1 Expression of *MT1* melatonin receptor (842 bp) in keratinocytes incubated with melatonin (10^{-3}, 10^{-6}, and 10^{-9} M) and next irradiated with UVB (30 and 60 mJ/cm^2) or UVA (15 J/cm^2). M. mass marker (100–1000 bp). (1) Keratinocytes, (2) keratinocytes + 30 mJ/cm^2, (3) keratinocytes + 10^{-3} M + 30 mJ/cm^2, (4) keratinocytes + 10^{-6} M + 30 mJ/cm^2, (5) keratinocytes + 10^{-9} M + 30 mJ/cm^2, (6) keratinocytes + 60 mJ/cm^2, (7) keratinocytes + 10^{-3} M + 60 mJ/cm^2, (8) keratinocytes + 15 J/cm^2, (9) keratinocytes + 10^{-3} M + 15 J/cm^2, (10) keratinocytes + 10^{-6} M + 15 J/cm^2, (11) keratinocytes + 10^{-9} M + 15 J/cm^2. Sequences of primers for nested PCR were taken from a work by Slominski et al. [35].

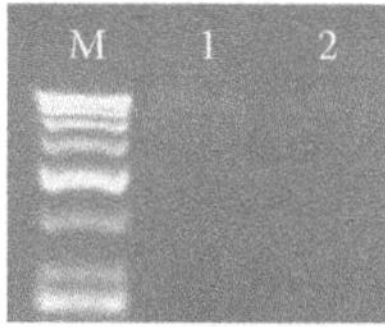

FIGURE 36.2 Expression of *MT1* melatonin receptor (842 bp) in keratinocytes incubated with melatonin (10^{-6} and 10^{-9} M) and irradiated with UVB. M. mass marker (50–1000 bp). (1) Keratinocytes + 10^{-6} M + 60 mJ/cm^2, (2) keratinocytes + 10^{-9} M + 60 mJ/cm^2. Sequences of primers for nested PCR were taken from a work by Slominski et al. [35].

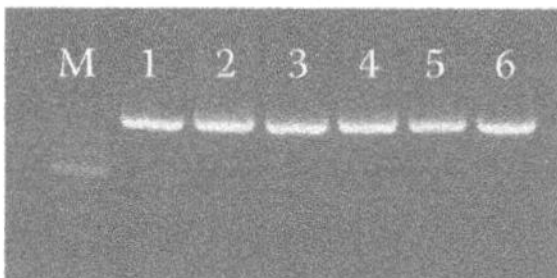

FIGURE 36.3 Expression of *MT1* melatonin receptor (842 bp) in fibroblasts incubated with melatonin (10^{-6} and 10^{-9} M) and next irradiated with UVB (30 and 60 mJ/cm^2) or UVA (15 J/cm^2). M. mass marker (100–1000 bp). (1) Fibroblasts, (2) fibroblasts + 30 mJ/cm^2, (3) fibroblasts + 10^{-6} M + 30 mJ/cm^2, (4) fibroblasts + 10^{-9} M + 30 mJ/cm^2, (5) fibroblasts + 10^{-6} M + 60 mJ/cm^2, (6) fibroblasts + 10^{-6} M + 15 J/cm^2. Sequences of primers for nested PCR were taken from a work by Slominski et al. [35].

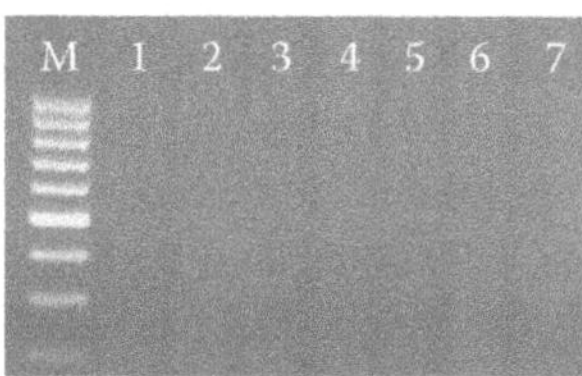

FIGURE 36.4 No expression of *MT1* melatonin receptor in fibroblasts incubated with melatonin (10^{-3} and 10^{-9} M) and next irradiated with UVB (30 and 60 mJ/cm^2) or UVA (15 J/cm^2). M. Mass marker (100–1000 bp). (1) Fibroblasts + 10^{-3} M + 30 mJ/cm^2, (2) fibroblasts + 60 mJ/cm^2, (3) fibroblasts + 10^{-3} M + 60 mJ/cm^2, (4) fibroblasts + 10^{-9} M + 60 mJ/cm^2, (5) fibroblasts + 15 J/cm^2, (6) fibroblasts + 10^{-3} M + 15 J/cm^2, (7) fibroblasts + 10^{-9} M + 15 J/cm^2. Sequences of primers for nested PCR were taken from a work by Slominski et al. [35].

Melatonin in pharmacological concentrations (10^{-3}–10^{-7} M) inhibited proliferation of human melanoma cells, i.e., SBCE2, WM-98, WM-164, and SKMEL-188 [33]. The oncostatic effect of melatonin on melanoma cells may involve its MT1 and MT2 receptors [36,54]. The expected oncostatic effect of exogenous melatonin on a BM melanoma cell line irradiated with UVB and UVA revealed that melatonin did not intensify cell damage processes but increased their survival rate in relation to cells that were only irradiated [55]. The increase in survival rate of melanoma cells as well as absence of *MT1* gene expression indicated protective effects of melatonin resulting from its antioxidant activity [53]. This mechanism may be confirmed by another study, in which melatonin inhibited apoptosis in prostate cancer cells exposed to ionizing radiation because of an increase in intracellular glutathione concentration [56]. Melatonin itself can act as a pro-oxidant and generate reactive oxygen species, both in normal and malignant cells [57]. The number of free radicals is, however, too small to produce oxidative stress or cell apoptosis but sufficient to activate transcription factor NFκB and cell proliferation [58].

36.2.2 The Influence of Melatonin on Normal and Malignant Cells Treated with Ionizing Radiation

In vitro, the protective effect of melatonin on cells exposed to ionizing radiation has been also investigated. Melatonin as well as its conjugate with α-lipoic acid decreased the level of lipid peroxidation in liposomes as well as the number of hemolyzed erythrocytes after exposition to γ radiation [59]. Melatonin at the concentration of 10^{-5} M protected fibroblasts exposed to an 8-Gy dose of X radiation from apoptosis, decreased levels of malondialdehyde, and increased the number of living cells by 30% in relation to cells that were only irradiated [60]. Among leukocytes isolated from the blood of patients treated with 300 mg melatonin and later exposed to a 1.5-Gy dose of X radiation, there was a decrease of about 60% in the number of cells with damaged chromosomes and micronuclei [61]. The addition of melatonin at a concentration of 2 mM to the culture medium 20 minutes before irradiation of lymphocytes with 1.5 Gy decreased the number of cells with damaged chromosomes and micronuclei by about 61% [62]. A study on HeLa S3 cells demonstrated that 30-minute incubation with melatonin at the concentration of 0.01 mM decreased the expression of transcription factor NFκB, which activates proinflammatory protein genes [63]. Melatonin protects normal cells but intensifies apoptosis in malignant cells. It is realized by means of the difference in regulation of p53 expression in these cells [64].

36.3 APPLICATION OF MELATONIN

The protective effect of melatonin on in vitro irradiated cells has been proven by in vivo studies. Melatonin applied to the skin prior to irradiation prevents the formation of erythema [43]. Even better results were obtained when melatonin was administered together with vitamins C and E. The above-mentioned substances acted synergistically and inhibited deactivation of antioxidant enzymes [65]. Administration of melatonin in rats prior to their whole-body exposure to ionizing radiation decreased the number of skin cells that undergo apoptosis [66]. Melatonin also prevented damage to the lens exposed to UVB radiation, because increased activity of antioxidant enzymes inhibited membrane lipid peroxidation and cell apoptosis [67,68]. Melatonin scavenged $O_2^{\bullet}$ radicals in the corneal epithelial cells irradiated with UVB [38]. Similarly, melatonin administered over a period of several days before the irradiation of the skull with γ rays decreased membrane lipid peroxidation and increased antioxidant enzyme activity in the rat lens [69].

With regard to its protective properties, melatonin is being considered as a possible cream ingredient [70,71]. However, the fact that the actual amount of melatonin reaching skin cells is insufficient to deactivate free radicals may become a problem [72]. Additionally, melatonin undergoes rapid degradation by the light. Administration of melatonin encapsulated in liposomes may overcome these obstacles. Carriers protect melatonin from photodegradation, facilitate transfer of melatonin into deeper skin layers, and allow its higher concentration in the skin [73,74]. Increase of the intracellular melatonin concentration by means of liposome carriers may increase its skin protective effect. Melatonin encapsulated in lipid nanoparticles is also applied onto skin in order to increase its concentration in blood serum [75].

36.4 SUMMARY

Melatonin was successfully used as a protective substance for the skin exposed to UVR, as well as compound protecting whole-body irradiated animals. In vitro studies enabled an understanding of the mechanisms of protective action of melatonin. Melatonin increases survival and decreases apoptosis of keratinocytes, fibroblasts, and leukocytes subjected to UVR as a result of scavenging of free radicals, as well as inhibits apoptotic proteins and lipid peroxidation. These processes may involve melatonin receptors. In studies on the effect of melatonin on cells exposed to ionizing radiation, melatonin decreases the number of cells with damaged DNA and inhibits cell membrane lipid peroxidation. Nowadays, studies are aimed at developing carriers that increase melatonin concentration in the skin and blood serum.

REFERENCES

1. Matta, J.L., Ramos, J.M., Armstrong, R.A., and H. D'Antoni. 2005. Environmental UV-A and UV-B threshold doses for apoptosis and necrosis in human fibroblasts. *Photochem Photobiol* 81:563–68.
2. Bernerd, F., and D. Asselinau. 1998. UVA exposure of human skin reconstructed in vitro induces apoptosis of dermal fibroblasts: subsequent connective tissue repair and implication in photoaging. *Cell Death Differ* 5:792–802.
3. Mass, P., Hoffman, K., Gabmichler, T., Altmeyer, P., and H.G. Mannherz. 2003. Premature keratinocyte death and expression of marker proteins of apoptosis in human skin after UVB exposure. *Arch Dermatol Res* 295:71–9.
4. Tada, A., Pereira, E., Beitner Johnson, D., Kavanagh, R., and Z.A. Abdel–Malek. 2002. Mitogen and ultraviolet-B-induced signaling pathways in normal human melanocytes. *J Invest Dermatol* 118:316–22.
5. Besaratinia, A., Kim, S., and G.P. Pfeifer. 2008. Rapid repair of UVA-induced oxidized purines and persistence of UVB-induced dipyrimidine lesions determine the mutagenicity of sunlight in mouse cells. *FASEB J* 22:2379–392.
6. Pacifico, A., Goldberg, L.H., Peris, K., Chimenti, S., Leone, G., and H.N. Ananthaswamy. 2008. Loss of CDKN2A and p14ARF expression occurs frequently in human nonmelanoma skin cancers. *Br J Dermatol* 158(2):291–97.
7. Greene, V.R., Johnson, M.M., Grimm, E.A., and J.A. Ellerhorst. 2009. Frequencies of NRAS and BRAF mutations increase from the radial to the vertical growth phase in cutaneous melanoma. *J Invest Dermatol* 129(6):1483–488.
8. D'Errico, M., Lemma, T., Calcagnile, A., de Santis, L.D., and E. Dogliotti. 2007. Cell type and DNA damage specific response to human skin cells to environmental agents. *Mutation Res* 614:37–47.
9. Van Laethem, A., Claerhout, S., Garmyn, M., and P. Agostinis. 2005. The sunburn cell: regulation of death and survival of the keratinocyte. *Int J Biochem Cell Biol* 37(8):1547–553.
10. Erb, P., Ji, J., Wernli, M., Kump, E., Glaser, A., and S.A. Buchner. 2005. Role of apoptosis in basal and squamous cell carcinoma formation. *Immunol Lett* 100(1):68–72.
11. Gupta, P.B., Kuperwasser, C., Brunet, J.P., et al. 2005. The melanocyte differentiation program predisposes to metastasis after neoplastic transformation. *Nat Genet* 37(10):1047–54.
12. Moysan, A., Marquis, I., Gaboriau, F., Santus, R., Dubertret, L., and P. Morlière. 1993. Ultraviolet A-induced lipid peroxidation and antioxidant defense systems in cultured human skin fibroblasts. *J Invest Dermatol* 100(5):692–98.
13. Wang, X.Y., and Z.G. Bi. 2006. UVB-irradiated human keratinocytes and interleukin-1α indirectly increase MAP kinase/AP-1 activation and MMP-1 production in UVA-irradiated dermal fibroblasts. *Chin Med J (Engl)* 119(10):827–31.
14. Van Laethem, A., Van Kelst, S., Lippens, S., et al. 2004. Activation of p38 MAPK is required for Bax translocation to mitochondria, cytochrome c release and apoptosis induced by UVB irradiation in human keratinocytes. *FASEB J* 18(15):1946–948.

15. Debacq–Chainiaux, F., Borlon, C., Pascal, T., et al. 2005. Repeated exposure of human skin fibroblasts to UVB at subcytotoxic level triggers premature senescence through the TGF-β1 signaling pathway. *J Cell Sci* 118(4):743–58.
16. Chi, C., Tanaka, R., Okuda, Y., et al. 2005. Quantitative measurements of oxidative stress in mouse skin induced by X-ray irradiation. *Chem Pharm Bull (Tokyo)* 53(11):1411–415.
17. Gollapalle, E., Wang, R., Adetolu, R., et al. 2007. Detection of oxidative clustered DNA lesions in X-irradiated mouse skin tissues and human MCF-7 breast cancer cells. *Radiat Res* 167(2):207–16.
18. Koike, M., Shiomi, T., and A. Koike. 2005. Identification of skin injury-related genes induced by ionizing radiator in human keratinocytes using cDNA microarray. *J Radiat Res* 46:173–84.
19. Kis, E., Szatmári, T., Keszei, M., et al. 2006. Microarray analysis of radiation response genes in primary human fibroblasts. *Int J Radiat Oncol Biol Phys* 66(5):1506–514.
20. Şener, G., Jahovic, N., Tosun, O., Atasoy, M.B., and B.Ç. Yeğen. 2003. Melatonin ameliorates ionizing radiation-induced oxidative organ damage in rats. *Life Sci* 74: 563–72.
21. Manda, K., Ueno, M., and K. Anzai. 2009. Cranial irradiation-induced inhibition of neurogenesis in hippocampal dentate gyrus of adult mice: attenuation by melatonin pretreatment. *J Pineal Res* 46: 71–8.
22. Yavuz, M.N., Yavuz, A.A., Ulku, C., et al. 2003. Protective effect of melatonin against fractionated irradiation-induced epiphyseal injury in a weanling rat model. *J Pineal Res* 35:288–94.
23. Pandi–Perumal, S.R., Srinivasan, V., and G.J.M. Maestroni. 2006. Melatonin: nature's most versatile biological signal? *FASEB J* 273(13):2813–838.
24. Allegra, M., Reiter, R.J., Tan, D.X., Gentile, C., Tesoriere, L., and M.A. Livrea. 2003. The chemistry of melatonin's interaction with reactive species. *J Pineal Res* 34(1):1–10.
25. Tomás–Zapico, C., and A. Coto–Montes. 2005. A proposed mechanism to explain the stimulatory effect of melatonin on antioxidative enzymes. *J Pineal Res* 39(2):99–104.
26. León, J., Acuña–Castroviejo, D., Escames, G., Tan, D.X., and R.J. Reiter. 2005. Melatonin mitigates mitochondrial malfunction. *J Pineal Res* 38:1–9.
27. Dziegiel, P., Murawska–Cialowicz, E., Jethon, Z., et al. 2003. Melatonin stimulates the activity of protective antioxidative enzymes in myocardial cells of rats in the course of doxorubicin intoxication. *J Pineal Res* 35:183–87.
28. Dziegiel, P., Suder, E., Surowiak, P., et al. 2002. Role of exogenous melatonin in reducing the nephrotoxic effect of daunorubicin and doxorubicin in the rat. *J Pineal Res* 33:95–100.
29. Fic, M., Podhorska–Okolow, M., Dziegiel, P., et al. 2007. Effect of melatonin on cytotoxicity of doxorubicin toward selected cell lines (human keratinocytes, lung cancer cell line A-549, laryngeal cancer cell line Hep-2). *In Vivo* 21(3):513–18.
30. Blask, D.E., Sauer, L.A., and R.T. Dauchy. 2002. Melatonin as a chronobiotic/anticancer agent: cellular, biochemical, and molecular mechanisms of action and their implications for circadian-based cancer therapy. *Curr Top Med Chem* 2:113–32.
31. Baturin, D.A., Alimova, I.N., Anisimov, V.N., et al. 2001. The effect of light regimen and melatonin on the development of spontaneous mammary tumors in HER-2/neu transgenic mice is related to a down-regulation of HER-2/neu gene expression. *Neuro Endocrinol Lett* 22(6):441–47.
32. Slominski, A., Wortsman, J., and D.J. Tobin. 2005. The cutaneous serotoninergic and melatoninergic system: securing a place under the sun. *FASEB J* 19:176–94.
33. Slominski, A., Pisarchik, A., Semak, I., et al. 2002. Serotoninergic and melatoninergic system are fully expressed in human skin. *FASEB J* 16:896–98.
34. Slominski, A., Fischer, T.W., Zmijewski, M.A., et al. 2005. On the role of melatonin in skin physiology and pathology. *Endocrine* 27:137–48.
35. Slominski, A., Pisarchik, A., Zbytek, B., Tobin, D.J., Kauser, S., and J. Wortsman. 2003. Functional activity of serotoninergic and melatoninergic system expressed in the skin. *J Cell Physiol* 196:144–53.
36. Fischer, T.W., Zmijewski, M.A., Zbytek, B., et al. 2006. Oncostatic effects of the indole melatonin and expression of its cytosolic and nuclear receptors in cultured human melanoma cell lines. *Int J Oncol* 29(3):665–72.
37. Fischer, T.W., Sweatman, T., Semak, I., Sayre, R.M., Wortsman, J., and A. Slominski. 2006. Constitutive and UV-induced metabolism of melatonin in keratinocytes and cell-free system. *FASEB J* 18:1564–566.
38. Ciuffi, M., Pisanello, M., Pagliai, G., et al. 2003. Antioxidant protection in cultured corneal cells and whole corneas submitted to UV-B exposure. *Photochem Photobiol* 71:59–68.
39. Fischer, T.W., Scholz, G., Knöll, B., Hipler, U.C., and P. Elsner. 2004. Melatonin suppresses reactive oxygen species induced by UV irradiation in leukocytes. *J Pineal Res* 37:107–12.

40. Saija, A., Tomaino, A., Trombetta, D., et al. 2002. Interaction of melatonin with model membranes and possible implications in its photoprotective activity. *Eur J Pharm Biopharm* 53:209–15.
41. Yamamoto, H.A., and P.V. Mohanan. 2001. Effects of melatonin on paraquat or ultraviolet light exposure-induced DNA damage. *J Pineal Res* 31(4):308–13.
42. Luchetti, F., Canonico, B., Curci, R., et al. 2006. Melatonin prevents apoptosis induced by UV-B treatment in U937 cell line. *J Pineal Res* 40:158–67.
43. Bangha, E., Elsner, P., and G.S. Kistler. 1997. Suppression of UV-induced erythema by topical treatment with melatonin (N-acetyl-5-methoxytryptamine). Influence of the application time point. *Dermatology* 195(3):248–52.
44. Izykowska, I., Cegielski, M., Gebarowska, E., et al. 2009. Effect of melatonin on human keratinocytes and fibroblasts subjected to UVA and UVB radiation in vitro. *In Vivo* 23(5):739–45.
45. Fischer, T.W., Zbytek, B., Sayre, R.M., et al. 2006. Melatonin increases survival of HaCaT keratinocytes by suppressing UV-induced apoptosis. *J Pineal Res* 40:18–26.
46. Fischer, T.W., Zmijewski, M.A., Wortsman, J., and A. Slominski. 2008. Melatonin maintains mitochondrial membrane potential and attenuates activation of initiator (casp-9) and effector caspases (casp-3/casp-7) and PARP in UVR-exposed HaCaT keratinocytes. *J Pineal Res* 44(4):397–407.
47. Cho, J.W., Kim, C.W., and K.S. Lee. 2007. Modification of gene expression by melatonin in UVB-irradiated HaCaT keratinocyte cell lines using a cDNA microarray. *Oncol Rep* 17(3):573–77.
48. Luchetti, F., Betti, M., Canonico, B., et al. 2009. ERK MAPK activation mediates the antiapoptotic signaling of melatonin in UVB-stressed U937 cells. *Free Radic Biol Med* 46(3):339–51.
49. Lee, K.S., Lee, W.S., Suh, S.I., et al. 2003. Melatonin reduces ultraviolet-B induced cell damages and polyamine levels in human skin fibroblasts in culture. *Exp Mol Med* 35(4):263–68.
50. Ryoo, Y.W., Suh, S.I., Mun, K.C., Kim, B.C., and K.S. Lee. 2001. The effect of the melatonin on ultraviolet-B irradiated cultured dermal fibroblasts. *J Dermatol Sci* 27:162–69.
51. Radogna, F., Paternoster, L., Albertini, M.C., et al. 2007. Melatonin antagonizes apoptosis via receptor interaction in U937 monocytic cells. *J Pineal Res* 43(2):154–62.
52. Radogna, F., Cristofanon, S., Paternoster, L., et al. 2008. Melatonin antagonizes the intrinsic pathway of apoptosis via mitochondrial targeting of Bcl-2. *J Pineal Res* 44:316–25.
53. Izykowska, I. 2010. Effect of melatonin on survival of human keratinocytes, fibroblasts and melanoma cells subjected to UV radiation. PhD diss., Wroclaw Medical University, Poland.
54. Kadekaro, A.L., Andrade, L.N., Floeter-Winter, L.M., et al. 2004. MT-1 melatonin receptor expression increases the antiproliferative effect of melatonin on S-91 murine melanoma cells. *J Pineal Res* 36(3):204–11.
55. Izykowska, I., Gebarowska, E., Cegielski, M., et al. 2009. Effect of melatonin on melanoma cells subjected to UVA and UVB radiation in in vitro studies. *In Vivo* 23(5):733–38.
56. Saintz, R.M., Reiter, R.J., Tan, D.X., et al. 2008. Critical role of glutathione in melatonin enhancement of tumor necrosis factor and ionizing radiation-induced apoptosis in prostate cancer cells in vitro. *J Pineal Res* 45(3):258–70.
57. Paternoster, L., Radogna, F., Accorsi, A., Albertini, M.C., Gualandi, G., and L. Ghibelli. 2009. Melatonin as a modulator of apoptosis in B-lymphoma cells. *Ann N Y Acad Sci* 1171:345–49.
58. Cristofanon, S., Uguccioni, F., Cerella, C., et al. 2009. Intracellular prooxidant activity of melatonin induces a survival pathway involving NF-κB activation. *Ann N Y Acad Sci* 1171:472–78.
59. Venkatachalam, S.R., Salaskar, A., Chattopadhyay, A., et al. 2006. Synthesis, pulse radiolysis, and in vitro radioprotection studies of melatoninolipoamide, a novel conjugate of melatonin and α-lipoic acid. *Bio Med Chem* 14:6414–419.
60. Kim, B.C., Shon, B.S., Ryoo, Y.W., Kim, S.P., and K.S. Lee. 2001. Melatonin reduces X-ray irradiation-induced oxidative damages in cultured human skin fibroblasts. *J Dermatol Sci* 26:194–200.
61. Vijayalaxmi, Reiter, R.J., Herman, T.S., and M.L. Meltz. 1996. Melatonin and radioprotection from genetic damage: In vivo/in vitro studies with human volunteers. *Mutat Res* 371:221–28.
62. Vijayalaxmi, Reiter, R.J., Sewerynek, E., Poeggeler, B., Leal, B.Z., and M.L. Meltz. 1995. Marked reduction of radiation-induced micronuclei in human blood lymphocytes pre-treated with melatonin. *Radiat Res* 143:102–06.
63. Mohan, N., Sadeghi, K., Reiter, R.J., and M.L. Meltz. 1995. The neurohormone melatonin inhibits cytokine, mitogen, and ionizing radiation-induced NF-κB. *Biochem Mol Biol Int* 37:1063–70.
64. Jang, S.S., Kim, W.D., and W.Y. Park. 2009. Melatonin exerts differential actions on X-ray radiation-induced apoptosis in normal mice splenocytes and Jurkat leukemia cells. *J Pineal Res* 47:147–55.

65. Dreher, F., Gabard, B., Schwindt, D.A., and H.I. Maibach. 1998. Topical melatonin in combination with vitamins E and C protects skin from ultraviolet-induced erythrema: a human study in vivo. *Br J Dermatol* 139:332–39.
66. Hussein, M.R., Abu-Dief, E.E., Abd el-Reheem, M.H., and A. Abd-Elrahamn. 2008. Ultrastructural evaluation of the radioprotective effects of melatonin against X-ray-induced skin damage in Albino rats. *Int J Exp Path* 86:45–55.
67. Anwar, M.M., and M.A. Moustafa. 2001. The effect of melatonin on eye lens of rats exposed to ultraviolet radiation. *Comp Biochem Physiol C Toxicol Pharmacol* 129:57–63.
68. Bardak, Y. 2000. Effect of melatonin on lenticular calcium and magnesium in rat exposed to ultraviolet radiation. *Ophthalmologica* 214:350–53.
69. Taysi, S., Memisogullari, R., Koc, M., et al. 2008. Melatonin reduces oxidative stress in the rat lens due to radiation-induced oxidative injury. *Int J Radiat Biol* 84(10):803–8.
70. Varvaresou, A., Tsirivas, E., Iakovou, K., et al. 2006. Development and validation of a reversed-phase ion-pair liquid chromatography method for the determination of magnesium ascorbyl phosphate and melatonin in cosmetic creams. *Anal Chim Acta* 573–574:284–90.
71. Fischer, T.W., Greif, C., Fluhr, J.W., Wigger-Alberti, W., and P. Elsner. 2004. Percutaneous penetration topically applied melatonin in a cream and alcoholic solution. *Skin Pharmacol Physiol* 17:190–94.
72. Nickel, A., and W. Wohlrab. 2000. Melatonin protects human keratinocytes from UVB radiation by light absorption. *Arch Dermatol Res* 292:366–68.
73. Dubey, V., Mishra, D., and N.K. Jain. 2007. Melatonin loaded ethanolic liposomes: physicochemical characterization and enhanced transdermal delivery. *Eur J Pharm Biopharm* 67:398–405.
74. Tursilli, R., Casolari, A., Iannuccelli, V., and S. Scalia. 2006. Enhancement of melatonin photostability by encapsulation in lipospheres. *J Pharm Biomed Anal* 40:910–14.
75. Priano, L., Esposti, D., Esposti, R., et al. 2007. Solid lipid nanoparticles incorporating melatonin as new model for sustained oral and transdermal delivery system. *J Nanosci Nanotechnol* 10:3696–601.

37 Melatonin and Oxidation

V. Haktan Ozacmak

CONTENTS

37.1 INTRODUCTION

Melatonin, a neurosecretory product of the pineal gland, was first isolated from bovine pineal tissue and was structurally distinguished as *N*-acetyl-5-methoxytryptamine in 1958.[1] Afterward, numerous reports have been announced to show various key physiological actions of melatonin. For instance, melatonin was found to be a sleep enhancer,[2] a chemical signal of light and darkness, and a regulator of photoperiod-dependent seasonal reproduction in some vertebrates. Both circadian rhythms and seasonal reproductive activities are closely regulated by the fluctuating endogenous melatonin signals. Thus, the daily and seasonally changing melatonin levels serve as a bio-clock and a bio-calendar in vertebrates.[3] Melatonin injection has effects on gonads, which are sometimes stimulating and sometimes inhibitory in some species, depending on the time of the day of the injection. This finding raised the hypothesis that the diurnal change in melatonin secretion acts as a timing signal coordinating endocrine and other internal events with the light/dark cycle of the external environment. Various reports have provided evidence supporting this observation. An interesting one is that in blind people with free-running circadian rhythms, injected melatonin entrains the rhythms.[4] The amphibian pineal tissue also contains the indole *N*-acetyl-5-methoxytryptamine, which is named as melatonin since it acts on melanophores, which results in lightening of the skin of tadpoles. On the other hand, in mammals, including humans, it appears not to play a physiological role in the regulation of skin color.[4] Subsequently, melatonin was found to be a potent, endogenously generated, and diet-derived free radical scavenger and broad-spectrum antioxidant.[5–7] In many lower life forms including unicellular organisms and several metazoans, it serves only as an antioxidant.[8] Melatonin is a direct scavenger of several reactive oxygen and nitrogen species (ROS/RNS) such as hydroxyl ($OH^{\bullet}$), superoxide anion ($O_2^{\bullet}$), nitric oxide ($NO^{\bullet}$), and peroxynitrite ($ONOO^{\bullet}$) radicals.[9] Unlike other antioxidants, melatonin does not undergo redox cycling, the ability of a molecule to undergo reduction and oxidation repeatedly. Redox cycling may allow other antioxidants (such as vitamin C) to regain their antioxidant properties. Melatonin, on the other hand, once oxidized, cannot be reduced to its former state because it forms several stable cnd-products upon reacting with free radicals. Therefore, it has been referred to as a terminal (or suicidal) antioxidant.[10] Furthermore, structurally different metabolites of melatonin appear to have free radical scavenging activity as well. The ability of melatonin and its metabolites to sequentially interact with ROS/RNS is referred to as the scavenging cascade reaction of melatonin.[10] The production of melatonin in the pineal gland of vertebrates shows an apparent circadian rhythm with its peak near the middle of the scotophase and basal levels during the photophase. The amount of melatonin synthesized in the pineal gland of mammals wanes with advanced age. In humans, melatonin production not only is diminished in the aged but also is significantly lower in many age-related diseases such as Alzheimer's disease[11,12] and cardiovascular disease.[13–16] As mentioned above, melatonin has pleiotropic bioactivities that are involved in several endocrinological and behavioral processes.[17,18] Chemically, melatonin is known to be a broad-spectrum antioxidant and an endogenous free radical scavenger acting through receptor-independent actions in vivo and in vitro. It can easily reach all cellular compartments since its molecular size is relatively small and it is an amphiphilic molecule.[6,19,20] In fact, melatonin is localized ubiquitously intracellularly in cytosolic, membrane, and nuclear compartments.[21,22] The highest melatonin concentrations among these compartments exist in mitochondria,[23] implying the possible involvement of its actions in situ in mitochondrial activities; for instance, majority of apoptotic signals have mitochondrial origin, and melatonin has well-known antiapoptotic effects.[24] ROS are generated in mitochondria at the highest production rate as well, and melatonin is a powerful antioxidant.[25] It has also been reported that melatonin can stimulate ATP synthesis.[26]

There is a substantial amount of evidence that melatonin may have a role in the biologic regulation of circadian rhythms, sleep, mood, reproduction, tumor growth, and aging. On the other hand, some unknowns and doubts still encompass the role of melatonin in human physiology and pathophysiology. Thus, understanding the metabolism of melatonin in depth will possibly help to explain the multiple functions of melatonin in organisms. Here, we focus on the oxidation process related to melatonin metabolism. Therefore, this review summarizes current knowledge about melatonin and oxidation.

37.2 MELATONIN BIOSYNTHESIS AND ITS METABOLITES

Melatonin is a hormone derived from tryptophan. The indolamine melatonin and the enzymes responsible for its synthesis from serotonin by *N*-acetylation and *O*-methylation are present in pineal parenchymal cells (Figure 37.1). The hormone is secreted by these cells into the blood and cerebrospinal fluid. It is also produced in other organs. Its synthesis takes place in the pineal gland, through a pathway in which the first steps are tryptophan hydroxylation and the subsequent decarboxylation thereof. The final reaction is the methylation of the *N*-acetyl-5-hydroxytryptamine[27]

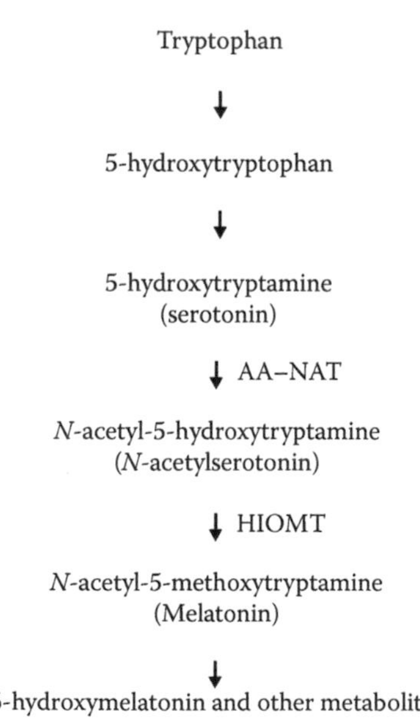

FIGURE 37.1 Formation and metabolism of melatonin. AA-NAT, arylalkilamine *N*-acetyltransferase; HIOMT, hydroxyindole *O*-methyltransferase.

immediately after the *N*-acetylation of 5-hydroxytryptamine (serotonin). Two enzymes are believed to play important roles in melatonin synthesis: arylalkilamine *N*-acetyltransferase (AA-NAT) and hydroxyindole *O*-methyltransferase (HIOMT). The rate-limiting enzyme in melatonin synthesis is classically known to be the pineal AA-NAT (serotonin N-acetyltransferase)[28] since the activity of AA-NAT exhibits the same circadian rhythm as does pineal melatonin level and since both the enzyme activity and pineal melatonin levels are suppressed during the photoperiod.[29–31] On the other hand, a number of recent reports have directly and indirectly shown that rather than AA-NAT, HIOMT might be a rate-limiting enzyme for melatonin synthesis.[32–36] It seems that HIOMT also participates in regulation of melatonin biosynthesis at night. Alternatively, but at lower flux rates, melatonin can be generated via *O*-methylation of serotonin and subsequent *N*-acetylation of 5-methoxytryptamine, or by *O*-methylation of tryptophan followed by decarboxylation and acetylation.[37] Unlike the original belief that melatonin was synthesized only in the pineal gland of vertebrates, studies have shown that it is produced in many extrapineal tissues and organs, such as the skin,[38] retina,[39] ciliary body,[40] lens,[41] brain,[42] lymphocytes,[43] placenta,[44] ovary,[45] testicle,[46] thymus,[47] airway epithelium,[48] bone marrow,[49,50] and gut.[51,52] Moreover, some extrapineal tissues appear to produce a larger amount of melatonin than that synthesized in the pineal gland. For instance, it is reported that melatonin generated from the gut is, at least, two orders of magnitude greater than that produced by the pineal gland.[52] It is estimated that keratinocytes have much higher levels of melatonin compared to the pinealocytes of rats or hamsters during the scotophase.[38] Elevated levels of melatonin have also been reported in the bone marrow, bile, and third ventricular fluid of rats and sheep.[49,53–55] However, melatonin in the extrapineal tissues seems not to contribute significantly to the melatonin circadian rhythm in the circulation since surgical or chemical pinealectomy lowers the circulating melatonin levels.[56] Thus, extrapineal melatonin does not act as a chemical signal of light/dark despite its large quantity. Rather, it probably serves as a protective mechanism of oxidative stress, considering especially the gut and skin, both of which are constantly exposed to stressors of the external environment (i.e., bacteria, parasites, UV, and toxins).

The pathways associated with melatonin synthesis are well established and have been known for more than three decades. Its catabolism, however, is not completely clarified, although it is known that the conjugation stages account for approximately 70% of an ingested amount.[57] Roughly 15% of the ingested dose is excreted untransformed, while the remaining is involved in catabolism associated with oxidative cleavage of the indole moiety. Melatonin in the circulation is rapidly metabolized in the liver by 6-hydroxylation followed by conjugation. Over 90% of the melatonin that present in the urine is in the form of 6-hydroxy conjugates and 6-sulfatoxymelatonin (6-hydroxymelatonin sulfate). The pathways by which the brain and some other organs metabolize melatonin are less understood but may involve cleavage of the indole nucleus.[4]

Melatonin is to be converted to more hydrophilic species for excretion via the kidney since it is a lipophilic molecule. It is catabolized to 6-hydroxymelatonin by the cytochrome P450 enzyme system in the liver, particularly by CYP1A1, CYP1A2, and CYP2C19. Then, 6-hydroxymelatonin is conjugated to sulfate by the action of sulfotransferase, forming 6-hydroxymelatonin sulfate, which is excreted in urine. It is believed that almost all of the 6-hydroxymelatonin is generated in the liver. However, recent studies suggest that some 6-hydroxymelatonin sulfate can be generated at extrahepatic sites as well. The cerebral cortex, kidney, and heart of rats, and skin keratinocytes produce and contain high levels of 6-hydroxymelatonin sulfate.[58,59] Additionally, 6-hydroxymelatonin sulfate can be formed by nonenzymatic processes, for instance, through an interaction with ROS/RNS. It is documented that melatonin interacts with $ONOO^•$, $OH^•$, or during UV irradiation, causing the formation of 6-hydroxymelatonin.[38]

Another metabolite of melatonin is 2-hydroxymelatonin, which is produced by melatonin interaction with ROS/RNS. 2-hydroxymelatonin and its keto tautomer, melatonin 2-indolinone, are oxidative products of melatonin's interaction with oxoferryl hemoglobin or $OH^•$.[60,61] In the presence of melatonin as a reductant, 2-hydroxymelatonin is also generated in vitro as an intermediate molecule in the process of oxidation of cytochrome C by H_2O_2, yielding another metabolite of melatonin,

N-acetyl-*N*-formyl-5-methoxykynuramine (AFMK).[62] In cell culture, UV-B irradiation induces keratinocytes to form 2-hydroxymelatonin.[38] It is approximated that 2-hydroxymelatonin present in urine is the 2% of the melatonin metabolized in mice.[63]

Cyclic 3-hydroxymelatonin is another oxidative melatonin metabolite. It is generated by the interaction of melatonin with OH•, ONOO•, 2, 2'-azino-bis (3-ethylbenzthiazilone-6-sulphonic acid) (ABTS) cation radical, or oxoferryl hemoglobin.[64–68]

Among metabolites of melatonin, AFMK and *N*-acetyl-5-methoxykynuramine (AMK) have appeared to draw more attention recently. Since its discovery as a melatonin metabolite in the rat brain three decades ago,[69] AFMK has been found to be formed not only enzymatically by indolamine 2,3-dioxygenase, but also via nonenzymatic processes such as interaction of melatonin with hydrogen peroxide (H_2O_2).[70] Pathways forming AFMK include melatonin being catalyzed by horseradish peroxidase and myeloperoxidase,[71–73] being metabolized by cytochrome C,[60] being oxidized by oxoferryl hemoglobin,[66] being irradiated by UV-B,[38] and interacting with $O_2^{\bullet-}$,[74] H_2O_2,[70] singlet oxygen,[75] carbonate radical, and ONOO•.[76] Moreover, upon activation by bacteria, virus, or lipopolysacchride, macrophages and neutrophils oxidize melatonin to form AFMK.[77–79] It is reported that AFMK is the only melatonin metabolite in the low-ranked species including unicellular organisms and small aquatic metazoans.[80] In mammals, it is detected in the retina and serum of rats, in cerebrospinal fluid,[81] in blood,[82] and in the urine of mice.[62] Interestingly, cerebrospinal fluid of meningitis patients contains very high levels of AFKM.[83] Some studies suggest that AFMK is the original metabolite of melatonin from the evolutionarily point of view and may be the primary metabolite produced in response to oxidative stress since melatonin undergoes oxidation with subsequent formation of AFMK when an organism is exposed to oxidative stress.[8] When deformylated by arylamineformamidase or hemoperoxidases or interacted with ROS/RNS, AFMK is metabolized to form AMK. AMK is present in cultured cells, serum of rats, and the urine of mice. It can be further metabolized by nonenzymatic processes. Its oligomers are produced once AMK interacts with ABTS cation radical.[84] When it reacts with ONOO•, resultant products are 3-acetamidomethyl-6-methoxycinnolinone and *N*-acetyl-5-methoxy-3-nitrokynuramine.[85]

Some minor melatonin metabolites are also known and found in vitro, such as 1-nitromelatonin and 1-nitrosomelatonin. However, whether they are generated in vivo remains to be elucidated. They are products of melatonin interaction with ONOO•, NO•, or nitrogen dioxide radical.[66,86,87]

AFMK has been suggested to be a primitive and primary metabolite of melatonin since it and its derivatives are the only measurable melatonin metabolites in plants and in numerous primitive organisms such as algae and metazoans.[8,80] In vertebrates, as mentioned earlier, a major portion of melatonin is believed to be metabolized by hepatic P450 mono-oxygenases followed by conjugation with sulfate, generating the main urinary metabolite 6-hydroxymelatonin sulfate. It is reported that only 37.1% of urinary melatonin metabolites in mice is 6-hydroxymelatonin sulfate.[63] Based on this study, it is speculated that either a major portion of melatonin is converted to unknown metabolites or urinary melatonin metabolites are distributed in the body. Further speculation is that the majority of melatonin is probably transformed to AFMK and its derivatives. The relatively low proportions of AFMK and AMK in urine may not represent their real production since they are not as hydrophilic as 6-hydroxymelatonin sulfate; thus, their urinary excretion rate is limited.[8] Moreover, in some tissues, melatonin is exclusively transformed to AFMK and its derivatives through oxidative cleavage, such as brain and leukocytes.[69,79] Some other tissues are likely to be the site generating AFMK, such as lung, skin, and red blood cells.[38,88] Among cellular organelles, mitochondria seem to be a major place for AFMK generation since melatonin and cytochrome C are abundant in mitochondria, and cytochrome C can use melatonin as its substrate to form AFMK.[62]

37.3 MELATONIN, FREE RADICALS, AND OXIDATION

Melatonin is a conserved molecule to a high degree. Photosynthetic prokaryotes, unicellular organisms, marine algae, and yeast have melatonin.[89–91] In these organisms, the primary function of melatonin is to defend against oxidative stress, while melatonin generated by pineal tissue in vertebrates exerts other functions mentioned already. Since the report of melatonin as a free radical scavenger and an antioxidant nearly two decades ago,[5] a substantial number of published studies have confirmed this observation in various experimental models. Melatonin defends strongly against toxic free radicals. Free radicals are chemical molecules that contain an unpaired electron in their outer orbital, which makes them very reactive and toxic. In other words, free radicals contain one or more electrons than their parent compounds. Vertebrates take a large amount of oxygen by respiration (i.e., inspiration). Up to 5% of this amount is converted to oxygen free radicals, namely, ROS. In healthy individuals, however, antioxidant enzymes produced endogenously counteract this amount of harmful free radicals. $O_2^{\bullet-}$ is generated by the addition of an electron to oxygen. $O_2^{\bullet-}$ is then reduced by superoxide dismutase to H_2O_2, which is not a free radical itself but very toxic. H_2O_2 can be reduced to $OH^{\bullet}$, one of the most harmful radicals. Melatonin is reported to be a very efficient neutralizer not only for the $OH^{\bullet}$ radical, but also for the other ROS and RNS. In free radical scavenging capacity, it is more effective than the well-known antioxidant, reduced glutathione (GSH). It is reported that melatonin stimulates glutathione peroxidase (GSH-Px) activity in neural tissue. This enzyme mediates the transformation of GSH to its oxidized form, the process of which results in conversion of H_2O_2 to H_2O, thus lowering the production of $OH^{\bullet}$. Moreover, melatonin is shown to be a more efficient scavenger of the peroxyl radical than is vitamin E. It lowers oxidative/nitrosative stress resulting from drugs, toxins, metals, and herbicides.[92]

From the chemical point of view, oxidation and reduction processes are complementary reactions described as the loss or gain, respectively, of one or more electrons by an atom or molecule. The term oxidation was originally used to express a reaction in which oxygen combines with an element or compound. Similarly, the term reduction was attributed to the removal of oxygen. In fact, when a compound combines with oxygen, it tends to give up electron(s) to the oxygen to form a chemical bond. The opposite events occur during the reduction process. Oxidation-reduction reactions are also called redox reactions. The number of electrons lost by one compound is equaled by the number gained by another compound. The substance losing electrons undergoes oxidation and is called an electron donor or reductant, since its lost electrons reduce the other substance. Conversely, the substance gaining electrons undergoes reduction and is named an electron acceptor or oxidant.

It is reported that endogenous indolamines generated from the essential aromatic amino acid tryptophan can function as substrates and mediators that are involved in electron transfer mechanisms and radical reactions. As an indolamine, melatonin is a powerful and effective radical scavenger. It selectively and efficiently scavenges reactive free radicals by donating electrons to these electrophilic compounds. In other words, melatonin, being an electron donor, undergoes oxidation during the neutralization of free radicals. For instance, melatonin is readily oxidized by the $OH^{\bullet}$ produced via the Fenton reagent ferrous sulfate and H_2O_2.[9] Highly electrophilic intermediates in the reaction of this study are riboflavin radical (R^-), $OH^{\bullet}$, and Fe^{3+}. Upon electron transfer by the electron donor, melatonin, occurs, the indolyl cation radical is generated, which is then rapidly converted to the kynuramine metabolite, AFMK. Formation of the indolyl cation radical results from the one-electron transfer reaction and partial oxidation of melatonin. Moreover, oxidation reactions occur in the biotransformation cascade of melatonin to its metabolites, which are also potent free radical scavengers, as mentioned below. However, melatonin is not subjected to redox cycling. Once oxidized, it does not undergo reduction, which is a feature differing from other antioxidants.

37.4 FUNCTIONS OF MELATONIN METABOLITES

Major metabolites of melatonin have also been reported to have potential activities. Besides having structural similarities with melatonin, 6-hydroxymelatonin also exerts a strong antioxidant activity. It reduces lipid peroxidation in the liver, brain, and muscle of rats subjected to oxidative stress.[93] 6-hydroxymelatonin protects against DNA damage via attenuating oxidative 8-hydroxy-2-deoxyguanosine generation induced by chromium.[94] It also reduces $OH^{\bullet}$ formed by the Fenton reagents, preventing DNA damage.[95] 6-hydroxymelatonin is reported to be beneficial in rat nephrotoxicity induced by cisplatin.[96] It prevents neurons and liver from toxicities resulting from cyanide, quinolinic acid, iron, and alpha-naphthylisothiocyanate.[97–100] The mechanism by which 6-hydroxymelatonin prevents tissue damage in these studies is reported to be involved with its direct free radical scavenging and antioxidant actions.[101,102] In addition, 6-hydroxymelatonin inhibits cytochrome C release from the mitochondria, suppresses caspase 3 activity, and stabilizes the mitochondrial membrane potential, therefore, preventing the cell death triggered by oxygen–glucose–serum deprivation in cultured neurons.[103] Another oxidative melatonin metabolite, cyclic 3-hydroxymelatonin, is present in the urine of rats and humans.[64] Its functions in organisms are unknown. Nevertheless, it reduces two ABTS cation radicals per molecule and prevents oxidative DNA damage induced by the Fenton reagents.[68,95] Interestingly, coexistence of cyclic 3-hydroxymelatonin and AFMK is common in the metabolic pathway of melatonin both in vitro and in vivo,[63] which probably implies that the cyclic 3-hydroxymelatonin may easily be transformed to AFMK. It is postulated that the ratio of the cyclic 3-hydroxymelatonin to AFMK may be an index for the level of the oxidative stress. This ratio could be used by organisms as a signal to adjust their antioxidative defense mechanisms (i.e., by either up- or downregulation of antioxidant enzymes).[8] Kynuramine metabolites of melatonin, namely, AFMK and AMK, have also been reported to exert some functions. They have similar structures, with AMK having one formyl group less. Various reports show the anti-inflammatory and immunoregulatory actions of AFMK and AMK. AMK inhibits the biosynthesis of prostaglandins,[104] while AFMK restrains the production of tumor necrosis factor-alpha and interleukin-8 in neutrophils and mononuclear cells of plasma. One of the important events in the cross-talking between neutrophils and monocytes is speculated to be the biosynthesis of AFMK during melatonin oxidation.[105] Gene expression of a proinflammatory enzyme, cyclo-oxygenase, is selectively inhibited by AFMK and AMK.[106] Various studies have also demonstrated the involvement of these metabolites with oxidative stress. AFMK is able to donate two electrons as a reductant.[107] One AFMK molecule can donate four or more electrons when interacting with reactive radicals.[108] Its antioxidant capacity appears to be very effective based on the published studies reporting that AFMK scavenges $O_2^{\bullet-}$ to a similar degree as melatonin,[109] reduces lipid peroxidation and oxidative DNA damage caused by oxidative stressors, and protects against H_2O_2 and amyloid beta-peptide-induced injury of neurons.[102,107,110,111] Regarding the scavenging ROS and impeding protein oxidation, AMK is more effective than is its precursor, AFMK.[112] Indirect antioxidant effects of AMK are also reported: inhibition of nitric oxide synthase activity and reduction of intracellular NO levels in neurons are caused by AMK.[113,114] Moreover, AMK enhances mitochondrial complex I activity that results in increased ATP production. These effects occur via decreased electron leakage and inhibition of opening of the mitochondrial permeability transition pore by AMK.[115,116]

37.5 CONCLUDING REMARKS

A substantial number of studies indicate that oxidation processes associated with both melatonin itself and some other molecules interacting with melatonin seem to account for possible multiple physiological functions of melatonin and its metabolites. Considering especially the scavenging cascade reaction provided by melatonin and its metabolites that sequentially interact with ROS/RNS, free radical scavenging and antioxidant properties are, at least, dependent upon biotransformation of molecules on the cascade, in which the oxidation reaction takes an important part. It appears that some actions of melatonin can be mediated and/or amplified by its metabolites (i.e., AFMK and AMK) which are the resultant products of melatonin oxidation.

REFERENCES

1. Lerner, Aaron B. 1958. Isolation of melatonin, a pineal factor that lightens melanocytes. *Journal of the American Chemical Society* 80: 2587.

2. Marczynski, Thaddeus J. 1964. Sleep induced by the administration of melatonin (5-methoxyn-acetyl-tryptamine) to the hypothalamus in unrestrained cats. *Experientia* 20: 435–37.
3. Reiter, Russel J. The melatonin rhythm: both a clock and a calendar. *Experientia* 49: 654–64.
4. Ganong, William F. 2005. Endocrine functions of the kidneys, heart, and pineal gland. In *Review of Medical Physiology*, ed. W.F. Ganong, 454–466. Singapore: McGraw–Hill.
5. Tan, Dun-Xian. 1993. Melatonin: a potent endogenous hydroxyl radical scavenger. *Endocrine Journal* 1: 57–60.
6. Tan, Dun-Xian. 2002. Chemical and physical properties and potential mechanisms: melatonin as a broad spectrum antioxidant and free radical scavenger. *Current Topics in Medicinal Chemistry* 2: 181–197.
7. Paredes, Sergio D. 2009. Phytomelatonin: a review. *Journal of Experimental Botany* 60(1): 57–69.
8. Tan, Dun-Xian. 2007. One molecule, many derivatives: a never-ending interaction of melatonin with reactive oxygen and nitrogen species? *Journal of Pineal Research* 42(1): 28–42.
9. Poeggeler, Burkhard. 1994. Melatonin—a highly potent endogenous radical scavenger and electron donor: new aspects of the oxidation chemistry of this indole accessed in vitro. *Annals of the New York Academy of Sciences* 738: 419–20
10. Tan, Dun-Xian. 2000. Significance of melatonin in anti oxidative defense system: reactions and products. *Biological Signals and Receptors* 9(3–4): 137–59.
11. Mishima, Kazuo. 1999. Melatonin secretion rhythm disorders in patients with senile dementia of Alzheimer's type with disturbed sleep-waking. *Biological Psychiatry* 45: 417–21.
12. Liu, Rong-Yu. 1999. Decreased melatonin levels in postmortem cerebrospinal fluid in relation to aging, Alzheimer's disease, and apolipoprotein E-epsilon4/4 genotype. *The Journal of Clinical Endocrinology and Metabolism* 84: 323–27.
13. Sakotnik, Andrea. 1999. Decreased melatonin synthesis in patients with coronary artery disease. *European Heart Journal* 20: 1314–7.
14. Altun, Armagan. 2002. Impaired nocturnal synthesis of melatonin in patients with cardiac syndrome X. *Neuroscience Letters* 327: 143–5.
15. Dominguez-Rodriguez, Alberto. 2002. Decreased nocturnal melatonin levels during acute myocardial infarction. *Journal of Pineal Research* 33: 248–252.
16. Yaprak, Mevlut. 2003. Decreased nocturnal synthesis of melatonin in patients with coronary artery disease. *International Journal of Cardiology* 89: 103–7.
17. Csernus, Valer. 2003. Biorhythms and pineal gland. *Neuro Endocrinology Letters* 6: 404–11.
18. Delagrange, Philippe. 2003. Therapeutic perspectives for melatonin agonists and antagonists. Journal of *Neuroendocrinology* 15(4): 442–8.
19. Rodriguez, Carmen. 2004. Regulation of antioxidant enzymes: a significant role for melatonin. *Journal of Pineal Research* 36: 1–9.
20. Allegra, Mario. 2003. The chemistry of melatonin's interaction with reactive species. *Journal of Pineal Research* 34: 1–10.
21. Menendez-Pelaez, Armando. 1993. Distribution of melatonin in mammalian tissues: the relative importance of nuclear versus cytosolic localization. *Journal of Pineal Research* 15: 59–69.
22. Costa, Ernane J. 1997. How melatonin interacts with lipid bilayers: a study by fluorescence and ESR spectroscopies. *FEBS Letters* 416: 103–6.
23. Martin, Miguel. 2000. Melatonin but not vitamins C and E maintains glutathione homeostasis in t-butyl hydroperoxide-induced mitochondrial oxidative stress. *The FASEB Journal* 14: 1677–9.
24. Andrabi, Shaida A. 2004. Direct inhibition of the mitochondrial permeability transition pore: a possible mechanism responsible for anti-apoptotic effects of melatonin. *The FASEB Journal* 18: 869–71.
25. Reiter, Russel J. 1999. Melatonin and tryptophan derivatives as free radical scavengers and antioxidants. *Advances in Experimental Medicine and Biology* 467: 379–87.
26. Leon, Josefa. 2004. Melatonin and mitochondrial function. *Life Sciences* 75: 765–90.
27. Axelrod, Julius. 1974. The pineal gland: a neurochemical transducer. *Science* 184: 1341–8.
28. Klein, David C. 1997. The melatonin rhythm-generating enzyme: molecular regulation of serotonin N-acetyltransferase in the pineal gland. *Recent Progress in Hormone Research* 52: 307–57.
29. Vollrath, Lutz. 1988. Response of pineal serotonin N-acetyltransferase activity in male guinea pigs exposed to light pulses at night. *Journal of Neural Transmission* 72: 55–66.
30. Foulkes, Nicholas S. 1997. Rhythmic transcription: the molecular basis of circadian melatonin synthesis. *Biology of the Cell* 89: 487–94.
31. Karolczak, Magdalena. 2005. The rhythm and blues of gene expression in the rodent pineal gland. *Endocrine* 27: 89–100.

32. Ceinos, Rosa M. 2004. Analysis of adrenergic regulation of melatonin synthesis in Siberian hamster pineal emphasizes the role of HIOMT. *Neurosignals* 13: 308–17.
33. Johnston, Jonathan D. 2004. Rhythmic melatonin secretion does not correlate with the expression of arylalkylamine N-acetyltransferase, inducible cyclic AMP early repressor, period1 or cryptochrome1 mRNA in the sheep pineal. *Neuroscience* 124: 789–95.
34. Ribelayga, Christophe. 2000. HIOMT drives the photoperiodic changes in the amplitude of the melatonin peak of the Siberian hamster. *American Journal of Physiology. Regulatory, Integrative and Comparative Physiology* 278: R1339–45.
35. Liu, Tiecheng. 2005. N-acetyltransferase is not the rate-limiting enzyme of melatonin synthesis at night. *Journal of Pineal Research* 39: 91–6.
36. Hardeland, Rüdiger. 2003. Non-vertebrate melatonin. *Journal of Pineal Research* 34: 233–41.
37. Hardeland, Rüdiger. 1993. The significance of the metabolism of the neurohormone melatonin: antioxidative protection and formation of bioactive substances. *Neuroscience and Biobehavioral Reviews* 17: 347–57.
38. Fischer, Tobias W. 2006. Constitutive and UV-induced metabolism of melatonin in keratinocytes and cell-free systems. *The FASEB Journal* 20: 1564–6.
39. Iuvone, P. Michael. 1983. Regulation of indoleamine N-acetyltransferase activity in the retina: effects of light and dark, protein synthesis inhibitors and cyclic nucleotide analogs. *Brain Research* 273: 111–9.
40. Martin, Xavier D. 1992. The ciliary body—the third organ found to synthesize indoleamines in humans. *European Journal of Ophthalmology* 2: 67–72.
41. Abe, Mitsushi. 1999. Detection of melatonin, its precursors and related enzyme activities in rabbit lens. *Experimental Eye Research* 68: 255–62.
42. Stefulj, Jasminka. 2001. Gene expression of the key enzymes of melatonin synthesis in extrapineal tissues of the rat. *Journal of Pineal Research* 30: 243–7.
43. Carrillo-Vico, Antonio. 2004. Evidence of melatonin synthesis by human lymphocytes and its physiological significance: possible role as intracrine, autocrine, and/ or paracrine substance. *The FASEB Journal* 18: 537–9.
44. Iwasaki, Shinya. 2005. Melatonin as a local regulator of human placental function. *Journal of Pineal Research* 39: 261–5.
45. Itoh, Masanori T. 1999. Melatonin, its precursors, and synthesizing enzyme activities in the human ovary. *Molecular Human Reproduction* 5: 402–8.
46. Tijmes, Matias. 1996. Melatonin in the rat testis: evidence for local synthesis. *Steroids* 61: 65–8.
47. Jimenez-Jorge, Silvia. 2005. Melatonin synthesis and melatonin-membrane receptor (MT1) expression during rat thymus development: role of the pineal gland. *Journal of Pineal Research* 39: 77–83.
48. Kvetnoy, Igor M. 1999. Extrapineal melatonin: location and role within diffuse neuroendocrine system. *The Histochemical Journal* 31: 1–12.
49. Tan, Dun-Xian. 1999. Identification of highly elevated levels of melatonin in bone marrow: its origin and significance. *Biochimica et Biophysica Acta* 1472: 206–14.
50. Conti, Ario. 2000. Evidence for melatonin synthesis in mouse and human bone marrow cells. *Journal of Pineal Research* 28: 193–202.
51. Huether, Gerald. 1992. Effect of tryptophan administration on circulating melatonin levels in chicks and rats: evidence for stimulation of melatonin synthesis and release in the gastrointestinal tract. *Life Sciences* 51: 945–53.
52. Huether, Gerald. 1993. The contribution of extrapineal sites of melatonin synthesis to circulating melatonin levels in higher vertebrates. *Experientia* 49: 665–70.
53. Tan, Dun-Xian. 1999. High physiological levels of melatonin in the bile of mammals. *Life Sciences* 65: 2523–9.
54. Skinner, Donal C. 1999. High melatonin concentrations in third ventricular cerebrospinal fluid are not due to Galen vein blood recirculating through the choroid plexus. *Endocrinology* 140: 4399–405.
55. Tricoire, Helene. 2002. Melatonin enters the cerebrospinal fluid through the pineal recess. *Endocrinology* 143: 84–90.
56. Vakkuri, Olli. 1985. Plasma and tissue concentrations of melatonin after midnight light exposure and pinealectomy in the pigeon. *Journal of Endocrinology* 105: 263–8.
57. Leone, Anna M. 1987. The isolation, purification, and characterisation of the principal urinary metabolites of melatonin. *Journal of Pineal Research* 4: 253–66.
58. Ma, Xiachao. 2005. Metabolism of melatonin by human cytochromes p450. *Drug Metabolism and Disposition* 33: 489–94.

59. Lahiri, Debomoy K. 2004. Age-related changes in serum melatonin in mice: higher levels of combined melatonin and 6-hydroxymelatonin sulfate in the cerebral cortex than serum, heart, liver and kidney tissues. *Journal of Pineal Research* 36: 217–23.
60. Horstman, Joseph A. 2002. Further insights into the reaction of melatonin with hydroxyl radical. *Bioorganic Chemistry* 30: 371–82.
61. Agozzino, Pasquale. 2003. Melatonin: structural characterization of its non-enzymatic mono-oxygenate metabolite. *Journal of Pineal Research* 35: 269–75.
62. Semak, Igor. 2005. A novel metabolic pathway of melatonin: oxidation by cytochrome C. *Biochemistry* 44: 9300–7.
63. Ma, Xiaochao. 2006. Urinary metabolites and antioxidant products of exogenous melatonin in the mouse. *Journal of Pineal Research* 40: 343–9.
64. Tan, Dun-Xian. 1998. A novel melatonin metabolite, cyclic 3-hydroxymelatonin: a biomarker of in vivo hydroxyl radical generation. *Biochemical and Biophysical Research Communications* 253: 614–20.
65. Zhang, Houwen. 1999. Reaction of peroxynitrite with melatonin: a mechanistic study. *Chemical Research in Toxicology* 12: 526–34.
66. Peyrot, Fabienne. 2002. Reactivity of peroxynitrite with melatonin as a function of pH and CO2 content. *European Journal of Organic Chemistry* 321: 1–10.
67. Tesoriere, Luisa. 2001. Oxidation of melatonin by oxoferryl hemoglobin: a mechanistic study. *Free Radical Research* 35: 633–42.
68. Tan, Dun-Xian. 2003. Mechanistic and comparative studies of melatonin and classic antioxidants in terms of their interactions with the ABTS cation radical. *Journal of Pineal Research* 34: 249–59.
69. Hirata, Fusao. 1974. In vitro and in vivo formation of two new metabolites of melatonin. The *Journal of Biological Chemistry* 249: 1311–3.
70. Tan, Dun-Xian. 2000. Melatonin directly scavenges hydrogen peroxide: a potentially new metabolic pathway of melatonin biotransformation. *Free Radical Biology and Medicine* 29: 1177–85.
71. Hardeland, Rüdiger. 2006. Melatonin. *The International Journal of Biochemistry and Cell Biology* 38: 313–6.
72. Silva, Sueli O. 2000. Myeloperoxidase-catalyzed oxidation of melatonin by activated neutrophils. *Biochemical and Biophysical Research Communications* 279: 657–62.
73. Ximenes, Valdecir F. 2001. Oxidation of melatonin and tryptophan by an HRP cycle involving compound III. *Biochemical and Biophysical Research Communications* 287: 130–4.
74. Hardeland, Rüdiger. 1995. On the primary functions of melatonin in evolution: mediation of photoperiodic signals in a unicell, photooxidation, and scavenging of free radicals. *Journal of Pineal Research* 18: 104–11.
75. de Almeida, Eduardo A. 2003. Oxidation of melatonin by singlet molecular oxygen (O2(1Dg)) produces N1-acetyl-N2-formyl-5-methoxykynurenine. *Journal of Pineal Research* 35: 131–7.
76. Hardeland, Rüdiger. 2003. Oxidation of melatonin by carbonate radicals and chemiluminescence emitted during pyrrole ring cleavage. *Journal of Pineal Research* 34: 17–25.
77. Rodrigues, Maria R. 2003. Interferon-gamma independent oxidation of melatonin by macrophages. *Journal of Pineal Research* 34: 69–74.
78. Silva, Sueli O. 2006. Melatonin and its kynurenin-like oxidation products affect the microbicidal activity of neutrophils. *Microbes and Infection/Institut Pasteur* 8: 420–5.
79. Silva, Sueli O. 2004. Oxidation of melatonin and its catabolites, N1-acetyl-N2-formyl-5-methoxykynuramine and N1-acetyl-5-methoxykynuramine, by activated leukocytes. *Journal of Pineal Research* 37: 171–5.
80. Poeggeler, B. 2001. Observations on melatonin oxidation and metabolite release by unicellular organisms and small aquatic metazoans. In *Actions and Redox Properties of Melatonin and other Aromatic Amino Acid Metabolites,* ed. R. Hardeland, 66–9. Gottingen: Cuvillier Verlag.
81. Rozov, Stanislav V. 2003. N1-acetyl-N2-formyl-5 methoxykynuramine is a product of melatonin oxidation in rats. *Journal of Pineal Research* 35: 245–50.
82. Harthe, Catherine. 2003. Radioimmunoassay of N-acetyl-N-formyl-5-methoxykynuramine (AFMK): a melatonin oxidative metabolite. *Life Sciences* 73: 1587–97.
83. Silva, Sueli O. 2005. High concentrations of the melatonin metabolite, N1-acetyl-N2-formyl-5-methoxykynuramine, in cerebrospinal fluid of patients with meningitis: a possible immunomodulatory mechanism. *Journal of Pineal Research* 39: 302–6.
84. Than, Ni N. 2006. Reactions of the melatonin metabolite N1-acetyl-5-methoxykynuramine (AMK) with the ABTS cation radical: identification of new oxidation products. *Redox Report* 11: 15–24.

85. Guenther, Anna L. 2005. Reactions of the melatonin metabolite AMK (N1-acetyl-5-methoxykynuramine) with reactive nitrogen species: formation of novel compounds, 3-acetamidomethyl-6-methoxycinnolinone and 3-nitro-AMK. *Journal of Pineal Research* 39: 251–60.
86. Peyrot, Fabienne. 2006. Melatonin nitrosation promoted by NO: 2; comparison with the peroxynitrite reaction. *Free Radical Research* 40: 910–20.
87. Peyrot, Fabienne. 2006. N-Nitroso products from the reaction of indoles with Angeli's salt. *Chemical Research in Toxicology* 19: 58–67.
88. Budu, Alexandre. 2007. N1-acetyl-N2-formyl-5-methoxykynuramine (AFMK) modulates the cell cycle of malaria parasites. *Journal of Pineal Research* 42(3): 261–6.
89. Manchester, Lucien C. 1995. Melatonin immunoreactivity in the photosynthetic prokaryote Rhodospirillum rubrum: implications for an ancient antioxidant system. *Cellular and Molecular Biology Research* 41: 391– 5.
90. Poeggeler, Burkhard. 1991. Pineal hormone melatonin oscillates also in the dinoflagellate Gonyaulax polyedra. *Die Naturwissenschaften* 78: 268–9.
91. Sprenger, Julia. 1999. Melatonin and other 5-methoxylated indoles in yeast: presence in high concentrations and dependence on tryptophan availability. *Cytologia* 64: 209–13.
92. Reiter, Russel J. 2008. Melatonin reduces oxidative/nitrosative stress due to drugs, toxins, metals, and herbicides. *Neuro Endocrinology Letters* 29: 609–13.
93. Hara, Masayuki. 1997. Administration of melatonin and related indoles prevents exercise-induced cellular oxidative changes in rats. *Biological Signals* 6: 90–100.
94. Qi, Wenbo. 2000. Increased levels of oxidatively damaged DNA induced by chromium(III) and H2O2: protection by melatonin and related molecules. *Journal of Pineal Research* 29: 54–61.
95. Lopez-Burillo, Silvia. 2003. Melatonin and its derivatives cyclic 3-hydroxymelatonin, N1-acetyl-N2-formyl-5-methoxykynuramine and 6-hydroxymelatonin reduce oxidative DNA damage induced by Fenton reagents. *Journal of Pineal Research* 34: 178–84.
96. Hara, Masayuki. 2001. Melatonin, a pineal secretory product with antioxidant properties, protects against cisplatin-induced nephrotoxicity in rats. *Journal of Pineal Research* 30: 129–38.
97. Maharaj, Deepa S. 2003. 6-Hydroxymelatonin protects against cyanide induced oxidative stress in rat brain homogenates. *Journal of Chemical Neuroanatomy* 26: 103–7.
98. Maharaj, Deepa S. 2005. 6-Hydroxymelatonin protects against quinolinic-acid-induced oxidative neurotoxicity in the rat hippocampus. *The Journal of Pharmacy and Pharmacology* 57: 877–81.
99. Calvo, Juan R. 2001. Characterization of the protective effects of melatonin and related indoles against alpha-naphthylisothiocyanate-induced liver injury in rats. *Journal of Cellular Biochemistry* 80: 461–70.
100. Maharaj, Deepa S. 2006. Melatonin and 6-hydroxymelatonin protect against iron-induced neurotoxicity. *Journal of Neurochemistry* 96: 78–81.
101. Matuszak, Zenon. 2003. Interaction of singlet molecular oxygen with melatonin and related indoles. *Photochemistry and Photobiology* 78: 449–55.
102. Liu, Xuwan. 2002. Melatonin as an effective protector against doxorubicin-induced cardiotoxicity. *American Journal of Physiology. Heart and Circulatory Physiology* 283: H254–63.
103. Duan, Qiuhong. 2006. Comparison of 6-hydroxylmelatonin or melatonin in protecting neurons against ischemia/reperfusion-mediated injury. *Journal of Pineal Research* 41: 351–7.
104. Kelly, Rodney W. 1984. N-acetyl-5-methoxy kynurenamine, a brain metabolite of melatonin, is a potent inhibitor of prostaglandin biosynthesis. *Biochemical and Biophysical Research Communications* 121: 372–9.
105. Silva, Sueli O. 2004. Neutrophils as a specific target for melatonin and kynuramines: effects on cytokine release. *Journal of Neuroimmunology* 156: 146–52.
106. Mayo, Juan C. 2005. Anti-inflammatory actions of melatonin and its metabolites, N1-acetyl-N2-formyl-5-methoxykynuramine (AFMK) and N1-acetyl-5-methoxykynuramine (AMK), in macrophages. *Journal of Neuroimmunology* 165: 139–49.
107. Tan, Dun-Xian. 2001. N1-acetyl-N2-formyl-5-methoxykynuramine, a biogenic amine and melatonin metabolite, functions as a potent antioxidant. *The FASEB Journal* 15: 2294–6.
108. Rosen, Joachim. 2006. Interactions of melatonin and its metabolites with the ABTS cation radical: extension of the radical scavenger cascade and formation of a novel class of oxidation products, C2-substituted 3-indolinones. *Journal of Pineal Research* 41: 374–81.
109. Maharaj, Deepa S. 2002. The identification of the UV degradants of melatonin and their ability to scavenge free radicals. *Journal of Pineal Research* 32: 257–61.

110. Burkhardt, Susanne. 2001. DNA oxidatively damaged by chromium(III) and H2O2 is protected by the antioxidants melatonin, N1-acetyl-N2-formyl-5-methoxykynuramine, resveratrol and uric acid. *The International Journal of Biochemistry and Cell Biology* 33: 775–83.
111. Onuki, Janice. 2005. Inhibition of 5-aminolevulinic acid-induced DNA damage by melatonin, N1-acetyl-N2-formyl-5-methoxykynuramine, quercetin or resveratrol. *Journal of Pineal Research* 38: 107–15.
112. Ressmeyer, Anna-Rebekka. 2003. Antioxidant properties of the melatonin metabolite N1-acetyl-5-methoxykynuramine (AMK): scavenging of free radicals and prevention of protein destruction. *Redox Report* 8: 205–13.
113. Entrena, Antonio. 2005. Kynurenamines as neural nitric oxide synthase inhibitors. *Journal of Medicinal Chemistry* 48: 8174–81.
114. Leon, Josefa. 2006. Inhibition of neuronal nitric oxide synthase activity by N1-acetyl-5-methoxy-kynuramine, a brain metabolite of melatonin. *Journal of Neurochemistry* 98: 2023–33.
115. Hardeland, Rüdiger. 2005. Antioxidative protection by melatonin: multiplicity of mechanisms from radical detoxification to radical avoidance. *Endocrine* 27: 119–30.
116. Acuna-Castroviejo, Dario. 2003. Mitochondrial regulation by melatonin and its metabolites. *Advances in Experimental Medicine and Biology* 527: 549–57.

Index

Page numbers followed by f and t indicate figures and tables, respectively.

F

G

H

I

J

K

L

M

N

O

P

Q

R

S

T